Textbook of Emergency General Surgery

Federico Coccolini • Fausto Catena
Editors

Textbook of Emergency General Surgery

Traumatic and Non-traumatic Surgical Emergencies

Volume I

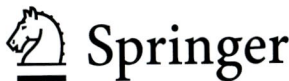

Editors
Federico Coccolini
General, Emergency and Trauma Surgery Dept.
Pisa University Hospital
Pisa, Italy

Fausto Catena
General and Emergency Surgery Dept.
Bufalini Hospital
Cesena, Italy

ISBN 978-3-031-22598-7   ISBN 978-3-031-22599-4   (eBook)
https://doi.org/10.1007/978-3-031-22599-4

© The Editor(s) (if applicable) and The Author(s), under exclusive license to Springer Nature Switzerland AG 2023

This work is subject to copyright. All rights are solely and exclusively licensed by the Publisher, whether the whole or part of the material is concerned, specifically the rights of translation, reprinting, reuse of illustrations, recitation, broadcasting, reproduction on microfilms or in any other physical way, and transmission or information storage and retrieval, electronic adaptation, computer software, or by similar or dissimilar methodology now known or hereafter developed.

The use of general descriptive names, registered names, trademarks, service marks, etc. in this publication does not imply, even in the absence of a specific statement, that such names are exempt from the relevant protective laws and regulations and therefore free for general use.

The publisher, the authors, and the editors are safe to assume that the advice and information in this book are believed to be true and accurate at the date of publication. Neither the publisher nor the authors or the editors give a warranty, expressed or implied, with respect to the material contained herein or for any errors or omissions that may have been made. The publisher remains neutral with regard to jurisdictional claims in published maps and institutional affiliations.

This Springer imprint is published by the registered company Springer Nature Switzerland AG
The registered company address is: Gewerbestrasse 11, 6330 Cham, Switzerland

Foreword

The concept of this textbook is very timely with the current existence and the future of general surgery being questioned by many in our current era of super-specialized surgical care. While specialization in elective fields can lead too safe, efficient, and effective care with high levels of patient satisfaction, its feasibility in acute care is questionable. Superspecialist surgeons working within very narrow fields in their daily routine practice are unlikely to be competent to manage all surgical emergencies outside of their expertise. Hospitals providing emergency general surgical service are also unlikely to be prepared to support and maintain dozens of specialist surgical rosters for the management of each individual organ or organ parts. This latter concept of many subspecialist general surgical rosters would also necessitate a second surgical triage system after the emergency department triage, which inadvertently would lead to further delay to definitive care of the acute surgical patients. These facts re-establish the concept of the generalist surgeon in our heavily specialized modern practice. Emergency general surgery practice for a broad spectrum of conditions combined with adequate elective surgical opportunities provides a viable option for surgeons dedicated to public/academic institutions with surgical training programs. This model provides excellent opportunities to maintain surgical skills, cost-effective for healthcare and ideal for resident training programs. The prolific book publishing Professors Catena and Coccolini have produced another Italian masterpiece, probably the most comprehensive one so far. This impressive textbook on emergency general surgery consists of more than 100 chapters with over 300 international contributors from an excess of 40 countries of all continents. After a generous first chapter of overarching concepts, the book covers the key anatomical regions such as head and neck, chest, abdomen, extremities, and soft tissue surgical conditions. Beyond being didactic, this work is also ultra-pragmatic by addressing all aspects of emergency general surgery in different age groups, complications of subspecialties including transplantation, communication principles, and ethical issues, just to mention a few. Considering the topic selection, the exceptional content, the contemporary illustration material, and latest references with evidence-based approach, this work will be an essential companion to all general surgical residents, acute care general surgeons, and subspecialists who occasionally need to deal with general surgical emergencies.

University of Newcastle Zsolt J. Balogh
Callaghan, Newcastle NSW Australia
John Hunter Hospital
New Lambton Heights NSW Australia

Foreword

At the beginning of 2020, the challenges raised by the Covid-19 pandemic induced an unprecedented public health crisis. More than 6.2 million people died because of Covid in the last two years, but road traffic injuries caused an estimated 1.3 million deaths worldwide in the last years, and more than 400,000 people die from homicide each year.

The World Society of Emergency Surgery (WSES) has been working on the Emergency General Surgery (EGS) organization since its foundation, collaborating with other societies for training and educational programs throughout the world. Management of emergency surgical patients with traumatic or non-traumatic acute conditions is a challenge and many countries have started a systematic effort in reorganizing EGS systems. Shortage of dedicated trained physicians, unfamiliarity with protocols, absence of dedicated teams, delay in surgery, and overcrowded emergency department and intensive care units may affect patient outcomes in unprepared systems.

In the last years many educational courses were developed and structured worldwide. But this book is a great opportunity to health professionals and undergraduate students learn more about EGS. The editors were very careful and intelligent to bring up various aspects of EGS, such as education, disease physiology, diagnosis, treatment, prognosis, and ethical issues. The authors are well-respected and recognized surgeons in their respective countries with extensive experience in EGS. I am very grateful to be a part of this project and it is an honor to write this preface, without prolonging too much, so that each reader can appreciate each of the chapters. And you can use this very comprehensive book to improve your clinical practice and better assist your patients.

Division of Trauma Surgery
University of Campinas,
Campinas, Brazil

Gustavo P. Fraga

Foreword

"The future belongs to preventive health care. This science, going hand in hand with curative health care will bring undoubted benefits to mankind."

N.I. Pirogov (1810–1881)

At present, the problem of diagnosis and treatment of surgical emergencies remain topical. The rapid development of high-tech surgical instruments and the spread of minimally invasive procedures have led to the emergence of unknown postoperative complications and new algorithms for managing such patients.

Gone are the days when S.P. Fedorov's statement "a great surgeon is recognizable by a large incision" was the motto for several generations of emergency surgeons. Today, modern surgeons have many high-tech instruments at their disposal for accurate and quick diagnoses as well as various alternative methods of surgery. In fact, this feature of modern medicine does not always benefit the patient. Indecision, the inability to make quick and correct decisions, lack of knowledge about the latest approaches of evidence-based medicine to treating certain diseases can devalue technological advances and lead to adverse events.

A doctor is the crucial element in the "science—human health" chain. Therefore, even in the era of digital technologies, neural networks, and artificial intelligence, an intelligent mind and skillful hands remain the principal instruments in the fight against illness and death.

I hope that every reader of this book, either a medical student or an experienced specialist, will discover not only something new, but also something useful, for example, a special feature of preoperative patient preparation, subtleties of operations, or equally important issues of postoperative management and rehabilitation of patients.

Sechenov Medical University Eduard A. Galliamov
Moskow, Russia

Foreword

The *Textbook of Emergency General Surgery: Traumatic and Non-traumatic Surgical Emergencies* is a comprehensive resource for surgeons throughout the world who provide emergent care for seriously ill and injured patients. The authors are authorities in their respective areas and represent experience and expertise. While the practice domain varies from civilian to military, country to country, and urban to rural, the common objective is to provide as optimal care as possible considering the surgeons' and hospitals' capabilities. Definitive care may require patient transfer to a more experience facility, despite the fact that the surgeon possesses the necessary skills. The first section of the book provides an overview of general principles that apply to initial evaluation and management of the patient requiring urgent care, including triage in mass casualty events. The next section covers the physiologic challenges in the critically ill and injured, including the important differences based on age and comorbidities. Prompt reversal of shock is a common problem in many of these patients that is important to prioritize in operative management. There is also a timely discussion of care during pandemics that we learned painfully during the unprecedented COVID-19 infection, impacting all authors of this text. Palliative and futile care are particularly relevant for emergent surgical challenges because there is frequently limited opportunity to discuss this topic with the patient before their event. The ensuing sections present topics based on anatomic location, literally from head to toe. These anatomic-based sections are complete covering emergent trauma and non-trauma topics, including life-threatening bleeding and infections. I congratulate the editors and authors on a spectacular resource document that highlights the essential role of emergency general surgeons who provide exemplary care 24 h a day/7 days a week throughout the year.

University of Colorado Ernest E. Moore
Denver, CA, USA

Foreword

The global burden of emergency surgery is very significant, and several issues need to be addressed in order to promote a global dialogue on what is the most appropriate way to conceive emergency surgery worldwide. Although minimal variations in the spectrum of emergency surgical diseases may be observed among and within countries, "essential" surgery in emergency should be viewed as a core group of services that can be delivered within the context of universal access.

Furthermore, the surgical capabilities required are not only those related to performing operations. Emergency surgical care also involves preoperative assessment, including the decision to operate; provision of safe anesthesia; and postoperative care. Even when patients do not need emergency surgical procedures, surgical providers often provide care and must be prepared to intervene operatively as complications arise or conditions deteriorate.

Finally, many hospitals worldwide continue to have logistic barriers associated with the application of evidence-based practice, leading to an overall poorer adherence to international guidelines and making them impractical to a large part of the world's clinicians.

In this scenario, a *Textbook of Emergency General Surgery* including both traumatic and non-traumatic surgical emergencies, written by experts from all continents can be very useful to promote global standards of care that can drive clinicians around the world by describing "reasonable" approaches to the management of emergency surgery diseases.

General Surgery
Macerata Hospital
Macerata, Italy

Massimo Sartelli

Preface

Emergency General Surgery (EGS) is the most widespread surgical discipline encompassing all traumatic and non-traumatic surgical emergencies. It is widely practiced throughout the entire world. Most general surgeons manage surgical emergencies during their daily activity. The emergency general surgeon may be the last surgeon able to deal with surgical emergencies in almost any region of the body in emergency setting, including traumatic and non-traumatic conditions.

The general emergency surgeon should be ideally trained to manage surgical and physiological derangements in all types of patients, from young and healthy to severely compromised. Currently, notwithstanding the worldwide spread of EGS and its importance along with its public health burdens, comprehensive and reliable textbooks have not been published yet.

This work represents the first in its field and is the result of worldwide participation. More than 250 authors from all continents contributed to the writing process with high-level chapters covering all the different topics. The work covers all aspects necessary for daily practice providing valuable assistance and sure help in handling even those rare and difficult situations.

High-quality photos and images clearly explain concepts giving a quick and effective tool to understand diseases and surgical techniques.

In addition, clear flowcharts will help surgeons around the world to rapidly evaluate and decide on the best strategy.

We devoted the past 2 years to this effort with the goal of improving patient care in a such difficult and widespread field.

This book is aimed at medical school students, residents, and specialists in general surgery, anesthesiology/intensive care, and emergency medicine.

Likewise, all residents and specialists in surgical and medical disciplines seeking to further their skills in the field of acute care surgery may find this textbook a useful guide.

We sincerely hope that it will be of help to all of you.

Enjoy it!

Pisa, Italy Federico Coccolini
Cesena, Italy Fausto Catena

Contents

Volume I

Part I   General Consideration

1 **History of Emergency General Surgery** 3
   Massimo Chiarugi

2 **General Approach to Emergency General Surgery** 9
   Patricia Correia Sousa Perissé and Antonio Marttos

3 **Evaluation of Traumatic and Nontraumatic Patients** 19
   Vitor F. Kruger and Gustavo P. Fraga

4 **Prioritizing Acute Care Surgery and Trauma Patients** 33
   R. Stephen Smith and Jessica E. Taylor

5 **Triage** 39
   Cordoba Mordehay, Ciro Paolillo, Federica Pitoni,
   and Klein Yoram

6 **Mass Casualties** 47
   Emmanouil Pikoulis, Anastasia Pikouli, and Athanasios
   Kalogeropoulos

7 **Point-of-Care Ultrasound for Emergency General Surgeons** . . . 63
   Bruno M. Pereira

8 **Systemic Response to Injury** 91
   Philip F. Dobson, Karen Muller, and Zsolt J. Balogh

9 **Coagulation and Thrombosis** 107
   Jonathan P. Meizoso, Hunter B. Moore, Angela Sauaia,
   and Ernest E. Moore

10 **Septic Shock** 127
   Sacha Rozencwajg and Philippe Montravers

11 **Hypovolemic Shock** 137
   Tyler J. Jones, Bishwajit Bhattacharya,
   and Kimberly A. Davis

12	**Principles of Perioperative Management in Acute Care Surgery**	147
	Oreste Romeo, Taylor A. Davidson, and Scott B. Davidson	
13	**Critical Care Medicine**	159
	Maria Di Matteo and Davide Corbella	
14	**Fluid and Blood Management in Traumatic and Non-traumatic Surgical Emergencies**	183
	Domien Vanhonacker, Michaël Mekeirele, and Manu L. N. G. Malbrain	
15	**Compartment Syndrome**	197
	Rao R. Ivatury	
16	**Antibiotic and Antimicotic Therapy**	219
	Marcelo A. F. Ribeiro Junior, Gabriela Tebar, and José Lucas Rodrigues Salgueiro	
17	**Pain Management**	243
	Etrusca Brogi and Francesco Forfori	
18	**Damage Control Surgery**	265
	Carlo Vallicelli and Federico Coccolini	
19	**Nutritional Support**	275
	Swathikan Chidambaram, En Lin Goh, and Mansoor Ali Khan	
20	**Palliative Care in the ICU**	285
	Mayur Narayan and Jeffry Kashuk	
21	**Immunosuppression in Surgical Patients**	313
	Hannah Groenen and Marja A. Boermeester	
22	**Pregnant Women**	331
	Pintar Tadeja	
23	**Geriatrics: Traumatic and Non-traumatic Surgical Emergencies**	347
	Kartik Prabhakaran and Rifat Latifi	
24	**Pediatrics**	367
	Matthew P. Landman and Denis Bensard	
25	**Cirrhotic Patients**	389
	Greg Padmore and Chad G. Ball	
26	**Management of Animal Bites: A Global Perspective**	401
	Saleh Abdel-Kader, Ihab M. Abbas, and Fikri M. Abu-Zidan	
27	**Burns, Inhalation, and Lightning Injury**	411
	Mariëlle Vehmeijer-Heeman and Edward Tan	

28	**Blast: Mechanisms of Injury and Implications upon Treatment**...	427
	Itamar Ashkenazi and Yoram Kluger	
29	**Major Bleeding Management and REBOA**..................	443
	Amelia Pasley, Victoria Sharp, Jason Pasley, and Megan Brenner	
30	**Robotics**..	457
	Giorgio Bianchi, Aleix Martínez-Pérez, and Nicola de'Angelis	
31	**Emergency and Trauma Surgery During Epidemia and Pandemia**...............................	471
	Belinda De Simone, Elie Chouillard, and Fausto Catena	
32	**Principles of Management of Surgical Complications**........	487
	Nikolaos Pararas, Anastasia Pikouli, Konstantinos Nastos, and Emmanouil Pikoulis	
33	**Iatrogenic Complications of Digestive Endoscopy**............	497
	Aleix Martínez-Pérez, Carmen Payá-Llorente, and Nicola de'Angelis	
34	**End-of-Life Care, Including the Role of Intensive Care in Tissue and Organ Donation**.......................	513
	Christopher James Doig and Kevin J. Solverson	
35	**Futility of Care and Palliative Care**.......................	523
	Paolo Malacarne and Silvia Pini	
36	**Communication in Emergency General Surgery**..............	531
	Evika Karamagioli	
37	**Patient Safety and Risk Management**......................	539
	Boris E. Sakakushev	
38	**Quality Evaluation in Emergency General Surgery**..........	569
	Michael Sugrue, Randal Parlour, Brendan Skelly, and Angus Watson	

Part II Head, Face and Neck

39	**Head and Brain Trauma**.................................	581
	Giacomo Bertolini, Luca Cattani, Corrado Iaccarino, Anna Fornaciari, and Edoardo Picetti	
40	**Emergency Surgical Access to the Neck**....................	605
	Iván Trostchansky and Fernando Machado	
41	**Face and Neck Infections**................................	623
	Alfons Mogedas, Mireia Pascua, and Xavier Guirao	

42	**Trauma to the Face**........................... 641
	Kerry P. Latham and Mark W. Bowyer
43	**Traumatic Neck Injuries** 651
	Rathnayaka M. Kalpanee D. Gunasingha and Mark W. Bowyer
44	**Management of Neck Surgery Complications** 665
	Giovanna Di Meo, Alessandro Pasculli, and Mario Testini

Part III Thorax and Mediastinum

45	**Emergency Surgical Access to the Thorax** 691
	Marc de Moya and Rebecca Mitchell
46	**Empyema**.. 703
	Linda C. Qu, Rahul Nayak, and Neil G. Parry
47	**Hemothorax and Pneumothorax**........................ 711
	David A. Spain, Ara Ko, and Jamie Tung
48	**Chest Trauma** 727
	Joseph M. Galante and Tanya N. Rinderknecht
49	**Thoracic Vascular Trauma**................................ 743
	G. Janssen, M. Khashram, S. Bhagvan, and I. Civil
50	**Resuscitative Thoracotomy** 753
	Ning Lu and Walter L. Biffl
51	**Cardiac Trauma and Tamponade** 765
	Lena M. Napolitano
52	**Management of Cardiothoracic Surgery Complications** 783
	Bernd Niemann, Ursula Vigelius-Rauch, and Andreas Hecker
53	**Acute Congenital and Acquired Heart Disease** 801
	Alessandro Leone, G. Murana, L. Di Marco, E. Angeli, L. Careddu, G. Gargiulo, and D. Pacini

Volume II

Part IV Abdomen

54	**Principles of Emergency and Trauma Laparotomy**........... 815
	S. Barbois and C. Arvieux
55	**Principles of Emergency and Trauma Laparoscopy** 833
	Felipe Vega-Rivera, Ignacio Alvarez-Valero, Fernando Pérez-Galaz, and Alberto Pérez Cantú-Sacal
56	**Esophageal Non-traumatic Emergencies** 855
	Luigi Bonavina, Emanuele Asti, and Tommaso Panici Tonucci

57	**Esophageal Trauma** 871
	Michael D. Kelly and Mircea Chirica
58	**Caustic Ingestion**. 877
	Mircea Chirica, Helene Corte, and Pierre Cattan
59	**Surgical Jaundice and Cholangitis** 889
	Aleksandar R. Karamarkovic, Jovan T. Juloski, and Vladica V. Cuk
60	**Biliary Colic and Acute Cholecystitis** 901
	Paola Fugazzola, Mario Improta, and Luca Ansaloni
61	**Hepatic Abscesses** 911
	Kyra N. Folkert, Sarah Khalil, and Robert Sawyer
62	**Spleen Non-traumatic Acute Surgical Conditions** 923
	Marco Ceresoli and Luca Degrate
63	**Acute Adrenal Conditions: Pheochromocytoma Emergencies** 935
	Gabriele Materazzi, Leonardo Rossi, and Piermarco Papini
64	**Nontraumatic Liver Hemorrhage** 949
	Amudan J. Srinivasan and Andrew B. Peitzman
65	**Acute Pancreatitis**. 969
	Ari Leppäniemi and Matti Tolonen
66	**Acute Appendicitis** 983
	Gaetano Gallo, Mauro Podda, Marta Goglia, and Salomone Di Saverio
67	**Acute Left Colonic Diverticulitis** 1001
	Massimo Sartelli
68	**Acute Mesenteric Ischemia** 1007
	Miklosh Bala and Asaf Kedar
69	**Upper Gastrointestinal Bleeding** 1017
	Helmut A. Segovia Lohse and Herald R. Segovia Lohse
70	**Gastric Outlet Obstruction** 1035
	Feibo Zheng, Liang Ha, and Yunfeng Cui
71	**Acute Lower Gastrointestinal Bleeding** 1049
	Muhammed A. Khalil Ali, Henry Bergman, Salomone Di Saverio, M. Adil Butt, and Ewen A. Griffiths
72	**Perforated Peptic Ulcer** 1067
	Delphina Yeo Boon Xue, Ramkumar Mohan, and Vishal G. Shelat
73	**Diagnosis and Management of Acute Small Bowel Obstruction** 1085
	Pepijn Krielen and Richard ten Broek

74	**Small Bowel Perforation**. 1095
	Dimitrios Damaskos, Anne Ewing, and Judith Sayers
75	**Small Bowel Diverticular Disease** 1103
	Carlos Yánez Benítez
76	**Large Bowel Obstruction**. 1117
	Tiffany Paradis, Tarek Razek, and Evan G. Wong
77	**Large Bowel Perforation** 1131
	V. Khokha
78	**Emergency Management of Abdominal Wall Hernia** 1143
	M. M. J. van Rooijen, J. F. Lange, and J. Jeekel
79	**Emergency Management of Internal Hernia** 1155
	David Czeiger, Julia Vaynshtein, Ivan Kukeev, and Gad Shaked
80	**Emergency Management Hiatal Hernia and Gastric Volvulus**. 1163
	Imtiaz Wani, G. M. Naikoo, and Nisar Hamdani
81	**Stoma-Related Surgical Emergencies**. 1175
	Arda Isik and Rajesh Ramanathan
82	**Inflammatory Bowel Disease** 1187
	Jeremy Meyer and Justin Davies
83	**Fulminant/Toxic Colitis** 1207
	Sanjay Marwah, Rajesh Godara, and Shouvik Das
84	**Clostridium Infections** 1227
	Giada Fasani, Angela Pieri, and Leonardo Pagani
85	**Bowel Parasitic Surgical Emergencies** 1253
	Ibrahima Sall, Magatte Faye, and Ibrahima Diallo
86	**Anorectal Emergencies**. 1263
	Antonio Tarasconi and Gennaro Perrone
87	**Gynaecological Surgical Emergencies**. 1283
	Robert Tchounzou, André Gaetan Simo Wambo, and Alain Chichom-Mefire
88	**Nontraumatic Urologic Emergencies** 1295
	Dyvon Walker, Rodrigo Donalisio da Silva, and Fernando J. Kim
89	**Non-Obstetric Abdominal Surgical Emergencies in Pregnancy and Puerperium**. 1307
	Goran Augustin
90	**Enterovesical and Enterogenital Fistulae** 1327
	Krishanth Naidu and Francesco Piscioneri

Contents

91 Enterocutaneous and Enteroatmospheric Fistulae 1337
Ashleigh Phillips, Eu Jhin Loh, and Francesco Amico

92 Complication of Bariatric Surgery 1351
Doron Kopelman and Uri Kaplan

93 Intra-Abdominal Hypertension and Abdominal Compartment Syndrome 1369
Tyler Lamb, Andrew W. Kirkpatrick, and Derek J. Roberts

94 Open Abdomen Management 1397
Pradeep Navsaria, Deidre McPherson, Sorin Edu, and Andrew Nicol

95 Liver Trauma 1415
Federico Coccolini, Camilla Cremonini, and Massimo Chiarugi

96 Splenic Trauma 1431
Tian Wei Cheng Brian Anthony, Carlo Vallicelli, and Fausto Catena

97 Bowel Trauma 1449
Carlos A. Ordoñez, Michael W. Parra, and Yaset Caicedo

98 Kidney and Urotrauma 1461
Federico Coccolini, Camilla Cremonini, and Massimo Chiarugi

99 Duodeno-Pancreatic and Extrahepatic Biliary Trauma 1483
Gennaro Perrone, Alfredo Annicchiarico, Elena Bonati, and Fausto Catena

100 Abdominal Vascular Trauma 1499
Franchesca J. Hwang, Jarrett E. Santorelli, Leslie M. Kobayashi, and Raul Coimbra

101 Genital and Anorectal Trauma 1513
Thobekile Nomcebo Shangase, Feroz Ganchi, and Timothy Craig Hardcastle

102 Pelvic Trauma 1527
Philip F. Stahel and Vincent P. Stahel

103 Ruptured Abdominal Aortic Aneurysm (rAAA) 1539
Tal M. Hörer

104 Visceral Artery Aneurysms 1553
Jonathan Parks and George C. Velmahos

105 Management of Complications Occurring After Pancreas Transplantation 1565
Fabio Vistoli, Emanuele Federico Kauffmann, Niccolò Napoli, Gabriella Amorese, and Ugo Boggi

106 Liver Transplant Complications Management 1581
Rami Rhaiem, Raffaele Brustia, Linda Rached,
and Daniele Sommacale

Part V   Extremities

107 Emergency Vascular Access to Extremities 1613
Frank Plani

108 Extremity Vascular Injuries........................... 1631
Viktor A. Reva and Adenauer Marinho de Oliveira Góes Junior

109 Extremities Trauma 1653
Ingo Marzi, Cora Rebecca Schindler, and Philipp Störmann

110 Extremity Compartment Syndrome 1663
Dominik A. Jakob, Elizabeth R. Benjamin,
and Demetrios Demetriades

111 Fasciitis... 1679
Yutaka Harima, Norio Sato, and Kaoru Koike

112 Bone Infections 1689
Luigi Branca Vergano and Mauro Monesi

Part VI   Soft Tissues

113 Necrotizing Soft Tissue Infection......................... 1715
Ashley A. Holly, Therese M. Duane, and Morgan Collom

114 Cutaneous and Subcutaneous Abscesses................... 1725
Jan Ulrych

115 Surgical Site Infections................................. 1737
A. Walker and M. Wilson

Part I

General Consideration

History of Emergency General Surgery

Massimo Chiarugi

1.1 Introduction

Mastering the art of surgery required centuries of endless improvement. The fathers of our profession managed to transform the evolution of knowledge in evolution of surgical care, finding a practical response to theoretical issues [1]. During the course of history, surgeons had to fight their way through the limits imposed by nature and the goal of their battle was to conquer physiology, technique, and time. All the progress of surgery, from ancient times to our present, focused on progressive ability to control these three key pillars and, with gradual proceeding, the development of one brought the others two factors to upgrade. This process took place in more than three millennia, starting from the religious roots of healers, through the pioneering studies of the great anatomists of Humanism, with an exceptional outbreak of possibilities and discoveries from the XIX century to our time [2–5]. The role of emergency general surgery (EGS) in this evolution is capital: as we are going to discuss in this chapter, most of the advances in the field are directly related to the response of medicine to war and emergency. In fact, the real beginning of surgery was in the necessity to face acute and emergency disease. Nevertheless, before the advent of a structured and evolute health care system, most procedures were at high risk of mortality and all surgery was to be considered as part of emergency setting. With the evolution of health care, surgery became progressively more and more like the integrated, precise, and effective medical science we know nowadays. However, even considering the outstanding advance of results in the last 50 years, the role of the emergency surgeon is yet to be definitively assessed.

In fact, emergency was more intended as the way the disease presents itself, than a specific setting requiring specific competences. Alongside with the increasing technical ability required and the arising possibilities coming from new discoveries, part of the duty of the general surgeon was reserved to the management of the emergency patients. However, the amount of specific knowledge and training required to perform complex procedures in specific anatomical districts fragmented the activity of the modern surgeon, weakening the synthetic ability to consider the peculiar characteristics of the patients requiring emergency procedures. At the same time, the conservative strategies acquired with the evolution of endoscopy and interventional radiology made some surgical abilities more complex to be trained or learned. Considering the three pillars mentioned above, a certain hypertrophy of technique and an almost unmanageable increasing in scientific physiology comprehension put the

M. Chiarugi (✉)
Emergency and Trauma Surgery Unit, Pisa University Hospital, Pisa, Italy
e-mail: massimo.chiarugi@unipi.it

hyperspecialized surgeon in a difficult situation: for several years, the emergency surgical patients were categorized and treated according to suboptimal criteria, borrowed from the elective setting.

In this chapter we are going to discuss from an historical perspective the progressive change in mentality and organization that allowed acute care surgery to be considered as an independent and comprehensive discipline, with specific competences and skills.

1.2 The Great Era of Surgery and the Origins of Emergency Model

The year 1846 can be considered the dawn of a Copernican revolution for surgeons: William Green Morton (1819–1868), dentist and physician, performed with John Collins Warren (1778–1856) the first public operation with ether anesthesia on a patient of the Massachusetts General Hospital. From that moment, in case we did not consider the natural and physiological resistance of tradition to innovation, a new concept of surgery arose. Alongside with chloroform and nitrous oxide, ether allowed painless interventions. The possibilities available to the genius of the great surgeons of that era increased drastically and procedures considered nearly impossible became reasonable options. The comprehension of physiology obtained by centuries of cadaver studies and medical research, along with the chance to access body districts until that moment inviolable, boosted surgical technique and surgery respectability to a level never seen before [6, 7].

However, if the conquer of time and the overcoming of technical limits became finally concrete options, on the other side, serious concern about infective complication and related mortality rates cooled down the enthusiasm: physiology and its pathological deranges were not under control. Surgery was increasing its feasibility and gaining respect in the scientific community, but a severe criticism on the insecurity of results inflamed the debate. It became clear that not only the procedure itself, but also the surgical environment, the ward, and the postoperatory management of patient were directly related with the outcomes. After the transformation of time management with anesthesia, technique was revolutionized by Joseph Lister (1827–1912), leading to a decisive improvement in physiology control: antiseptic method and phenol sterilization for instruments and wounds were the first practical applications to surgery of Pasteur's bacteria theory. After years of violent skepticism, well symbolized by the tragic destiny of Ignac Semmelweiss (1818–1965), Lister's methods were accepted and even perfectionated by the end of the XIX century. Following the endorsement of legends of surgery, such as Emil Kocher (1841–1917) and William Steward Halsted (1852–1922), the results of these techniques were published at the tenth International Congress of Medicine of 1890, in Berlin. From antisepsis, the active destruction of pathogens involved in potential infective processes with phenol, surgeons made then a gradual shift to asepsis, creating adequate facilities and sterilizing instruments easier to be cleaned and sanitized.

Strong of unforeseen positive results, the cultural momentum could not be more powerful. The variety of results obtained was so wide that every surgical school started to focus on specific fields. From the second half of the XIX century, the establishment of specialistic surgical branches produced the first tear in the univocal conception of a unified discipline: every anatomical district required specific techniques and specific skills.

Moreover, emergency was an abstract concept, derived from the type of presentation of the pathology: the procedure proposed was not necessarily different from the one performed in nonurgent conditions. Emergency influenced the practical organization of the intervention and the related increase in mortality and complications, not the technical performance. However, embryonal signs of emergency surgery independence sporadically appeared. In 1904, William S. Halsted (1852–1922) himself declared "Every important hospital should have on its resident staff of surgeons at least one who is well and able to deal with any emergency that may arise", thus acknowledging the peculiarity of the discipline and that the increasing volume of specialistic notions was shifting the surgeons towards an approach not always at ease with emergency.

The experience of the battlefield became fundamental to the process of emancipation of emergency and trauma surgery. The conflicts arose all over Europe, and in the United States, forced the field surgeons to give a proof of the latest improvements in a contest far more different from the organized city hospitals.

Already at the begin of XIX century, during the Napoleonic Wars, Dominique-Jean Larrey (1766–1842) introduced a rudimental concept of triage, understanding the capital importance of time management way beyond the operative time. He created the first system of battlefield evacuation with the introduction of *ambulances volantes* (flying ambulances), proposing the necessity of patient's centralization.

These improvements started to appear also in other parts of the world, pushed by eminent members of surgical history. Among the others, Nikolay Pirigov (1810–1881), Russian army surgeon, showed a pioneering scientific attitude: he considered war as an epidemic of trauma and systematically promoted the concept of triage in rescue organization. Considered one of the first to use anesthetic agents on the battlefield, Pirigov also proposed an osteoplastic method for foot amputation, opening emergency and trauma to a conservative and not only demolitive approach. Following on his footsteps, Vera Gedroits (1870–1932), first woman professor of surgery, described the beneficial effect of early celiotomy in combat wounds to the abdomen, setting the basis for the actual conception of trauma laparotomy. Probably one of the most modern minds on emergency and trauma surgery organization was Vladimir Oppel (1872–1932). Studying the mortality and return-to-duty rates of the Russian army, he theorized the necessity of "the right operation for the right patient at the right location at the right time". Again, it became clear that the time factor in emergency setting was different from the one in the city hospitals: the availability of medical facilities closer to the combat action, able to stabilize the wounded, was a key issue in improving care quality as well as dedicated guidelines for casualty management. Moreover, the improvements were based on data analysis, setting the bases for the development of a contemporary scientific approach to emergency and trauma.

World War I and World War II allowed further development of these concepts, tragically validating the theory with catastrophic numbers of casualties.

The creation of the Mobile Army Surgical Hospitals (MASH) during the Korean War completed the process of a modernization of field surgery, introducing the progressive transport of the patient from primary stabilization to more complex care. Moreover, the wide diffusion of antibiotics permitted a significant reduction of infective complications and, therefore, general mortality.

The improvement of results and the new awareness of the strict dependency between time and outcome created the model for a new branch of surgery, with specific technique and new attention towards the physiological complexity of the emergency patient. From military experience, it became evident that a unified approach to the surgical patient, borrowed from the daily experience in the operatory room, was no more admittable. In the same fashion, a change in the organization of the civilian emergency health care begin to be required.

1.3 Emergency Management in Modern Times

It became clear from the modern war experience that the organization of civilian emergency surgery was involving not only medical aspects, but also logistical and structural ones. The first major revolution was dedicated to trauma care. From the late '50s, in the US, a first coordinated system of accreditation for trauma centers started to appear, basing on the available facilities and on treatment possibilities. In 1969, in Maryland, a police helicopter was use for the transport of patient from the injury scene to the hospital, suggesting that a prompt centralization to a center dedicated to trauma could lead to better outcomes. Progressively, in the '70s, the evacuation of the traumatized patient changed from reaching the closest hospital available to stabilization and transport to specialized trauma center [8].

Unlike in war settings, the civilian scenario is rarely presenting with scarcity of resources and large numbers of victims. If we exclude mass casualties, the process of triage in normal conditions is based on the evaluation of the best possible treatment for one or a small number of patients, according to severity of injury and presenting status. This decision-making process needed to be supported by shared and evidenced-based opinions: in 1976, simultaneously with the creation of a quality review program for designed trauma centers, the American College of Surgeons (ACS) promoted a first set of guidelines for stratification of injury severity, basing on anatomical and physiological criteria. The following 25 years brought several improvements to the first proposed flowcharts, gradually reaching the structure of organization we know nowadays.

However, the change did not involve only structural organization, but also scientific approach: already in 1938, the American Association for Traumatic Surgery was created (name change later in American Association for the Surgery of Trauma—AAST), showing the birth of a precocious attention to the matters specifically connected with the traumatic pathology. The US national registers allowed the analysis of large amounts of data, leading to progressive improvement of guidelines and, ultimately, of quality of care. At the same time, the combined upgrading of military and civilian technology brought surgical and acute care technique to ameliorate.

The three pillars discussed above were again modified by the progressive awareness of the peculiarity of emergency: the connection between time and physiology became more and more clear with the introduction of concepts such as the golden hour and the lethal triad; standard surgical technique was apparently dominated by decades of experience and practice. This process, however, was principally applied only to trauma for the second half of XX century: the emergency surgery part of acute care was a sort of nobody's land, where heterogeneous specialized skills were used to perform only a variation on the elective surgery theme. This identity crisis was further increased by the development of conservative techniques, able to replace in the long run some of the procedures traditionally managed by the emergency surgeon.

Conversely, the need of a structured emergency system was increasing. Trauma was not the only silent epidemic: with an estimated five million people dying every year from injuries, 900,000 deaths happen from illnesses under the jurisdiction of the acute surgeon. If the great majority of these deaths occur in the low- and medium-income countries, the magnitude of the problem involves the most evolute health care systems, too. In fact, while medical facilities and surgical resources are reduced or –in a best-case scenario- kept at the same levels, the progressive oldening of the population and the very characteristics of the health care system cause a constant increase in the demand for urgent services and providers. Moreover, the growing clinical complexity of the patients and the necessity of both intensive and sub-intensive care units begin to require professionals trained with skills going beyond pure surgery.

This perception was clear in Europe since the '70s: the different epidemiology of trauma and the different organization of health care brought a precocious awareness of the problems related to emergency surgery and surgical invasive care. In 1973, in Milan, a first congress of Emergency Surgery and Surgical Intensive Care was held. In the following years, a tenacious will of collaboration allowed to overcome the political divisions of the European continent and to start a coordinated effort to create common spaces of discussion. In the '90s, facilitated by the new economic cooperation among EU countries, association of emergency professionals begin to set shared standards for quality of care. In this spirit, EAES (European Association of Emergency Surgery) was created: the project of an international partnership, strongly promoted since the '70s by the futuristic vision of Vittorio Staudacher (1913–2005) and Louis F. Hollender (1922–2011), became reality under the first presidency of Enrico Cavina (1936). The association later changed its name in EATES (European Association for Trauma and Emergency Surgery).

The need for cooperation among trauma, emergency surgery, and critical care became progressively a priority, and at the turn of the millennium, the medical community involved in emergency surgery focused its activity on rediscussing the paradigms of acute care surgery. In 2003, AAST, ACS, the Eastern Trauma Society, and the Western Trauma Society proposed to codify trauma surgery, emergency general surgery, and acute surgical care under the unified field of acute care surgery (ACS). In 2007, closing a process started in 2004, EATES and ETS (European Trauma Society) merged to create ESTES (European Society for Trauma and emergency Surgery). In the same year, the World Society of Emergency Surgery (WSES) was created, with the intention to develop an international scientific cooperation able to understand the different needs of the different socioeconomic settings where acute care surgery is required. At the same time, strong effort was made worldwide to define the curriculum required for an acute care surgery expert, with the idea of creating a certification with a specific educational program, encompassing both clinical and surgical aspects and touching competences in more distant fields, such as neurosurgery, orthopedics, burn care, and pediatric surgery.

1.4 Future Perspectives of Acute Care Surgery

The XXI century brought important challenges for the emergency surgeon. The great effort for reformation of the first decade of the 2000s is only the first part of a revolution that involves health care in every part of the world.

If we analyze again the three pillars of surgery (time, physiology, and technique), we can easily recognize that the struggle for improvement still involves these key factors. However, in a time of liquid categories, the interdependence of the three is more than ever evident. Technique is no more a matter of mere surgical skills, but is also represented by the facilities available, the chances at disposition, and the ability to choose among different treatments, where surgery is only one of the possibilities. On the other side, technique is still a capital issue when it comes to the difficult relationship between training in elective setting and training in emergency setting. In fact, the acute care surgeon's competences should encompass all districts, beyond the modern concept of hyper-specialization, but, at the same time, the skills required in emergency setting are slightly different from those required in elective activity. Time is not only a key point in the management of the urgent patient, but it is also a parameter of the efficiency of a system and of access to care. Physiology is interlaced not only with time, but also with technique: different strategies, from conservative approach to damage control surgery, have enormous influence on outcomes and must be chosen from our toolbox only with a clear understanding of the pro and cons. Moreover, the peculiar physiology of the urgent surgical patient is also a matter of resources: 20% of accesses in the US are for urgent EGS conditions, accounting however for the 25% of total inpatients costs. The emergency general surgery patient, in fact, has an eight-fold increased risk of mortality when compared to the same procedure in elective setting, a higher rate of readmission and complications, and a significative change of care discontinuity after discharge. For all these reasons, alongside with trauma, emergency surgery, and surgical critical care, it has been proposed to include elective general surgery and surgical rescue within the definition of EGS.

Physiology and its study comprehend also the scientific effort dedicated to EGS. The collection of data, the analysis of results, and the derived literature are crucial to the continuous upgrading process. To overcome the extreme difficulty of creating randomized trials in such a heterogeneous field, international registers are a possible solution to obtain data from different settings and to create cohorts of patients with adequate numerosity. With the same spirit, the production of guidelines coming from common effort of different scientific societies is a strong way to increase the coherence of EGS performance and, thus, of resulting data.

A certain attention must be given also to all facilities and professionals involved in EGS. The Sars-CoV-2 pandemic showed how fragile and yet interconnected is the global health care system: a significative endeavor should be dedicated protecting and strengthening sensible resources, such as emergency and acute care. The lessons learned from this dramatic experience should be treasured and guide our future attitude towards the organization of health systems: equity and quality of care must be protected at all costs.

1.5 Conclusion

EGS and its perception changed during the ages of medical progress. Despite being part of the very core of medical science, it has almost lost its identity during the era of hyper-specialization. However, the strong effort put in its renovation and the consequent results show that the history of EGS, more than the development of a framework, is the history of how we perceive the challenges of health. Renovation and evolution are directly connected with the ability of a system to change and to accept the peculiar challenges of its times.

References

1. Lyu HG, Najjar P, Havens JM. Past, present, and future of emergency general surgery in the USA. Acute Med Surg. 2018;5(2):119–22. https://doi.org/10.1002/ams2.327. PMID: 29657721; PMCID: PMC5891107.
2. Mackersie RC. History of trauma field triage development and the American College of Surgeons criteria. Prehosp Emerg Care. 2006;10(3):287–94. https://doi.org/10.1080/10903120600721636. PMID: 16801263.
3. Wright JR Jr, Schachar NS. Necessity is the mother of invention: William Stewart Halsted's addiction and its influence on the development of residency training in North America. Can J Surg. 2020;63(1):E13–9. https://doi.org/10.1503/cjs.003319. PMID: 31944636; PMCID: PMC7828946.
4. Catena F, Moore F, Ansaloni L, Leppäniemi A, Sartelli M, Peitzmann AB, Biffl W, Coccolini F, Di Saverio S, Simone BD, Pisano M, Moore EE. Emergency surgeon: "last of the mohicans" 2014-2016 editorial policy WSES- WJES: position papers, guidelines, courses, books and original research; from WJES impact factor to WSES congress impact factor. World J Emerg Surg. 2014;9(1):14. https://doi.org/10.1186/1749-7922-9-14. Erratum in: World J Emerg Surg 2014;9(1):25. PMID: 24484743; PMCID: PMC3913950.
5. Søreide K. Emergency surgery over 111 years: are we still at a crossroads or ready for emergency surgery 2.0? Scand J Trauma Resusc Emerg Med. 2015;23:107. https://doi.org/10.1186/s13049-015-0189-9. PMID: 26689822; PMCID: PMC4687313.
6. Knowlton LM, Minei J, Tennakoon L, Davis KA, Doucet J, Bernard A, Haider A, Scherer LRT 3rd, Spain DA, Staudenmayer KL. The economic footprint of acute care surgery in the United States: implications for systems development. J Trauma Acute Care Surg. 2019;86(4):609–16. https://doi.org/10.1097/TA.0000000000002181. PMID: 30589750; PMCID: PMC6433481.
7. Kutcher ME, Peitzman AB. A history of acute care surgery (emergency surgery). In: Di Saverio S, Catena F, Ansaloni L, Coccolini F, Velmahos G, editors. Acute care surgery handbook. Cham: Springer; 2017. https://doi.org/10.1007/978-3-319-15341-4_2.
8. Barnett R. Crucial interventions: an illustrated treatise on the principles & practice of nineteenth-century surgery. London: Thames & Hudson; 2015. isbn-10:9780500518106.

General Approach to Emergency General Surgery

Patricia Correia Sousa Perissé and Antonio Marttos

2.1 Introduction

The definition of acute abdomen is an acute episode of abdominal pain, within less than a week, related to an intra-abdominal, thoracic, or systematic pathology that requires urgent intervention such as surgery.

Acute abdomen has a potential surgical nature and immediate management is required. The workup starts with a history, physical examination, labs, and imaging studies [1].

During the history, the abdominal pain description, onset, progression, duration, radiation, severity grade, and location (may signal a localized or diffuse process), associated with the additional symptoms such as nausea, vomiting, hematemesis/hematochezia, loss of appetite, diarrhea, or constipation and the patient's past medical history, will help the surgeon to determine the differential diagnosis and the patient's initial treatment.

An attentive and organized physical examination is essential for the patient's accurate diagnosis and treatment. The sequence begins with a general inspection and abdominal inspection, four quadrants auscultation, percussion, and finishes with palpation (See details on the physical examination section).

The patient's history and physical examination remain the mainstays of determining the accurate diagnosis and starting a proper and timely therapy. The labs and imaging studies are used to confirm the suspicions [1]. Depending on the diagnosis, the patient could be submitted to laparoscopy, laparotomy, or clinical management [1].

The abdominal pain's evaluation must be precise and careful; many diseases can present the symptom and be managed without surgery (See examples in the differential diagnosis section).

Imaging like X-Ray, CT, ultrasonography, and MRI may help the surgeon determine the diagnosis and management [2].

As a general principle, the specific treatment during an emergency is oriented by the organ(s) affected, the relative speed at which clinical symptoms progress and worsen, and the underlying physiological stability of the patient.

P. C. S. Perissé (✉)
Miami University Miller School of Medicine, Miami, FL, USA

Division of Trauma and Surgical Critical Care, Miami, FL, USA

A. Marttos
William Lehman Injury Research Center, Miami, FL, USA

Division of Trauma and Surgical Critical Care, Miami, FL, USA

Dewitt Daughtry Department of Surgery, University of Miami Miller School of Medicine, Miami, FL, USA
e-mail: amarttos@med.miami.edu

> **Learning Goals**
> - Explain the acute abdomen history, clinical presentation, physical exam, management, and evaluation
> - Identify surgical cases of acute abdomen
> - Describe differential diagnosis for the acute abdomen.

2.1.1 Epidemiology

The acute abdomen's main cause is nonspecific abdominal pain (24–44.3%), followed by acute appendicitis (15.9–28.1%), acute biliary disease (2.9–9.7%), and bowel obstruction or diverticulitis in elderly patients. Two-thirds of the children with acute abdomen may have association with acute appendicitis, representing the number one surgical pathology within this population. The patients between ages 30 and 69 years old experienced an increase of 6.3% [3].

Addiss et al. [4] describe the relation between sex and race with the appendicitis prevalence. In his study, Males presented higher rates of appendicitis than females for all age groups (overall ratio 1.4:1), and Whites had 1.5 times increased risk than non-Whites.

The Bologna guidelines describe the epidemiology of adhesive small bowel obstruction as one of the leading causes of surgical emergencies requiring emergent surgery. Small bowel obstruction was the indication for 51% of all emergency laparotomies in the UK. Even with the advent of laparoscopic surgery, intra-abdominal adhesions remain a significant cause of SBO, accounting for 65% of cases.

Feliciano et al. [5] Mc Graw describe that approximately 15% of hospital admissions for acute abdominal pain in the USA are due to small and large bowel obstructions, and approximately 20% of cases need surgical care.

Meagher et al. describe that trauma injuries are the leading cause of death for Americans aged 1–44 years and the third leading cause of death overall.

Feliciano et al. [5] describe that injury deaths have risen over the period from 2000 to 2016 in the USA, from 52 per 100.000 in 2000 to 72 per 100.000 in 2016.

2.1.2 Etiology

The main causes associated with surgical acute abdomen are hemorrhage, infection, perforation, vascular occlusion, obstruction, and trauma.

2.1.3 Classification

Surgical acute abdomen can be classified by cause: Hemorrhage, infection, perforation, vascular occlusion, obstruction, and trauma [6].

Trauma injury is divided into blunt (direct impact with an object sudden deceleration) and penetrating injuries. Splenic injury is the most frequent lesion after blunt trauma, followed by liver and kidney involvement. In penetrating abdominal injuries, hollow visceral organs are most frequently affected [5, 7].

2.1.4 Pathophysiology

The pathophysiology of the acute abdomen is beyond the scope of this chapter, being associated to the acute abdomen causes described in the etiology section, as well as the pain components: visceral and parietal [6].

Visceral nerves are part of the autonomic nervous system and are sensitive to ischemia, inflammation, and mechanical distention.

Visceral pain is vague and poorly localized in the epigastrium, periumbilical region, or hypogastrium, depending on its localization. The pain originating from the foregut structures such as the stomach, liver, pancreas, and gallbladder radiates to the epigastrium. The stimulus originating from the midgut structures such as the small bowel and appendix radiates to the periumbilical area, and the pain originating from hindgut structures such as the large bowel and rectum radiates to the lower abdomen.

Parietal pain corresponds to the segmental nerve roots innervating the peritoneum and tends to be sharper and better localized. Referred pain is localized by the patient in a distant site from the cause of the stimulus. For example, a patient with diaphragm inflammation may present pain in the shoulders, or a patient with cholecystitis may present pain radiated to the right scapula.

Visceral pain can be felt as referred because visceral and parietal afferent nerve fibers share spinal cord segments.

2.2 Diagnosis

Despite the etiology involved with the acute abdomen, every case's evaluation shall be initiated by the history and physical examination that remain the mainstay to diagnosis. Labs and imaging exams are important to confirm the diagnosis.

The acute abdomen is a challenging clinical scenario with a great surgical potential, requiring a prompt workup. Its sequence follows the usual order of history, physical examination, labs, and imaging studies. The most important part of evaluation remains a thorough history and meticulous physical examination. Labs and imaging studies are directed by the findings collected with the history and physical examination [2, 3, 8, 9].

2.2.1 Clinical Presentation

2.2.1.1 History

The principal chief complaint is abdominal pain followed by fever, nausea, vomiting, anorexia, constipation, blood per rectum, jaundice, UTI symptoms, pelvic pain, suspected pregnancy, anuria, or a history of accident or injury.

The initial admission of the stable patient shall initiate with a scrupulous history, focusing on abdominal pain description, onset, progression, duration, radiation, severity grade, location (may signal a localized or diffuse process), additional symptoms such as nausea, vomiting, hematemesis/hematochezia, loss of appetite, diarrhea, or constipation, and the patient's past medical history. This initial approach is crucial to determine the differential diagnosis and the patient's initial treatment.

The intensity and severity of the abdominal pain are related with the grade of tissue damage. Sudden onset of excruciating pain suggests ischemia or organ perforation. Inflammatory or infectious conditions may present pain that worsens during hours [2].

The location and radiation of the pain are important clues to diagnosis. Solid organ visceral pain is related in the quadrant of the involved organ (Table 2.1):

A careful history must identify associated symptoms such as nausea, vomiting, diarrhea,

Table 2.1 Relation between pain location and organ injury - Adapted from [6, 10]

Right hypochondrium	Epigastrium	Left hypochondrium
Gallbladder, liver, duodenum, right kidney upper portion, pancreas, small intestine, ascending/transverse colon	Stomach, lower part of esophagus, descending aorta, first part of duodenum/small intestine, and pancreas head	Stomach, pancreas, spleen, liver, left kidney upper portion, small intestine, transverse/descending colon
Right flank	**Umbilical region**	**Left flank**
Right kidney, ascending colon, and parts of small intestine	Small intestine, transverse portion of the colon, aorta	Left kidney, descending colon, small intestine
Right iliac fossa	**Hypogastrium**	**Left iliac fossa**
Appendix, ureter, cecum, fallopian tube, ovary, spermatic cord	Bladder, uterus	Ureter, sigmoid portion, ovary, fallopian tube, spermatic cord

melena, hematemesis, hematochezia, hematuria, constipation, massive abdominal distention, and bloody diarrhea, because they are important clues to the diagnosis. Vomiting may occur due to many reasons such as ileus, mechanical obstruction, and severe abdominal pain. Constipation may be related with mechanical obstruction or ileum. Massive distention may be related with bowel ischemia or perforation. Bloody diarrhea may be related with mesenteric ischemia.

The past medical history offers for the surgeon details about previous illnesses or diagnosis that can be related with the present illness.

Medications and gynecologic history will help the surgeon to find relations with medications that can cause or mask the symptoms, discover an ectopic pregnancy, or other gynecologic cause for the pain. Steroids and NSAIDs are related with GI hemorrhage; and narcotics may cause constipation and bowel obstruction.

Social history focuses on drug use, alcohol abuse, and sexual activity.

2.2.2 Physical Examination

An attentive and organized physical examination is essential to a patient's accurate diagnosis and treatment protocol. The sequence begins with a general inspection and abdominal inspection, four quadrants auscultation, percussion, and finishes with palpation.

General inspection may identify pallor, cyanosis, jaundice, and diaphoresis. The identification of abnormalities in the patient's position such as lying very still on bed and the maintenance of the knees and hips flexed on bed may indicate peritonitis.

Abdominal inspection may address the abdomen contouring, possible distentions, scaphoid appearance, any mass effect, pulsatile masses, hernias, operative scars, skin erythema, edema, and ecchymosis.

Auscultation can provide information about gastrointestinal tract and vascular system. A hyperactive bowel sound suggests enteritis or ischemic intestine while an absent bowel sound suggests ileus, a high-pitched sound is common in mechanical bowel obstruction, and bruits are heard in cases of 70–90% arterial stenosis and arteriovenous fistula.

Percussion is used to assess for bowel distention, free abdominal air, ascitic fluid graduation, or to detect the presence of peritoneal inflammation.

Palpation provides many information about the case severity, location of the injury, presence of peritonitis, identify the presence of a mass or organomegaly, and voluntary and involuntary guarding. Palpation of radial and femoral arteries is mandatory for every examination.

Digital rectal examination is also mandatory in all patients with acute abdominal pain to check for the presence of mass, intraluminal blood, or pelvic pain.

Pelvic examination should be performed in all women who present infraumbilical pain [2, 3, 8].

There are many abdominal signs during the physical examination that suggest a specific cause to the acute abdomen (Table 2.2):

2.2.3 Tests

Hemoglobin, white blood cell count with differential, electrolyte, blood urea nitrogen and creatinine, urinalysis, amylase, lipase, bilirubin total and direct, alkaline phosphatase, serum aminotransferase, serum lactate levels, stool for ova and parasites, C. difficile culture and toxin assay, ECG, ABG (PaO_2, $PaCO_2$, PH, BE, HCO_3, Base excess, Lactate), panel, bilirubin, GGT, blood glucose levels, CRP, Troponin, HBV, HCV, blood culture (fever), urine culture (fever), and BHCG (female) [3].

2.2.3.1 Imaging
- Abdominal Ultrasound (intra-abdominal effusion, inflammation of the abdominal viscus, gallstones, hydronephrosis, HIDA (cholecystitis), FAST(trauma)) [11–15].
- CT and abdomen x-ray: Ischemia or inflammation of the abdominal viscus, intra-abdominal effusion, and free air. Erect x-ray

Table 2.2 Acute abdomen signs - Adapted from [2, 6]

Pathology	Sign	Definition
Acute appendicitis	Rovsing sign	Pain at McBurney point when compressing the colon retrogradely from the left lower abdomen
	Mc-Burney sign	Pain at McBurney point during direct compression (right iliac fossa)
Appendicitis with retrocecal abscess	Iliopsoas sign	Elevation and extension of leg against resistance creating pain
Acute cholecystitis	Murphy sign	Pain caused by inspiration while applying pressure to Murphy point
Acute hemorrhagic pancreatitis	Grey Turner sign	Local areas of discoloration around umbilicus and flanks
Cholangitis	Charcot triad	Intermittent right upper abdominal pain, jaundice, and fever
Hemoperitoneum	Kehr sign	Left shoulder pain when supine and pressure placed on left upper abdomen
Pelvic inflammation (especially pelvic appendicitis)	Obturator sign	Flexion with external rotation of thigh while supine creates hypogastric pain
Peritoneal inflammation	Blumberg sign	Transient abdominal wall rebound tenderness
Retroperitoneal bleeding	Cullen sign	Periumbilical bruising

Table 2.3 Acute abdomen differential diagnosis - Adapted from [6, 9, 13, 14, 19–23]

Inflammation/Infection	Acute appendicitis, diverticulitis, cholecystitis, acute peritonitis, acute pyelonephritis, acute pancreatitis, chorioamnionitis, psoas, hepatic or diverticular abscess, and Meckel's diverticulitis	
Perforation	Acute peptic ulcer (most important), Boerhaave syndrome, perforated diverticulum, perforated gastrointestinal cancer	
Vascular occlusion	Ovarian torsion, testicular torsion, MALT, ischemic colitis, mesenteric thrombosis or embolism, Buerger disease, and strangulated hernias	
Obstruction	Adhesions in small or large bowels, sigmoid volvulus, cecal volvulus, incarcerated hernias, inflammatory bowel disease, gastrointestinal malignant neoplasm, and intussusception	
Trauma	Liver rupture, kidney damage, spleen laceration, hemoperitoneum, post-traumatic GI perforations	
Nonsurgical	Cardiovascular	Acute coronary syndrome, endocarditis, pericarditis, myocarditis, aortic dissection, aortic aneurysm rupture
	Respiratory	Pneumonia, pleuritis, empyema, pneumothorax, pulmonary thromboembolism
	Esophageal	Esophageal rupture, spasm, and esophagitis
	Pelvic region	Torsion of spermatic cord, epididymitis, hemorrhoids and anal fistula, tubo-ovarian abscess
	Endocrine	Acute adrenal insufficiency, diabetes ketoacidosis, hyperthyroidism, porphyria, uremia, and hereditary Mediterranean fever
	Hematologic	Sickle cell crisis, acute leukemia, other blood dyscrasias

shows pneumoperitoneum with free gas under the diaphragm [13, 14, 16].
- MRI for specific hollow viscus damage cases.
- Angiography (Ischemic acute abdomen and bleeding localization during an abdominal trauma) [15, 17]

Differential Diagnosis [18]
Acute abdomen differential diagnosis may be related to the etiology of acute abdomen (Table 2.3):

2.3 Treatment

The acute abdomen treatment involves pain killers, antiemetics, management of dehydration, hypovolemia and acidosis, evaluation, and maintenance of kidneys and liver functions.

2.3.1 Medical Treatment

The first step in acute abdomen management is the evaluation of the patient's vital signs together with airway (A), breathing (B), circulation (C), and consciousness. The emergency treatment is provided based on the determination of abnormal vital signs and the diagnosis of the disease. The early recognition of the patient who presents abdominal sepsis is essential for an effective treatment. The prompt administration of fluids, titrated to the clinical response and sometimes vasopressor agents (if the fluid resuscitation fails), is used to resuscitation. The goal is the maintenance of the mean arterial pressure of 65 mmHg during the first 6 h of treatment.

The early approach to the patient involves the use of cardiac monitor, pulse oximetry, monitoring HR, RR and BP, ECG, Glasgow Coma Scale, IV saline, analgesia (IV titrated narcotic analgesia), antiemetic, tetanus immunization (trauma), antibiotics, urine output, ERCP (Cholangitis), and barium enema (volvulus) [3, 11, 24, 25].

2.3.1.1 Trauma Victims: ABCDE
Unstable patients: Fluid resuscitation: Crystalloids fluids 20–30 mL/kg, Blood resuscitation(trauma), avoid hypothermia, monitoring HR, BP (keep the systolic pressure greater than 90 mmHg or a shock index less than 1 (HR/SBP)), warm fluid and blood before the administration to the patient.

– Blunt trauma: Patients with no indications of intra-abdominal injury requiring surgery or CT evaluation, stable, may be observed with serial abdominal examinations.

The Eastern Association for the Surgery of Trauma analyses patients managed without surgery after penetrating abdominal trauma. The guideline does not indicate routine laparotomy in hemodynamically stable patients with abdominal stab wounds without signs of peritonitis or diffuse abdominal tenderness and stable patients presenting abdominal gunshot wounds if the wounds are tangential and there are no peritonitis signs.

Patients presenting penetrating abdominal trauma and managed nonoperatively are discharged, in most cases, after 24 h of observation if the history and abdominal examination demonstrate patient hemodynamic stability, minimal tenderness, and no signs of viscus damage or peritonitis [5, 7, 26].

2.3.2 Surgical Treatment

The laparotomic or video-laparoscopic surgery is indicated to diagnose or to treat, and the main indications besides trauma are: Peritonitis, intra-abdominal organ perforation, certain intra-abdominal infection, intra-abdominal organ necrosis, internal bleeding, and total bowel obstruction. Diagnostic laparoscopy can be used to evaluate diaphragmatic lacerations and peritoneal penetration.

Penetrating trauma: Indications for immediate laparotomy (LAP) include hemodynamic instability, evisceration, peritonitis, or impalement. Selective nonoperative management of stable, asymptomatic patients has been demonstrated to be safe. Adjunctive diagnostic testing-ultrasonography, computed tomography, local wound exploration, diagnostic peritoneal lavage, and laparoscopy are often used to identify significant injuries requiring operative management. However, prospective studies indicate that these tests frequently lead to nontherapeutic laparotomies and are not cost-effective [1, 2, 22, 27–29].

2.3.3 Prognosis

In general, the acute abdomen is indicative of emergency treatment, and in the past, the patient would be taken directly to the operating room. The general approach to emergencies related to general surgery changed with the medical advances, the use of technology, and the increased knowledge about damage control. These approach modifications allow patients who are victims of abdominal trauma and other causes of the acute abdomen to be treated without surgeries, with excellent recoveries. Today, CT scans and the US are used to support the diagnosis and allow the surgeon to know what to expect during surgery. This technology avoids unnecessary surgery in patients with medical causes of an acute abdomen. The surgeon plays a fundamental role during the acute abdomen management, and their conduct depends on the hemodynamic patient's state. Stable patients permit imaging studies to be obtained, but unstable patients need immediate surgical intervention. The prognosis is dependent on the abdomen's acute cause.

Patterson JW, Kashyap S, and Dominique E demonstrated that complicated intra-abdominal infections presented an overall mortality of 9.2% [18].

Cardiovascular diseases, poor overall status, hemodynamic instability, comorbidities, and advanced age are factors of a poor prognosis in an acute abdomen.

Patients presenting acute abdomen due to cardiovascular diseases (myocardial infarction, mesenteric arterial occlusion, nonobstructive mesenteric ischemia, and aortic aneurysm rupture) or intestinal necrosis due to ileal strangulation have a high mortality and morbidity rates.

High-volume centers typically have better acute abdomen outcomes than low volume centers.

Dos and Don'ts

Dos
- Stabilization of the patient's vital signs is a priority and crystalloid's solutions should be used.
- Patients who are hemodynamically unstable or who have diffuse abdominal tenderness should be taken emergently for laparotomy. Also, patients who are hemodynamically stable with an unreliable clinical examination (i.e., brain injury, spinal cord injury, intoxication, or need for sedation or anesthesia) should have a further diagnostic investigation done for intraperitoneal injury or undergo exploratory laparotomy.

Don't
- A routine laparotomy is not indicated in hemodynamically stable patients with abdominal stab wounds without signs of peritonitis or diffuse abdominal tenderness (away from the wounding site) in centers with surgical expertise.
- The unstable patient is not a candidate for an immediate CT.

Take-Home Messages
- The history and physical examination remain the mainstay to diagnosis. Labs and imaging exams are important to confirm the diagnosis.
- A focused history, physical examination and detection of instability on the vital signs and the fast management with adequate treatment, labs, and imaging exams are critical to an accurate diagnosis.
- The intensity and severity of the abdominal pain are related with the grade of tissue damage.
- The knowledge of acute abdomen differential diagnosis is crucial for the accurate treatment.
- The knowledge of the protocols of penetrating and blunt abdominal trauma management is important to avoid unnecessary laparotomies.

Questions

1. What is the acute abdomen definition?
   A. Abdominal pain that lasts one day.
   B. Abdominal pain that presents nausea and vomiting.
   C. **Acute episode of abdominal pain, within less than a week, related to an intra-abdominal, thoracic, or systematic pathology that requires urgent intervention such as surgery.**
   D. Any abdominal pain.
2. What is essential to acute abdomen diagnosis?
   A. Ultrasonography
   B. CT scan
   C. X ray
   D. **History and Physical examination**
3. What is the acute abdomen classification by etiology?
   A. **Hemorrhage, infection, perforation, vascular occlusion, obstruction, and trauma.**
   B. Inflammation, hemorrhage, perforation, vascular obstruction.
   C. Hemorrhage, infection, vascular occlusion, and trauma.
   D. Hemorrhage, trauma, obstruction, and dehydration.
4. What are examples of differential diagnosis?
   A. **Appendicitis, cholecystitis, and ovarian abscess.**
   B. Appendicitis, cholangitis, and pneumonia.
   C. Appendicitis, urinary tract infection, and bowel obstruction.
   D. Appendicitis, diverticulitis, and hepatitis.
5. What are the gold standard imaging tests related to the initial acute abdomen approach?
   A. CT scan and urinalysis
   B. **Ultrasonography and blood tests**
   C. X-ray and Ct scan
   D. X-ray and ultrasonography.
6. What are examples that can mimic an acute abdomen?
   A. **Lower lobe pneumonia**
   B. Tonsillitis
   C. Pharyngitis
   D. Laryngitis.
7. What are examples of surgical treatment indications?
   A. Sickle cell anemia crisis
   B. Uremia
   C. Porphyria
   D. **Cholangitis**
8. What are examples of non-surgical treatment indications?
   A. Strangulated hernia
   B. Ovarian abscess
   C. **Hepatitis**
   D. Perforated gastric ulcer.
9. What are examples of factors of poor prognosis in acute abdomen?
   A. **Cardiovascular diseases, poor overall status, hemodynamic instability, comorbidities, and advanced age are factors of a poor prognosis in an acute abdomen**
   B. Age, the presence of urinary infection, and race.
   C. Religious beliefs and age.
   D. Race and the presence of urinary infection.
10. What is considered a laparotomy indication.
    A. **Patient's hemodynamic instability.**
    B. Any episode of abdominal trauma
    C. Hematuria
    D. Any acute abdomen

References

1. Sartelli M, et al. 2013 WSES guidelines for management of intra-abdominal infections. World J Emerg Surg. 2013;8(1):1–29.
2. Mayumi T, et al. The practice guidelines for primary care of acute abdomen 2015. Jpn J Radiol. 2016;34(1):80–115.

3. Grundmann RT, et al. The acute (surgical) abdomen-epidemiology, diagnosis and general principles of management. Zeitschrift fur Gastroenterologie. 2010;48(6):696–706.
4. Addiss DG, et al. The epidemiology of appendicitis and appendectomy in the United States. Am J Epidemiol. 1990;132(5):910–25.
5. Feliciano DV, et al., editor. Trauma, 9th ed. McGraw Hill; 2020.
6. Sabiston, textbook of surgery. 20th ed. 2016. p. 1121–1137.
7. Biffl WL, Leppaniemi A. Management guidelines for penetrating abdominal trauma. World J Surg. 2015;39(6):1373–80.
8. Gans SL, Pols MA, Stoker J, Boermeester MA, Expert Steering Group. Guideline for the diagnostic pathway in patients with acute abdominal pain. Dig Surg. 2015;32(1):23–31. https://doi.org/10.1159/000371583. Epub 2015 Jan 28.
9. Vasilescu A, Occhionorelli S, Venara A, Vereczkei A, Vettoretto N, Vlad N, Walędziak M, Yilmaz TU, Yuan KC, Yunfeng C, Zilinskas J, Grelpois G, Catena F. Prospective Observational Study on acute Appendicitis Worldwide (POSAW). World J Emerg Surg. 2018;13:19. https://doi.org/10.1186/s13017-018-0179-0. PMID: 29686725; PMCID: PMC5902943.
10. Leppäniemi A, Tolonen M, Tarasconi A, Segovia-Lohse H, Gamberini E, Kirkpatrick AW, Ball CG, Parry N, Sartelli M, Wolbrink D, van Goor H, Baiocchi G, Ansaloni L, Biffl W, Coccolini F, Di Saverio S, Kluger Y, Moore E, Catena F. 2019 WSES guidelines for the management of severe acute pancreatitis. World J Emerg Surg. 2019;14:27. https://doi.org/10.1186/s13017-019-0247-0. PMID: 31210778; PMCID: PMC6567462.
11. Broek T, Richard PG, et al. Bologna guidelines for diagnosis and management of adhesive small bowel obstruction (ASBO): 2017 update of the evidence-based guidelines from the world society of emergency surgery ASBO working group. World J Emerg Surg. 2018;13(1):1–13.
12. Ripollés T, Sebastián-Tomás JC, Martínez-Pérez MJ, Manrique A, Gómez-Abril SA, Torres-Sanchez T. Ultrasound can differentiate complicated and uncomplicated acute colonic diverticulitis: a prospective comparative study with computed tomography. Abdom Radiol (NY). 2021;46(8):3826–34. https://doi.org/10.1007/s00261-021-03060-5. Epub 2021 Mar 25. PMID: 33765176.
13. Laméris W, van Randen A, Bipat S, Bossuyt PM, Boermeester MA, Stoker J. Graded compression ultrasonography and computed tomography in acute colonic diverticulitis: meta-analysis of test accuracy. Eur Radiol. 2008;18(11):2498–511. https://doi.org/10.1007/s00330-008-1018-6. Epub 2008 Jun 4. PMID: 18523784.
14. Mattson B, Dulaimy K. The 4 quadrants: acute pathology in the abdomen and current imaging guidelines. Semin Ultrasound CT MR. 2017;38(4):414–23. https://doi.org/10.1053/j.sult.2017.02.006. Epub 2017 Feb 20. PMID: 28865530.
15. Vauth C, Englert H, Fischer T, Kulp W, Greiner W, Willich SN, Stroever B, von der Schulenburg JMG. Sonographic diagnosis of "acute abdomen" in children and adults. GMS Health Technol Assess. 2005;1:Doc08. PMID: 21289929; PMCID: PMC3011316.
16. Heiken JP, Katz DS, Menu Y. Emergency radiology of the abdomen and pelvis: imaging of the non-traumatic and traumatic acute abdomen. Dis Abdom Pelvis. 2018–2021 (2018):123–143.
17. Koizumi M, Takada T, Kawarada Y, Hirata K, Mayumi T, Yoshida M, Sekimoto M, Hirota M, Kimura Y, Takeda K, Isaji S, Otsuki M, Matsuno S, JPN. JPN guidelines for the management of acute pancreatitis: diagnostic criteria for acute pancreatitis. J Hepatobiliary Pancreat Surg. 2006;13(1):25–32. https://doi.org/10.1007/s00534-005-1048-2. PMID: 16463208; PMCID: PMC2779365.
18. Patterson JW, Kashyap S, Dominique E. Acute abdomen. 2021.
19. You H, et al. The management of diverticulitis: a review of the guidelines. Med J Aust. 2019;211(9):421–7.
20. Swanson SM, Strate LL. Acute colonic diverticulitis. Ann Intern Med. 2018;168(9):ITC65–80. https://doi.org/10.7326/AITC201805010. Erratum in: Ann Intern Med. 2020 May 5;172(9):640. PMID: 29710265; PMCID: PMC6430566.
21. Hecker A, Uhle F, Schwandner T, Padberg W, Weigand MA. Diagnostics, therapy and outcome prediction in abdominal sepsis: current standards and future perspectives. Langenbecks Arch Surg. 2014;399(1):11–22. https://doi.org/10.1007/s00423-013-1132-z. Epub 2013 Nov 2. PMID: 24186147.
22. Luther B, Mamopoulos A, Lehmann C, Klar E. The ongoing challenge of acute mesenteric ischemia. Visc Med. 2018;34(3):217–23. https://doi.org/10.1159/000490318. Epub 2018 Jun 18. PMID: 30140688; PMCID: PMC6103345.
23. Krishnamoorthi R, Ramarajan N, Wang NE, Newman B, Rubesova E, Mueller CM, Barth RA. Effectiveness of a staged US and CT protocol for the diagnosis of pediatric appendicitis: reducing radiation exposure in the age of ALARA. Radiology. 2011;259(1):231–9. https://doi.org/10.1148/radiol.10100984. Epub 2011 Jan PMID: 21324843.
24. Sartelli M, et al. 2017 WSES guidelines for management of intra-abdominal infections. World J Emerg Surg. 2017;12:29.
25. Cristaudo AT, Jennings SB, Hitos K, Gunnarsson R, DeCosta A. Treatments and other prognostic factors in the management of the open abdomen: a systematic review. J Trauma Acute Care Surg. 2017;82(2):407–18. https://doi.org/10.1097/TA.0000000000001314. PMID: 27918375.
26. Como JJ, et al. Practice management guidelines for selective nonoperative management of penetrating abdominal trauma. J Trauma Acute Care Surg. 2010;68(3):721–33.

27. Catena F, et al. Bowel obstruction: a narrative review for all physicians. World J Emerg Surg. 2019;14(1):1–8.
28. Kobayashi L, Coimbra R, Goes AMO Jr, Reva V, Santorelli J, Moore EE, Galante JM, Abu-Zidan F, Peitzman AB, Ordonez CA, Maier RV, Di Saverio S, Ivatury R, De Angelis N, Scalea T, Catena F, Kirkpatrick A, Khokha V, Parry N, Civil I, Leppaniemi A, Chirica M, Pikoulis E, Fraga GP, Chiarugi M, Damaskos D, Cicuttin E, Ceresoli M, De Simone B, Vega-Rivera F, Sartelli M, Biffl W, Ansaloni L, Weber DG, Coccolini F. American Association for the Surgery of Trauma-World Society of Emergency Surgery guidelines on diagnosis and management of abdominal vascular injuries. J Trauma Acute Care Surg. 2020;89(6):1197–211. https://doi.org/10.1097/TA.0000000000002968. PMID: 33230049.
29. Andersson M, Kolodziej B, Andersson RE. Validation of the appendicitis inflammatory response (AIR) score. World J Surg. 2021;45(7):2081–91. https://doi.org/10.1007/s00268-021-06042-2. Epub 2021 Apr 6. PMID: 33825049; PMCID: PMC8154764.

Evaluation of Traumatic and Nontraumatic Patients

Vitor F. Kruger and Gustavo P. Fraga

3.1 Trauma Patient

3.1.1 Introduction

> **Learning Goals**
> Understand the need for initial care for traumatized patients—based on adequate prehospital triage, teamwork, interdisciplinary communication, and decision making in critically ill patients for better outcomes.

The improvement in the quality of emergency medical service (EMS) care has decreased polytrauma mortality. Haas et al. [1] reported that in major trauma patients who were not referred to trauma centers, mortality increased by 30% compared to those who were referred. The organization of trauma systems means that high-energy polytrauma cases are admitted to trauma rooms more frequently; therefore, planning is essential for reception.

The reception must be done at the trauma bay at the emergency department (ED), but evaluation of the trauma patient starts at the scene, by identifying the mechanism of trauma and providing prehospital care, which are determinant to quickly refer the "right patient, to the right hospital." At the ED, sufficient space, materials, and equipment for endotracheal intubation or difficult airway, chest drainage, and ultrasound must be available. Crystalloid solutions must be warmed, and blood products must be organized, checked, and easily available. Multidisciplinary and multiprofessional staff must be prepared, trained for their role, and properly supplemented with personal protective equipment.

Information about the patient, vital signs at the scene, and trauma kinematics are part of the primary survey; therefore, adequate and clear communication between the EMS and hospital team is essential.

The importance of leadership, human factors, and crew resource management in trauma care has recently been recognized [2]. Trauma teams must be trained in technical and nontechnical skills. Capacity in interpersonal communication, teamwork, decision making, leadership, task management, and situational awareness have major influences on the effectiveness of the team and the best outcome for the patients.

The concept of leadership is complex and includes multidimensional behaviors involving communication, efficiency, and safety actions. Leadership styles are divided into two main categories: directive and empowering [2].

In the former, the leader explicitly instructs subordinates on which tasks to perform. It is more

---

V. F. Kruger · G. P. Fraga (✉)
Division of Trauma Surgery, University of Campinas, Campinas, Brazil

effective when tasks are simple, or if the leader is the only member with expertise. However, empowering leadership is more effective with complex tasks [3].

Based on the empowering leadership-style, the concept of a trauma team leader (TTL) and trauma team members (TTM) is essential in the primary survey of major trauma. In this model, the TTL becomes a facilitator and responsibilities are delegated, allowing the TTM to make decisions while the TTL focuses on team communication and coordination.

Traditionally, the TTL is a surgeon who coordinates the primary survey and ensures adherence to ATLSÒ guidelines; however, this has been questioned. Currently, nonsurgeon TTLs with training in emergency medicine have emerged with technical and nontechnical capabilities. The available evidence suggests that there is no significant difference in outcomes with either a surgeon or a nonsurgeon TTL [4].

In addition to emergency physicians and surgeons, trauma teams must be formed by nursing teams for initial care; however, must understand that for the subsequent management of trauma patient, medical teams such as hematologists, radiologists, anesthetists, vascular surgeons and ICU teams must be involved in the care. The team briefing and "trauma alert" should involve all members when major trauma is expected.

3.1.2 Diagnosis

The primary survey is based on physiology and not on anatomical injuries. To quickly assess the patient's physiological condition and vital functions, we can simply ask the patient's name or what had happened at the scene and immediate evaluation of the airway, ventilation, perfusion, and neurological status can be performed. An appropriate response suggests that the airway is patent, ventilation is not severely impaired, and there is perfusion to maintain a level of consciousness; however, an inappropriate response suggests abnormalities, justifying evaluation and urgent treatment (Fig. 3.1) [5].

Another purpose of identifying immediate life-threatening injuries is for a global assessment in a few seconds that includes the patient's interaction with the examiner, ventilatory effort, and skin perfusion [6].

The primary survey has a linear and sequential progression; however, many of these activities

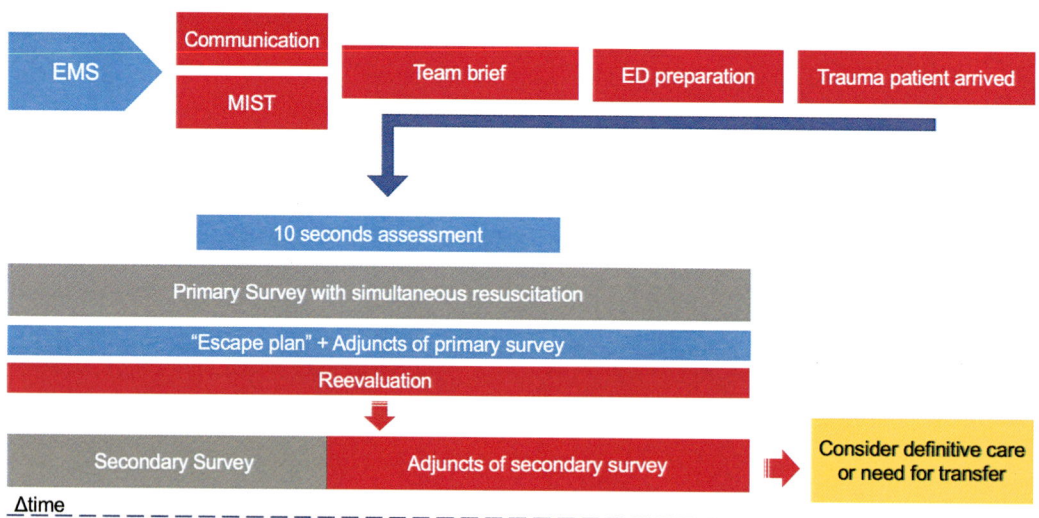

Fig. 3.1 Initial assessment and management of Trauma patients

occur simultaneously. It is mandatory to reassess the patient frequently to identify, treat, or anticipate potential problems.

3.1.3 Treatment

The priority in all trauma patients is the airway, ensuring adequate oxygenation and ventilation. Despite not being the main cause of death in trauma, airway compromise is the situation that kills the fastest [5]. When the patient has airway involvement, regardless of the cause, the priority is to clear it and make it safe.

In trauma patients, regardless of the anatomy, the airway is always to be considered as difficult. The two main factors that may represent an indication for a definitive airway in traumatized patients are oxygenation (hypoxia and hypoventilation) and failure to protect; however, multiple factors may be present, which makes the decision to intubate less straightforward [7]. If intubation is decided on, the best technique in trauma, in which previous fasting is not considered, is rapid sequence intubation with direct laryngoscopy [7].

Rapid sequence intubation consists of preoxygenation and the use of specific medications to facilitate orotracheal intubation. The concept of preoxygenation has three goals: raise O_2 saturation to the nearest 100%; increase the oxygen supply in the alveoli, instead of nitrogen; and optimize oxygenation of the bloodstream, avoiding catastrophic scenarios due to a drop in saturation and hypoxia [8].

Midazolam and fentanyl induce rapid unconsciousness; however, they induce hypotension in trauma patients, leading to a worsening of perfusion. Other medications that can be used in traumatized patients include etomidate and ketamine. The former does not affect blood pressure or intracranial pressure, and the current literature does not provide any contraindications for its use, concluding that although relative adrenal insufficiency can occur after use, it does not change mortality [9]. Ketamine is an anesthetic with sympathomimetic action and has been suggested for use in trauma patients with hemodynamic instability. Cohen et al. [10] concluded in their study that in patients with severe traumatic brain injury, induction with ketamine caused no significant effect on cerebral perfusion pressure. Furthermore, succinylcholine is recommended as the neuromuscular blockade agent [7].

Supra-glottic devices may be useful in facilitating ventilation and oxygenation in nonsuccessful endotracheal intubation and/or in emergency situations [7].

Life-threatening situations due to impaired ventilation depends on rapid diagnosis and decision making; for example, tension pneumothorax, which has a clinical diagnosis, does not require imaging and can be managed initially by rapidly applying finger decompression thoracostomy or needle catheter decompression in the fifth interspace, slightly anterior to the midaxillary line [5, 11]. Open pneumothorax requires prompt closure with a three-point large dressing, followed by chest drainage. Attention should be paid to simple pneumothorax, especially in patients undergoing general anesthesia or receiving positive pressure ventilation without having a chest tube inserted, which can lead to tension pneumothorax [5].

Hemorrhage is the main cause of preventable death in trauma. Recognizing the presence of shock, identifying the probable source, and initiating treatment are the goals of the primary survey. Resuscitation is not a substitute for definitive bleeding control [5]. In scenarios with exsanguinating external hemorrhage, the cABC sequence is emphasized, initiating the primary assessment by seeking and treating severe hemorrhages. Adjuncts, such as the use of tourniquets, decrease mortality in these patients [12].

Several resources are used to recognize shock in the trauma bay. Initial careful physical examination and monitoring to evaluate early manifestations, such as tachycardia and cutaneous vasoconstriction, must be done while keeping in mind that delayed hypotension can occur. Blood samples and complementary studies must be also correctly interpreted.

The initial interpretation of hemoglobin and hematocrit requires attention, and massive blood loss may produce only a slight drop in their concentration [13]. Among its limitations of use are hemodilution by crystalloids and trauma patients who lose whole blood and require time for compensatory mechanisms to move interstitial fluids.

Arterial blood gas analysis measuring excess base and lactate is the gold standard laboratory test for assessing perfusion and trauma survival. Base excess (BE) is defined to reflect the buildup of acids by determining how much base it would take to neutralize the acid blood pH. A BE below −6 is related to a high probability of occult hemorrhagic shock, a need for massive transfusion, higher rates of complications, and mortality [14, 15].

Trauma team members should be familiar with extended focused trauma ultrasound (eFAST) as a propaedeutic tool in the trauma bay. In addition to the conventional exam sites (perihepatic, perisplenic, pericardial, and retrovesical space), the anterior parasternal spaces of the 3–8 interspace and the pulmonary bases must be evaluated [16].

Signs suggestive of pneumothorax are absence of sling pleura on mode B and bar code or beach sign on mode M [16]. For hemothorax, an anechoic collection or free fluid in the chest cavity is suggestive. Its sensitivity and specificity are greater than those of chest X-rays for pneumothorax and hemothorax [17].

Chest and pelvic radiography in the trauma bay are useful for recognizing sources of bleeding in unstable patients. Chest x-ray, for example, can lead to a suspicion of a large hemothorax in addition to being sensitive for suspected traumatic aortic injury [18]. On the other hand, pelvic x-ray can identify severe pelvic fractures [19].

Patients with complex pelvic trauma, with massive blood loss and who are hemodynamically unstable, should undergo placement of a pelvic binder device immediately to produce a temporary fixation, even under the minimal diagnostic suspicion of mechanical pelvic instability [19].

Damage control resuscitation must be performed early during major trauma. This rational and current concept includes limited use of crystalloid, early activation of a massive transfusion protocol (MTP), high proportions of blood components, use of tranexamic acid, and permissive hypotension [20].

Large volumes of crystalloid in blunt trauma increase morbidity, length of stay in intensive care, mechanical ventilation days, bloodstream infections, abdominal compartment syndrome, acute respiratory distress syndrome, and multiple organ failure [21]. Ley et al. [22] concluded that 1.5 L or more of crystalloid was an independent risk factor for mortality. Excessive resuscitation with crystalloids should be avoided.

To achieve hemostasis, blood products are preferred for resuscitating patients with hemorrhagic shock. Delays in activating the delivery of blood products have been associated with increased time for hemostasis and increased mortality [23]. In the military setting, it has already been shown that high proportions of pRBCs, plasma, and platelets reduce mortality. The PROPPR clinical study [24] evaluated mortality in the proportions 1:1:1 and 1:1:2 and concluded that more patients achieved hemostasis in the 1:1:1 group (86.1% vs. 78.1%), with a lower mortality rate due to exsanguination in 24 h.

Whole blood, a military method of transfusion, has been widely studied since the last decade. Duschenne et al. [25] found lower incidence of acute respiratory distress syndrome, days of mechanical ventilation, and amount of blood components transfused in trauma patients who used whole blood; however, the authors concluded that the survival of patients transfused with whole blood is like that of patients transfused with components [25, 26].

Trauma coagulopathy is present in up to 25% of trauma patients with ISS > 15 admitted to the trauma bay. It is important to understand that coagulopathy is multifactorial and complex and involves interaction between hemostasis, perfusion, and systemic inflammatory response. It is related to endogenous factors, such as hyperfibrinolysis, platelet dysfunction, and endotheliopathy, but it can also be aggravated by exogenous factors, such as metabolic acidosis, hemodilution, and hypothermia [27]. Early diagnosis and prevention are mandatory. Conventional laboratory tests for coagulation are not reliable and take time to obtain results. The use of viscoelastic tests (for example TEG®, ROTEM®) demonstrates real-time platelet dysfunction, hyperfibrinolysis, and clot strength, offering the possibility of personalized transfusion.

Gonzales et al. [28] studied related viscoelastic testing and mortality, comparing the use of TEG® and conventional laboratory tests, concluding that the 28-day mortality in the TEG® group was lower than that in the conventional-tests group (19.6% vs. 36.4%), in addition to the rational use of plasma and platelets in the TEG group.

Tranexamic acid blocks hyperfibrinolysis by preventing the transformation of plasminogen into plasmin and plays a fundamental role in coagulopathy. The prospective studies CRASH-2 and 3 [29, 30] concluded that the administration of tranexamic acid with bolus dose of 1 g infused in 10 min, followed by an intravenous infusion of 1 g in 8 h, within 3 h of trauma, reduced mortality in patients with extracranial and intracranial bleeding.

It has been established that the creation and promotion of a MTP benefits trauma patients, with reduced mortality, morbidity, or use of blood components, and cost savings [20]. Careful activation of MTP is essential for the rational and early use of blood components. The literature has attempted to validate scores for the activation of this protocol. Among them, the ABC score, created in 2009 by Nunez [31], uses non-laboratory and non-weighted parameters and is easy to calculate at the bedside. Four parameters are used: penetrating trauma, systolic blood pressure ≤ 90 mmHg, heart rate > 120 bpm on admission, and positive FAST. Each item, when present, is worth one point, and it was concluded that the presence of two points would already be the trigger for initiating the MTP protocol, with the highest accuracy among the scores [31]. Attention should be paid to ionic calcium during massive transfusions. This ion is essential for platelet function. Acute hypocalcemia is a common complication of massive transfusion, and low levels are associated with increased mortality [32].

Hybrid operating rooms for patients with major trauma are currently being developed. They offer the ability to concomitantly perform advanced angiographic and operative hemostasis techniques, focusing on early control of hemorrhage and decreasing morbidity and mortality [33]. These rooms have computed tomography (CT) scans, angiography, an operating room structure, and advanced devices. Procedures such as acquisition of whole-body CT, angio-embolization, resuscitative endovascular balloon occlusion of the aorta (REBOA), and immediate surgery can be performed in the hybrid room at admission, without transferring the patient.

Techniques for the temporary control of non-compressible hemorrhage, such as REBOA, should be used in major trauma. The literature places REBOA as the method of choice, in comparison to thoracotomies, for aortic clamping in severely hypotensive patients with a pulse; however, complications of perfusion of the extremities have been reported, requiring further studies [34, 35].

Permissive hypotension is a strategy for penetrating and blunt trauma, except in patients with severe traumatic brain injury. This strategy consists of maintaining sufficient blood pressure for perfusion of essential organs. Li et al. [36], in an experimental study with animals, concluded that the time limit for permissive hypotension was 90 min, maintaining a mean arterial pressure (MAP) between 50 and 60 mmHg.

Glasgow coma scale (GCS) is a quick, simple, and objective method for determining the level of consciousness [5]. Every effort must be made during initial care to ensure the prevention of secondary brain injury, including oxygenation and perfusion as the main principles. Neurosurgeons should be informed immediately after the diagnosis of the injury. The measurement of the optic nerve sheath by ultrasound in a trauma bay can identify an increase in intracranial pressure in severe traumatic brain injury. Thickening of more than 5 mm can be used to identify intracranial pressure (ICP) > 20 mmHg with a sensitivity of 96% and specificity of 94% [37].

In a recent study using a German trauma database of 15,230 patients, Weuster et al. studied accidental hypothermia in traumatized patients and concluded that although hypothermia occurs regularly, recording the central temperature is still a challenge, and patients with severe hypothermia have high sepsis rates, multiple organ failure, and mortality [38]. Every effort should be made to avoid hypothermia: the trauma bay temperature should be appropriate; and warmed air blankets and heated fluid must be used.

3.2 Nontraumatic Patient

3.2.1 Introduction

> **Learning Goals**
> Understand the need for initial care for nontrauma patients, triage based on priority patients, ED communication, rapid surgeon assessment, rapid ability to diagnose sepsis, guided resuscitation, large broad antibiotic therapy, and effective control of source of contamination and revascularization of ischemic viscera or resection.

Acute nontraumatic surgical emergencies include acute abdomen, gastrointestinal bleeding, and soft tissue infections and visceral ischemia. A multicenter study evaluating 4553 patients with septic intra-abdominal complications over 4 months concluded that morbidity and mortality are higher when these patients are poorly managed in the emergency department [39].

The experience with traumatic emergencies must be extrapolated to nontraumatic emergencies. Efforts to improve the triage system must be carried out to develop a quality improvement tool [40]. Globally, numerous daily surgical consultations are carried out at emergency departments, making an efficient triage protocol mandatory, based on admission parameters and rapid assessment by the surgeon. The World Society of Emergency Surgery (WSES) proposes the use of a color triage system for nontraumatic surgical emergencies, aiming for surgical resolution in a timely manner (see dedicated chapter) [40].

Initial care for acute nontraumatic surgical emergencies follows the same priorities as traumatic emergencies. Leaderships with technical and nontechnical skills are the same. Communication, teamwork, decision making, task management, and situational awareness are essential for decision-making, early diagnosis, and surgical treatment, if necessary. As with trauma, the availability of resources and prior communication between those involved are essential.

The cornerstone of effective care for acute nontraumatic emergencies is based on early diagnosis, resuscitation, antibiotic therapy, and effective control of the source of contamination or ischemic viscera revascularization or resection [40].

3.2.2 Diagnosis

Systematic anamnesis and physical examination must be performed during the initial evaluation. The evolution of the disease, family history, comorbidities, use of medications, and previous surgical procedures are part of the evaluation. Physical examination of a collaborative patient is mandatory. Signs of systemic inflammatory response should be actively sought, including fever, tachycardia, and tachypnea. Abdominal tenderness suggests peritonitis, and signs of hypoperfusion and diminished levels of consciousness are indicative of sepsis (Fig. 3.2).

According to the SEPSIS-3 consensus [41], sepsis is defined as life-threatening organ dysfunction caused by an uncontrolled host response to infection. Shock in general and Septic shock in particular is defined as cellular, metabolic, and perfusion abnormalities and it is associated with an increased risk of mortality. Clinically, patients with septic shock present with requiring vasopressors to maintain MAP >65 mmHg or a worse perfusion with measured serum lactate >2 mmol/L, in the absence of hypovolemia.

The Quick Sequential Organ Failure Assessment (qSOFA) is a tool used to identify patients at risk for sepsis (see septic shock chapter). Although it does not have diagnostic value, it is accurate in predicting mortality in the emer-

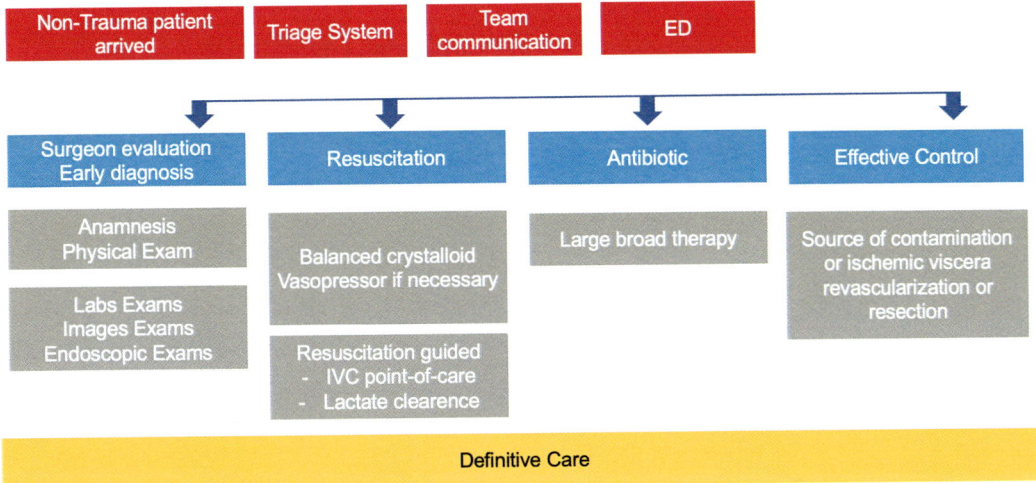

Fig. 3.2 Initial assessment and management of nontrauma patients

gency department [42]. This short version of the SOFA-score does not require weighted arterial blood gas parameters and can be performed at the bedside, as it only includes the respiratory rate, level of consciousness, and blood pressure. A score >2 is related to higher mortality (Fig. 3.3) [41].

Abdominal sepsis represents a host systemic inflammatory response to intra-abdominal infections and is a dynamic process of varying severity. Some of the factors that influence the prognosis of these patients are elderly, malnutrition, pre-existing diseases, prolonged length of stay with nosocomial infections, immunosuppression, diffuse peritonitis without contamination control, and septic shock [43].

Prognostic scores that assess severity, and create a therapeutic proposal for complicated abdominal diseases, have been validated and should be part of the primary survey and decision making in acute nontraumatic surgical emergencies.

The WSES Sepsis Severity Score includes clinical conditions on admission, delay in controlling contamination, source of abdominal infection, acquisition of infection, and patient risk factors. This score shows high sensitivity and specificity as predictors of mortality (Fig. 3.4) [43].

3.2.3 Treatment

In trauma patients, every effort should be made to recognize and stop the bleeding; however, in acute nontraumatic surgical urgency, the entire team must actively recognize sepsis and perform early resuscitation.

Fluids in resuscitation therapy aim to correct microvascular dysfunction. If delayed, this dysfunction leads to irreversible tissue hypoxia and multiple organ failure [44]. Balanced crystalloid solutions are the first line, requiring at least 30 mL/kg in the first 3 h [41]. Guided therapeutic goals and continuous reevaluation of the patient are mandatory during resuscitation. The rational use of fluids can be based on physiological parameters such as urine output, heart rate, and blood pressure; however, currently, some dynamic variables used to predict fluid responsiveness are suggested.

Inferior vena cava diameter variation (collapse or dilation) has been suggested for guiding resuscitation and to assess the need for fluids [45]. An echocardiography at the point-of-care allows for a more detailed assessment of hemodynamics [46]. Serum lactate level, despite being an indirect test for measuring tissue perfusion, is important in the evolution of the patient's resus-

Fig. 3.3 SOFA Score (Sepsis-related Organ Failure Assessment)

PaO_2/FiO_2 (mmHg)	SOFA score
<400	1
<300	2
<200 and mechanically ventilated	3
<100 and mechanically ventilated	4
Glasgow coma scale	
13–14	1
10–12	2
6–9	3
<6	4
Mean arterial pressure OR administration of vasopressors required	SOFA score
MAP <70 mm/Hg	1
dop ≤5 or dob (any dose)	2
dop >5 OR epi ≤0.1 OR nor ≤0.1	3
dop >15 OR epi >0.1 OR nor >0.1	4
Bilirubin (mg/dl) [µmol/L]	
1.2–1.9 [>20–32]	1
2.0–5.9 [33–101]	2
6.0–11.9 [102–204]	3
>12.0 [>204]	4
Platelets × $10^3/\mu l$	
<150	1
<100	2
<50	3
<20	4
Creatinine (mg/dl) [µmol/L] (or urine output)	
1.2–1.9 [110–170]	1
2.0–3.4 [171–298, 305]	2
3.5–4.9 [300–440] (or <500 ml/d)	3
>5.0 [>440] (or <200 ml/d)	4

Fig. 3.4 WSES sepsis severity score for patients with complicated Intra-abdominal infections [43]

Clinical condition at the admission	
·Severe sepsis (acute organ dysfunction) at the admission	3 score
· Septic shock (acute circulatory failure characterized by persistent arterial hypotension. It always requires vasopressor agents) at the admission	5 score
Setting of acquisition	
· Healthcare associated infection	2 score
Origin of the IAIs	
· Colonic non-diverticular perforation peritonitis	2 score
· Small bowel perforation peritonitis	3 score
· Diverticular diffuse peritonitis	2 score
· Post-operative diffuse peritonitis	2 score
Delay in source control	
· Delayed initial intervention [Preoperative duration of peritonitis (localized or diffuse) > 24 h)]	3 score
Risk factors	
· Age>70	2 score
· Immunosuppression (chronic glucocorticoids, immunosuppresant agents, chemotherapy, lymphatic diseases, virus)	3 score

citation. The literature concludes that the mortality of patients with septic shock and resuscitation guided by early lactate clearance is minor [47].

Maintenance of hypotension (MAP <65 mmHg) after fluid-optimized resuscitation should be treated with vasopressor medications. The use of these medications has been established in the early therapy of sepsis, with norepinephrine as the first-line vasopressor [48]. The rapid initiation of broad-spectrum antimicrobial therapy improves the outcomes of patients with severe infections [41].

The diagnosis of acute nontraumatic surgical emergencies is based on a progressive approach that depends on the capacity and resources available and starts with examination and laboratory tests, up to more complex imaging examinations.

When available, radiography or ultrasonography can be performed to assist in diagnosis. In places with more resources, the use of CT with the use of intravenous contrast should be indicated, especially in cases of diagnostic doubt, where more information is required by the surgeon, or if possible, less invasive intervention, such as interventional radiology, should be performed.

Delay in recognizing and controlling infection reduces survival rates; therefore, the attending physician for acute nontraumatic surgical emergencies must be judicious and avoid excess complementary exams, and similar to trauma, definitive treatment should not be delayed. After thorough investigation, most cases evolve into unequivocal diagnoses [40].

Control of the source of infection as well as revascularization or resection of ischemic viscera must be performed as early as possible. Surgical consultation for an appropriately timed operation is mandatory. Inappropriate delay in performing surgical procedures in some diseases can result in worse outcomes.

Take-Home Messages

- The primary survey for traumatic and nontraumatic surgical emergencies is based on patient physiology.
- Traumatic and nontraumatic surgical emergencies must be performed by empowering leadership and using multidisciplinary teams.
- In trauma patients, it is necessary to recognize the presence of shock, identify its source, and initiate treatment after obtaining a clear airway.
- In nontraumatic acute surgical emergencies, treatment is based on early sepsis diagnosis, resuscitation, antibiotic therapy, effective control of the source of contamination, and ischemic viscera revascularization or resection by surgeons.
- The experience with traumatic emergency triage tools, protocols, and prognoses scores must be extrapolated to nontraumatic emergencies.

Questions

1. Answer the wrong sentence about primary survey:
   A. Evaluation of the trauma patient starts at the scene, by identifying the mechanism of trauma and providing prehospital care, which are determinants to quickly refer the "right patient, to the right hospital."
   B. At the ED, sufficient space, materials, and equipment for endotracheal intubation or difficult airway, chest drainage, and ultrasound must be available. Crystalloid solutions must be warmed, and blood products must be organized, checked, and easily available.
   C. Multi-professional staff must be prepared, trained for their role, and properly supplemented with personal protective equipment.
   D. **There is no role of importance of leadership, human factors, and crew resource management in trauma care. Recently, it has been recognized that trauma attendance is an individual ability and is focused only on skill techniques.**
2. Answer the right sentence about primary survey:
   A. Primary survey is based only on anatomical injuries.
   B. **To quickly assess the patient's physiological condition and vital functions, we can simply ask the patient's name or what had happened at the scene and immediate evaluation of the airway, ventilation, perfusion, and neurological status can be performed.**
   C. It is not mandatory to reassess the patient frequently to identify, treat, or anticipate potential problems.
   D. The primary survey there is no priority to identifying immediate life-threatening injuries and all attendants must make individual decisions.
3. About the airway and trauma, answer the correct sentence:
   A. Airway is not the priority in all trauma patients. Circulation and neurologic status are the situations that kill fastest on primary survey.
   B. Supraglottic devices can never be useful to facilitate ventilation and oxygenation in emergency situations of unsuccessful endotracheal intubation.
   C. In trauma patients, regardless of the anatomy, the airway is always considered easy.
   D. **Rapid sequence intubation consists of preoxygenation and the use of specific medications to facilitate orotracheal intubation.**

4. About rapid sequence intubation, answer the correct sentence:
   A. Midazolam and fentanyl induce rapid unconsciousness; however, they induce hypertension in trauma patients, improving the perfusion.
   B. Etomidate and Ketamine cannot be used in trauma patients with severe TBI, usually increase and worse intracranial pressure.
   C. Succinylcholine is not recommended as the neuromuscular blockade agent because of the long half-life.
   D. **Ketamine is an anesthetic with sympathomimetic action and has been suggested for use in trauma patients with hemodynamic instability.**
5. About ventilation in trauma patients at emergency department, answer the false sentence:
   A. Life-threatening situations due to impaired ventilation depend on rapid diagnosis and decision making, for example, tension and open pneumothorax.
   B. Open pneumothorax requires prompt closure with a three-point large dressing, followed by chest drainage.
   C. **Tension pneumothorax does require imaging and can be managed initially by rapidly applying finger decompression thoracostomy or needle catheter decompression in the fifth interspace, slightly anterior to the midaxillary line.**
   D. Attention should be paid to simple pneumothorax, especially in patients undergoing general anesthesia or receiving positive pressure ventilation without having a chest tube inserted.
6. About shock in trauma patients, answer the false sentence:
   A. Recognizing the presence of shock, identifying the probable source, and initiating treatment are the goals of the primary survey.
   B. In settings with exsanguinating external hemorrhage, among the goals of the primary survey is identified and controlled during severe hemorrhage. Adjuncts, such as the use of tourniquets, decrease mortality in these patients.
   C. Initial careful physical examination and monitoring to evaluate early manifestations, such as tachycardia and cutaneous vasoconstriction, must be done while keeping in mind that hypotension can occur delayed.
   D. **The initial interpretation of hemoglobin and hematocrit is the gold-standard laboratory exam, because blood loss always produces a huge drop in their concentration.**
7. About the initial evaluation in trauma patients, answer the false sentence:
   A. Trauma team members should be familiar with extended focused trauma ultrasound (eFAST) as a propaedeutic tool in the trauma bay. Its sensitivity and specificity are greater than those of chest X-rays for pneumothorax.
   B. **Large volumes of crystalloid in blunt trauma decrease morbidity, length of stay in intensive care, mechanical ventilation days, bloodstream infections, abdominal compartment syndrome, acute respiratory distress syndrome.**
   C. Damage control resuscitation must be performed early during major trauma.

D. Tranexamic acid blocks hyperfibrinolysis by preventing the transformation of plasminogen into plasmin and plays a fundamental role in coagulopathy.
8. Answer the false sentence:
   A. Efforts to improve the triage system must be carried out to develop a quality improvement tool in the emergency department.
   B. The cornerstone of effective care for acute nontraumatic emergencies is based on early diagnosis, resuscitation, antibiotic therapy, and effective control of the source of contamination.
   C. **Systematic anamnesis and physical examination play no role during the initial evaluation. CT-scan or ultrasound always should be done first.**
   D. Septic shock is defined as cellular, metabolic, and perfusion abnormalities and is associated with an increased risk of mortality.
9. About infection in trauma patients, answer the false sentence:
   A. Signs of systemic inflammatory response should be actively sought, including fever, tachycardia, and tachypnea. Abdominal tenderness suggests peritonitis, and signs of hypoperfusion and diminished levels of consciousness are indicative of sepsis.
   B. Quick Sequential Organ Failure Assessment (qSOFA) is a tool used to identify patients at risk for sepsis; it is accurate in predicting mortality in the emergency department.
   C. Abdominal sepsis represents a host systemic inflammatory response to intra-abdominal infections and is a dynamic process of varying severity. Some of the factors that influence the prognosis of these patients are: elderly, malnutrition, preexisting diseases, prolonged length of stay with nosocomial infections, immunosuppression, diffuse peritonitis without contamination control, and septic shock.
   D. **Delay in recognizing and controlling infection improve survival rates; therefore, definitive treatment should not be delayed.**
10. About shock in trauma patients, answer the correct sentence:
    A. Balanced colloids solutions are the first line in resuscitation therapy aimed to correct microvascular dysfunction.
    B. **Inferior vena cava diameter variation (collapse or dilation) has been suggested for guiding resuscitation and for assessing the need for fluids.**
    C. Serum lactate level, despite being an indirect test for measuring tissue perfusion, is not important in the evolution of the patient's resuscitation.
    D. Maintenance of hypotension (MAP <65 mmHg) after fluid-optimized resuscitation should be treated with vasopressor medications, with vasopressin as the first-line medication.

References

1. Haas B, Stukel TA, Gomez D, Zagorski B, De Mestral C, Sharma SV, et al. The mortality benefit of direct trauma center transport in a regional trauma system: a population-based analysis. J Trauma Acute Care Surg. 2012;72(6):1510–7.
2. Ford K, Menchine M, Burner E, et al. Leadership and teamwork in trauma and resuscitation. West J Emerg Med. 2016;17(5):549–56.
3. Pearce CL, Sims HP Jr. Vertical versus shared leadership as predictors of the effectiveness of change management teams: an examination of aversive, directive, transactional, transformational, and empowering

leader behaviors. Group Dyn Theory Res Pract. 2002;6(2):172–97.
4. Hajibandeh S, Hajibandeh S. Who should lead a trauma team: surgeon or non-surgeon? A systematic review and meta-analysis. J Inj Violence Res. 2017;9(2):107–16.
5. American College of Surgeons Committee on Trauma. Advanced Trauma Life Support (ATLS®) student manual, 10th ed. Chicago; 2018.
6. Thies K, Gwinnutt C, Driscoll P, et al. The European trauma course—from concept to course. Resuscitation. 2007;74(1):135–41.
7. Mayglothling J, Duane TM, Gibbs M, McCunn M, Legome E, Eastman AL, Whelan J, Shah KH, Eastern Association for the Surgery of Trauma. Emergency tracheal intubation immediately following traumatic injury: an Eastern Association for the Surgery of Trauma practice management guideline. J Trauma Acute Care Surg. 2012;73(5 Suppl 4):S333–40.
8. Campbell IT, Beatty PC. Monitoring preoxygenation. Br J Anaesth. 1994;72:3–4.
9. Erdoes G, Basciani RM, Eberle B. Etomidate—a review of robust evidence for its use in various clinical scenarios. Acta Anaesthesiol Scand. 2014;58(4):380–9.
10. Cohen L, Athaide V, Wickham ME, Doyle-Waters MM, Rose NG, Hohl CM. The effect of ketamine on intracranial and cerebral perfusion pressure and health outcomes: a systematic review. Ann Emerg Med. 2015;65(1):43–51.
11. Inaba K, Branco BC, Eckstein M, et al. Optimal positioning for emergent needle thoracostomy: a cadaver-based study. J Trauma. 2011;71:1099–103.
12. Kragh JF Jr, Walters TJ, Baer DG, Fox CJ, Wade CE, Salinas J, Holcomb JB. Survival with emergency tourniquet use to stop bleeding in major limb trauma. Ann Surg. 2009;249(1):1–7.
13. Zehtabchi S, Sinert R, Goldman M, Kapitanyan R, Ballas J. Diagnostic performance of serial haematocrit measurements in identifying major injury in adult trauma patients. Injury. 2006;37(1):46–52.
14. Juern J, Khatri V, Weigelt J. Base excess: a review. J Trauma Acute Care Surg. 2012;73(1):27–32.
15. Rutherford EJ, Morris JA, Reed GW, Hall KS. Base deficit stratifies mortality and determines therapy. J Trauma. 1992;33:417–23.
16. Hefny AF, Kunhivalappil FT, Paul M, Almansoori TM, Zoubeidi T, Abu-Zidan FM. Anatomical locations of air for rapid diagnosis of pneumothorax in blunt trauma patients. World J Emerg Surg. 2019;14:44.
17. Kirkpatrick AW, Sirois M, Laupland KB, Liu D, Rowan K, Ball CG, et al. Hand-held thoracic sonography for detecting post-traumatic pneumothoraces: the extended focused assessment with sonography for trauma (EFAST). J Trauma. 2004;57:288–95.
18. Ekeh AP, Peterson W, Woods RJ, Walusimbi R, Nwuneli N, Saxe JM, et al. Is chest x-ray an adequate screening tool for the diagnosis of blunt thoracic aortic injury? J Trauma. 2008;65:1088–92.
19. Coccolini F, Stahel PF, Montori G, Biffl W, Horer TM, Catena F, et al. Pelvic trauma: WSES classification and guidelines. World J Emerg Surg. 2017;12:5.
20. Cannon JW, Khan MA, Raja AS, Cohen MJ, Como JJ, Cotton BA, et al. Damage control resuscitation in patients with severe traumatic hemorrhage: a practice management guideline from the Eastern Association for the Surgery of Trauma. J Trauma Acute Care Surg. 2017;82(3):605–17.
21. Kasotakis G, Sideris A, Yang Y, de Moya M, Alam H, King DR, et al. Aggressive early crystalloid resuscitation adversely affects outcomes in adult blunt trauma patients: an analysis of the Glue Grant database. J Trauma Acute Care Surg. 2013;74(5):1215–22.
22. Ley EJ, Clond MA, Srour MK, Barnajian M, Mirocha J, Margulies DR, et al. Emergency department crystalloid resuscitation of 1.5 L or more is associated with increased mortality in elderly and nonelderly trauma patients. J Trauma. 2011;70(2):398–400.
23. Meyer DE, Vincent LE, Fox EE, O'Keeffe T, Inaba K, Bulger E, et al. Every minute counts: time to delivery of initial massive transfusion cooler and its impact on mortality. J Trauma Acute Care Surg. 2017;83(1):19–24.
24. Holcomb JB, Tilley BC, Baraniuk S, Fox EE, Wade CE, Podbielski JM, et al; PROPPR Study Group. Transfusion of plasma, platelets, and red blood cells in a 1:1:1 vs a 1:1:2 ratio and mortality in patients with severe trauma: the PROPPR randomized clinical trial. JAMA. 2015;313(5):471–82.
25. Duchesne J, Smith A, Lawicki S, Hunt J, Houghton A, Taghavi S, et al. Single institution trial comparing whole blood vs balanced component therapy: 50 years later. J Am Coll Surg. 2021;232(4):433–42.
26. Seheult JN, Anto V, Alarcon LH, Sperry JL, Triulzi DJ, Yazer MH. Clinical outcomes among low-titer group O whole blood recipients compared to recipients of conventional components in civilian trauma resuscitation. Transfusion. 2018;58(8):1838–45.
27. Giordano S, Spiezia L, Campello E, Simioni P. The current understanding of trauma-induced coagulopathy (TIC): a focused review on pathophysiology. Intern Emerg Med. 2017;12(7):981–91.
28. Gonzalez E, Moore EE, Moore HB, Chapman MP, Chin TL, Ghasabyan A, et al. Goal-directed hemostatic resuscitation of trauma-induced coagulopathy: a pragmatic randomized clinical trial comparing a viscoelastic assay to conventional coagulation assays. Ann Surg. 2016;263(6):1051–9.
29. CRASH-2 Collaborators, Roberts I, Shakur H, Afolabi A, Brohi K, Coats T, Dewan Y, et al. The importance of early treatment with tranexamic acid in bleeding trauma patients: an exploratory analysis of the CRASH-2 randomised controlled trial. Lancet. 2011;377(9771):1096–101, 1101.e1–2.
30. CRASH-3 Trial Collaborators. Effects of tranexamic acid on death, disability, vascular occlusive events and other morbidities in patients with acute traumatic brain injury (CRASH-3): a randomised, placebo-controlled trial. Lancet. 2019;394(10210):1713–23.

31. Nunez TC, Voskresensky IV, Dossett LA, Shinall R, Dutton WD, Cotton BA. Early prediction of massive transfusion in trauma: simple as ABC (assessment of blood consumption)? J Trauma. 2009;66(2):346–52.
32. Magnotti LJ, Bradburn EH, Webb DL, Berry SD, Fischer PE, Zarzaur BL, et al. Admission ionized calcium levels predict the need for multiple transfusions: a prospective study of 591 critically ill trauma patients. J Trauma. 2011;70(2):391–7.
33. Kinoshita T, Yamakawa K, Matsuda H, Yoshikawa Y, Wada D, Hamasaki T, et al. The survival benefit of a novel trauma workflow that includes immediate whole-body computed tomography, surgery, and interventional radiology, all in one trauma resuscitation room: a retrospective historical control study. Ann Surg. 2019;269(2):370–6.
34. Brenner M, Inaba K, Aiolfi A, DuBose J, Fabian T, Bee T, et al; AAST AORTA Study Group. Resuscitative endovascular balloon occlusion of the aorta and resuscitative thoracotomy in select patients with Hemorrhagic shock: early results from the American Association for the Surgery of Trauma's Aortic Occlusion in Resuscitation for Trauma and Acute Care Surgery Registry. J Am Coll Surg. 2018;226(5):730–740.
35. Saito N, Matsumoto H, Yagi T, Hara Y, Hayashida K, Motomura T, et al. Evaluation of the safety and feasibility of resuscitative endovascular balloon occlusion of the aorta. J Trauma Acute Care Surg. 2015;78(5):897–904.
36. Li T, Zhu Y, Hu Y, Li L, Diao Y, Tang J, et al. Ideal permissive hypotension to resuscitate uncontrolled hemorrhagic shock and the tolerance time in rats. Anesthesiology. 2011;114(1):111–9.
37. Rajajee V, Vanaman M, Fletcher JJ, Jacobs TL. Optic nerve ultrasound for the detection of raised intracranial pressure. Neurocrit Care. 2011;15(3):506–15.
38. Weuster M, Brück A, Lippross S, Menzdorf L, Fitschen-Oestern S, Behrendt P, et al.; Trauma Register DGU. Epidemiology of accidental hypothermia in polytrauma patients: an analysis of 15,230 patients of the trauma register DGU. J Trauma Acute Care Surg. 2016;81(5):905–912.
39. Sartelli M, Chichom-Mefire A, Labricciosa FM, Hardcastle T, Abu-Zidan FM, Adesunkanmi AK, et al. The management of intra-abdominal infections from a global perspective: 2017 WSES guidelines for management of intra-abdominal infections. World J Emerg Surg. 2017;12:29.
40. Kluger Y, Ben-Ishay O, Sartelli M, Ansaloni L, Abbas AE, Agresta F, et al. World Society of Emergency Surgery Study Group initiative on timing of acute care surgery classification (TACS). World J Emerg Surg. 2013;8(1):17.
41. Rhodes A, Evans LE, Alhazzani W, Levy MM, Antonelli M, Ferrer R, et al. Surviving sepsis campaign: international guidelines for management of sepsis and septic shock: 2016. Intensive Care Med. 2017;43(3):304–77.
42. Freund Y, Lemachatti N, Krastinova E, Van Laer M, Claessens YE, Avondo A, et al.; French Society of Emergency Medicine Collaborators Group. Prognostic accuracy of Sepsis-3 criteria for in-hospital mortality among patients with suspected infection presenting to the emergency department. JAMA. 2017;317(3):301–308.
43. Sartelli M, Abu-Zidan FM, Catena F, Griffiths EA, Di Saverio S, Coimbra R, et al. Global validation of the WSES sepsis severity score for patients with complicated intra-abdominal infections: a prospective multicentre study (WISS study). World J Emerg Surg. 2015;10:61.
44. Esteban A, Frutos-Vivar F, Ferguson ND, Peñuelas O, Lorente JA, Gordo F, et al. Sepsis incidence and outcome: contrasting the intensive care unit with the hospital ward. Crit Care Med. 2007;35:1284–9.
45. Abu-Zidan FM. Optimizing the value of measuring inferior vena cava diameter in shocked patients. World J Crit Care Med. 2016;5(1):7–11.
46. Cecconi M, De Backer D, Antonelli M, Beale R, Bakker J, Hofer C, et al. Consensus on circulatory shock and hemodynamic monitoring. Task force of the European Society of Intensive Care Medicine. Intensive Care Med. 2014;40(12):1795–815.
47. Jansen TC, van Bommel J, Schoonderbeek FJ, Sleeswijk Visser SJ, van der Klooster JM, et al.; LACTATE Study Group. Early lactate-guided therapy in intensive care unit patients: a multicenter, open-label, randomized controlled trial. Am J Respir Crit Care Med. 2010;182(6):752–761.
48. Avni T, Lador A, Lev S, Leibovici L, Paul M, Grossman A. Vasopressors for the treatment of septic shock: systematic review and meta-analysis. PLoS One. 2015;10(8):e0129305.

Further Reading

Advanced Trauma Life Support (ATLS®), 10th ed.
European Trauma Course: (ETC®). The team approach.
Emergency Surgery Course (ESC®) manual.

Prioritizing Acute Care Surgery and Trauma Patients

R. Stephen Smith and Jessica E. Taylor

Learning Goals
Access to resuscitation bays, operating rooms, and interventional suites is limited. A rational and well-developed approach to prioritize patient care is essential. After review of this chapter the learner will gain an understanding of the need to optimally utilize hospital resources and the necessity of prioritizing patients based on acuity, underlying pathology, and improving outcomes.

Dos and Don'ts
Do
- Understand that the operating room and procedure suites are a limited resource that must be utilized optimally for global healthcare.
- Develop and practice a system of prioritization based on objective criteria (anatomic, physiologic, pathologic) of patient acuity.
- Educate surgeons, other physicians, nurses, and other staff regarding the institution's prioritization plan and the rationale for having such a plan.

Don't
- Deviate from an accepted prioritization plan unless circumstances are extraordinary.
- Incorporate nonmedical criteria (financial, political, administrative) into the prioritization plan as this will undermine the credibility of the prioritization process.
- Allow prioritization plans to be relegated to the category of a forgotten, unused policy.

4.1 Introduction

Globally, healthcare systems deal on a regular basis with a mismatch between available resources and the needs of patients. This situation has been consistent for some time, but has been made even more severe by the recent COVID 19 pandemic. The hospital portal of entry for most patients with trauma and emergency surgical issues is the Emergency Department. Prioritization of patients in this area of the hospital is critical. This concept is well known in

R. S. Smith (✉) · J. E. Taylor
University of Florida, Gainesville, FL, USA
e-mail: Steve.Smith@surgery.ufl.edu;
Robert.Smith@surgery.ufl.edu;
Jessica.Taylor@surgery.ufl.edu

trauma centers where patients are assigned a level of priority based on anatomic and physiologic factors such as airway compromise, hypotension, the requirement for blood transfusions, Glasgow Coma Scale score, or wounding mechanism (gunshot wounds) or the location of a penetrating injury (trunk) [1]. Since these patients receive assignment to a special category, they, by definition, are prioritized to earlier procedural and operative treatment. In the absence of physiologic or anatomic indications of life-threatening injury, high-risk mechanisms of injury (motor cycle crashes, high speed automobile crashes, falls) are criteria for giving a patient priority in initial assessment. Mass casualty and disaster scenarios must be approached from a different perspective [1]. The inclination and design of many civilian healthcare systems is to expend tremendous amounts of resources on individual patients with critical illness. This paradigm is inappropriate in the mass casualty scenario when a philosophy of "the greatest good for the greatest number" must be followed. In effect, this means that patients with little chance of survival would have a lower priority for operation than patients with less severe injuries who can be saved with fewer resources.

Rapid access to operative treatment of seriously ill and injured patients is well recognized as the primary determinant of a favorable outcome for a patient with a life-threatening condition [2]. Because of the particular equipment and expertise required for surgical patients, the operating room is the most obvious example of an area that requires a systematic approach to provide care to patients in a timely manner. The operating room is a very frequent and critical "bottleneck" in the provision of patient care. This problem is further complicated by the increasing specialization of surgeons, operative teams, and operating rooms. Does the patient require an open or minimally invasive approach? Increasingly, specialty surgical care is best performed in purpose designed suites, i.e., hybrid operating rooms, minimally invasive suites, that may not be optimal for other types of surgical care. This process is more complicated in patients who have multiple conditions that require operative treatment. For example, a polytrauma patient who requires operative intervention by trauma surgery, orthopedics, and neurosurgery presents a significant challenge. The effective surgeon must take all aspects of care into account to provide thoughtful prioritization of surgical care. While focused efforts have been performed to streamline the decision making process by the creation of evidence-based protocols and algorithms, sound clinical judgement is irreplaceable and remains the most effective tool [3–11].

4.2 Trauma

In simple terms, patients with the greatest risk to life and limb should have the highest priority for operative or nonoperative treatment (Table 4.1). Prioritization may include the triage of multiple patients for access to the treatment or the prioritization of injuries in a single polytrauma patient to determine the most appropriate order of therapeutic intervention for various injuries. A well-accepted guide to triage and prioritization is the ABCDE approach forwarded by the American College of Surgeons Advanced Trauma Life Support Course [1]. This concept mandates the treatment of patients based on the maintenance of an adequate airway, assuring adequate ventilation and oxygenation, maintenance of adequate circulation through the control of hemorrhage coupled with fluid and blood resuscitation, and treatment of severe neurologic injury. For example, an obstructed airway treated with endotracheal intubation or crichothyroidectomy will take precedence over placement of a tube thoracoscopy for

Table 4.1 Characteristics of injured patients indicating high priority

Airway compromise
Respiratory insufficiency or failure
Hemorrhage
Hemodynamic instability (shock)
Requirement for transfusion to maintain blood pressure
Truncal gunshot wounds
Severe traumatic brain injury (Glasgow coma scale score < 9)

hemopneumothorax. Similarly, control of severe hemorrhage from a Grade V splenic laceration will have priority over placement of an intracranial pressure monitor in a patient with a Glasgow Coma Score of 8. This is not to say that there should be any delay in treatment of a life-threating injury, but instead provides a rational and logical method to allow prioritization. In many mature trauma programs, injuries of these types may be treated in an almost simultaneous manner.

Immediate access to the operating room is essential for critically injured patients, since significant delay will lead to increased morbidity and mortality. Prior to transportation of a critically injured patient to the operating room, interventional radiology suite, or ICU, a number of interventions should be performed to stabilize the patient. The priority of treatment should be focused on maintaining a definitive airway, respiration, and perfusion of vital organs. Initial evaluation and resuscitation, including procedures such as establishment of an endotracheal tube and tube thoracostomy, are usually performed in the trauma bay or the emergency department. Tourniquets and pelvic binders are important, life-saving techniques to control ongoing hemorrhage. Establishment of vascular access, potentially including intraosseus infusion devices, is frequently performed in the pre-hospital setting and in the emergency department. Initial volume resuscitation, including blood products via a massive transfusion protocol, should be initiated as soon as hemorrhagic shock is suspected [1].

A useful rule of thumb is that a patient who requires emergent operative or procedural treatment should have access to a fully equipped and staffed operating room within 1 h. This degree of hospital capability requires significant and consistent commitment from the entire operative team including surgeons, anesthesiologists, nurses, operating room technicians and, very importantly, hospital administration. Consistent performance improvement processes must be in place to provide ongoing and timely monitoring of prioritization decisions and operating room availability.

4.3 Emergency General Surgery

It is estimated that 1.5–2% of deaths globally are caused by conditions, other than trauma, that require emergency general surgical treatment [3, 4]. The majority of these disease entities involve an intra-abdominal process (Table 4.2) [3–11]. A difference between common emergency general surgery procedures and trauma exists. The majority of emergency general surgery interventions can undergo initial nonoperative stabilization through the administration of volume, antibiotics, pressors, or blood products [2–8]. This permits the surgeon the luxury of additional time to more fully assess and initially resuscitate these types of patients (Table 4.3).

An incarcerated hernia may lead to strangulation, which is a true surgical emergency. An incarcerated hernia may be a long-term condition in some patients, but chronicity should not reduce the surgeon's level of concern. An incarcerated hernia that suddenly causes a change in symptomatology such as bowel obstruction, overlying skin changes, increasing lactic acidosis, or the onset of sepsis should alert the surgeon to possible strangulation. A strangulated hernia is an emergency that requires immediate operative

Table 4.2 Common indications for high priority emergency general surgery

Acute appendicitis
Acute cholecystitis/cholangitis
Incarcerated/strangulated hernia
Bowel obstruction
Gastrointestinal perforation
Gastrointestinal hemorrhage
Fulminate colitis
Necrotizing soft tissue infection

Table 4.3 Prioritization of emergency general surgery procedures

Category 1: Emergent operation required within 2 h to preserve life or limb
Category 2: Urgent operation required between 2 and 6 h
Category 3: Operation required between 6 and 24 h
Category 4: Operations that may be delayed based on initial medical treatment or subsequent or "second look" procedures

intervention, preferably within 2 h. An incarcerated hernia without obvious characteristics of strangulation should be repaired within 24 h, if at all possible.

Acute appendicitis remains are the common general surgery emergency. A delay in treatment for greater than 24 h increases the risk of perforation, peritonitis, or abscess formation. Early administration of antibiotics can temporize or treat appendicitis, but the goal of surgical prioritization should be removal within 24 h of onset of symptoms. Acute cholecystitis is quite common, and cholecystectomy is the most common abdominal operation performed in developed countries. Acute cholecystitis is best treated with cholecystectomy within 24 h. The course of acute cholecystitis can be ameliorated with the administration of antibiotics and operation may be safely delayed for several days if the patient demonstrates a favorable response to antibiotics. Conversely, if the patient exhibits evidence of worsening sepsis or cholangitis, immediate intervention is indicated. In patients with bile duct obstruction secondary to choledocholithiasis, many centers and surgeons prefer to "clear the duct" with endoscopic (ERCP) removal of common bile duct stones prior to performance of cholecystectomy. Symptomatic cholelithiasis is not an emergency and may be treated on an elective basis [11].

Intestinal obstructions may be caused by adhesive disease, hernia, volvulus, intussusception, or parasites. Small bowel obstruction secondary to adhesive disease is usually treated successfully by nonoperative management and is rarely a surgical emergency. It is acceptable to wait for improvement for a period of 24 h prior to operative treatment. An exception to this general rule is evidenced by imaging of a closed loop obstruction. This finding represents a true surgical emergency that may lead to extensive bowel strangulation and necrosis. A prior history of a bariatric surgical procedure makes this unfortunate finding more likely. Operative intervention should ideally begin within 2 h to minimize the risk of bowel loss. Volvulus is frequently identified by imaging. Procedural intervention should proceed within a few hours. Evidence of potential strangulation secondary to volvulus mandates immediate operative intervention.

Complications of peptic ulcer disease include perforation and bleeding. Perforated ulcers produce peritonitis and may initiate hypovolemia and/or sepsis. The treatment of a perforated ulcer is operative and should be accomplished as soon as possible, but certainly within 24 h. Preoperative stabilization with nasogastric suction, volume resuscitation, and antibiotics facilitates an urgent rather than an emergent approach in most cases. Upper gastrointestinal hemorrhage usually responds well to medical management, endoscopic interventions, or angiographic embolization. Therefore, the need for emergent operative intervention is relatively uncommon. Perforation and bleeding from colonic diverticular disease are relatively common in developed countries. The majority of early diverticular perforations respond well to nonoperative antibiotic therapy. Urgent or emergent (within 6 h) operative intervention is usually reserved for Hinchey class 4 disease and evidence of sepsis. Colonic hemorrhage may present with severe hemorrhage requiring immediate operation, but a more measured approach is usually the case. Operation within 6 h may be required, but is uncommon. Fulminant colitis secondary to Clostridium difficile is increasing in frequency. Colitis that progresses despite adequate medical management, including appropriate antibiotic coverage, is an indication for urgent operative treatment [2–11].

The incidence of necrotizing soft tissue infections is increasing, particularly in populations where diabetes and obesity are prevalent. This is a life-threatening condition. While initial resuscitation and antibiotic administration are critical, early urgent operative debridement is essential and absolutely necessary for successful treatment [2].

Questions
1. Which of the following patients has the highest priority for the operating room?
   A. 24 year old man with suspected acute appendicitis of 12 h duration.

B. 49 year old woman with a 3 day history of right upper quadrant pain. Ultrasound identifies cholelithiasis without evidence of cholecystitis
   C. **17 year old man (stable vital signs) with the history of a gunshot wound of the abdomen 15 min prior to arrival at the hospital. FAST exam is positive for fluid in Morison's pouch**
   D. 57 year old diabetic man with the history of a perirectal abscess of 16 h duration
2. Which of the following conditions is an indication for the highest level of trauma team activation?
   A. A 32 year old woman brought from the field with bilateral femur fractures, stable vital signs.
   B. A 39 year old man brought to the hospital by ambulance with suspected flail chest from blunt trauma, vital signs stable, SaO_2 93% with 2 L of oxygen by nasal cannula
   C. **A 51 year old woman with an open book pelvic fracture transferred from another hospital, transfused 4 units of whole blood due to hypotension (82/48 mmHg)**
   D. A 16 year old man with the history of a 5 min loss of consciousness after a motorcycle crash, Glasgow Coma Scale score = 14.
3. Which of the following patients mandates the highest priority of operative intervention?
   A. A 78 year old man who presents with nausea, vomiting, and abdominal distention with the history of recurrent small bowel obstruction secondary to adhesive disease.
   B. **A 46 year old woman with a previous Roux - N - Y gastric bypass for obesity who presents with abdominal pain and CT findings consistent with an internal hernia.**
   C. A 13 year old girl who presents with an 8 h history of right lower quadrant pain and anorexia.
   D. A 53 year old man with acute pancreatitis and choledocholithiasis.

References

1. Advanced Trauma Life Support, student course manual, 10th ed. Chicago: American College of Surgeons; 2018. isbn: 78-0-9968262-3-5.
2. Dellinger RP, Levy MM, Rhodes A, et al. Surviving sepsis campaign: International guidelines for management of severe sepsis and septic shock, 2012. Intensive care Med. 2013;39:165–228. https://doi.org/10.1007/s00134-012-2769-8.
3. Catena F, Biffl W, De Simone B, et al. Emergency general surgeons: the special forces of general surgery (the Navy Seals paradigm). World J Emerg Surg. 2020;15:11. https://doi.org/10.1186/s13017-020-0293-7.
4. Saunders DI, Murray D, Pichel AC, et al. Variations in mortality after emergency laparotomy: the first report of the UK emergency laparotomy network. Br J Aneasth. 2012;109:368–75.
5. Catena F, Moore EE. Emergency surgery, acute care surgery and the boulevard of broken dreams. World J Emerg Surg. 2009;4:4. https://doi.org/10.1186/1749-7922-4-4.
6. Catena F, Moore EE. World Journal of Emergency Surgery (WJES), World Society of Emergency Surgery (WSES) and the role of emergency surgery in the world. World J Emerg Surg. 2007;2:3.
7. Barazanchi A, Bhat S, Palmer-Neels K, et al. Evaluating and improving current risk prediction tools in emergency laparotomy. J Trauma Acute Care Surg. 2020;89:382–7.
8. Sorenson LT, Malaki A, Wille-Jorgenson P, et al. Risk factors in mortality and post-operative complications after general surgery. J Gastrointest Surg. 2007;11:903–10.
9. Eugene N, Oliver CM, Bassett MG, et al. Development and internal validation of a novel risk model for adult patients undergoing emergency laparotomy surgery: the National Emergency Laparotomy Risk audit model. Br J Anasth. 2018;121:739–48.
10. Srikumar G, Eglinton T, MacCormick AD. Development of the general surgery prioritization tool implemented in New Zealand in 2018. Health Policy. 2020;124:1043–9. https://doi.org/10.1016/j.healthpol.2020.07.018.
11. Solans-Domenech M, Adam P, Tebe C, et al. Developing a universal tool for the prioritization of patients waiting elective surgery. Health Policy. 2013;113:118–26.

Triage

Cordoba Mordehay, Ciro Paolillo, Federica Pitoni, and Klein Yoram

5

> **Learning Goals**
> After completing this chapter, participants will have a clear understanding of the triage system and structure and how the content may be applied in their work environment. Participants will also develop an appreciation international development that forms the basis of emergency department triage in Australia, USA, and England. They will also be able to identify factors influencing consistency of triage in that context.

Triage is the process of defining the priority of patients' management according to the severity of their clinical condition and the available resources [1]. The term comes from the French verb trier, meaning to separate, sort, shift, or select.

A triage system is the essential framework by which all incoming emergency patients are evaluated according to their condition using a standard rating scale. It's the first point of public contact with the hospital. Urgency refers to the need for time-critical intervention—it is not synonymous with severity. Three phases of triage have emerged in modern healthcare system. First, **prehospital triage** in order to dispatch ambulance and prehospital care resources. Second, **triage at scene** by first clinician attending the patient. Thirst, **triage on arrival at ED** or receiving Hospital. In modern Emergency Departments (EDs), triage officers, usually nurses appropriately educated, evaluate patients who present for disorders and prioritize them. ED triage systems work to identify the most urgent cases to make so that they could receive priority treatment, followed by the less urgent cases.

The triage system should have three characteristics:

Speed: triage access-coding time must be rapid

Accuracy: all potentially critically ill patients must be identified

Organization: an organized patient processing system that supports assessment, treatment, and disposition.

The concept of prioritizing by prognosis is not new and is described in the Edwin Smith papyrus dated from the seventeenth century B.C [2]. The modern concept of triage is attributed

---

C. Mordehay · K. Yoram (✉)
Department Surgery B and Division of Trauma and Critical Care Surgery, Sheba Medical Center, Ramat Gan, Israel
e-mail: moti.cordoba@sheba.gov.il;
yoram.klein@sheba.health.gov.il

C. Paolillo · F. Pitoni
Emergency Department, University and Hospital Trust—Ospedale Borgo Trento, Verona, Italy
e-mail: federica.pitoni@aovr.veneto.it

to Dominique Jean Larrey, who was a surgeon of Napoleon Bonaparte's Imperial Guard throughout the Napoleonic Wars. Larrey established a categorical rule for the triage of war casualties, treating the wounded according to the observed gravity of their injuries and the urgency for medical care, regardless of their rank or nationality [3].

Since Larrey's time, the concept of triage has evolved. Though the main process still relies on clinical assessment and physiological findings, the use of computerized algorithm-based system is evolving, making triage much more sophisticated.

Triage is one of the most common tasks in the professional life of the acute care surgeon. We are prioritizing our tasks on an hourly basis.

There are several situations in which the acute care surgeons need to practice the principles of triage. We need this process for prioritizing the patients in the emergency department (ED), to schedule imaging studies, to make timing decisions regarding surgical interventions (this subject will be discussed in a dedicated chapter), admitting patients to units with limited number of beds (i.e., ICU), and to manage mass casualty incidents.

The triage process should be done repeatedly and should be based on the clinical condition of the patient, the pathophysiology of the medical conditions, the needed interventions, the prognosis, and the available resources.

Table 5.1 Emergency Severity Index

Level 1	Patient requires immediate life-saving intervention
Level 2	Patient is in a high risk situation, is disoriented, in severe pain, or vitals are in danger zone
Level 3	Multiple resources are required to stabilize the patient, but vitals are not in the danger zone
Level 4	One resource is required to stabilize the patient
Level 5	The patient don't require any resources to be stabilized

5.1 Triage Scales

Almost all of ED in the developed world use five-tier triage scales for categorizing people who are seeking assessment and treatment in hospital EDs. The five categories triage is more precise and reliable when compared with the older triage systems (three or four category). Several methods of 5-level triage are in use. For example, the Emergency Severity Index, (Table 5.1) developed in the United States (1999), designates the most acutely ill patients as level 1 (highest level) or 2 and uses the number of resources a patient needs to determine levels 3 to 5 (lowest level). The Manchester Triage Scale, used widely in Great Britain and in North of Europe, uses 52 algorithms based on the patient's sign and symptoms to determine the triage. The Canadian Triage and Acuity Scale uses an extensive list of clinical descriptors to place patients in one of 5 triage levels. Each level has an associated time required for physician assessment, with all level 1 patients needing to be treated immediately. All the triage systems have the same purpose: early identification of physiological abnormality and risk factors for poor outcome and consequently activation of focused ongoing medical assessment and investigation.

5.2 Triage in the ED

Every patient in the ED can be categorized to one of three options. The patient might need urgent intervention, admission to one of the hospital departments, or he can be safely discharged home. In a crowded modern ED, the prompt identification of the critically ill patient who needs urgent intervention is crucial. This should be based on a quick clinical inspection and detection of overt signs of physiological distress. On top of the traditional vital signs of heart rate, pulse oximetry, and blood pressure, the triage officer must prioritize patients with dyspnea, signs of skin hypoperfusion (pallor, diaphoresis, mottling), restlessness, and agonizing abdominal pain. The practical meaning of this process is that these patients should be placed immediately in a monitored environment, and the most senior physician available should approach him immediately, regardless of the load of other patients in the ED, or other tasks that the physician is occupied with.

5.3 Pain Assessment at Triage

Pain is the most common symptom reported by patients who present to the ED. Pain assessment must remain at the forefront of the triage. Without pain assessment, the provision of appropriate analgesia at triage is not possible. Pain is an important issue for a number of reasons. First, it ensures that a patient's pain is evaluated and managed at the earliest opportunity. Patient anxiety is reduced, and communication is improved. The patient's pain is to be assessed at triage for helping to determine the urgency with which that patient is to be seen.

There are three main types of pain assessment tools (Table 5.2):

Verbal descriptor scales
Visual analogue scales
Pain behavior tools

Even though the patient's self-report is regarded as the gold standard for measuring pain, it is unrealistic to expect that only the patient's subjective assessment will be taken into consideration during this process. By the same reason, it is inappropriate that the triage practitioners make their own subjective assessment of the patient's pain in isolation. An expert nurse at triage should consider other factors that may be influencing the patient's assessment of his pain (facial expressions and physiological parameters, for example). Musculoskeletal pain can be effectively reduced through simple measures such as rest, ice, compression, and elevation (RICE). The administration of pharmacological agents within the triage area needs to be supported by institutional policies and procedures and should be considered by individual departments, considering the physical organization of the triage area and the ability to reevaluate, monitoring the patients.

5.3.1 Triage Trauma Assessment

By the field triage to triage at Emergency Department

In the first half of life, more Americans die from injuries and violence—such as motor vehicle crashes, suicide, or homicides. This makes injury the leading cause of death among persons aged 1-44. (CDC)

The development of field triage criteria paralleled the development of trauma centers, ('70/'90) including the concept of bypassing closer facilities in favor of those with enhanced capabilities for treating severely injured patients. A trauma center is an acute-care facility that has made preparations and achieved certain resource and personnel standards to provide care for severely injured patients such as car accident injuries, gunshot wounds, traumatic brain injuries, stab wounds, serious falls, and blunt trauma. In addi-

Table 5.2 Pain Assessment Scale

Simple Descriptive Pain Intensity Scale[1]						
No pain	Mild pain		Moderate pain	Severe pain	Very severe pain	Worst possible pain
0–10 Numeric Pain Intensity Scale[1]						
0	1	2	3	4	5	6	7	8	9	10
No pain		Moderate pain								Worst possible pain
Visual Analog Scale (VAS)[2]						
No pain						Pain as bad as it could possibly be

tion to 24-h ED care, such a facility ensures access to surgeons, anesthesiologists, other physician specialists, and nurses and life support equipment needed to treat severely injured persons. Trauma patients should be allocated based on clinical urgency. There are specific mechanisms of injury associated with risk of life-threatening injury that need to be incorporated in triage decisions. Examples include vehicle rollover, death of same-vehicle occupant, ejection from a vehicle, and fall from a height greater than three meters. All victims of trauma should be allocated a triage category according to their objective clinical urgency. As with other clinical situations, this will include consideration of high-risk history as well as brief physical assessment (general appearance ± physiological observations). Although individual departments may have policies that provide for immediate team responses to patients meeting certain criteria (Trauma Team), these patients should still be allocated an objective triage category according to their clinical presentation.

5.3.2 Triage Decision-Making

Triage decision isn't easy to perform. It's a multilevel three-step process. The first challenge is to evidence the main symptom or sign referred by patients and the care workers. The second step is to determine priority following information allowed. That information should be integrated with information that are discriminator of specific condition (for example severe pain or chest pain).

Physiological abnormalities are known risk factors for poor outcomes. Timely responses to abnormal clinical findings have been shown to reduce morbidity and mortality in critically ill patients.

The most common triage scales consider respiratory rate, saturation, pulse, blood pressure, level of consciousness, and temperature (Table 5.3).

The Manchester Triage System consists of 53 presentations most with five priorities—one to five—making a total of 258 presentation–priority combinations. After the choice of the adequate symptoms of presentation, the nurse at triage should consider appropriate disposition (resuscitation room, or minor treatment area, for example).

Triage is a rapid and focused encounter in which information are gathered, but it's also a dynamic process and should be undertaken periodically on all patients while they are waiting for treatment. Any change in status can be identified and the triage category can be modified if necessary.

Table 5.3 Adult Physiological Predictors for Australian Triage Scale

	Category 1 Immediate	Category 2 10 min	Category 3 30 min	Category 4 60 min	Category 5 120 min
Airway	Obstructed/partially obstructed	Patent	Patent	Patent	Patent
Breathing	Severe respiratory distress/absent respiration/hypoventilation	Moderate respiratory distress	Mild respiratory distress	No respiratory distress	No respiratory distress
Circulation	Severe haemodynamic compromise/absent circulation Uncontrolled haemorrhage	Moderate haemodynamic compromise	Mild haemodynamic compromise	No haemodynamic compromise	No haemodynamic compromise
Disability	GCS <9	GCS 9–12	GCS >12	Normal GCS	Normal GCS

5.4 Triage for Imaging Studies

The modern practice of acute care surgery demands an extensive use of imaging studies. It is now relatively rare to proceed to urgent surgery without advance imaging, mostly computerized tomography (CT). The most common exception is of cause an abdominal trauma patient with signs of hemorrhagic shock and positive FAST. Recent years' developments in percutaneous interventions and in nonoperative management mandate the use of CT in patients with conditions that traditionally would have been taken directly to an obligatory surgery (clinically suspected appendicitis, diffuse peritonitis, etc.). The extensive use of CT creates a situation in which the patients should be prioritized to urgent imaging studies, especially CT. Triage patients for urgent CT should be based on the pathophysiology of the suspected problem, the presumed speed of potential deterioration, and the significance of the imaging results to decision making. In general terms, the most urgent study is a head CT for suspected intracranial injury in an unconscious patient. The pathophysiology of increased intracranial pressure can cause a rapid deterioration towards a disastrous herniation, sometimes within minutes, and the imaging results may lead to an emergency lifesaving intervention, such as an evacuation of epidural hematoma. The next priority is a CT for localizing of acute bleeding, in patients who arrive to the ED in hemorrhagic shock that was responsive for initial resuscitation. The next level of urgency is for patients with suspected ischemia, such as mesenteric ischemia, bowel obstruction with suspected strangulation, or limb arterial occlusion. In most circumstances, ischemic changes can deteriorate to an irreversible state within 6–8 h from the beginning of the ischemia. Since in most cases there is also a patient's delay before arriving to medical care, there is a narrow window of opportunity for a salvage procedure that is dependent on the results of the imaging study. The fourth priority is diagnosis of an infection source in septic patients. The imaging study in these cases can lead to a timely interventional infection source control. All other case, such as acute appendicitis or diverticulitis without clinical signs of sepsis, can be safely delayed until more urgent exams will be completed.

5.5 Triage to the Intensive Care Unit (ICU)

The rapid expansion in the medical knowledge and technology has allowed us to treat critically ill patients who didn't survive in the past. Naturally, this evolution increased the need for ICU resources. The practical meaning is that there is a daily competition over available ICU beds—in other words, the acute care surgeon needs to prioritize the patients who are candidates for ICU. In general, admissions to the ICU can be divided into two categories. The first and most important is the clinical condition and the severity of the organ dysfunction. The main purpose is supporting the failing vital systems. For example, a patient with perforate diverticulitis and septic shock. The second category is admission due to anticipation for rapid deterioration based on the pathophysiology and the natural history of the disease, for example—a patient with acute pancreatitis and high risk for deterioration based on one of the prognostic scores (Ranson, apache, Glasgow, etc.). While admission to the ICU is mandatory in the first category, admissions of patients with the second category indication should be prioritized based on the available resources and the condition of other candidates.

5.6 Triage in Mass Casualty Incidents (MCI)

MCI is one of the most challenging situations that the acute care surgeon needs to manage. The main mission is to save the maximum number of salvageable patients. This task cannot be accomplished without an ongoing process of triage. The process is starting in the field by the emergency services personnel. The victims in the field should be divided into those who need an emergency intervention (mostly managing compromised airway and control of external bleeding) and need to be urgently transferred to a hospital (mostly patients with suspected intracranial injury, or with uncontrolled bleeding) and those who can be temporarily delayed in the field. The next level of triage regards the transfer destination. Basically, there are three options: the nearest medical center, the most appropriate center in the area that has the facilities to deal with the suspected specific injury (for example patients with signs of severe head injury to a hospital with neurosurgical capabilities), and off-area transfer to a remote center in order to avoid overwhelming of the areas' medical resources. The factors that dictate the choice of the transfer destinations are the location of the incident, the magnitude of the incident, the available prehospital medical resources, and the available hospitals' resources in the area. The next stage is done by the hospital triage officer at the entrance to the emergency department. Every hospital is required to establish MCI plan in which different admission sites are prepared. The admission sites are usually critical, lying down patients and walking patients. The only mission of the triage officer is to send the patient to the appropriate admission site based on a brief clinical assessment. This should be done within seconds in order to avoid the creation of a bottleneck at the entrance. As the patient is assigned to an admission site and is evaluated by a medical team, the same triage principles that were described earlier in the chapter should be used in order to cope with the imbalance between the medical needs and the available resources in MCI.

> **Do and Dont's**
> - All patients in the waiting room must be reassessed by the Triage Nurse once the triage time has expired.
> - The level and quality of care that is delivered to the community should not be driven by administrative or organizational criteria, but by clinical criteria.

> **Take-Home Messages**
> - A triage system is the essential structure by which all incoming emergency patients are prioritized using a standard rating scale.
> - A five-tier triage scale is a valid and reliable method for categorizing ED patients.
> - Triage scales must be sensitive enough to capture novel presentations of high acuity

> **Questions**
> 1. What is triage:
>   A. **is the process of immediate assessment of all patients who present to the Emergency Department**
>   B. is a process of immediate assessment of older patients who present to the Emergency Department
>   C. is a process of immediate assessment of wounded patients who present to the Emergency Department
>   D. is a process of immediate assessment only of critical patients who present to the Emergency Department
> 2. Who perform the triage?
>   A. **an experienced nurse in triage decision making**
>   B. an experienced nurse
>   C. an emergency physician
>   D. an experienced nurse in critical care
> 3. Emergency Triage scales:
>   A. must be specific enough to capture novel presentations of high acuity.
>   B. the scale must be very difficult to apply by emergency nurses
>   C. the Australian Triage system has three levels of acuity
>   D. **the application of the scale must be independent of the nurse performing the role**

4. Five-tier triage scales are:
   A. equal to three-tier scales
   B. **more reliable than three- or four-tier scales**
   C. equal to four-tier scales
   D. depend on the nurse
5. In an Emergency Department triage system, 'urgency' refers to:
   A. the complexity of the patient's condition at a particular point in time
   B. **the clinical features of the patient's condition**
   C. severity of diseases
   D. the number of patients admitted in Emergency Department

References

1. Kluger Y, Ben-Ishay O, Sartelli M, et al. World Society of Emergency Surgery Study Group initiative on Timing of Acute Care Surgery classification (TACS). World J Emerg Surg. 2013;8:17.
2. van Middendorp JJ, Sanchez GM, Burridge AL. The Edwin Smith papyrus: a clinical reappraisal of the oldest known document on spinal injuries. Eur Spine J. 2010;19:1815–23.
3. Skandalakis PN, Lainas P, Skandalakis JE, Mirilas P. 'To afford the wounded speedy assistance': Dominique Jean Larrey and Napoleon. World J Surg. 30(8):1392–9.

Further Reading

Australian College of Emergency Medicine. Guidelines on the implementation of the Australian Triage Scale in Emergency Departments. Australian College of Emergency Medicine; 2018. www.acemc.org.au.

Bullard MJ, Unger B, et al. Revision to the Canadian Emergency Department Triage and Acuity Scale (CTAS) adult guideline. CJEM. 2008;10(2):136–51.

Emergency Triage Education Kit. Triage workbook. Australian Government. Department of Health and Aging. 2009.

Kuriyama A, Urushidani S, Nakayam T. Five-level emergency triage systems: variation in assessment of validity. Emerg Med J. 2017;34(11):703–10.

Mackway-Jones K, Marsden J, Windle J. Emergency triage. Manchester Triage Group. 3rd ed. Wiley Blackwell.

Tsai LH, Huang CH, Su YC. Comparison of prehospital triage and five-level triage system at the emergency department. Emerg Med J. 2017;34(11):720–5.

Mass Casualties

6

Emmanouil Pikoulis, Anastasia Pikouli, and Athanasios Kalogeropoulos

6.1 Introduction

Disasters can happen suddenly worldwide. From Haiti Earthquake to World Trade Center Attack, disasters result in mass casualties. Healthcare professionals assume responsibility of providing medical care to patients. Unlike everyday provision of medicine, in disasters the healthcare providers need to adapt their practice to a large number of casualties, and at the same time, integrate their response to a multiservice disaster framework. For this reason, the healthcare providers need to understand the principles of disaster medicine and receive training in the disaster management. The realization of the special circumstances, under which medicine is practiced in mass casualties incidents, has forged the development of specialized training courses in medical management of mass casualty incidents.

> **Learning Goals**
> - Define and understand what is a mass casualty incident.
> - Acknowledge the different types of disasters.
> - Understand how communities can prepare themselves and respond to disasters.
> - Understand how the medical service can approach a mass casualty incident in a structured framework.
> - Acknowledge how medical service can be deployed at the scene of a mass casualty incident.

6.1.1 Terminology and Definitions

Humans from the very beginning of their existence to this world were confronted with **incidents** challenging the function and sustainability of their habitat. Sometimes these incidents overwhelmed the capacity of local communities in manpower and resources, in order to be effectively constrained. Whenever an incident mandates extraordinary resources, because of the location, the number of patients, the severity, and the type of live casualties, it is defined as a **major incident** [1].

Major incidents result from causal events of a natural or man-made origin, which are called

E. Pikoulis (✉)
Faculty of Medicine, Third Department of Surgery, Attikon General Hospital, National and Kapodistrian University of Athens (NKUA), Athens, Greece
e-mail: mpikoul@med.uoa.gr

A. Pikouli
Faculty of Medicine, National and Kapodistrian University of Athens (NKUA), Athens, Greece

A. Kalogeropoulos
Orthopaedics and Trauma, Sonnenhofspital, Bern, Switzerland

hazards. Whenever major incidents happen in a human habitat, they may have a severe impact to the function of the local community and they often result in human losses, failure of technological infrastructure, and destruction of the surrounding environment. These major incidents are defined as **disasters**, so as to be differentiated from incidents, which take place in remote areas without impact to the human society [2]. Disasters may be the result of various natural phenomena, man-made events, or they may be the result of hybrid incidents. Irrespective of the cause, they always refer to a disruption of normal function of the local society, which lacks the human and material resources to respond effectively, and for this reason, an external assistance for recovery is needed [3].

Not all communities share the same risk of a disaster. As **risk** is defined as the probability of a hazardous event to take place in a specific region, in a specific time period and has a negative effect on people, systems, and assets. The risk is depicted as the synergic function of the hazards, the exposure of humans/infrastructure as well as the vulnerability of those exposed and it can be estimated through the formula in Fig. 6.1.

The **vulnerability** depicts how much susceptible to damage or disruption is a society after a disaster. There are many factors affecting the vulnerability of a society (Table 6.1) [4, 5].

Last but not the least, when the number and severity of casualties after a major incident

Table 6.1 Factors affecting vulnerability of a society to disasters

Vulnerability factors		
1. Physical factors	1.1	Low quality of structural infrastructure
	1.2	Lack of land use control
	1.3	Lack of city planning
2. Social factors	2.1	Gender discrimination
	2.2	Social discrimination
	2.3	Degradation of public health system
	2.4	Social marginalization
	2.5	Disability
	2.6	Age related
	2.7	Psychological factors
	2.8	Population growth
	2.9	Transition in cultural practices
	2.10	War and civil strife
	2.11	Lack of awareness and information
3. Economic factors	3.1	Rapid urbanization
	3.2	Trade and international voyages
	3.3	Technological and industrial development
	3.4	Poverty
4. Environmental factors	4.1	Climate change
	4.2	Changes in habitats
	4.3	Deforestation
	4.3	Environmental degradation
	4.4	Poor environmental management
	4.5	Interaction with wildlife

Fig. 6.1 Risk Assessment

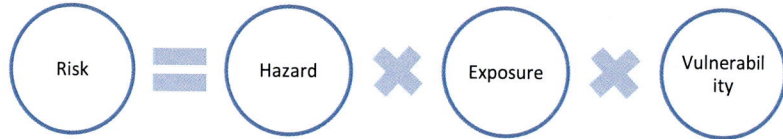

exceed the capacity of emergency medical services, then the event is described as a **mass casualty incident (MCI or MASCAL)** [6].

6.2 Diagnosis

6.2.1 Classification

6.2.1.1 Classification of Disasters
Disasters can be classified into natural disasters, when the causal event is a natural phenomenon, and man-made disasters, when the human factor is the cause and hybrid incidents [3]. Since there is a plethora of etiological events resulting to a MCI, the response of healthcare services should acquire an "**all hazard approach**" structure.

6.2.1.2 Natural Disasters
Natural disasters are categorized to geophysical, meteorological, hydrological, climatological, biological, and extraterrestrial [7] (Fig. 6.2). Among most disastrous natural phenomena are the earthquakes, floods, tsunamis, wildfires, and volcanos.

Earthquakes are very disastrous natural phenomena, resulting into one million deaths the last 20 years. The number of earthquakes every year is estimated approximately to 500,000, most of them are located in the Pacific Ring of Fire. Risk factors of their impact are the magnitude, the depth, and the proximity to the human habitat. Due to increasing urbanization and technological infrastructure, the number of casualties and deaths is raised to thousands [8].

Tsunamis are giant waves, occurring in oceans. They are usually the result of earthquakes and they have an enormous human and social impact. From eighteenth to twenty-first century, approximately 420.000 people lost their lives and thousands others were injured or went missing because of the tsunamis. Vulnerable communities are those who lack the appropriate defense infrastructure, resistant buildings, and effective evacuation lines based on early warning systems [9].

Floods are usually caused by massive rainfall, deforestation, and melting of snow. They present the highest frequency (40%) as well as mortality rates among other disasters [10]. The affected population is located in lowlands, close to water

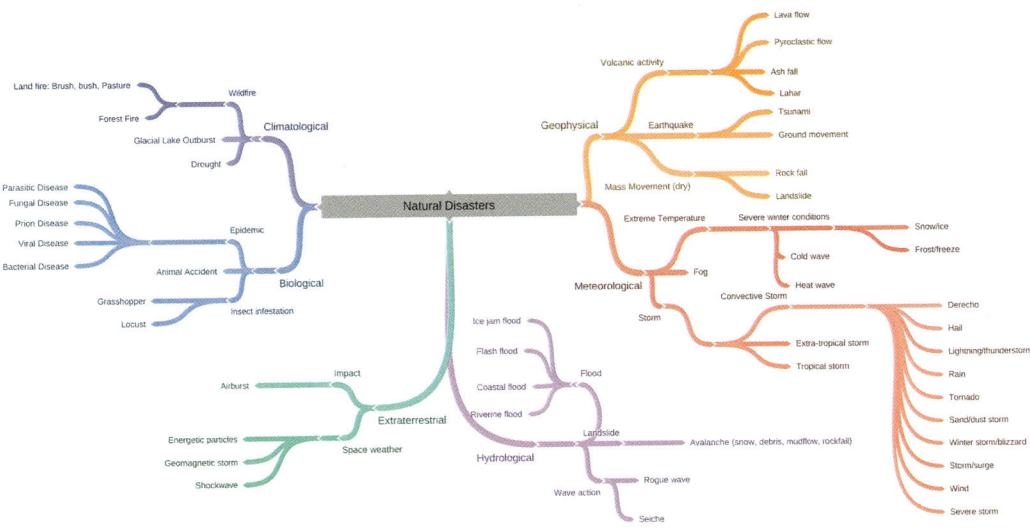

Fig. 6.2 Classification of natural disasters

reservoirs or downhill from a dam. Most communities experience a flood within 6 h after heavy rainfall, which is provoked by sudden release of debris dam, commonly known as flash floods [11].

The active **volcanos** are about 1.500 worldwide, affecting potentially 500 million people, who reside close to them. Most active volcanoes are found on the Pacific Ring of Fire. During the last 300 years, 270.000 people lost their lives due to volcanic eruptions [12].

Wildfires can be initiated by natural causes such as lightening, volcanoes, dry climate, or human causes such as arson, cigarettes, controlled burning, and power line arcs. Up to 90% of wildfires are attributed to human activity. Among documented hazards during a wildfire are thermal burns, smoke, the dust, hazardous chemicals, falls, heat related illnesses, fatigue, cuts, electrocution, animal bites, unstable structures, and rhabdomyolysis [13].

6.2.1.3 Technological Disasters

Technological disasters are less frequent than the natural disasters, but they are equally disastrous, since they often occur near human habitat and thus have a high impact on human losses and property damage. They are classified to industrial accidents, transport accidents, and miscellaneous accidents [7] (Fig. 6.3). Especially in cases where chemical, biological, radiological, and nuclear agents (CBRN) are involved, it is of paramount importance to assure that a thorough procedure of zoning the incident, decontamination, triage, and treatment is provided [14].

6.2.2 Disaster Cycle

Disasters usually occur suddenly to a region, which often is unprepared to absorb the magnitude of such events. For this reason, local communities should prepare their emergency response services to respond quickly and effectively.

All disastrous phenomena share a common cyclical pattern, commonly referred to as the disaster cycle (Fig. 6.4). The cycle is composed of four reactionary stages: (1) preparedness (organize and prepare for disasters in coordination of emergency response agencies) (2) response (respond to disaster to save lives and preserve property), (3) recovery (support individuals and communities to return to normality), and (4) mitigation (develop means and ways to reduce the negative effects of disasters).

Emergency medical services should participate in each stage of the cycle. In the preparatory phase, healthcare professionals should take part in the mitigation and preparedness phase at a local, private office, or hospital level. When the hazard strikes, they facilitate the medical response to mass casualties, and after the disaster, they participate in the recovery phase [15, 16].

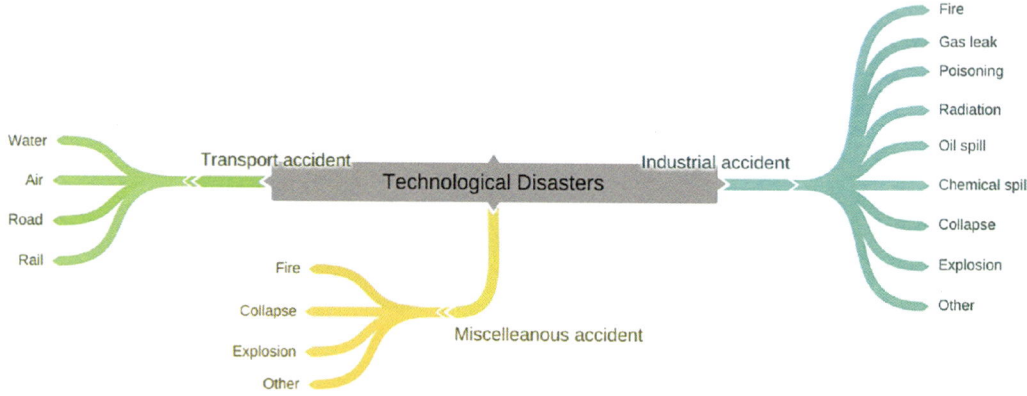

Fig. 6.3 Classification of technological disasters

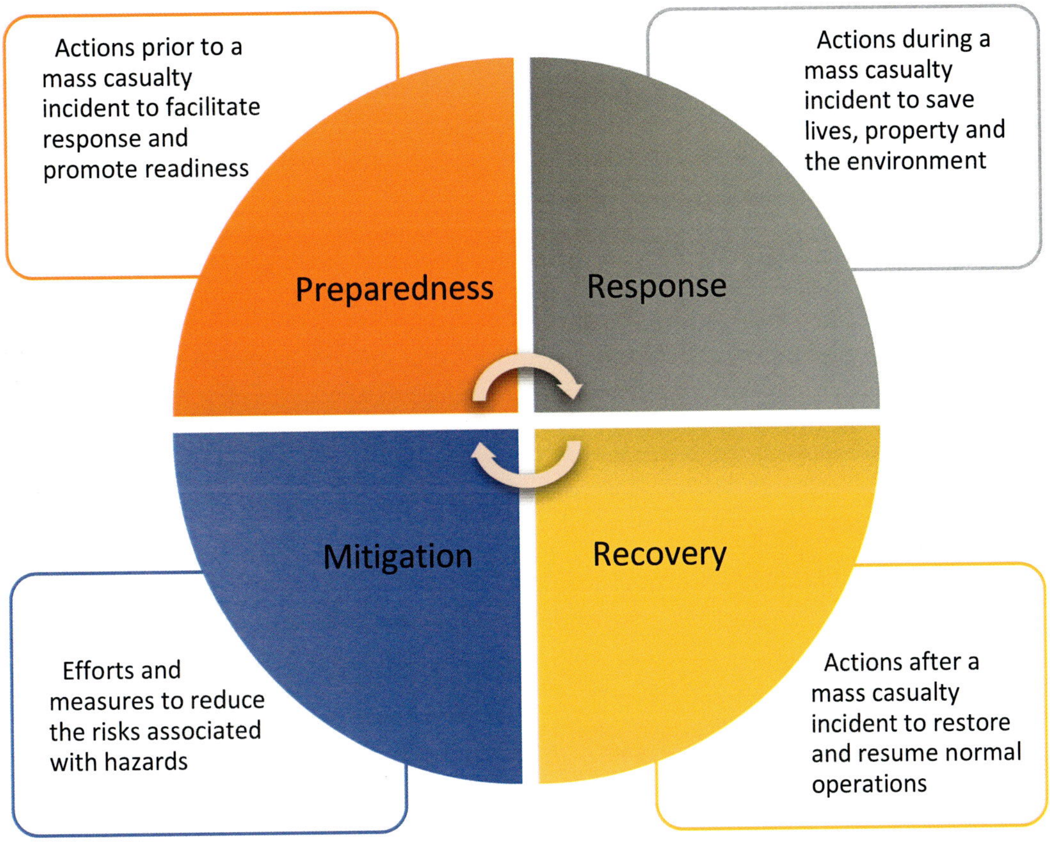

Fig. 6.4 Disaster Cycle

6.3 Treatment

6.3.1 Medical Response to Mass Casualty Incidents

6.3.1.1 All Hazard Approach
Because there is a plethora of disasters resulting in mass casualty incidents, it is of paramount importance that the medical service facilitates an all-hazard approach irrespective of the hazard type, in order to respond quickly and effectively. The prioritization of actions can be structured as followed in Fig. 6.5 [17].

6.3.1.2 Initial Actions at Scene
Usually, the initial response of the medical service to a MCI consisted of a double-crewed ambulance. The senior healthcare provider assumes the role of the medical incident commander (MIC) and the assistant, the role of communication officer (CO). The crew should approach the incident with (1) safety, (2) estab-

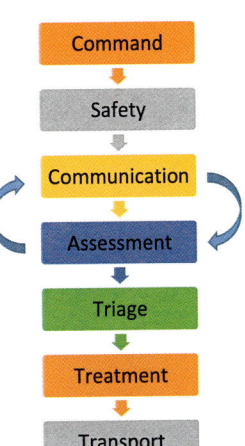

Fig. 6.5 CSCATTT Approach

lish control by cordoning the scene, (3) assess the area for hazards, and (4) initiate communication with the medical control center by transmitting a message. Under no circumstances should the first crew undertake (5) triage, treatment, and transport measures, unless it is found in remote area, where extrication as well as transport may require prolonged time. Otherwise, the provision of care may compromise the organizational set up of the medical service at early stages of the response with disastrous consequences later on. The phrase "Safety, Control then ACT" summarizes the first actions (Fig. 6.6) [18].

After a rapid scene assessment, the MIC is responsible for delivering information from the scene to the control center in a structured way. The METHANE structure is an established framework for conveying important information from a MCI (Fig. 6.7). At the beginning of the METHANE report, the MIC should give his call sign and either set the MCI as "standby" or "declared". Then the exact location is provided as grid reference, providing the road name as well as naming a nearby landmark. The "type of incident" provides information over the mechanism of injury and an estimate of magnitude. The hazards may be more than one and may appear new hazards because of the dynamic character of a disaster. By setting a one-way access and egress to the incident, it is granted a safe and fast route to the scene for the emergency services. At the first report, the MIC provides an estimate of the number of casualties; as the scene matures, more updated messages are provided with information concerning the severity and type of injury. Last but not the least, the MIC delivers information over the emergency services, which have already responded at scene and provide an estimate of required human and material resources [19].

If the major incident is already declared, then the message becomes "ETHANE". As soon as the scene matures, the MIC is required to provide updated information at predetermined time intervals in the form of "HANE" (JESIP).

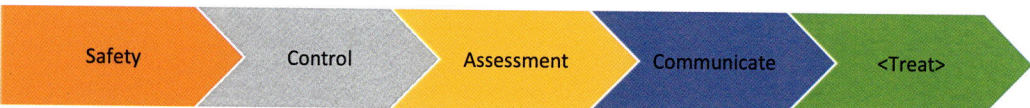

Fig. 6.6 Initial Actions at Scene

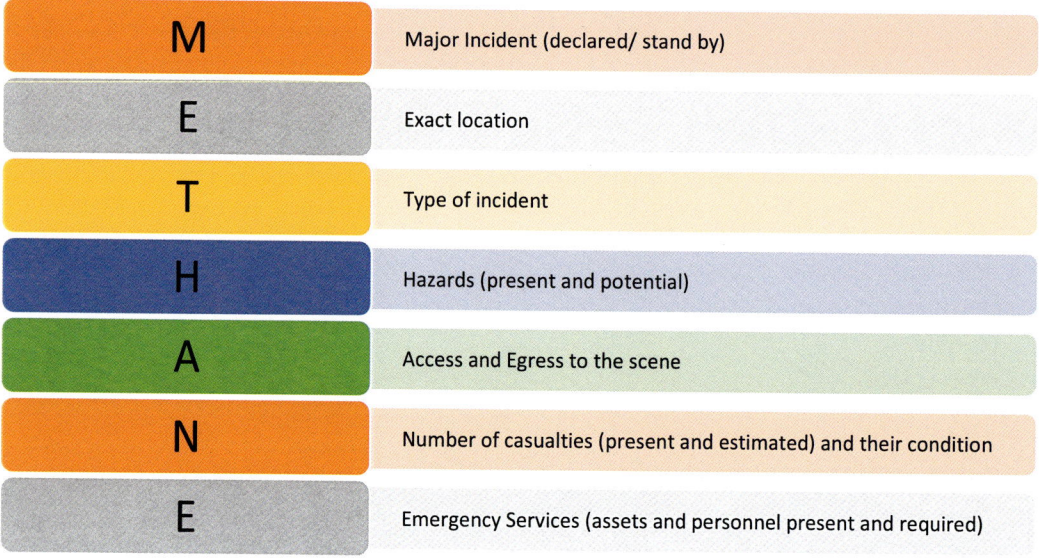

Fig. 6.7 METHANE report

6.3.1.3 Command - Control

The first ambulance at scene deploys a medical incident command post (MICP). The effective management of the incident requires an established vertical line of authority within the medical service, defined as the **command** line, and a horizontal line of authority across various emergency response services at scene, depicted as the **control** line.

The overall responsibility of the incident lies on the **Incident Command**, who is supported by command staff and general staff (Fig. 6.8). The command staff may be deployed in the incident command post/center. Whenever the incident is within the jurisdiction of one service, the incident command is run by one single service. However, when the incident mandates an interdisciplinary management, then a unified command center is deployed [20].

As the incident matures and more healthcare providers respond to scene, the command structure of the medical service is expanding and more key roles are allocated (Fig. 6.9).

In a multiagency setting, the communication and coordination among various services are challenging. For this reason, one agency should assume the role of moderator (incident control), in order to assure a smooth cooperation and minimize overlapping or deficiencies. Depending on the type of hazard, different agencies are responsible for the **Incident control**. In offshore disasters, the coast guard is responsible for the overall control, whereas wildfires or chemical spills are within responsibility of the fire service. The police service usually assumes the overall control in urban settings or in man-made disasters.

The incident usually occupies a wide area. In order to secure the area and support emergency response services' movement, cordons are placed to stratify different areas of action. The **inner cordon** encircles the hazard, the hot/bronze/operational area, and it is denoted with tape. Movement across cordons is limited only to those authorized to act forwardly. Individuals are tagged at check-in and check-out points and documented in log lists. Since the scene is dynamic, the inner cordon can be extended or reduced. The **outer cordon** separates the warm/silver/tactical area from the cold/gold/strategic area. Access across outer cordon is granted only to individuals, who participate in the disaster response. In the warm/silver/tactical zone, the medical service can deploy an **Incident Command Post (ICP)**, where the medical incident commander (MIC) liaises with other commanders and works together with command staff to manage the MCI. In proximity but also in a safe distance from the hazard, the **Casualty Clearing Station (CCS)** is deployed, where medical care is provided to casualties. Casualties are evacuated from the hot zone to the CCS. In case that a MCI covers a very wide area, the patients can be transferred to the nearby **Trauma Stabilization Points (TSP)** temporarily, and after an initial sta-

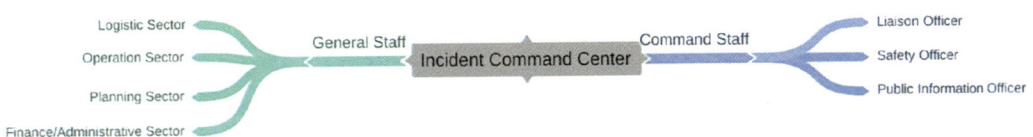

Fig. 6.8 Incident Command System (ICS) structure

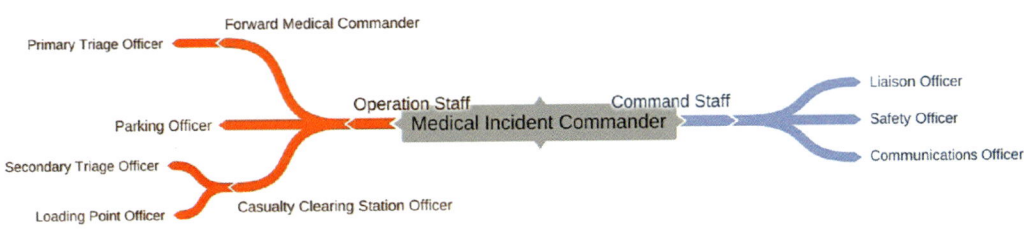

Fig. 6.9 Medical Service Command Structure

bilization, they can be transported to CCS for further advanced care (Fig. 6.10). After the clinical stabilization of patients and the provision of suitable treatment, the casualties are transferred to the **Loading Point**, in order to be loaded to ambulances and transported to hospitals. Uninjured survivors or casualties with very minor injuries are accompanied to **Survivor Resting Area (SRA)**, and after a short period of monitoring for possible underlying injuries, they are discharged home. Ambulances enter into the warm area via a designated entry point (**Access**), after stationing at the **Parking Point**, they are mobilized upon demand to the Loading Point, where they are loaded with casualties, and via a designated exit point (**Egress**), they are heading to the suitable hospital (Fig. 6.11) [21].

6.3.1.4 Safety

The safety depicts the (1) personal safety measures, (2) the safety for others (colleagues and survivors), and (3) the scene safety. The personal protective equipment should be comfortable to the healthcare provider, durable for a long period of medical response, and functional so as not to compromise the provision of high quality medical care. Protective equipment should include a helmet, a visual and a hearing protection, proper clothing and tabard for identification, and hand and foot protection (Fig. 6.12) [18].

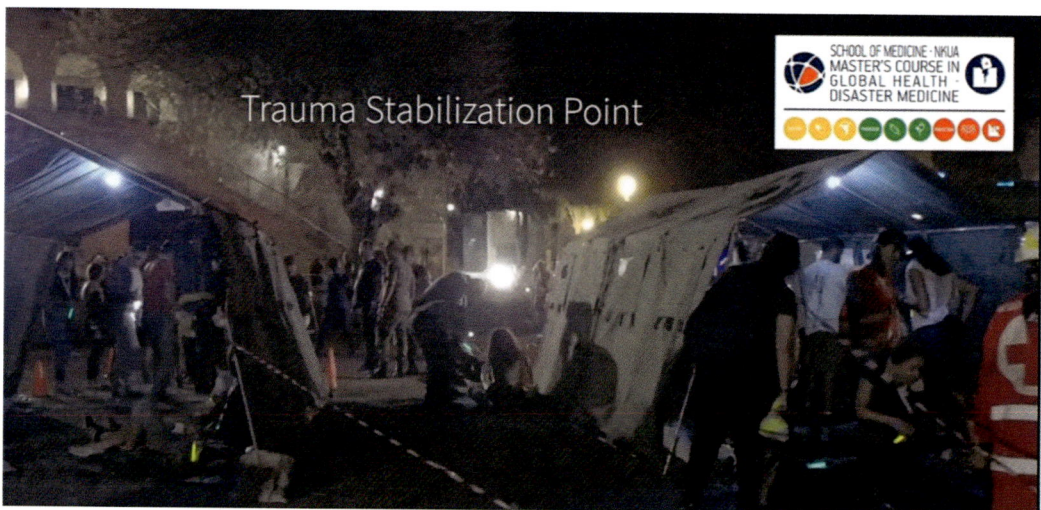

Fig. 6.10 Trauma Stabilization Point in a large-scale MCI scenario (with permission)

Fig. 6.11 Medical Service Layout

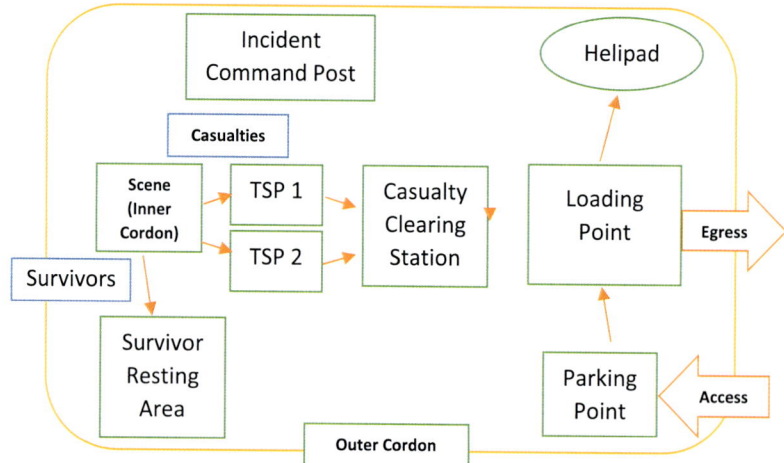

6 Mass Casualties

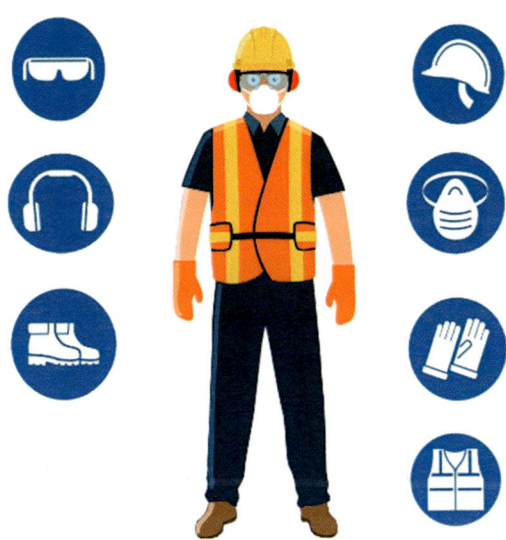

Fig. 6.12 Minimum Personal Protective Equipment

Table 6.2 Methods of communicating information from scene

Communication methods	
1	Radios (traditional analogue, TETRA)
2	Telephone (land lines, cellular, internet, satellite)
3	Whistles, hand signals
4	Runners
5	Loud hailers, tannoy system
6	Broadcasting (television, radio, social media)
7	Data transmission, telemedicine

6.3.1.5 Communication

Communication is crucial for the effective management of a MCI. The information should be accurate, complete, and transmitted in a timely fashion. Common reasons of problematic communication are the lack of information, lack of coordination, and lack of confirmation of the received information. Various communication methods can be incorporated, depending on the situation (Table 6.2).

6.3.1.6 Assessment

At scene, the MIC should assess the surrounding area and gather information, which will facilitate a quick and effective medical response. The important information is framed in the METHANE report (Fig. 6.7). Because of the dynamic nature of mass casualty incidents, the assessment should be repeated in predetermined intervals or after notable events. Thus, the ongoing assessment should include information for new or imminent hazards, a possible change in access or egress, an updated number of casualties, their sustained injuries as well as their severity and information over required human and material resources. All these can be grouped as part of the previous framework, commonly referred as "HANE" report [18].

6.3.1.7 Triage

In a major incident, the high influx of injured patients necessitates a sorting process in order to categorize the casualties according to their needs [22]. During disaster management, triage takes place in different levels and it is adjusted to different decision making processes. At the first level, triage focuses on the **priority of treatment (T)** in order to provide the greatest good for the greatest number of patients [23]. There are different triage methods; two widely used protocols in disaster response are the simple triage and rapid treatment (START) and the Triage Sieve/Short [21, 24]. Triage sieve and START triage are performed at the field as a primary sorting method to classify casualties for care towards the CCS. As soon as the primary care is delivered, the Triage short and the Reverse Trauma Score (RVS) are utilized to upgrade or downgrade priority of care in the CCS, depending on the evolution of the clinical situation. When casualties are stabilized, a sorting process starts to determine the **priority of transport (P)** out of the scene (Fig. 6.13).

6.3.1.8 Treatment

The treatment of casualties is carried out across all different zones, from the scene of the major incident to the definitive care facility. At the beginning, minutes after the MCI, care is provided at a basic level by bystanders. Once healthcare professionals arrive at scene and the medical service is deployed, advanced medical care is provided in the Casualty Clearing Station. During the transport to the hospital, healthcare professionals provide suitable medical care to keep the patient stabilized, until the ambulance reached the hospital. At the emergency department, a patient-centered approach is applied, following ATLS principles (Fig. 6.14) [25].

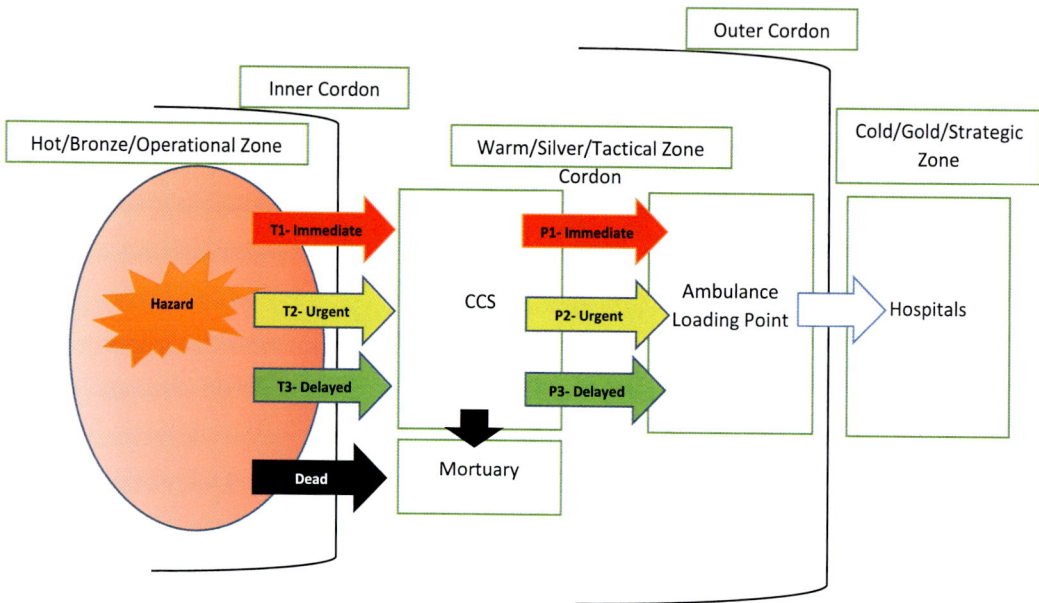

Fig. 6.13 Scheme depicting sorting for treatment and transport

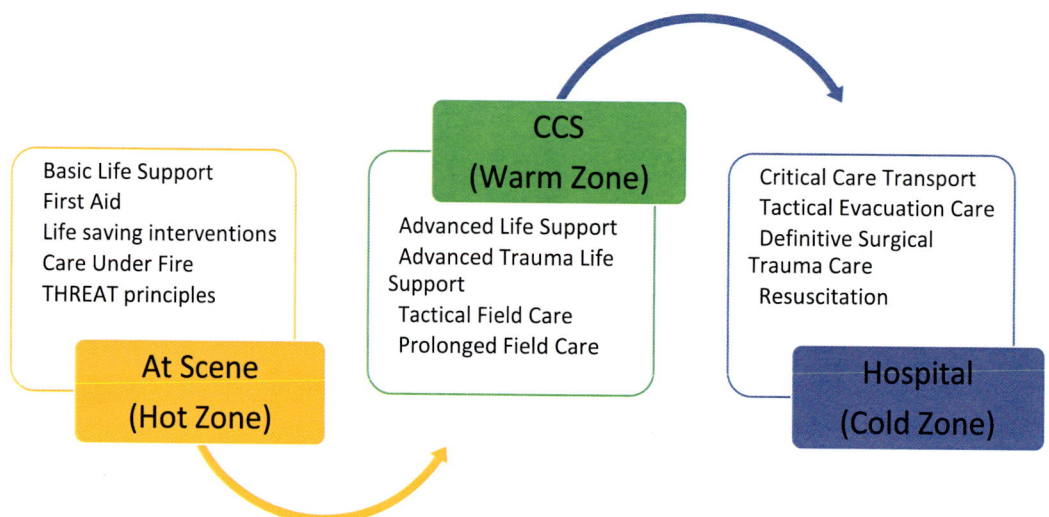

Fig. 6.14 Levels of medical care

At war or in conflict zones, prehospital care is modified in order to comply with the special safety circumstances. The different levels of care follow the principles of Tactical Combat Casualty Care (TCCC), where Care Under Fire (CUF) is provided, whenever there is an exchange of fire. At that point, it's important to (1) return effective fire towards the threat, (2) provide tactical transport of casualty to an area with cover, and (3) control with tourniquet any massive external hemorrhage. As soon as the casualty is evacuated away from the hot zone, to an area of relative security in warm zone, healthcare providers can initiate Tactical Field Care following the MARCHE algorithm. First, the massive hemorrhage is addressed, then the airway control, the support of respirations, the management of circulation, the prevention of hypothermia and at the end "everything else" such as the management of soft tissue injuries, and the administration of medications follow. En route to the hospital is provided the Tactical Evacuation Care, until the patient reaches a definitive care facility. In case of a delayed extrication from the scene, the medical care can follow the Prolonged Field Care principles to ensure a high quality care, until a medical evacuation is possible [26, 27].

A special type of a MCI are the active shooter mass casualties. Because of the rapid changing environment, as in conflict zones, the response in the hot zone follows the THREAT principles. Law enforcement officers have to suppress the threat (T), then to control the external hemorrhage (H), to rapidly extricate the casualty to safety (RE), to assure assessment by medical providers (A), and to provide transport to definitive care (T) [28].

6.3.1.9 Transport

As a rule of thumb, the priority of evacuation should follow the priority of treatment. However, this is not always feasible, since the vehicles are not always available or the transport means at scene are not suitable for all casualties. In case that the casualties require specialized treatment, they should be evacuated accordingly to specialized centers. As a mnemonic rule of thumb, healthcare providers can use the 4 R's: Right Patient, Right Mean of Transport, Right Hospital, and Right Time. Possible delays result in worse outcomes [29]. As a preferred evacuation mean to a MASCAL is the ambulance, because medical care is provided during the transport (MEDEVAC). In case that ambulances are unavailable, other vehicles can be considered for casualties with light injuries, who can be evacuated without medical care during transport (CASEVAC). The casualties who do not require specialized care may be transported to the nearest healthcare center, because a high number of casualties can be evacuated with limited ambulance resources in repeated short rounds [30]. In international missions or in civilian-military cooperation disaster response, a "9-Liner message" for a helicopter MEDEVAC request may be required (Fig. 6.15).

6.3.2 Medical Training for Mass Casualties

A key element to a successful response to a MCI is the quick deployment of the medical service, because many critically injured casualties will

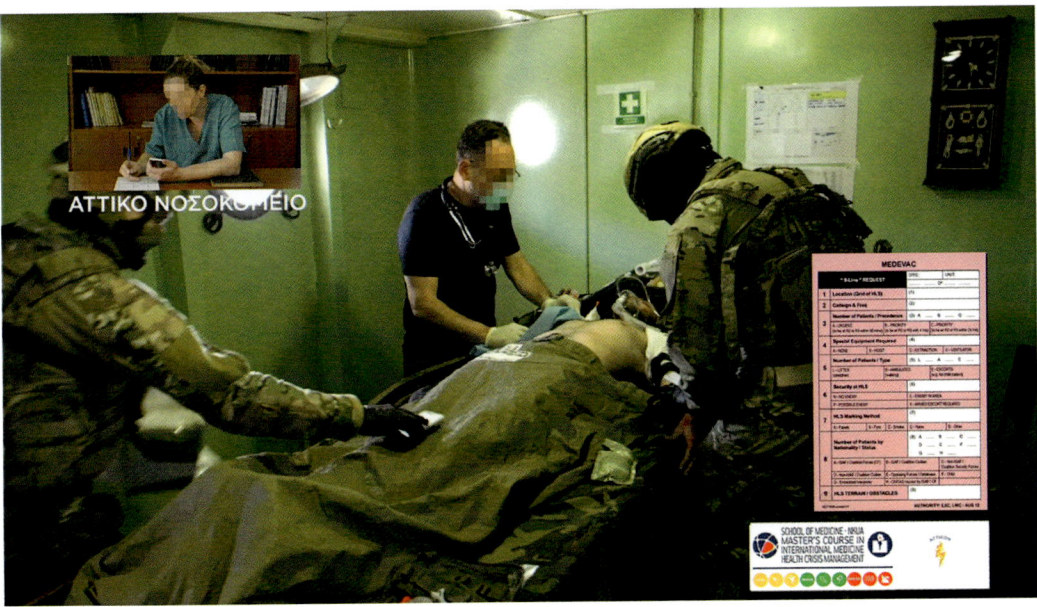

Fig. 6.15 9-Liner for MEDEVAC request in Military- Civilian MCI response (with permission)

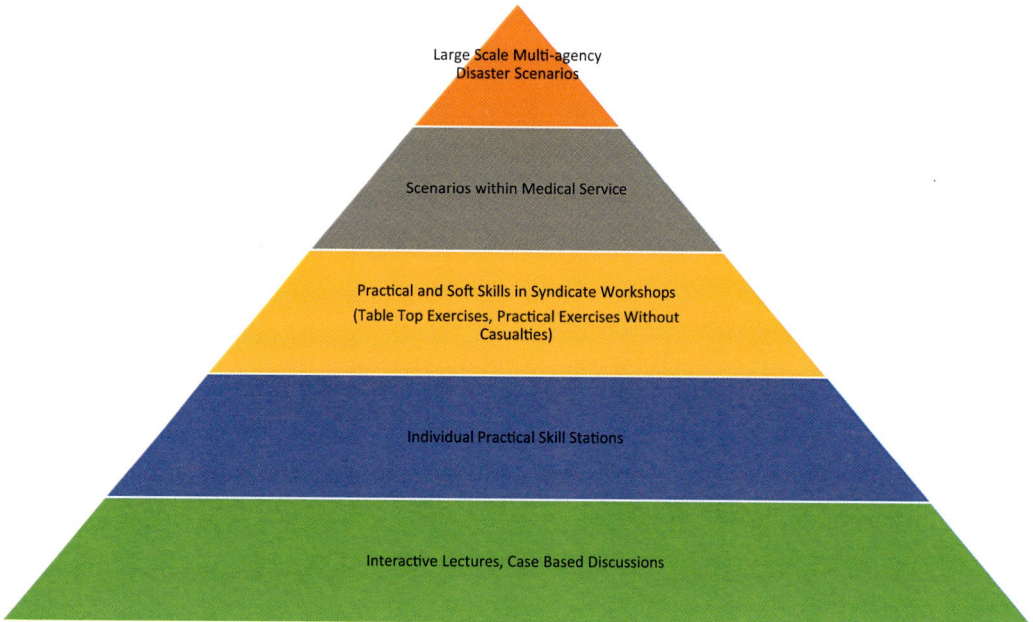

Fig. 6.16 MCI Training for healthcare professionals

succumb to their injuries in the first 4 h [31]. Medical training for mass casualties should include various adult training methodologies spanning from interactive case-based lectures and practical workshops to large-scale pre-/in-hospital scenarios as well as multiagency MASCAL disaster scenarios. All possible medical units should be involved in disaster response scenarios, from prehospital medics to specialized ICU personnel (Fig. 6.16) [32]. Through an holistic interdisciplinary training, the healthcare provider will advance not only his technical skills in austere environment, but also his interprofessional cognitive skills under stress conditions, both of them are important on MCI response [33, 34]. After each MCI training, a debriefing process should focus on lessons learned and provide constructive feedback to healthcare providers on personal performance as individuals and on team's performance holistically as units [35].

Dos and Don'ts
- Do acknowledge that effective MCI management necessitates knowledge base far greater than medicine.
- Do respond to the scene of a MCI with an "all-hazard approach" algorithm.
- Do acknowledge that suitable deployment of medical service at scene is equally important with provision of medical care.
- Don't initiate triage, treatment, and transport if you are the only medical asset at scene.
- Don't act alone in a multidisciplinary disaster response.
- Don't neglect the need for specialized training in disaster medicine.

Take-Home Messages

- Disasters occur every day worldwide. Failure to plan in advance, it is planning for failure in managing the mass casualties.
- The medical service participation to disaster management should be holistic and integrated to all stages of disaster cycle.
- The medical response to a MCI should be all-hazard oriented.
- The framework of actions to a MCI is elaborated by the "CSCATTT" acronym.
- The important information from scene should be structured with the "METHANE" message.
- The casualties are sorted for priority of treatment and priority of transport.
- The provided medical care in different zones spans from life-saving procedures in hot zone, to advanced life support in warm zone and critical care transport/evacuation care en route to the hospital.

Multiples Choice Questions

1. Which of the following disasters presents the highest frequency as well as mortality rates?
   A. Earthquakes
   B. Volcanos
   C. Wildfires
   D. Floods
   Correct Answer: D

2. Which of the following is more possible to be described as a mass casualty incident?
   A. A collision between a school bus and a car with 5 casualties
   B. A fire in a factory with chemicals during working hours
   C. Accident at sea with two casualties
   D. A fire in remote residence, where a family lives
   Correct Answer: B

3. Who has the overall control in the hot zone?
   A. Municipal Authorities
   B. Police service
   C. Nongovernmental Organizations
   D. Medical service
   Correct Answer: B

4. An ambulance with two healthcare providers has responded to the scene of a MCI. Which action should not be initiated, until more assistance arrives?
   A. Command – Control
   B. Communication
   C. Assessment
   D. Triage
   Correct Answer: D

5. Which of the following has priority for healthcare providers at the scene of a major incident?
   A. Survivors' safety
   B. Scene safety
   C. Personal safety
   D. Equipment's safety
   Correct Answer: C

6. During a disaster response to a MCI, the medical incident commander wants to inform the control center over the situation at scene. Which structured message will be used?
   A. METHANE
   B. CSCATTT
   C. MIST
   D. 9 Liner
   Correct Answer: A

7. Which of the following will the Primary Triage Officer utilize to sort the casualties?
   A. Triage Sieve
   B. Triage Sort
   C. Reverse Trauma Score
   D. Glasgow Coma Scale
   Correct Answer: A

8. The walking survivors with no injuries should be accompanied to:
   A. Survivor Resting Area
   B. Casualty Clearing Station
   C. Media Centre
   D. Debriefing Station
   Correct Answer: A
9. When the external massive hemorrhage should be initially addressed?
   A. During primary triage
   B. During secondary triage
   C. At the casualty clearing station
   D. During evacuation phase
   Correct Answer: A
10. Which of the following andragogic methods should be included in the training process for a mass casualty incident?
    A. Lectures and practical workshops
    B. Practical Exercises Without Casualties
    C. Interdisciplinary large scale MCI scenarios
    D. All of the above
    Correct Answer: D

References

1. Tintinalli JE, Stapczynski JS, Ma OJ, Cline DM, Cydulka RK, Meckler GD. Chapter 6. Disaster preparedness and response. In: Tintinalli's emergency medicine. 7th ed. New York: McGraw-Hill; 2011.
2. United Nations International Strategy for Disaster Reduction. http://www.unisdr.org/we/inform/terminology.org.master.com/texis/master/search/mysite.txt?q¼disaster+preparedness&order¼r&id¼60413a1214953850&cmd¼xml. Accessed 28 Apr 2021.
3. Shaluf IM. Disaster types. Disaster Prev Manag. 2007;16:704–17.
4. Lowe D, Ebi KL, Forsberg B. Factors increasing vulnerability to health effects before, during and after floods. Int J Environ Res Public Health. 2013;10(12):7015–67.
5. Smolinski MS, Hamburg MA, Lederberg J. Committee on emerging microbial threats to health in the 21st century. Microbial threats to health in the United States: emergence, detection and response. Washington, DC: National Academy Press; 2003.
6. Mackway-Jones K. Major incident medical management and support: the practical approach at the scene/Advanced Life Support Group. 3rd ed. West Sussex: Wiley-Blackwell; 2012.
7. Guha-Sapir D, Hoyois P, Below R. Annual disaster statistical review 2015: the numbers and trends. Brussels: CRED; 2016.
8. Rosenberg M. Haiti death toll could reach 300,000: preval. Reuters; 2010. https://www.reuters.com/article/us-quake-haiti-deathtoll-idUKTRE61L01P20100222. Accessed 28 Apr 2021.
9. Llewellyn M. Floods and tsunamis. Surg Clin North Am. 2006;86:557–78.
10. Noji E. Natural disaster management. In: Auerbach P, editor. Wilderness medicine: management of wilderness and environmental emergencies. 3rd ed. St Louis: Mosby; 1995. p. 644–63.
11. Kalogeropoulos A, Pikouli A. Natural disasters: medical management. In: Pikoulis E, Doucet J, editors. Hot topics in acute care surgery and trauma. Cham: Springer Nature; 2021. p. 433–50.
12. European Space Agency. Volcanoes. 2009. http://www.esa.int/Our_Activities/Observing_the_Earth/Space_for_our_climate/Volcanoes. Accessed 28 Apr 2021.
13. Corey C, Dalsey L. Wildland fire fighting safety and health. NIOSH science blog. National Institute of Occupational Safety and Health. Archived on 13 July 2012. https://blogs.cdc.gov/niosh-science-blog/2012/07/13/wildlandfire/. Accessed 28 Apr 2021.
14. Ramesh AC, Kumar S. Triage, monitoring, and treatment of mass casualty events involving chemical, biological, radiological, or nuclear agents. J Pharm Bioallied Sci. 2010;2(3):239–47.
15. de Boer J. Order in chaos: modeling medical management in disasters. Eur J Emerg Med. 1999;6(2):141–8.
16. Pikoulis E, Pikouli A, Pavlidou E. Principles of disaster medicine. In: Pikoulis E, Doucet J, editors. Emergency medicine, trauma and disaster management: from prehospital to hospital care and beyond. Cham: Springer Nature; 2021. p. 3–10.
17. National Ambulance Resilience Unit (NARU). Major incident initial action cards. V.1.2. 2015. https://naru.org.uk/documents/major-incident-initial-action-cards/. Accessed 28 Apr 2021.
18. Russell RJ. The approach to a major incident. J R Army Med Corps. 2000;146:8–12.
19. Joint Emergency Services Interoperability Programme (JESIP). https://www.jesip.org.uk/. Accessed 28 Apr 2021.
20. US Department of Homeland Security. National Incident Management System. 2008. https://www.fema.gov/pdf/emergency/nims/NIMS_core.pdf. Accessed 28 Apr 2021.
21. Russell R, Bess A. Clinical guidelines for operations, change 3. Joint Service Publication (JSP) 999. Ministry of Defense UK. 2012.
22. Robertson-Steel I. Evolution of triage systems. Emerg Med J. 2006;23(2):154–5.
23. Frykberg ER. Triage: principles and practice. Scand J Surg. 2005;94:272–8.

24. Kahn CA, Schultz CH, Miller KT, et al. Does START triage work? An outcomes assessment after a disaster. Ann Emerg Med. 2009;54(3):424–30.
25. Kluger Y, Coccolini F, Catena C, Ansaloni L. WSES handbook of mass casualties incidents management. Cham: Springer Nature; 2020.
26. Lenhart M, Savitsky E, Eastridge B. Combat Casualty Care Lessons Learned from OEF and OIF. Office of the Surgeon General. Department of the Army. United States. V. Borden Institute (U.S.). 2012.
27. Remick K, Elster E. Management of combat casualties. In: Pikoulis E, Doucet J, editors. Emergency medicine, trauma and disaster management: from prehospital to hospital care and beyond. Cham: Springer Nature; 2021. p. 485–500.
28. Jacobs LM, Wade DS, McSwain NE, Butler FK, Fabbri WP, Eastman AL, Rotondo M, Sinclair J, Burns KJ. The Hartford consensus: THREAT, a medical disaster preparedness concept. J Am Coll Surg. 2013;217(5):947–53.
29. Gough LB, Painter DM, Hoffman LA, Caplan JR, Peters AC, Cipolle DM. Right patient, right place, right time: field triage and transfer to level I trauma centers. Am Surg. 2020;86(5):400–6.
30. Dean MD, Nair SK. Mass-casualty triage: distribution of victims to multiple hospitals using the SAVE model. Eur J Oper Res. 2014;238(1):363–73.
31. Frykberg E, Tepas JJ III, Alexander R. The 1983 Beirut Airport terrorist bombing. Injury patterns and implications for disaster management. Am Surg. 1989;55:134–41.
32. Pikoulis E, Pikoulis A, Kalogeropoulos A. Intensive care for emergency surgeons: mass casualties. In: Picetti E, Pereira BM, Razek T, Narayan M, Kashuk JL, editors. Intensive care for emergency surgeons. Cham: Springer Nature; 2019.
33. Exadaktylos A. The importance of education and training in disaster management: an overview. In: Pikoulis E, Doucet J, editors. Emergency medicine, trauma and disaster management: from prehospital to hospital care and beyond. Cham: Springer Nature; 2021. p. 591–8.
34. Pikoulis E, Karamagioli E, Kalogeropoulos A, Pikoulis A, Lykoudis P, Remick K, Malone D, Kushner A, Domres B, Leppäniemi A, Exadaktylos A, Elster E, Rich N. When the going gets tough, the tough get going: improving the disaster preparedness of health care providers: a single center's 4-year experience. Disaster Med Public Health Prep. 2022;16(2):520–30.
35. Broadmann Maeder M. The value of training: debriefing. In: Pikoulis E, Doucet J, editors. Emergency medicine, trauma and disaster management: from prehospital to hospital care and beyond. Cham: Springer Nature; 2021. p. 599–606.

Further Reading

Kluger Y, Coccolini F, Catena C, Ansaloni L. WSES handbook of mass casualties incidents management. Cham: Springer Nature; 2020.

Mackway-Jones K. Major incident medical management and support: the practical approach at the scene. Advanced Life Support Group. 3rd ed. West Sussex: Wiley-Blackwell. 2012.

Pikoulis E, Doucet J. Emergency medicine, trauma and disaster management: from prehospital to hospital care and beyond. Cham: Springer Nature; 2021.

Russell R, Bess A. Clinical guidelines for operations, change 3. Joint Service Publication (JSP) 999. Ministry of Defense UK. 2012.

Point-of-Care Ultrasound for Emergency General Surgeons

Bruno M. Pereira

Learning Goals
The main learning goals of this chapter are: (1) to demonstrate the broad use of POCUS on the field of the Emergency General Surgeon (EGS), (2) give basic and advanced principles for EGS education and training on POCUS, (3) stimulate POCUS daily use on EGS.

7.1 Introduction

7.1.1 Point-of-Care Ultrasound Significance of Use for Emergency General Surgeons

The routine use of portable ultrasound in medical practice has enabled the development of a new patient assessment format at the bedside.

B. M. Pereira (✉)
Masters Program in Health Applied Sciences, Vassouras University, Vassouras, RJ, Brazil

General Surgery Residency Program Santa Casa de Campinas, Campinas, Brazil

Terzius College, Campinas, Brazil

Grupo Surgical, Campinas, Brazil

World Society of the Abdominal Compartment, Antwerp, Belgium

Brazilian College of Surgeons, São Paulo, Brazil
e-mail: dr.bruno@gruposurgical.com.br

Expanding into different medical specialties such as emergency medicine, intensive care, and so on, general surgery was not left out. Currently, many possibilities of point-of-care ultrasound (POCUS) are acceptable in the field of surgery, expanding fast as technologies advance, and with it, surgeons' training and qualification on this new propaedeutic and decision aid method.

Among the vast repertoire of possibilities, we highlight the usefulness of POCUS in assessing volemic status, diagnosis of acute postoperative dyspnea, rapid assessment of trauma patients, circulatory shock, assistance in procedures, postoperative analgesia, and many others. It is not difficult to anticipate that modern surgeons, especially those connected to trauma and surgical emergencies, are undoubtedly desired in training with ultrasound at the bedside, since their use assists in the decision process, is noninvasive, low cost, can be repeated easily, and therefore has the potential to improve morbidity and mortality. Year after year, as technology becomes cheaper, hundreds of surgeons will have access to POCUS daily use and certainly better quality of treatment will be offered. POCUS is no longer the future. Different technologies are reaching the market at lightning speed. Lightweight portable Wi-Fi devices are now available with high-definition capabilities. With this technology, it is easy to reach out your patient anywhere and improve diagnosis timeframe as well as delivery of care.

© The Author(s), under exclusive license to Springer Nature Switzerland AG 2023
F. Coccolini, F. Catena (eds.), *Textbook of Emergency General Surgery*,
https://doi.org/10.1007/978-3-031-22599-4_7

Acute and critical surgical patients are the ones who benefit most from this tool.

In the Emergency Medicine field, a recent study showed that POCUS potentially influenced and modified management and treatment in 45% of cases [1]. Cardiac and pulmonary POCUS was among the most useful applications, especially in patients with cardiopulmonary complaints and in those with abnormal vital signs. In general surgery until the present data, the number of publications that study the use of ultrasound in daily practice is relatively low; however, the ascending curve is remarkable, proving that awareness of surgeons to POCUS is in fact raising.

This chapter arrives at a perfect moment where POCUS is becoming the great device to help surgeons on the decision-making, diagnostic, and treatment processes. Worth to stress that training surgeons in the use of POCUS on the daily basis clinical practice does not diminish the need of the radiologist opinion when indicated. In case of any doubts during POCUS execution, the radiologist must be consulted for further discussion. With the content presented here, we expect to bring to light the importance of POCUS on the General Surgery field and how its use can change your practice.

7.1.2 Ultrasound Concepts and Principles

Sound waves are organized mechanical vibrations, originated from a determined source, traveling through a medium that may be solid, liquid, or gas. In ultrasound, the vibrating source is the piezoelectric crystals located into the transducers, which transform the electrical stimulus into mechanical energy in the form of sound waves through a conductive medium (gel, tissues, and body fluids) (Table 7.1).

All sound waves oscillate at a specific frequency, or number of vibrations or cycles per second. Human hearing extends to a maximum frequency of about 20,000 cycles per second (20 KHz), while the majority of ultrasonic applications utilize frequencies between 500,000 and 10,000,000 cycles per second (500 KHz–10 MHz), the reason why ultrasound frequencies are not heard by humans (Fig. 7.1).

The sound wave is transmitted by the conducting means and can suffer attenuation, refraction, and reflection in the path, due to the difference between the acoustic impedances of each one of them. When there is no difference in impedance between two media, there will be no reflection. The wave that returns to the transducer is captured, processed in a variation of grey tones between black (hypoechogenic—liquid medium) and white (hyperechogenic—solid medium), and reproduced as an image on the device's screen.

Table 7.1 Acoustic impedance

Acoustic impedance	
Bone	2000–4000
Soft tissue	1540
Fat	1300
Lungs	300–1000
Air	344
Water	1498

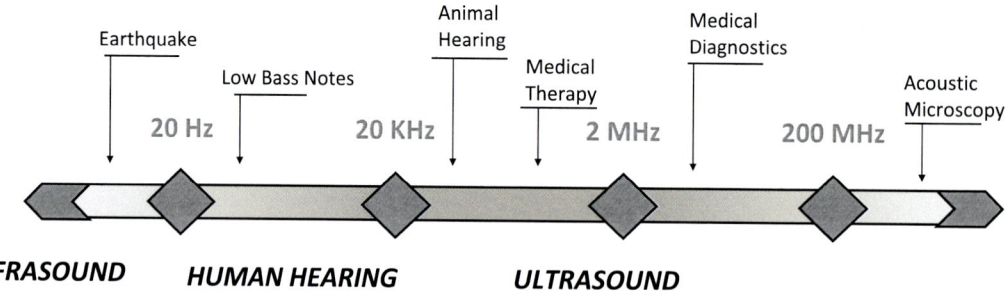

Fig. 7.1 Sound frequency scale

7.1.3 Transducers and Controls

For general surgery purposes, three types of transducers will be most used:

- Linear array (higher frequencies): Used for superficial tissues such as muscles, vessels, and ocular ultrasound. May also be used for lungs.
- Curvilinear array (intermediate frequencies): Commonly used to perform the FAST exam (Focused Assessment Sonography for Trauma), but they serve multiple other uses such as visualization of abdominal viscera, deep vessels, and lungs.
- Phased array (lower frequencies): Used for echocardiography and dynamic measurements of the inferior vena cava (Fig. 7.2).

Correct transducer handling is critical for excellent POCUS performance.

The initial step is to properly locate the position of the objective of the examination on the device's screen. The precaution in keeping the image of interest focused from the middle to the upper third of the screen to optimize the image and detect artifacts is a basic action that must always be exercised. An important tip is to use the depth control to adjust the image to fit the size of the screen and keep the focus control in the same range as the objective of the study. Another basic and mandatory action is to pay attention to the upper mark that appears on the screen indicating the right or left side of the structure. This marking that normally appears in the factory setup to the left of the screen may come in different colors or shapes depending on the manufacturer. This mark can appear as a circle (blue, green, red…) or in a letter format or the specific brand of the device. It is also important to check that the transducer index (mark that determines the transducer direction in accordance with the screen marking) is facing the same side of this symbol on the screen, either right or left. Keep in mind the mnemonic *PART* (**p**ressure, **a**lignment, **r**otation, and **t**ilt) when performing POCUS exam in order to get better image quality. Pressure fits for the pressure applied to the surface of the patient's body, alignment for lateral deviation of the transducer, rotation for spinning the transducer on the same axis (looking for a transversal or longitudinal ultrasound window), and tilt for the angulation between the transducer and the skin.

There are several available controls on ultrasound devices that allow general adjustments and measurements. As to date, there are many manufactures producing different types of consoles, including those with tablet or cell phone interaction. There is no sense to explain each one of those here; however, some commands are mandatory and equivalent to all types of consoles and

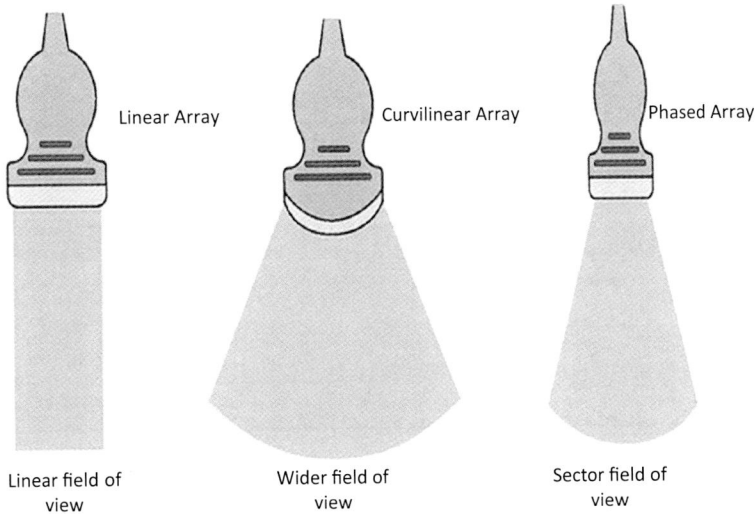

Fig. 7.2 Types of transducers

platforms. Thus, the main controls that must be mastered by the emergency general surgeon and other physicians working at the emergency scenarios are:

- B (brightness) mode: traditional two-dimensional US imaging mode.
- M (movement) mode: represents a one-dimensional image over time. Used for specific measurements and to evaluate structures with high mobility.
- Measure: Opens the measurement option and calculation tab.
- Freeze: freezes the image, making it possible to measure and store the images.
- Gain: increases the intensity of the image.
- Sectorial gain: Represented by the acronym TGC (time gain compensation), it adjusts the gain independently in the upper, middle, and lower thirds of the screen.
- Zoom: allows the enlargement of the image to make detailed measurements or more detailed visualization.
- Depth: controls the depth of the viewing field.
- Focus: Must be adjusted in the range of the structure of interest.

7.2 Diagnosis: Pocus Daily Application for the Emergency General Surgeon

7.2.1 E-Fast and Rush

Many trauma patients have injuries that are not apparent on the primary examination. This patient population may also present distracting lesions or altered level of consciousness due to the acute hypoperfusion state. Therefore, significant abdominal and thoracic bleeding can occur without obvious warning signs. It is true that other adverse scenarios can also occur, such as hypertensive pneumothorax and cardiac tamponade, but bleeding is still the first cause of preventable death in trauma. Here is where POCUS, not only FAST, can really help. The aim of FAST is to quickly identify free fluid (blood) in the perito- neal cavity, pericardial space, or pleural spaces, nevertheless expanding to POCUS in trauma, making use of other protocols such as RUSH (**R**apid **U**ltrasound for **S**hock and **H**ypotension) or HIMAP (**H**eart, **I**VC, **M**orison Pouch, **P**ulmonary, a coordination to run RUSH correctly); much more information can be extracted from the critical patient by the emergency general surgeons (EGS). Soon EGS will be no longer performing the FAST (or E-FAST) exam. Protocols that can gather as much information as possible in order to offer outstanding quality of care at the same speed of the E-FAST will certainly be preferred by EGS.

The RUSH protocol, for instance, adds four acoustic windows to the E-FAST exam and excludes the subxiphoid acoustic window as two of the windows included give much better view and understanding from the heart than the subxiphoid window.

Below are found the 9-ultrasound windows of the RUSH protocol, so it could serve as a stimulus for EGS to consider whether or not its use is worth.

1. Parasternal long cardiac view
2. Apical four-chamber cardiac view
3. Inferior vena cava view
4. Morison's with hemothorax view
5. Splenorenal with hemothorax view
6. Bladder view
7. Aortic slide views
8. Right pulmonary view
9. Left pulmonary view

FAST exam is a propaedeutic tool that adds to the examination of trauma critical patients and does not replace the need for x-rays in the emergency room or the need for CT-scan when indicated on the hemodynamically stable patient.

Although ultrasound is not 100% sensitive to identify various bleeds, it is undoubtedly an almost perfect way to recognize free intraperitoneal fluid in hypotensive patients who eventually need an emergency surgical intervention or for the diagnosis of cardiac injuries in penetrating trauma. Recently, studies have shown that POCUS is easy to learn and equivalent to or better than chest X-ray to identify a hemothorax or pneumothorax in trauma [2, 3].

It is worth to mention that the E-FAST exam must follow an order of execution according to the risk of severity of the injuries as follows: (1) Subxiphoid window, (2) Right upper quadrant, (3) Left Upper quadrant, (4) Pelvic window, (5) Pulmonary windows (Fig. 7.3).

7.2.1.1 Practical Key Considerations

Penetrating Cardiac Trauma

POCUS performed by doctors working in the emergency setting significantly reduces mortality in patients with penetrating cardiac injuries with a very high sensitivity value for diagnosis [4]. Many patients with stab wounds to the heart do not suffer significant blood loss due to the sealing of the pericardium that prevents active bleeding into the chest or mediastinum; on the other hand, this sealing allows the evolution of bleeding into the pericardium. Once cardiac tamponade symptoms develop, clinical decompensation occurs quickly resulting in signs of shock and ultimately cardiac arrest. The "classic" signs of the Beck triad are not commonly present and are difficult to appear mainly in patients suffering from severe trauma who have another source of bleeding. The key to the treatment of penetrating chest trauma is to identify a developing pericardial effusion as early as possible, before tamponade and cardiac arrest occur. All patients with penetrating chest injury should be screened for potential pericardial bleeding. If pericardial fluid is present, it is understood that there is cardiac injury until proven otherwise. A positive pericardial effusion on POCUS may suggest an indication for immediate surgical pericardial window for decompression before proceeding to definitive care as demonstrated by Pereira BM and colleagues in 2013 [5].

Blunt Cardiac Trauma

Blunt cardiac trauma is relatively uncommon. Most patients who suffer severe cardiac injury, such as rupture of the ventricular wall or chordae tendineae, die quickly. Even with this concept, authors stress the importance of performing POCUS in all patients with significant blunt chest trauma. Myocardial rupture causes an important and rapid pericardial tamponade, which will be easily recognized during point-of-care cardiac

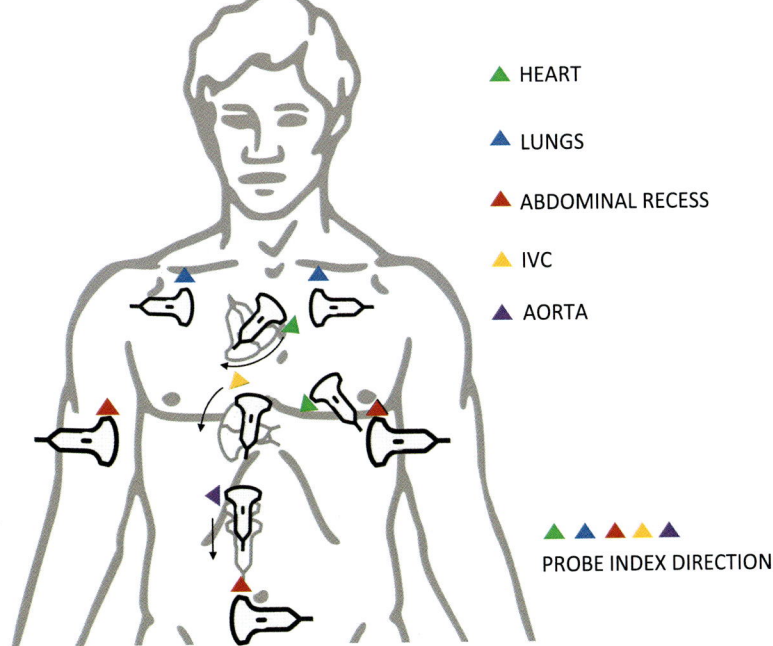

Fig. 7.3 RUSH Protocol

evaluation. Severe global ventricular dysfunction can also be seen during RUSH exam, most likely the result of severe acidosis and hypovolemic shock caused by blunt cardiac trauma. In conclusion, although cardiac rupture resulting from blunt trauma is rare, the POCUS cardiac examination must be performed in all patients with significant blunt trauma, especially those who are hypotensive.

Performing the Pericardic Window

There are two different ways to look at the heart on the POCUS exam when searching for pericardial effusion. Further heart echography windows with complimentary content will be discussed ahead in Sect. 7.2.3. Usually, only one form is sufficient for the evaluation of pericardial fluid. However, it is important to know both windows, since one of the windows can be easily obtained in a given patient and the other impossible, or vice versa.

Subxyphoid window (FAST): Place the probe on the subxiphoid topography with the index marker towards the patient's right side or right shoulder. Angle the probe to the left shoulder. This window shows the right ventricle immediately adjacent to the left lobe of the liver. A pericardial effusion will be easily recognized between the liver and the heart. By increasing the depth, the chances of obtaining a good image improve.

Paraesternal longitudinal axis (RUSH): Position the probe just to the left of the sternum bone at the height of the 4°/5° intercostal space, directly over the heart. This window shows the anterior and posterior pericardium. By sliding the probe towards the cardiac apex, a good exposure of the apex is observed. This window requires less depth and is easier to obtain in uncooperative patients.

Blunt Abdominal Trauma

Intraperitoneal bleeding after blunt trauma is common. It is usually the result of an injury to the liver or spleen, which is difficult to diagnose by physical examination alone. Either RUSH or FAST exam is an ideal initial screening modality for the early identification of intraperitoneal blood since it is fast, safe, and sensitive and can be repeated as indicated or changes in the patient's clinical/hemodynamic status.

Penetrating Abdominal Trauma

Although many studies have limited FAST analysis to blunt abdominal trauma, its use in penetrating abdominal trauma is equally sensitive when it comes to detecting hemoperitoneum. In addition, it can be used to assist in the critical decision of the initial priority in the treatment of patients with multiple penetrating injuries or an unknown projectile trajectory. In a few minutes, the FAST/RUSH exam allows the EGS to direct and concentrate his initial efforts according to the presence of fluid in the cardiac, chest, and/or intraperitoneal window.

Chest Trauma: Hemothorax

Bleeding in the pleural space is common in both blunt and penetrating trauma. Simply draining the chest usually treats 80% of these conditions. Approximately 200 mL of liquid in the pleural cavity is required before the hemothorax can be detected using a simple chest x-ray. POCUS, in turn, is hypersensitive for the detection of fluid in the pleural space and can identify as little as 20 mL in this same space. Recent evidence [2] has already shown that point-of-care ultrasonography is equivalent to chest X-ray in detecting hemothorax in the trauma setting and has also been shown to be a much faster procedure, taking about 1 min versus 15 min for chest radiography. POCUS can be used during the initial minutes of the trauma assessment, to determine if chest tube placement is urgently needed and to confirm chest tube placement. This approach saves valuable time in the management of an unstable trauma patient.

Chest Trauma: Pneumothorax

Using POCUS to assess the presence of a pneumothorax is a relatively new concept. Pneumothoraxes are common in trauma and more than half are not diagnosed on a chest radiograph in the supine position.

Using ultrasound to diagnose a hidden pneumothorax is critical in situations where lack of this diagnosis could result in significant deterioration, especially patients who require positive pressure ventilation or helicopter transport. The use of ultrasound has been widespread even in situations of catastrophes or incidents with multiple victims, when the diagnosis of a pneumothorax prior to boarding victims in fixed-wing aircraft (airplanes) makes a lot of difference in the patient's prognosis.

Computed Tomography (CT) has many advantages over POCUS, but the purpose and performing timing is different. In a trauma scenario, one exam does not exclude the other or vice-versa; nevertheless, in the impossibility of performing a CT scan for several reasons (hemodynamic instability, unavailability of the CT scanner, and others), POCUS remains a watershed moment in the critical decision to treat trauma victims.

Performing the Abdominal and Thoracic Windows

Abdominal and lower thoracic window: When a patient is in the supine position, the areas of greatest reflection where fluids usually accumulate are the Morison space (located between the right liver and kidney—upper right side), the splenorenal space (located between the spleen and kidney—upper left side), and the topography posterior to the bladder in the male and the *Douglas pouch* (posterior to the uterus) in women. These three echography windows are paramount when searching for intra-abdominal free fluids and the basis for FAST and RUSH exam. Extending both upper echography windows is acceptable and recommended to investigate free intrathoracic fluid.

Right coronal window and oblique intercostal window: It is the easiest abdominal window to get a good picture of Morison's space. To obtain this window, position the probe on the middle axillary line at the height of the 8th to 11th intercostal space with the index marker facing the cephalic position. This position offers a coronal view of the interface between the liver and the right kidney. It is important to follow the lower edge of the liver caudally until a good image is obtained. Both transverse and longitudinal windows can be obtained here.

Free fluid is usually seen in Morison's space or along the lower edge of the liver, and around the lower tip of the liver, shadow of the ribs may be prominent when the index marker is pointed directly at the cephalic position. These acoustic shadows can be minimized by slightly rotating the probe counterclockwise, so that the index marker is pointed at the posterior axilla, presenting an intercostal oblique view.

Slide the probe cephalically to get a view of the diaphragm and look for the presence of pleural effusion. Pleural fluid appears as a black triangle just above the diaphragm. In addition, this window can reveal free intraperitoneal fluid superior to the liver (between the liver and the diaphragm) and around the tip of the liver lobe.

Left coronal window and oblique intercostal window: This is often the most difficult abdominal window to obtain on fresh-trained hands. Place the probe in the axillary-posterior line at the level of the sixth to ninth intercostal space with the index marker pointed at cephalic position, thus producing a coronal observation. From this position, the interface between the spleen and left kidney can be found. Free fluid is regularly seen around the spleen or at the space between spleen and diaphragm. To avoid the acoustic shadows of the ribs, and to get a better view of the spleen, slide the probe cephalically and rotate it slightly clockwise, producing an intercostal oblique view, so that the spleen (not the kidney) is then observed. The index marker will be pointed towards the posterior armpit. This window will allow good images of the lower tip and the upper surface of the spleen, where free intraperitoneal fluid is expected to be present. The diaphragm will also be seen in this window, just above the spleen. Pleural effusion will appear as a black stripe or in a triangle shape just above the diaphragm.

Pelvic window: This is the reflection of the peritoneal space that free fluid is most likely present on POCUS examination. It is a good tactic to obtain both longitudinal and transverse windows of the pelvis. If the longitudinal window is performed for the first time, it is often easier to understand the anatomy and obtain better images. Place the probe on the midline with the index marker in a cephalic position just above the pubic bone.

Check if the probe position is correct; in fact, placing the probe on the pubis and noting the bone acoustic shadow in the image is a good tip as a starting point. From this position, sliding the probe slightly for cephalic topography, a good longitudinal pelvic view is observed. The bladder is found cephalad to the pubic bone and can usually be observed even if almost empty. The full bladder takes the shape of a balloon and it is not uncommon to see bilateral ureteral flow. When the patient is already with a bladder catheter, the visualization of the bladder becomes even easier with the visualization of the catheter's balloon. The lower angle of the bladder marks the border between the intraperitoneal space (left side of the image) and the real pelvic structures (right side of the image). Free fluid can also be seen around the edges of the uterus.

To obtain a transverse window, simply rotate the probe 90°. In the transverse pelvic window, free fluid can be seen posterior to the bladder or uterus, or adjacent to the edges of the full bladder.

Anterior thoracic window: When using ultrasound to assess the presence of a pneumothorax, the probe is usually placed over the anterior chest in the third or fourth intercostal space with the median clavicle line. This is a starting point and a likely place to find a pneumothorax when the patient is in supine position. Subsequent images can be taken on any part of the chest wall if there is a concern about a very small pneumothorax.

A small, high frequency linear probe (7–10 MHz) can be used for this exam, but a standard curvilinear abdominal probe also works well in the absence of the first. The most important part about this exam is to decrease the depth setting, so that the ultrasound image shows a maximum depth of 4 cm. The probe is placed in a longitudinal position with the index marker point in the cephalic position.

In this orientation, the acoustic shadows of the ribs can be used to help locate the pleural space. It is preferable to adjust the probe linearly to two prominent ribs, one on each side of the image. It is important to "anchor" the probe and hold it firmly when looking at the sliding movement of the visceral pleura against the parietal pleura. If the "slip signal" is not present, a pneumothorax is highly likely. Contralateral comparison of the rib cage can be useful. In M mode, observe the presence of the "shore sign" (normal) or "stratosphere sign" (pneumothorax) as an auxiliary predictor for the diagnosis of pneumothorax (Fig. 7.4).

RUSH		HIMAP	
PUMP	LV Contratility, RV Strains, Tamponade	H	Heart
		I	IVC
TANK	IVC variations, Leaks, Tank Compromise	M	Morrison's Pouch/FAST
		A	Aorta + Deep Veins
PIPE	Aneurisms, DVT, Aortic Dissection	P	Pneumothorax, Pulm Edema

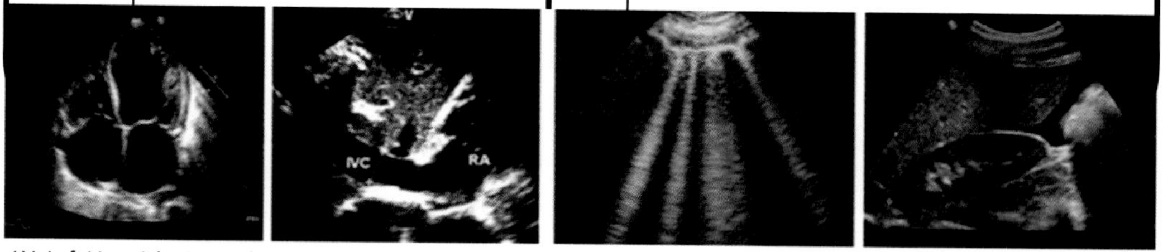

LV: Left Ventricle, RV: Right Ventricle: IVC: Inferior Vena Cava

Fig. 7.4 RUSH/HIMAP

When POCUS is important for the EGS on a trauma case?

- Hemodynamically unstable patients, when the cause of hypotension is not clear.
- Patients who need an emergency procedure at the bedside.
- Patients in a community or rural hospital who need to be transferred to a trauma center. Assisting in the decision of pericardiocentesis in the presence of a pericardial effusion, in helping to consider blood transfusion early in the presence of a significant hemoperitoneum, in assisting in the decision to proceed with chest drainage in the presence of a hemothorax or pneumothorax, especially when transporting aeromedical is planned.
- Intoxicated patients who can be observed and reexamined.
- Patients presenting with multiple penetrating injuries or an uncertain trajectory, especially when the injury affects the thoracoabdominal topography.
- Patients with an important trauma mechanism, but with no indication or impossibility for CT scan.
- Careful reassessment with POCUS exam is demanded. Sensitivity of the serial exam can significantly decrease in the presence of aggressive resuscitation or administration of intravenous crystalloid solutions along the first hours of trauma.

7.2.2 Heart

The use of cardiac qualitative POCUS by EGS in the emergency scenario has a different focus than the examination performed by the cardiologist at the outpatient clinic. It is a concise examination, with specific objectives, adapted to specific needs and a basis for making decisions that can often save lives [6]. It is usually performed quickly (10.5 ± 4.2 min) and does not involve measurements or doppler use most of the times, as the examination in the emergency room or ICU bed involves some challenges:

- Dyspneic patients may not tolerate proper positioning.
- Swollen patients offer greater difficulty in obtaining images.
- The presence of a surgical wound can hinder the correct positioning of the transducer.
- The presence of subcutaneous emphysema can be an obstacle to the passage of sound waves (great difference in impedance between the media).
- Inadequate lighting level for the examination.
- Emergency situations requiring rapid decision-making.

The ideal transducer is the sectorial one, as it is more anatomic to be located between intercostal spaces, avoiding the blocking of sound waves by the ribs, and has an adequate frequency (3–5 MHz). Some positioning techniques can be used to improve images, but there are limitations from each patient:

- Abduction of the left arm increases the space between the costal arches, facilitating the positioning of the transducer.
- Supine position facilitates viewing in the subcostal window.
- Left lateral decubitus prevents the lung from overlapping between the heart and the chest wall.
- Lung forced inspiration and Valsalva's maneuver may improve acoustic windows visualization.

7.2.2.1 Performing the Cardiac Pocus

For the ultrasound examination of the heart, it is essential to know the main windows and their correlation with the corresponding anatomic structures.

Left Ventricular Longitudinal Parasternal Window (PLVE) or Long Axis

It is usually obtained at the height of the fourth left intercostal space, adjacent to the sternum. The index marker on the transducer must face the right shoulder and with movements in the cephalic or caudal direction, the image is obtained.

In this window, the left ventricle (LV) is viewed in the longitudinal direction. Aortic valve, aortic root (Ao), descending aorta, mitral valve, right ventricle (RV), the interventricular septum, papillary muscle, coronary sinus, and the pericardium are also viewed.

This acoustic window is useful for assessing qualitative LV contractility and evaluating ejection fraction, the pericardium, aortic and mitral valve, aortic root, and left atrium. The PLVE window is not suitable for estimating the size of the right ventricle.

Left Ventricular Transverse Parasternal Window (PTVE) or Short Axis

The PTVE window or short axis is obtained at the same point as the PLVE window (the fourth left intercostal space adjacent to the sternum); however, the position of the index mark must be turned towards the patient's left shoulder, viewing the left ventricle in a cross section.

With angulation movements in the cephalic for the caudal direction, the aortic valve (central), tricuspid valve (medial), pulmonary valve (lateral), and right and left ventricle (basal, papillary, and apical portion) are visualized.

In this cut, qualitative LV contractility, ejection fraction, assessing the RV/LV ratio (important for the diagnosis of right overload), assessing valves, and pericardium can be estimated.

Apical Window

The image in the apical window is obtained at the point of the ictus cordis, usually lateral and inferior to the left nipple on man.

The index marker should be turned to 3 o'clock to obtain the apical window 4 chambers. From this image, the transducer can be tilted in the cephalic direction, towards the heart base vessels, showing the image of the aortic valve, then called the 5-chamber apical window. In the 4-chamber apical window, there is a left atrium, left ventricle, mitral valve, right atrium, right ventricle, and tricuspid valve. In the 5-chamber window, the aortic valve is observed, in addition to the structures seen in the 4-chamber window [6].

The apical window is used to assess global and segmental contractility, chamber volume and size, mitral and tricuspid anatomy, pericardial effusion, and the RV/LV ratio.

Subcostal Window

The subcostal window (subxyphoid FAST window) is best obtained with the patient in the supine position, with the transducer positioned below the xiphoid process, at an acute angle with the skin and directed towards the precordium. The index marker should be directed to the patient's left shoulder.

The cut allows you to view the four chambers, the inferior vena cava, and the pericardial space.

It is useful in the evaluation of pericardial effusion, oscillation of the inferior vena cava in the respiratory cycle, and size of the chambers, being the best window to assess defects of the interatrial septum.

Preload Evaluation

Having assessment to cardiac preload in a patient with circulatory shock is extremely important. With POCUS use on daily practice of the EGS, the management and diagnosis of the cause of shock is much easier. When assuming that a patient has a reduced preload, he can be a "responder" or "non-responder" to volume infusion. For example, a patient with a hypocontractile left ventricle and a distended inferior vena cava, which does not oscillate with breathing, may suggest cardiogenic shock and fluid therapy would not be indicated. A patient with a hypercontractile left ventricle, reduced vena cava with reduced diameter, which oscillates more than 50% of its diameter with breathing, and a history of vomiting and diarrhea suggests hypovolemia and the chosen therapy must be fluid infusion.

It is clear that the preload assessment starts with a previous history and clinical context of each case, physical examination, and evaluation of a set of ultrasound parameters, such as pulmonary ultrasound, echocardiogram, RUSH/E-FAST, among others. The EGS have usually three scenarios that will mostly work: (1) the emergency room, (2) operating theatre, and

(3) ICU. Each of those has its peculiarity reason why clinical history and physical assessment are most important. POCUS comes to add on clinical decision and decision-making. Could not stress less, the importance of POCUS on the daily clinical practice of the EGS.

The measurement should be performed 2 or 3 cm from the junction of the inferior vena cava to the right atrium. To better assess the oscillation in the respiratory cycle, M-Mode is preferably used.

Patients on mechanical ventilation and using vasodilators have an increase in diameter and less oscillation of the inferior vena cava; however, even in patients on spontaneous ventilation, the measurement has a greater correlation with PVC in cases where the diameter is reduced and the oscillation is greater than 50%.

Contractile Function Evaluation

The value of qualitative assessment of contractile function in hypotensive patients is already well defined in the medical literature [7]. In a prospective observational study, the qualitative analysis of the ejection fraction performed by doctors in the emergency department with the quantitative analysis performed by cardiologists is compared. There was agreement in 84% of cases, showing that trained physicians can estimate the ejection fraction qualitatively with accuracy.

Assessment of the Right Ventricle

The right ventricle is a less thick muscular chamber and smaller than the left ventricle. When there is a sharp increase in afterload, it is unable to generate greater pressure, dilating. Chronically, it may show a thickening of your wall. There is no absolute ultrasound criterion to differentiate between acute and chronic cor pulmonale, but thickening of the ventricular wall and high pulmonary artery pressure (usually above 60 mmHg) suggest chronicity.

Overload of Right Chambers in Pulmonary Embolism

In patients with overload signs of the right chambers, several diagnoses can be considered, such as: chronic obstructive pulmonary disease with cor pulmonale, pulmonary embolism, mechanical ventilation with elevated parameters, acute respiratory distress syndrome, acute right heart failure, among others. In these cases, there is great difficulty in differentiating an acute event (mainly pulmonary embolism) in a patient who already has chronic RV dysfunction. Although some characteristics favor chronicity (thickened RV walls, pulmonary pressure above 60 mmHg), they do not exclude a new event in patients with chronic overload of the right chambers. These are not rare cases on the postoperative scenario. Thus, the POCUS diagnosis of deep vein thrombosis in the lower limbs contributes to the diagnosis of pulmonary embolism.

Visualization of a thrombus in the right cavities is not a common finding; however, it seals the diagnosis of pulmonary embolism when present.

Baseline RV hypokinesia accompanied by apical hyperkinesia (McConnell's sign) is not an exclusive sign of pulmonary embolism and may be present in patients with pulmonary hypertension in the absence of embolism [8].

Cardiac Tamponade

Pericardial effusion as mentioned on the E-FAST/RUSH section is the accumulation of effluents in the pericardial sac. It can be blood, exudative, or transudative in origin and its evolution to compromise cardiac function depends on the volume of the stroke, pressure exerted in the cardiac chambers, and the installation time. Smaller, sudden onset strokes can easily evolve into tamponade, while slow strokes may contain large amounts of volume with little hemodynamic repercussion.

Initially, the accumulation of fluid occurs in the posterior region of the LV, progressing to the anterior region of the RV and, later, involving the whole heart. Acute pericardial effusions over 1 cm are classified as severe cardiac tamponade.

In some cases, there may be an operator misinterpretation between pleural effusion and pericardial effusion. In pericardial effusions, fluid is observed between the left atrium and the descending aorta on the PLVE axis, which does not happen in pleural effusions. Cardiac tamponade occurs when there is compression of the cardiac chambers by the effusion, preventing the diastolic filling of them, leading to a drop in cardiac output and, consequently, hypotension and shock. The main POCUS findings of cardiac tamponade are described below:

- Diastolic collapse of the Right Atrium: movement of the atrial wall into the cavity at the end of diastole. It is the most sensitive sign, but it is not specific for tamponade (it can occur in hypovolemic patients).
- The most specific sign is the diastolic collapse of the right ventricle. The movement of the ventricular wall into the cavity at the end of diastole.
- The swinging heart sign is observed in massive acute spills. The heart "sways" from side to side, due to greater mobility within the fluid-filled pericardial sac.
- Lower Vena Cava Dilatation occurs due to increased pericardial pressure. Venous return is reduced, resulting in distension and absence of oscillation.

7.2.3 Lungs

Until the 1980s, the chest was considered "inaccessible" to ultrasound, a paradigm that was broken mainly with the works of Lichtenstein and collaborators [9–11].

There is nothing specific in pulmonary ultrasound for EGS, nonetheless the general surgeon who knows how to perform pulmonary and cardiac POCUS undoubtedly has a great advantage when dealing with the critical surgical patient. These advantages are numerous, starting with the diagnosis of pneumothorax but not being restricted to this. Excluding the trauma scenarios, knowing how to interpret the Blue protocol, identifying a lung with consolidation, presence of fluid, or even atelectasis is an unprecedented advantage in the surgical critical patient management. Not infrequently, we encountered severe patients in this specific period being treated for septic shock and who actually had either a mixed shock or a cardiogenic shock. In these cases, POCUS played a fundamental role in saving their lives.

7.2.3.1 Performing Pulmonary Pocus

The transducer used in pulmonary ultrasound is the curvilinear, of low frequency (3–5 MHz), as it allows the visualization of superficial and deep structures with adequate quality for the identification of the pathologies investigated. The linear transducer can also be used to search for some pulmonary changes; however, the use of the curvilinear transducer is useful in all cases.

Start with the patient in the supine position. In the BLUE Protocol (Bed Lung Ultrasound in Emergency), Lichtenstein didactically proposed 3 reference points in each hemithorax for the study of the lung, called: upper BLUE point, lower BLUE point, and PLAPS point (Posterolateral Alveolar or Pleural Syndromes). Pulmonary scanning is done cranio-caudally, anteroposterior, transversely, and longitudinally to the costal arches [13]. There are 6 basic principles of pulmonary ultrasound, as follows:

1. In the chest, air and water interpose, generating specific ultrasound signals, patterns, and artifacts.
2. The lung is the bulkiest organ, so defining study points/regions allows for a standardized analysis.
3. All signs and artifacts start at the pleural line, the reference point in the study.
4. The artifacts generated are patterns of normality or specific pathologies.
5. The lung is a vital organ that moves, so the dynamic analysis provided by ultrasound is essential, with the pleural side being the basic dynamic signal of normality.
6. All serious changes are located superficially in the region of the pleural line, creating an acoustic window for pulmonary ultrasound.

Following the principles described by Lichtenstein, it is possible to identify and describe some ultrasound signals that will help EGS to characterize the main pulmonary syndromes.

7.2.3.2 Normal Lung

Bat Sign

Image formed with a transducer positioned transversely to the coastal arches. We observed the acoustic shadow of the two costal arches and, between these, a hyperechogenic line, generated by the pleurae.

Pleural Slip, A-Lines, and Seashore Sign

These define the normal surface of the lung. It indicates air movement and sliding of the parietal and visceral pleurae (see also E-FAST/RUSH section). The A lines represent the reverberation of the pleural signal. In M mode, a pattern is identified as seashore sign.

Lines B (Comet Tail)

Line B is a vertical "comet's tail" artifact, originating from the pleural line, until the end of the screen, coinciding with the pleural sliding and erasing the A lines. The finding of up to 2 B lines between 2 coastal arcs is considered normal pattern. This artifact is commonly evident in the lung bases where there is greater pulmonary vascularization.

7.2.3.3 Abnormal Findings: Pleural Effusion

Sharp Signal and Sinusoidal Signal

To search for pleural effusion, the transducer is placed at the PLAPS point, posterior and as close to the diaphragmatic line as possible. In the presence of pleural effusion, an anechoic image is identified within a quadrant, this one delimited by the shadows of the coastal arches, the parietal pleura, and the visceral pleura. In M mode, the visceral pleura draws a sinusoidal image by its movement towards the parietal pleura during the respiratory cycle.

7.2.3.4 Abnormal Findings: Alveolar Syndromes

Flap Sign and Hepatization

These are signs seen in pulmonary consolidations. The deepest edges of the consolidations are juxtaposed with aerated lung tissue, giving an ultrasonographic pattern of "shredded tissue", like irregular hyperechogenic images in the lung tissue. Pulmonary consolidation makes the lung tissue visible to the US as a massive organ (echogenicity similar to the liver), hence the term tissue-like sign.

7.2.3.5 Abnormal Findings: Interstitial Syndromes

Lung Rocket Sign

Three or more B lines between 2 ribs are considered pathological and the presence of a large number of B lines is called the Lung Rocket sign, a sign of interstitial syndrome (Acute Lung Edema, SARA) with 93% accuracy [10]. The number of B lines is related to the severity of interstitial involvement and the presence of confluent B lines is related to the "ground glass" pattern of computed tomography.

7.2.3.6 Abnormal Findings: Pneumothorax

Lung Point and Stratosphere Signal or Bar Code

The absence of pleural sliding with exclusive A lines (absence of B lines) suggests pneumothorax, with a sensitivity of 95% and a negative predictive value of 100%. In M mode, the pneumothorax generates a pattern called the stratosphere or bar code. The visualization of the pulmonary point, the intersection of the pneumothorax with the normal lung, is a suggestive sign of pneumothorax.

7.2.4 Adding Point-of-Care Ecography and Lung Pocus in EGS Practice

7.2.4.1 Acute Respiratory Distress Evaluation

In 2008, a study evaluated the benefit of pulmonary POCUS in patients with acute respiratory failure admitted to an ICU, concluding that pulmonary POCUS helps in the faster diagnosis of patients in acute respiratory failure [12].

The Blue Protocol

The proposed algorithm defines 8 presentation profiles, correlating with 6 pathologies seen in 97% of patients admitted to intensive care units, including surgical patients.

Below the profiles A, A′, B, B′, A/B, C, PLAPS and normal profile, are described:

- Profile A has the ultrasound pattern as the presence of A lines anteriorly and bilaterally in the chest, associated with sliding of the pleura (isolated B lines may be present); Profile A defines the normal lung. When associated with DVT (deep vein thrombosis), it makes the diagnosis of Pulmonary Embolism with 99% specificity. Associated with the PLAPS profile in the absence of DVT suggests the diagnosis of Pneumonia (specificity of 96%). In the case of profile A and the absence of DVT and PLAPS, respiratory distress will possibly be diagnosed as severe asthma or decompensated COPD (specificity 97%).
- Profile A′ presents the profile A with pleural sliding and no lung point (p point); Profile A′ with absence of B lines suggests Pneumothorax, requiring the identification of the lung point as a conclusive sign. The stratosphere signal or bar code in M mode corroborates the diagnosis.
- Profile B designates a pattern with more than 3 B lines (B+), anteriorly in the chest, associated with sliding of the pleura (isolated lines A may be present); Profile B is the representation of the patient with Acute Lung Edema (specificity 95%).
- Profile B′ presents the profile B with abolished pleural sliding; Profile B′ is related to the diagnosis of Pneumonia with 100% specificity.
- Profile A/B represents the predominant presence of B + lines in one hemithorax and A lines in the other hemithorax, anteriorly to the chest; The A/B Profile (unilateral lung Rocket) is also related to Pneumonia with 100% specificity.
- Profile C represents the pattern of anterior alveolar consolidation (shred sign or tissue-like sign); Profile C defined as anterior pulmonary consolidation also suggests pneumonia (99% specificity).
- PLAPS (posterolateral alveolar and/or pleural syndrome), pleural and/or posterolateral alveolar syndrome, is the presence of pleural effusion and / or posterior alveolar consolidations.
- The Normal Profile is the association of Profile A without the PLAPS Profile (Flowchart 7.1).

7.2.4.2 Shock Evaluation

The assessment of a patient with hypotension and hypoperfusion is a challenge for the EGS in multiple different scenarios. For this specific critical situation, a POCUS algorithm was proposed— The FALLS protocol (*Fluid Administration Limited by Lung Sonography*) [10].

The Falls Protocol

Obstructive Shock

The first step in the FALLS protocol is to visualize the cardiac window, with immediate identification of a potential Cardiac Tamponade. Once this is ruled out, the visualization of the right cardiac chambers must be the next step. In the case of dilation, paradoxical movement of the septum suggests Pulmonary Embolism. The next step, once no diagnosis is sealed, is the anterior chest search for the abolished pleural sliding and presence of A lines (Profile A′ of the Blue Protocol) for diagnosis of Hypertensive Pneumothorax. The absent of B lines, the stratosphere signal in M mode, and the identification of the Lung point confirm the diagnosis of pneumothorax and the shock state is possibly secondary to this find.

Cardiogenic Shock

Disregarding the signs of pathologies associated with obstructive shock, it follows to identify signs of interstitial syndrome. This is characterized by the presence of Lung Rockets, 3 or more B Lines between 2 coastal arches. In the Blue Protocol, the visualization of interstitial syndrome, anterior, bilateral, and pleural sliding, defines Profile B, with a sensitivity of 97% and

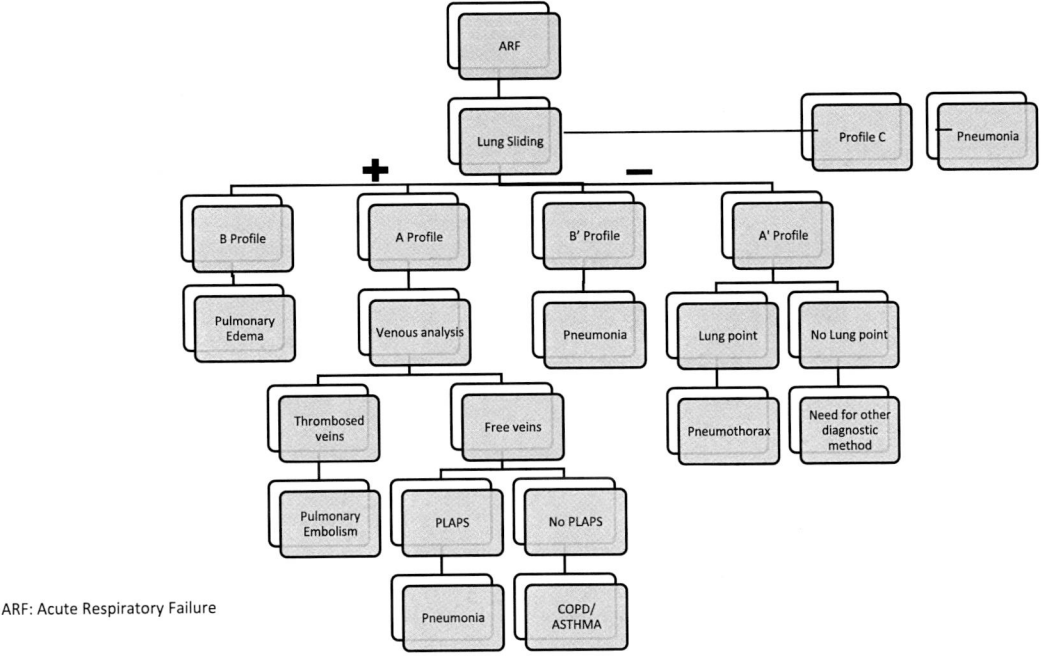

Flowchart 7.1 Blue Protocol—Algorithm for the assessment of acute respiratory failure using pulmonary ultrasound. (Adapted from Lichtenstein et al.)

specificity of 95% of the diagnosis of Acute Pulmonary Edema (APE). This picture of shock and APE is directly associated with left heart failure and cardiogenic shock.

The absence of Profile B (anterior, bilateral Lung Rockets) discards cardiogenic shock.

Hypovolemic Shock

Once the diagnoses of obstructive and cardiogenic shock are ruled out, the next step is to view Profile A again (Lines A and pleural sliding). There is a direct correlation between Profile A and pulmonary capillary pressure below 18 mmHg, with a specificity of 93% and a positive predictive value of 97%. A patient in circulatory shock who has a Profile A is called FALLS Responder. This patient can and needs volume replacement. At this point, the FALLS protocol is characterized by a therapeutic test. Fluids are administered with monitoring of hemodynamics and pulmonary ultrasound. During fluid replacement, you can also look for possible causes of shock (hemorrhage, sepsis, etc.). Patients who, after volume infusion, present hemodynamic improvement while maintaining Profile A′ are defined in the FALLS protocol as hypovolemic shock regardless of the cause. The main cause of hypovolemic shock in such cases is the Hemorrhagic Shock.

Worth to stress that complimentary protocols are useful as mentioned above. The FAST and RUSH exams can be performed depending on the picture you and your patients are found in. For example, the FAST/RUSH exams are perfect to be executed at the emergency room when the FALLS protocol is the best option to evaluate the surgical/clinical and trauma patient at the ICU. However, there is nothing on literature against the concomitant use of FALLS and RUSH for instance. FAST is specific for trauma and its sensitivity is higher if performed earlier on the trauma scenario. FAST potentially loses its sensibility after fluid resuscitation.

Distributive Shock

If during hemodynamic replacement there is no hemodynamic improvement, hypervolemia will result, particularly with lung tissue overload.

Pulmonary capillary pressures above 18 mmHg will result in the pattern changing from Profile A to Profile B, with the appearance of Lung Rockets. Interstitial edema is a stage prior to pulmonary edema, and the FALLS protocol is an early marker of hypervolemia. At this point in the algorithm, volume replacement ends and the shock diagnosis is characterized by vasoplegic, as the other causes of shock have been ruled out. The main cause of vasoplegic shock is the Septic Shock (Flowchart 7.2).

7.2.5 Vascular

The main blood vessels in the cervical topography, lower limbs, and abdomen of critical surgical patients can be assessed by POCUS. The diagnosis of deep venous thrombosis (DVT), abdominal aortic aneurysm, or anatomic variations can be done in a few minutes or even seconds in the hands of a trained surgeon in bedside ultrasound. Most ultrasound examinations are conclusive through the B-mode (gray scale) associated or not with mechanical compression of the vessel with the transducer (compressive ultrasound).

For the evaluation of blood vessels in the superficial and deep systems of the cervical region and limbs, the linear transducer is preferably used, which allows high-resolution images through the use of higher frequencies waves. Curvilinear transducers provide images with lower resolution. On the other hand, it presents advantages in the evaluation of deeper structures or in the examination of obese or swollen critical patients [13].

7.2.5.1 Performing Vascular POCUS

Ultrasonography of peripheral vessels must be initiated by the transverse plane, in which the vessels appear on the screen as anechoic tubular, round, or oval structures. Enlarged lymph nodes or collections can initially be confused with vessels; however, the vessels extend in the cranial and caudal directions, while other structures have restricted dimensions in the dynamic evaluation. The difficulty in identifying vessels in the transversal plane may be related to hypovolemia, to the collapse of the vein walls caused by the excess pressure applied to the transducer, or even to the agenesis or hypoplasia of the vessels in rare cases.

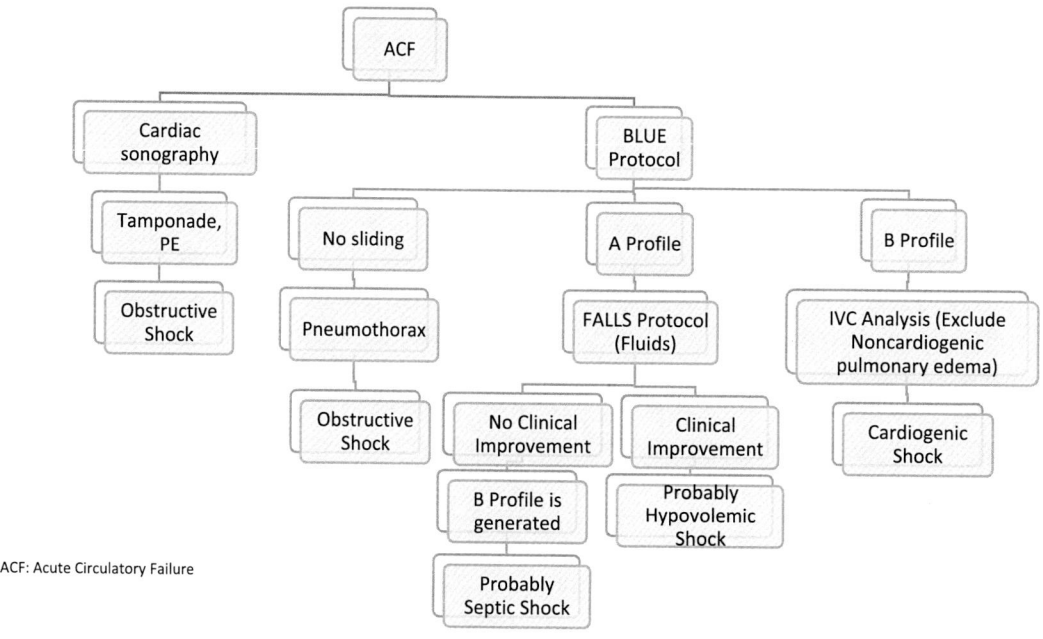

ACF: Acute Circulatory Failure

Flowchart 7.2 Falls Protocol. (Adapted from Lichtenstein et al.)

After identification, the vessel must be centered on the screen. Then the depth of the assessment of the equipment must be adjusted so that the region of interest is demonstrated in an appropriate size. Finally, you can fine-tune the focus and gain of the device. It is important to note that the index marker must be directed to the screen mark already explained in the first section of this chapter. The light to moderate compression of the transducer over a vein usually overcomes its low internal pressure causing the anterior and posterior walls to completely obliterate its light. The collapse of the vessel lumen by external compression virtually excludes the diagnosis of thrombosis.

Sagittal (Transversal)/Longitudinal Plane

After evaluating the vessels in the axial plane, transducer can be rotated 90° on its axis, seeking the sagittal/longitudinal plane of the vessel. Acquiring this image can be difficult for inexperienced sonographers. In addition, compressive ultrasound performed on the sagittal/longitudinal axis of the vessel should be performed with special attention, as the loss of the vessel image can be falsely interpreted as the collapse of the vein.

Color Doppler Mode

In rare situations, the ultrasound diagnosis at the bedside performed using the B-mode (gray scale) and/or by compressive ultrasound may be inconclusive. In such cases, it may be necessary to complement the exam with the color or amplitude Doppler mode. Through Doppler, it is possible to identify the blood flow inside the vessels.

Assessment of Deep Venous Thrombosis (DVT)

The clinical diagnosis of DVT shows multiple false positive and negative results, which justifies the use of complementary diagnostic methods in all patients with moderate or high probability of DVT. In most circumstances, ultrasonography is the main complementary method for the diagnosis of DVT due to its availability, safety and, above all, high accuracy in the diagnosis of venous thrombosis. As with any test, it is best evaluated in conjunction with other clinical or laboratory data.

Cervical Zone Examination Technique

Deep cervical vessels are easily assessed in the axial plane, with linear transducers. Most of the times, it is easy to access and possible to perfectly visualize the cervical anatomy. Compressive ultrasound is useful to confirm the Internal Jugular Vein. Doppler mode is usually unnecessary.

Upper Limb Examination Technique

The search for thrombi in the upper limbs and cervical regions in critically ill patients is important because up to 20% of those of massive embolisms originate from the subclavian or jugular veins. The B-mode POCUS obtains images of excellent quality of the superficial and deep veins of the upper limbs. The identification of the subclavian vein in its axial plane must be performed with the transducer positioned in the longitudinal direction, with its cranial portion over the clavicle. After identifying the vessel, the transducer can be rotated 90° on its axis in which the subclavian vein can be evaluated in its sagittal plane. The subclavian veins are not easily compressible, so it is essential to identify the gauge variation related to the cardiac and respiratory cycles since the spontaneous collapse of the vein most of the times excludes the presence of a thrombus inside. The plasticity of these vessels is normally decreased in patients on mechanical ventilation, which should not be interpreted as thrombosis.

Lower Limb Examination Technique

Venous thrombosis evaluation of the lower limbs consists of searching for signs of compression or direct visualization of the thrombus in vessels most commonly involved in the genesis of pulmonary embolism. The vast majority comes from the venous system of the lower limbs. The impossibility of complete compression of the vein, visualized by the B-mode, has good sensitivity in the detection of deep venous thrombosis. The compression movement of the vessel must be careful not to cause displacement of the thrombus and new embolization episode.

When the two-point evaluation technique (inguinal and popliteal region) is compared with the complete evaluation of the venous network of the lower limbs for deep venous thrombosis, there was agreement of specificity and sensitivity between the methods; thus, the evaluation of deep venous thrombosis of the lower limbs using the two-point technique is suggested.

The examination of DVT research in the lower limbs is initiated by the identification of the superficial venous system in the axial plane. The depth of the equipment is then adjusted to include the deep venous system, located below the deep fascia. It is not uncommon for inexperienced EGS to misinterpret the great saphenous vein and its tributaries as part of the deep venous system.

Once the deep venous system has been identified, the image popularly known as "Mickey's" (Walt Disney) head must be obtained, formed by the femoral veins and arteries and the cross of the great saphenous vein. Descending the scan on the caudal direction, the duplication of the femoral artery in its superficial and deep branches is identified. Just below, the duplication of the common femoral vein occurs. In most exams, it is not possible to identify the femoral vein distal to the adductor muscle channel or Hunter's channel. The examination is completed by compressive ultrasound of the popliteal vein, performed with flexion and external rotation of the knee.

Due to the depth of the venous system of the lower limbs, except in the case of extensive thrombosis, the identification or exclusion of the thrombus may be difficult on B-mode. Compressive ultrasonography of the common femoral veins, the proximal region of the superficial and deep femoral veins, and the popliteal vein shows sensitivity and specificity greater than 95% to the diagnosis of DVT of the lower limbs [14].

Superficial Venous Thrombosis or Thrombophlebitis

Superficial thrombophlebitis, also called superficial venous thrombosis (SVT), is a pathological condition characterized by the presence of a thrombus in the lumen of a superficial vein, accompanied by inflammatory reaction of adjacent tissues.

Thrombophlebitis usually occurs after puncture of vessels of the superficial venous system in the arms or in the cervical region. Its diagnosis saves time and resources.

POCUS diagnosis of thrombophlebitis is usually simple, since the thrombus in these cases is quite echogenic due to the presence of gases related to the infection.

Abdominal Aortic Aneurysm

Abdominal aortic aneurysms (AAA) are segmental dilatations of the infrarenal abdominal aorta, with a diameter ≥ 3 cm. The risk factors involved with AAA rupture are diameter >5.5 cm, growth >0.5 cm in 6 months, smoking habit, female gender, and uncontrolled hypertension.

Typical signs of rupture occur in only half of the cases of rupture and are: abdominal distension, acute abdominal pain, back pain, ecchymosis in the flank region, hemodynamic instability.

In asymptomatic patients, ultrasonography is the method of choice for diagnosis because it presents sensitivity and specificity close to 100% when the cut-off point of 3 cm (LaRoy) is used. In symptomatic cases, CT is essential for preoperative planning. In hemodynamically unstable cases, confirmatory imaging is not mandatory, especially if there is a known history of aortic aneurysm. However, POCUS in the emergency room or in the operating theater can be performed quickly and confirm or exclude alternative diagnoses.

Ultrasonographic diagnosis of aortic aneurysm is usually quite simple by identifying the dilation of a segment of the aorta, which is fusiform in most cases, but can be saccular. When conditions are favorable, it is possible to identify details such as thickening of the vessel wall and differentiate mural thrombi from residual light by ultrasonography. Signs of impending rupture are asymmetry and broken calcifications. In cases of rupture, it is possible to identify a collection in the retroperitoneal space, on the left. In the dissection of the aorta, a mobile echogenic flap separates two channels. In such cases, the investigation must be completed in the thoracic aorta.

7.2.5.2 The IVC

One of the frequent uses of POCUS in today's EGS practice is for the assessment of blood volume and fluid-responsiveness by assessing the diameters of the inferior vena cava. The use of static parameters (such as central venous pressure) is very imprecise, and the pulse pressure variation (ΔPP) requires arterial access and some prerequisites that limit its usefulness. The Lower Vena Cava (IVC) begins at the level of the navel and ends at the xiphoid process. As in the vessels of the upper limbs, their caliber varies greatly with the cardiac and respiratory cycles, especially in patients breathing spontaneously. In this situation, the complete collapse of the IVC can be identified, which most of the times exclude thrombosis. In intubated patients, the variation in IVC caliber is less intense, and compression of IVC against the spine may be necessary to adequate fluid responsiveness evaluation or thrombosis diagnosis.

POCUS allows a noninvasive assessment of the preload, through the visualization of the inferior vena cava (IVC). In spontaneous breathing, inspiration results in a reduction in intrathoracic pressure, increasing venous return and, thus, decreasing the IVC diameter. In mechanical ventilation, the opposite happens. Inhalation leads to an increase in intrathoracic pressures, making venous return difficult, while passive expiration reduces these pressures, with an increase in venous return and a reduction in IVC diameter. Mechanical ventilation measurements can be integrated into the distensibility index (ID = (VCI max − VCI min)/VCI min) In any case, both in spontaneous and mechanical ventilation, the greater variation in IVC during the respiratory cycle increases the probability that patients are "dependent on preload" and, therefore, potentially fluid-responsive.

A systematic review with a recent meta-analysis [15] proposed to evaluate the real results and potential causes of heterogeneity. In general, the use of the variation in the diameter of the vena cava was able to predict response to the volume test with 73% sensitivity, 82% specificity, and area under the 0.85 ROC curve. However, there is a great deal of heterogeneity between studies and, apparently, 85% of this heterogeneity is due to the variation in mechanical ventilation parameters. In 2019, another study recommended that dIVC should be used with caution when critically ill patients on controlled mechanical ventilation display normal right ventricular function in combination with abnormal left ventricular systolic function [16]. These data expose one of the limitations of applying the IVC dynamics as a predictor of response to volume testing.

7.2.6 Ocular Nerve Sheath (ONS) POCUS

Ocular Nerve Sheath (ONS) POCUS has been used in the evaluation of intracranial hypertension (ICH) subsequent to trauma and other etiologies by EGS as an adjunct to physical examination. The gold standard method for diagnosing ICH is done through the insertion of an intraventricular catheter that allows the monitoring of intracranial pressure (ICP). However, it is an invasive method, not immediate and associated with complications such as infection, bleeding, and neurological dysfunction.

The optic canal, located in the minor wing of the sphenoid bone, receives the optic nerve (cranial nerve II) from the intraorbital region, bringing afferents from the retina. This nerve is surrounded by a meningeal sheath consisting of dura mater, arachnoid, and pia mater. The CSF content is present throughout the subarachnoid space and reflects the PIC. Due to the anatomic relationship of the optic nerve complex with the entire cerebral subarachnoid space, an increase in ICP results in distention of the sheath and consequently an increase in its thickness, thus the diameter of the optic nerve sheath (ONS) directly translates to ICP [17].

7.2.6.1 Ocular Ultrasound and Assessment ONS

A high frequency linear transducer (7–10 MHz) is used and ultrasound is configured to view structures up to 5–6 cm deep. The transducer is placed on the closed eyelid after generous application of gel.

The optic nerve is identified as a hypoechoic structure traversing along a regular course behind the eyeball. For measurement, a vertical line is drawn from the junction between the optic nerve and the eyeball. This line is for reference only and should be 3 mm long. Once the 3 mm length is established, a horizontal line is drawn through the nerve. This second line provides the measurement of the optic nerve sheath in mm.

7.2.7 POCUS for Intra-abdominal Hypertension

With the increased use of ultrasound as a bedside modality in both emergency and critical care patients, it is paramount to consider point-of-care ultrasound (POCUS) as an adjuvant tool for IAH and management of fluid strategies.

For patients with IAP greater than grade I, decompression of intraluminal content is recommended. The WSACS medical management algorithm advises placement of a nasogastric tube (NGT) as the first step. Passing a NGT under direct ultrasound (US) guidance with the probe on the epigastrium, allowing direct visualization of air artefact when air is insufflated through the NGT is a good example of using POCUS for IAH. A 100 per cent accuracy was observed when using US to determine NGT placement and positioning [18]; however, it should be remembered that esophageal placement may result in a false positive sign. POCUS is also useful more or less on the third day of admission when gastric content may be visualized, thus allowing the physician to remove the NGT.

POCUS may also be used to evaluate bowel movements and colonic content. This is useful during daily assessment of postoperative patients and nutrition could be initiated earlier than usual due to detectable bowel movements. Likewise, POCUS may be used to detect colonic material, thus guiding the physician on the need for further enemas to decompress the colon. These findings may also facilitate early recognition of bowel wall edema, a consequence of extravasation from fluid resuscitation. Theoretically, this may help early management decisions regarding patient fluid balances and targets. POCUS may also be used in the first 2 steps of the second stage of the WSACS medical management algorithm, being used to identify moderate to large amounts of free intra-abdominal fluid. In cirrhotic patients with acute ascites, ultrasound for guided paracentesis is considered a mandatory safety step.

The use of POCUS can be extended in patients with severe acute pancreatitis and IAH, providing valuable information in the assessment of fluid balance and guiding further therapeutic management. POCUS is helpful in assessing the inferior vena cava for volume status and fluid response and/or cardiac function with bedside transthoracic echocardiography. The use of POCUS during first 3 days of admission improved clinical performance in IAH scenarios and fluid management. Furthermore, POCUS can be used to evaluate abdominal wall compliance and detecting whether there is abdominal wall movement. Lastly, POCUS can be used for optimization of systemic/regional perfusion through assessment of renal/hepatic artery and porto-venous flow (Fig. 7.5).

7.2.8 Central Venous Access

The central venous access technique by anatomic reference, which is still widely performed worldwide, is easy to be performed when applied correctly, but recent literature demonstrates that the safety of ultrasound-guided venous access at the bedside is greater [19]. It is also worth mentioning that up to 9% of the population has anatomic abnormalities that can hinder the procedure,

7.2.8.1 Obtaining a Central Venous Access with POCUS

There are several different ways of ultrasound-guided central venous access: the transverse position (also known as short axis) and the longitudinal position (long axis). There is also a dynamic way (visualization of the vessel and the needle during the puncture) and a static way (previous visual-

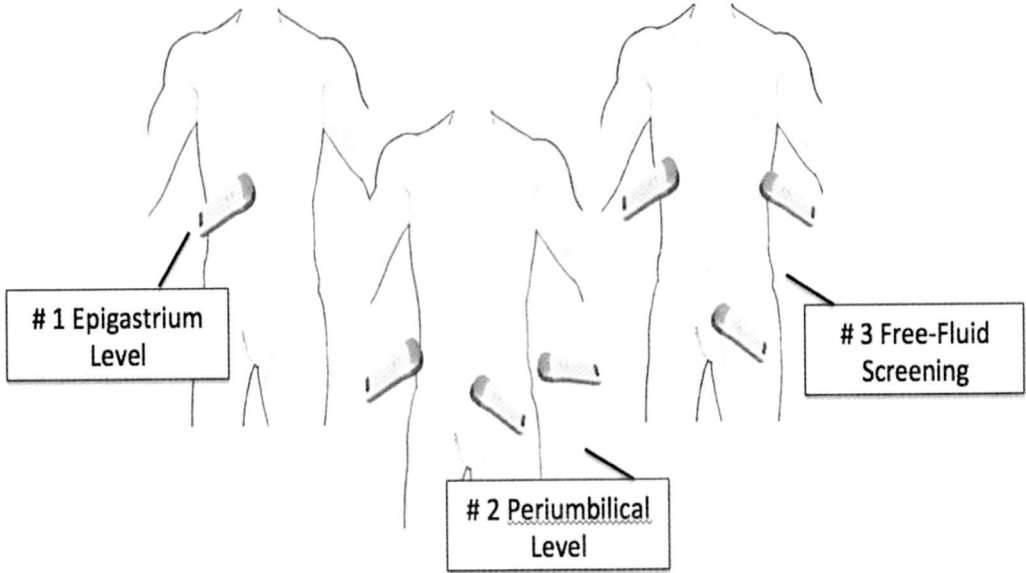

Fig. 7.5 Probe position to access the different POCUS windows

ization of the vessel to provide a mark for the puncture optimal site).

POCUS should be used prior to the puncture for local assessment of possible complications such as the presence of intraluminal thrombi and/or unfavorable anatomy.

When used by a qualified physician, there is no absolute contraindication for its use. According to a Cochrane 2015 review [20, 21], guided puncture of the internal jugular vein, for instance, reduces the number of complications by 71% and the risk of inadvertent arterial puncture by 72%. The number of attempts is reduced, with the chance of success on the first attempt being increased to 57%.

Mode B must be selected, with the possibility of using the probe both on the transverse axis and on the longitudinal axis for venous puncture. On the transverse axis, the image is perpendicular to the course of the vessel and the vascular structure appears as an anechoic circle to be centered on the screen, with a hyperechoic point that corresponds to the needle when already inside the vessel. The longitudinal axis is perpendicular to the course of the vessel. It will appear as a long anechoic image, with the presence of the stem and tip of the needle in a hyperechoic image, as the needle is advanced into the vessel. On the transverse puncture, the probe must advance with the needle along the puncture, as this avoids underestimating the depth with minimized risks for puncturing the posterior wall of the vessel. With the longitudinal axis, the trained EGS is able to see the entire needle during puncture as well as the passage of the indwelling wire.

7.2.8.2 Dynamic Versus Static Technique

The dynamic technique can be performed by a professional or two simultaneously. On this technique, the EGS must dominate the process with both hands, one holding the probe and the other the syringe.

The static technique in turn uses ultrasound to determine the location of the vessel and its patency and the structures that surround it and delimit the puncture site. Important to stress that in both techniques previous study of the vessel and its anatomy is important. The difference between both techniques is that in this case, ultrasound is only used to demarcate the location of the procedure, whereas in dynamics the progression of the needle is seen in real time, a technique that has proven to be superior in the literature.

7.2.8.3 Internal Jugular Vein POCUS Access

If tolerable, the patient should be positioned in Trendelenburg, which allows for greater venous engorgement and reduces the risk of gas embolism at the time of puncture. Although a cervical rotation is necessary to facilitate the use of a probe, it should be minimized as far as possible, as the greater the rotation, the greater the possibility that there will be an overlap of the internal jugular vein with the carotid artery. Also, this rotation is contraindicated in trauma. The operator should be positioned at the patient's bedside with the ultrasound device positioned right in front of him, in a way that allows his easy viewing during the entire procedure. As mentioned, the anatomy must be studied before preparing the patient, allowing the EGS the change of site if necessary. On the transversal axis, the index of the probe must be positioned to the operator's left, corresponding to the patient's left and the images to the left of the screen. Ideally, the location to be chosen for the puncture is the one in which the jugular vein is lateral to the carotid artery, which in the unguided method generally corresponds to the apex of the anterior cervical triangle.

7.2.8.4 Subclavian Vein POCUS Access

Subclavian vein puncture demands higher operator training due to the proximity to the lung and the impossibility of compression in the case of an inadvertent arterial puncture. On this site, the technique is challenging by the presence of the clavicle, which makes it difficult to visualize the image.

In the literature, there are three possible techniques for its approach: infraclavicular (proximal), axillary vein (infraclavicular but laterally), and supraclavicular. Direct visualization of the subclavian vein is possible, positioning the probe over the supraclavicular topography visualizing the vein in a longitudinal way. Before the procedure, all anatomic structures must be identified—clavicle, pleural line, vein, and subclavian artery.

7.2.8.5 Femoral Vein POCUS Access

For patients who require prolonged venous access, femoral access is not an interesting choice due to its increased risk of infection. However, the distance from the cervical and pulmonary structures reduces the risk of major complications, and the relative constant anatomy allows this access to be punctured quickly blindly using the arterial pulse as an anatomic guide. However, in situations of significant hypotension and cardiac arrest, this puncture becomes impossible without the use of ultrasound. The risk of inadvertent arterial puncture is also not low, since the femoral vein becomes deeper than the artery as it advances distally.

The puncture must be performed with the lower limb slightly rotated externally, which reduces the overlap of the femoral artery over the femoral vein, keeping the vein medially positioned. Due to the proximity of the femoral artery, ultrasound confirmation of the indwelling wire inside the desired vessel must be done prior to vascular dilation in order to avoid inadvertent dilation of the artery.

7.2.9 Paracentesis

Paracentesis is the most efficient way to confirm the presence of ascites, diagnose its cause, and determine whether the fluid is infected. It is a simple procedure, usually performed at the bedside, which consists of inserting a needle into the peritoneal cavity to remove ascitic fluid. Paracentesis can be diagnostic and/or therapeutic.

POCUS-guided paracentesis increases safety and also allows for a smaller number attempts to succeed.

7.2.9.1 Performing POCUS Paracentesis

Place the patient in a sitting position with the headboard elevated at 30°/45°. Search the abdomen with the probe of the ultrasound device and choose the best site for puncture, based on the one with the lowest risk of injury to intra-abdominal organs and higher hyperechoic finding.

Perform the guided puncture either on the long axis or on the short axis—according to your practice after preparing the puncture site with aseptic technique and local analgesia.

7.2.10 Pericardiocentesis

Pericardiocentesis is the term used for the puncture and aspiration of a certain fluid contained in the pericardium. This is a life-saving procedure on the presence of cardiac tamponade, for example, even in complications of acute Stanford A type aortic dissection or when cardiothoracic surgery is not immediately available.

Cardiac tamponade is a time-dependent life-threatening condition, which therefore requires immediate diagnosis and treatment. The diagnosis of cardiac tamponade is based on the triad of clinical findings (the 3D's): (1) Decreased arterial blood pressure, (2) Distended Jugular veins, (3) Distant heart sounds.

However, some studies have shown that the association of these classic findings is observed in only a minority of patients with cardiac tamponade.

7.2.10.1 Performing POCUS Pericardiocentesis

Position the patient in a semi-reclined position at an angle of 30°–45°. This position brings the heart closer to the anterior chest wall. The supine position is an acceptable alternative. In Emergency, pericardiocentesis is indicated when the patient is hemodynamically unstable and unable to be transferred to the operating room.

Make sure the patient has at least one established venous access, receives supplemental oxygen, and is connected to a pulse and cardiac oximetry monitor. If time permits, placing a nasogastric tube to decompress the stomach and decrease the risk of gastric perforation is recommended.

Identify anatomic landmarks, scan with POCUS device probe through the subxyphoid window or transthoracic window, and choose a location for insertion of the needle. The most commonly used sites are the left sternal-costal margin or the subxiphoid approach.

7.2.11 Thoracocentesis

Thoracentesis is a diagnostic surgical procedure used to elucidate diseases and dysfunctions that affect the pleural space, providing an improper accumulation of fluid in this cavity, which can cause functional changes in pulmonary and cardiac mechanics.

7.2.11.1 Performing POCUS Thoracocentesis

Place the patient in a sitting position with the back facing the operator. Use a linear array to locate the pleural effusion, and once infection and analgesia cautions are taken, the procedure can be performed. Usually with direct vision, the surgical procedure is with no difficulties and the extract sample of pleural effusion is sent to analysis. Same anatomy rules for chest drain work for thoracocentesis and therefore superior costal board is the preferred site for puncture.

7.2.12 Decision Making Assistance

POCUS is an excellent device on the diagnostic EGS armamentarium as demonstrated so far, but not restricted to diagnosis only. Innumerous are the possibilities of POCUS use on EGS decision making assistance such as abdominal distension, abdominal pain, and fever, which are the common complications encountered after surgical operations. In the patients with abdominal distention, bowel distention or ascites can be easily detected for instance, the same for extra-abdominal complications. As mentioned by Abu-Zidan et al. [22], POCUS stands for: Physiology, On spot clinical decision tool, Clinical examination extension, Unique and expanding tool, Safe repeatable tool.

Bellow, we present some of the applications of POCUS on decision making and surgical complications [22–27]:

- Identification of atelectasis.
- Recognition of free fluid. However, POCUS cannot differentiate between different types of fluid (urine, bile, ascites, or blood). In such case, POCUS is still useful guiding paracentesis of intra-abdominal fluid for further investigation with low risk of complications.
- Detection of free intraperitoneal air. Air is a strong reflector for the ultrasound waves giving increased echogenicity under the abdominal fascia. Three are the POCUS findings for free intraperitoneal air: enhanced peritoneal stripe sign, shifting phenomenon, and reverberation artefact.
- Small bowel obstruction POCUS identification includes increased loop dimensions, increased wall thickness (greater than 3 mm), increased intestinal contents, increased or decreased peristaltic movements, enlarged and visible valvulae connivences (greater than 2 mm), and collapsed colonic lumen. These six findings are important to differentiate mechanical obstruction from functional obstruction. Dilated small bowel loops, full of gas and fluid, without peristalsis associated with colonic gas, fluid, or feces may be considered as postoperative paralytic ileus.
- Identification of hernias, intussusception, ascariasis, foreign bodies, and tumors is also possible with POCUS and adequate training.
- Detection of acute appendicitis, acute cholecystitis, acute diverticulitis, and the differential diagnosis of obstructive kidney stones is safe to be performed by the EGS. Different techniques may be used for different diagnostic searches, including the graded compression technique.
- Chest tube placement, follow-up, and removal. A step-by-step approach for ultrasound-guided chest tube drainage is already proposed. Safety is improved with the use of POCUS.
- Soft tissue complications can easily be identified and treated with POCUS.

7.2.13 Transversus Abdominal Plane (TAP) Block

The TAP Block is a modality of regional anesthesia used with good results in abdominal surgeries, such as cesarean section, laparotomies, appendectomy, inguinal/abdominal wall hernias, bariatric surgery, among others. When done with the aid of POCUS, it allows very precisely to locate the abdominal structures and injections of smaller doses of local anesthetics between the transverse abdomen and internal oblique muscles.

Usually, the TAP Block is performed on either before or immediately after surgery, at the midaxillary line bilaterally, but this approach can change depending on the procedure and the side of intervention. When bilaterally done, 10 mL of Ropivacaine or Bupivacaine 0.5% on each side is sufficient for excellent analgesia and good postoperative recover [27–29].

7.2.14 POCUS-Guided Quadratus Lumborum Block

Quadratus Lumborum (QL) Block has only recently been described. There are some reports of its usefulness as an analgesic technique after abdominal surgery with excellent results in postoperative pain control, being used even in chronic pain. The QL muscle originates from the lower border of the 12 costal arch and in the transverse processes of the four upper lumbar vertebrae and has its insertions in the inner lip of the iliac crest and in the ileo-lumbar ligament. The QL muscle is covered by the transverse fascia (TF) and the thoraco-lumbar fascia, which share a common embryonic origin. The TF divides into two slides at the diaphragm level and continues as the lower diaphragmatic fascia and endothoracic fascia [30–32] (Fig. 7.6).

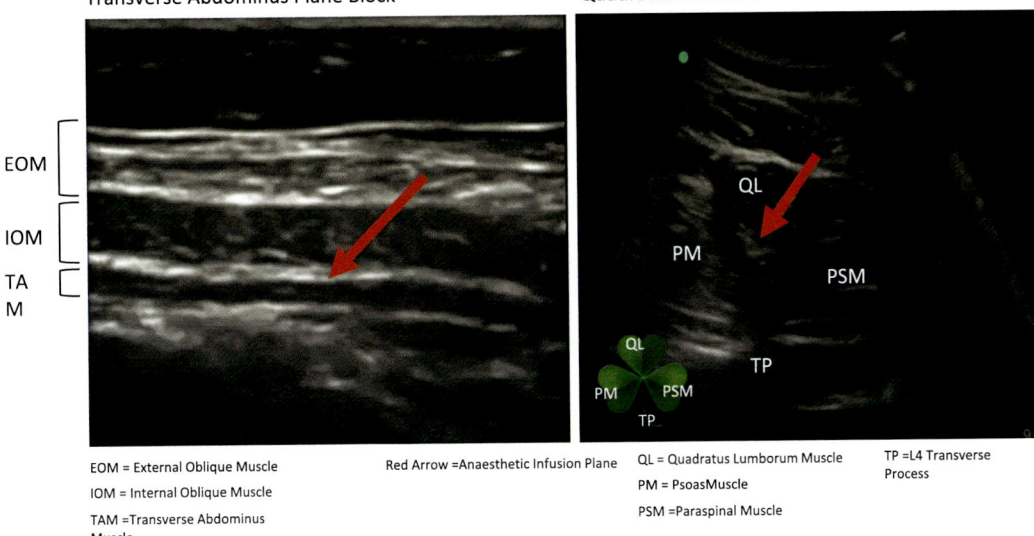

Fig. 7.6 TAP and QL Block Pictures

Dos and Don'ts

Dos

- Flourish your interest in POCUS. The application of these techniques by EGS is no longer the future. It is the present.
- Daily training is very important to bring you confidence and technical dexterity.
- Using POCUS daily will undoubtedly bring benefits to your patient and quality to your practice. Do it everyday!

Don'ts

- Don't let the technology scare you away from the immeasurable benefit that POCUS can bring you.
- Don't try it before having proper training. Misunderstanding POCUS information could be dangerous and discouraging.

Take-Home Message

POCUS in the Emergency General Surgery field is no longer the future, it is the present. Practice it every day and improve your practice for good.

Multiple Choice Questions

1. On the POCUS Basics, the mnemonic *PART* stands for:
   A. **Pressure, Alignment, Rotation, and Tilt**
   B. Patient, Acute, Reason, and Testing
   C. Penetration, Acoustic, Reverberation, and Time
   D. Performance, Action, Resources, and Tactics
2. Which of those below is not part of the RUSH protocol:
   A. Parasternal long cardiac view
   B. Aortic slide views
   C. Splenorenal with hemothorax view
   D. **Ocular Nerve Sheath view**
3. When POCUS is most important for the EGS on a trauma case? Mark the TRUE answer.
   A. Hemodynamically stable patients, when the cause of hypotension is clear
   B. **Patients who need an emergency procedure at the bedside**
   C. Conscious patients who can remember all the trauma history and have no pain complain

D. When EGS has taken the decision to take the patient to the OR
4. The following windows are pattern for POCUS heart evaluation, except:
   A. PTVE
   B. Apical
   C. **Sternal Wishbone**
   D. Subcostal
5. The Lung Rocket sign is an abnormal fining commonly seen in:
   A. Pneumothoraxes
   B. Pleural effusions
   C. **Interstitial syndromes**
   D. Alveolar syndromes
6. ONS POCUS are found to be normal in adults when measurement is:
   A. **<5 mm**
   B. 5 mm
   C. =5 mm
   D. Between 4.5 and 6 mm
7. Which one below is the best answer?
   A. POCUS can't be used on ACS cases
   B. POCUS is not useful in IAH Grade I
   C. POCUS is useful to recognize different types of intra-abdominal fluids
   D. **POCUS is useful either on diagnosis and or treatment of IAH**
8. Regarding the use of POCUS and the central venous access. Mark the correct answer:
   A. Supraclavicular site isn't an option
   B. Femoral site should be the first option
   C. Subclavian site is an impossible option
   D. **Jugular site is an easier site for beginners**
9. The TAP Block is the infusion of local anesthetics in between:
   A. **The transverse abdomen and internal oblique muscles**
   B. The transverse abdomen and the peritoneum
   C. The internal oblique and the external oblique muscles
   D. The external oblique muscle and anterior abdominal fascia
10. When followed the correct procedure, the QL Block can begin analgesic effects in:
    A. About 3 min after the infusion of local anesthetic
    B. **About 5 min after the infusion of local anesthetic**
    C. About 7 min after the infusion of local anesthetic
    D. About 10 min after the infusion of local anesthetic

References

1. Goldsmith AJ, Shokoohi H, Loesche M, Patel RC, Kimberly H, Liteplo A. Point-of-care ultrasound in morbidity and mortality cases in emergency medicine: who benefits the most? West J Emerg Med. 2020;21(6):172–8.
2. Chan KK, Joo DA, McRae AD, Takwoingi Y, Premji ZA, Lang E, Wakai A. Chest ultrasonography versus supine chest radiography for diagnosis of pneumothorax in trauma patients in the emergency department. Cochrane Database Syst Rev. 2020;7(7):CD013031.
3. Jang T, Kryder G, Sineff S, Naunheim R, Aubin C, Kaji AH. The technical errors of physicians learning to perform focused assessment with sonography in trauma. Acad Emerg Med. 2012;19(1):98–101.
4. Rozycki GS, Feliciano DV, Davis TP. Ultrasound as used in thoracoabdominal trauma. Surg Clin North Am. 1998;78(2):295–310. https://doi.org/10.1016/s0039-6109(05)70314-5. Erratum in: Surg Clin North Am 1998 Dec;78(6).
5. Pereira BM, Nogueira VB, Calderan TR, Villaça MP, Petrucci O, Fraga GP. Penetrating cardiac trauma: 20-y experience from a university teaching hospital. J Surg Res. 2013;183(2):792–7.
6. Levitov A, Frankel HL, Blaivas M, Kirkpatrick AW, Su E, Evans D, Summerfield DT, Slonim A, Breitkreutz R, Price S, McLaughlin M, Marik PE, Elbarbary M. Guidelines for the appropriate use of bedside general and cardiac ultrasonography in the evaluation of critically ill patients-part II: cardiac ultrasonography. Crit Care Med. 2016;44(6):1206–27.
7. Moore CL, Rose GA, Tayal VS, Sullivan DM, Arrowood JA, Kline JA. Determination of left ventricular function by emergency physician echocar-

diography of hypotensive patients. Acad Emerg Med. 2002;9(3):186–93.
8. Mediratta A, Addetia K, Medvedofsky D, Gomberg-Maitland M, Mor-Avi V, Lang RM. Echocardiographic diagnosis of acute pulmonary embolism in patients with McConnell's sign. Echocardiography. 2016;33(5):696–702.
9. Lichtenstein DA. Current misconceptions in lung ultrasound: a short guide for experts. Chest. 2019;156(1):21–5.
10. Lichtenstein DA. BLUE-protocol and FALLS-protocol: two applications of lung ultrasound in the critically ill. Chest. 2015;147(6):1659–70.
11. Lichtenstein DA. Whole body ultrasonography in the critically ill. Springer; 2010.
12. Lichtenstein DA, Mezière GA. Relevance of lung ultrasound in the diagnosis of acute respiratory failure: the BLUE protocol. Chest. 2008;134(1):117–25.
13. Pedraza García J, Valle Alonso J, Ceballos García P, Rico Rodríguez F, Aguayo López MÁ, Muñoz-Villanueva MDC. Comparison of the accuracy of emergency department-performed point-of-care-ultrasound (POCUS) in the diagnosis of lower-extremity deep vein thrombosis. J Emerg Med. 2018;54(5):656–64.
14. Lensing AW, Prandoni P, Brandjes D, Huisman PM, Vigo M, Tomasella G, Krekt J, Wouter Ten Cate J, Huisman MV, Büller HR. Detection of deep-vein thrombosis by real-time B-mode ultrasonography. N Engl J Med. 1989;320(6):342–5.
15. Si X, Xu H, Liu Z, Wu J, Cao D, Chen J, Chen M, Liu Y, Guan X. Does respiratory variation in inferior vena cava diameter predict fluid responsiveness in mechanically ventilated patients? A systematic review and meta-analysis. Anesth Analg. 2018;127(5):1157–64.
16. Zhang H, Zhang Q, Chen X, Wang X, Liu D, Chinese Critical Ultrasound Study Group (CCUSG). Respiratory variations of inferior vena cava fail to predict fluid responsiveness in mechanically ventilated patients with isolated left ventricular dysfunction. Ann Intensive Care. 2019;9(1):113.
17. Wilson CL, Leaman SM, O'Brien C, Savage D, Hart L, Jehle D. Novice emergency physician ultrasonography of optic nerve sheath diameter compared to ophthalmologist fundoscopic evaluation for papilledema. J Am Coll Emerg Physicians Open. 2021;2(1):e12355.
18. Pereira BM, Pereira RG, Wise R, Sugrue G, Zakrison TL, Dorigatti AE, Fiorelli RK, Malbrain MLNG. The role of point-of-care ultrasound in intra-abdominal hypertension management. Anaesthesiol Intensive Ther. 2017;49(5):373–81.
19. Arnold MJ, Jonas CE, Carter RE. Point-of-care ultrasonography. Am Fam Physician. 2020;101(5):275–85.
20. Brass P, Hellmich M, Kolodziej L, Schick G, Smith AF. Ultrasound guidance versus anatomical landmarks for internal jugular vein catheterization. Cochrane Database Syst Rev. 2015;1(1):CD006962.
21. Brass P, Hellmich M, Kolodziej L, Schick G, Smith AF. Ultrasound guidance versus anatomical landmarks for subclavian or femoral vein catheterization. Cochrane Database Syst Rev. 2015;1(1):CD011447.
22. Abu-Zidan FM, Cevik AA. Diagnostic point-of-care ultrasound (POCUS) for gastrointestinal pathology: state of the art from basics to advanced. World J Emerg Surg. 2018;13:47.
23. Carroll PJ, Gibson D, El-Faedy O, Dunne C, Coffey C, Hannigan A, Walsh SR. Surgeon-performed ultrasound at the bedside for the detection of appendicitis and gallstones: systematic review and meta-analysis. Am J Surg. 2013;205:102–8.
24. Sharif S, Skitch S, Vlahaki D, Healey A. Point-of-care ultrasound to diagnose appendicitis in a Canadian emergency department. CJEM. 2018;20(5):732–5.
25. Pereira J, Bass GA, Mariani D, et al. Surgeon-performed point-of-care ultrasound for acute cholecystitis: indications and limitations: a European Society for Trauma and Emergency Surgery (ESTES) consensus statement. Eur J Trauma Emerg Surg. 2020;46:173–83.
26. Menegozzo CAM, Utiyama EM. Steering the wheel towards the standard of care: proposal of a step-by-step ultrasound-guided emergency chest tube drainage and literature review. Int J Surg. 2018;56:315–9.
27. Nooitgedacht J, Haaksma M, Touw HRW, Tuinman PR. Perioperative care with an ultrasound device is as Michael Jordan with Scotty Pippen: at its best! J Thorac Dis. 2018;10(12):6436–41. https://doi.org/10.21037/jtd.2018.12.82.
28. Peltrini R, Cantoni V, Green R, Greco PA, Calabria M, Bucci L, Corcione F. Efficacy of transversus abdominis plane (TAP) block in colorectal surgery: a systematic review and meta-analysis. Tech Coloproctol. 2020;24(8):787–802.
29. Gao T, Zhang JJ, Xi FC, Shi JL, Lu Y, Tan SJ, Yu WK. Evaluation of transversus abdominis plane (TAP) block in hernia surgery: a meta-analysis. Clin J Pain. 2017;33(4):369–75.
30. Dhanjal S, Tonder S. Quadratus lumborum block. In: StatPearls. Treasure Island: StatPearls Publishing; 2020.
31. Ueshima H, Otake H, Lin JA. Ultrasound-guided quadratus lumborum block: an updated review of anatomy and techniques. Biomed Res Int. 2017;2017:2752876.
32. Akerman M, Pejčić N, Veličković I. A review of the Quadratus lumborum block and ERAS. Front Med (Lausanne). 2018;5:44.

Further Reading

Acute Care Surgery Book, vol. 1. Chapter 19. General aspects. Non-gastrointestinal and critical care emergencies. Springer; 2017.
Intensive Care for Emergency Surgeons. Chapter 16. Hot topics in acute care surgery and trauma. Springer; 2019.

Systemic Response to Injury

Philip F. Dobson, Karen Muller, and Zsolt J. Balogh

8.1 Introduction

Learning Goals
- To understand the effects of traumatic injury to tissues and cells and pro-inflammatory and anti-inflammatory mechanisms.
- To understand the concept, the source, and effect of DAMPs in the pathogenesis of systemic inflammation associated with trauma.
- To understand how non-modifiable factors such as age and injury severity, as well as modifiable factors such as shock resuscitation, medication, and surgery, may affect the body's response to trauma.

8.1.1 The Burden of Trauma

Traumatic injury is the leading cause of injury in people under the age of 35 and accounts for 4.4 million deaths worldwide each year, which is 8% of all deaths [1, 2]. If not fatal, trauma can also cause a significant degree of disability with consequence to the patient and society at bio-psycho-social levels. This has been commonly described as "disability-adjusted life-years" (DALY) in an effort to quantify the years of life lost in poor health [3]. Unintentional injuries affect a significant proportion of young people with flow effects to their families, workplace, and world economy. Males are also more likely to be affected than females at an approximate ratio of 2:1. Low-income countries carry a significant proportion of this global injury burden which is only expected to increase with population growth and a mismatch in industrialization and safety provisions in these countries. Road traffic-related injuries (RTRI) are the cause for the vast majority of these trauma and the death rate due to RTRI is 3 times higher in low-income countries than high-income countries [4]. Even in high income countries, fatal and non-fatal trauma disproportionally affect people from poorer economic backgrounds. People from poorer economic backgrounds are also more likely to be malnourished or have co-morbidities such that their systemic response to injury is proportionally more significant and more likely to be fatal. The term and concept of polytrauma describe the disease in response to injury, which is

P. F. Dobson · K. Muller · Z. J. Balogh (✉)
Department of Traumatology, John Hunter Hospital and University of Newcastle,
Newcastle, NSW, Australia
e-mail: Philip.Dobson@health.nsw.gov.au;
Karen.Muller@health.nsw.gov.au;
Zsolt.Balogh@health.nsw.gov.au

associated with homeostatic disturbance, systemic inflammatory response, and dysfunction of uninjured organs [5]. The current consensus definition of polytrauma is based on significant injuries affecting at least 2 body regions, with physiological compromise and risk of organ dysfunction in uninjured organs [6, 7]. Patients sustaining polytrauma are at higher risk of morbidity and mortality than the summation of the expected outcomes of each individual injury [8].

8.1.2 Physiological Effects of Trauma

The human body's response to trauma is dependent on the severity of traumatic insult. An isolated stab wound causing haemorrhagic shock from a large vessel injury, or blunt polytrauma such as that seen in high speed car crashes, are two very different mechanisms of mechanical trauma but both will lead to a cascade of pathophysiological effects that constitute systemic inflammatory response syndrome (SIRS). Aside from these examples of mechanical trauma, cellular damage can also occur with thermal injuries and with localized ischaemic and reperfusion injuries. Traumatic shock can cause widespread tissue hypoperfusion and ischemia, the effects of which are compounded by protective mechanisms such as compensatory tachycardia and the stress hormone response, leading to direct and indirect cellular compromise [9]. Early initiation of appropriate resuscitation to restore microcirculation in this scenario attenuates the deleterious downstream effects of the physiological response to severe trauma. The intensity and impact on the organism vary depending on severity of injury and patient characteristics such as age, genetic makeup, and co-morbidities. Apart from primary prevention, even modern trauma care has no control over these non-modifiable factors, but SIRS can be attenuated by careful resuscitation and appropriate choice of medication, surgical interventions, and the timing and the invasiveness of the latter. Patient recovery following trauma is enhanced by taking steps to minimize systemic hyper-inflammation and by promoting reparative, anti-inflammatory processes. This chapter will summarize the pathophysiological mechanisms that underlie SIRS and the various patient and treatment-related factors which can augment it.

8.2 Modern Concepts on Systemic Response to Trauma

8.2.1 Cellular Damage

The human immune system, both innate and adaptive, is able to recognize invading pathogens such as bacteria, fungi, and viruses and mount appropriate immune responses quickly. The body is adept at distinguishing "self" from "non-self", and in normal homeostasis, cell turnover and death occur via mechanisms such as apoptosis (controlled cell death) and autophagy in which dying cells are engulfed and broken down in a controlled manner. However, in injury, cell membranes in traumatized tissue are disrupted and cellular contents, which the immune system is naïve to, are released into the systemic circulation, provoking an inflammatory response in which the body recognizes these antigens as pathogenic and a state of "injured versus intact self" ensues [10]. Damaged cells may also become necrotic if they sustain damage beyond their repair capabilities. This process involves changes in cellular shape, expansion of organelles within and de-condensation of nuclear chromatin, and ultimately cell lysis [11]. The subsequent immune response that occurs is designed to clear damaged cells and tissue in an effort to restore the body to its normal pre-injury state. Release of damage-associated molecular patterns (DAMPs), intra-cellular components such as nuclear DNA, histones, mitochondrial DNA, and mitochondrial peptides into the systemic circulation occurs when cellular membrane damage or necrosis occurs [10, 12]. DAMPs are molecules, which are normally not exposed to the surveillance of the innate immune system and are thought to be significant mediating molecules to trigger the innate immune system in response to trauma, via cellular, and humoral mechanisms. Examples of the better characterized DAMPS beyond nucleic acids include high mobility box protein (HMGB1), cardiolipid, uric acid, mitochondrial inner membrane proteins, S100A proteins and histones, heat shock proteins, and even adenosine tri-phosphate (ATP) [12, 13]. In traumatic injury, the immune system may also be exposed to pathogen-associated molecular patterns (PAMPs) from infectious agents such as bacteria, fungi, or viruses [14]. In addition to this, neutrophils and other immune cells which are activated in response to tissue injury release inflammatory mediators such as interleukins and DAMPs, the overall effects of which is vigorous activation of the innate immune system [15, 16]. In response to DAMPs/PAMPs, the complement system is activated resulting in release of potent humoral factors, C3a, C5a, and C5b-9, the serum concentrations of which correlate with severity of inflammation [17, 18]. This further enhances the inflammatory response with further production, mobilization and extravasation of immune cells with delayed apoptosis, release of tumour necrosis factor, and interleukins such as IL-1α, IL-1β, and IL-6, the overall effects of which are to generate the systemic response frequently termed SIRS [13, 19, 20]. SIRS is a uniform response to polytrauma and clinically characterized by physiological derangements such as elevated heart rate, hypothermia or hyperthermia, tachypnoea, and changes in numbers of circulating white blood cells. While SIRS mobilizes the resources of the host and is essential for survival, if it is uncontrolled it can lead to severe secondary organ damage even in uninjured organs, and can result in lethal complications like sepsis and postinjury multiple organ failure [21].

8.2.2 Pro-inflammatory and Anti-inflammatory Responses

In addition to intra-cellular components being released following tissue trauma via cellular damage and necrosis, platelets become activated by circulating pro-inflammatory mediators as well as through activation of the clotting cascade. The serine protease system which is made up of the complement, coagulation, and kinin cascade is rapidly activated following trauma due to detection of DAMPs and PAMPs, and the effects of this system are intensified in acidotic patients. Leukocytes also release microvesicles which enhances leukocyte adhesion, systemic inflammation, and activation of the clotting system [20]. Activated platelets release additional pro-inflammatory mediators, further stimulating the immune response [22]. Pro-inflammatory cytokines also cause upregulation of neutrophil activity, which via the release of proteases, cause further cellular damage, not just of already injured tissues, but also to otherwise healthy tissues and organs [23, 24]. Simultaneously activated protective mechanisms to maintain homeostatic control over SIRS exist, predominantly via the release of anti-inflammatory cytokines such as transforming growth factor beta, interleukin 10, and cytokine antagonists, which serve to tether the activity of pro-inflammatory cells and mediators [25]. The compensatory anti-inflammatory response syndrome (CARS) is intense and can result in prolonged immunosuppression following traumatic injury [26]. The processes of SIRS and CARS are believed to occur simultaneously [27]. Depending on the level of pro-inflammatory stimulus, these protective factors may serve to entirely suppress systemic inflammation and return the body to a normal physiological state, or persistent inflammation, immunosuppression, and catabolism syndrome (PICS) may occur [28]. Suppressing DAMPs (SAMPs) are also produced by activated leukocytes and macrophages when injury occurs. In parallel to the pro-inflammatory response caused by the release of DAMPs, SAMPs trigger anti-inflammatory processes. SAMPs such as prostaglandin E2 and AnxA1 have been shown to promote CARS [29]. The prolonged nonspecific innate immune response that occurs during the SIRS response delays adequate adaptive immune response, which also creates vulnerability to pathogens and ensuing sepsis. Circulating pathogens stimulate the inflammatory response further, perpetuating the systemic response, putting the host at risk of sepsis, and multiple organ failure. The high susceptibility to infection following severe trauma has been attributed to the immunosuppressive effects of CARS [27]. CARS is thought to be a homeostatic process designed to prevent damage to organs distant from the site of injury caused by SIRS. The magnitude of CARS tends to be proportional to SIRS, which means that patients with more severe SIRS are more likely to develop secondary infections [30]. This is further confounded by changes in the adaptive immune system in which a change in balance from T-helper cell type Th1, to a Th2 type immune response occurs in conjunction with reduced T cell function following trauma and suppression of T cell effector functions. In addition, reduced generation of cytokines and an increased number of myeloid derived suppressor cells occur, as does decreased expression of HLA-DR in macrophages contributing to the suppressed immune response in trauma [13, 28]. If a severe enough traumatic insult occurs, an imbalance can occur with regard to the inflammatory response and the mechanisms that counter this, leading to prolonged SIRS and increased risk of multiple organ failure. Increased levels of DAMPs systemically have been shown to positively correlate with morbidity and mortality in animals and humans which have been subject to traumatic or surgical insults. Conversely, in vivo studies have shown that the use of antibodies or small molecules to block DAMPs leads to a reduction in the incidence of organ failure and sepsis.

The stress response to trauma incudes activation of the hypothalamus-pituitary-adrenal axis, leading to release of dehydroepiandrosterone (DHEA), its sulphated ester DHEAS, and cortisol from the adrenal glands. Cortisol release initially mobilizes existing neutrophil granulocytes from the bone marrow, but in general it inhibits the immune responses, both innate and adaptive, the effects of which is designed to be anti-inflammatory. However, following severe trauma and the sustained SIRS that can follow, DHEAS levels fall and a resultant increased ratio of cortisol to DHEA occurs, which is associated with increased risk of infection [31, 32].

Traumatic brain injury contributes to SIRS, not just directly from the effects of cellular damage, but also indirectly through parasympathetic and sympathetic pathways. Local cellular damage activates neutrophils, platelets, and the complement system [33]. Activation of the sympathetic pathway heightens SIRS via its effects on the adrenal glands, and subsequent steroid and catecholamine release. Activation of the parasympathetic nervous system, in addition, also inhibits the immune system. The integrity of the blood brain barrier is compromised by endothelial damage caused by pro-inflammatory cytokines and allows further inflammatory mediators to enter contributing to further neuro inflammation and neuronal damage and loss [34].

8.2.3 Mitochondria

Mitochondria are found in all nucleated mammalian cells and most eukaryotic cells. The functions of mitochondria are numerous and include energy production for all cellular processes in the form ATP via the process of oxidative phosphorylation, cell metabolism via the citric acid cycle, calcium homeostasis, iron-sulphur cluster biogenesis, apoptosis, and the urea cycle. The most commonly accepted evolutionary theory of mitochondrial existence is one of endosymbiosis by which mitochondria are thought to have arisen following the engulfment of a bacterial endosymbiont or α-proteobacterium by a precursor of the modern eukaryotic cell, most likely an Archeabacterium [35]. Mitochondria contain their own 16,596 base pair circular genome, which is present in cells in multiple copies. A mammalian cell contains around 1000–10,000 copies of the mitochondrial genome [36] with around 6–10 copies contained within protein complexes called nucleoids [37] which exist in abundance within mitochondria.

Cellular damage, such as that which occurs in trauma, due to tissue damage or hypoxia, leads to the sustained release of cell-free mitochondrial DNA (cf-mtDNA) into the systemic circulation [38, 39]. Traumatic release of mtDNA stimulates the innate immune response via Toll-like receptor 9 (TLR-9) and plays a significant role in the development of the inflammatory response following injury [40, 41]. mtDNA shares some characteristics of bacterial DNA, such as its circular form and high concentration of unmethylated CpG islands, and this is thought to contribute to the potent immune-stimulatory effect [12]. Severe trauma leads to high concentrations of mtDNA being released from tissues, and several studies have demonstrated an association between cf-mtDNA and post-traumatic complications, with a positive correlation between cf-mtDNA concentration, injury severity, and mortality [39, 42, 43]. In addition to mtDNA contained within mitochondria, mitochondria also contain several other DAMPs such as transcription factor A (TFAM), Cytochrome c, N-formyl-peptides, and adenosine triphosphate (ATP). Mitochondrial DAMPs such as mtDNA activate leukocytes and are also thought to contribute to increased endothelial permeability during systemic inflammation [44].

Metabolically active cells with higher energy requirements (brain, striated muscle, liver) usually contain more mitochondria. While platelets contain approximately 4 mitochondria per cell, skeletal muscle cells contain approximately 5000 mitochondria per cell, which suggests that skeletal muscle trauma is likely to lead to release of a large number of cf-mtDNA and consequently a larger inflammatory response than low-energy bone or skin injuries where mitochondrial content is less [45]. However, the anatomical origin of cf-mtDNA remains unknown. The fact that increasing plasma concentrations of mt-DNA occur after trauma and surgical interventions means it is likely that living functional cells at the site of injury are likely to be the source via an active secretion process. SIRS has been shown to be associated with increased levels of cf-mtDNA and its return to baseline levels correlates with subsequent clinical recovery adding further credence to this theory. A secondary source of mt-DNA is also thought to arise from secondary active release of mt-DNA by immune cells and platelets which are drawn into the zone of injury, which explains the continued increase in plasma mtDNA concentration in the days following injury, despite a subsidence in cell necrosis markers [44]. Delayed reperfusion of injured tissue may also contribute to increasing serum concentrations of mtDNA following injury, as mtDNA sequestered in injured tissue is released [40, 46, 47].

Further cellular injury occurs in relation to excessive reactive oxygen species (ROS) production secondary to tissue hypoxia [47]. ROS produced by mitochondria are a natural by-product of aerobic respiration and they usually occur during the process of oxidative phosphorylation during reactions involving oxygen molecules and electron transfer. Although ROS are known to act as important signalling molecules within cells, they are also potentially harmful and consequently, cells have evolved several anti-oxidative mechanisms to counteract their potentially damaging effects. In normal physiology, a balance between creation and scavenging of ROS exists [48]. When excessive production of ROS occurs such as in severe tissue injury, protective mechanisms are overburdened, and mitochondria begin to swell and lyse. Oxidized mtDNA accumulates in cell cytosol and can trigger further cell injury. Following injury, post shock hypermetabolism and a hypercatabolic state occur which are associated with increased oxygen consumption, mitochondrial activity, and ROS production. Apoptosis of inflammatory cells is attenuated contributing to prolongation of their activity [49–51].

The prevalent role of mitochondria in SIRS means that mitochondrial DAMPs may be important therapeutic targets to reduce the immune response to trauma [38]. Therapeutics to counteract increased ROS production associated with trauma is also a theoretical possibility.

8.2.4 Neutrophil Extracellular Traps

Neutrophils are an ancient component of the innate immune system, and one of the first lines of defence against invading pathogens. These fully differentiated cells migrate to areas of infection or inflammation in response to local cytokine release where they have the capability of engulfing pathogens [52]. More recent discoveries have shed light on the ability of neutrophils to form neutrophil extracellular traps (NETs) which represent an additional weapon in the innate immune systems arsenal. NETs have been shown to be present within the blood of patients who have sustained trauma, as well as in other disease states such as sepsis, appendicitis, pre-eclampsia, necrotizing fasciitis, systemic lupus erythematous, and cancer [44, 53–55]. They are capable of trapping gram-negative and gram-positive organisms, in addition to fungi. NET formation has been proposed via different methods, one via "netosis" in which NET formation occurs when neutrophil death occurs, and one in which viable neutrophils actively produce NETs. NETS are web-like structures, formed from chromatin derived from DNA, in addition to histones and proteins. NETosis is thought to occur in trauma in response to circulating DAMPs and platelet activation. The process contributes to systemic inflammation and risk of MOF in which NETs compromise blood flow and precipitate thrombus formation within the microcirculation. cf-mtDNA has been shown to stimulate NET production directly, which has the potential to be a self-perpetuating process, with subsequent cellular damage leading to release of more cf-mtDNA. Interestingly, NETs produced by viable neutrophils contain only mtDNA, whereas those produced by "netosis" contain a mixture of nuclear and mitochondrial DNA [53, 56].

8.2.5 DNA

Nucleic acids from DNA and RNA are also released into the circulation following tissue damage or cell necrosis caused by trauma [57, 58]. Toll-like receptors (TLRs) are evolutionary conserved pattern recognition receptors (PRR) which usually detect microbial products mediate inflammatory response in relation to these particles, triggering the innate immune response [13]. Cell-free DNA (cfDNA) can be released by various host cells such as neutrophils and macrophages, as well as certain strains of bacteria. Increased levels of circulating cfDNA occur within the first 24 h of trauma, and increased levels of circulating nuclear DNA have been shown to correlate with leukocyte gene expression and clinical outcomes [58]. cfDNA also has prothrombotic effects; NETS which are made up of DNA strands, histones and antimicrobial proteins, stimulate thrombus formation. The procoagulant effects of DNA binding proteins such as histones and HMGB1 which are released into the circulation after cell death are believed to be involved in the pathogenesis of trauma-associated coagulopathy [13].

8.3 Patient Factors

8.3.1 Age

For any given level of severity of trauma, increased age has been shown to be an independent risk factor for mortality and worse prognosis, not just in humans but also in animal models. In humans, the relation of age to poorer prognosis persists even when outcome measures are adjusted for patient co-morbidities [59]. The mechanism for the impaired healing response to traumatic insults observed in older people is poorly understood, although it is thought to be related to a combination of impaired physiological reserve, in addition to a heightened SIRS, and possible impairment in the body's ability to produce anti-inflammatory cytokines. Inflammageing is a term used to describe the phenomenon of persistent low grade levels of inflammation observed in elderly people and it has been speculated that the associated heightened level of baseline cytokines contributes to the heightened response to trauma, either because of the relatively increased circulating concentrations of cytokines that ensue, or because of immune system "priming" by the elevated baseline cytokine levels [60, 61]. Mitochondrial DNA (mtDNA) mutations are known to accumulate with advancing age. Accumulating evidence suggests that these may be intrinsic to the ageing process [36]. These mtDNA mutations may play a role in the exaggerated SIRS, either because they contribute to the reduced cellular and tissue physiological reserve and impaired reparative mechanisms, or because mutations within mtDNA released into the systemic circulation from damaged cells cause an enhanced immune response. In addition to these factors, due to a decline in effectiveness of the innate and adaptive immune system response, an increasing vulnerability to pathogens occurs with advancing age [62]. Age-associated changes in ACTH and cortisol secretion, leading to relative glucocorticoid excess, also attenuate the stress response and contribute to an impaired ability to recover from traumatic insults. Dehydroepiandrosterone (DHEA), secreted by the adrenal glands, acts to enhance immune function, but decreases significantly with advancing age, falling to approximately 30% of peak values in women and 20% in men by the age of 70–80 [63]. The increased ratio of cortisol to DHEA in older patients may contribute to inflammageing and the exaggerated inflammatory response to trauma [31].

8.3.2 Genetic Predisposition

The inflammatory responses evoked by a particular injury pattern can vary dramatically between patients. While factors such as age are clearly significant, the systemic response to injury is also heavily influenced by genetic factors, with some patients being predisposed to more severe adverse outcomes after trauma than others. Susceptibility to SIRS following trauma also appears to be affected by ethnicity with one study showing that in patients admitted to ICU with ISS >15, Caucasians were significantly more likely to develop SIRS than their African American counterparts [64]. This finding may relate to variations in genetic polymorphisms between patients. Some cytokine genetic polymorphisms of IL-1β, IL-6, and TNF-α have been shown to be linked to inflammatory disease processes such as sepsis, pneumonia and arthritis [65]. Certain polymorphisms in the promoter region of the TNF-α gene are associated with increased production of TNF-α. This in conjunction with some polymorphisms of TNF-β have been associated with an increased incidence of sepsis and poorer outcome after major trauma, burns, and sepsis. Some polymorphisms within the IL-6 allele confer a survival advantage in patients suffering with post-operative sepsis and reduced IL-6 levels during inflammatory processes. Conversely, other polymorphisms of the IL-6 allele predispose to increased mortality and organ dysfunction in SIRS [66]. Stimulation of human blood cultures with bacterial antigens invokes varying responses in IL-10 production depending on the IL-10 haplotype present within the allele [67]. The development of sepsis following trauma has also been shown to be more likely with particular interferon-γ alleles. In addition, polymorphisms within regulatory genes are thought to affect cytokine release, including promotors of IL-6, IL-10, and IL-18 [66].

8.3.3 Co-morbidities

Diabetes poses a huge health care burden and patients affected by it have been shown to have worse outcomes in acute illnesses, regardless of the severity of the initial illness [68]. Higher complication rates have been shown to occur in patients with acute stroke, myocardial infarctions, and in cardiothoracic surgery, when compared to patients without diabetes [69–71]. In the context of trauma, a retrospective analysis compared almost 12,500 diabetic patients admitted to trauma centres and matched these by age, sex, and ISS to a patient group of equal number without diabetes. The study showed that patients affected by diabetes were associated with a higher number of days spent on ICU and on ventilation, with a significantly higher complication rate (23.0% in diabetes group vs 14.0% in the non-diabetes group [OR 1.80; 95% confidence interval, 1.69–1.92]). This included infectious and non-infectious complications. However, the mortality rate and overall length of hospital stay were not significantly different [72]. Hyperglycaemia is thought to attenuate the innate immune response, with consequent impairment of cellular function including impairment of cellular adhesion, chemotaxis, phagocytosis, and oxidative burst [73, 74]. Glycaemic control in critically ill patients has been shown to reduce the incidence of infection, sepsis, renal failure, number of days requiring ventilatory support, and mortality [75, 76].

Patients with background adrenal insufficiency are not able to mount normal responses to trauma, and acute adrenal insufficiency can also occur as a result of trauma. Haemorrhagic shock has been shown to be associated with hyperacute adrenal insufficiency (HAI) and mortality [77]. Approximately half of patients with moderate to severe traumatic brain injuries also demonstrate adrenal insufficiency [78]. In the context of septic shock, treatment of adrenal insufficiency is associated with improved outcomes [79]. However, in trauma, although adrenal insufficiency is a recognized phenomenon and the degree of impairment has been shown to correlate with ISS, there are no high-quality studies to demonstrate a survival benefit in adrenal replacement therapy in patients who have sustained significant trauma. However, consideration and assessment of adrenal function should be made in the context of trauma, and when deemed appropriate, adrenal replacement therapy should be considered.

8.4 Surgical and Resuscitative Factors

8.4.1 Surgery

Surgery causes injury to local tissue with a consequent release of mtDNA and other DAMPs from damaged cells and subsequent further release due to cell necrosis [80]. A move towards damage control orthopaedics occurred many years ago, in an effort to curtail the increased SIRS associated with the traumatic insult of surgery in addition to that caused by the initial injury [81]. Early total care was deemed to only be appropriate in patients who were haemodynamically normal with no signs of significant physiological compromise, with some evidence suggesting that more severely injured patients were at increased risk of acute lung injury when this strategy was implemented [82]. However, in more recent years, evidence suggests that damage control orthopaedics does not appear to be superior to early total care except from situations of extremis. These advances have been aided by better resuscitative strategies which improve patient's physiological reserve prior to surgical intervention such as improved haemostatic resuscitation techniques and lung protective ventilation, which helps to prevent pressure-induced lung injury. Surgery, however, should still be appropriately timed simultaneously or shortly after initial efforts to restore microcirculation. Higher concentrations of mtDNA have been identified in patients undergoing major pelvic surgery when compared to minimally invasive surgery [80]. Elevated levels of mtDNA have also been identified in patients who have undergone cardiopulmonary bypass surgery, and high quantities of mtDNA occur in femoral reamings from patients undergoing femoral intramedullary nail fracture fixation [44]. Even endotracheal intubation is associated with increased concentrations of mtDNA in throat lavage, with higher concentrations evident in patients who report throat discomfort or pain following intubation [83]. Higher concentrations of mtDNA have been shown to be associated with post-operative complications [84]. Careful surgical planning is imperative when dealing with polytrauma patients. For example when dealing with a mangled extremity with significant soft tissue damage and fractures, attempts at surgical reconstruction will lead to a prolonged inflammatory response secondary to ongoing DAMPs and mtDNA release, whereas limb amputation will lead to quicker resolution of systemic inflammation. Likewise, removal of necrotic tissue and the released mtDNA within it curtail persistent release of immunostimulatory factors into the systemic circulation. The nature of the surgery will determine the overall effect on the systemic response and must be considered carefully to avoid a significant second hit, especially in patients who have poor physiological reserve or in those individuals who have not been adequately resuscitated.

8.4.2 Medication

Various therapies, some of which are in common use, and modifications to current treatments can modulate the systemic response to injury. These include drugs such as tranexamic acid, and hydrocortisone, as well as fluids and blood products used for volume resuscitation. Toll like receptors (TLRs) play an important role in the detection of invading pathogens and in DAMP detection. Opioids offer powerful analgesic effects, but are well known to suppress natural killer cell activity via opioid receptor activation and TLR4 signalling, the effects of which are to impair innate immunity activity against pathogens [85]. Volatile anaesthetic agents have also been shown to modulate TLR2 and TLR4 function, with isoflurane and sevoflurane both attenuating TLR4 function. Recent work has demonstrated that while sevoflurane effects TLR2 function, isoflurane, propofol, and dexmedetomidine do not when used at normal concentrations [86].

Tranexamic acid is now used routinely in trauma following the results of the CRASH-2 trial which demonstrated a survival benefit when tranexamic acid was used early in traumatic injury [87]. Tranexamic acid competitively inhibits the conversion of plasminogen to plasmin, the downstream effect of which is to inhibit fibrin degradation. Plasmin is a stimulator of the complement arm of the immune system and fibrin degradation products provoke the inflammatory response further. The reduced production of these factors secondary to the use of tranexamic acid is likely to dampen SIRS and may be key in the pathophysiological mechanisms leading to the reduced mortality rates associated with its use. The results of the recent PATCH trial, designed to assess the effects of tranexamic acid given in the pre-hospital setting vs placebo, will be of significant interest.

The use of steroids in trauma is not routinely recommended, although one RCT reported that systemic hydrocortisone significantly reduced the rates of hospital acquired pneumonia and the number of days requiring mechanical ventilation [88]. In contrast to these findings, the CRASH-1 study demonstrated that steroids increased mortality when administered to patients who had sustained head injuries, a finding which is thought to be related to the systemic immunosuppressive effects of steroids [89].

Prophylactic antibiotics have been shown to reduce the risk of respiratory tract infections in critically ill trauma patients, when combined with selective gut decontamination, although no significant reduction in mortality was observed in this study [90]. In trauma patients who have sustained open fractures, antibiotics have been shown to significantly reduce infection rates [91].

Many different targets for treatment have been designed to inhibit the effects of pro-inflammatory mediators, but their results in clinical practice have not been convincing. For example, recombinant human-activated protein C and drotrecogin-α have failed to show significant effects in clinical trials [92]. Prostaglandin E1, intended to suppress neutrophil activity, showed no significant effect on mortality in patients with sepsis or respiratory failure [93]. Antioxidants designed to minimize damage caused by free radicals and ROS in trauma have shown some promise [94].

8.4.3 Traumatic Shock Resuscitation

There has been an increased focus on the early use of blood products for volume resuscitation following trauma in recent years, rather than the use of large volumes of crystalloid or colloid fluids. Massive transfusion protocols vary between trauma units, but in general a balanced resuscitation strategy is favoured in terms of blood product administration. The Pragmatic Randomized Optimal Platelet and Plasma Ratios (PROPPR) Trial was an RCT which aimed to establish the optimal ratio of transfused blood products in trauma. The study randomized 680 haemorrhagic patients and to either 1:1:1 or 1:1:2 (plasma, platelets, red blood cells) transfusion protocols. The study found that exsanguination, the predominant cause of death within the first 24 h, was significantly decreased in the 1:1:1 group (9.2% vs 14.6%; [95% CI, −10.4% to −0.5%]; $p = 0.03$). More haemostasis was also achieved in the 1:1:1 group also (86% vs 78%, respectively; $p = 0.006$) [95]. Plasma transfusion in trauma has also been shown to be beneficial in restoring damaged glycolax. High concentrations of catecholamine release associated with significant trauma result in redistribution of blood flow, platelet activation, and release of procoagulant and profibrinolytic factors from the endothelium. These factors can lead to direct damage of endothelium and the endothelial glycolax which protects the endothelium and helps to maintain its barrier function. This is also why the vasoconstrictive effects of some inotropes can potentially have a damaging effect on glycolax. Circulating levels of syndecan-1 and heparan sulfate are proportionally related to the amount of glycolax damage which occurs.

Glycolax damage has been shown to be associated with reduced thrombin generation, coagulopathy, and death. Early resuscitation using plasma rather than lactated Ringer's solution has been shown to be beneficial in glycolax restoration in animal models. Clinical studies in humans also suggest that plasma transfusion restores glycolax in patients with haemorrhagic shock, with plasma syndecan-1 levels being found to decrease following resuscitation with plasma [96].

Early volume replacement is beneficial as it optimizes blood pressure, end organ perfusion, and tissue oxygenation, which all serve to limit acidosis at the tissue level and therefore the perpetuation of SIRS. Early restoration of endothelial glycolax associated with plasma transfusion also appears to be beneficial in attenuating the deleterious effects of trauma, as described. The use of a restrictive blood transfusion strategy rather than liberal transfusion of red blood cells is advocated after the initial resuscitation phase on the ICU, as this has been shown to be associated with a lower risk of infection and mortality in surgical and critically ill patients [97, 98]. Some studies have also shown that the use of blood products which have been stored for 14 days or more is associated with higher risk of infection [99, 100].

Many traumatologists advocate the use of a permissive hypotensive strategy, with an aim to maintain systolic blood pressure in the region of 90 mm Hg in the early phase of trauma, the purpose of which is to allow clot formation and stabilization. However, prolonged periods of hypotension impair end organ perfusion and once haemostasis has been achieved, efforts should be made to restore blood pressure. Alternatives to blood products for fluid resuscitation can have adverse effects on patient physiology due to their stimulatory effects on the immune system. Starch for example has been shown to cross endothelia which has been damaged by SIRS, the effects of which can be deleterious [101]. The use of normal saline has also been shown to be associated with higher mortality rates than Hartmann's solution or albumin. The use of crystalloid solutions for volume replacement in trauma patients should be limited as much as possible, with an aim to replace lost volume with blood products, ideally limiting the use of crystalloid to 1 L at most in the early stages following traumatic injury. Activation of neutrophils and increased expression of adhesion molecules have been shown to occur with exposure to crystalloid and artificial colloid solutions in a dose responsive manner, although human albumin solutions do not appear to have the same effect [102]. Lactated Ringer's solution is associated with increased systemic inflammation, vascular permeability, and lung injury after haemorrhagic shock, compared to resuscitation with fresh whole blood in an animal model [103]. Clinical studies in humans have also shown that in patients requiring massive transfusion, using crystalloids to packed red blood cells at a ratio greater than 1.5:1 is independently associated with a higher risk of MOF, ARDS, and abdominal compartment syndrome [104]. In another animal model of haemorrhagic shock, resuscitation with normal saline has been shown to significantly increase endothelial permeability and leukocyte rolling and adhesion when compared to lactated Ringer's solution, but restoration of endothelial glycolax was not restored with either. The work suggested that administration of normal saline actually contributed to ongoing shedding of the endothelial glycolax [105].

However, despite the apparent clear advantages of blood products in traumatic shock resuscitation, there are some associated risks with massive blood transfusion in which the entirety of patients circulating blood volume can sometimes be replaced with what is essentially allogenic graft material. The potential deleterious immune-modulatory characteristics of blood transfusion are consistently reported as an independent predictor of postinjury complications such as sepsis, MOF, and poor outcomes [98]. Allogenic transfusions can have several additional negative effects on postinjury homeostasis, which include but not limited to a shift to the left in the oxygen dissociation curve, acid-base imbalance, hypothermia, hypocalcaemia, and coagulopathy. These adverse effects are predictable and partially preventable with proactive care and optimized conditions. Transfusion-related complications should be monitored for and dealt with appropriately.

Dos and Don'ts

Do
- Avoid exacerbation of SIRS with early, effective resuscitation.
- Aim to restore microcirculatory function with balanced blood and blood component resuscitation instead of focusing on gross indicators of central circulation
- Judicious, well-timed, and measured surgical interventions, which reduce blood loss, eliminate contamination, and curtail further release of DAMPs, are essential parts of early resuscitation

Don't
- Do not use crystalloid solutions in excess in trauma resuscitation to restore blood pressure
- Do not use medications which may impair the immune response or exacerbate SIRS, if they can be avoided

Avoid unnecessary, non-essential surgery, which adds to the tissue damage and homeostatic derangement instead of controlling those

Take-Home Messages
- Trauma causes a significant burden of death and disability, particularly in younger and more disadvantaged populations.
- Polytrauma is a unique disease in response to severe mechanical injury characterized by tissue injury to multiple body regions, physiological compromise, systemic inflammatory response, and dysfunction of even uninjured organ systems
- The injured "self" via DAMPs is a key underlying mechanism of SIRS and pathological responses in polytrauma.
- Appropriately attenuating SIRS to trauma with traumatic shock resuscitation, medications, transfusions, and surgery can improve outcomes and recovery times for patients affected by major trauma.

Multiple Choice Questions

1. Opioids and volatile anaesthetic agents impair the function of the innate immune system via attenuation of which toll-like receptor?
   A. TLR2
   B. **TLR4**
   C. TLR6
   D. TLR8

2. Tranexamic acid work by what mechanism?
   A. Promotion of intrinsic pathway
   B. Promotion of extrinsic pathway
   C. **Inhibition of conversion of plasminogen to plasmin**
   D. Promotion of fibrin degradation

3. Effective strategies in the routine care of trauma patients may include?
   A. Pressure controlled ventilation, transfusion as required in ratios of 1:1:1 (plasma, platelets red blood cells), routine use of systemic hydrocortisone
   B. Volume controlled ventilation, transfusion ratio of 1:1:2, recombinant activated protein C
   C. **Volume controlled ventilation, transfusion ratio of 1:1:1, opiates for pain control**
   D. Pressure controlled ventilation, transfusion ration of 1:2:1, tranexamic acid

4. The systemic response to trauma includes the following:
   A. **Increased ratio of cortisol to DHEA**
   B. Inhibition of serine protease system
   C. Impaired leukocyte adhesion
   D. Reduction in circulating complement factors

5. Which of the following is true:
   A. Mitochondria consume reactive oxygen species via the process of oxidative phosphorylation
   B. Trauma without infection does not cause formation of neutrophil extracellular trap formation (NET)

C. **Circulating levels of syndecan-1 and heparan sulfate are proportionally related to the amount of glycolax damage**
D. The use of vasoconstrictive inotropes can help to prevent endothelial glycolax damage

6. Which of the following are false
   A. Levels of DHEA decrease with advancing age contributing to an exaggerated inflammatory response
   B. The degree of adrenal impairment has been shown to correlate with Injury Severity Score, and evidence has shown that adrenal replacement therapy provides no survival advantage in severe trauma
   C. **Suppressing DAMPS (SAMPs) such as E2 and AnxA1 inhibit the compensatory anti-inflammatory response (CARS)**
   D. Decreased expression of HLA-DR in macrophages occurs during the systemic response to trauma, contributing to impaired immune function

7. Regarding trauma patients with diabetes which is true?
   A. **They will have a higher number of days spent in ICU and complication rate**
   B. They will have a higher mortality rate and overall length of stay in hospital
   C. Hypoglycaemia is thought to attenuate the innate immune response
   D. Good glycaemic control has minimal effects on rates of infection and sepsis

8. Polymorphisms in which of these genes may be associated with an increased survival advantage in patients with inflammatory disease processes?
   A. TNF-α
   B. TBF-β
   C. **IL-6**
   D. IL-1β

9. cfDNA increases in the first 24 h of trauma and has been shown to correlate with leukocyte gene expression, clinical outcomes, and also has prothrombotic effects. cfDNA can be released by:
   A. Neutrophils
   B. Macrophages
   C. Bacteria
   D. **All of the above**

10. Which is true of neutrophils?
    A. They migrate to areas of infection or inflammation in response to temperature
    B. **They can form NETS (Neutrophil extracellular traps) from both nuclear and mitochondrial DNA**
    C. They are one of the richest cells in mitochondria
    D. Neutrophils are not fully differentiated cells

11. The physiological response to trauma:
    A. **Depends on the severity and type of traumatic insult**
    B. Cannot be mitigated by haemostatic resuscitation
    C. Rarely occurs in thermal injuries
    D. Will not vary with genetic makeup

References

1. Injuries and violence. World Health Organization; 2021. https://www.who.int/news-room/fact-sheets/detail/injuries-and-violence.
2. Søreide K. Epidemiology of major trauma. Br J Surg. 2009;96(7):697–8.
3. Haagsma JA, Graetz N, Bolliger I, Naghavi M, Higashi H, Mullany EC, et al. The global burden of injury: incidence, mortality, disability-adjusted life years and time trends from the global burden of disease study 2013. Inj Prev. 2016;22(1):3–18.
4. World Health Organization. Global status report on road safety 2018: summary. Geneva: World Health Organization; 2018.
5. Keel M, Trentz O. Pathophysiology of polytrauma. Injury. 2005;36(6):691–709.
6. Butcher N, Balogh Z. Update on the definition of polytrauma. Eur J Trauma Emerg Surg. 2014;40(2):107–11.
7. Pape H-C, Lefering R, Butcher N, Peitzman A, Leenen L, Marzi I, et al. The definition of poly-

7. trauma revisited: an international consensus process and proposal of the new 'Berlin definition'. J Trauma Acute Care Surg. 2014;77(5):780–6.
8. Butcher N, Balogh ZJ. AIS> 2 in at least two body regions: a potential new anatomical definition of polytrauma. Injury. 2012;43(2):196–9.
9. Lenz A, Franklin GA, Cheadle WG. Systemic inflammation after trauma. Injury. 2007;38(12):1336–45.
10. Pugin J. How tissue injury alarms the immune system and causes a systemic inflammatory response syndrome. Ann Intensive Care. 2012;2(1):1–6.
11. Berghe TV, Vanlangenakker N, Parthoens E, Deckers W, Devos M, Festjens N, et al. Necroptosis, necrosis and secondary necrosis converge on similar cellular disintegration features. Cell Death Differ. 2010;17(6):922–30.
12. Zhang Q, Raoof M, Chen Y, Sumi Y, Sursal T, Junger W, et al. Circulating mitochondrial DAMPs cause inflammatory responses to injury. Nature. 2010;464(7285):104–7.
13. Relja B, Land WG. Damage-associated molecular patterns in trauma. Eur J Trauma Emerg Surg. 2020;46(4):751–75.
14. Bianchi ME. DAMPs, PAMPs and alarmins: all we need to know about danger. J Leukoc Biol. 2007;81(1):1–5.
15. Manson J, Thiemermann C, Brohi K. Trauma alarmins as activators of damage-induced inflammation. J Br Surg. 2012;99(Supplement_1):12–20.
16. Kovtun A, Messerer DA, Scharffetter-Kochanek K, Huber-Lang M, Ignatius A. Neutrophils in tissue trauma of the skin, bone, and lung: two sides of the same coin. J Immunol Res. 2018;2018:8173983.
17. Burk A-M, Martin M, Flierl MA, Rittirsch D, Helm M, Lampl L, et al. Early complementopathy after multiple injuries in humans. Shock. 2012;37(4):348–54.
18. Hecke F, Schmidt U, Kola A, Bautsch W, Klos A, Kohl J. Circulating complement proteins in multiple trauma patients-correlation with injury severity, development of sepsis, and outcome. Crit Care Med. 1997;25(12):2015–24.
19. Hirsiger S, Simmen H-P, Werner CM, Wanner GA, Rittirsch D. Danger signals activating the immune response after trauma. Mediat Inflamm. 2012;2012:315941.
20. Huber-Lang M, Lambris JD, Ward PA. Innate immune responses to trauma. Nat Immunol. 2018;19(4):327–41.
21. Baue AE, Durham R, Faist E. Systemic inflammatory response syndrome (SIRS), multiple organ dysfunction syndrome (MODS), multiple organ failure (MOF): are we winning the battle? Shock. 1998;10(2):79–89.
22. Golebiewska EM, Poole AW. Platelet secretion: from haemostasis to wound healing and beyond. Blood Rev. 2015;29(3):153–62.
23. Fujishima S, Aikawa N. Neutrophil-mediated tissue injury and its modulation. Intensive Care Med. 1995;21(3):277–85.
24. Wang J. Neutrophils in tissue injury and repair. Cell Tissue Res. 2018;371(3):531–9.
25. Seok J, Warren HS, Cuenca AG, Mindrinos MN, Baker HV, Xu W, et al. Inflammation and host response to injury, large scale collaborative research program. Genomic responses in mouse models poorly mimic human inflammatory diseases. Proc Natl Acad Sci U S A. 2013;110(9):3507–12.
26. Adib-Conquy M, Cavaillon J-M. Compensatory anti-inflammatory response syndrome. Thromb Haemost. 2009;101(1):36–47.
27. Ward NS, Casserly B, Ayala A. The compensatory anti-inflammatory response syndrome (CARS) in critically ill patients. Clin Chest Med. 2008;29(4):617–25, viii.
28. Gentile LF, Cuenca AG, Efron PA, Ang D, McKinley BA, Moldawer LL, et al. Persistent inflammation and immunosuppression: a common syndrome and new horizon for surgical intensive care. J Trauma Acute Care Surg. 2012;72(6):1491.
29. Land WG. Use of DAMPs and SAMPs as therapeutic targets or therapeutics: a note of caution. Mol Diagn Ther. 2020;24(3):251–62.
30. Hotchkiss RS, Monneret G, Payen D. Immunosuppression in sepsis: a novel understanding of the disorder and a new therapeutic approach. Lancet Infect Dis. 2013;13(3):260–8.
31. Butcher SK, Killampalli V, Lascelles D, Wang K, Alpar EK, Lord JM. Raised cortisol: DHEAS ratios in the elderly after injury: potential impact upon neutrophil function and immunity. Aging Cell. 2005;4(6):319–24.
32. Wade C, Lindberg J, Cockrell J, Lamiell J, Hunt M, Ducey J, et al. Upon-admission adrenal steroidogenesis is adapted to the degree of illness in intensive care unit patients. J Clin Endocrinol Metabol. 1988;67(2):223–7.
33. Lu J, Goh SJ, Tng P, Deng YY, Ling E-A, Moochhala S. Systemic inflammatory response following acute traumatic brain injury. Front Biosci. 2009;14(1):3795–813.
34. Meisel C, Schwab JM, Prass K, Meisel A, Dirnagl U. Central nervous system injury-induced immune deficiency syndrome. Nat Rev Neurosci. 2005;6(10):775–86.
35. Lane N, Martin W. The energetics of genome complexity. Nature. 2010;467(7318):929–34.
36. Trifunovic A, Larsson NG. Mitochondrial dysfunction as a cause of ageing. J Intern Med. 2008;263(2):167–78.
37. Holt IJ, He J, Mao CC, Boyd-Kirkup JD, Martinsson P, Sembongi H, et al. Mammalian mitochondrial nucleoids: organizing an independently minded genome. Mitochondrion. 2007;7(5):311–21.
38. Tuboly E, McIlroy D, Briggs G, Lott N, Balogh ZJ. Clinical implications and pathological associations of circulating mitochondrial DNA. Front Biosci (Landmark Ed). 2017;22(6):1011–22.
39. Simmons JD, Lee YL, Mulekar S, Kuck JL, Brevard SB, Gonzalez RP, et al. Elevated levels of

plasma mitochondrial DNA DAMPs are linked to clinical outcome in severely injured human subjects. Ann Surg. 2013;258(4):591–6; discussion 6–8.
40. Xie L, Liu S, Cheng J, Wang L, Liu J, Gong J. Exogenous administration of mitochondrial DNA promotes ischemia reperfusion injury via TLR9-p38 MAPK pathway. Regul Toxicol Pharmacol. 2017;89:148–54.
41. Gu X, Wu G, Yao Y, Zeng J, Shi D, Lv T, et al. Intratracheal administration of mitochondrial DNA directly provokes lung inflammation through the TLR9-p38 MAPK pathway. Free Radic Biol Med. 2015;83:149–58.
42. Gu X, Yao Y, Wu G, Lv T, Luo L, Song Y. The plasma mitochondrial DNA is an independent predictor for post-traumatic systemic inflammatory response syndrome. PLoS One. 2013;8(8):e72834.
43. Yamanouchi S, Kudo D, Yamada M, Miyagawa N, Furukawa H, Kushimoto S. Plasma mitochondrial DNA levels in patients with trauma and severe sepsis: time course and the association with clinical status. J Crit Care. 2013;28(6):1027–31.
44. Thurairajah K, Briggs GD, Balogh ZJ. The source of cell-free mitochondrial DNA in trauma and potential therapeutic strategies. Eur J Trauma Emerg Surg. 2018;44(3):325–34.
45. Boudreau LH, Duchez AC, Cloutier N, Soulet D, Martin N, Bollinger J, et al. Platelets release mitochondria serving as substrate for bactericidal group IIA-secreted phospholipase A2 to promote inflammation. Blood. 2014;124(14):2173–83.
46. Hu Q, Ren H, Ren J, Liu Q, Wu J, Wu X, et al. Released mitochondrial DNA following intestinal ischemia reperfusion induces the inflammatory response and gut barrier dysfunction. Sci Rep. 2018;8(1):1–11.
47. Granger DN, Kvietys PR. Reperfusion injury and reactive oxygen species: the evolution of a concept. Redox Biol. 2015;6:524–51.
48. Zorov DB, Juhaszova M, Sollott SJ. Mitochondrial reactive oxygen species (ROS) and ROS-induced ROS release. Physiol Rev. 2014;94(3):909–50.
49. Stowe DF, Camara AKS. Mitochondrial reactive oxygen species production in excitable cells: modulators of mitochondrial and cell function. Antioxid Redox Signal. 2009;11(6):1373–414.
50. Ogunbileje JO, Porter C, Herndon DN, Chao T, Abdelrahman DR, Papadimitriou A, et al. Hypermetabolism and hypercatabolism of skeletal muscle accompany mitochondrial stress following severe burn trauma. Am J Physiol Endocrinol Metab. 2016;311(2):E436–E48.
51. Kroemer G, Galluzzi L, Brenner C. Mitochondrial membrane permeabilization in cell death. Physiol Rev. 2007;87(1):99–163.
52. Amulic B, Cazalet C, Hayes GL, Metzler KD, Zychlinsky A. Neutrophil function: from mechanisms to disease. Annu Rev Immunol. 2012;30:459–89.
53. Yousefi S, Mihalache C, Kozlowski E, Schmid I, Simon HU. Viable neutrophils release mitochondrial DNA to form neutrophil extracellular traps. Cell Death Differ. 2009;16(11):1438–44.
54. McIlroy DJ, Jarnicki AG, Au GG, Lott N, Smith DW, Hansbro PM, et al. Mitochondrial DNA neutrophil extracellular traps are formed after trauma and subsequent surgery. J Crit Care. 2014;29(6):1133.e1–5.
55. Papayannopoulos V. Neutrophil extracellular traps in immunity and disease. Nat Rev Immunol. 2018;18(2):134–47.
56. Brinkmann V, Reichard U, Goosmann C, Fauler B, Uhlemann Y, Weiss DS, et al. Neutrophil extracellular traps kill bacteria. Science. 2004;303(5663):1532–5.
57. Gögenur M, Burcharth J, Gögenur I. The role of total cell-free DNA in predicting outcomes among trauma patients in the intensive care unit: a systematic review. Crit Care. 2017;21(1):14.
58. Stortz JA, Hawkins RB, Holden DC, Raymond SL, Wang Z, Brakenridge SC, et al. Cell-free nuclear, but not mitochondrial, DNA concentrations correlate with the early host inflammatory response after severe trauma. Sci Rep. 2019;9(1):13648.
59. Lehmann R, Beekley A, Casey L, Salim A, Martin M. The impact of advanced age on trauma triage decisions and outcomes: a statewide analysis. Am J Surg. 2009;197(5):571–5.
60. Ferrucci L, Fabbri E. Inflammageing: chronic inflammation in ageing, cardiovascular disease, and frailty. Nat Rev Cardiol. 2018;15(9):505–22.
61. Franceschi C, Capri M, Monti D, Giunta S, Olivieri F, Sevini F, et al. Inflammaging and anti-inflammaging: a systemic perspective on aging and longevity emerged from studies in humans. Mech Ageing Dev. 2007;128(1):92–105.
62. Shaw AC, Goldstein DR, Montgomery RR. Age-dependent dysregulation of innate immunity. Nat Rev Immunol. 2013;13(12):875–87.
63. Yiallouris A, Tsioutis C, Agapidaki E, Zafeiri M, Agouridis AP, Ntourakis D, et al. Adrenal aging and its implications on stress responsiveness in humans. Front Endocrinol. 2019;10:54.
64. NeSmith EG, Weinrich SP, Andrews JO, Medeiros RS, Hawkins ML, Weinrich MC. Demographic differences in systemic inflammatory response syndrome score after trauma. Am J Crit Care. 2012;21(1):35–41.
65. Kany S, Vollrath JT, Relja B. Cytokines in inflammatory disease. Int J Mol Sci. 2019;20(23):6008.
66. Giannoudis P, Van Griensven M, Tsiridis E, Pape H. The genetic predisposition to adverse outcome after trauma. J Bone Joint Surg. 2007;89(10):1273–9.
67. Eskdale J, Gallagher G, Verweij CL, Keijsers V, Westendorp RG, Huizinga TW. Interleukin 10 secretion in relation to human IL-10 locus haplotypes. Proc Natl Acad Sci. 1998;95(16):9465–70.
68. Umpierrez GE, Isaacs SD, Bazargan N, You X, Thaler LM, Kitabchi AE. Hyperglycemia: an independent marker of in-hospital mortality in patients

69. Pulsinelli WA, Levy DE, Sigsbee B, Scherer P, Plum F. Increased damage after ischemic stroke in patients with hyperglycemia with or without established diabetes mellitus. Am J Med. 1983;74(4):540–4.
70. Malmberg K, Rydén L, Hamsten A, Herlitz J, Waldenström A, Wedel H. Mortality prediction in diabetic patients with myocardial infarction: experiences from the DIGAMI study. Cardiovasc Res. 1997;34(1):248–53.
71. Thourani VH, Weintraub WS, Stein B, Gebhart SS, Craver JM, Jones EL, et al. Influence of diabetes mellitus on early and late outcome after coronary artery bypass grafting. Ann Thorac Surg. 1999;67(4):1045–52.
72. Ahmad R, Cherry RA, Lendel I, Mauger DT, Service SL, Texter LJ, et al. Increased hospital morbidity among trauma patients with diabetes mellitus compared with age- and injury severity score–matched control subjects. Arch Surg. 2007;142(7):613–8.
73. Geerlings SE, Hoepelman AI. Immune dysfunction in patients with diabetes mellitus (DM). FEMS Immunol Med Microbiol. 1999;26(3–4):259–65.
74. Calvet HM, Yoshikawa TT. Infections in diabetes. Infect Dis Clin North Am. 2001;15(2):407–21, viii.
75. van den Berghe G, Wouters P, Weekers F, Verwaest C, Bruyninckx F, Schetz M, et al. Intensive insulin therapy in critically ill patients. N Engl J Med. 2001;345(19):1359–67.
76. Finney SJ, Zekveld C, Elia A, Evans TW. Glucose control and mortality in critically ill patients. JAMA. 2003;290(15):2041–7.
77. Stein DM, Jessie EM, Crane S, Kufera JA, Timmons T, Rodriguez CJ, et al. Hyperacute adrenal insufficiency after hemorrhagic shock exists and is associated with poor outcomes. J Trauma Acute Care Surg. 2013;74(2):363–70.
78. Cohan P, Wang C, McArthur DL, Cook SW, Dusick JR, Armin B, et al. Acute secondary adrenal insufficiency after traumatic brain injury: a prospective study. Crit Care Med. 2005;33(10):2358–66.
79. Annane D, Sébille V, Charpentier C, Bollaert PE, François B, Korach JM, et al. Effect of treatment with low doses of hydrocortisone and fludrocortisone on mortality in patients with septic shock. JAMA. 2002;288(7):862–71.
80. McIlroy DJ, Bigland M, White AE, Hardy BM, Lott N, Smith DW, et al. Cell necrosis-independent sustained mitochondrial and nuclear DNA release following trauma surgery. J Trauma Acute Care Surg. 2015;78(2):282–8.
81. Roberts CS, Pape H-C, Jones AL, Malkani AL, Rodriguez JL, Giannoudis PV. Damage control orthopaedics: evolving concepts in the treatment of patients who have sustained orthopaedic trauma. JBJS. 2005;87(2):434–49.
82. Pape H-C, Hildebrand F, Pertschy S, Zelle B, Garapati R, Grimme K, et al. Changes in the management of femoral shaft fractures in polytrauma patients: from early total care to damage control orthopedic surgery. J Trauma Acute Care Surg. 2002;53(3):452–62.
83. Puyo CA, Peruzzi D, Earhart A, Roller E, Karanikolas M, Kollef MH, et al. Endotracheal tube-induced sore throat pain and inflammation is coupled to the release of mitochondrial DNA. Mol Pain. 2017;13:1744806917731696.
84. Sandler N, Kaczmarek E, Itagaki K, Zheng Y, Otterbein L, Khabbaz K, et al. Mitochondrial DAMPs are released during cardiopulmonary bypass surgery and are associated with postoperative atrial fibrillation. Heart Lung Circulation. 2018;27(1):122–9.
85. Maher DP, Walia D, Heller NM. Suppression of human natural killer cells by different classes of opioids. Anesth Analg. 2019;128(5):1013.
86. Mitsui Y, Hou L, Huang X, Odegard KC, Pereira LM, Yuki K. Volatile anesthetic sevoflurane attenuates toll-like receptor 1/2 activation. Anesth Analg. 2019;131(2):631–9.
87. Olldashi F, Kerçi M, Zhurda T, Ruçi K, Banushi A, Traverso MS, et al. Effects of tranexamic acid on death, vascular occlusive events, and blood transfusion in trauma patients with significant haemorrhage (CRASH-2): a randomised, placebo-controlled trial. Lancet. 2010;376(9734):23–32.
88. Roquilly A, Mahe PJ, Seguin P, Guitton C, Floch H, Tellier AC, et al. Hydrocortisone therapy for patients with multiple trauma: the randomized controlled HYPOLYTE study. JAMA. 2011;305(12):1201–9.
89. CRASH Trial Collaborators. Final results of MRC CRASH, a randomised placebo-controlled trial of intravenous corticosteroid in adults with head injury—outcomes at 6 months. Lancet. 2005;365(9475):1957–9.
90. D'Amico R, Pifferi S, Leonetti C, Torri V, Tinazzi A, Liberati A. Effectiveness of antibiotic prophylaxis in critically ill adult patients: systematic review of randomised controlled trials. BMJ. 1998;316(7140):1275–85.
91. Gosselin RA, Roberts I, Gillespie WJ. Antibiotics for preventing infection in open limb fractures. Cochrane Database Syst Rev. 2004;2004(1):CD003764.
92. Bernard GR, Vincent J-L, Laterre P-F, LaRosa SP, Dhainaut J-F, Lopez-Rodriguez A, et al. Efficacy and safety of recombinant human activated protein C for severe sepsis. N Engl J Med. 2001;344(10):699–709.
93. Vassar M, Fletcher M, Perry C, Holcroft JW. Evaluation of prostaglandin E1 for prevention of respiratory failure in high risk trauma patients: a prospective clinical trial and correlation with plasma suppressive factors for neutrophil activation. Prostaglandins Leukot Essent Fat Acids. 1991;44(4):223–31.
94. Collier BR, Giladi A, Dossett LA, Dyer L, Fleming SB, Cotton BA. Impact of high-dose antioxidants on outcomes in acutely injured patients. J Parenter Enter Nutr. 2008;32(4):384–8.

95. Holcomb JB, Tilley BC, Baraniuk S, Fox EE, Wade CE, Podbielski JM, et al. Transfusion of plasma, platelets, and red blood cells in a 1:1:1 vs a 1:1:2 ratio and mortality in patients with severe trauma: the PROPPR randomized clinical trial. JAMA. 2015;313(5):471–82.
96. Schött U, Solomon C, Fries D, Bentzer P. The endothelial glycocalyx and its disruption, protection and regeneration: a narrative review. Scand J Trauma Resusc Emerg Med. 2016;24(1):1–8.
97. Bochicchio GV, Napolitano L, Joshi M, Bochicchio K, Meyer W, Scalea TM. Outcome analysis of blood product transfusion in trauma patients: a prospective, risk-adjusted study. World J Surg. 2008;32(10):2185.
98. Malone DL, Dunne J, Tracy JK, Putnam AT, Scalea TM, Napolitano LM. Blood transfusion, independent of shock severity, is associated with worse outcome in trauma. J Trauma Acute Care Surg. 2003;54(5):898–907.
99. Koch CG, Li L, Sessler DI, Figueroa P, Hoeltge GA, Mihaljevic T, et al. Duration of red-cell storage and complications after cardiac surgery. N Engl J Med. 2008;358(12):1229–39.
100. Andreasen JJ, Dethlefsen C, Modrau IS, Baech J, Schonheyder HC, Moeller JK, et al. Storage time of allogeneic red blood cells is associated with risk of severe postoperative infection after coronary artery bypass grafting. Eur J Cardiothorac Surg. 2011;39(3):329–34.
101. Zarychanski R, Abou-Setta AM, Turgeon AF, Houston BL, McIntyre L, Marshall JC, et al. Association of hydroxyethyl starch administration with mortality and acute kidney injury in critically ill patients requiring volume resuscitation: a systematic review and meta-analysis. JAMA. 2013;309(7):678–88.
102. Rhee P, Wang D, Ruff P, Austin B, DeBraux S, Wolcott K, et al. Human neutrophil activation and increased adhesion by various resuscitation fluids. Crit Care Med. 2000;28(1):74–8.
103. Makley AT, Goodman MD, Friend LAW, Deters JS, Johannigman JA, Dorlac WC, et al. Resuscitation with fresh whole blood ameliorates the inflammatory response after hemorrhagic shock. J Trauma. 2010;68(2):305–11.
104. Neal MD, Hoffman MK, Cuschieri J, Minei JP, Maier RV, Harbrecht BG, et al. Crystalloid to packed red blood cell transfusion ratio in the massively transfused patient: when a little goes a long way. J Trauma Acute Care Surg. 2012;72(4):892–8.
105. Torres LN, Chung KK, Salgado CL, Dubick MA, Torres Filho IP. Low-volume resuscitation with normal saline is associated with microvascular endothelial dysfunction after hemorrhage in rats, compared to colloids and balanced crystalloids. Crit Care. 2017;21(1):160.

Coagulation and Thrombosis

Jonathan P. Meizoso, Hunter B. Moore, Angela Sauaia, and Ernest E. Moore

9.1 Introduction

Learning Goals
- Describe the spectrum of trauma-induced coagulopathy, including epidemiology and pathophysiology.
- Understand various methods to diagnose trauma-induced coagulopathy, including clinical and laboratory parameters.
- Manage patients with trauma-induced coagulopathy using goal-directed hemostatic resuscitation, viscoelastic hemostatic assay-guided resuscitation, and adjunctive therapies, including fibrinogen supplementation, prothrombin complex concentrate, and tranexamic acid.

Trauma-induced coagulopathy (TIC) refers to a syndrome characterized by dysregulated coagulation as a direct consequence of severe tissue injury and shock. There is no standard clinical or laboratory-based definition for TIC. The natural history of TIC ranges from an early hypocoagulable state to a late hypercoagulable state, with unique presentations and host of complications within each phenotype. The first pathologic report of these temporal changes in coagulation after severe injury was documented by Innes and Sevitt in the 1960s [1]. However, it was not until 1982 that TIC was implicated as a cause of early mortality in trauma patients in a report that found that half of hemorrhage-related deaths occurred after mechanical hemorrhage control [2]. It has subsequently been established that trauma-related preventable deaths occur within hours and are generally due to uncontrolled hemorrhage [3–10] while those that occur late are due to hypercoagulability [11]. In this chapter, we will discuss the epidemiology, etiology, and patho-

J. P. Meizoso (✉)
Divisions of Trauma, Surgical Critical Care, and Burns, DeWitt Daughtry Family Department of Surgery, Ryder Trauma Center | Jackson Memorial Hospital, University of Miami Leonard M. Miller School of Medicine, Miami, FL, USA
e-mail: jpmeizoso@miami.edu

H. B. Moore
Division of Transplant Surgery, Department of Surgery, University of Colorado Denver, Denver, CO, USA
e-mail: hunter.moore@cuanschutz.edu

A. Sauaia
Schools of Public Health and Medicine, University of Colorado Denver, Denver, CO, USA
e-mail: angela.sauaia@cuanschutz.edu

E. E. Moore
Department of Surgery, Ernest E. Moore Shock Trauma Center at Denver Health, University of Colorado Denver, Denver, CO, USA
e-mail: ernest.moore@dhha.org

physiologic mechanisms believed to be associated with TIC. Additionally, we will describe current methods for diagnosing TIC clinically and best practices for the management of TIC in patients with life-threatening hemorrhage.

9.1.1 Epidemiology

Massive hemorrhage comprises approximately 25% of all-cause mortality after trauma [12–20] and 40–80% of preventable or potentially preventable deaths [21]. Of these hemorrhagic deaths, about 25% likely have a TIC component with an associated 35–50% mortality [22, 23]. Understanding the time course and causes of these deaths is essential in understanding the effect of TIC and how modifying this effect can lead to improved patient outcomes. Most deaths occurring immediately after injury were due to nonsurvivable injuries [3, 13]. In these instances, primary prevention is the only available treatment. However, deaths early after injury and up to 24 h are overwhelmingly due to traumatic brain injury (TBI) and uncontrolled hemorrhage, with the latter being responsible for most of the preventable deaths and occurring usually between 3 and 6 h postinjury [3, 6–8, 24–31] (Fig. 9.1). Deaths occurring later during the hospitalization, including those within and after the first week, are largely due to multiple organ failure (MOF) [3]. Targeted interventions to mitigate early (within 24 h) and late deaths have the potential to prevent or lessen the morbidity and mortality associated with life-threatening hemorrhage.

9.1.2 Etiology

The "lethal triad" of metabolic acidosis, hypothermia, and coagulopathy was originally stressed as the underlying cause of life-threatening hemorrhage after trauma, where one component of the triad begets the next and the so-called "bloody vicious cycle" ensues [2]. It is now known that the two major risk factors for TIC are hemorrhagic shock and tissue injury, with the severity of TIC increasing when both factors are present

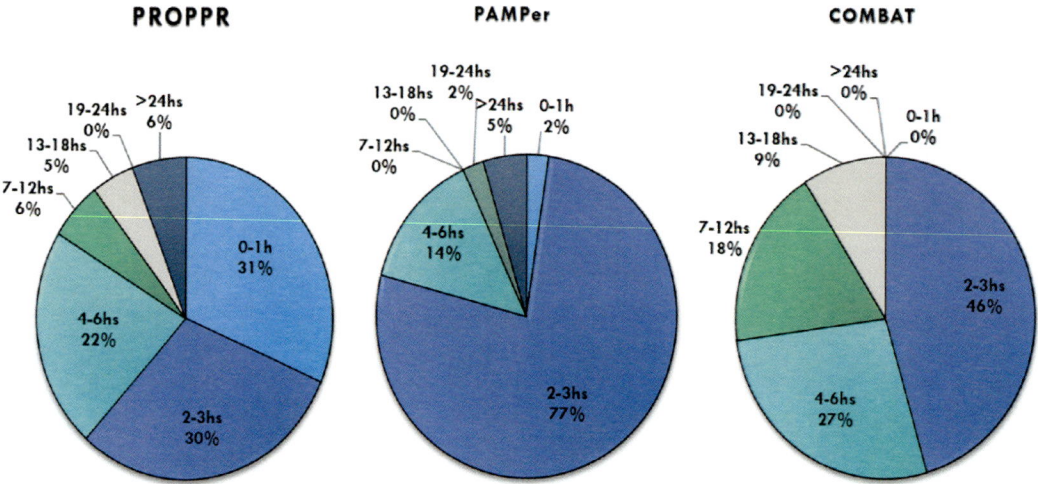

Fig. 9.1 Distribution of all hemorrhagic deaths over time in three randomized controlled trials. For PROPPR (*n* = 680), time zero was the time of randomization in-hospital. Entry criteria were transfusion of >1 unit of blood products and Assessment of Blood Consumption score > 1 or physician's prediction of massive transfusion need. For PAMPer (*n* = 501), time zero was the time of scene arrival. Entry criteria were air transportation and systolic blood pressure (SBP) < 70 mmHg or SBP < 90 mmHg plus heart rate > 108 beats per minute. For COMBAT (*n* = 144), time zero was the time of emergency medical services dispatch. Entry criteria were ground transportation and SBP < 70 mmHg or SBP < 90 mmHg plus heart rate > 108 beats per minute. Among patients requiring ≥1 unit of red blood cells/24 h, 85% of hemorrhagic deaths in PAMPer and 50% in COMBAT occurred in ≤6 h

[32, 33]. Several other risk factors have since been identified that either promote the development or contribute to the worsening of TIC, including prolonged prehospital transport time, metabolic acidosis, hypocalcemia, hypothermia, prehospital crystalloid infusion, and the severity of TBI, although shock is usually present when TIC develops after severe TBI [34–39]. These risk factors contribute to the pathophysiology of TIC by disrupting the complex interconnected coagulation and inflammation systems described below. It should be noted that presence of these risk factors and other objective evidence of TIC (e.g., laboratory values) does not necessarily result in massive hemorrhage. Life-threatening bleeding can be absent in a substantial number of patients who appear coagulopathic based on laboratory values and risk factors [40].

9.2 Pathophysiology

The mechanisms underlying which patients develop TIC and how those coagulation disturbances are corrected with treatment are topics of immense interest with many unanswered questions. TIC can be divided broadly into early and late TIC, and the two categories are not mutually exclusive. Significant overlap exists and patients can exhibit features of each phenotype simultaneously. In general, early TIC generally occurs within 6–24 h of injury and is characterized by profound hypocoagulability with inadequate hemostasis and the potential for uncontrolled life-threatening hemorrhage and recalcitrant hemorrhagic shock. Late TIC, which generally occurs after the first 24 h, is characterized by a hypercoagulable state that is associated with large vessel [e.g., venous thromboembolism (VTE)] and small vessel [e.g., acute respiratory distress syndrome (ARDS), MOF] thrombosis. The time points used to define early and late TIC correlate well with the epidemiology of trauma deaths, where early deaths are due to life-threatening hemorrhage and late deaths are due to MOF (see Sect. 9.1.1. "Epidemiology" above). The point at which an individual patient transitions from early to late TIC, however, is difficult to identify due to the dynamic changes occurring related to that individual's level of tissue injury and degree of hemorrhagic shock, as well as the treatment strategies employed. The dominant mechanisms related to this transition from a hypocoagulable to a hypercoagulable state involve disorders of platelet function, thrombin generation, and fibrinolysis, which are driven by tissue injury and shock and promote endothelial cell and immune system activation, which will be discussed further in the following sections.

9.2.1 Early TIC

As described above, the two main drivers of early TIC are hemorrhagic shock and tissue injury (Fig. 9.2). Shock results in cellular hypoxia in the microcirculation, which subsequently leads to metabolic acidosis due to anaerobic metabolism. The effect of shock on TIC is compounded by the presence of tissue injury [32, 33], and resuscitation with crystalloid solutions or unbalanced blood product transfusion leads to hemodilution and dysfunction of remaining coagulation factors. The net result of acidosis has several implications for coagulation. Viscoelastic testing data demonstrate that acidosis slows the rate of fibrin polymerization and decreases clot strength [41]. Acidosis is also associated with decreased platelet counts and aggregation, decreased thrombin generation, increased fibrinogen consumption, decreased factor V and IX activity, and deranges conventional coagulation tests [42–44]. Furthermore, metabolic by-products may impair thrombin generation and promote fibrinolysis. Two other results of hemorrhagic shock that may affect TIC are activation of protein C and hypocalcemia. Hypoperfusion results in the possibly maladaptive response of activation of the anticoagulant protein C as well as reduced levels of plasminogen activator inhibitor-1 (PAI-1), further augmenting the hypocoagulable state [22, 36, 37, 39, 45]. However, the central role of activated protein C in TIC has been questioned. More recent data suggest that overwhelming tissue plasminogen activator (tPA) release from the activated endothelium, rather than a relative defi-

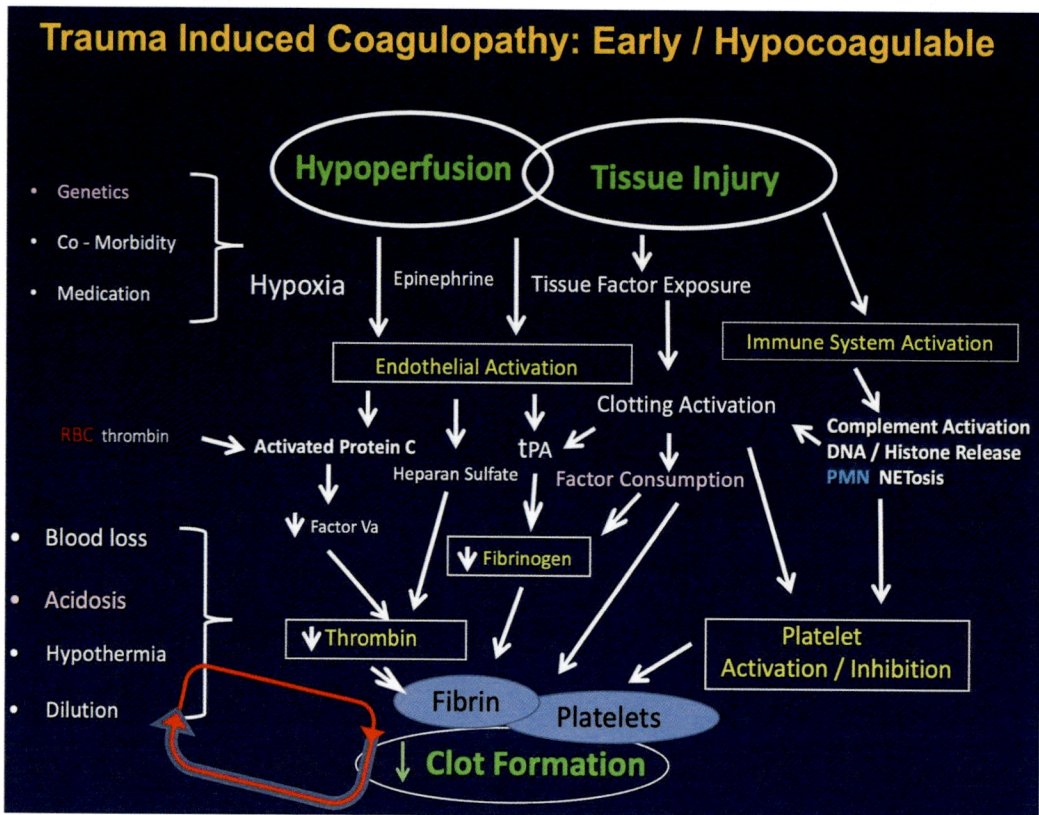

Fig. 9.2 Mechanisms of Early Trauma-Induced Coagulopathy

ciency of PAI-1 secondary to activated protein C, is the primary mechanism driving the hyperfibrinolytic phenotype of early TIC [46, 47]. Hypocalcemia secondary to hemorrhagic shock has recently been implicated in TIC [39]. Calcium is integral in the formation and stabilization of fibrin polymerization sites on the endothelial surface and is also necessary for platelet-dependent functions [48]. Platelets and endothelial cells are the two key players in hemostasis according to the cell-based model of hemostasis [49] (Fig. 9.3); their dependence on calcium for normal function underscores the important role of hypocalcemia in the pathophysiology of TIC.

Tissue injury ultimately results in activation of the coagulation system via tissue factor, which complexes to factor VIIa and leads to thrombin generation and formation of a fibrin-rich clot [50]. This occurs after tissue injury results in endothelial cell disruption and exposure of the basement membrane where tissue factor resides.

The development of TIC and a maladaptive hypocoagulable response is related to the severity of tissue injury [22, 23, 33, 35] including the release of damage-associated molecular patterns (DAMPs), which stimulate inflammation and may render platelets hyporesponsive, further worsening the coagulopathy [51, 52]. Finally, the specific organ injured may play a role in the progression of TIC as well (e.g., tPA-rich pancreas), although further study is required to determine the real world implications of this.

Another pathophysiologic mechanism that plays a role in the development or progression of TIC is the so-called endotheliopathy of trauma (EOT). EOT is the loss of the normal protective barrier provided by the endothelium as a consequence of hemorrhagic shock and tissue injury [53]. This results in endothelial activation with shedding of the anticoagulant heparan sulfate ectodomain of syndecan-1, as well as leukocyte activation, loss of endothelial barrier function,

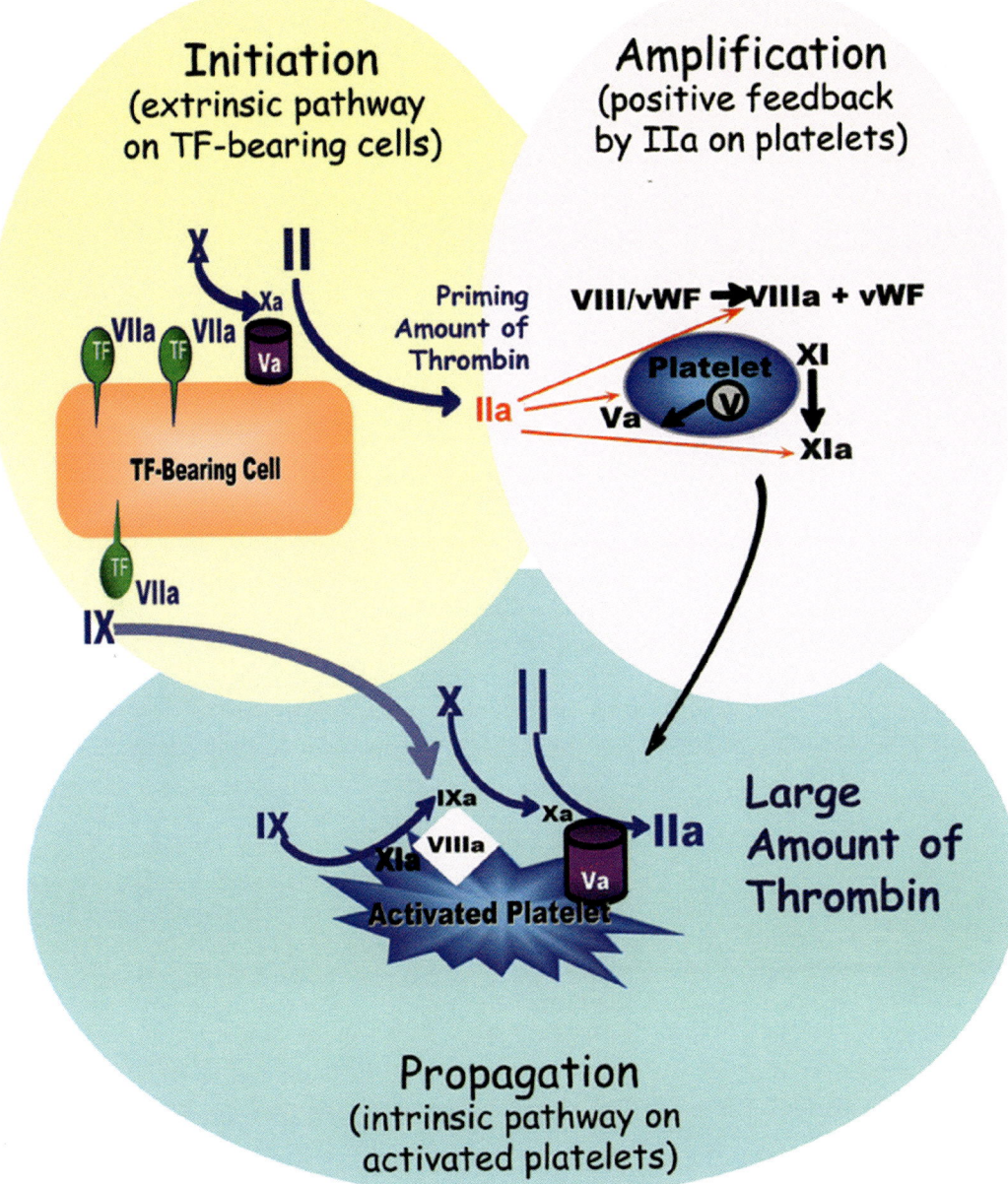

Fig. 9.3 Cell-based Model of Hemostasis. Initiation occurs on tissue factor (TF)-bearing cells as the factor VIIa/TF complex activates factor X. Factor Xa binds to its cofactor, factor Va, and activates small amounts of thrombin. Thrombin generated on the TF-bearing cell amplifies the procoagulant response by activating additional coagulation factors and platelets. The large burst of thrombin required for formation of a fibrin clot is generated on platelet surfaces during the propagation phase. (Source: Hoffman M. Cell-mediated hemostasis. In: Moore HB, Neal MD, Moore EE, editors. Trauma Induced Coagulopathy. 2nd ed. Springer; 2020). (Reprinted by permission from [the Licensor]: [Journal Publisher])

and resultant clinical coagulopathy with both micro- and macro-vascular thrombosis. The presence of circulating syndecan-1, a marker for endothelial glycocalyx shedding, is associated with inflammation, coagulopathy, and death in early TIC [54–56]. Furthermore, activation of the thrombin-thrombomodulin system occurs in early TIC and may diminish the protective effects of the endothelial barrier [36, 45]. Finally, current evidence suggests that EOT may be at least partially reversed by plasma transfusion [53, 57–60], potentially by reducing circulating levels of proteins from damaged endothelium [61, 62], and possibly explaining the improved clinical outcomes reported after plasma transfusion [6, 7]. There is some evidence that tranexamic acid (TXA) may also partially curtail EOT [63, 64].

Deficiencies in both platelet number and function are also central problems in early TIC, with at least 50% of injured patients having some form of platelet dysfunction [65–67]. Paradoxically, most patients with TIC have normal platelet counts albeit with impaired aggregation [68, 69]. This phenomenon, termed "platelet exhaustion," is likely driven by shock, tissue injury, endothelial release of TF, platelet activating factor, and von Willebrand factor [70–72]; this results in a cadre of circulating platelets that are unable to participate in primary hemostasis.

Thrombin generation is likely insufficient early after injury and appears to occur in up to 17% of patients [73], resulting in clots composed of thick fibrin fibers that have diminished stability and are more prone to fibrinolysis. This insufficient thrombin generation is driven by shock, acidosis, hypothermia, and insufficient coagulation factor levels, either from dilution or consumption [74–77]. However, prospective randomized data suggest that severely injured patients present with >64% activity of coagulation factors [6]. In fact, thrombin generation is significantly higher in trauma patients compared to noninjured patients, and in those without TIC, despite lower levels of coagulation proteins [78, 79]. However, low thrombin generation in severely injured patients is associated with three-fold and four-fold higher odds of 30-day mortality and massive transfusion, respectively [73].

Fibrinogen is normally cleaved by thrombin to form fibrin monomers, which are then cross-linked by factor XIIIa and polymerize to form a stable fibrin-rich clot that is protected from fibrinolysis [80]. Additionally, fibrinogen binds with high affinity to the glycoprotein IIb/IIIa receptor on platelets and thereby facilitates platelet aggregation to increase clot strength [81]. Virtually all circulating fibrinogen is derived from the liver and can increase up to 20 times physiologic levels during the acute phase response [82, 83]. Despite being the most abundant coagulation protein in the circulation [84], fibrinogen is also the first coagulation factor to become depleted after major hemorrhage [85, 86] by various mechanisms, including dilution, consumption, hypothermia, and acidosis [86–89]. Increased circulating plasmin levels during hemorrhagic shock, likely secondary to overwhelming tPA release with inadequate levels of PAI-1, result in hyperfibrinolysis and further fibrinogen degradation [47, 76, 86, 90]. Clinically, hypofibrinogenemia is associated with increased injury severity and base deficit, underscoring the importance of tissue injury and shock to its pathophysiology, and is an independent predictor of 24-h and 28-day mortality in severely injured patients [91–93]. This has led to European guidelines calling for early fibrinogen supplementation in patients with massive hemorrhage if fibrinogen levels are below 1.5 g/L [94].

Finally, dysregulated fibrinolysis plays a key role in early TIC. The spectrum of postinjury fibrinolysis ranges from hyperfibrinolysis to fibrinolysis shutdown, the latter being more frequently associated with late TIC [11]. Hyperfibrinolysis occurs in approximately 20% of seriously injured patients at admission and is associated with hemorrhagic shock [11, 95–98]. Postinjury, hyperfibrinolysis is characterized by elevated tPA levels, PAI-1 depletion, platelet dysfunction, and loss of fibrinolytic inhibitors and regulators of clot breakdown [47, 91, 93, 99–104]. Hyperfibrinolysis is associated with mortality from hemorrhage [11, 98]. Fibrinolysis shutdown represents the other end of the postinjury fibrinolysis spectrum and is present in 50-60% of severely injured patients at admission [11, 98]. These patients present with evidence of prior fibrinolysis activation (e.g., elevated D-dimer) and have low systemic levels of fibrinolysis [97]. This phenomenon has been described in other pathologies (e.g., viral infection) [105, 106] and is associated with 2- to 6-fold higher mortality from micro- and macrovascular thrombosis in trauma patients [107].

9.2.2 Late TIC

The progression of hemorrhagic shock leads to a transition from an early hypocoagulable state (i.e., early TIC) to a later hypercoagulable state (i.e., late TIC). This transition is mediated by prothrombotic changes and fibrinolysis shutdown, which leads to organ damage via thrombin generation, occlusion of the microvascular circulation, and ultimately MOF [11, 108]. Tissue injury likely promotes late TIC through increased thrombin generation and resultant fibrin formation via histone release and a myosin-mediated pathway, where myosin binds to factors Xa and Va, increasing the ability to create prothrombinase and, therefore, thrombin [50, 109]. The downstream effects of endotheliopathy also play a significant role in late TIC. Circulating markers of the shed glycocalyx are associated with vascular thrombosis, organ failure, and death in late TIC [54–56]. Furthermore, EOT-associated persistently elevated levels of structurally ultra-large vWF and impaired clearance of vWF by ADAMTS13 are associated with a prothrombotic and proinflammatory state and contribute to late TIC [70, 110].

As in early TIC, platelet dysfunction and disordered fibrinolysis play a central role in the pathophysiology of late TIC. Platelets are predominantly involved in the hypercoagulable state seen in late TIC via an immune-mediated pathway [67, 111]. High circulating levels of platelet-leukocyte aggregates as a result of platelet activation are associated with a procoagulant milieu via release of platelet factor 4, tissue factor, fibrinogen, and factor Xa [69]. Other mechanisms by which platelets promote hypercoagulability include signaling via toll-like receptor 4, platelet ballooning, monocyte recruitment by platelet-derived high mobility group protein B1, and neutrophil extracellular trap formation, all of which are associated with a proinflammatory state and hypercoagulability [112–114]. Platelet dysfunction has also been implicated as a central player in postinjury VTE and MOF [65–67].

Most patients transition to a hyperfibrinolytic state after severe injury [115]. This is likely secondary to a surge in PAI-1 that occurs approximately 2 h postinjury in an effort to suppress hyperfibrinolysis via elevated tPA and results in fibrinolysis shutdown in most patients by 12 h [116]. However, this adaptive response is pathologic if it persists for longer than 24 h. Fibrinolysis shutdown is associated with significantly higher mortality than physiologic fibrinolysis [97, 117, 118]. Death in patients with fibrinolysis shutdown is secondary to TBI and MOF [11]. Finally, persistent fibrinolysis shutdown (defined as shutdown lasting >24 h) is also associated with significantly higher mortality when compared to patients whose state of fibrinolysis shutdown resolves [115, 116, 119, 120].

9.3 Diagnosis

9.3.1 Early TIC

Early TIC is characterized clinically by life-threatening hemorrhage [89, 121, 122]. Conventional coagulation tests aid in the laboratory diagnosis of early TIC. These standard tests include platelet count, prothrombin time/international normalized ratio (PT/INR), activated partial thromboplastin time (aPTT), and the Clauss assay to measure functional fibrinogen levels. Historically, PT/INR was used for the diagnosis of TIC as PT prolongation is present in a quarter of severely injured patients [22, 23] and is associated with four-fold higher mortality than patients without PT/INR prolongation. However, conventional coagulation tests have significant limitations, including the time it takes to receive actionable results, inability to assess fibrinolytic function, and the fact that PT/INR may be abnormal despite normal clotting factor activity [123, 124].

The resurgence of viscoelastic hemostatic assays (VHAs) has significantly improved our

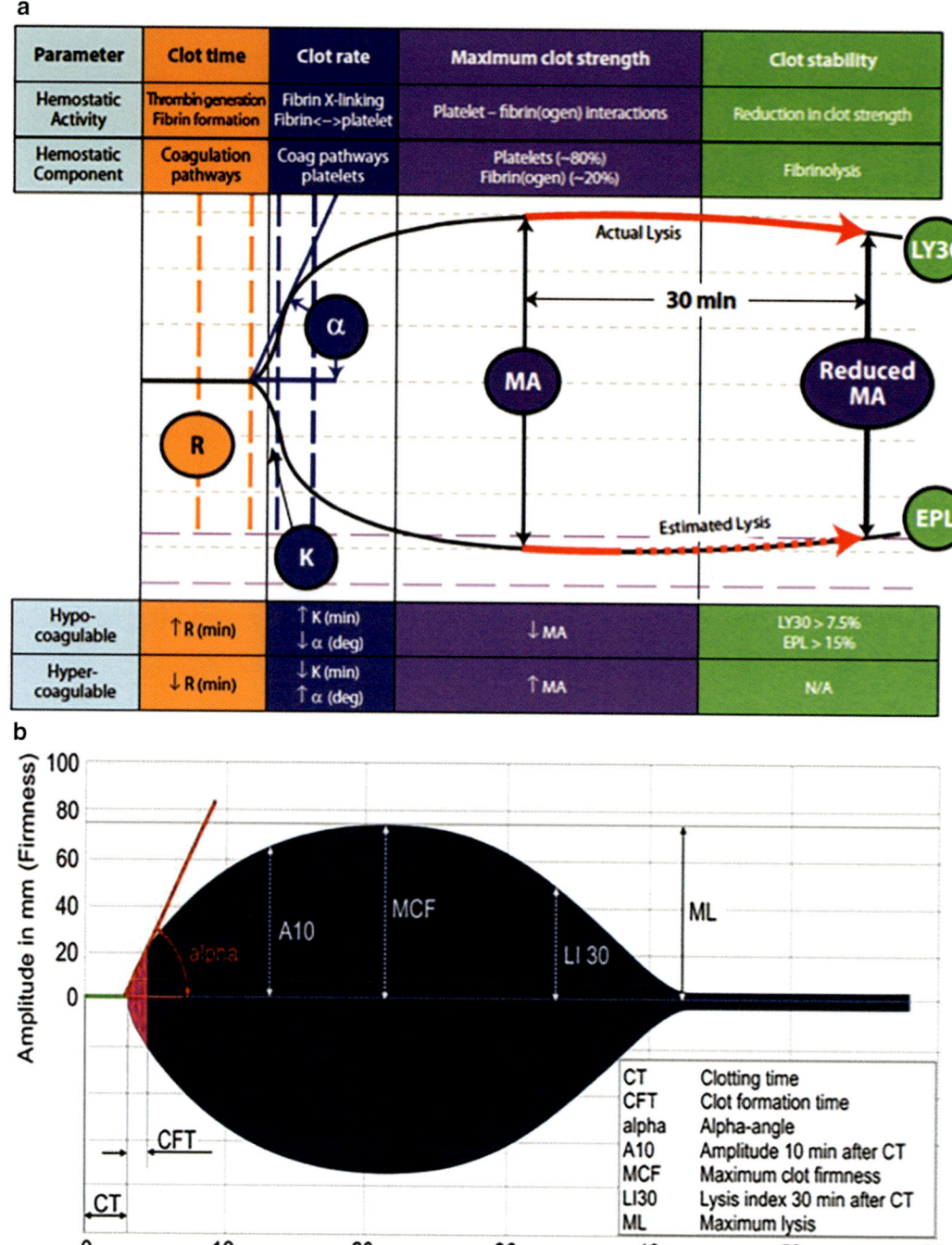

Fig. 9.4 Viscoelastic hemostatic assays. Examples of thrombelastography and rotational thromboelastometry readouts. Panel (**a**) illustrates the typical curve produced by thrombelastography. Panel (**b**) demonstrates the typical curve produced by rotational thromboelastometry

ability to detect TIC in severely injured patients. VHAs offer several benefits over conventional coagulation tests. They provide assessment of whole blood clot formation and fibrinolysis in real time in a single readout (Fig. 9.4). Actionable data are available earlier, with the newest VHAs providing results within 5 min [121, 125, 126]. VHAs also correspond to specific blood component requirements, massive transfusion, and mortality better than conventional coagulation tests [127–130]. In a United States-based randomized controlled trial, VHAs used to guide resuscitation in severely injured trauma patients were associated with decreased mortality compared to conventional coagulation tests [25]. While the recent ITACTIC study [131] conducted in Europe reported no differences in clinical outcomes of resuscitation guided by VHAs or conventional coagulation tests, there were some methodological issues. Indeed, the VHA transfusion thresholds in the ITACTIC were based on the same thresholds for conventional testing used in the control group, thereby creating a circular logic that resulted in the two groups being treated similarly. The appropriate conclusion from the ITACTIC study is that resuscitation based on the VHA thresholds set in their study did not offer benefit over conventional tests guidance, but the study does not offer evidence for different, outcome-based VHA resuscitation thresholds. The major limitations to VHA use are cost and reproducibility in older versions [132]; however, it is currently recommended that VHAs replace conventional coagulation tests for the diagnosis of TIC [121].

Despite the availability of various laboratory tests to diagnose TIC, the clinical status of the patient should ultimately drive decision-making. In the absence of clinical coagulopathy (e.g., overt bleeding, need for surgery, or other interventional procedures for hemorrhage control), abnormal values on conventional coagulation tests or VHAs should not be corrected empirically.

9.3.2 Late TIC

In contrast to early TIC, where the diagnosis is made using a combination of clinical and laboratory parameters, the diagnosis of late TIC is largely clinical. The clinical presentation of late TIC is characterized by VTE, ARDS, and MOF largely mediated by fibrinolysis shutdown [11, 98, 119], with those who develop severe early TIC being at greatest risk of developing late TIC. Various prior works have identified risk factors for the development of VTE after trauma [133]. These include age [134–137], immobility [134, 135], history of VTE [135], spinal cord injury [135, 136], coma [135, 138], pelvic fractures [135, 138], lower extremity fractures [135–137], repair of lower extremity major venous injuries [135, 137], blood transfusions [136, 138], and surgery [137, 138]. While no single laboratory measurement is available for the diagnosis of a hypercoagulable state, a hypercoagulable VHA is associated with stroke [139] and VTE, despite appropriate thromboprophylaxis [140–146]. Fibrinolysis shutdown may further identify patients at risk for thrombotic events.

9.4 Treatment

The highest priority in the management of patients with life-threatening hemorrhage is mechanical hemorrhage control. This is accomplished using direct pressure, tourniquet application, and ultimately surgical or other interventional hemorrhage control. Prevention also plays an important role in the management of these patients. Prevention programs, like the American College of Surgeons Committee on Trauma Stop the Bleed program, have trained thousands of civilians and healthcare providers on the basic principles of hemorrhage control [147, 148]. The resuscitative endovascular balloon occlusion of the aorta (REBOA) device is a useful adjunct in certain patients. The second priority is reversing shock as this is a dominant factor in prolonging TIC. In addition to hemorrhage control, goal-directed hemostatic resuscitation, restoration of clotting homeostasis, and consideration of damage control resuscitation [25, 149] and damage control surgery techniques [150, 151] to accomplish this are top priorities in the management of patients with life-threatening hemorrhage.

Goal-directed hemostatic resuscitation is a central tenet in the management of patients in hemorrhagic shock (Fig. 9.5). Although international guidelines vary [94, 152–156], most emphasize that a balanced blood product resuscitation with high ratios of plasma to packed red

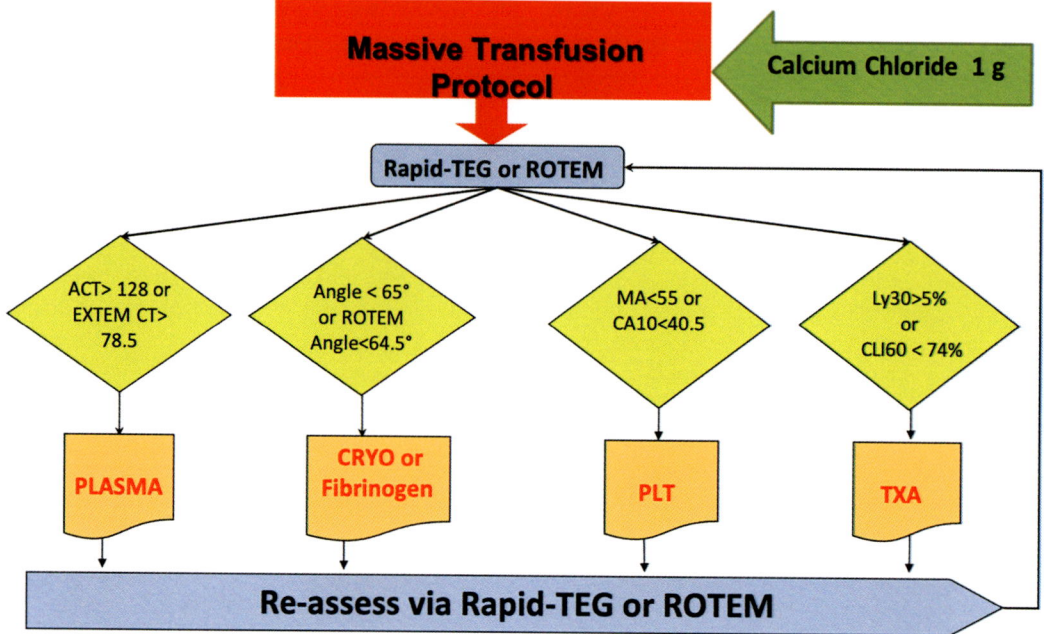

Fig. 9.5 Goal-directed algorithm for hemostatic resuscitation in patients at risk of severe bleeding. Example of an institutional protocol using goal-directed hemostatic resuscitation based on viscoelastic hemostatic assay results. (With permission)

blood cells is a superior approach compared to high volumes of crystalloid. Large volume crystalloid resuscitation is associated with hemodilution of coagulation factors and antifibrinolytic proteins [157], hyperfibrinolysis [95], and ultimately exacerbation of TIC with significant effects on outcomes. The optimal ratio of plasma to packed red blood cell transfusion is debated; however a ratio of at least 1:2 (plasma: packed red blood cells) is recommended [24, 158]. The Pragmatic, Randomized Optimal Platelet and Plasma Ratios (PROPPR) trial, a multicenter randomized trial conducted at 12 North American level I trauma centers including 680 severely injured patients randomized to either 1:1 vs. 1:2 ratios of plasma to packed red blood cells, found no overall survival benefit in the 1:1 group compared to 1:2; however, shorter time to hemostasis was achieved with a 1:1 strategy [24]. Ultimately, early empiric blood product resuscitation for all patients in hemorrhagic shock is required to avoid worsening of coagulopathy. US guidelines emphasize the importance of plasma in massive transfusion protocols as an effective volume expander with added beneficial effects on endothelial function and mortality [154]. Prehospital plasma has been associated with decreased mortality in patients with blunt trauma and prolonged transport times in a multicenter randomized controlled trial [6, 7], although its beneficial effect does not extend to patients in an urban setting with short transport times [6]. Plasma may also have positive effects on the restoration of endothelial function and reversal of EOT [53, 57–60] as evidenced by lower circulating levels of syndecan-1 in patients receiving early plasma transfusion [61, 62].

As previously mentioned, fibrinogen is the most abundant coagulation protein in the circulation. However, it is also the first to reach critically low levels in patients with hemorrhagic shock. Therefore, European guidelines stress the need for early supplementation with fibrinogen and prothrombin complex concentrate for adequate restoration of clotting function [94]. These guidelines recommend fibrinogen supplementation to maintain a fibrinogen level > 1.5 g/L. The data suggest that high ratios of fibrinogen or cryoprecipitate to packed red blood cells should be maintained to improve survival in patients with hemorrhagic shock [159], particularly in those receiving >4 units of red blood cells [88]. Randomized clinical trials are currently underway to determine the effects of empiric fibrinogen administration (ClinicalTrials.gov Identifiers: NCT01475344, NCT02344069, NCT02203968, NCT03304899, NCT03780894, NCT02745041, NCT04149171, NCT02864875, NCT04704869, NCT04534751).

TXA is an antifibrinolytic agent commonly used as a resuscitative adjunct in the massively hemorrhaging patient. TXA was found in the Clinical Randomization of an Antifibrinolytic in Significant Haemorrhage (CRASH)-2 trial, an international multicenter randomized controlled trial with over 20,000 patients with or at risk of significant bleeding, to be associated with lower all-cause mortality and mortality from hemorrhage compared to placebo [160]. These findings led to rapid adoption of TXA in massive transfusion protocols at trauma centers throughout the world, despite the fact that only half of the patients in CRASH-2 required a blood transfusion and less than half required an operation, raising questions about the actual injury severity of these patients. A subsequent analysis of CRASH-2 reported that it must be given to patients within 3 h of injury or else mortality in patients receiving TXA actually increases [14]. Other studies have identified potential beneficial effects of TXA in select subpopulations. The Study of Tranexamic Acid during Air and Ground Medical Transport (STAAMP) trial found no significant difference in 30-day mortality between patients receiving TXA versus placebo except in patients with severe shock, defined as a systolic blood pressure < 70 mmHg, who received TXA within 1 h postinjury [161]. CRASH-3 also identified a survival benefit in patients who received TXA with mild and moderate, but not severe, TBI [162]. Similarly, patients with moderate to severe TBI without hemorrhagic shock who received TXA had no significant improvement in favorable neurologic outcome at 6 months or 28-day mortality compared to those who did not receive TXA [163]. An additional concern with the administration of TXA in patients with TIC is the development of VTE. CRASH-2 and CRASH-3 did not identify an increased risk of VTE among patients receiving TXA [160, 162]; however, those studies had low overall rates of transfusion and surgery and may not accurately represent the massively hemorrhaging trauma patient. Others have identified an association between TXA and a higher incidence of VTE events [164–166], including the recent HALT-IT trial where a significant increase in VTE was reported in patients who received a high-dose 24-h TXA infusion for gastrointestinal bleeding [167]. Given the significant potential consequences of administering TXA to patients with TIC, particularly the possibility of thrombotic events, we recommend avoiding TXA in patients with fibrinolysis shutdown and administering it to patients at high risk of or with evidence of hyperfibrinolysis on VHA [168, 169].

Dos and Don'ts
- Do establish control of mechanical bleeding as soon as possible.
- Do reverse shock with high plasma to packed red blood cell ratios (at least 1:2).
- Do use VHAs to guide hemostatic resuscitation.
- Do consider early supplementation of fibrinogen using fibrinogen concentrate or cryoprecipitate, particularly in patients receiving >4 units of packed red blood cells.
- Do employ damage control resuscitation and damage control surgery strategies, as appropriate.
- Do consider tranexamic acid in patients within 3 h of injury with evidence of hyperfibrinolysis on VHA testing.
- Do not infuse high volumes of crystalloid fluids.
- Do not administer TXA in patients with viscoelastic evidence of fibrinolysis shutdown.

Take-Home Messages
- TIC is a clinical syndrome in severely injured patients with significant associated morbidity and mortality that is characterized by early hypocoagulability and late hypercoagulability.
- Hemorrhagic shock, tissue injury, platelet dysfunction, inadequate thrombin generation, hypofibrinogenemia, endotheliopathy, and disordered fibrinolysis all play a role in both early and late TIC.
- The diagnosis of early TIC is made with a combination of clinical and laboratory parameters. Late TIC is largely a clinical diagnosis, characterized by thrombotic events including VTE, ARDS, and MOF.
- Management of patients with TIC includes surgical hemorrhage control, goal-directed hemostatic resuscitation, limitation of crystalloid use, and consideration of adjunctive therapies, including fibrinogen, prothrombin complex concentrate, and tranexamic acid.

Questions
1. What factor in the endothelium initiates clot formation?
   A. syndecan
   B. **tissue factor**
   C. fibrin
   D. histones
2. Death from bleeding occurs most frequently at?
   A. 0–2 h
   B. **2–4 h**
   C. 4–6 h
   D. 6–8 h
3. The leading preventable cause of death is due to?
   A. brain injury
   B. coagulopathy
   C. **uncontrolled bleeding**
   D. multiple organ failure
4. Tranexamic acid binds to which protein to inhibit fibrinolysis?
   A. tissue plasminogen activator
   B. plasmin
   C. fibrin
   D. **plasminogen**
5. The first factor to be reduced following hemorrhage is?
   A. **Factor 1 (fibrinogen)**
   B. Factor II
   C. Factor V
   D. Factor VII
6. Thrombelastography measurement of clot strength?
   A. ACT
   B. angle
   C. **MA**
   D. LY30
7. Thrombelastography measurement of fibrinolysis?
   A. ACT
   B. angle
   C. MA
   D. **LY30**
8. What is the definition of a massive transfusion?
   A. >4 U RBC/1 h
   B. >6 U RBC/6 h
   C. >10 U RBC/24 h
   D. **all**
9. The most important cell in the cell-based model of hemostasis is?
   A. RBC
   B. PMN
   C. **platelet**
   D. macrophage
10. Tissue factor binds to which activated clotting factor to initiate clot formation?
    A. Factor II
    B. Factor V
    C. **Factor FVII**
    D. Factor VIII

References

1. Innes D, Sevitt S. Coagulation and fibrinolysis in injured patients. J Clin Pathol. 1964;17:1–13.
2. Kashuk JL, Moore EE, Millikan JS, Moore JB. Major abdominal vascular trauma—a unified approach. J Trauma. 1982;22(8):672–9.
3. Tisherman SA, Schmicker RH, Brasel KJ, Bulger EM, Kerby JD, Minei JP, et al. Detailed description of all deaths in both the shock and traumatic brain injury hypertonic saline trials of the Resuscitation Outcomes Consortium. Ann Surg. 2015;261(3):586–90.
4. Eastridge BJ, Mabry RL, Seguin P, Cantrell J, Tops T, Uribe P, et al. Death on the battlefield (2001–2011): implications for the future of combat casualty care. J Trauma Acute Care Surg. 2012;73(6 Suppl 5):S431–7.
5. Fox EE, Holcomb JB, Wade CE, Bulger EM, Tilley BC, PROPPR Study Group. Earlier endpoints are required for hemorrhagic shock trials among severely injured patients. Shock. 2017;47(5):567–73.
6. Moore HB, Moore EE, Chapman MP, McVaney K, Bryskiewicz G, Blechar R, et al. Plasma-first resuscitation to treat haemorrhagic shock during emergency ground transportation in an urban area: a randomised trial. Lancet. 2018;392(10144):283–91.
7. Sperry JL, Guyette FX, Brown JB, Yazer MH, Triulzi DJ, Early-Young BJ, et al. Prehospital plasma during air medical transport in trauma patients at risk for hemorrhagic shock. N Engl J Med. 2018;379(4):315–26.
8. Sauaia A. Epidemiology of hemorrhagic deaths. In: Moore HB, Neal MD, Moore EE, editors. Trauma induced coagulopathy. 2nd ed. Springer; 2020.
9. Kalkwarf KJ, Drake SA, Yang Y, Thetford C, Myers L, Brock M, et al. Bleeding to death in a big city: an analysis of all trauma deaths from hemorrhage in a metropolitan area during 1 year. J Trauma Acute Care Surg. 2020;89(4):716–22.
10. Trunkey DD. Trauma. Accidental and intentional injuries account for more years of life lost in the U.S. than cancer and heart disease. Among the prescribed remedies are improved preventive efforts, speedier surgery and further research. Sci Am. 1983;249(2):28–35.
11. Moore HB, Moore EE, Gonzalez E, Chapman MP, Chin TL, Silliman CC, et al. Hyperfibrinolysis, physiologic fibrinolysis, and fibrinolysis shutdown: the spectrum of postinjury fibrinolysis and relevance to antifibrinolytic therapy. J Trauma Acute Care Surg. 2014;77(6):811–7; discussion 7.
12. Sobrino J, Shafi S. Timing and causes of death after injuries. Proc (Bayl Univ Med Cent). 2013;26(2):120–3.
13. Sauaia A, Moore FA, Moore EE, Moser KS, Brennan R, Read RA, et al. Epidemiology of trauma deaths: a reassessment. J Trauma. 1995;38(2):185–93.
14. CRASH-2 Trial Collaborators. The importance of early treatment with tranexamic acid in bleeding trauma patients: an exploratory analysis of the CRASH-2 randomised controlled trial. Lancet. 2011;377(9771):1096–101.
15. Kahl JE, Calvo RY, Sise MJ, Sise CB, Thorndike JF, Shackford SR. The changing nature of death on the trauma service. J Trauma Acute Care Surg. 2013;75(2):195–201.
16. Shackford SR, Mackersie RC, Holbrook TL, Davis JW, Hollingsworth-Fridlund P, Hoyt DB, et al. The epidemiology of traumatic death. A population-based analysis. Arch Surg. 1993;128(5):571–5.
17. Callcut RA, Kornblith LZ, Conroy AS, Robles AJ, Meizoso JP, Namias N, et al. The why and how our trauma patients die: a prospective multicenter Western Trauma Association study. J Trauma Acute Care Surg. 2019;86(5):864–70.
18. Evans JA, van Wessem KJ, McDougall D, Lee KA, Lyons T, Balogh ZJ. Epidemiology of traumatic deaths: comprehensive population-based assessment. World J Surg. 2010;34(1):158–63.
19. Soreide K, Kruger AJ, Vardal AL, Ellingsen CL, Soreide E, Lossius HM. Epidemiology and contemporary patterns of trauma deaths: changing place, similar pace, older face. World J Surg. 2007;31(11):2092–103.
20. Oyeniyi BT, Fox EE, Scerbo M, Tomasek JS, Wade CE, Holcomb JB. Trends in 1029 trauma deaths at a level 1 trauma center: impact of a bleeding control bundle of care. Injury. 2017;48(1):5–12.
21. Teixeira PG, Inaba K, Hadjizacharia P, Brown C, Salim A, Rhee P, et al. Preventable or potentially preventable mortality at a mature trauma center. J Trauma. 2007;63(6):1338–46; discussion 46–7.
22. Brohi K, Singh J, Heron M, Coats T. Acute traumatic coagulopathy. J Trauma. 2003;54(6):1127–30.
23. MacLeod JB, Lynn M, McKenney MG, Cohn SM, Murtha M. Early coagulopathy predicts mortality in trauma. J Trauma. 2003;55(1):39–44.
24. Holcomb JB, Tilley BC, Baraniuk S, Fox EE, Wade CE, Podbielski JM, et al. Transfusion of plasma, platelets, and red blood cells in a 1:1:1 vs a 1:1:2 ratio and mortality in patients with severe trauma: the PROPPR randomized clinical trial. JAMA. 2015;313(5):471–82.
25. Gonzalez E, Moore EE, Moore HB, Chapman MP, Chin TL, Ghasabyan A, et al. Goal-directed Hemostatic resuscitation of trauma-induced coagulopathy: a pragmatic randomized clinical trial comparing a viscoelastic assay to conventional coagulation assays. Ann Surg. 2016;263(6):1051–9.
26. Roberts I, Shakur H, Coats T, Hunt B, Balogun E, Barnetson L, et al. The CRASH-2 trial: a randomised controlled trial and economic evaluation of the effects of tranexamic acid on death, vascular occlusive events and transfusion requirement in bleeding trauma patients. Health Technol Assess. 2013;17(10):1–79.
27. Moore EE, Moore FA, Fabian TC, Bernard AC, Fulda GJ, Hoyt DB, et al. Human polymerized hemoglobin for the treatment of hemorrhagic shock when blood

28. Roberts DJ, Harzan C, Kirkpatrick AW, Dixon E, Grondin SC, McBeth PB, et al. One thousand consecutive in-hospital deaths following severe injury: has the etiology of traumatic inpatient death changed in Canada? Can J Surg. 2018;61(3):150–2.
29. Arslan ED, Kaya E, Sonmez M, Kavalci C, Solakoglu A, Yilmaz F, et al. Assessment of traumatic deaths in a level one trauma center in Ankara, Turkey. Eur J Trauma Emerg Surg. 2015;41(3):319–23.
30. Holcomb JB, del Junco DJ, Fox EE, Wade CE, Cohen MJ, Schreiber MA, et al. The prospective, observational, multicenter, major trauma transfusion (PROMMTT) study: comparative effectiveness of a time-varying treatment with competing risks. JAMA Surg. 2013;148(2):127–36.
31. Holcomb JB, Moore EE, Sperry JL, Jansen JO, Schreiber MA, Del Junco DJ, et al. Evidence-based and clinically relevant outcomes for hemorrhage control trauma trials. Ann Surg. 2021;273(3):395–401.
32. Frith D, Goslings JC, Gaarder C, Maegele M, Cohen MJ, Allard S, et al. Definition and drivers of acute traumatic coagulopathy: clinical and experimental investigations. J Thromb Haemost. 2010;8(9):1919–25.
33. Niles SE, McLaughlin DF, Perkins JG, Wade CE, Li Y, Spinella PC, et al. Increased mortality associated with the early coagulopathy of trauma in combat casualties. J Trauma. 2008;64(6):1459–63; discussion 63–5.
34. Kutcher ME, Howard BM, Sperry JL, Hubbard AE, Decker AL, Cuschieri J, et al. Evolving beyond the vicious triad: differential mediation of traumatic coagulopathy by injury, shock, and resuscitation. J Trauma Acute Care Surg. 2015;78(3):516–23.
35. Maegele M, Lefering R, Yucel N, Tjardes T, Rixen D, Paffrath T, et al. Early coagulopathy in multiple injury: an analysis from the German trauma registry on 8724 patients. Injury. 2007;38(3):298–304.
36. Brohi K, Cohen MJ, Ganter MT, Matthay MA, Mackersie RC, Pittet JF. Acute traumatic coagulopathy: initiated by hypoperfusion: modulated through the protein C pathway? Ann Surg. 2007;245(5):812–8.
37. Cohen MJ, Brohi K, Ganter MT, Manley GT, Mackersie RC, Pittet JF. Early coagulopathy after traumatic brain injury: the role of hypoperfusion and the protein C pathway. J Trauma. 2007;63(6):1254–61; discussion 61–2.
38. Moore HB, Tessmer MT, Moore EE, Sperry JL, Cohen MJ, Chapman MP, et al. Forgot calcium? Admission ionized-calcium in two civilian randomized controlled trials of pre-hospital plasma for traumatic hemorrhagic shock. J Trauma Acute Care Surg. 2020;88(5):588–96.
39. Ditzel RM Jr, Anderson JL, Eisenhart WJ, Rankin CJ, DeFeo DR, Oak S, et al. A review of transfusion- and trauma-induced hypocalcemia: is it time to change the lethal triad to the lethal diamond? J Trauma Acute Care Surg. 2020;88(3):434–9.
40. Chang R, Fox EE, Greene TJ, Swartz MD, DeSantis SM, Stein DM, et al. Abnormalities of laboratory coagulation tests versus clinically evident coagulopathic bleeding: results from the prehospital resuscitation on helicopters study (PROHS). Surgery. 2018;163(4):819–26.
41. Engstrom M, Schott U, Romner B, Reinstrup P. Acidosis impairs the coagulation: a thromboelastographic study. J Trauma. 2006;61(3):624–8.
42. Martini WZ, Pusateri AE, Uscilowicz JM, Delgado AV, Holcomb JB. Independent contributions of hypothermia and acidosis to coagulopathy in swine. J Trauma. 2005;58(5):1002–9; discussion 9–10.
43. Martini WZ, Holcomb JB. Acidosis and coagulopathy: the differential effects on fibrinogen synthesis and breakdown in pigs. Ann Surg. 2007;246(5):831–5.
44. Marumo M, Suehiro A, Kakishita E, Groschner K, Wakabayashi I. Extracellular pH affects platelet aggregation associated with modulation of store-operated Ca(2+) entry. Thromb Res. 2001;104(5):353–60.
45. Cohen MJ, Call M, Nelson M, Calfee CS, Esmon CT, Brohi K, et al. Critical role of activated protein C in early coagulopathy and later organ failure, infection and death in trauma patients. Ann Surg. 2012;255(2):379–85.
46. Cap A, Hunt BJ. The pathogenesis of traumatic coagulopathy. Anaesthesia. 2015;70(Suppl 1):96–101, e32–4.
47. Chapman MP, Moore EE, Moore HB, Gonzalez E, Gamboni F, Chandler JG, et al. Overwhelming tPA release, not PAI-1 degradation, is responsible for hyperfibrinolysis in severely injured trauma patients. J Trauma Acute Care Surg. 2016;80(1):16–23; discussion 23–5.
48. Weisel JW, Litvinov RI. Mechanisms of fibrin polymerization and clinical implications. Blood. 2013;121(10):1712–9.
49. Hoffman M, Monroe DM 3rd. A cell-based model of hemostasis. Thromb Haemost. 2001;85(6):958–65.
50. Gando S. Tissue factor in trauma and organ dysfunction. Semin Thromb Hemost. 2006;32(1):48–53.
51. Vulliamy P, Kornblith LZ, Kutcher ME, Cohen MJ, Brohi K, Neal MD. Alterations in platelet behavior after major trauma: adaptive or maladaptive? Platelets. 2021;32(3):295–304.
52. Neal MD. The great platelet paradox: evolution of platelet contribution to hemostasis, inflammation, and thrombosis after injury. Blood Adv. 2020;4(11):2556.
53. Kozar RA, Pati S. Syndecan-1 restitution by plasma after hemorrhagic shock. J Trauma Acute Care Surg. 2015;78(6 Suppl 1):S83–6.
54. Johansson PI, Stensballe J, Rasmussen LS, Ostrowski SR. A high admission syndecan-1 level, a marker of endothelial glycocalyx degradation, is associated with inflammation, protein C depletion, fibrinolysis, and increased mortality in trauma patients. Ann Surg. 2011;254(2):194–200.

55. Gonzalez Rodriguez E, Ostrowski SR, Cardenas JC, Baer LA, Tomasek JS, Henriksen HH, et al. Syndecan-1: a quantitative marker for the endotheliopathy of trauma. J Am Coll Surg. 2017;225(3):419–27.
56. Ban K, Peng Z, Pati S, Witkov RB, Park PW, Kozar RA. Plasma-mediated gut protection after Hemorrhagic shock is lessened in Syndecan-1−/− mice. Shock. 2015;44(5):452–7.
57. Pati S, Matijevic N, Doursout MF, Ko T, Cao Y, Deng X, et al. Protective effects of fresh frozen plasma on vascular endothelial permeability, coagulation, and resuscitation after hemorrhagic shock are time dependent and diminish between days 0 and 5 after thaw. J Trauma. 2010;69(Suppl 1):S55–63.
58. Kozar RA, Peng Z, Zhang R, Holcomb JB, Pati S, Park P, et al. Plasma restoration of endothelial glycocalyx in a rodent model of hemorrhagic shock. Anesth Analg. 2011;112(6):1289–95.
59. Haywood-Watson RJ, Holcomb JB, Gonzalez EA, Peng Z, Pati S, Park PW, et al. Modulation of syndecan-1 shedding after hemorrhagic shock and resuscitation. PLoS One. 2011;6(8):e23530.
60. Peng Z, Pati S, Potter D, Brown R, Holcomb JB, Grill R, et al. Fresh frozen plasma lessens pulmonary endothelial inflammation and hyperpermeability after hemorrhagic shock and is associated with loss of syndecan 1. Shock. 2013;40(3):195–202.
61. Gruen DS, Brown JB, Guyette FX, Vodovotz Y, Johansson PI, Stensballe J, et al. Prehospital plasma is associated with distinct biomarker expression following injury. JCI Insight. 2020;5(8):e135350.
62. Fitzgerald ML, Wang Z, Park PW, Murphy G, Bernfield M. Shedding of syndecan-1 and -4 ectodomains is regulated by multiple signaling pathways and mediated by a TIMP-3-sensitive metalloproteinase. J Cell Biol. 2000;148(4):811–24.
63. Prudovsky I, Carter D, Kacer D, Palmeri M, Soul T, Kumpel C, et al. Tranexamic acid suppresses the release of mitochondrial DNA, protects the endothelial monolayer and enhances oxidative phosphorylation. J Cell Physiol. 2019;234(11):19121–9.
64. Diebel ME, Martin JV, Liberati DM, Diebel LN. The temporal response and mechanism of action of tranexamic acid in endothelial glycocalyx degradation. J Trauma Acute Care Surg. 2018;84(1):75–80.
65. Kutcher ME, Redick BJ, McCreery RC, Crane IM, Greenberg MD, Cachola LM, et al. Characterization of platelet dysfunction after trauma. J Trauma Acute Care Surg. 2012;73(1):13–9.
66. Tweardy DJ, Khoshnevis MR, Yu B, Mastrangelo MA, Hardison EG, Lopez JA. Essential role for platelets in organ injury and inflammation in resuscitated hemorrhagic shock. Shock. 2006;26(4):386–90.
67. Ding N, Chen G, Hoffman R, Loughran PA, Sodhi CP, Hackam DJ, et al. Toll-like receptor 4 regulates platelet function and contributes to coagulation abnormality and organ injury in hemorrhagic shock and resuscitation. Circ Cardiovasc Genet. 2014;7(5):615–24.
68. Kornblith LZ, Kutcher ME, Redick BJ, Calfee CS, Vilardi RF, Cohen MJ. Fibrinogen and platelet contributions to clot formation: implications for trauma resuscitation and thromboprophylaxis. J Trauma Acute Care Surg. 2014;76(2):255–6; discussion 62–3.
69. Zipperle J, Altenburger K, Ponschab M, Schlimp CJ, Spittler A, Bahrami S, et al. Potential role of platelet-leukocyte aggregation in trauma-induced coagulopathy: ex vivo findings. J Trauma Acute Care Surg. 2017;82(5):921–6.
70. Kornblith LZ, Robles AJ, Conroy AS, Hendrickson CM, Calfee CS, Fields AT, et al. Perhaps it's not the platelet: ristocetin uncovers the potential role of von Willebrand factor in impaired platelet aggregation following traumatic brain injury. J Trauma Acute Care Surg. 2018;85(5):873–80.
71. Starr NE, Matthay ZA, Fields AT, Nunez-Garcia B, Callcut RA, Cohen MJ, et al. Identification of injury and shock driven effects on ex vivo platelet aggregometry: a cautionary tale of phenotyping. J Trauma Acute Care Surg. 2020;89(1):20–8.
72. Plautz WE, Matthay ZA, Rollins-Raval MA, Raval JS, Kornblith LZ, Neal MD. Von Willebrand factor as a thrombotic and inflammatory mediator in critical illness. Transfusion. 2020;60(Suppl 3):S158–66.
73. Cardenas JC, Rahbar E, Pommerening MJ, Baer LA, Matijevic N, Cotton BA, et al. Measuring thrombin generation as a tool for predicting hemostatic potential and transfusion requirements following trauma. J Trauma Acute Care Surg. 2014;77(6):839–45.
74. Meng ZH, Wolberg AS, Monroe DM 3rd, Hoffman M. The effect of temperature and pH on the activity of factor VIIa: implications for the efficacy of high-dose factor VIIa in hypothermic and acidotic patients. J Trauma. 2003;55(5):886–91.
75. Wolberg AS, Meng ZH, Monroe DM 3rd, Hoffman M. A systematic evaluation of the effect of temperature on coagulation enzyme activity and platelet function. J Trauma. 2004;56(6):1221–8.
76. Martini WZ. Coagulopathy by hypothermia and acidosis: mechanisms of thrombin generation and fibrinogen availability. J Trauma. 2009;67(1):202–8; discussion 8–9.
77. Floccard B, Rugeri L, Faure A, Saint Denis M, Boyle EM, Peguet O, et al. Early coagulopathy in trauma patients: an on-scene and hospital admission study. Injury. 2012;43(1):26–32.
78. Woolley T, Gwyther R, Parmar K, Kirkman E, Watts S, Midwinter M, et al. A prospective observational study of acute traumatic coagulopathy in traumatic bleeding from the battlefield. Transfusion. 2020;60(Suppl 3):S52–61.
79. Dunbar NM, Chandler WL. Thrombin generation in trauma patients. Transfusion. 2009;49(12):2652–60.
80. Muszbek L, Bereczky Z, Bagoly Z, Komaromi I, Katona E. Factor XIII: a coagulation factor with multiple plasmatic and cellular functions. Physiol Rev. 2011;91(3):931–72.

81. Kononova O, Litvinov RI, Blokhin DS, Klochkov VV, Weisel JW, Bennett JS, et al. Mechanistic basis for the binding of RGD- and AGDV-peptides to the platelet integrin alphaIIbbeta3. Biochemistry. 2017;56(13):1932–42.
82. Tennent GA, Brennan SO, Stangou AJ, O'Grady J, Hawkins PN, Pepys MB. Human plasma fibrinogen is synthesized in the liver. Blood. 2007;109(5):1971–4.
83. Levy JH, Szlam F, Tanaka KA, Sniecienski RM. Fibrinogen and hemostasis: a primary hemostatic target for the management of acquired bleeding. Anesth Analg. 2012;114(2):261–74.
84. Mosesson MW. Fibrinogen and fibrin structure and functions. J Thromb Haemost. 2005;3(8):1894–904.
85. Hiippala ST, Myllyla GJ, Vahtera EM. Hemostatic factors and replacement of major blood loss with plasma-poor red cell concentrates. Anesth Analg. 1995;81(2):360–5.
86. Schlimp CJ, Schochl H. The role of fibrinogen in trauma-induced coagulopathy. Hamostaseologie. 2014;34(1):29–39.
87. Wohltmann CD, Franklin GA, Boaz PW, Luchette FA, Kearney PA, Richardson JD, et al. A multicenter evaluation of whether gender dimorphism affects survival after trauma. Am J Surg. 2001;181(4):297–300.
88. Nunns GR, Moore EE, Stettler GR, Moore HB, Ghasabyan A, Cohen M, et al. Empiric transfusion strategies during life-threatening hemorrhage. Surgery. 2018;164(2):306–11.
89. Moore HB, Moore EE, Chapman MP, Huebner BR, Einersen PM, Oushy S, et al. Viscoelastic tissue plasminogen activator challenge predicts massive transfusion in 15 minutes. J Am Coll Surg. 2017;225(1):138–47.
90. Raza I, Davenport R, Rourke C, Platton S, Manson J, Spoors C, et al. The incidence and magnitude of fibrinolytic activation in trauma patients. J Thromb Haemost. 2013;11(2):307–14.
91. Rourke C, Curry N, Khan S, Taylor R, Raza I, Davenport R, et al. Fibrinogen levels during trauma hemorrhage, response to replacement therapy, and association with patient outcomes. J Thromb Haemost. 2012;10(7):1342–51.
92. McQuilten ZK, Wood EM, Bailey M, Cameron PA, Cooper DJ. Fibrinogen is an independent predictor of mortality in major trauma patients: a five-year statewide cohort study. Injury. 2017;48(5):1074–81.
93. Inaba K, Karamanos E, Lustenberger T, Schochl H, Shulman I, Nelson J, et al. Impact of fibrinogen levels on outcomes after acute injury in patients requiring a massive transfusion. J Am Coll Surg. 2013;216(2):290–7.
94. Spahn DR, Bouillon B, Cerny V, Duranteau J, Filipescu D, Hunt BJ, et al. The European guideline on management of major bleeding and coagulopathy following trauma: fifth edition. Crit Care. 2019;23(1):98.
95. Cotton BA, Harvin JA, Kostousouv V, Minei KM, Radwan ZA, Schochl H, et al. Hyperfibrinolysis at admission is an uncommon but highly lethal event associated with shock and prehospital fluid administration. J Trauma Acute Care Surg. 2012;73(2):365–70; discussion 70.
96. Schochl H, Frietsch T, Pavelka M, Jambor C. Hyperfibrinolysis after major trauma: differential diagnosis of lysis patterns and prognostic value of thrombelastometry. J Trauma. 2009;67(1):125–31.
97. Moore HB, Moore EE, Chapman MP, Hansen KC, Cohen MJ, Pieracci FM, et al. Does tranexamic acid improve clot strength in severely injured patients who have elevated fibrin degradation products and low fibrinolytic activity, measured by thrombelastography? J Am Coll Surg. 2019;229(1):92–101.
98. Moore HB, Moore EE, Liras IN, Gonzalez E, Harvin JA, Holcomb JB, et al. Acute fibrinolysis shutdown after injury occurs frequently and increases mortality: a multicenter evaluation of 2,540 severely injured patients. J Am Coll Surg. 2016;222(4):347–55.
99. Cardenas JC, Matijevic N, Baer LA, Holcomb JB, Cotton BA, Wade CE. Elevated tissue plasminogen activator and reduced plasminogen activator inhibitor promote hyperfibrinolysis in trauma patients. Shock. 2014;41(6):514–21.
100. Moore HB, Moore EE, Huebner BR, Dzieciatkowska M, Stettler GR, Nunns GR, et al. Fibrinolysis shutdown is associated with a fivefold increase in mortality in trauma patients lacking hypersensitivity to tissue plasminogen activator. J Trauma Acute Care Surg. 2017;83(6):1014–22.
101. Davenport RA, Guerreiro M, Frith D, Rourke C, Platton S, Cohen M, et al. Activated protein C drives the hyperfibrinolysis of acute traumatic coagulopathy. Anesthesiology. 2017;126(1):115–27.
102. Moore HB, Moore EE, Chapman MP, Gonzalez E, Slaughter AL, Morton AP, et al. Viscoelastic measurements of platelet function, not fibrinogen function, predicts sensitivity to tissue-type plasminogen activator in trauma patients. J Thromb Haemost. 2015;13(10):1878–87.
103. Bouma BN, Mosnier LO. Thrombin activatable fibrinolysis inhibitor (TAFI) at the interface between coagulation and fibrinolysis. Pathophysiol Haemost Thromb. 2003;33(5–6):375–81.
104. Fraser SR, Booth NA, Mutch NJ. The antifibrinolytic function of factor XIII is exclusively expressed through alpha(2)-antiplasmin cross-linking. Blood. 2011;117(23):6371–4.
105. Wright FL, Vogler TO, Moore EE, Moore HB, Wohlauer MV, Urban S, et al. Fibrinolysis shutdown correlation with thromboembolic events in severe COVID-19 infection. J Am Coll Surg. 2020;231(2):193–203.e1.
106. Meizoso JP, Moore HB, Moore EE. Fibrinolysis shutdown in COVID-19: clinical manifestations, molecular mechanisms, and therapeutic implications. J Am Coll Surg. 2021;232(6):995–1003.
107. Moore HB, Moore EE, Neal MD, Sheppard FR, Kornblith LZ, Draxler DF, et al. Fibrinolysis shutdown in trauma: historical review and clinical implications. Anesth Analg. 2019;129(3):762–73.

108. Hardaway RM, Mc KD. Intravascular thrombi and the intestinal factor of irreversible shock. Ann Surg. 1959;150(2):261–5.
109. Deguchi H, Sinha RK, Marchese P, Ruggeri ZM, Zilberman-Rudenko J, McCarty OJT, et al. Prothrombotic skeletal muscle myosin directly enhances prothrombin activation by binding factors Xa and Va. Blood. 2016;128(14):1870–8.
110. Dyer MR, Plautz WE, Ragni MV, Alexander W, Haldeman S, Sperry JL, et al. Traumatic injury results in prolonged circulation of ultralarge von Willebrand factor and a reduction in ADAMTS13 activity. Transfusion. 2020;60(6):1308–18.
111. Vogel S, Bodenstein R, Chen Q, Feil S, Feil R, Rheinlaender J, et al. Platelet-derived HMGB1 is a critical mediator of thrombosis. J Clin Invest. 2015;125(12):4638–54.
112. Vulliamy P, Gillespie S, Armstrong PC, Allan HE, Warner TD, Brohi K. Histone H4 induces platelet ballooning and microparticle release during trauma hemorrhage. Proc Natl Acad Sci U S A. 2019;116(35):17444–9.
113. Dyer MR, Chen Q, Haldeman S, Yazdani H, Hoffman R, Loughran P, et al. Deep vein thrombosis in mice is regulated by platelet HMGB1 through release of neutrophil-extracellular traps and DNA. Sci Rep. 2018;8(1):2068.
114. Stark K, Philippi V, Stockhausen S, Busse J, Antonelli A, Miller M, et al. Disulfide HMGB1 derived from platelets coordinates venous thrombosis in mice. Blood. 2016;128(20):2435–49.
115. Roberts DJ, Kalkwarf KJ, Moore HB, Cohen MJ, Fox EE, Wade CE, et al. Time course and outcomes associated with transient versus persistent fibrinolytic phenotypes after injury: a nested, prospective, multicenter cohort study. J Trauma Acute Care Surg. 2019;86(2):206–13.
116. Moore HB, Moore EE, Gonzalez E, Huebner BR, Sheppard FR, Banerjee A, et al. Reperfusion shutdown: delayed onset of fibrinolysis resistance after resuscitation from Hemorrhagic shock is associated with increased circulating levels of plasminogen activator Inhibitor-1 and postinjury complications. Blood. 2016;128:206.
117. Gall LS, Vulliamy P, Gillespie S, Jones TF, Pierre RSJ, Breukers SE, et al. The S100A10 pathway mediates an occult hyperfibrinolytic subtype in trauma patients. Ann Surg. 2019;269(6):1184–91.
118. Cardenas JC, Wade CE, Cotton BA, George MJ, Holcomb JB, Schreiber MA, et al. TEG lysis shutdown represents coagulopathy in bleeding trauma patients: analysis of the PROPPR cohort. Shock. 2019;51(3):273–83.
119. Meizoso JP, Karcutskie CA, Ray JJ, Namias N, Schulman CI, Proctor KG. Persistent fibrinolysis shutdown is associated with increased mortality in severely injured trauma patients. J Am Coll Surg. 2017;224(4):575–82.
120. Leeper CM, Neal MD, McKenna CJ, Gaines BA. Trending fibrinolytic dysregulation: fibrinolysis shutdown in the days after injury is associated with poor outcome in severely injured children. Ann Surg. 2017;266(3):508–15.
121. Holcomb JB, Minei KM, Scerbo ML, Radwan ZA, Wade CE, Kozar RA, et al. Admission rapid thrombelastography can replace conventional coagulation tests in the emergency department: experience with 1974 consecutive trauma patients. Ann Surg. 2012;256(3):476–86.
122. Ives C, Inaba K, Branco BC, Okoye O, Schochl H, Talving P, et al. Hyperfibrinolysis elicited via thromboelastography predicts mortality in trauma. J Am Coll Surg. 2012;215(4):496–502.
123. McCully SP, Fabricant LJ, Kunio NR, Groat TL, Watson KM, Differding JA, et al. The international normalized ratio overestimates coagulopathy in stable trauma and surgical patients. J Trauma Acute Care Surg. 2013;75(6):947–53.
124. Stettler GR, Moore EE, Moore HB, Nunns GR, Coleman JR, Colvis A, et al. Variability in international normalized ratio and activated partial thromboplastin time after injury are not explained by coagulation factor deficits. J Trauma Acute Care Surg. 2019;87(3):582–9.
125. Kelly JM, Rizoli S, Veigas P, Hollands S, Min A. Using rotational thromboelastometry clot firmness at 5 minutes (ROTEM((R)) EXTEM A5) to predict massive transfusion and in-hospital mortality in trauma: a retrospective analysis of 1146 patients. Anaesthesia. 2018;73(9):1103–9.
126. Barrett CD, Moore HB, Vigneshwar N, Dhara S, Chandler J, Chapman MP, et al. Plasmin TEG rapidly identifies trauma patients at risk for massive transfusion, mortality and hyperfibrinolysis: a diagnostic tool to resolve an international debate on TXA? J Trauma Acute Care Surg. 2020;89(6):991–8.
127. Coleman JR, Moore EE, Sauaia A, Samuels JM, Moore HB, Ghasabyan A, et al. Untangling sex dimorphisms in coagulation: initial steps toward precision medicine for trauma resuscitation. Ann Surg. 2020;271(6):e128–30.
128. Pezold M, Moore EE, Wohlauer M, Sauaia A, Gonzalez E, Banerjee A, et al. Viscoelastic clot strength predicts coagulation-related mortality within 15 minutes. Surgery. 2012;151(1):48–54.
129. Nystrup KB, Windelov NA, Thomsen AB, Johansson PI. Reduced clot strength upon admission, evaluated by thrombelastography (TEG), in trauma patients is independently associated with increased 30-day mortality. Scand J Trauma Resusc Emerg Med. 2011;19:52.
130. Plotkin AJ, Wade CE, Jenkins DH, Smith KA, Noe JC, Park MS, et al. A reduction in clot formation rate and strength assessed by thrombelastography is indicative of transfusion requirements in patients with penetrating injuries. J Trauma. 2008;64(2 Suppl):S64–8.
131. Baksaas-Aasen K, Gall LS, Stensballe J, Juffermans NP, Curry N, Maegele M, et al. Viscoelastic haemostatic assay augmented protocols for major trauma

131. haemorrhage (ITACTIC): a randomized, controlled trial. Intensive Care Med. 2021;47(1):49–59.
132. Holbrook TL, Hoyt DB, Anderson JP. The importance of gender on outcome after major trauma: functional and psychologic outcomes in women versus men. J Trauma. 2001;50(2):270–3.
133. Meizoso JP, Proctor KG. Venous thromboembolism after trauma. In: Moore HB, Moore EE, Neal MD, editors. Trauma induced coagulopathy. 2nd ed. Springer; 2021.
134. Sevitt S, Gallagher N. Venous thrombosis and pulmonary embolism. A clinico-pathological study in injured and burned patients. Br J Surg. 1961;48:475–89.
135. Shackford SR, Davis JW, Hollingsworth-Fridlund P, Brewer NS, Hoyt DB, Mackersie RC. Venous thromboembolism in patients with major trauma. Am J Surg. 1990;159(4):365–9.
136. Geerts WH, Code KI, Jay RM, Chen E, Szalai JP. A prospective study of venous thromboembolism after major trauma. N Engl J Med. 1994;331(24):1601–6.
137. Knudson MM, Ikossi DG, Khaw L, Morabito D, Speetzen LS. Thromboembolism after trauma: an analysis of 1602 episodes from the American College of Surgeons National Trauma Data Bank. Ann Surg. 2004;240(3):490–6; discussion 6–8.
138. Meizoso JP, Karcutskie CA 4th, Ray JJ, Ruiz X, Ginzburg E, Namias N, et al. A simplified stratification system for venous thromboembolism risk in severely injured trauma patients. J Surg Res. 2017;207:138–44.
139. Sumislawski JJ, Moore HB, Moore EE, Swope ML, Pieracci FM, Fox CJ, et al. Not all in your head (and neck): stroke after blunt cerebrovascular injury is associated with systemic hypercoagulability. J Trauma Acute Care Surg. 2019;87(5):1082–7.
140. Brill JB, Badiee J, Zander AL, Wallace JD, Lewis PR, Sise MJ, et al. The rate of deep vein thrombosis doubles in trauma patients with hypercoagulable thromboelastography. J Trauma Acute Care Surg. 2017;83(3):413–9.
141. Kashuk JL, Moore EE, Sabel A, Barnett C, Haenel J, Le T, et al. Rapid thrombelastography (r-TEG) identifies hypercoagulability and predicts thromboembolic events in surgical patients. Surgery. 2009;146(4):764–72; discussion 72–4.
142. Secemsky EA, Rosenfield K, Kennedy KF, Jaff M, Yeh RW. High burden of 30-day readmissions after acute venous thromboembolism in the United States. J Am Heart Assoc. 2018;7(13):e009047.
143. Van Haren RM, Valle EJ, Thorson CM, Jouria JM, Busko AM, Guarch GA, et al. Hypercoagulability and other risk factors in trauma intensive care unit patients with venous thromboembolism. J Trauma Acute Care Surg. 2014;76(2):443–9.
144. Coleman JR, Kay AB, Moore EE, Moore HB, Gonzalez E, Majercik S, et al. It's sooner than you think: blunt solid organ injury patients are already hypercoagulable upon hospital admission—results of a bi-institutional, prospective study. Am J Surg. 2019;218(6):1065–73.
145. Chapman BC, Moore EE, Barnett C, Stovall RT, Biffl WL, Burlew CC, et al. Hypercoagulability following blunt solid abdominal organ injury: when to initiate anticoagulation. Am J Surg. 2013;206(6):917–22; discussion 22–3.
146. Gary JL, Schneider PS, Galpin M, Radwan Z, Munz JW, Achor TS, et al. Can thrombelastography predict venous thromboembolic events in patients with severe extremity trauma? J Orthop Trauma. 2016;30(6):294–8.
147. Goolsby C, Jacobs L, Hunt RC, Goralnick E, Singletary EM, Levy MJ, et al. Stop the bleed education consortium: education program content and delivery recommendations. J Trauma Acute Care Surg. 2018;84(1):205–10.
148. Rossaint R, Bouillon B, Cerny V, Coats TJ, Duranteau J, Fernandez-Mondejar E, et al. The STOP the bleeding campaign. Crit Care. 2013;17(2):136.
149. Holcomb JB, Jenkins D, Rhee P, Johannigman J, Mahoney P, Mehta S, et al. Damage control resuscitation: directly addressing the early coagulopathy of trauma. J Trauma. 2007;62(2):307–10.
150. Moore EE. Staged laparotomy for the hypothermia, acidosis, and coagulopathy syndrome. Am J Surg. 1996;172(5):405–10.
151. Stone HH, Strom PR, Mullins RJ. Management of the major coagulopathy with onset during laparotomy. Ann Surg. 1983;197(5):532–5.
152. Etchill E, Sperry J, Zuckerbraun B, Alarcon L, Brown J, Schuster K, et al. The confusion continues: results from an American Association for the Surgery of Trauma survey on massive transfusion practices among United States trauma centers. Transfusion. 2016;56(10):2478–86.
153. The National Blood Authority's patient blood management guideline: module 1. Critical bleeding/massive transfusion; 2011. https://www.blood.gov.au/system/files/documents/pbm-module1_0.pdf.
154. Cryer HG, Nathens AB, Bulger EM, et al. American College of Surgeons trauma quality improvement program massive transfusion guidelines; 2014. https://www.facs.org/-/media/files/quality-programs/trauma/tqip/transfusion_guidelines.ashx.
155. Joint United Kingdom (UK) Blood transfusion and tissue transplantation services professional advisory committee. Transfusion management of major haemorrhage. Handbook of transfusion medicine, 5th ed. 2014. https://www.transfusionguidelines.org/transfusion-handbook/7-effective-transfusion-in-surgery-and-critical-care/7-3-transfusion-management-of-major-haemorrhage.
156. Miyata S, Ikatura A, Ueda Y, et al. Transfusion guidelines for the patients with massive bleeding. Jpn J Transfus Cell Ther. 2019;65(1):21–92.
157. Moore HB, Moore EE, Gonzalez E, Wiener G, Chapman MP, Dzieciatkowska M, et al. Plasma is the physiologic buffer of tissue plasminogen activator-mediated fibrinolysis: rationale for plasma-first resuscitation after life-threatening hemorrhage. J Am Coll Surg. 2015;220(5):872–9.

158. Borgman MA, Spinella PC, Perkins JG, Grathwohl KW, Repine T, Beekley AC, et al. The ratio of blood products transfused affects mortality in patients receiving massive transfusions at a combat support hospital. J Trauma. 2007;63(4):805–13.
159. Itagaki Y, Hayakawa M, Maekawa K, Saito T, Kodate A, Honma Y, et al. Early administration of fibrinogen concentrate is associated with improved survival among severe trauma patients: a single-centre propensity score-matched analysis. World J Emerg Surg. 2020;15:7.
160. CRASH-2 trial collaborators. Effects of tranexamic acid on death, vascular occlusive events, and blood transfusion in trauma patients with significant haemorrhage (CRASH-2): a randomised, placebo-controlled trial. Lancet 2010;376(9734):23-32.
161. Guyette FX, Brown JB, Zenati MS, Early-Young BJ, Adams PW, Eastridge BJ, et al. Tranexamic acid during prehospital transport in patients at risk for hemorrhage after injury: a double-blind, placebo-controlled, randomized clinical trial. JAMA Surg. 2020;156(1):11–20.
162. CRASH-3 Trial Collaborators. Effects of tranexamic acid on death, disability, vascular occlusive events and other morbidities in patients with acute traumatic brain injury (CRASH-3): a randomised, placebo-controlled trial. Lancet. 2019;394(10210):1713–23.
163. Rowell SE, Meier EN, McKnight B, Kannas D, May S, Sheehan K, et al. Effect of out-of-hospital tranexamic acid vs placebo on 6-month functional neurologic outcomes in patients with moderate or severe traumatic brain injury. JAMA. 2020;324(10):961–74.
164. Myers SP, Kutcher ME, Rosengart MR, Sperry JL, Peitzman AB, Brown JB, et al. Tranexamic acid administration is associated with an increased risk of posttraumatic venous thromboembolism. J Trauma Acute Care Surg. 2019;86(1):20–7.
165. Johnston LR, Rodriguez CJ, Elster EA, Bradley MJ. Evaluation of military use of tranexamic acid and associated thromboembolic events. JAMA Surg. 2018;153(2):169–75.
166. Valle EJ, Allen CJ, Van Haren RM, Jouria JM, Li H, Livingstone AS, et al. Do all trauma patients benefit from tranexamic acid? J Trauma Acute Care Surg. 2014;76(6):1373–8.
167. HALT-IT Trial Collaborators. Effects of a high-dose 24-h infusion of tranexamic acid on death and thromboembolic events in patients with acute gastrointestinal bleeding (HALT-IT): an international randomised, double-blind, placebo-controlled trial. Lancet. 2020;395(10241):1927–36.
168. Moore EE, Moore HB, Gonzalez E, Sauaia A, Banerjee A, Silliman CC. Rationale for the selective administration of tranexamic acid to inhibit fibrinolysis in the severely injured patient. Transfusion. 2016;56(Suppl 2):S110–4.
169. Moore HB, Moore EE, Huebner BR, Stettler GR, Nunns GR, Einersen PM, et al. Tranexamic acid is associated with increased mortality in patients with physiological fibrinolysis. J Surg Res. 2017;220:438–43.

Further Reading

Cryer HG, Nathens AB, Bulger EM, et al. American College of Surgeons trauma quality improvement program massive transfusion guidelines. 2014. https://www.facs.org/-/media/files/quality-programs/trauma/tqip/transfusion_guildelines.ashx.

Gonzalez E, Moore EE, Moore HB, et al. Goal-directed hemostatic resuscitation of trauma-induced coagulopathy: a pragmatic randomized clinical trial comparing a viscoelastic assay to conventional coagulation assays. Ann Surg. 2016;263(6):1051–9.

Holcomb JB, Tilley BC, Baraniuk S, et al. Transfusion of plasma, platelets, and red blood cells in a 1:1:1 vs a 1:1:2 ratio and mortality in patients with severe trauma: the PROPPR randomized clinical trial. JAMA. 2015;313(5):471–82.

Moore EE, Moore HB, Kornblith L, et al. Trauma-induced coagulopathy. Nat Rev Dis Primers. 2021;7:30.

Moore HB, Gando S, Iba T, et al. Defining trauma-induced coagulopathy with respect to future implications for patient management: communication from the SSC of the ISTH. J Thromb Haemost. 2020;18(3):740–7.

Septic Shock

10

Sacha Rozencwajg and Philippe Montravers

10.1 Introduction

Learning Goals
- **Diagnosis of septic shock** can be challenging. It relies on early identification of sepsis with the qSOFA score and presence of a hypotension or abnormal lactate levels despite adequate fluid resuscitation.
- **Source identification is based on adequate imaging** (e.g., chest X-ray, abdominal CT-scan) **and microbiological samples.** At least two sets of blood cultures are recommended prior to antimicrobial therapy to increase the chance of pathogen identification.
- **Restoration of adequate tissue perfusion + initiation of an empirical antimicrobial therapy + source control** are the cornerstone of treatment.

10.1.1 Definition of Sepsis and Septic Shock

In 2016, the Third International Consensus Definition for Sepsis and Septic Shock (Sepsis-3) published an updated definition for sepsis and septic shock [1]. The definition encompasses three severity states:

- **Infection**
- **Sepsis**: infection + SOFA score ≥ 2
- **Septic shock**: sepsis with persisting hypotension requiring vasopressors to maintain a mean arterial pressure (MAP) ≥ 65 mmHg and having a serum lactate level > 2 mmol/L (18 mg/dL) despite adequate volume resuscitation.
- *Infection* is defined as the state resulting in the invasion by, and multiplication of, microorganisms. It is typically suspected in case of fever and symptoms related to the infection site (e.g., lungs, urine, skin).
- *Sepsis* is defined as a life-threatening organ dysfunction resulting from dysregulated host

S. Rozencwajg
Département d'Anesthésie-Réanimation, CHU Bichat-Claude Bernard, GHU Nord, APHP, Paris, France

Université Paris Cité, Paris, France
e-mail: sacha.rozencwajg@aphp.fr

P. Montravers (✉)
Département d'Anesthésie-Réanimation, CHU Bichat-Claude Bernard, GHU Nord, APHP, Paris, France

Université Paris Cité, Paris, France

INSERM UMR 1152, Paris, France
e-mail: philippe.montravers@aphp.fr

Table 10.1 Sepsis-related Organ Failure Assessment (SOFA) score

System	SOFA score 0	SOFA score 1	SOFA score 2	SOFA score 3	SOFA score 4
Respiration					
PaO_2/FiO_2, mmHg (kPa)	≥400 (≥53.3)	<400 (<53.3)	<300 (<40)	<200 (<26.7) with respiratory support	<100 (<13.3) with respiratory support
Coagulation					
Platelets, ×10³/μL	≥150	<150	<100	<50	<20
Liver					
Bilirubin, mg/dL (μmol/L)	<1.2 (<20)	1.2–1.9 (20–32)	2.0–5.9 (33–101)	6.0–11.9 (102–204)	≥12.0 (≥204)
Cardiovascular[a]					
	MAP ≥70 mmHg	MAP <70 mmHg	Dopamine <5 or dobutamine (any dose)	Dopamine 5.1–15 or epinephrine ≤0.1 or norepinephrine ≤0.1	Dopamine >15 or epinephrine >0.1 or norepinephrine >0.1
Central nervous system					
Glasgow coma score		13–14	10–12	6–9	<6
Renal					
Creatinine, mg/dL (μmol/L) Urine output, mL/day	<1.2 (<110)	1.2–1.9 (110–170)	2.0–3.4 (171–299)	3.5–4.9 (300–440) <500	≥5.0 (≥440) <200

responses to infection. The definition of sepsis relies on the suspicion of an infection with organ dysfunctions assessed by a **Sepsis-related Organ Failure Assessment (SOFA) score ≥ 2**. The SOFA score (Table 10.1), used to evaluate the degree of organ dysfunction [2], has been widely used in intensive care units (ICUs) for over 20 years.

- *Septic shock* is defined as sepsis with circulatory, cellular, and metabolic abnormalities. The combination of a clinical criteria (i.e., hypotension requiring vasopressor to maintain a MAP above 65 mmHg) and a biological criteria (i.e., serum lactate level > 2 mmol/L) had the best value to discriminate septic shock from other diagnosis.

10.1.2 Pathophysiology

Sepsis is classically characterized by a dysregulated response from a host to infection. The precise mechanisms leading to sepsis-induced organ failure are not fully understood and remain an active area of scientific investigation. Figure 10.1 illustrates the main mechanisms responsible for sepsis and septic shock.

From a macrocirculatory point of view, septic shock can be defined as the instauration and perpetuation of a **mismatch between tissue perfusion and its metabolic requirements** [3]. The three main causes for this imbalance are (1) the **"relative hypovolemic state"** caused by the increased capillary permeability due to endothelial injury [4], (2) the global **vasodilatory state** [5] due to hyporesponsiveness to endogenous vasoconstrictors [6, 7], and (3) the **inflammation-induced cardiac dysfunction** [8].

From a microcirculatory point of view, sepsis induces alterations of microcirculatory perfusion related to endothelial dysfunctions and injuries combined with coagulation disorders, including microvascular clotting, activation of proinflammatory mediators, as well as blood and tissular phagocytes and immunity cells. These multiple targets result in an **alteration of oxygen extraction** capacities at the cellular level [9, 10] and a **dysregulation of the blood flow distribution**

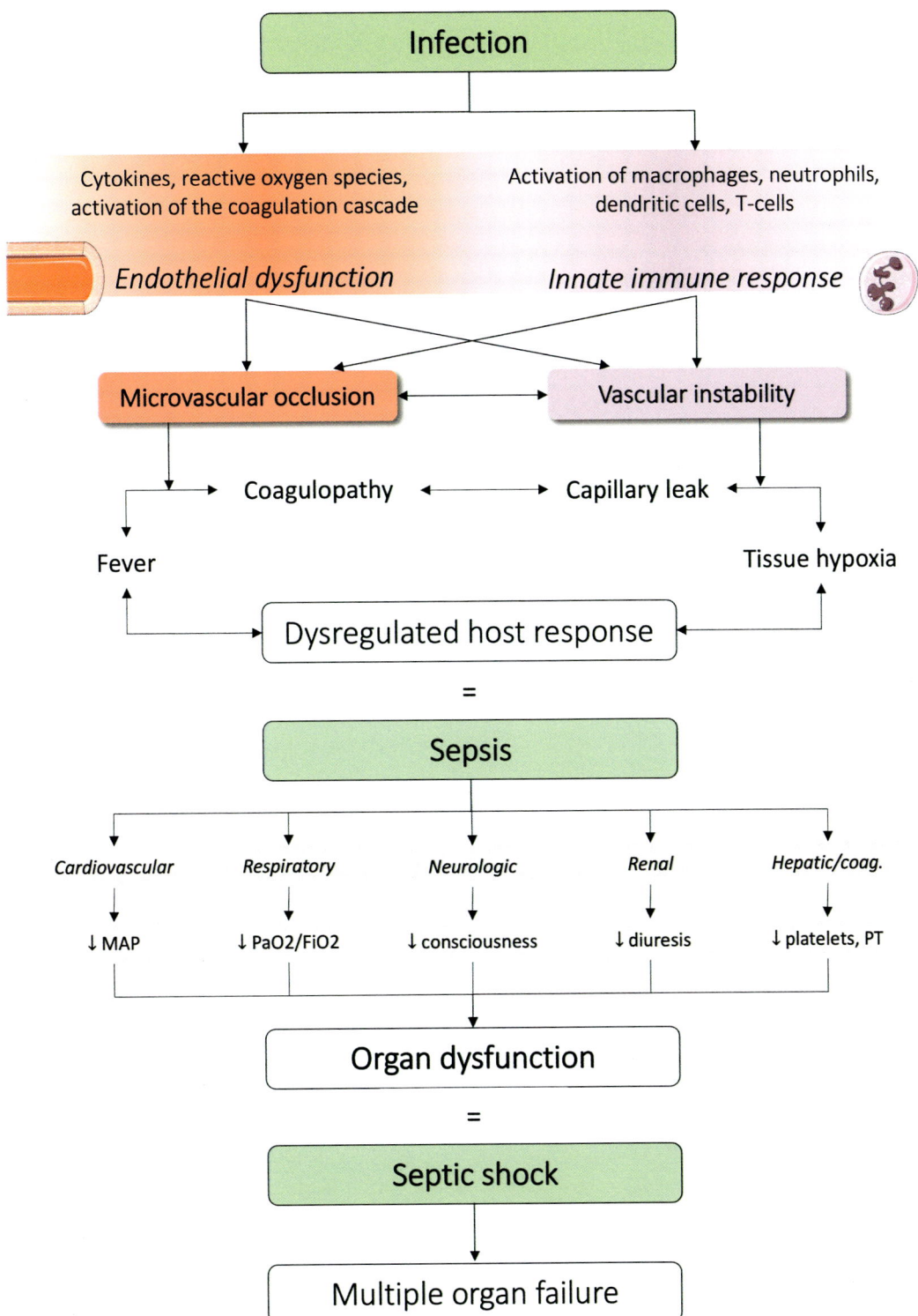

Fig. 10.1 Summary of main mechanisms leading to sepsis and organ dysfunction. *FiO$_2$* inspired fraction of oxygen, *MAP* mean arterial pressure, *PaO$_2$* arterial pressure of oxygen, *PT* prothrombin time

explaining the relative debt in the tissular metabolic requirement. These microcirculatory perfusion impairments lead to organ failure, and in the most severe cases, to death.

10.1.3 Epidemiology

Of septic patients admitted to ICUs worldwide [11], the three most common sources of infection are the **lungs** (60%), **abdomen** (18%), and bloodstream (15%). There is a **predominance of Gram-negative bacterial** infections which are responsible for **two thirds of the documented infections**, the other third being Gram-positive microorganisms. Additionally, fungal infections account for less than 16% of isolated microorganisms. The most common Gram-negative pathogens are enterobacteriaceae (with *Klebsiella* species constituting 27% and *Escherichia coli* 25%) and non-fermenting Gram-negative bacilli (*Pseudomonas aeruginosa* representing 24% and Acinetobacter spp. 11%). *Staphylococcus aureus* (15%) and *Streptococcus* species (7%) are the most common Gram-positive organisms.

10.2 Diagnosis

10.2.1 Screening for Sepsis

Clinical diagnosis relies on (1) the infection site-specific symptoms and (2) the host response signs.

Organ/site-specific symptoms are developed later in specific chapters.

Host response symptoms and signs may vary in terms of presence and intensity. Patients often present to the emergency department with several of the following signs: general malaise, fever or hypothermia, altered mental state, tachycardia or tachypnea, decreased capillary refill time, mottled skin, cold extremities, and arterial hypotension (which is a late sign). None of these signs are sufficiently specific, but the combination of them may help the clinician identify patients at risk of sepsis. In addition, clinical presentation is often misleading in elderly patients. To improve and to accelerate the identification of sepsis, the **quick SOFA** (qSOFA) has been proposed as a practical screening tool or an alert sign. This score comprises three items (1 point per criterion):

- **altered mentation** (Glasgow Coma Scale < 15)
- **systolic blood pressure ≤ 100 mmHg**
- **respiratory rate ≥ 22/min**

This score is a simple and effective tool to screen patients for sepsis and is directly linked with the prognosis: patients with a qSOFA score of 3 had a 23% risk of death, and patients with an infection who had a qSOFA score ≥ 2 accounted for 70% of in-hospital deaths [12].

10.2.2 The Place for Biomarkers

Researchers and physicians have been eager to identify a biomarker with a high sensitivity, high specificity, speed, and the ability to function as a diagnostic, a prognostic, and a follow-up tool – with no success so far. Several "routine labs" are helpful to help identify sepsis, such as leukocytosis (white blood count >12 G/L) or leucopenia (white blood count <4 G/L) and should as such be defined as biomarkers.

C-reactive protein (CRP) and procalcitonin (PCT) are inflammatory markers both elevated in any inflammation state. They have been extensively used and studied over the last decade to help differentiate sepsis from a noninfectious severe state.

C-reactive protein is elevated in several physiological situations, such as aging or pregnancy, and in many noninfectious pathological situations, such as rheumatoid arthritis or burns. Nevertheless, despite its **low diagnostic specificity** [13] and the **absence of correlation with the degree of systemic inflammation** [14], CRP is the most widely used surrogate biomarker for sepsis. In the specific context of postabdominal surgery, Facy et al. found a positive correlation between CRP levels and postsurgical infections [15].

Procalcitonin has been developed as a potential sepsis identification biomarker in several situations. However, several pathological situations led to false positive results, such as scheduled non-septic surgery, cardiopulmonary bypass, noninfectious systemic inflammation, or acute renal failure. **Further investigations are needed to determine its usefulness** and to compare the cost-effectiveness of PCT with other markers [16].

For the reasons presented above, **guidelines do not recommend the use of biomarkers alone for the diagnosis of sepsis or septic shock**.

10.3 Management

The Surviving Sepsis Campaign (SSC) provides updated guidelines on sepsis and septic shock recognition and management [17] and highlights the need for simultaneous collaboration between emergency medicine physicians, infectious disease specialists, and surgeons with three main determinants:

1. Early recognition
2. Early treatment
3. Quality of the medical and surgical management

10.3.1 Early Recognition

The SCC guidelines emphasize the need for early recognition and early treatment of septic shock for improving the prognosis for these patients [18–20]. Therefore, experts recommend that "hospitals and hospital systems have a performance improvement program for sepsis, including sepsis screening for acutely ill, high-risk patients". As an example, creation of a "sepsis team" decreases the time to antibiotics and fluids administration [21].

10.3.2 Early Management

Management of septic shock patients is detailed in the next chapters and summarized in Fig. 10.2. In short, septic shock requires a rapid identification of the infection source, resuscitation, antimicrobial therapy, and the control of the source through surgical or percutaneous techniques or the removal of any foreign body suspected of infection.

10.3.2.1 Identification of the Source

This includes a full clinical exam, adequate imaging (e.g., ultrasound, echocardiography, computed tomography scan without delaying the management), and **microbiological cultures as soon as possible** in order to identify the possible pathogens responsible for septic shock. On top of site-specific cultures, **two sets of aerobic and anaerobic blood cultures** should be drawn prior to any antimicrobial therapy without delaying it. Indeed, their performance is associated with an increased proportion of pathogen identification, a shorter delay for adequate anti-infective therapy, and antimicrobial de-escalation [22, 23].

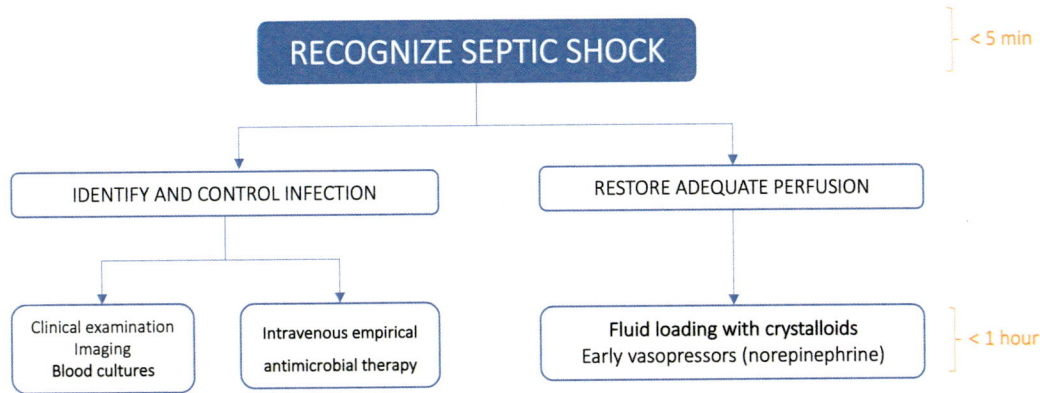

Fig. 10.2 Schematic representation of septic shock early management

10.3.2.2 Resuscitation

SSC Guidelines Regarding Resuscitation Targets

Septic shock resuscitation means rapidly restoring tissue perfusion with fluid therapy and vasopressors. The main goals of resuscitation are as follows:

- a **MAP ≥ 65 mmHg**
- an adequate urine output (>0.5 mL/kg/h)
- a **normalization of capillary refill time** (≤3 s) **and lactatemia** (≤2 mmol/L)

Fluid Resuscitation

The SCC guidelines recommend that "*at least 30 mL/kg of intravenous crystalloid fluid be given within the first 3 h*". The amount of fluid that should be administered remains controversial [24, 25]. The current approach aims at limiting the amount of fluid administered to patients who are "truly" hypovolemic (i.e., dehydrated)—such as older patients or patients with minimal oral intake or nausea/vomiting. Indeed, an excess in fluid loading has been proven to be deleterious in retrospective studies [26, 27].

Crystalloids are the first choice for fluid resuscitation, whether they are unbalanced (0.9% sodium chloride) or balanced (e.g., Lactated Ringer, Hartmann's...) crystalloids. **There is little to no place for colloids** in the initial resuscitation, as several studies have shown an increased risk of acute kidney injury when using hydroxyethyl starch [28, 29] (which is no longer approved by the Food and Drug Administration for sepsis) and no benefit of albumin [30, 31].

Vasoactive Agents

After the early phase of septic shock, only about 50% of patients will respond to fluid challenge (so called "fluid-responders"), which means that additional fluid loading will not increase cardiac output. Combined with the risk of fluid overload, vasopressors are often required to restore an adequate MAP. **Norepinephrine is the first-choice vasopressor**. Dobutamine should only be used in ICU after further hemodynamic and echocardiographic assessment. The ideal timing for starting norepinephrine is still debated, but there is a current trend in using norepinephrine early to prevent a prolonged hypotension and fluid overload, as reported in a recent survey [32].

Monitoring

The initial monitoring of patients in septic shock consists of **reassessment of signs of hypoperfusion** (MAP, capillary refill time, urinary output, and lactate) **and fluid responsiveness**. Fluid responsiveness in ICU may be assessed using the echocardiographic measure of stroke volume after a fluid challenge or other dynamic parameters under mechanical ventilation. During the initial resuscitation, mostly happening in the emergency department, passive leg raising is a simple and effective way to assess the need for fluid loading, as recently reported in a meta-analysis [33].

10.3.3 Antimicrobial Therapy and Control of the Source of Infection

Antimicrobial therapy and controlling the source of infection are the cornerstones of managing these severe patients. The quality and timing of these two therapeutic arms are the only potential ways to improve the prognosis. Many clinical investigations have demonstrated increased morbidity and mortality rates in case of inadequate and/or delayed management of both anti-infective therapy and source control. Nevertheless, the equation **"appropriate antibiotic agents" + "adequate source control"** may be difficult to solve in a constraining timeframe. Choice of antimicrobial therapy must be based on suspected microorganisms (e.g., *Enterobacteriaceae* for intra-abdominal infections), regional/national ecology for community-acquired infections, and local hospital epidemiology and susceptibility for healthcare-associated infections. Underdosing of anti-infective agents is frequent in critically ill patients. To limit this risk, the first dose must not be adapted to the renal function for hydrophilic antibiotics with renal clearance (betalactams, aminoglycosides, glycopeptides...). Therapeutic drug monitoring should be adapted to renal clearance from day 2 [34]. **Source control should never be delayed**. The patient is never too sick for surgery or drainage after achieving hemodynamic stabilization of shock.

10.4 Prognosis

10.4.1 Mortality and Risk Factors

Patients with septic shock criteria have an overall mortality rate of approximately 40%.

Risk factors for mortality in sepsis and septic shock can be classified into three categories:

- Host risk factors
- Pathogen and infection type risk factors
- Management risk factors

Figure 10.3 summarizes the different risk factors identified in multicenter studies [35–40].

10.4.2 Long-term Outcomes

Patients with septic shock suffer long-term consequences from post-sepsis syndrome [41] and post-intensive care syndrome [42]. These two syndromes are responsible for several impairments:
A more rapid **cognitive decline** has been identified in patients suffering from sepsis as compared to a matched population [43];

New **functional limitations** that are often a consequence of ICU-acquired muscle weakness which can persist for years [44];

Depression, posttraumatic stress disorder (PTSD), or general anxiety are reported in 30 to 40% of sepsis survivors [45];

Hospital readmissions are also increased [46] as patients present an increased risk for **cardiovascular disease** [47];

In the long term, **persisting or definitive organ impairments** are also described following multiple organ failure, such as renal or respiratory chronic dysfunction following acute renal failure or acute respiratory distress syndrome.

10.5 Conclusion

Septic shock is a condition that follows a dysregulated interaction between a pathogen and a host. Timely and adequate management are the key determinants for the improvement of the prognosis of this life threatening syndrome. An early recognition and treatment of septic shock is essential to maximize chances of survival. The triptych of septic shock management is resuscitation/antimicrobial therapy/control of the source. Among survivors, many patients suffer from long-term neurocognitive impairments, new functional disabilities, and mental illnesses linked to post-sepsis syndrome or post-ICU syndrome.

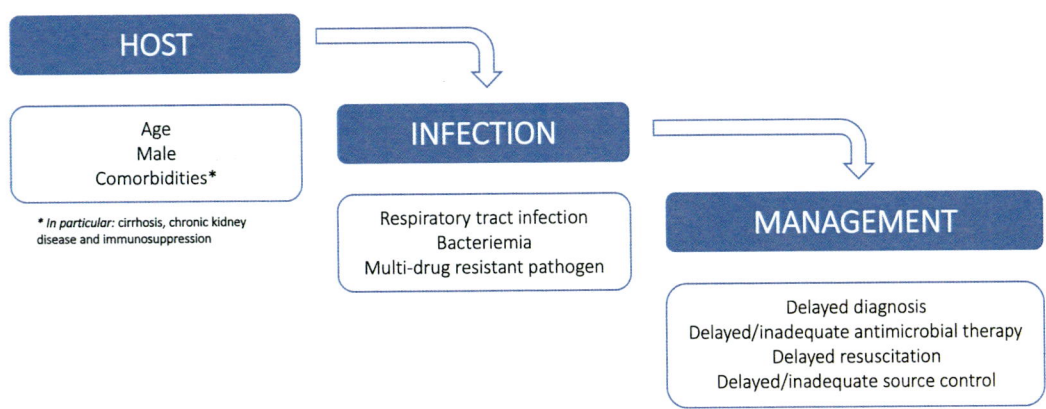

Fig. 10.3 Risk factors for mortality in patients with sepsis and septic shock

Dos and Don'ts

Dos

- Think of simple tactics (and the most frequent diseases)
- Follow the SCC guidelines
- Ask for help (a team effort is always valuable)
- Consider local epidemiology in terms of source of infection and main pathogens
- Use full dose of anti-infective agents for the first 24 hours

Don'ts

- Miss the diagnosis of septic shock (overdiagnosis is rare)
- Delay source control
- Waste time in poorly relevant tests and pending radiological examination
- Experiment new approaches except in case of labeled protocols or approved investigations

Take-Home Messages

- Septic shock follows a **dysregulated interaction** between a pathogen and a host.
- It is defined as sepsis with a **refractory hypotension or hyperlactatemia**.
- **Early recognition and treatment** is essential to maximize chances of survival.
- Management's triptych is **resuscitation/antimicrobial therapy/control of the source**.
- Many survivors suffer from **long-term neurocognitive impairments**, new functional disabilities, and mental illnesses linked to post-sepsis syndrome or post-ICU syndrome.

MCQ

1. **What are the three components of the quick SOFA (qSOFA)?**
   A. Altered mental state, high respiratory rate, fever
   B. High respiratory rate, low mean arterial pressure, fever
   C. Altered mental state, low systolic blood pressure, fever
   D. Altered mental state, low systolic blood pressure, high respiratory rate
   E. Low systolic blood pressure, high respiratory rate, fever

2. **Regarding C-reactive protein and procalcitonin, which of the following proposition(s) is(are) true?**
   A. One biomarker is mandatory for the positive diagnosis of septic shock
   B. Both have a good prognosis value in surgical patients
   C. PCT could be used to reduce the duration of antibiotics
   D. PCT could be used to identify multidrug-resistant bacteria
   E. PCT is a biomarker of fungal sepsis

3. **Which exam(s) may help reduce inadequate antimicrobial therapy?**
   A. PCT
   B. Urine sample
   C. Computed tomography scanner
   D. Ultrasound
   E. Blood cultures

4. **Which of the following objective(s) is(are) part of the resuscitation guidelines?**
   A. Mean arterial pressure (MAP) ≥ 65 mmHg
   B. Normalization of lactataemia
   C. Normalization of leucytosis
   D. Normalization of capillary refill time
   E. Normalization of oxygenation

5. Which of the following fluids should be used for initial resuscitation?
   A. Normal saline
   B. Lactated Ringer
   C. Albumin
   D. Packed red blood cells
   E. Hydroxyethyl starch

Answers: 1. D; 2. B and C; 3. E; 4. A, B, and D; 5. A and B

References

1. Singer M, Deutschman CS, Seymour CW, et al. The third international consensus definitions for sepsis and septic shock (Sepsis-3). JAMA. 2016;315(8):801–10.
2. Vincent J-L, Moreno R, Takala J, Willatts S, De Mendonça A, Bruining H, Reinhart CK, Suter PM, Thijs LG. The SOFA (Sepsis-related Organ Failure Assessment) score to describe organ dysfunction/failure. Intensive Care Med. 1996;22:707–10.
3. Pool R, Gomez H, Kellum JA. Mechanisms of organ dysfunction in sepsis. Crit Care Clin. 2018;34:63–80.
4. Tyml K, Wang X, Lidington D, Ouellette Y. Lipopolysaccharide reduces intercellular coupling in vitro and arteriolar conducted response in vivo. Am J Physiol Heart Circ Physiol. 2001;281:H1397–406.
5. Landry DW, Oliver JA. The pathogenesis of vasodilatory shock. N Engl J Med. 2001;345:588–95.
6. Pleiner J, Mittermayer F, Schaller G, Marsik C, MacAllister RJ, Wolzt M. Inflammation-induced vasoconstrictorhyporeactivity is caused by oxidative stress. J Am Coll Cardiol. 2003;42:1656–62.
7. Sharawy N. Vasoplegia in septic shock: do we really fight the right enemy? J Crit Care. 2014;29:83–7.
8. Habimana R, Choi I, Cho HJ, Kim D, Lee K, Jeong I. Sepsis-induced cardiac dysfunction: a review of pathophysiology. Acute Crit Care. 2020;35:57–66.
9. Bateman RM, Sharpe MD, Ellis CG. Bench-to-bedside review: microvascular dysfunction in sepsis—hemodynamics, oxygen transport, and nitric oxide. Crit Care. 2003;7:359–73.
10. Bateman R, Sharpe M, Sibbald W, Gill R, Ellis C. Effect of a maldistribution of microvascular blood flow on capillary O2 extraction in sepsis. Crit Care. 2002;6:P133.
11. Vincent J-L, Sakr Y, Singer M, et al. Prevalence and outcomes of infection among patients in intensive care units in 2017. JAMA. 2020;323:1478.
12. Seymour CW, Liu VX, Iwashyna TJ, et al. Assessment of clinical criteria for sepsis: for the third international consensus definitions for sepsis and septic shock (Sepsis-3). JAMA. 2016;315:762.
13. Wu C-C, Lan H-M, Han S-T, Chaou C-H, Yeh C-F, Liu S-H, Li C-H, Blaney GN, Liu Z-Y, Chen K-F. Comparison of diagnostic accuracy in sepsis between presepsin, procalcitonin, and C-reactive protein: a systematic review and meta-analysis. Ann Intensive Care. 2017;7(1):91.
14. Ryoo SM, Han KS, Ahn S, et al. The usefulness of C-reactive protein and procalcitonin to predict prognosis in septic shock patients: a multicenter prospective registry-based observational study. Sci Rep. 2019;9(1):657.
15. Facy O, Paquette B, Orry D, Binquet C, Masson D, Bouvier A, Fournel I, Charles PE, Rat P, Ortega-Deballon P. Diagnostic accuracy of inflammatory markers as early predictors of infection after elective colorectal surgery: results from the IMACORS study. Ann Surg. 2016;263:961–6.
16. Cousin F, Ortega-Deballon P, Bourredjem A, Doussot A, Giaccaglia V, Fournel I. Diagnostic accuracy of procalcitonin and C-reactive protein for the early diagnosis of intra-abdominal infection after elective colorectal surgery: a meta-analysis. Ann Surg. 2016;264:252–6.
17. Rhodes A, Evans LE, Alhazzani W, et al. Surviving sepsis campaign: international guidelines for management of sepsis and septic shock: 2016. Intensive Care Med. 2017;43:304–77.
18. Dellinger RP. The future of sepsis performance improvement. Crit Care Med. 2015;43:1787–9.
19. Damiani E, Donati A, Serafini G, Rinaldi L, Adrario E, Pelaia P, Busani S, Girardis M. Effect of performance improvement programs on compliance with sepsis bundles and mortality: a systematic review and meta-analysis of observational studies. PLoS One. 2015;10:e0125827.
20. Gatewood MO, Wemple M, Greco S, Kritek PA, Durvasula R. A quality improvement project to improve early sepsis care in the emergency department. BMJ Qual Saf. 2015;24:787–95.
21. Hayden GE, Tuuri RE, Scott R, Losek JD, Blackshaw AM, Schoenling AJ, Nietert PJ, Hall GA. Triage sepsis alert and sepsis protocol lower times to fluids and antibiotics in the emergency department. Am J Emerg Med. 2016;34:1–9.
22. Levy MM, Dellinger RP, Townsend SR, et al. The surviving sepsis campaign: results of an international guideline-based performance improvement program targeting severe sepsis. Intensive Care Med. 2010;36:222–31.
23. Garnacho-Montero J, Gutiérrez-Pizarraya A, Escoresca-Ortega A, Corcia-Palomo Y, Fernández-Delgado E, Herrera-Melero I, Ortiz-Leyba C, Márquez-Vácaro JA. De-escalation of empirical therapy is associated with lower mortality in patients with severe sepsis and septic shock. Intensive Care Med. 2013;40:32–40.
24. Marik PE, Byrne L, van Haren F. Fluid resuscitation in sepsis: the great 30 mL per kg hoax. J Thorac Dis. 2020;12:S37–47.

25. Byrne L, Van Haren F. Fluid resuscitation in human sepsis: time to rewrite history? Ann Intensive Care. 2017;7:4.
26. Maitland K, Kiguli S, Opoka RO, et al. Mortality after fluid bolus in African children with severe infection. N Engl J Med. 2011;364:2483–95.
27. For the FEAST Trial Group, Maitland K, George EC, et al. Exploring mechanisms of excess mortality with early fluid resuscitation: insightsfrom the FEAST trial. BMC Med. 2013;11:68.
28. Schortgen F, Lacherade J-C, Bruneel F, Cattaneo I, Hemery F, Lemaire F, Brochard L. Effects of hydroxyethylstarch and gelatin on renal function in severe sepsis: a multicentre randomised study. Lancet. 2001;357:911–6.
29. Perner A, Haase N, Guttormsen AB, et al. Hydroxyethyl starch 130/0.42 versus Ringer's acetate in severe sepsis. N Engl J Med. 2012;367:124–34.
30. SAFE Study Investigators, Finfer S, McEvoy S, Bellomo R, McArthur C, Myburgh J, Norton R. Impact of albumin compared to saline on organ function and mortality of patients with severe sepsis. Intensive Care Med. 2011;37:86–96.
31. Caironi P, Tognoni G, Masson S, et al. Albumin replacement in patients with severe sepsis or septic shock. N Engl J Med. 2014;370:1412–21.
32. Scheeren TWL, Bakker J, De Backer D, et al. Current use of vasopressors in septic shock. Ann Intensive Care. 2019;9:20.
33. Monnet X, Marik P, Teboul J-L. Passive leg raising for predicting fluid responsiveness: a systematic review and meta-analysis. Intensive Care Med. 2016;42:1935–47.
34. Timsit J-F, Bassetti M, Cremer O, et al. Rationalizing antimicrobial therapy in the ICU: a narrative review. Intensive Care Med. 2019;45:172–89.
35. Vincent J-L. International study of the prevalence and outcomes of infection in intensive care units. JAMA. 2009;302:2323.
36. Shankar-Hari M, Harrison DA, Ferrando-Vivas P, Rubenfeld GD, Rowan K. Risk factors at index hospitalization associated with longer-term mortality in adult sepsis survivors. JAMA Netw Open. 2019;2:e194900.
37. Kumar A, Roberts D, Wood KE, et al. Duration of hypotension before initiation of effective antimicrobial therapy is the critical determinant of survival in human septic shock*. Crit Care Med. 2006;34:1589–96.
38. Kumar A, Ellis P, Arabi Y, et al. Initiation of inappropriate antimicrobial therapy results in a fivefold reduction of survival in human septic shock. Chest. 2009;136:1237–48.
39. Kadri SS, Lai YL, Warner S, et al. Inappropriate empirical antibiotic therapy for bloodstream infections based on discordant in-vitro susceptibilities: a retrospective cohort analysis of prevalence, predictors, and mortality risk in US hospitals. Lancet Infect Dis. 2021;21:241–51.
40. Seymour CW, Gesten F, Prescott HC, Friedrich ME, Iwashyna TJ, Phillips GS, Lemeshow S, Osborn T, Terry KM, Levy MM. Time to treatment and mortality during mandated emergency care for Sepsis. N Engl J Med. 2017;376:2235–44.
41. Mostel Z, Perl A, Marck M, Mehdi SF, Lowell B, Bathija S, Santosh R, Pavlov VA, Chavan SS, Roth J. Post-sepsis syndrome—an evolving entity that afflicts survivors of sepsis. Mol Med. 2020;26:6.
42. Harvey MA, Davidson JE. Postintensive care syndrome: right care, right now… and later. Crit Care Med. 2016;44:381–5.
43. Iwashyna TJ, Ely EW, Smith DM, Langa KM. Long-term cognitive impairment and functional disability among survivors of severe sepsis. JAMA. 2010;304:1787–94.
44. Brummel NE, Balas MC, Morandi A, Ferrante LE, Gill TM, Ely EW. Understanding and reducing disability in older adults following critical illness. Crit Care Med. 2015;43:1265–75.
45. Rabiee A, Nikayin S, Hashem MD, Huang M, Dinglas VD, Bienvenu OJ, Turnbull AE, Needham DM. Depressive symptoms after critical illness: a systematic review and meta-analysis. Crit Care Med. 2016;44:1744–53.
46. Prescott HC, Langa KM, Iwashyna TJ. Readmission diagnoses after hospitalization for severe sepsis and other acute medical conditions. JAMA. 2015;313:1055.
47. Ou S-M, Chu H, Chao P-W, Lee Y-J, Kuo S-C, Chen T-J, Tseng C-M, Shih C-J, Chen Y-T. Long-term mortality and major adverse cardiovascular events in sepsis survivors. A nationwide population-based study. Am J Respir Crit Care Med. 2016;194:209–17.

Hypovolemic Shock

11

Tyler J. Jones, Bishwajit Bhattacharya, and Kimberly A. Davis

11.1 Introduction

> **Learning Goals**
> - Understand the etiology and pathophysiology of hypovolemic shock.
> - Development of an evaluation and treatment strategy for hypovolemic shock.

11.1.1 Epidemiology

The overall annual incidence of shock is approximately 0.3–0.7 per 1000 patients with roughly 30% of cases being attributed to hypovolemic shock [1]. Hypovolemic shock can be divided into hemorrhagic and nonhemorrhagic shock. Hemorrhagic shock is the most common type of hypovolemic shock and overall shock in adults, while nonhemorrhagic hypovolemic shock is the most common in children [2, 3]. Nonhemorrhagic hypovolemia is a common entity encountered by the acute care surgeon. In this chapter we shall focus exclusively on nonhemorrhagic hypovolemic shock.

T. J. Jones (✉) · B. Bhattacharya · K. A. Davis
Division of General Surgery, Trauma and Surgical Critical Care, Department of Surgery, Yale School of Medicine, New Haven, CT, USA
e-mail: t.jones@yale.edu;
bishwajit.bhattacharya@yale.edu;
kimberly.davis@yale.edu

11.1.2 Etiology

Nonhemorrhagic hypovolemic shock is secondary to decreased intravascular volume from extracellular fluid loss. This can be due to a wide variety of causes. The following are common reasons for water and/or sodium loss [4]:

- Gastrointestinal loss-vomiting, diarrhea, external drainage via high output from stomas and fistulae or nasogastric decompression
- Renal loss-osmotic diuresis (i.e., secondary to hyperglycemia), diuretic and medication effect, renal tubular acidosis, interstitial diseases, and other salt-wasting nephropathies, hypoaldosteronism
- Integumentary loss-excessive sweating, exposure in hot climates, heat stroke, burns, dermatologic conditions such as Stevens-Johnson syndrome, or burns
- Third-spacing-systemic inflammatory response, pancreatitis, bowel obstruction, postoperative, venous obstruction, crush injuries, cirrhosis, and hypoalbuminemia (Table 11.1)

11.1.3 Pathophysiology

Shock is a state in which the delivery of oxygen and other substrates to end organs and the removal of metabolites are insufficient to maintain normal aerobic metabolism. The associated

Table 11.1 Hypovolemic shock etiology

Source	Clinical scenario
Gastrointestinal losses	High output ostomy, gastroenteritis, nasogastric decompression
Renal losses	Iatrogenic diuresis, osmotic diuresis, renal tubular acidosis
Integumentary loss	Burn, heat exposure, open abdomen
Third spacing	Pancreatitis, liver cirrhosis, bowel obstruction

tissue hypoperfusion activates a systemic cascade to compensate for inadequate oxygen delivery and by-product removal. Hypovolemic shock is the result of decreased intravascular volume which is sensed by the aortic arch and carotid body baroreceptors and results in increased sympathetic output. This, in turn, results in increased cardiac output and peripheral vasoconstriction. If the cause of the hypovolemia is left untreated, this vasoconstriction can worsen peripheral tissue hypoperfusion, thereby decreasing clearance of metabolites and worsening the overall state of shock. Other intrinsic compensatory mechanisms to counteract hypovolemia include activation of both the hypothalamus and posterior pituitary by the baroreceptors in the aortic arch and carotid body to secrete antidiuretic hormone as well as activation of the renin-angiotensin-aldosterone axis by juxtaglomerular cells in the kidney which leads to increased serum aldosterone. Combined, these mechanisms result in decreased renal excretion of both sodium and water to both conserve intravascular volume and preserve blood pressure.

Emergency general surgery patients may also experience an inflammatory response due the underlying disease process causing tissue damage or secondary to tissue ischemia and reperfusion. A surge of pro-inflammatory cytokines are released from macrophages and monocytes—namely TNF-α interleukin, IL-6, and IL-8—and there is also a downregulation of anti-inflammatory cytokines. This inflammatory cascade also results in the release of nitric oxide which causes the endothelium to become more permeable [5]. This results in tissue edema and thereby compromises oxygen delivery. This cytokine-generated cascade of events results in a systemic inflammatory response syndrome. The volume loss due to leakage can result in decreased circulatory volume that needs to be replaced.

11.2 Diagnosis

11.2.1 Clinical Presentation

The clinical presentation of nonhemorrhagic hypovolemic shock is variable. Patients can present with a broad spectrum of symptoms, physical exam findings, alterations in vital signs, and laboratory derangements.

The symptoms experienced are related to the underlying cause of the volume depletion, decreased intravascular volume, electrolyte abnormalities, the resultant hemodynamic compromise, or a combination of the above. Decreased intravascular volume can cause patients to experience polydipsia, anxiety, lethargy, confusion, fatigue, dizziness, oliguria, and myalgias. Electrolyte disturbances such as hypokalemia and hypocalcemia can lead to muscle spasms and/or pain. Hyponatremia and hypernatremia can cause a spectrum of neurologic manifestations from confusion and lethargy to seizures and coma. The resultant shock and acidosis can lead to tachypnea, cold hands and feet, and chest and/or abdominal pain in addition to previously mentioned symptoms.

In patients with nonhemorrhagic hypovolemic shock, no single physical exam finding has been proven to be sensitive or specific for diagnosis. However, there are classic physical exam findings which, while nonspecific, can raise the suspicion of hypovolemia in the appropriate clinical scenario. The most rudimentary physical exam finding is the lack of moisture of the skin and mucous membranes. Specific sites to evaluate for moisture are the mucous membranes of the mouth and tongue as well as the skin of the axilla. Another physical exam finding suggestive of hypovolemia is decreased skin turgor. Under normal conditions, the skin will maintain its elasticity or turgor when pinched, but in hypovolemic patients it sometimes loses this property (tents) and does not retract back to its original position due to interstitial fluid loss. This is best assessed in the presternal skin and medial thighs [6].

Patients with hypovolemic shock have significant alterations in their hemodynamics. Hypovolemia causes a decreased preload which decreases cardiac filling pressures and stroke volume leading to a compensatory increase in heart rate to maintain cardiac output combined with an increased peripheral vascular resistance. Initially, this results in an increased diastolic blood pressure and therefore narrowed pulse pressure. As the degree of hypovolemia increases, the compensatory mechanisms become less able to overcome the decreased circulatory volume. This manifests initially as postural hypotension, a finding that is much more pronounced in hemorrhagic shock, but also seen in hypovolemic shock from fluid loss. Patients with greater than 20% intravascular volume loss may have normal blood pressure and heart rate in the supine or seated position, but exhibit hypotension and compensatory tachycardia upon standing. Once intravascular volume is decreased by about 30–40%, these homeostatic mechanisms are no longer able to overcome the volume loss, hypotension and associated hypoperfusion become more pronounced, and shock ensues [4]. Elderly patients maybe in shock at higher blood pressures compared to younger patients due to changes in their cardiovascular system. Older patients should be considered in shock at higher blood pressure thresholds with some literature considering 110 mmHg as a cutoff [7].

11.2.2 Diagnostics

As with physical exam findings and hemodynamic alterations, there are no laboratory values or aberrations that are sensitive or specific to hypovolemic shock. In general, laboratory evaluation of patients with suspected hypovolemia should include measurement of serum metabolic panel/electrolytes, complete blood count, lactic acid level, arterial blood gas, osmolality, coagulation factors, albumin, and glucose level. Urine studies including urinalysis, osmolality, and urine chemistry (electrolytes, creatinine, and urea nitrogen) should also be obtained. Some of the abnormalities are discussed below.

While serum BUN and creatinine are not a reliable measure of renal function in all patients, serial determinations, trends, and ratios can be utilized to assess patients with hypovolemia. In patients with normal kidney function, the serum BUN to creatinine ratio is usually around 10:1. In cases of hypovolemia, serum BUN increases more substantially than does creatinine, so this ratio is often greater than 20:1. Of note, this is influenced heavily by both urea production and excretion and may be abnormal in patients with GI tract hemorrhage due to resorption of blood from the GI tract.

There are no distinct serum electrolyte abnormalities that suggest hypovolemia; however, certain derangements can suggest one cause of hypovolemia over another. For instance, patients who are hypovolemic may have hypernatremia, hyponatremia, or eunatremia. Hypernatremia in the setting of hypovolemia is most often caused by primary loss of free water (i.e., diarrhea, vomiting, diabetes insipidus, skin losses). Hyponatremia in the setting of hypovolemia is due to combined sodium and free water loss with net sodium loss exceeding water loss such as the case of diarrhea or vomiting in which the loss is replaced with plain water ingestion or hypotonic intravenous fluid replacement [8–10]. Alterations in potassium levels are also seen in hypovolemic states, with hypokalemia being more common than hyperkalemia due to loss of potassium from the urine or gastrointestinal secretions.

Depending on the cause of hypovolemia, metabolic acid-base disturbances can also be seen. Metabolic acidosis is more common than metabolic alkalosis. Metabolic acidosis can occur with severe diarrhea or high output stomas or fistulae or third space losses due to inflammatory and/or infectious processes. When patients progress to the point of hypovolemic shock, anaerobic respiration increases leading to metabolic and lactic acidosis [11]. However, metabolic alkalosis can be seen in the setting of severe upper gastrointestinal volume loss or usage of certain diuretics. It is important to note that arterial pH may be normal in the setting of metabolic derangements due to acute respiratory compensation.

Biochemical parameters such as base deficit and lactic acid can be indicative of hypoperfusion, but have their limitations. In the case of base deficit, the values maybe altered by iatrogenic intervention. Crystalloids are typically of low pH and are hyperchloremic. As patients are resuscitated with such fluids, the base deficit can be "driven" negative and inaccurately suggest under resuscitation, particularly with the use of isotonic saline [12]. Similarly, lactic acid levels can be measured, but a distinction must be made between lactic acidemia and lactic acidosis. Lactic acid levels can be elevated as stress response and resolve as the response abates. The rate of clearance of lactic acid also is variable and may not be predicted by volume resuscitation [13].

Urine sodium, osmolality, creatinine, and even urinalysis can be altered by multiple intrinsic and extrinsic changes associated with hypovolemia. Urine sodium is often reduced in patients with hypovolemia. Fractional excretion of sodium (FENa)—which can be calculated from the urine and serum sodium and urine and serum creatinine levels—can be used to assess the cause of acute kidney injury. FENa of <1% is suggestive of hypovolemia as a cause of acute kidney injury. Urinalysis is often normal in the setting of hypovolemia because there is usually no intrinsic renal pathology with isolated hypovolemia [14]. Resuscitation of hypovolemic shock requires the ability to accurately assess the volume status of the patient. Urine output can be indicator of intravascular status; however, acutely ill patients may have acute kidney injury due to the inflammatory cascade that is independent of prerenal factors (Table 11.2).

Vital signs such as tachycardia and hypotension are basic parameters to evaluate volume status. However, in the inflammatory state these parameters can be altered regardless of volume status due to cytokine cascade [5, 15]. Arterial blood pressure should be closely monitored in all patients with suspected hypovolemia. Initially, systolic blood pressure is preserved and diastolic may even be increased due to increased systemic vascular resistance, leading to a narrow pulse pressure. Orthostatic vital signs should also be measured if clinically feasible as another evaluation of postural hypotension secondary to possible hypovolemia. Postural hypotension is defined as a drop in systolic blood pressure >20 mmHg, diastolic blood pressure >10 mmHg within 3 min of standing when compared with a blood pressure measurement while in a sitting or supine position [4].

Table 11.2 Resuscitation parameter and limitations

Parameter	Limitations
Hemodynamic parameters	Confounded by systemic inflammation regardless of volume status
Urine output	Acute kidney injury-related decreased output independent of prerenal factors
Base deficit	Iatrogenicallly altered by crystalloid resuscitation
Lactic acid	Elevated secondary to stress response

Measurements of central venous volumes to determine volume status can aid in the diagnosis of hypovolemia. Historically, central venous and pulmonary artery catheter assessment was used to help differentiate the etiology of shock. The classic constellation of hemodynamic parameters seen in hypovolemic shock includes a decreased central venous pressure, stable to decreased pulmonary capillary wedge pressure (PCWP), decreased cardiac output, increased systemic vascular resistance, and stable to decreased mixed venous oxygen saturation. However, the routine use of pulmonary artery catheters has decreased in the modern era due to multiple RCTs showing no benefit in decreasing mortality, ICU, or overall length of stay [16].

CVP determination via central venous catheter or PAC has been used to estimate volume status by using it as a surrogate measure of preload. Specifically, it has been used as a trend to assess responsiveness to volume resuscitation. There are many factors which limit its utility to estimate volume status including but not limited to right-sided heart failure, mechanical ventilation, and poor chest wall compliance. Due to these reasons, CVP measurement has largely fallen out of favor as well [17].

Ultrasonography and echocardiography—while user-dependent—have emerged as useful bedside adjuncts in the assessment of volume status in patients. On ultrasound, the inferior vena cava can be easily visualized. Variations in the diameter of the IVC with respiration can serve as surrogate for intravascular volume and predict fluid responsiveness. A 12–18% variation in mechanically ventilated patients and 50% in spontaneously breathing patients are considered predictive of fluid responsiveness. However, there are limitations to the use measuring the IVC to predict fluid responsiveness. In certain clinical scenarios involving vasodilatory shock, fluid responsiveness is not as accurately predicted. The presence of increased abdominal pressure and elevated and positive end-expiratory pressure (PEEP) may confound IVC diameter. Furthermore, since bedside ultrasound is user-dependent, formal echocardiography may be beneficial to guide clinical assessment in scenarios in which high-quality bedside ultrasound assessment is not possible [18–25].

There are few radiographic modalities that assess for hypovolemic shock. Plain films and cross-sectional imaging can be used to workup certain causes of hypovolemic shock; however, they have limited utility in the diagnosis and evaluation of responsiveness to treatment.

11.2.3 Differential Diagnosis

The differential diagnosis for hypovolemic shock primarily includes the other types of shock, recognizing that shock can be and often is multifactorial. For instance, concurrent septic and hypovolemic shock can be seen in the case of severe or fulminant Clostridium difficile colitis. Global assessment focused on ruling out causes of distributive, obstructive, cardiogenic, and/or hemorrhagic shock should be undertaken prior to settling on a diagnosis of hypovolemic shock.

11.3 Treatment

11.3.1 Medical Treatment

Effective treatment of hypovolemic shock requires a two-pronged approach. The first goal is to correct the hypovolemic shock—regardless of whether or not the cause has been determined—followed by determining and treating the underlying cause to prevent recurrence or worsening of the shock. Emergency general surgeons encounter many disease processes that result in hypovolemic shock. Significant gastrointestinal losses due to ostomy losses, gastrointestinal decompression in cases of intestinal obstruction or postoperative ileus, or inflammatory processes such as pancreatitis which result in significant third spacing of fluid are all common causes of hypovolemia in emergency general surgery patients. Recognition of the cause of volume loss is one key aspect of treatment.

Treatment of hypovolemia requires replenishment of volume lost. Standard treatment is to replace volume loss with crystalloids fluid to ultimately restore intravascular volume. Crystalloids administered are generally hypotonic solutions and do not remain within the intravascular space and eventually "leak" into the interstitial space. Less than 25% of infused saline are retained in the intravascular fluid compartment 1 h after infusion [26]. However, the entire volume of iso-oncotic colloid (most commonly either 5% albumin or 25% albumin) is retained with the intravascular space after 1 h. Colloids have the theoretical advantage of better intravascular retention due to an increase in intravascular oncotic pressure and have been shown to achieve hemodynamic targets with lower volumes; however, there is no advantage in overall patient outcomes with a colloid-based approach. In fact, in some patient subpopulations such as patients with severe traumatic brain injuries resuscitation with albumin have been shown to have worse outcomes compared to crystalloids resuscitation [27]. Volume replacement with albumin may be beneficial in some subsets of patients such as liver cirrhosis patients with large volume ascites loss (>5 L), by theoretically increasing the intravascular oncotic pressure and volume with a lower sodium load than crystalloid [28].

11.3.2 Surgical Treatment

Surgical treatment of nonhemorrhagic cause of hypovolemic shock is focused on treating the underlying condition and therefore limited. Gastrointestinal causes of hypovolemia such as high output fistulae and bowel obstructions may require operative interventions such as takedown of the fistulae, lysis of adhesions to relieve the obstruction, and/or bowel resection. Insensible fluid loss from severe burns and other dermatologic conditions such as Stevens-Johnson syndrome may require debridement and wound coverage to prevent ongoing insensible fluid loss.

11.3.3 Prognosis

The prognosis for hypovolemic shock depends upon a complex interplay etiology of hypovolemic shock and patient comorbidities. Several assessment tools such as the Sequential Organ Failure Assessment (SOFA) Score or Acute Physiology and Chronic Health Evaluation (APACHE) II score tools are available to help quantify the severity of critical illness in a patient and thereby predict mortality [29]. Other tools available to the emergency general surgeon include risk calculators to predict outcomes of patients preoperatively. These tools can help guide discussions with patients and families regarding realistic expectations.

Replacement of depleted volume is essential to restoring intravascular volume. However, the excessive fluid resuscitation can be detrimental. Crystalloids are generally hypotonic and 'leak' into the interstitial space within an hour. This accumulation of fluid in the interstitial space eventually results in many complications including sequestering of fluids in the lungs and other soft tissues. Excessive resuscitation can result in abdominal (and even rarely extremity) compartment syndrome. Major risk factors are large volume resuscitation, management with an open body cavity, core hypothermia, coagulopathy requiring component therapy, severe sepsis or septic shock, critical illness in the setting of cirrhosis or other liver failure accompanied by large volume ascites, mechanical ventilation, and PEEP greater than 10 cmH_2O pressure [30, 31]. Intra-abdominal pressure increases and results in a constellation of findings and physiological derangements. These include decreased venous return resulting in decreased cardiac output causing end organ perfusion compromise demonstrated with hypotension, decreased urine output. Increase in intra-abdominal pressure also results in decreased thoracic compliance causing increased airway pressures (Fig. 11.1). Immediate decompression is required to relieve the pressure, often resulting in an open abdomen that may not be primarily closed. In some settings, abdominal compartment syndrome caused by excessive ascites from both inflammatory state and fluid resuscitation—such as burn patients and patients with severe pancreatitis—paracentesis, may have some utility to relieve the pressure without a laparotomy.

Fig. 11.1 Abdominal compartment syndrome. (1) Position the patient supine with HOB flat. (2) Patient should be calm, not agitated and ensure that abdominal muscle contractions are absent. (3) Level transducer at the iliac crest in line with the midaxillary line and zero the transducer. (4) Clamp the urinary drainage tubing distal to the specimen port. (5) Clean specimen port with chlorhexidine wipes and attach the end of the pressure tubing. (6) Turn stop cock off to the patient, activate fast-flush mechanism while drawing up 20–25 mL of NS. (7) Turn stopcock off to the NS bag and open to the patient, instill NS into the bladder for 10–15 s. (8) Wait 30–60 s before obtaining a measurement. Obtain at end expiration and record. (9) When measurement is complete, reposition patient and remove clamp from the tubing. (10) Deduct the amount of instilled NS from UOP. (Dept.ynhh.org/sicu/educational-opportunities.aspx)

11 Hypovolemic Shock

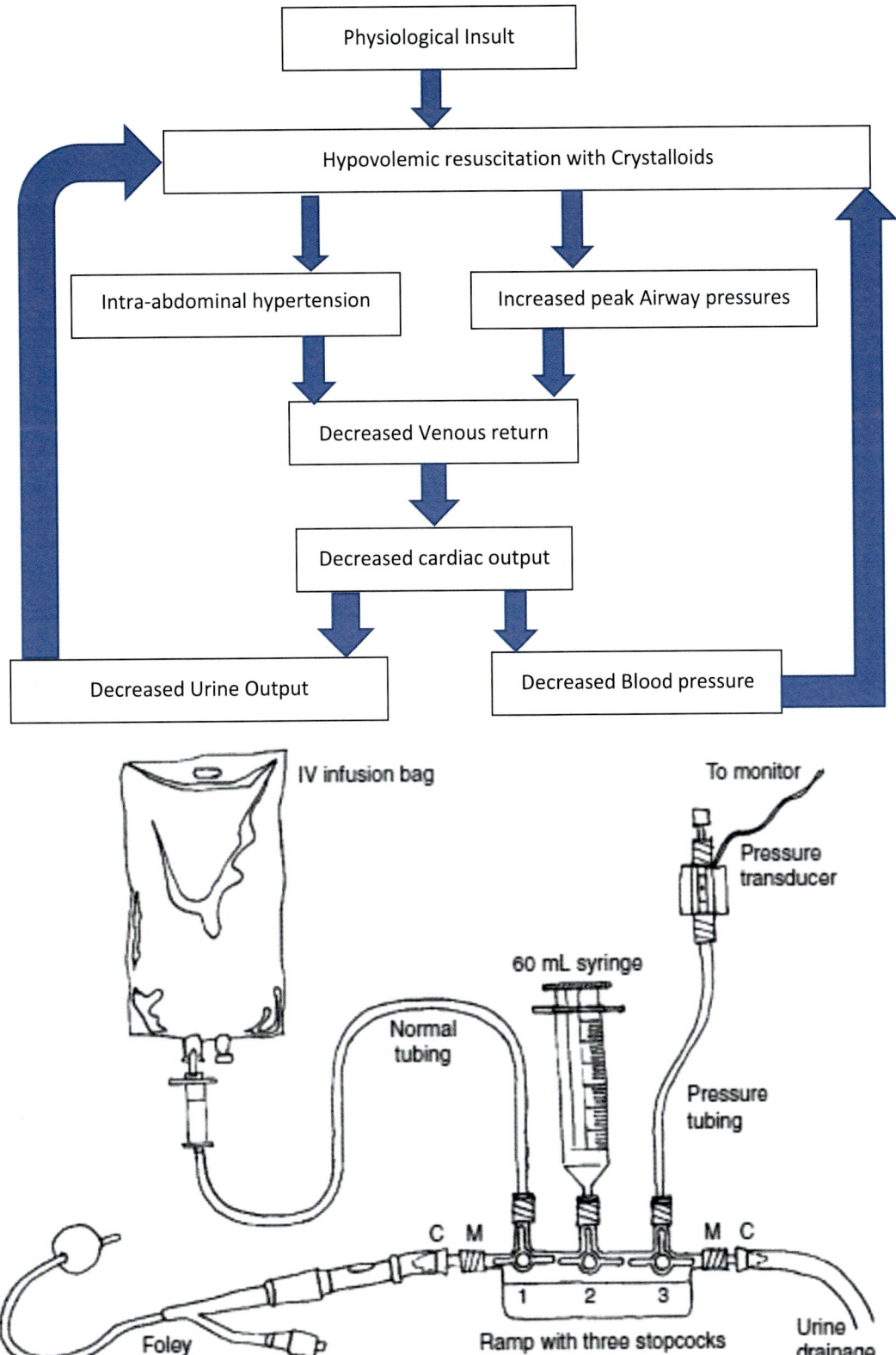

Dos and Don'ts

Hypovolemic shock needs to be correctly identified as a first step and distinguished from other types of shock. Whereby the optimal treatment for hemorrhagic shock is identifying and stopping the source of blood loss combined with blood volume replacement, in nonhemorrhagic hypovolemic shock, blood transfusion is rarely necessary. Volume replacement for hypovolemic shock should be judicious to avoid complications of excessive leakage of fluids from the capillaries into the interstitial space. Monitoring resuscitative response with physiological response and dynamic monitoring with ultrasound can help reduce excessive fluid resuscitation.

Take-Home Messages

- Hypovolemic shock is a common entity encountered in the practice of emergency general surgery.
- Volume resuscitation and recognition of the underlying cause are key to optimal outcomes.
- Excessive resuscitation is detrimental to patients and must be avoided.
- Judicious fluid resuscitation combined with adjuncts can help prevent these pitfalls.

Multiple Choice Questions

1. Nonhemorrhagic hypovolemic shock can be caused by the following:
   A. Gastrointestinal losses
   B. Osmotic diuresis
   C. Insensible losses
   D. All of the above
   Correct answer: D

2. Physical exam findings suggestive of hypovolemic shock include:
   A. Decreased skin turgor
   B. Dry mucosal membranes
   C. Cool extremities
   D. All of the above
   Correct answer: D

3. The use of a Swan-Ganz catheter to direct resuscitation can be beneficial to:
   A. Differentiate etiology of shock
   B. Predict adequate preload
   C. Decide optimal resuscitation fluid
   D. Provide a survival advantage
   Correct answer: A

4. The optimal central venous pressure (CVP) for goal directed therapy is:
   A. 0–5 mmHg
   B. 6–10 mmHg
   C. 11–15 mmHg
   D. Unknown
   Correct answer: D

5. Base deficit correction can be confounded by the following:
   A. Saline infusion
   B. Shock
   C. Hemorrhagic shock
   D. Hypothermia
   Correct answer: A

6. Abdominal compartment syndrome is characterized by the following:
   A. Hypotension
   B. Increased Peak airway pressures
   C. Oliguria
   D. All of the above
   Correct answer: D

7. Geriatric patients can be in shock at a blood pressure threshold below:
   A. 110 mmHg
   B. 120 mmHg
   C. 130 mmHg
   D. 160 mmHg
   Correct answer: A

8. The treatment of abdominal compartment syndrome is:
   A. Diuresis
   B. Paralysis
   C. Abdominal decompression
   D. Paracentesis
   Correct answer: C

9. One hour after administration of 1 L of NS, which percentage will remain intra-vascular?
    A. 90%
    B. 60%
    C. Less than 25%
    D. 40%

    Correct answer: C

10. Which of the following is true regarding resuscitation fluids for hypovolemic shock?
    A. Colloids are the fluid of choice for resuscitation
    B. Crystalloids are the fluid of choice for resuscitation
    C. Colloid resuscitation provides a survival advantage
    D. Crystalloids and colloids should be administered in a 1:1 ratio

    Correct answer: B

References

1. Taghavi S, Askari R. Hypovolemic shock [Updated 2020 Jul 20]. In: StatPearls [Internet]. Treasure Island: StatPearls Publishing; 2021. https://www.ncbi.nlm.nih.gov/books/NBK513297/.
2. Mbevi G, Ayieko P, Irimu G, Akech S, English M, Clinical Information Network Authors. Prevalence, aetiology, treatment and outcomes of shock in children admitted to Kenyan hospitals. BMC Med. 2016;14(1):184. Published 2016 Nov 16. https://doi.org/10.1186/s12916-016-0728-x.
3. Cannon JW. Hemorrhagic shock. N Engl J Med. 2018;378(4):370–9. https://doi.org/10.1056/NEJMra1705649. PMID: 29365303.
4. Gitz Holler J, Jensen HK, Henriksen DP, Rasmussen LM, Mikkelsen S, Pedersen C, Lassen AT. Etiology of shock in the emergency department: a 12-year population-based cohort study. Shock. 2019;51(1):60–7.
5. Koo EG, Lai LM, Choi GY, Chan MT. Systemic inflammation in the elderly. Best Pract Res Clin Anaesthesiol. 2011;25(3):413–25.
6. McGee S, Abernethy WB 3rd, Simel DL. The rational clinical examination. Is this patient hypovolemic? JAMA. 1999;281(11):1022–9. https://doi.org/10.1001/jama.281.11.1022. PMID: 10086438.
7. Brown JB, Gestring ML, Forsythe RM, Stassen NA, Billiar TR, Peitzman AB, Sperry JL. Systolic blood pressure criteria in the National Trauma Triage Protocol for geriatric trauma: 110 is the new 90. J Trauma Acute Care Surg. 2015;78(2):352–9.
8. Hendy A, Bubenek-Turconi ŞI. The diagnosis and hemodynamic monitoring of circulatory shock: current and future trends. J Crit Care Med (Targu Mures). 2016;2(3):115–23. Published 2016 Aug 10. https://doi.org/10.1515/jccm-2016-0018.
9. Crandall ML, Maier RV. Shock. Elsevier; 2004. p. 245–249. isbn:9780124755703. https://doi.org/10.1016/B0-12-475570-4/01191-4. https://www.sciencedirect.com/science/article/pii/B0124755704011914.
10. Rose BD. New approach to disturbances in the plasma sodium concentration. Am J Med. 1986;81(6):1033–40. https://doi.org/10.1016/0002-9343(86)90401-8. PMID: 3799631.
11. Rose BD, Post TW. Clinical physiology of acid-base and electrolyte disorders. 5th ed. New York: McGraw-Hill; 2001. p. 749.
12. Kaplan LJ, Philbin N, Arnaud F, Rice J, Dong F, Freilich D. Resuscitation from hemorrhagic shock: fluid selection and infusion strategy drives unmeasured ion genesis. J Trauma. 2006;61(1):90–7; discussion 97–8.
13. Bakker J, Postelnicu R, Mukherjee V. Lactate: where are we now? Crit Care Clin. 2020;36(1):115–24.
14. Miller TR, Anderson RJ, Linas SL, Henrich WL, Berns AS, Gabow PA, Schrier RW. Urinary diagnostic indices in acute renal failure: a prospective study. Ann Intern Med. 1978;89(1):47–50. https://doi.org/10.7326/0003-4819-89-1-47. PMID: 666184.
15. Lenz A, Franklin GA, Cheadle WG. Systemic inflammation after trauma. Injury. 2007;38(12):1336–45.
16. Rajaram SS, Desai NK, Kalra A, Gajera M, Cavanaugh SK, Brampton W, Young D, Harvey S, Rowan K. Pulmonary artery catheters for adult patients in intensive care. Cochrane Database Syst Rev. 2013;2013(2):CD003408.
17. Marik PE, Baram M, Vahid B. Does central venous pressure predict fluid responsiveness? A systematic review of the literature and the tale of seven mares. Chest. 2008;134:172–8.
18. Zengin S, Al B, Genc S, Yildirim C, Ercan S, Dogan M, Altunbas G. Role of inferior vena cava and right ventricular diameter in assessment of volume status: a comparative study: ultrasound and hypovolemia. Am J Emerg Med. 2013;31(5):763–7. https://www.sciencedirect.com/science/article/pii/S0735675712005384.
19. Zengin S, Al B, Genc S, Yildirim C, Ercan S, Dogan M, Altunbas G. Role of inferior vena cava and right ventricular diameter in assessment of volume status: a comparative study: ultrasound and hypovolemia. Am J Emerg Med. 2013;31(5):763–7.
20. Carr BG, Dean AJ, Everett WW, Ku BS, Mark DG, Okusanya O, Horan AD, Gracias VH. Intensivist bedside ultrasound (INBU) for volume assessment in the intensive care unit: a pilot study. J Trauma. 2007;63(3):495–502.
21. Unluer EE, Evrin T, Katipoglu B, Bayata S. A bedside ultrasound technique for fluid therapy monitoring in severe hypovolemia: tissue Doppler imaging of the

right ventricle. Interv Med Appl Sci. 2017;9(4):212–4. https://akjournals.com/view/journals/1646/9/4/article-p212.xml. Accessed 26 Mar 2021.
22. Bentzer P, Griesdale DE, Boyd J, MacLean K, Sirounis D, Ayas NT. Will this hemodynamically unstable patient respond to a bolus of intravenous fluids? JAMA. 2016;316(12):1298–309. https://doi.org/10.1001/jama.2016.12310. PMID: 27673307.
23. Airapetian N, Maizel J, Alyamani O, Mahjoub Y, Lorne E, Levrard M, et al. Does inferior vena cava respiratory variability predict fluid responsiveness in spontaneously breathing patients? Crit Care. 2015;19:400.
24. Barbier C, Loubieres Y, Schmit C, Hayon J, Ricome JL, Jardin F, et al. Respiratory changes in inferior vena cava diameter are helpful in predicting fluid responsiveness in ventilated septic patients. Intensive Care Med. 2004;30(9):1740–6.
25. Feissel M, Michard F, Faller JP, Teboul JL. The respiratory variation in inferior vena cava diameter as a guide to fluid therapy. Intensive Care Med. 2004;30(9):1834–7.
26. Falk JL, Rackow EC, Weil MH. Colloid and crystalloid fluid resuscitation. Acute Care. 1983–1984;10(2):59–94.
27. Caironi P, Tognoni G, Masson S, Fumagalli R, Pesenti A, Romero M, Fanizza C, Caspani L, Faenza S, Grasselli G, Iapichino G, Antonelli M, Parrini V, Fiore G, Latini R, Gattinoni L, ALBIOS Study Investigators. Albumin replacement in patients with severe sepsis or septic shock. N Engl J Med. 2014;370(15):1412–21.
28. Umgelter A, Reindl W, Wagner KS, Franzen M, Stock K, Schmid RM, Huber W. Effects of plasma expansion with albumin and paracentesis on haemodynamics and kidney function in critically ill cirrhotic patients with tense ascites and hepatorenal syndrome: a prospective uncontrolled trial. Crit Care. 2008;12(1):R4.
29. Ho KM. Combining sequential organ failure assessment (SOFA) score with acute physiology and chronic health evaluation (APACHE) II score to predict hospital mortality of critically ill patients. Anaesth Intensive Care. 2007;35(4):515–21.
30. Han K, Lee JM, Achanta A, et al. Emergency surgery score accurately predicts the risk of post-operative infection in emergency general surgery. Surg Infect (Larchmt). 2019;20(1):4–9.
31. Luckianow GM, Ellis M, Governale D, Kaplan LJ. Abdominal compartment syndrome: risk factors, diagnosis, and current therapy. Crit Care Res Pract. 2012;2012:908169. https://doi.org/10.1155/2012/908169.

Further Reading

Brown JB, Gestring ML, Forsythe RM, Stassen NA, Billiar TR, Peitzman AB, Sperry JL. Systolic blood pressure criteria in the National Trauma Triage Protocol for geriatric trauma: 110 is the new 90. J Trauma Acute Care Surg. 2015;78(2):352–9.

Caironi P, Tognoni G, Masson S, Fumagalli R, Pesenti A, Romero M, Fanizza C, Caspani L, Faenza S, Grasselli G, Iapichino G, Antonelli M, Parrini V, Fiore G, Latini R, Gattinoni L, ALBIOS Study Investigators. Albumin replacement in patients with severe sepsis or septic shock. N Engl J Med. 2014;370(15):1412–21.

Marik PE, Baram M, Vahid B. Does central venous pressure predict fluid responsiveness? A systematic review of the literature and the tale of seven mares. Chest. 2008;134:172–8.

Principles of Perioperative Management in Acute Care Surgery

12

Oreste Romeo, Taylor A. Davidson, and Scott B. Davidson

12.1 Introduction

The acute care surgeon will often face complex management decisions during the initial 72 h of treatment. The role of the surgeon remains undoubtedly central to navigating the patient through all phases of care into excellent outcomes. Through the process of surgical care, the patient's physiology is taxed to tolerate the surgical insult and to heal the operative site. Optimization of the physiologic baseline thus becomes imperative to achieve successful outcomes. Preparing a patient for surgery and the immediate postoperative management can present a daunting array of physiologic and metabolic derangements. This endeavor can be overwhelming and circumstances may not allow for the immediate assistance of critical care consultants or other subspecialists. The emergent surgical and trauma patient requires attention to additional physiologic and biologic factors that must be addressed. Preoperative risk stratification and risk factor modification, while useful in elective surgery, may be of limited utility to the surgeon embarking on emergent intervention. However, several well-established guidelines, i.e., balanced resuscitation with massive transfusion protocol (MTP), Surviving Sepsis Campaign (SSC), and Acute Respiratory Distress Syndrome Network (ARDSnet), can be readily incorporated into this framework and assist the surgeon in preparation and resuscitation.

There are multiple approaches to the management and care of complex and critically ill patients. We have found that assessment mirroring that of the traumatically injured patient can be utilized in any patient, is pragmatic, and allows the surgeon to institute a thorough care plan throughout the perioperative timeframe.

A primary survey is performed, followed by a secondary survey where each body system is assessed, incorporating the physical exam, laboratory, and radiologic findings pertinent to that system. The management plan then follows to address any abnormalities of that system. This sequential approach allows for the assimilation of large amounts of data while minimizing the risk of missing critical information. What follows is a brief review of the shock states that may be encountered by the practicing general surgeon. Next is a summary of some of the common endpoints of resuscitation. These endpoints can be utilized throughout the perioperative course and serve to minimize injury to key organ systems. The challenge of this chapter is to provide a practical framework from which to assess and manage these most complex patients.

O. Romeo (✉) · S. B. Davidson
Bronson Methodist Hospital, Surgical Critical Care and Trauma Surgery, Kalamazoo, MI, USA
e-mail: romeoo@bronsonhg.org; Davidsos@Bronsonhg.org

T. A. Davidson
Lake Erie College of Osteopathic Medicine, Greensburg, PA, USA
e-mail: tadavi@umich.edu

> **Learning Goals**
> - Recognition and treatment of the common types of perioperative shock whenever present
> - Recognition and treatment of the multiple perioperative abnormalities that the emergency general surgeon and trauma surgeon may encounter
> - Early identification of physiological derangements of the different organ systems and their timely correction
> - Awareness of endocrine emergencies and appropriate corrective therapies

12.2 Shock Etiology

In the many scenarios facing the surgeon, none is more demanding than that dominated by the core physiological instability of the shock states. The ultimate recovery of the surgical patient hinges as much on the appropriate and timely interventions apt at restoring the physiologic integrity in the ICU as it does on appropriately planned and expeditiously performed procedures in the operating room. Cuthbertson in 1942 was the first to describe two distinct phases of the metabolic shift that occurs after major trauma and later recognized this to be a common denominator of all shock states [1]. He characterized "ebb" and "flow" phases of posttraumatic metabolic alterations. The "ebb" phase, early and shorter in nature, is associated with reduced total body expenditure and increased urinary nitrogen wasting in addition to a surge in the release of neuroendocrine hormones and an increased sympathetic flow response. In contrast, the "flow" phase occurs after resuscitation from a state of shock. This leads to increased metabolic turnover, activation of the innate immune system, and induction of the hepatic acute phase response.

Shock is defined as inadequate delivery of oxygen at the cell level with a secondary metabolic shutdown and eventual multiorgan dysfunction syndrome. Prompt recognition is the paramount first step in affording intervention towards mitigation and its early reversal. The acute care surgeon may encounter several types of shock, with septic and hemorrhagic as the most common. Lawrence categorizes shock as follows: [2].

Hypovolemic shock (hemorrhagic, nonhemorrhagic) results from reduced intravascular volume, leading to reduced preload and cardiac output (CO).

Distributive shock (septic, neurogenic, anaphylactic, adrenal crisis) results from excessive vasodilatation of the peripheral vasculature, leading to impaired distribution of blood flow.

Cardiogenic shock results from sudden failure of the cardiac pump function as seen in acute MI, valve rupture, or arrhythmias.

Obstructive shock results from impaired blood flow in the cardiopulmonary circuit. Common causes include tension pneumothorax, pericardial tamponade, and massive pulmonary emboli.

Structured scores and quality initiatives have been created to facilitate early recognition. Resuscitative endpoints, especially for the hemorrhagic and septic categories most crucial to the acute care and trauma surgeon, will be emphasized in this chapter.

12.3 Priorities and Endpoints of Resuscitation

No single endpoint exists to gauge successful physiologic resuscitation of the acutely ill. A complete discussion of the many parameters used as endpoints is beyond the scope of this chapter. Trending endpoints, as often as every 1–2 h, can guide titration of therapies for optimal outcome. Successful achievement is marked by elimination of acidosis with restoration of aerobic metabolism. Lactate and base deficit have both been shown to be useful in the initial quantification of the shock state and as a gauge to ongoing resuscitative efforts. Decreases in elevated lactate levels during treatment are universally associated with improved outcome in critically ill patients and can provide an early and objective assessment of the response to therapy [3]. Failure to decrease elevated lactate within 48 h correlates with increased mortality [4]. Persistent elevation in the base deficit (up to 96 h) is a marker for ongoing resuscitation requirements and can be present despite normalized vital signs and urine output. Of note, lactate levels can remain elevated in patients with impaired clearance such as liver dysfunction, cardiac surgery, and sepsis. Patients positive for alcohol and drugs may demonstrate elevations in both markers. Urine output as a marker of end organ perfusion remains one of the clinically reliable endpoints, though variable based on patient's preexisting conditions. A urinary output of 0.5 cc/kg/h is a general threshold in the adult patient. Cardiac indices such as right ventricular end diastolic volume index (RVEDI) correlate best with cardiac preload, but requires placement of a pulmonary artery catheter. Evidence shows that interventions to increase RVEDI result in improved gut perfusion restoration and decreased rate of organ failure. The FloTrac™ device attaches to the arterial line to provide advanced hemodynamic parameters, including stroke volume (SV), stroke volume variance (SVV), mean arterial pressure (MAP), systemic vascular resistance (SVR), and continuous cardiac output (CCO). These parameters update every 20 s and do not require central venous catheterization, although the patient must be intubated. Point of care ultrasound (POCUS) has rapidly expanded our bedside diagnostic capability. It allows for noninvasive determination of preload through visualization of inferior vena cava diameter and right ventricular filling. This modality is subject to patient size, anatomy, and user expertise.

12.4 Primary Survey

History and physical exam are paramount in the initial evaluation of the acutely ill surgical patient. The "AMPLE" history as outlined in Advanced Trauma Life Support (ATLS) can identify key components essential to further management. **A**llergies with attention to anaphylactic reactions, IV contrasts, and antibiotic problems are most pertinent [5]. **M**edications with a focus on anticoagulants, cardiac, diabetic, and steroids are salient. **P**ast medical and surgical history provides surgical context and helps to assess risk. **L**ast oral intake relates to aspiration risk for intubation or possibly sedation if further diagnostic workup is contemplated, such as interventional radiologic procedures. **E**vents in these patients would focus on the presentation, duration, onset, and severity of the illness.

12.4.1 Pulmonary

Assessment of the patient in need of intubation must be determined promptly. Usually, emergent endotracheal intubation is indicated in the following scenarios:

- Hypoxemic respiratory failure despite maximum maneuvers such as noninvasive positive pressure support.
- Hypercapnic ventilatory respiratory failure leading to respiratory acidosis and increased work of breathing.
- Upper airway obstruction of the pharynx by the tongue or foreign body, or secretions or edema from massive resuscitation (i.e., burns).
- Shock or hemodynamic instability associated with altered mental status and increased work of breathing.
- Clinical conditions with risk for airway compromise such as stroke, Glasgow Coma Scale (GCS) less than 8, drug overdose, or severe agitation preventing medical intervention.

Asking the patient to speak, auscultating the neck and chest, noting respiratory rate, and use of accessory muscles of breathing are fast and effective. Evaluation of pulse oximetry, CXR and arterial blood gases augment the exam. Once the decision is made to proceed with a definitive airway, defined as intubation of the trachea by either the nasal or the oral route, preparation is immediate. Preoxygenation by nasal cannula or mask is maintained, suction and intubating equipment gathered. Rapid sequence intubation is the technique that induces immediate unresponsiveness with an induction agent and muscular relaxation with a neuromuscular blocking agent. Commonly used induction agents include Etomidate, Ketamine, and Propofol. Neuromuscular blocking agents (NMBAs) must always be preceded by sedatives to ensure the patient is not aware of the paralysis. NMBAs include Succinylcholine, a depolarizing agent, and Vecuronium and Rocuronium, which are non-depolarizing agents.

Ventilator settings will vary based on the patient's altered physiology and underlying disease states. However, specific parameters are recommended by ARDSnet [6] (Table 12.1).

Table 12.1 ARDS network mechanical ventilation protocol summary [6]

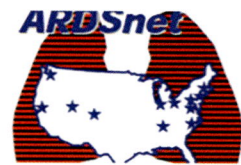

NIH NHLBI ARDS Clinical Network
Mechanical Ventilation Protocol Summary

INCLUSION CRITERIA: Acute onset of
1. $PaO_2/FiO_2 \leq 300$ (corrected for altitude)
2. Bilateral (patchy, diffuse, or homogeneous) infiltrates consistent with pulmonary edema
3. No clinical evidence of left atrial hypertension

PART I: VENTILATOR SETUP AND ADJUSTMENT
1. Calculate predicted body weight (PBW)
   Males = 50 + 2.3 [height (inches) - 60]
   Females = 45.5 + 2.3 [height (inches) -60]
2. Select any ventilator mode
3. Set ventilator settings to achieve initial V_T = 8 ml/kg PBW
4. Reduce V_T by 1 ml/kg at intervals $\leq$ 2 hours until V_T = 6ml/kg PBW.
5. Set initial rate to approximate baseline minute ventilation (not > 35 bpm).
6. Adjust V_T and RR to achieve pH and plateau pressure goals below.

pH GOAL: 7.30-7.45
Acidosis Management: (pH < 7.30)
If pH 7.15-7.30: Increase RR until pH > 7.30 or $PaCO_2$ < 25 (Maximum set RR = 35).

If pH < 7.15: Increase RR to 35.
If pH remains < 7.15, V_T may be increased in 1 ml/kg steps until pH > 7.15 (Pplat target of 30 may be exceeded).
May give $NaHCO_3$
Alkalosis Management: (pH > 7.45) Decrease vent rate if possible.

I: E RATIO GOAL: Recommend that duration of inspiration be $\leq$ duration of expiration.

PART II: WEANING
A. Conduct a SPONTANEOUS BREATHING TRIAL daily when:
   1. $FiO_2 \leq 0.40$ and PEEP $\leq$ 8.
   2. PEEP and $FiO_2 \leq$ values of previous day.
   3. Patient has acceptable spontaneous breathing efforts. (May decrease vent rate by 50% for 5 minutes to detect effort.)
   4. Systolic BP $\geq$ 90 mmHg without vasopressor support.
   5. No neuromuscular blocking agents or blockade.

OXYGENATION GOAL: PaO_2 55-80 mmHg or SpO_2 88-95%
Use a minimum PEEP of 5 cm H_2O. Consider use of incremental FiO_2/PEEP combinations such as shown below (not required) to achieve goal.

Lower PEEP/higher FiO2

FiO_2	0.3	0.4	0.4	0.5	0.5	0.6	0.7	0.7
PEEP	5	5	8	8	10	10	10	12

FiO_2	0.7	0.8	0.9	0.9	0.9	1.0		
PEEP	14	14	14	16	18	18-24		

Higher PEEP/lower FiO2

FiO_2	0.3	0.3	0.3	0.3	0.3	0.4	0.4	0.5
PEEP	5	8	10	12	14	14	16	16

FiO_2	0.5	0.5-0.8	0.8	0.9	1.0	1.0		
PEEP	18	20	22	22	22	24		

PLATEAU PRESSURE GOAL: $\leq$ 30 cm H_2O
Check Pplat (0.5 second inspiratory pause), at least q 4h and after each change in PEEP or V_T.
If Pplat > 30 cm H_2O: decrease V_T by 1ml/kg steps (minimum = 4 ml/kg).
If Pplat < 25 cm H_2O and V_T < 6 ml/kg, increase V_T by 1 ml/kg until Pplat > 25 cm H_2O or V_T = 6 ml/kg.
If Pplat < 30 and breath stacking or dys-synchrony occurs: may increase V_T in 1ml/kg increments to 7 or 8 ml/kg if Pplat remains $\leq$ 30 cm H_2O.

B. **SPONTANEOUS BREATHING TRIAL (SBT):**
If all above criteria are met and subject has been in the study for at least 12 hours, initiate a trial of UP TO 120 minutes of spontaneous breathing with $FiO2 \leq 0.5$ and PEEP $\leq$ 5:
  1. Place on T-piece, trach collar, or CPAP $\leq$ 5 cm H_2O with PS $\leq$ 5
  2. Assess for tolerance as below for up to two hours.
      a. $SpO_2 \geq 90$: and/or $PaO_2 \geq 60$ mmHg
      b. Spontaneous $V_T \geq 4$ ml/kg PBW
      c. RR $\leq$ 35/min
      d. pH ≥ 7.3
      e. No respiratory distress (distress= 2 or more)
         ➢ HR > 120% of baseline
         ➢ Marked accessory muscle use
         ➢ Abdominal paradox
         ➢ Diaphoresis
         ➢ Marked dyspnea
  3. If tolerated for at least 30 minutes, consider extubation.
  4. If not tolerated resume pre-weaning settings.

Definition of UNASSISTED BREATHING
(Different from the spontaneous breathing criteria as PS is not allowed)

1. Extubated with face mask, nasal prong oxygen, or room air, OR
2. T-tube breathing, OR
3. Tracheostomy mask breathing, OR
4. CPAP less than or equal to 5 cm H_2O without pressure support or IMV assistance.

NIH-NHLBI ARDS Network

12.4.2 Cardiovascular

Perhaps the most intimidating perioperative scenario facing the emergency surgeon is the patient in shock. The cardiovascular system plays a central role in the initial evaluation and ongoing resuscitation of patients suffering from shock. No single marker or test exists to direct therapy in these complex scenarios. The clinician must incorporate clinical exam findings, resuscitative endpoints, physiologic parameters, and imaging techniques to guide intervention.

Clinical assessment of vital signs, mental status, capillary refill, jugular vein distention, breath sounds, skin temperature, and pallor can provide useful clues as to potential etiology of the shock state. Early intervention is crucial and resuscitation measures can start at this point without the delay of more complex diagnostic studies. One must recognize that compensatory mechanisms, age, medications, and overall health complicate the diagnosis. Hypotension does not necessarily equal shock. Similarly, normotension does not mean that all tissue beds are adequately perfused, and the patient is not at risk.

The classification of hemorrhagic shock incorporated into (ATLS) has proved to be essential in caring for this patient population. This classification offers the ability to recognize early or late phases of hemorrhagic shock by allowing an estimation of losses, identifying traits of stability, and prompting corrective action [5] (Table 12.2).

Patients in Class I or II shock may respond to crystalloid resuscitation. If ongoing blood loss has been controlled, blood products may not be required. Patients in Class III and IV shock should be resuscitated with a balanced component blood product regimen where packed red cells, plasma, and platelets are provided in a 1:1:1 ratio [7]. This regimen coupled with damage control surgery and a goal systolic blood pressure of 90 mmHg until hemorrhage is controlled is the basis for the current damage control resuscitation. This regimen can be tailored to the patient's coagulation profile utilizing the viscoelastic assays thromboelastography (TEG) or thromboelastometry (ROTEM). End points of resuscitation are followed to guide fluid and blood product administration as care progresses into the critical care unit postsurgical or radiologic intervention.

12.4.3 Renal

Perioperative acute kidney injury (AKI) is defined as sudden and often unanticipated decline in renal function that occurs within hours to days of surgery. It is associated with up to a tenfold increase in mortality, reduced long-term survival, and increased development of chronic kidney disease with subsequent need for hemodialysis. Most commonly, this is due to renal hypoperfusion or systemic inflammation that occurs as a direct response to surgery, although multiple factors may contribute [8]. The Acute Kidney Injury Network (AKIN) defines AKI as any of the following within 48 h: increased serumCr × 1.5, serumCr increase 0.3 mg/dL or more, or urine output less than 0.5 mL/kg/h for more than 6 h [9].

Table 12.2 Advanced trauma life support hypovolemic shock classifications [5]

Parameter	Class I	Class II (Mild)	Class III (Moderate)	Class IV (Severe)
Blood loss (%)	<15	15–30	30–40	>40
Heart rate	<100	100–120	120–140	>140
Blood pressure	Normal	Normal	Decreased	Greatly decreased
Pulse pressure	Normal–increased	Decreased	Decreased	Decreased
Respiratory rate	14–20	20–30	30–40	>35
Urine output (mL/h)	>30	20–30	5–15	Minimal
Glasgow Coma Scale (GCS)	Normal	Normal	Decreased	Decreased
Base deficit	0 to −2 mEq/L	−2 to −6 mEq/L	−6 to −10 mEq/L	−10 mEq/L or less
Need for blood products	Monitor	Possible	Yes	Massive transfusion

ATLS® Advanced Trauma Life Support Student Course Manual, 10th ed. American College of Surgeons, 2018

Goal-directed therapy is recommended when AKI develops. Utilization and optimization of endpoints of resuscitation should be instituted; this may require transfer to a critical care unit and possible invasive procedures. Early consultation with nephrology has been shown to lessen chronic kidney disease. Renal replacement therapy may be instituted in cases of refractory fluid overload, severe hyperkalemia (K+ >6.5 mEq/L), signs of uremia, and severe metabolic acidosis (pH < 7.1).

12.4.4 Gastrointestinal

Use of nasogastric decompression tubes preoperatively in the emergent general surgery patient is selective. Patients with bowel obstruction, high-grade ileus, or at high risk for emesis with aspiration require decompression. These tubes may facilitate early institution of enteral feeding as well. Routine use of nasogastric tubes after abdominal surgery to hasten resolution of postoperative ileus, diminish aspiration risk from gastric contents, improve patient comfort, protect intestinal anastomoses, or shorten hospital stay is not recommended [10].

Surgical patients at severe risk for stress ulceration are those on mechanical ventilation for more than 48 hours and coagulopathy. Additional high risk factors include traumatic brain injury, spinal cord injury, burns, greater than one week in the ICU, steroid use, and past history of gastrointestinal (GI) bleeding [11]. Multiple prophylactic regimens exist for stress ulceration. When compared to histamine 2 blockers, proton pump inhibitors were shown to be more protective against GI bleeding [12].

Early enteral nutrition in the postoperative phase of care is highly beneficial. Advantages include better glycemic control, improved anastomotic integrity, and reduced infectious morbidity [13]. While several systematic reviews have favored post-pyloric feeding over gastric feeding, a large multicenter randomized control study by Davies failed to show a preferential route [14].

12.4.5 Endocrine

In both the diabetic and nondiabetic populations, hyperglycemia in the perioperative period is an independent marker of poor surgical outcomes such as delayed wound healing, increased infection rates, increased hospital length of stay, and increased hospital mortality. Van den Berghe demonstrated that an intensive insulin therapy (IIT) regimen targeting a blood glucose (BG) of 80–110 mg/dL reduced in-hospital mortality by 34% compared to a standard therapy target of 180–200 mg/dL in surgical ICU patients [15]. Due to concerns for hypoglycemia utilizing IIT, several societies now support moderating the target BG. The Society for Critical Care Medicine (SCCM) recommends BG < 150 mg/dL [16], and the American College of Physicians recommends BG 140–200 mg/dL [17].

Acute adrenal insufficiency may require attention in the emergent surgical patient. Preoperatively, any patient who is taking more than 20 mg/day of prednisone or its equivalent, or any patient on glucocorticoids who has clinical Cushing's syndrome should be considered adrenal insufficient due to decreased function of the hypothalamic-pituitary-adrenal axis (HPA). For minor procedures, patients should take their usual morning dose with no extra supplementation. For moderate stress procedures, the morning dose should be supplemented with hydrocortisone 50 mg IV immediately pre-op and 25 mg of hydrocortisone every 8 h for 24 h. Return to usual dose thereafter. For major operative procedures, the usual morning dose is supplemented with hydrocortisone 100 mg IV preinduction of anesthesia and 50 mg every 8 h for 24 h. The dose should then be tapered by half per day to maintenance dose [18].

Adrenal insufficient critically ill patients can be difficult to identify due to lack of specific signs and symptoms. Of particular concern is the patient with refractory shock (systolic BP <90 mmHg), despite adequate fluid resuscitation and vasopressor therapy. The decision to utilize steroid therapy is usually made clinically, as testing for HPA function is of limited value in critically ill patients. Current recommendations are for hydrocortisone 200–400 mg/day in divided doses [19].

12.4.6 Hematologic

Bleeding in the acute care and trauma patient can present overtly or subtly. The etiology of perioperative hemorrhage is often multifactorial and can include blood loss, hemodilution, acquired platelet dysfunction, coagulation factor consumption, hypothermia, activation of fibrinolytic pathways, and prescribed oral anticoagulants [20]. An awareness of the more common coagulopathies, their assessment, and treatment is indispensable in managing these patients. Thromboelastography (TEG) and thromboelastometry (ROTEM) are both point of care assays that are rapid and measure the complex interactions of different coagulation elements not appreciated by the slower, isolated coagulation parameters such as the prothrombin time (PT), activated partial thromboplastin time (aPTT), or the international normalized ratio (INR) [21]. An example of a TEG assay curve is illustrated in Fig. 12.1.

Acute traumatic coagulopathy (ATC) is an impairment in hemostasis with self-sustaining activation of the fibrinolytic system indepen-

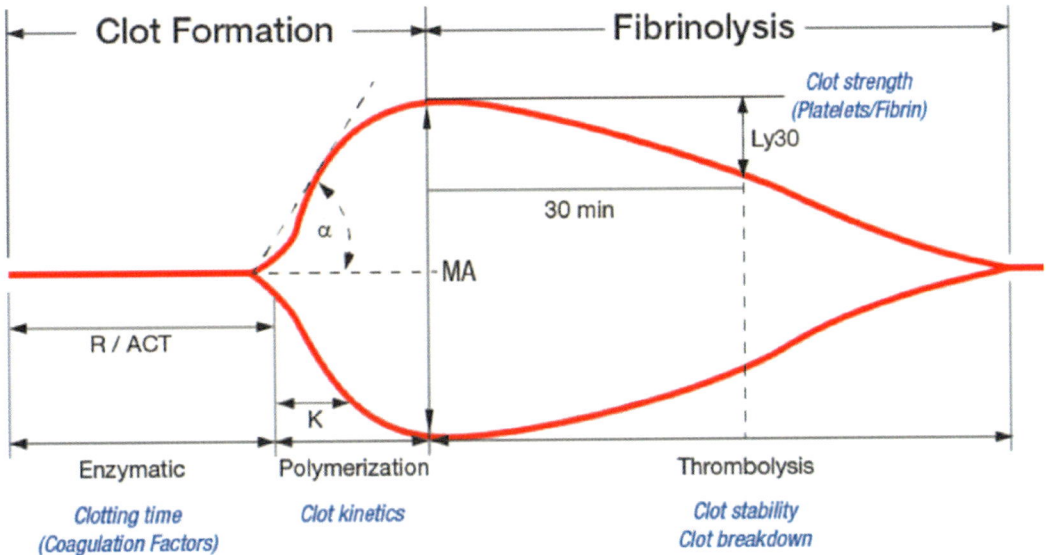

Fig. 12.1 TEG Assay Curve Demonstrating Normal Coagulation Profile [22]. (TEG® hemostasis analyzer tracing image used by permission of Haemonetics Corporation. TEG® and Thrombelastograph® are registered trademarks of Haemonetics Corporation in the US, other countries or both)

dent of hypothermia, acidosis, and hemodilution [23]. Management of major bleeding requires repair of the underlying cause after surgery or trauma, volume resuscitation with blood products, and diagnosis and management of ongoing coagulopathy.

Disseminated Intravascular Coagulopathy (DIC) is the systemic activation of the coagulative pathways, leading to generation and deposition of fibrin and microvascular thrombi. There is potential for end organ damage and can occur with trauma, sepsis, or amniotic fluid emboli. If not corrected, an additional consumptive state with compounding consumptive coagulopathy features will lead to exhaustion of platelets, coagulation proteins, and accelerated fibrinolysis with continued or worsening bleeding. The hallmark of DIC is fibrinolysis; regardless of other parameters, there will be evidence of breakdown products of fibrinogen [24].

A multitude of therapies have recently emerged with new indications for anticoagulant therapy. The risk of bleeding versus thromboembolism must be balanced in the acute care setting and trauma. High-risk patients such as those with a mechanical mitral valve, atrial fibrillation with mitral valve disease, or history of thromboembolism should be placed on intravenous heparin therapy while off warfarin. Prothrombin complex (PCC) provides the benefit of reversal while limiting volume administration that is associated with plasma reversal. This has been especially advantageous in high-risk reversal situations such as intracranial hemorrhage and intra-abdominal bleeding. The direct oral anticoagulants (DOACs) reversibly inhibit coagulation factors. There are multiple agents available on the market, some of which have specific reversal agents, but not always readily available. Early consultation with pharmacy services is essential.

12.4.7 Infectious

The Surviving Sepsis Campaign defines sepsis as life-threatening organ dysfunction caused by a dysregulated host response to infection. Septic shock is a subset of sepsis with circulatory and cellular or metabolic dysfunction, associated with a higher risk of mortality. Patients with sepsis face a mortality rate of 25–30% and patients with septic shock face a 40–60% mortality rate. Surgical patients make up one third of all sepsis cases, and the incidence of sepsis among patients undergoing emergency surgery is twice that of patients undergoing elective operations. Risk factors include male gender, age greater than 50 years, pancreatic or small intestine procedures, American Society of Anesthesiologists (ASA) physical status class 3–5, and a partially or a totally dependent functional status [25, 26].

Treatment and fluid resuscitation should begin immediately. The goal is to increase cardiac output and improve end organ perfusion [27] (Fig. 12.2).

Obtain blood cultures and lactate levels, begin fluid resuscitation immediately and complete within 3 h. Empiric broad-spectrum antibiotics are started immediately to cover all potential pathogens. At least two sets of blood cultures (aerobic and anaerobic) should be taken prior to antibiotic therapy, but therapy should not be delayed in order to obtain cultures. Antimicrobial therapy should be narrowed once the pathogen and its sensitivities are identified or discontinued if no infection is established. Vasopressors should be started within the first hour to achieve a MAP of greater than 65 mmHg if blood pressure is not restored after initial fluid therapy. The SCCM recommends hydrocortisone 50 mg IV every 6 h, only in the case of vasopressor resistant shock [19].

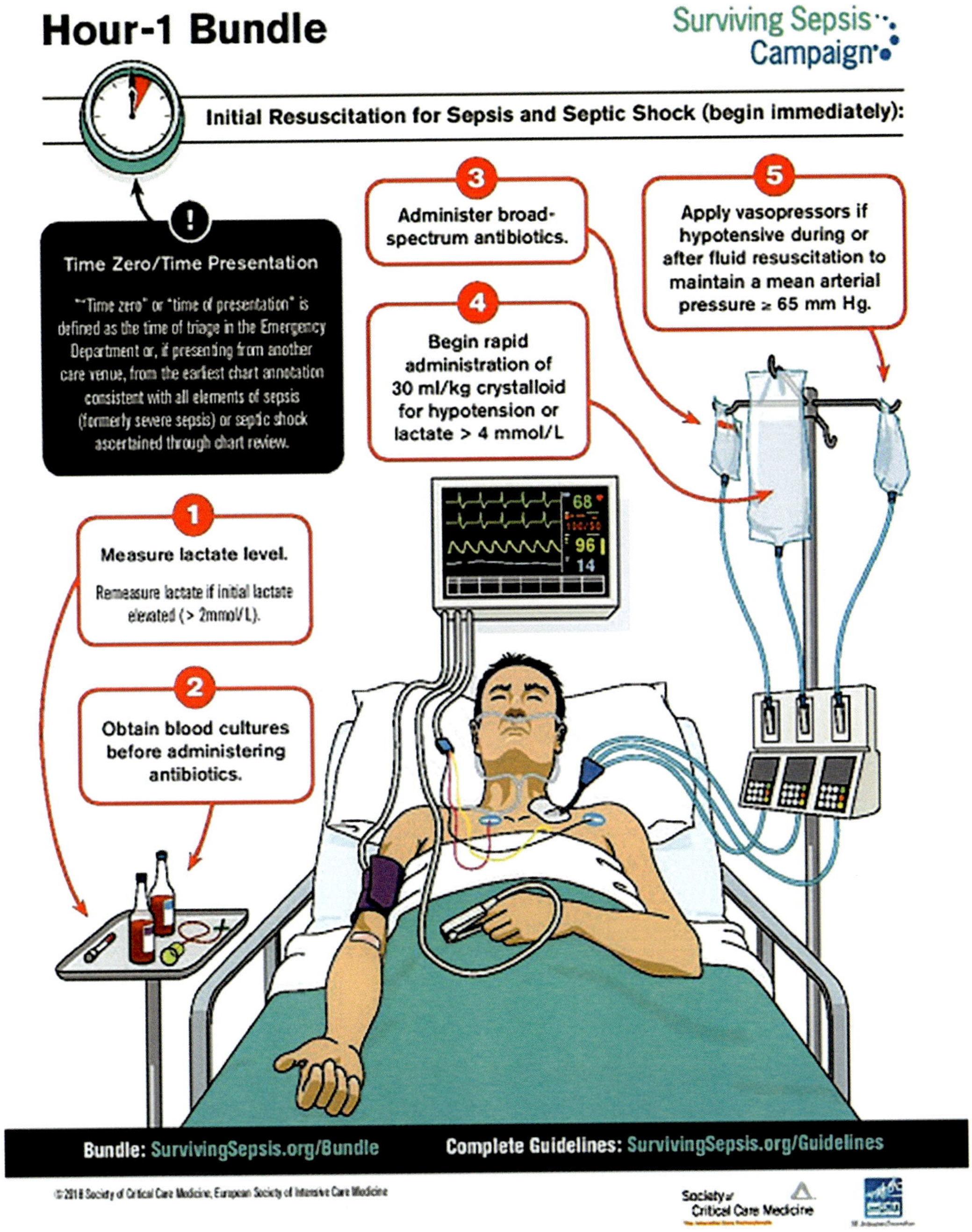

Fig. 12.2 Surviving Sepsis Campaign Guidelines for Management of Sepsis and Septic Shock [28] (Reproduced with permission from survivingsepsis.org. Copyright©2019 the Society of Critical Care Medicine and the European Society of Intensive Care Medicine)

Dos and Don'ts

Dos
- Early establishment of definitive airway if indicated
- Early attention to heart rate, blood pressure, respiratory rate, and mental status
- Prompt assessment of lactic acid, base deficit, pH, and TEG parameters
- Timely blood cultures and antibiotic therapy where applicable

Don'ts
- Delay in evaluation and care
- Over or under resuscitate as guided by trends in the endpoints of resuscitation
- Overlook adrenal insufficiency and blood glucose levels

Take-Home Messages
- Follow the ABC's of resuscitation
- Early treatment of hemorrhagic shock with a balanced ratio of blood products
- Early implementation of Surviving Sepsis Campaign Bundle
- Timely implementation of the ARDS Network protocol

Multiple Choice Questions

1. Which of the following sedative agents has the adverse effect of hypotension and should not be used in patients with hemodynamic instability?
   A. Ketamine
   B. Etomidate
   C. **Propofol**
   D. Rocuronium

2. Which of the following sedative agents causes adrenal insufficiency and should not be administered as a continuous infusion?
   A. Propofol
   B. Ketamine
   C. Midazolam
   D. **Etomidate**

3. Renal replacement therapy is indicated in which of the following cases?
   A. Severe hypokalemia
   B. Severe metabolic alkalosis
   C. **Severe metabolic acidosis**
   D. Urine output <0.5 cc/kg/h

4. Despite its variability, based on the patient's preexisting conditions, urine output can serve as a clinical marker of end organ perfusion. The urinary output of the adult being resuscitated should reach:
   A. **0.5 cc/kg/h**
   B. 1.0 cc/kg/h
   C. 0.75 cc/kg/h
   D. 0.25 cc/kg/h

5. A 62 year old female recently diagnosed with breast cancer underwent port placement 3 days ago. The incision is erythematous and indurated. Her blood pressure is 90/60 mmHg, temperature 100.5 °F, heart rate 95 bpm, respirations 22. Fluid resuscitation should begin with:
   A. 50 cc/kg normal saline in the first 5 h
   B. 30 cc/kg normal saline in the first 5 h
   C. **30 cc/kg lactated ringers in the first 3 h**
   D. 30 cc/kg colloid in the first 3 h

6. An ICU patient requires fluid resuscitation and shows little improvement after 48 h. Which of the following parameters suggests increased mortality?
   A. Increased urine output after resuscitation
   B. **Elevated lactate levels**
   C. Increased right ventricular end diastolic volume index
   D. Base deficit of −4 mEq/L

7. A 42 year old male involved in a motor vehicle collision is brought to the ED via ambulance. Over the course of the exam, you see increasing work of

breathing and accessory muscle use. His temperature is 98.6 °F, heart rate 110 bpm, respirations 23, and oxygen saturation 90%. Which of the following next steps in management is most appropriate at this time?
   A. Begin empiric antibiotic therapy
   B. Perform imaging studies
   C. Start 30 cc/kg lactated ringers
   D. **Consider endotracheal intubation**
8. A surgical ICU patient with a blood glucose of 195 does not have a medical history of diabetes mellitus. In order to reduce in-hospital mortality, postoperative management:
   A. **Should incorporate insulin therapy to achieve a blood glucose of <150 mg/dL**
   B. Is already controlling his blood glucose within the target range of 180–200 mg/dL
   C. Does not require insulin therapy because the patient is not diabetic
   D. Should incorporate insulin therapy to achieve a blood glucose of <190 mg/dL
9. Which of the following is not a risk factor for sepsis?
   A. Male gender
   B. ASA PS class 3–5
   C. **Gallbladder procedures**
   D. Totally dependent functional status
10. Patients in Class III and Class IV hypovolemic shock should be resuscitated with which of the following regimens?
    A. PRBCs, plasma, and platelets in a 2:1:1 ratio
    B. **PRBCs, plasma, and platelets in a 1:1:1 ratio**
    C. Crystalloid IVFs only
    D. Crystalloid IVF and PRBCs

References

1. Cuthbertson DP. Post-shock metabolic response. Lancet. 1942;239(6189):433–7.
2. Evans C, Bauman ZM, Cooper C, Capella JM. Surgical shock. In: Essentials of general surgery and surgical specialties. 6th ed. Philadelphia: Wolters Kluwer; 2019.
3. Vincent JL, Silva AQE, Couto L Jr, Taccone FS. The value of blood lactate kinetics in critically ill patients: a systematic review. Crit Care. 2016;20(1):257.
4. Mikulaschek A, Henry SM, Donovan R, Scalea TM. Serum lactate is not predicted by anion gap or base excess after trauma resuscitation. J Trauma. 1996;40(2):218–22.
5. ATLS®. Advanced trauma life support student course manual, 10th ed. American College of Surgeons; 2018.
6. National Heart, Lung and Blood Institute, Acute Respiratory Distress Syndrome Network (NHLBI ARDS Network). http://www.ardsnet.org.
7. Holcomb JB, Tilley BC, Baraniuk S, et al. Transfusion of plasma, platelets, and red blood cells in a 1:1:1 vs. a 1:1:2 ratio and mortality of patients with severe trauma: the PROPPR randomized clinical trial. JAMA. 2015;313(5):471–81.
8. Rodriguez JD, Hilthe CC. Perioperative acute kidney injury. StatPearls [Internet] 2020. Treasure Island: StatPearls Publishing; 2021. PMID: 32491609.
9. Mehta RL, Kellum JA, Shah SV, Molitoris BA, Ronco C, Warnock DG, Levin A. Acute kidney injury network: report of an initiative to improve outcomes in acute kidney injury. Crit Care. 2007;11(2):R31. https://doi.org/10.1186/cc5713.
10. Verma R, Nelson RL. Prophylactic nasogastric decompression after abdominal surgery. Cochrane Database Syst Rev. 2007;2007(3):CD004929. https://doi.org/10.1002/14651858.CD004929.
11. Cook DJ, Fuller HD, Guyatt GH, Marshall JC, Leasa D, Hall R, Winton TL, Rutledge F, Todd TJR, Roy P, Lacroix J, Griffith L, Willan A. Risk factors for gastrointestinal bleeding in critically ill patients. JAMA. 1994;330(6):377–81.
12. Barkun AN, Bardou M, Pham CQD, Martel M. Proton pump inhibitors vs. histamine 2 receptor antagonists for stress-related mucosal bleeding prophylaxis in critically ill patients: a meta-analysis. Am J Gastroenterol. 2012;107(4):507–20.
13. Cresci GAM, MacGregor JM, Harbison SP. Surgical nutrition. In: Essentials of general surgery and surgical specialties. 6th ed. Philadelphia: Wolters Kluwer; 2019.
14. Davies AR, Morrison SS, Bailey MJ, Bellomo R, Cooper DJ, Doig GS, Finfer SR, Heyland DK. A multicenter, randomized controlled trial comparing early

nasojejeunal with nasogastric nutrition in critical illness. Crit Care Med. 2012;40(8):2342–8.
15. Van den Berghe G, Wouters P, Weekers F, Verwaest C, Ferdinande P, Lauwers P, Bouillon R. Intensive insulin therapy in critically ill patients. N Engl J Med. 2001;345(19):1359–67.
16. Jacobi J, Bircher N, Krinsley J, Agus M, Braithwaite S, Deutschman C, Freire A, Geehan D, Kohl B, Nasraway SA, Rigby M, Sands K, Schallom L, Taylor B, Umpierrez G, Mazuski J, Schenemann H. Guidelines for the use of an insulin infusion for the management of hyperglycemia in critically ill patients. Crit Care Med. 2012;40(12):3251–76.
17. Qaseem A, Humphrey LL, Chou R, Snow V, Shekelle P. Use of intensive insulin therapy for the management of glycemic control in hospitalized patients: a clinical practice guideline from the American College of Physicians. Ann Intern Med. 2011;154(4):260–7.
18. Hamrahian AH, Roman S, Milan S. The management of the surgical patient taking glucosteroids. In: UpToDate, Post TW (editor). Waltham; 2021. Accessed 29 Apr 2021.
19. Kaufman DA. Glucocorticoid therapy in septic shock in adults. In: UpToDate, Post TW (editor). Waltham; 2021. Accessed 29 Apr 2021.
20. Ghadimi K, Levy JH, Welsby IJ. Perioperative management of the bleeding patient. Br J Anaesth. 2016;117(suppl 3):iii18–30.
21. Tanaka KA, Bader SO, Gorlinger K. Novel approaches in management of perioperative coagulopathy. Curr Opin Anaesthesiol. 2014;27(1):72–80.
22. TEG® hemostasis analyzer tracing image used by permission of Haemonetics Corporation. TEG® and Thrombelastograph® are registered trademarks of Haemonetics Corporation in the US, other countries or both.
23. Brohi K, Singh J, Heron M, Coats T. Acute trauma coagulopathy. J Trauma. 2003;54(6):1127–30.
24. Levi M, Toh CH, Thacil J, Watson HG. Guidelines for the diagnosis and management of disseminated intravascular coagulation. Br J Haematol. 2009;145(1):24–33.
25. Rhodes A, Evans LE, Alhazzani W, et al. Surviving sepsis campaign: international guidelines for management of sepsis and septic shock 2016. Crit Care Med. 2017;45(3):486–552.
26. Gabriel V, Grigorian G, Nahmias J, Pejcinovska M, Smith M, Sun B, Won E, Bernal N, Barrios C, Schubl SD. Risk factors for post-operative sepsis and septic shock in patients undergoing emergency surgery. Surg Infect (Larchmt). 2019;20(5):367–72.
27. Levy MM, Evans LE, Rhodes A. The surviving sepsis campaign bundle: 2018 update. Crit Care Med. 2018;46(6):997–1000.
28. Copyright©2019 the Society of Critical Care Medicine and the European Society of Intensive Care Medicine. Reproduced with permission from survivingsepsis.org.

Further Reading

ATLS®. Advanced trauma life support student course manual, 10th ed. American College of Surgeons; 2018.

Hamrahian AH, Roman S, Milan S. The management of the surgical patient taking glucosteroids. In: UpToDate, Post TW (editor). Waltham; 2021. Accessed 29 Apr 2021.

Holcomb JB, Tilley BC, Baraniuk S, et al. Transfusion of plasma, platelets, and red blood cells in a 1:1:1 vs. a 1:1:2 ratio and mortality of patients with severe trauma: the PROPPR randomized clinical trial. JAMA. 2015;313(5):471–81.

Rhodes A, Evans LE, Alhazzani W, et al. Surviving sepsis campaign: international guidelines for management of sepsis and septic shock 2016. Crit Care Med. 2017;45(3):486–552.

Soni NJ, Arntfield R, Kory P. Point-of-care ultrasound. 2nd ed. Philadelphia: Elsevier; 2020.

Critical Care Medicine

13

Maria Di Matteo and Davide Corbella

> **Learning Points**
> After reading this chapter, you should be able to:
> - Define Critical Care Medicine and its role in the setting of Emergency General Surgery
> - Describe different ICU models and their logistics, technological, and workforce need
> - Discuss the principles of management of critically ill EGS patients, focusing on respiratory support.

13.1 Introduction

Critical Care Medicine (CCM) is a relatively new branch of medicine whose primary focus is treating a patient with the need for invasive organ support or at high risk of needing one.

This situation is an anomaly in the medicine panorama. It accounts for the fact that the definition of critical care medicine is "operative and instrumental." In contrast with other branches of medicine, it does not focus its interests on treating a single and specific organ- or system-specific disease, but on restoring normal physiology to "gain time" to recover. It focuses on restoring physiologic balance and the process of how to treat the patient rather than on the pathology he may suffer. In contrast, organ- or system-specific failures are still a prerogative of other areas of medicine.

In 2017, the World Federation of Societies of Intensive and Critical Care Medicine (WFSICCM) came out with this definition: "Intensive care, also known as critical care, is a multidisciplinary and interprofessional specialty dedicated to the comprehensive management of patients having, or at risk of developing, acute, life-threatening organ dysfunction." [1] This definition sums up the different ones given by national or international learned societies (Table 13.1 reports some definitions of CCM and ICUs). Clearly, every "intensive care physician" should conform to local legislation and be aware of the requirements mandatory in his jurisdiction. The intensive care physician must undergo a specific training and certification in Critical Care. He should be able to diagnose, manage, monitor, intervene, arbitrate, and individualize the Care to each critically ill patient affected by single or multiple health care issues [6, 7]. Lastly, the intensive care physician is the coordinator and leader of the multidisciplinary and often multispecialty approach to the critically ill patient [4, 6–8].

M. Di Matteo · D. Corbella (✉)
NeuroTrauma Intensive Care Unit, Department of Anesthesia, Emergency and Critical Care, Azienda Socio Sanitaria Territoriale Papa Giovanni XXIII, Bergamo, Italy
e-mail: mdimatteo@asst-pg23.it; dcorbella@asst-pg23.it

Table 13.1 Definitions of intensive care unit and critical care medicine

Author	Year	Definition
Society of Critical Care Medicine [2]	1999	ICU serves as a place for monitoring and care of patients with potentially severe physiological instability requiring technical and/or artificial life support. The level of care in an ICU is greater than that available on the floor or intermediate care unit
European Society of Intensive Care Medicine [3]	2011	The ICU is a distinct organizational and geographic entity for clinical activity and care, operating in cooperation with other departments integrated in a hospital. The ICU is preferably an independent unit or department that functions as a closed unit under the full medical responsibility of the ICU staff in close concert with the referring medical specialists. It has a defined geographical location concentrating the human and technical resources, such as manpower, professional skills and competencies, technical equipment, and the necessary space
World Federation of Societies of Intensive and Critical Care Medicine [1]	2016	Intensive care, also known as critical care, is a multidisciplinary and interprofessional specialty dedicated to the comprehensive management of patients having, or at risk of developing, acute, life-threatening organ dysfunction. Intensive care uses an array of technologies that provide support to failing organ systems, particularly the lungs, cardiovascular system, and kidneys
College of Intensive Care Medicine of Australia and New Zealand [4]	2016	An Intensive Care Unit (ICU) is a specially staffed and equipped, separate, and self-contained area of a hospital dedicated to the management of patients with life-threatening illnesses, injuries and complications, and monitoring of potentially life-threatening conditions
Weil [5]	2009	[The ICU is] the commitment to dedicated care, on site, by physicians and specially trained professional nurses and technicians with preparedness for immediate lifesaving interventions for the most seriously ill and injured

13.2 Who Is the Critical Care Patient?

The critical patient is a patient having or at risk of developing acute, life-threatening organ dysfunction [9]. Therefore, the Surgical Intensive Care Unit (SICU) provides constant monitoring, organ support, and possibly emergency interventions to unstable, severely, or potentially severely ill patients in the perioperative setting [10].

Trauma and acute care surgical patients are very different from those presented in the non-acute care setting, and they more often require ICU admission [11, 12]. The lack of preoperative evaluation and optimization exposes these patients to a greater risk of death and complications. In addition, EGS patients present with acute physiologic derangements, requiring aggressive and timely resuscitation even before a definitive diagnosis. When the EGS patients arrive in the ICU, they may need ongoing optimization of tissue perfusion and further investigations/surgery before definitively correcting the "anatomic" disturbances [13].

13.2.1 The Critical Emergency Surgery Patient

EGS patients represent a unique population with the highest rate of death and complications [14, 15]. Recent studies have shown that EGS patients are six to eight times more likely to die than patients undergoing the same procedure electively [16]. Approximately half of EGS patients experience a postoperative complication [17].

The patient group is highly heterogeneous; therefore, the need for observation and intensive Care will vary [18]. In general, EGS patients are older, have a high fragility incidence, a reduced physiologic reserve, and are significantly more acutely ill at admission [19].

Unsurprisingly, the risk of perioperative death is higher in the elderly emergency laparotomy patient than in younger patients [20]. Green et al. reported an overall mortality of 45%, with 12% intraoperative complications and 70% postoperative complications (including myocardial infarction, wound infection, hematoma, and sepsis) in octogenarians undergoing EGS [21].

Apart from age, several factors can explain the increased risk of death following EGS, among which are the inability to optimize preoperative status before surgery and the time-sensitivity of the pathology. Nevertheless, Havens et al. showed that EGS patients have a worse outcome than non-EGS (NEGS) patients, even after controlling for preoperative variables and different procedure type [16].

A possible explanation can be found in the severe physiologic derangement associated with the acute disease: the physiology of EGS patients differs considerably from that of patients undergoing elective procedures, mainly due to the presence of shock. Indeed, while in NEGS cases, large-volume blood loss and fluid shifts might be anticipated but not yet present, bleeding or infection in EGS patients often results in substantial effective fluid loss already in place at the time of presentation [22].

Privette et al. identify a subgroup of EGS patients with higher acuity, the "acute care surgery" (ACS) patients [23]. The authors defined ACS patients as nonelective, nontrauma patients with significantly altered physiology requiring ICU admission, specific operative interventions, or both. ACS patients were more similar to trauma patients than to elective or EGS patients. They more likely required multiple operations, had longer hospital and ICU stay, higher mortality, and need for post-discharge rehabilitation. Moreover, Lissauer et al. demonstrated that ACS patients need more ICU resources than other general surgical patients: they have longer ICU lengths of stay and more frequently require mechanical ventilation and continuous renal replacement therapy [12, 24]. They do represent a distinct population.

13.2.2 The Critical Trauma Patient

According to the Trauma ICU Prevalence Project (TRIPP study), trauma patients have high medical acuity, presenting a wide breadth of pathology and requiring different interventions [25]. While no consensus definition for "polytrauma" has been recognized, generally accepted definitions use an Injury Severity Score (ISS) of greater than 15 to 17 or an Abbreviated Injury Scale (AIS) of greater than 2 in at least two body regions [26].

The TRIPP study provided a representation of patient types, injuries, and conditions in ICUs caring for trauma patients. According to this prevalence study, trauma patients can present with multiple high-intensity diagnoses (septic shock, 10.2%; multiple organ failure, 5.58%; adult respiratory distress syndrome, 4.38%). Hemorrhagic shock was present in a high proportion of patients (11.6% of trauma patients and 6.55% of all patients). A wide range of traumatic injuries was documented: head, neck, and thoracic injuries predominated, but spine, orthopedic, vascular, and intra-abdominal injuries were also prevalent. Over 69% of the trauma patients had a major operation, illustrating the ongoing surgical nature of trauma and the importance of surgical subspecialty care at trauma centers. Median ICU length of stay was 9 days; 30-day mortality was 11.2% [25].

Trauma patients present with anatomic and physiologic derangements requiring prompt identification and treatment. Correcting the physiologic derangement is the primary goal, while definitive correction of the anatomic disturbances is usually postponed until physiologic stabilization occurs. Following initial resuscitation and possibly damage control surgery, trauma patients presenting to the ICU may be far from stable with ongoing resuscitative needs and injuries still requiring definitive repair. This group of patients presents unique challenges for the ICU physician, including determining resuscitation endpoints and managing early post-resuscitation complications [27]. Trauma resuscitation has evolved from a one-size-fits-all approach to one tailored to patient physiology [28].

Virtually all critically injured patients require some degree of physiologic support on arrival to the ICU. It is essential to assess active bleeding and the extent of unresolved shock since these two factors will guide ongoing resuscitation [28, 29].

13.2.3 Stratification of Patients

The critical care patient is defined as a patient at risk of or with ongoing organ support. This generic and highly unspecific statement can be applied to an almost moribund trauma patient as well as to an elective surgical patient after an uneventful procedure. In order to compare those two patients, two main artifices have been explored: the use of Severity of Illness Scoring Systems (SISS) and the Nursing Workload Score (NWS).

The SISSs [30] are scoring systems that predict the mortality (usually at discharge from the ICU or hospital) according to the characteristics of the patient (e.g., age, diagnosis of admission, modality of admission, comorbidities, derangement of physiologic parameters at admission or in the first 24-h stay in ICU). The aims of the SISSs are well-described by their main characteristics: the calibration and the discrimination ability [31]. Discrimination defines the probability that a test will correctly discriminate between two alternatives. In the case of SISS, it helps to identify the patient who eventually will die correctly. A SISS with excellent discrimination may have some role at the patient level when counseling the family or triggering a revision over the therapeutic ceiling. Calibration is the degree to which the predicted probability generated by a model agrees with the actual event rate observed in a population, i.e., the ability of a model to correctly stratify groups of patients accordingly to their observed incidence of death. This characteristic is helpful when comparing two different populations, for example, if higher mortality is just the effect of a more critical population. SISSs are affected by several flaws intrinsic to the way they are built. Internal validity can be severely affected by the clinician withholding or withdrawing a treatment accordingly to the SISS. This leads to the classical scenario of the self-fulfilling prophecy that creates artificial overconfidence in a model specificity and negative predictive value [32]. The external validity can be even more challenging as the outcome can be a function of the resources and expertise available to treat the patient (e.g., a high-volume academic center vs. a rural ICU) or the implementation of an effective treatment in a previously untreatable disease.

NWS are used to classify patients according to the demand of assistance and program the number of nurses a unit needs. Cullen et al. [33] in 1974 described the Therapeutic Intervention Scoring System (TISS), a 57-items score to describe the nurse workload. Every item is a typical nurse activity in ICU, and the score is the sum of those activities done in 24 h. This score is the archetype of the NWS and correlated with costs, need for nurse units, and mortality because patients with a higher severity show a higher need for assistance. The idea is to quantify the time spent by the nurse in personal activities through the record of specific activities. The negative side is that to score 57 or 76 items is time-consuming, so a simplified version, the TISS-28, with only 28-items, was developed in 1996 [34]. The Nine Equivalents of Nursing Manpower Score is a furthermost simplification of the TISS-28 [35], considering only nine items comprehensive of the 28 items of the TISS-28. 40–50 NEMS points are the maximum "amount of work" a nurse can deliver, and six of those items are directly related to the organ failure a patient can suffer in ICU. This substantial overlap between nursing workload and the number and severities of organ failures (a proxy of the severity of the patient) is the basis for the definition of Level of Care (LoC). LoC is defined as the relationship between the severity of the illness of the patient and the nurse-to-patient ratio [36]. LoC can be high, intermediate, and low (see Table 13.2), and the number of patients a nurse can attend is related to their LoC [37].

Table 13.2 Set of criteria to define the Level of Care

High level of care	mR, mRc, mRd, mRcd, mC,
Major criteria	mCr, mCd, mCrd, mRC, mRCd
Minor criteria	mrc, mrd, mcd, mrcd
Low level of care	m, mr, mc, md, r, c, d

m basic monitoring, *R* mechanical ventilation, *r* noninvasive respiratory support, *C* more than two vasoactive drugs on continuous perfusion, *c* only one vasoactive drug on continuous perfusion, *d* dialysis

13.3 What Is an ICU?

The WFSICCM definition [1] of ICU is: "An intensive care unit is an organized system for the provision of care to critically ill patients that provides intensive and specialized medical and nursing care, an enhanced capacity for monitoring, and multiple modalities of physiologic organ support to sustain life during a period of acute organ system insufficiency. Although an ICU is based in a defined geographic area of a hospital, its activities often extend beyond the walls of the physical space to include the emergency department, hospital ward, and follow-up clinic." According to human, technological, and organizational resources, this dense statement defines ICUs with a lesser role for technological ones. ICU is a matter of workflow rather than the place where it happens or the devices used. Several national societies pose the benchmarks for ICUs. Since 2001, the Society of Critical Care Medicine (SCCM) has classified ICUs focusing on the concept of "model," who delivers the care, and "level," how invasive and complex care can be [6]. Those definitions reflected different, regionalized, local stories that brought to the creation of ICUs and mirrored locally available resources.

13.3.1 ICUs Models

ICU model defines who is in charge of the critically ill patient and has the privileges to admit and discharge patients from ICU [6].

In the open model, every physician can admit to ICU, and those patients are under his direct care. Those physicians have compelling responsibilities in the hospital (i.e., operating rooms, outpatient clinic, or general ward) and did not receive specific training in critical care medicine. The intensivist, if available, is consulted only at the discretion of the admitting physician.

In the transitional model, the patient is admitted under the care of a nonintensivist physician, but intensivist consultation is mandatory, at least once during the ICU stay.

In the closed ICU model, only the intensivist has the privileges to admit and discharge patients. All the patients admitted to the ICU are under the direct care of an intensivist.

These models can be subclassified as high-intensity staffing if an intensivist is 24 h available and low-intensity staffing if the intensivist is not always available [38].

The classification of ICUs has a historical origin. In 1991, the SCCM published the data from a survey upon ICU organization and staffing [39, 40]. Those data comprised 40% of all ICUs from the United States. They showed a wide variety of management and organizational structure, with just 22% of units fulfilling the criteria for a closed one. Since then, compelling evidence suggested increased patient outcome [41] (reduced mortality [38], length of hospital/ICU stay [38], adherence to guidelines, and best medical practice [42]) when mainly intensivists staffed ICUs. In 2001 SCCM favored the model of an ICU with extensive, if not exclusive, presence of intensivists to reduce mortality, length of stay, and costs and increase the overall quality of work [6]. Subsequent evidence pointed out that "an intensivist-led, high-intensity team is an integral part of effective care delivery in the ICU and can lead to improved outcomes" [43] as several studies showed to fail an improvement in outcomes of a strictly closed with 24/7 onsite intensivist coverage.

One of the main drives for those studies was to overcome the shortages of intensivists and reduce costs. In 2011, the European Society of Critical Care (ESICM) rolled out the essential requirement for ICUs regarding structural and organizational aspects, coming to a different solution [3]. ESICM stated that ICUs should be staffed only by intensivists with a recognized and certified intensive care curriculum. All the other physicians participating in the care of critically ill patients should be considered a consultant. However, how an ICU is physician-staffed is often a matter of available resources. In a low-resource setting, it is more likely that the ICU will have physician and nurse staffing from different backgrounds.

Moreover, the recent COVID-19 pandemic with the tremendous surge of critically ill respiratory patients forced to stretch medical and nurse expertise. Several institutions promoted remote consultation by intensivists and highly protocolized bundles of care taken over by nonintensivist [44]; others stretched resources as much as possible, and physicians and nurses with non-ICU backgrounds were implemented [45] to run ICUs. Despite the lack of solid evidence, this stepping back from the model of high-intensity staffing might have led to less-than-optimal results, as suggested by a striking difference in mortality favoring patients transferred to ICUs not overwhelmed by the inflow of patients from those treated locally with the available resources [46].

13.3.2 ICUs Levels

ICU level refers to the ability to provide specialized care to critically ill patients with increasing complexity of monitoring and treatment. Definitions are usually at the nation or regional level and consider the resources available on the territory and peculiarities such as underpopulated areas, remote areas, or large academic centers. Several scientific societies [1, 3, 6, 43], national societies, and governmental regulatory authorities [4, 8] defined the ICUs level, pointing out: how they should be staffed, what type of monitoring and organ support must be available, what type, and for how long they should be able to treat critically ill patients, what is their role in the community they sit. Every intensivist should be aware of the specific requirement in the area where he works.

The usual classification is in three levels, from the most basic level I to the most advanced Level III.

A level I ICU sits in a small, not specialistic, hospital. It should be able to provide essential monitoring and basic cardiovascular and ventilatory support for a short period. The unit must have a protocol for transferring and referring more complex patients to secondary or tertiary ICUs. Medical staffing can be challenging as few certified intensivists are usually willing to work full-time in small centers. However, at least the medical director should be a certified intensivist [3, 4, 8]. Ideally, the level I ICU is in an underpopulated area or is a small clinic in an urban center dealing mainly with postsurgical patients or critically ill patients with basic needs. As a rule, they treat patients who need a short period of stabilization or patients for whom the treatment in the community they live out outweighs the advantages of a transfer in a center capable of more advanced monitoring and treatment options [8]. To maintain sufficient clinical skills, the minimal number of mechanically ventilated patients is not established, but one hundred can be considered a reasonable number [4].

A level II ICU provides a high standard of general ICU care for a prolonged period of time [1, 3, 4, 8]. It should be capable of delivering care to a patient requiring complex multisystem life support like mechanical ventilation, continuous renal replacement therapy, invasive cardiovascular monitoring, and essential invasive cardiovascular support. A level II ICU is a designated area in a medium-large hospital that treats definitively the critically ill patients referred to that hospital. Transfer of patients happens when there is no appropriate specialty within the hospital. The ICU should have a protocol in place to refer for admission and consultation patients to tertiary centers capable of neurosurgery, cardiothoracic surgery, transplant, burn, and advanced pediatric care. Despite the shortage of intensivists, a Level II ICU should be staffed only by certified intensivists [3]. A caseload of at least 200 mechanically ventilated patients per annum is advisable to maintain a high level of clinical expertise and provide adequate clinical exposure and education to staff [4].

A level III ICU is a tertiary referral unit for intensive care patients and should provide complex multisystem life support for an indefinite time [3, 4, 6, 8]. A level III ICU should sit in a tertiary referral hospital center, have academic and research commitment, and give specialized and definitive care to subspecialty patients (i.e., neuro-trauma, cardiovascular, pediatric, transplant, ECMO, and burns patients). Physicians with privileges to work there should be certified intensivists and, possibly, formally trained in the subspecialty they practice. It is difficult to identify a minimal caseload of complex patients per annum to maintain enough clinical exposure. If 400 mechanically ventilated patients can be enough to retain enough high-level skills in complex patients [4], this number can be less critical when a tertiary center is dedicated to specific pathologies (e.g., liver transplant unit, neuro-trauma, cardiothoracic unit) or to specific treatment (e.g., ECMO center, bone marrow transplant unit).

13.3.3 ICU Workforce

13.3.3.1 Physicians

Physician staffing of ICUs is driven by local legislation, the availability of physicians trained in Intensive Care, recommendation by the national or international societies of CCM, and the ICU level. As a general rule, the majority of societies recommend that the higher the level of the ICU, the higher the share of intensive care-trained physicians [1, 4, 6, 8]. However, ESICM [3] suggests that only intensive care-certified physicians should practice in ICU, if possible.

The training and core curriculum of an intensivist is highly variable at the national level. The SCCM rolled out the first list of competencies an intensivist should have in 1992 [7]. Since that benchmarking paper, the core curriculum has become a competency-based one in several countries. In 2003, Competency-Based Training in Intensive Care medicinE (CoBaTrICE) was founded to create the first unified European curriculum in CCM. The main focus was to standardize the competencies an intensivist should have at an international level in the EU area and provide a reliable and unified assessment through the institution of a mandatory exit exam, the European Diploma of Intensive Care (EDIC). However, the training program is still very variable between countries [47]. CCM is considered: a primary specialty with direct access after undergraduate training in some countries (i.e., Sweden and Switzerland), in other, is a multidisciplinary 'supra-specialty' with access from several primary specialties to a standard national core curriculum for CCM (e.g., USA, Germany, Ireland), in other is just a piece of another specialty (e.g., Denmark,

Germany) or a dual joint certification, usually anesthesia and CCM (e.g., France, Italy). A formal national system for quality assurance of CCM training exists in the majority of the European countries, as well as some form of mandatory exit evaluation. Despite the presence of a well-recognized international standard, all EU countries are different, and the mandatory examination can range from an informal evaluation (e.g., Turkey) to a national exam (e.g., France) or a mandatory pass of the EDAIC (e.g., Denmark, Ireland).

A few papers investigate the optimal number of patients a single physician can manage (patient-to-intensivist ratio, PIR). Gershengorn et al. [48] evaluated the possible relationship between the PIR and mortality and found a U-shaped curve with a nadir of mortality for a PIR between 7 and 8. The authors argue that a PIR lower than seven probably does not assure enough exposure to the intensivist to keep him proficient in treating complex patients. On the contrary, a PIR higher than eight just overwhelms the intensivist and increases mortality.

13.3.3.2 Nurses

Nurse staffing should be provided by nurses with specific training in CCM and emergency medicine, giving rise to the critical care nurse (CCN) [1, 3, 4, 8, 43, 49] The prominent role of CCN in emergency medicine and critical care has been recognized since the first experiences in Pittsburg in the '60s. As Safar stated [50], "we discovered nursing in this area required special skills not ordinarily available in the average hospital nurse." Hence, they provided advanced training to them in mechanical ventilation and hemodynamic monitoring. Nurse education evolved from a secondary level to a tertiary level almost everywhere in the world [51, 52]. The peculiarity of the work in an ICU requires a post-tertiary (e.g., master or Ph.D.) education or, at least, some informal training in ICU while working under supervision. A recent survey in the EU [53] showed that 70% of European countries have a formal post-tertiary program to educate CCN and that 54% of the European Countries surveyed recognized CCNs as specialized and highly skilled health care professional workers. Despite acknowledging the importance of the CCNs, the training programs were highly variable, ranging from a 240-h course to a 2-years theoretical and practical course. The survey pointed out the lack of standardization between and inside countries regarding how teaching was provided, the students assessed, and the qualification awarded. The education of CCN cannot be overemphasized as, probably, even limited education programs on specific issues, like mechanical ventilation, may reduce strong outcomes as mortality, length of stay in ICU, or ventilator acquired pneumonia [54].

National and international societies defined the number of nurses and the share with a post-tertiary education an ICU should have [1, 3, 4, 8, 55]. The LoC drives the planning of nurses' unit need because different levels need a different nurse-to-patient ratio. A patient with a high LoC needs a nurse-to-patient ratio of 1:1 or 1:2. At the same time, the 1:3 or 1:4 nurse-to-patient ratio can suffice for those with a lower or intermediate LoC [36].

13.3.3.3 Allied Health Care Professionals

Other professional figures have flanked physicians and nurses since the first experiences of ICU. Several national and international guidelines define the work in ICU as a "teamwork" [3, 4, 6, 8]. Intensivists and CCN have as a primary task to coordinate other healthcare workers in multidisciplinary or interdisciplinary care, in which team members work in parallel but maintain strict disciplinary boundaries. In 2018, Donovan et al. [56], on behalf of the SCCM, defined interprofessional care as "the care provided by a team of healthcare professionals with overlapping expertise and an appreciation for the unique contribution of other team members, working as partners in achieving a common goal." This vision goes beyond the classical teamwork to embrace a different definition of the team as "a cohesive group with shared team identity, clarity, interdependence, integration, and shared responsibility" [57]. This definition emphasizes the team over its members or the sum of them. A team-based approach demonstrated an impact on major outcomes: adherence to bungles and guidelines, reduction of cost and mortality, better end-of-life decisions, ICU rounds, and handover [56].

An ICU team can be formed by: intensivist, nonintensivist physicians, CCN, advanced practice providers (APP), clinical pharmacists, respiratory care practitioners, rehabilitation specialists, dietitians, social workers, case managers, and spiritual care providers [1, 3, 4, 6, 8, 56]. Few of those professional characters have demonstrated an impact on the outcome of the patients.

APP such as nurse practitioners and physician assistants are used with more frequency as a shortcoming to the lack of intensivists. Several studies showed no differences in strong outcomes like mortality or length of hospital stay when comparing units staffed with APPs or physicians in training [56, 58, 59]. However, the evidence was weak due to their academic single-center population, retrospective design, and failure to control for intensivist staffing models. However, those studies showed longer ICU length of stay and nonhome discharge.

Clinical pharmacists have had a longer presence in ICU teams and are common in several countries [3, 4, 8]. In 2000, SCCM defined in a position paper [60] how a critical care pharmacy service should be organized and the requirements for a clinical pharmacist to work in the ICU. Several studies reviewed the impact of clinical pharmacists on ICU outcome [61], in particular: increased adherence to specific interdisciplinary bundles, reduction of adverse events, and costs.

Respiratory care Practitioners have a central role in intubated but also for non-intubated patients. Their presence contributes specifically to the optimal provision of spontaneous breathing trials, early mobility, implementation of PAD guidelines, and ABCDEF bundles [56].

Rehabilitation therapists have a fundamental role in improving and speeding up functional and cognitive impairment in critical care patients. Their work has been demonstrated to be safe, feasible, and to have a positive effect in the following areas: decreased ICU and hospital lengths of stay, shorter duration of delirium, better functional outcomes at hospital discharge, and more ventilator-free days, reduced delirium incidence, assessment and management of dysphagia, facilitation of communication, and management of patients with tracheotomies and adherence to the ABCDEF bundle.

13.3.4 ICU Service: Operational Requirement

Quality healthcare is defined as care that is "safe, effective, efficient, equitable, timely and patient-centered" [62]. National and International guidelines [1, 3, 4, 8, 63] pose benchmarking standard of logistics, equipment, design, and technological need of an ICU as well as other operational requirements related to the development of human resources and organization. Material requirements are related to the level and model of the ICU and, most importantly, to the resources available, i.e., the availability of monitoring or expensive invasive procedure (like ECMO or continuous renal replacement therapy) is different between high, middle, and low-income countries. We will briefly overview the operational requirements related to work organization and human resources. Whereas they are still related to the available recourses, there is a cultural background that health care providers and managers should adopt and adapt to their local environment. This cultural background is founded on the concept of clinical audit, i.e., a means to find out if the healthcare provided is in line with the best standards. This is achieved by identifying how the service is performing and where improvement could be made. Quality Improvement is the ultimate step. It is the "combined and unceasing efforts of everyone –to make changes that will lead to better patient outcome (health), better system performance (care) and better professional development (learning)" [64]. Several guidelines [1, 3, 4, 8] address this goal and define some tools an ICU should have to reach it, and in some cases, they are mandatory to accredit an ICU. The most cited are: a continuous medical education system with staff nurses and physicians that have a protected time to meet the educational demands of the unit and protected time for the unit itself to continue education; mandatory participation in a national or international audit system with revision of cases, treatment, ICU performances and comparison of results with other units; a morbidity and mortality program; structured handover and clinical rounds; the participation in research and development activities; a dedicated interprofessional group for the implementation of multidisciplinary bundles; a post-ICU clinic in order to continue test long- and middle-term patients' outcome [65].

13.4 General Principle of Management

Table 13.3 reports the general principle of monitoring and respiratory management in trauma and EGS patients.

Table 13.3 Principle of monitoring and respiratory management in trauma and EGS patients

Principle of respiratory management in trauma and EGS patients
Adequacy of blood flow and oxygen delivery to tissues is the primary goal of monitoring
Basic vital signs (HR, BP, UO) should be monitored in all EGS patients; nevertheless they can miss low CO states
Focused echocardiography allows rapid, noninvasive, point-of-care assessment of the hemodynamic status
Pulse oximetry and respiratory rate should be monitored in all EGS patients
Capnography provides essential information on both ventilation and perfusion
Principle of respiratory management in trauma and ECGS patients
LPV is recommended in EGS patients at risk of ARDS
EGS patients with postoperative ARDS should be managed according to the ARDSnet guidelines
Prone positioning can be used safely in trauma and EGS patients with severe ARDS
In the setting of respiratory failure and IAH, IAP monitoring is essential, and oesophageal pressure should be considered
Prevention of lung injury is a cornerstone in the management of trauma patients
Optimal ventilation strategy varies according to lesional status and phase of treatment of trauma
Both LPV and OLV may have a role in the ventilation strategy of trauma patients
PEEP can be safely applied in the management of ARDS following TBI
When ICP is increased, the control of PaCO₂ takes priority on LPV

EGS emergency general surgery, *HR* heart rate, *BP* blood pressure, *UO* urine output, *CO* cardiac output, *LPV* lung protective ventilation, *ARDS* acute respiratory distress syndrome, *IAH* intra-abdominal hypertension, *IAP* intra-abdominal pressure, *OLV* open-lung ventilation, *PEEP* positive end-expiratory pressure, *TBI* traumatic brain injury, *ICP* intracranial pressure, *PaCO₂* arterial partial pressure of carbon dioxide

13.4.1 Monitoring

The ICU provides a place for monitoring and care of patients with potentially severe physiologic instability, such as EGS patients. The critical endpoint is oxygen supply to tissues according to their metabolic needs. Therefore, both oxygenation and perfusion must be monitored in the implementation of any resuscitation strategy [66].

Despite this high acuity of ICU patients described in the TRIPP study, 'monitoring' was the reason for ICU admission for 16.6% of non-trauma surgical patients [25].

Trauma and EGS patients are prone to hemodynamic instability. Several complications may occur, so they must be monitored with various modalities, invasive and noninvasive, to detect any deterioration promptly.

13.4.1.1 Hemodynamic Monitoring

The importance of hemodynamic monitoring was highlighted in 2020 by the American Association for the Surgery of Trauma (AAST).

The AAST underlines a delicate balance between hypovolemia/hypoperfusion and volume overload, which is equally associated with complications [67].

Current practice in EGS patients involves the assimilation of multiple endpoints of resuscitation into an overall assessment. Resuscitative endpoints should be tracked in real-time, and, as they approach a normal range, resuscitation is titrated not to overshoot euvolemia [67].

Heart rate, blood pressure, and urine output are basic vital signs that should be monitored in all trauma and nontrauma EGS patients. However, they can easily miss low cardiac output (CO) states and are of limited value in the surgical ICU [68] or trauma settings [69]. Evidence of persistent hypoperfusion could be found in 80% of critically traumatized patients, despite the normalization of their vital signs [70]. Hence, different markers of low CO states have been evaluated: shock index, biomarkers like serum lactate or the oxygen saturation in superior vena cava, invasive or minimally invasive CO monitoring, and functional hemodynamic monitoring like echocardiography. Focused echocardiography may allow rapid, noninvasive, point-of-care assessment of hemodynamic status, providing valuable information on the etiology of shock and assessing response to therapeutic interventions [71, 72]. Hemodynamic monitoring is addressed in other chapters of this book.

13.4.1.2 Respiratory Monitoring

Pulse oximetry, airway patency, and respiratory rate should be monitored in all surgical patients. Patients with hypothermia, hypotension, hypovolemia, or peripheral vascular disease, or receiving vasoconstrictive medications may have inaccurate pulse oximetry readings.

Some patients will arrive in ICU already extubated; nevertheless, they still need respiratory monitoring since postoperative pulmonary complications (PPCs) can occur. Postoperative pain and immobility may lead to decreased cough, clearance of secretions, and an inability to recruit alveoli. Monitoring pain score is essential since appropriate pain control and early mobilization are critical in preventing pulmonary complications [73].

All patients under mechanical ventilation benefit from capnography measurement because the presence of $ETCO_2$ implies adequate ventilation and perfusion; an acute decrease in $ETCO_2$ is a life-threatening emergency, representing a sudden decrease in one or both of these parameters. Frequent causes in the postoperative setting include a pulmonary embolus, low cardiac output state, or disconnection from the ventilator.

Outside the ICU, continuous monitoring of oximetry and capnography may allow the detection of pathophysiologic abnormalities earlier in postoperative patients, but the evidence for improved clinical outcomes remains weak [74].

Other respiratory monitoring techniques can include arterial blood gas analysis and imaging studies, such as chest x-ray or lung ultrasounds. In ventilated patients, monitoring respiratory mechanics may be relevant as well.

13.4.1.3 Neurologic Monitoring

A focused neurologic examination should follow every acute care surgical procedure. After anesthesia, patients should return to their preoperative level of consciousness and exhibit no lateralizing signs. In the immediate postoperative period, depressed mental status with nonfocal findings most commonly represents persistent anesthetic drug effects or under-resuscitation. If there is no improvement after the appropriate time, imaging may be required.

Besides clinical examination, additional monitoring may be required in trauma or emergency surgical patients (ICP, EEG, $SjvO_2$, $PtbO_2$, and TCD) [75–79].

13.4.2 Organ Function Support

Hemodynamic support (i.e., fluid therapy and vasoactive drugs) and coagulation support are addressed in other chapters. We will focus on respiratory support in the general trauma and surgical patients and special populations as the patients with an open abdomen treatment or a severe traumatic brain injury.

13.4.2.1 Respiratory Support

Postoperative pulmonary complications (PPC)—such as atelectasis, pneumonia, respiratory insufficiency- are frequent causes of morbidity and mortality after EGS [80, 81].

According to current literature, patients undergoing major abdominal EGS are the surgical patients with the highest risk of developing PCCs [82, 83].

Emergency surgery confers a two-to-six-fold increase in the risk of PPCs compared to elective surgery [84]. In the ALPINE study, 48% of patients undergoing emergency laparotomy developed a PPC, with respiratory failure being the most common one [85]. The development of PPCs after EGS has been associated with prolonged hospital stay and increased death rate [86]. Advanced age, abnormal BMI (<21 kg/m [6] or >30 kg/m [6]), upper or upper/lower incision, and multiple procedures have been associated with increased risk for PPCs [86].

Incidence of acute respiratory distress syndrome (ARDS) after trauma has been reported in 12–25% of injured patients [87]. While studies differ on the mortality attributable to ARDS in trauma patients, with some reporting no increase in mortality in patients experiencing ALI [88], injured patients with ARDS and MOF have mortality rates as high as 50–80% [89].

Multivariable predictors of ARDS after trauma include subject age, Acute Physiology and Chronic Health Evaluation II Score, injury severity score, the presence of blunt traumatic injury, pulmonary contusion, massive transfusion, and flail chest injury (area under the receiver operator characteristic curve 0.79) [90].

13.4.2.2 Ventilation

Emergency General Surgery

There has been increasing evidence that a lung-protective ventilation (LPV) strategy is associated with reduced postoperative pulmonary complications (PPCs), mainly derived from studies on elective abdominal surgery [91]. According to the ALPINE study [85], a recent prospective multicentre observational study, only 4.9% of patients undergoing emergency laparotomy were ventilated using the LPV strategy. In contrast, most patients received a median tidal volume of 8 mL/kg ideal body weight (IBW), a PEEP of 5 cm H_2O, and a median peak inspiratory pressure (PIP) of 20 cm H_2O. The study revealed that almost half of these patients developed a PPC and that PIP, increased FiO_2, and age were significantly associated with it [85].

There is a lack of evidence regarding the best ventilator settings in the specific setting of emergency surgery. However, optimizing mechanical ventilation with protective ventilation is essential to minimize VILI in patients at risk of ARDS undergoing surgical procedures.

Moreover, evidence supports the benefit of lung-protective ventilation strategies in high-risk surgical patients, including EGS patients.

Patients undergoing EGS may present with ARDS or develop this syndrome postoperatively.

The incidence of ARDS in the postoperative period is relatively low, but the impact of ARDS on patient outcomes is significant. The postoperative development of ARDS is associated with prolonged hospitalization, longer duration of mechanical ventilation, increased intensive care unit length of stay, high morbidity, and mortality [91]. EGS patients with postoperative ARDS should be managed according to the ARDSnet guidelines [92].

Despite prone positioning being a major intervention in severe ARDS [92], clinicians remain uncertain whether ARDS patients in the postoperative period of abdominal surgery should be turned prone because of the risk of abdominal complications. Recently, the SAPRONADONF trial demonstrated that the prone position of ARDS patients after abdominal surgery was not associated with an increased rate of surgical complication with clear benefit in terms of oxygenation [93].

Postoperative strategies to decrease the risk of respiratory complications include: head-up or sitting position, encouragement of deep breathing exercises, early mobilization, intensive physiotherapy, incentive spirometry, airway toilette, careful fluid management, and adequate opioid-sparing analgesia. However, high-quality evidence for these strategies is lacking.

Noninvasive positive pressure ventilation (NIMV) or Continuous Positive Airway Pressure (CPAP) can be used to treat early mild ARDS. However, their role as prophylactic measures is unclear in patients with previously healthy lungs at risk of ARDS [94].

Early recognition of underlying respiratory infections and pneumonia should include identifying the causative pathogens, early empiric antibiotic therapy, and subsequent de-escalation to directed therapy in patients with sepsis.

Intra-abdominal Hypertension

EGS patients present several recognized risk factors for intra-abdominal hypertension (IAH), especially in patients with a BMI > 30 kg/m^2, admitted to the ICU after emergency abdominal surgery or with a diagnosis of pancreatitis [95].

There is an association between IAH and respiratory failure due to the effects of IAH on respiratory mechanics (decrease in lung volumes, respiratory system, but especially chest wall system compliance and increase in airway pressures) and gas exchange (increased dead-space ventilation, intrapulmonary shunt, and lung edema) [96].

The presence of IAH may add to the development of VILI. Optimal ventilator management of patients with ARDS and IAH should include the following:

- Intra-abdominal, oesophageal pressure, and hemodynamic monitoring;
- Lung protective ventilation;
- Deep sedation with or without neuromuscular paralysis in severe ARDS.
- Open abdomen in selected patients with severe abdominal compartment syndrome [97].

Abdominal-thoracic pressure transmission is around 50% [98]. While keeping driving pressures within safe limits, higher plateau pressures than normally considered might be acceptable [99]. Regli et al. [97] suggest the following correction: corrected target plateau pressure = target plateau pressure − 7 + IAP (mmHg) * 0.7.

Higher positive end-expiratory pressure (PEEP) levels are often required to avoid alveolar collapse, but the optimal PEEP in these patients is still unknown. Some authors suggest setting a PEEP (in cm H_2O) equals IAP value (in mmHg) or using esophageal pressure in the most challenging case of IAH and concomitant ARDS [100].

During recruitment maneuvers, higher opening pressures may be required while closely monitoring oxygenation and the hemodynamic response.

Adjunctive therapies to consider are neuromuscular blocking agents that can reduce IAP and improve oxygenation, negative fluid balance, ascites drainage, and laparostoma [101].

Prone positioning cannot be routinely recommended for IAH patients. However, it may reduce IAP and improve oxygenation in patients with IAH and ARDS if a free-hanging abdomen is assured and no IAP increase is documented [102].

Open Abdomen

Patients with an open abdomen (OA) after trauma and nontrauma EGS are usually subjected to prolonged mechanical ventilation, likely due to the need for repeated revision of the laparostoma. Although most patients with an OA have underlying conditions that mandate intubation and mechanical ventilation, the presence of OA does not require intubation per se. Several papers showed that by maintaining negative subdiaphragmatic pressures (a factor that prevents rapid loss of volume during expiration), respiratory musculature can compensate for the loss of the abdominal wall integrity [103].

There are no guidelines or weaning protocols to guide respiratory management, particularly the feasibility of extubating patients with an OA. Taveras et al. demonstrated the feasibility of early extubation in trauma, and EGS patients managed with an OA, possibly decreasing VAP rates with minimal risk of extubation failure [104].

However, patients with OA have a significant risk of developing ARDS early in their ICU course. A lung-protective approach is recommended, and extubation of such patients should be done cautiously.

Trauma

The incidence of ARDS in severely injured trauma patients is still significant, with figures approaching 10–30% and intubation rates ranging from 25 to 75% in the specific context of chest trauma [90]. Trauma-related ARDS is a relatively infrequent ARDS risk factor (only 5% of ARDS), and it is associated with lowered mortality rates compared to other causes of ARDS [105]. Nevertheless, the development of ARDS after severe trauma has been associated with significant increases in morbidity and mortality beyond baseline severity of illness [106].

Prevention of lung injury before the onset of ARDS should be considered a cornerstone in managing patients with chest trauma. Optimal pain control and early application of positive end-expiratory pressure (PEEP) can improve the outcome of trauma patients at risk of respiratory deterioration [107, 108].

Factors predisposing multiple trauma patients to respiratory failure are not fully understood. Several scoring systems have been developed to identify patients at risk for pulmonary complications, such as the Lung Organ Failure Score [109] or the Watkins predictive model [90]. While these scores seem to have limited value in the early identification of ARDS, the Thoracic Trauma Severity score [110] seems to be preferable since it predicts both early and delayed ARDS in almost half of the trauma patients with lung contusion [111].

ARDS after trauma may differ from other forms of ARDS. Two distinct patterns have been described: early-onset (days 1–2) ARDS that is associated with higher severity of chest trauma, more severe hypotension, and increased red blood cell transfusion requirement, and late-onset (days 4–5) ARDS where pneumonia, sepsis, and multiorgan dysfunction are the main culprits.

In the setting of trauma, ARDS may occur because of different mechanisms:

1. Direct thoracic injury;
2. Secondary mechanisms induced by trauma, such as fat embolism, transfusion-related lung injury, activation of local and systemic inflammatory mechanisms, or sepsis;
3. Mechanical ventilation: ventilator-induced lung injury (VILI) and ventilator-associated pneumonia (VAP) [112].

Many thoracic injuries can lead to respiratory impairment because they compromise gas exchange, chest-wall mechanic, or both [112]. Pulmonary contusions are well known to evolve towards respiratory failure, usually after a free interval of 24–48 h. A pulmonary contusion surface of 20% of the overall parenchyma was documented as a robust predictive threshold for ARDS (positive predictive values 80%) [113].

Despite current progress in ARDS management, only a limited body of high-quality evidence is available on the best strategy in the specific setting of chest trauma-related ARDS. Two ventilatory strategies are frequently adopted in this context: lung-protective ventilation (LPV) and open-lung ventilation (OLV).

LPV forms the basis of respiratory support, and most experts strongly recommend its use [112].

The ARDSNet protocol includes tidal volumes (VT) of 6–8 mL/kg of PBW, standardized PEEP/FiO$_2$ ratios based on oxygenation, and avoidance of elevation of plateau pressure beyond 30 cm H$_2$O [114].

Trauma is one of the recognized risk factors for ARDS. LPV strategies have never been studied explicitly in chest trauma with associated ARDS, especially in the flail chest. Trauma patients represent only 8–13% of the cohorts of the principal ARDS trials [114–119]. Although reducing mortality by using LPV strategies in patients at risk for ARDS has been well documented, LPV is not always applied in trauma patients, especially regarding VT [120]. Interestingly, Plurad et al. [121] demonstrated that the restrictive transfusion policies and ventilation strategies that potentially limit elevations in early peak inspiratory pressures are associated with the decreased incidence of late posttraumatic ARDS observed in the last decades.

OLV seems a reasonable strategy, and it has been more extensively studied in trauma. However, high PEEP may be associated with hemodynamic compromise and significant stress and strain to the heterogeneous lung parenchyma of the trauma patient [116]. Moreover, the OLV strategy is not applicable in the case of air leaks (tracheobronchial rupture, bronchopleural fistula).

In the delicate and heterogeneous trauma setting, it seems necessary to determine the optimal ventilation strategy according to lesional status and phase of treatment.

After the PROSEVA trial demonstrated a mortality benefit using prone positioning in ARDS [122], the 2017 ATS/ESICM/SCCM international consensus guidelines for ARDS management made a strong recommendation for prone positioning in severe ARDS [92].

Of note, exclusion criteria of the PROSEVA trial pertinent to the trauma population included ICP >30, unstable fractures of the spine, femur, or pelvis, burn >20% TSBA, facial trauma, and recent sternotomy or anterior chest tube presence with active air leak [122]. Nevertheless, there is increasing evidence that prone positioning can be used safely with similar oxygenation benefits in trauma and EGS patients [93, 99].

Alternative methods of mechanical ventilation have been studied in ARDS related to chest trauma, such as airway pressure release ventilation (APRV), high-frequency oscillatory ventilation (HFOV), high-frequency percussive ventilation (HFPV), high-frequency jet ventilation (HFJV), or independent lung ventilation.

APRV is a pressure-limited, time-cycled mode of ventilation where a CPAP is applied, with intermittent releases to allow for convective CO$_2$ removal. APRV allows unrestricted spontaneous breathing in any phase of the mechanical ventilation, and APVR showed significant benefit on oxygenation [123] in a cohort of trauma patients, but many issues remain unanswered. Andrews et al. [124] showed a reduction in mortality using early APRV. At the same time, Maung et al. [125] found that APRV increased the duration of mechanical ventilation when compared to conventional ventilation in trauma patients with respiratory failure.

HFOV, a mode characterized by the high-frequency application of minimal tidal volumes, may have some physiological benefit in cases of chest trauma. However, its use is not recommended due to the higher mortality rate observed with HFO in ARDS not related to trauma [117].

HFPV seems an acceptable temporary ventilation strategy in specific cases, such as refractory pulmonary contusions or broncho-pleural disruption.

HFJV may have a role only as a temporary and rescue strategy in the setting of traumatic tracheobronchial rupture during the initial management while waiting for emergent surgical repair.

Independent lung ventilation (ILV) is a complex strategy suitable in rare refractory cases of unilateral chest trauma. The asymmetry in lung pathology, resulting in different compliances between the two lungs, provides the rationale for ILV. ILV has been proposed to ventilate the diseased lung while avoiding hyperinflation in the normal lung, thus improving the ventilation/perfusion matching in each lung [126].

Despite the fear of the hemorrhagic risk, ECMO has to be considered a rescue strategy since it may improve survival [127]. Heparin-free ECMO is a safe and valid option in patients with a high risk of bleeding [128].

Traumatic brain injury (TBI) represents a challenging situation since the ventilatory management goals for lung and brain injury may conflict. Respiratory failure develops in up to one-third of patients suffering from a severe head injury, and it fulfills ARDS criteria in 8% of patients with head abbreviated injury score (AIS) of 4 or greater [129].

In isolated brain injury, a degree of vulnerability is still present in the lung tissue secondary to the proinflammatory state, and high tidal volumes [130] ventilation aggravates it.

High levels of PEEP can increase intrathoracic pressure with a detrimental effect on cerebral venous drainage and cerebral perfusion. However, in case of decreased lung compliance, the transmission of intrathoracic pressure to the cranium is reduced, with a minor effect on cerebral perfusion. Therefore, in the case of ARDS and TBI, PEEP can be safely applied, provided the volume status and mean arterial pressure are maintained.

There is a general lack of good quality clinical studies upon the best strategies to ventilate TBI patients. In 2020, a large consensus conference from the ESICM [131] failed to reach a consensus on several topics and came out with expert-determined recommendations. As a general rule, patients without an Intracranial Pressure Elevation should receive a protective lung strategy. In case TBI and acute lung injury are present together with increased intracranial pressure, the control of $PaCO_2$ takes the priority, even if higher tidal volumes, which can lead to pulmonary injury, are required.

> **Take-Home Message**
> - An Intensive Care Unit (ICU) is an organized system that provides specialized medical and nursing care for comprehensive management of patients having, or at risk of developing, acute, life-threatening organ dysfunction.
> - ICU model (open, transitional, or closed) defines who is in charge of the critically ill patient and, as a general rule, the higher the level of the ICU, the higher the share of intensive care trained physicians should be.
> - ICU level refers to the ability to provide specialized care to critically ill patients with increasing complexity of monitoring and treatment.
> - ICU provides a place for monitoring and care of patients with potentially severe physiologic instability, such as EGS patients.
> - There is limited high-quality evidence on the best strategy in the setting of respiratory failure occurring after EGS and trauma. The ventilation strategy should be adapted to lesional status and phase of treatment.

> **Dos and Don'ts**
> **Do**
> - Do admit to ICU only patients with potentially severe physiologic instability, such as EGS patients.
> - Do optimize resource and personnel especially in high volume admission flux.
>
> **Don't**
> - Do not overwhelm the HUB ICU; whenever possible use the step down.
> - Do not forget to organize the HUB-SPOKE step down protocols.

> **Multiple-Choice Questions**
> 1. One of the following characteristics is not in the definition of critical care medicine:
>   A. It is focused on the treatment of patients requiring mechanical ventilation; (Correct Answer)
>   B. The main focus of CCM is restoring normal, or close to normal, physiology;
>   C. It is a multidisciplinary and interprofessional specialty dedicated to the comprehensive management of patients having, or at risk of developing, acute, life-threatening organ dysfunction;

D. CCM is driven by a multidisciplinary and multispecialty approach to critically ill patients.
2. What is\are the main characteristics of a Severity of Illness Scoring System:
   A. Calibration ability;
   B. Discrimination ability;
   C. All the previous; (Correct Answer)
   D. None of them.

3. A level II ICU should transfer a patient who needs:
   A. Mechanical ventilation for a prolonged period;
   B. Continuous renal replacement therapy for acute renal failure;
   C. Invasive monitoring of Cardiac Output by a pulmonary artery catheter;
   D. Invasive monitoring of the Intracranial Pressure. (Correct Answer)

4. In the ICU multidisciplinary team can be present:
   A. Respiratory therapist;
   B. Advanced Care Providers;
   C. Clinical Pharmacist;
   D. All the above. (Correct Answer)

5. What is an "open model" ICU:
   A. It is an ICU where every physician with privileges, even without intensive care training, can admit to ICU, and those patients are under his direct care; (Correct Answer)
   B. It is an ICU where relatives can visit the patients whenever they want;
   C. It is an ICU where only intensivists have privileges to admit and discharge patients in ICU;
   D. It is an ICU where the patient is admitted under the care of a nonintensivist, but intensivist consultation is mandatory.

6. Which one of the following is the correct statement regarding monitoring of EGS patients?
   A. Heart rate, blood pressure, and urine output can always identify low CO states;
   B. Pulse oximetry and respiratory rate monitoring is not required in surgical patients;
   C. There is a delicate balance between hypovolemia and volume overload, which are both equally associated with complication; (Correct Answer)
   D. Focused echocardiography cannot be implemented in EGS setting.

7. Ventilator setting after EGS (choose the correct statement):
   A. Can be easily protocolized according to current high-level evidence in literature
   B. Is critical to minimize VILI in patients at risk of ARDS undergoing surgical procedures; (Correct Answer)
   C. Always follows the LPV strategy according to recent surveys
   D. Should never be managed according to the ARDSnet guidelines.

8. Postoperative strategies to decrease the risk of respiratory complications do not include:
   A. Head-up or sitting position and early mobilization
   B. Intensive physiotherapy and incentive spirometry
   C. Generous fluid administration; (Correct Answer)
   D. Adequate opioid-sparing analgesia.

9. EGS patients with intra-abdominal hypertension (choose the correct statement):
   A. Are not at risk of respiratory failure
   B. May require higher PEEP levels, even though optimal PEEP is still unknown; (Correct Answer)
   C. Should never undergo prone positioning
   D. Should not receive lung protective ventilation.

10. ARDS after trauma (choose the correct statement):
    A. May occur because of different mechanisms, only early (1–2 days) after trauma
    B. Is not related to the extent of pulmonary contusion
    C. May require prone positioning, which can be used safely; (Correct Answer)
    D. Cannot benefit from lung protective ventilation.
11. Respiratory failure in TBI patients (choose the correct statement):
    A. Is a rare complication in this setting
    B. Can be easily managed like other forms of respiratory failure
    C. Cannot benefit from PEEP
    D. Is a challenging a situation since the ventilatory management goals for lung and brain injury may conflict. (Correct Answer)

References

1. Marshall JC, Bosco L, Adhikari NK, Connolly B, Diaz JV, Dorman T, Fowler RA, Meyfroidt G, Nakagawa S, Pelosi P, Vincent J-L, Vollman K, Zimmerman J. What is an intensive care unit? A report of the task force of the World Federation of Societies of Intensive and Critical Care Medicine. J Crit Care. 2017;37:270–6.
2. Guidelines for intensive care unit admission, discharge, and triage. Task force of the American College of Critical Care Medicine, Society of Critical Care Medicine. Crit Care Med. 1999;27:633–638.
3. Valentin A, Ferdinande P, ESICM Working Group on Quality Improvement. Recommendations on basic requirements for intensive care units: structural and organizational aspects. Intensive Care Med. 2011;37:1575–87.
4. CICM—professional documents. https://www.cicm.org.au/Resources/Professional-Documents#Policies. Accessed 16 Jan 2021.
5. Ristagno G, Weil MH. History of critical care medicine: the past, the present and the future. In: Gullo A, Lumb PD, Besso J, Williams GF, eds. Intensive and critical care medicine: WFSICCM World Federation of Societies of Intensive and Critical Care Medicine. Milano: Springer Milan, 2009:3–17. https://doi.org/10.1007/978-88-470-1436-7_1. Accessed 22 Sept 2021.
6. Brilli RJ, Spevetz A, Branson RD, Campbell GM, Cohen H, Dasta JF, Harvey MA, Kelley MA, Kelly KM, Rudis MI, St Andre AC, Stone JR, Teres D, Weled BJ, American College of Critical Care Medicine Task Force on Models of Critical Care Delivery. The American College of Critical Care Medicine Guidelines for the Definition of an Intensivist and the Practice of Critical Care Medicine. Critical care delivery in the intensive care unit: defining clinical roles and the best practice model. Crit Care Med. 2001;29:2007–19.
7. Guidelines for the definition of an intensivist and the practice of critical care medicine. Guidelines Committee; Society of Critical Care Medicine. Crit Care Med. 1992;20:540–542.
8. Guidelines for the provision of intensive care services V2 | The Faculty of Intensive Care Medicine. https://www.ficm.ac.uk/standards-research-revalidation/guidelines-provision-intensive-care-services-v2. Accessed 16 Jan 2021.
9. Ghaffar S, Pearse RM, Gillies MA. ICU admission after surgery: who benefits? Curr Opin Crit Care. 2017;23:424–9.
10. Rohrig SAH, Lance MD, Faisal Malmstrom M. Surgical intensive care—current and future challenges? Qatar Med J. 2019;2019:3.
11. Lyu HG, Najjar P, Havens JM. Past, present, and future of emergency general surgery in the USA. Acute Med Surg. 2018;5:119–22.
12. Weissman C, Klein N. The importance of differentiating between elective and emergency postoperative critical care patients. J Crit Care. 2008;23:308–16.
13. Giannoudi M, Harwood P. Damage control resuscitation: lessons learned. Eur J Trauma Emerg Surg. 2016;42:273–82.
14. Ozdemir BA, Sinha S, Karthikesalingam A, Poloniecki JD, Pearse RM, Grocott MPW, Thompson MM, Holt PJE. Mortality of emergency general surgical patients and associations with hospital structures and processes. Br J Anaesth. 2016;116:54–62.
15. Pearse RM, Moreno RP, Bauer P, Pelosi P, Metnitz P, Spies C, Vallet B, Vincent J-L, Hoeft A, Rhodes A, European Surgical Outcomes Study (EuSOS) group for the Trials groups of the European Society of Intensive Care Medicine and the European Society of Anaesthesiology. Mortality after surgery in Europe: a 7 day cohort study. Lancet. 2012;380:1059–65.
16. Havens JM, Peetz AB, Do WS, Cooper Z, Kelly E, Askari R, Reznor G, Salim A. The excess morbidity and mortality of emergency general surgery. J Trauma Acute Care Surg. 2015;78:306–11.
17. Kassin MT, Owen RM, Perez SD, Leeds I, Cox JC, Schnier K, Sadiraj V, Sweeney JF. Risk factors for 30-day hospital readmission among general surgery patients. J Am Coll Surg. 2012;215:322–30.
18. Cihoric M, Toft Tengberg L, Bay-Nielsen M, Bang Foss N. Prediction of outcome after emergency high-risk intra-abdominal surgery using the surgical Apgar score. Anesth Analg. 2016;123:1516–21.

19. Parmar KL, Law J, Carter B, Hewitt J, Boyle JM, Casey P, Maitra I, Farrell IS, Pearce L, Moug SJ, ELF Study Group. Frailty in older patients undergoing emergency laparotomy: results from the UK observational emergency laparotomy and frailty (ELF) study. Ann Surg. 2021;273:709–18.
20. Hajibandeh S, Hajibandeh S, Antoniou GA, Antoniou SA. Meta-analysis of mortality risk in octogenarians undergoing emergency general surgery operations. Surgery. 2021;169:1407–16.
21. Green G, Shaikh I, Fernandes R, Wegstapel H. Emergency laparotomy in octogenarians: a 5-year study of morbidity and mortality. World J Gastrointest Surg. 2013;5:216–21.
22. McCunn M, Dutton RP, Dagal A, Varon AJ, Kaslow O, Kucik CJ, Hagberg CA, McIsaac JH, Pittet J-F, Dunbar PJ, Grissom T, Vavilala MS. Trauma, critical care, and emergency care anesthesiology: a new paradigm for the "acute care" anesthesiologist? Anesth Analg. 2015;121:1668–73.
23. Privette AR, Evans AE, Moyer JC, Nelson MF, Knudson MM, Mackersie RC, Callcut RA, Cohen MJ. Beyond emergency surgery: redefining acute care surgery. J Surg Res. 2015;196:166–71.
24. Lissauer ME, Galvagno SM, Rock P, Narayan M, Shah P, Spencer H, Hong C, Diaz JJ. Increased ICU resource needs for an academic emergency general surgery service*. Crit Care Med. 2014;42:910–7.
25. Michetti CP, Fakhry SM, Brasel K, Martin ND, Teicher EJ, Newcomb A, TRIPP Study Group. Trauma ICU prevalence project: the diversity of surgical critical care. Trauma Surg Acute Care Open. 2019;4:e000288.
26. Butcher N, Balogh ZJ. AIS>2 in at least two body regions: a potential new anatomical definition of polytrauma. Injury. 2012;43:196–9.
27. Shere-Wolfe RF, Galvagno SM, Grissom TE. Critical care considerations in the management of the trauma patient following initial resuscitation. Scand J Trauma Resusc Emerg Med. 2012;20:68.
28. Harris T, Davenport R, Mak M, Brohi K. The evolving science of trauma resuscitation. Emerg Med Clin North Am. 2018;36:85–106.
29. Kirkpatrick AW, Ball CG, D'Amours SK, Zygun D. Acute resuscitation of the unstable adult trauma patient: bedside diagnosis and therapy. Can J Surg. 2008;51:57–69.
30. Lemeshow S, Le Gall JR. Modeling the severity of illness of ICU patients. A systems update. JAMA. 1994;272:1049–55.
31. Alba AC, Agoritsas T, Walsh M, Hanna S, Iorio A, Devereaux PJ, McGinn T, Guyatt G. Discrimination and calibration of clinical prediction models: users' guides to the medical literature. JAMA. 2017;318:1377–84.
32. McCracken DJ, Lovasik BP, McCracken CE, Frerich JM, McDougal ME, Ratcliff JJ, Barrow DL, Pradilla G. The intracerebral hemorrhage score: a self-fulfilling prophecy? Neurosurgery. 2019;84:741–8.
33. Cullen DJ, Civetta JM, Briggs BA, Ferrara LC. Therapeutic intervention scoring system: a method for quantitative comparison of patient care. Crit Care Med. 1974;2:57–60. http://pubmed.ncbi.nlm.nih.gov/4832281/. Accessed 1 Sept 2021.
34. Miranda DR, de Rijk A, Schaufeli W. Simplified Therapeutic Intervention Scoring System: the TISS-28 items—results from a multicenter study. Crit Care Med. 1996;24:64–73.
35. Reis Miranda D, Moreno R, Iapichino G. Nine equivalents of nursing manpower use score (NEMS). Intensive Care Med. 1997;23:760–5.
36. Miranda DR, Langrehr D. National and Regional Organisation. In: Miranda DR, Williams A, Loirat PH, editors. Management of intensive care: guidelines for better use of resources. Developments in critical care medicine and anesthesiology. Dordrecht: Springer Netherlands; 1990. p. 83–102. https://doi.org/10.1007/978-94-009-2043-9_4. Accessed 1 Sept 2021.
37. Iapichino G, Radrizzani D, Bertolini G, Ferla L, Pasetti G, Pezzi A, Porta F, Miranda DR. Daily classification of the level of care. A method to describe clinical course of illness, use of resources and quality of intensive care assistance. Intensive Care Med. 2001;27:131–6.
38. Pronovost PJ, Angus DC, Dorman T, Robinson KA, Dremsizov TT, Young TL. Physician staffing patterns and clinical outcomes in critically ill patients: a systematic review. JAMA. 2002;288:2151–62.
39. Groeger JS, Guntupalli KK, Strosberg M, Halpern N, Raphaely RC, Cerra F, Kaye W. Descriptive analysis of critical care units in the United States: patient characteristics and intensive care unit utilization. Crit Care Med. 1993;21:279–91.
40. Groeger JS, Strosberg MA, Halpern NA, Raphaely RC, Kaye WE, Guntupalli KK, Bertram DL, Greenbaum DM, Clemmer TP, Gallagher TJ. Descriptive analysis of critical care units in the United States. Crit Care Med. 1992;20:846–63.
41. Wilcox ME, Chong CAKY, Niven DJ, Rubenfeld GD, Rowan KM, Wunsch H, Fan E. Do intensivist staffing patterns influence hospital mortality following ICU admission? A systematic review and meta-analyses. Crit Care Med. 2013;41:2253–74.
42. Hanson CW, Deutschman CS, Anderson HL, Reilly PM, Behringer EC, Schwab CW, Price J. Effects of an organized critical care service on outcomes and resource utilization: a cohort study. Crit Care Med. 1999;27:270–4.
43. Weled BJ, Adzhigirey LA, Hodgman TM, Brilli RJ, Spevetz A, Kline AM, Montgomery VL, Puri N, Tisherman SA, Vespa PM, Pronovost PJ, Rainey TG, Patterson AJ, Wheeler DS, Task Force on Models for Critical Care. Critical care delivery: the importance of process of care and ICU structure to improved outcomes: an update from the American College of Critical Care Medicine Task Force on Models of Critical Care. Crit Care Med. 2015;43:1520–5.

44. Harris GH, Baldisseri MR, Reynolds BR, Orsino AS, Sackrowitz R, Bishop JM. Design for implementation of a system-level ICU pandemic surge staffing plan. Crit Care Explor. 2020;2:e0136.
45. Zangrillo A, Gattinoni L. Learning from mistakes during the pandemic: the Lombardy lesson. Intensive Care Med. 2020;46(8):1622–3.
46. Guillon A, Laurent E, Godillon L, Kimmoun A, Grammatico-Guillon L. Inter-regional transfers for pandemic surges were associated with reduced mortality rates. Intensive Care Med. 2021;47(7):798–800.
47. CoBaTrICE Collaboration. The educational environment for training in intensive care medicine: structures, processes, outcomes and challenges in the European region. Intensive Care Med. 2009;35:1575–83.
48. Gershengorn HB, Harrison DA, Garland A, Wilcox ME, Rowan KM, Wunsch H. Association of intensive care unit patient-to-intensivist ratios with hospital mortality. JAMA Intern Med. 2017;177:388–96.
49. McKinley S, Elliott D. Twenty-five years of critical care nursing scholarship in Australia. Aust Crit Care. 2013;26:7–11.
50. Safar P, Dekornfeld TJ, Pearson JW, Redding JS. The intensive care unit. A three year experience at Baltimore city hospitals. Anaesthesia. 1961;16:275–84.
51. Kerlin MP, Costa DK, Kahn JM. The Society of Critical Care Medicine at 50 years: ICU organization and management. Crit Care Med. 2021;49:391–405.
52. Xu Y, Xu Z, Zhang J. The nursing education system in the People's Republic of China: evolution, structure and reform. Int Nurs Rev. 2000;47:207–17.
53. Endacott R, Jones C, Bloomer MJ, Boulanger C, Ben Nun M, Lliopoulou KK, Egerod I, Blot S. The state of critical care nursing education in Europe: an international survey. Intensive Care Med. 2015;41:2237–40.
54. Guilhermino MC, Inder KJ, Sundin D. Education on invasive mechanical ventilation involving intensive care nurses: a systematic review. Nurs Crit Care. 2018;23:245–55.
55. Perioperative and intensive care management of the surgical patient—ClinicalKey. https://www-clinicalkey-com.ospbg.clas.cineca.it/#!/content/book/3-s2.0-B9780702072475000050?indexOverride=GLOBAL. Accessed 7 Jan 2021.
56. Donovan AL, Aldrich JM, Gross AK, Barchas DM, Thornton KC, Schell-Chaple HM, Gropper MA, Lipshutz AKM, University of California, San Francisco Critical Care Innovations Group. Interprofessional care and teamwork in the ICU. Crit Care Med. 2018;46:980–90.
57. Reeves S, Lewin S, Espin S, Zwarenstein M. Interprofessional teamwork for health and social care. Hoboken: Wiley; 2011.
58. Scherzer R, Dennis MP, Swan BA, Kavuru MS, Oxman DA. A comparison of usage and outcomes between nurse practitioner and resident-staffed medical ICUs. Crit Care Med. 2017;45:e132–7.
59. Kawar E, DiGiovine B. MICU care delivered by PAs versus residents: do PAs measure up? JAAPA. 2011;24:36–41.
60. Rudis MI, Brandl KM. Position paper on critical care pharmacy services. Society of Critical Care Medicine and American College of Clinical Pharmacy Task Force on Critical Care Pharmacy Services. Crit Care Med. 2000;28:3746–50.
61. Erstad BL, Haas CE, O'Keeffe T, Hokula CA, Parrinello K, Theodorou AA. Interdisciplinary patient care in the intensive care unit: focus on the pharmacist. Pharmacotherapy. 2011;31:128–37.
62. Baker A. Crossing the quality chasm: a new health system for the 21st century. BMJ. 2001;323:1192.
63. Papali A, Adhikari NKJ, Diaz JV, Dondorp AM, Dünser MW, Jacob ST, Phua J, Romain M, Schultz MJ. Infrastructure and organization of adult intensive care units in resource-limited settings. In: Dondorp AM, Dünser MW, Schultz MJ, editors. Sepsis management in resource-limited settings. Cham: Springer; 2019. http://www.ncbi.nlm.nih.gov/books/NBK553820/. Accessed 13 July 2021.
64. Batalden PB, Davidoff F. What is "quality improvement" and how can it transform healthcare? Qual Saf Health Care. 2007;16:2–3.
65. Modrykamien AM. The ICU follow-up clinic: a new paradigm for intensivists. Respir Care. 2012;57:764–72.
66. Kipnis E, Ramsingh D, Bhargava M, Dincer E, Cannesson M, Broccard A, Vallet B, Bendjelid K, Thibault R. Monitoring in the intensive care. Crit Care Res Pract. 2012;2012:473507.
67. Martin ND, Codner P, Greene W, Brasel K, Michetti C, AAST Critical Care Committee. Contemporary hemodynamic monitoring, fluid responsiveness, volume optimization, and endpoints of resuscitation: an AAST Critical Care Committee Clinical Consensus. Trauma Surg Acute Care Open. 2020;5:e000411.
68. Celoria G, Steingrub JS, Vickers-Lahti M, Teres D, Stein KL, Fink M, Friedmann P. Clinical assessment of hemodynamic values in two surgical intensive care units. Effects on therapy. Arch Surg. 1990;125:1036–9.
69. Convertino VA, Ryan KL, Rickards CA, Salinas J, McManus JG, Cooke WH, Holcomb JB. Physiological and medical monitoring for en route care of combat casualties. J Trauma. 2008;64:S342–53.
70. Abou-Khalil B, Scalea TM, Trooskin SZ, Henry SM, Hitchcock R. Hemodynamic responses to shock in young trauma patients: need for invasive monitoring. Crit Care Med. 1994;22:633–9.
71. Nagre AS. Focus-assessed transthoracic echocardiography: implications in perioperative and intensive care. Ann Card Anaesth. 2019;22:302–8.
72. Cowie BS. Focused transthoracic echocardiography in the perioperative period. Anaesth Intensive Care. 2010;38:823–36.

73. Britt LD, Trunkey DD, Feliciano DV. Acute care surgery. Principles and practice. In: Acute care surgery. Principles and practice. Vol. The perioperative management of the acute care surgical patient. Springer; 2007. p. 67–83.
74. Lamberti JP. Respiratory monitoring in general care units. Respir Care. 2020;65:870–81.
75. Kochanek PM, Carney N, Adelson PD, Ashwal S, Bell MJ, Bratton S, Carson S, Chesnut RM, Ghajar J, Goldstein B, Grant GA, Kissoon N, Peterson K, Selden NR, Tasker RC, Tong KA, Vavilala MS, Wainwright MS, Warden CR, American Academy of Pediatrics-Section on Neurological Surgery, American Association of Neurological Surgeons/Congress of Neurological Surgeons, Child Neurology Society, European Society of Pediatric and Neonatal Intensive Care, Neurocritical Care Society, Pediatric Neurocritical Care Research Group, Society of Critical Care Medicine, Paediatric Intensive Care Society UK, Society for Neuroscience in Anesthesiology and Critical Care, World Federation of Pediatric Intensive and Critical Care Societies. Guidelines for the acute medical management of severe traumatic brain injury in infants, children, and adolescents—second edition. Pediatr Crit Care Med. 2012;13 Suppl 1:S1–S82.
76. Carney N, Totten AM, O'Reilly C, Ullman JS, Hawryluk GWJ, Bell MJ, Bratton SL, Chesnut R, Harris OA, Kissoon N, Rubiano AM, Shutter L, Tasker RC, Vavilala MS, Wilberger J, Wright DW, Ghajar J. Guidelines for the management of severe traumatic brain injury, fourth edition. Neurosurgery. 2017;80:6–15.
77. Hawryluk GWJ, Aguilera S, Buki A, Bulger E, Citerio G, Cooper DJ, Arrastia RD, Diringer M, Figaji A, Gao G, Geocadin R, Ghajar J, Harris O, Hoffer A, Hutchinson P, Joseph M, Kitagawa R, Manley G, Mayer S, Menon DK, Meyfroidt G, Michael DB, Oddo M, Okonkwo D, Patel M, Robertson C, Rosenfeld JV, Rubiano AM, Sahuquillo J, Servadei F, et al. A management algorithm for patients with intracranial pressure monitoring: the Seattle International Severe Traumatic Brain Injury Consensus Conference (SIBICC). Intensive Care Med. 2019;45:1783–94. https://link.springer.com/epdf/10.1007/s00134-019-05805-9. Accessed 1 Sept 2020.
78. Chesnut RM, Temkin N, Videtta W, Petroni G, Lujan S, Pridgeon J, Dikmen S, Chaddock K, Barber J, Machamer J, Guadagnoli N, Hendrickson P, Aguilera S, Alanis V, Bello Quezada ME, Bautista Coronel E, Bustamante LA, Cacciatori AC, Carricondo CJ, Carvajal F, Davila R, Dominguez M, Figueroa Melgarejo JA, Fillipi MM, Godoy DA, Gomez DC, Lacerda Gallardo AJ, Guerra Garcia JA, la Fuente Zerain G, Lavadenz Cuientas LA, et al. Consensus-Based Management Protocol (CREVICE Protocol) for the treatment of severe traumatic brain injury based on imaging and clinical examination for use when intracranial pressure monitoring is not employed. J Neurotrauma. 2020;37:1291–9.
79. Chesnut R, Aguilera S, Buki A, Bulger E, Citerio G, Cooper DJ, Arrastia RD, Diringer M, Figaji A, Gao G, Geocadin R, Ghajar J, Harris O, Hoffer A, Hutchinson P, Joseph M, Kitagawa R, Manley G, Mayer S, Menon DK, Meyfroidt G, Michael DB, Oddo M, Okonkwo D, Patel M, Robertson C, Rosenfeld JV, Rubiano AM, Sahuquillo J, Servadei F, et al. A management algorithm for adult patients with both brain oxygen and intracranial pressure monitoring: the Seattle International Severe Traumatic Brain Injury Consensus Conference (SIBICC). Intensive Care Med. 2020;46:919–29.
80. Tengberg LT, Cihoric M, Foss NB, Bay-Nielsen M, Gögenur I, Henriksen R, Jensen TK, Tolstrup M-B, Nielsen LBJ. Complications after emergency laparotomy beyond the immediate postoperative period—a retrospective, observational cohort study of 1139 patients. Anaesthesia. 2017;72:309–16.
81. McCoy CC, Englum BR, Keenan JE, Vaslef SN, Shapiro ML, Scarborough JE. Impact of specific postoperative complications on the outcomes of emergency general surgery patients. J Trauma Acute Care Surg. 2015;78:912–8; discussion 918–919.
82. Fernandez-Bustamante A, Frendl G, Sprung J, Kor DJ, Subramaniam B, Martinez Ruiz R, Lee J-W, Henderson WG, Moss A, Mehdiratta N, Colwell MM, Bartels K, Kolodzie K, Giquel J, Vidal Melo MF. Postoperative pulmonary complications, early mortality, and hospital stay following non-cardiothoracic surgery: a multicenter study by the Perioperative Research Network Investigators. JAMA Surg. 2017;152:157–66.
83. Canet J, Gallart L, Gomar C, Paluzie G, Vallès J, Castillo J, Sabaté S, Mazo V, Briones Z, Sanchis J, ARISCAT Group. Prediction of postoperative pulmonary complications in a population-based surgical cohort. Anesthesiology. 2010;113:1338–50.
84. Miskovic A, Lumb AB. Postoperative pulmonary complications. Br J Anaesth. 2017;118:317–34.
85. Watson X, Chereshneva M, Odor PM, Chis Ster I, Pan-London Perioperative Audit and Research Network (PLAN), Cecconi M. Adoption of lung protective ventilation IN patients undergoing emergency laparotomy: the ALPINE study. A prospective multicentre observational study. Br J Anaesth 2018;121:909–917.
86. Serejo LGG, da Silva-Júnior FP, Bastos JPC, de Bruin GS, Mota RMS, de Bruin PFC. Risk factors for pulmonary complications after emergency abdominal surgery. Respir Med. 2007;101:808–13.
87. Rubenfeld GD, Caldwell E, Peabody E, Weaver J, Martin DP, Neff M, Stern EJ, Hudson LD. Incidence and outcomes of acute lung injury. N Engl J Med. 2005;353:1685–93.
88. Treggiari MM, Hudson LD, Martin DP, Weiss NS, Caldwell E, Rubenfeld G. Effect of acute lung injury and acute respiratory distress syndrome on outcome

89. Holland MC, Mackersie RC, Morabito D, Campbell AR, Kivett VA, Patel R, Erickson VR, Pittet J-F. The development of acute lung injury is associated with worse neurologic outcome in patients with severe traumatic brain injury. J Trauma. 2003;55:106–11.
90. Watkins TR, Nathens AB, Cooke CR, Psaty BM, Maier RV, Cuschieri J, Rubenfeld GD. Acute respiratory distress syndrome after trauma: development and validation of a predictive model. Crit Care Med. 2012;40:2295–303.
91. Serpa Neto A, Hemmes SNT, Barbas CSV, Beiderlinden M, Biehl M, Binnekade JM, Canet J, Fernandez-Bustamante A, Futier E, Gajic O, Hedenstierna G, Hollmann MW, Jaber S, Kozian A, Licker M, Lin W-Q, Maslow AD, Memtsoudis SG, Reis Miranda D, Moine P, Ng T, Paparella D, Putensen C, Ranieri M, Scavonetto F, Schilling T, Schmid W, Selmo G, Severgnini P, Sprung J, et al. Protective versus conventional ventilation for surgery: a systematic review and individual patient data meta-analysis. Anesthesiology. 2015;123:66–78.
92. Fan E, Del Sorbo L, Goligher EC, Hodgson CL, Munshi L, Walkey AJ, Adhikari NKJ, Amato MBP, Branson R, Brower RG, Ferguson ND, Gajic O, Gattinoni L, Hess D, Mancebo J, Meade MO, McAuley DF, Pesenti A, Ranieri VM, Rubenfeld GD, Rubin E, Seckel M, Slutsky AS, Talmor D, Thompson BT, Wunsch H, Uleryk E, Brozek J, Brochard LJ, American Thoracic Society, European Society of Intensive Care Medicine, and Society of Critical Care Medicine. An official American Thoracic Society/European Society of Intensive Care Medicine/Society of Critical Care Medicine clinical practice guideline: mechanical ventilation in adult patients with acute respiratory distress syndrome. Am J Respir Crit Care Med. 2017;195:1253–63.
93. Gaudry S, Tuffet S, Lukaszewicz A-C, Laplace C, Zucman N, Pocard M, Costaglioli B, Msika S, Duranteau J, Payen D, Dreyfuss D, Hajage D, Ricard J-D. Prone positioning in acute respiratory distress syndrome after abdominal surgery: a multicenter retrospective study: SAPRONADONF (Study of Ards and PRONe position After abDOmiNal surgery in France). Ann Intensive Care. 2017;7:21.
94. Ireland CJ, Chapman TM, Mathew SF, Herbison GP, Zacharias M. Continuous positive airway pressure (CPAP) during the postoperative period for prevention of postoperative morbidity and mortality following major abdominal surgery. Cochrane Database Syst Rev. 2014;2014:CD008930.
95. Smit M, Koopman B, Dieperink W, Hulscher JBF, Hofker HS, van Meurs M, Zijlstra JG. Intra-abdominal hypertension and abdominal compartment syndrome in patients admitted to the ICU. Ann Intensive Care. 2020;10:130.
96. Ranieri VM, Brienza N, Santostasi S, Puntillo F, Mascia L, Vitale N, Giuliani R, Memeo V, Bruno F, Fiore T, Brienza A, Slutsky AS. Impairment of lung and chest wall mechanics in patients with acute respiratory distress syndrome: role of abdominal distension. Am J Respir Crit Care Med. 1997;156:1082–91.
97. Regli A, Pelosi P, Malbrain MLNG. Ventilation in patients with intra-abdominal hypertension: what every critical care physician needs to know. Ann Intensive Care. 2019;9:52.
98. De Keulenaer BL, De Waele JJ, Powell B, Malbrain MLNG. What is normal intra-abdominal pressure and how is it affected by positioning, body mass and positive end-expiratory pressure? Intensive Care Med. 2009;35:969–76.
99. Voggenreiter G, Aufmkolk M, Stiletto RJ, Baacke MG, Waydhas C, Ose C, Bock E, Gotzen L, Obertacke U, Nast-Kolb D. Prone positioning improves oxygenation in post-traumatic lung injury—a prospective randomized trial. J Trauma. 2005;59:333–41; discussion 341–343.
100. Tonetti T, Cavalli I, Ranieri VM, Mascia L. Respiratory consequences of intra-abdominal hypertension. Minerva Anestesiol. 2020;86:877–83.
101. De Keulenaer B, Regli A, De Laet I, Roberts D, Malbrain MLNG. What's new in medical management strategies for raised intra-abdominal pressure: evacuating intra-abdominal contents, improving abdominal wall compliance, pharmacotherapy, and continuous negative extra-abdominal pressure. Anaesthesiol Intensive Ther. 2015;47:54–62.
102. Kirkpatrick AW, Pelosi P, De Waele JJ, Malbrain ML, Ball CG, Meade MO, Stelfox HT, Laupland KB. Clinical review: intra-abdominal hypertension: does it influence the physiology of prone ventilation? Crit Care. 2010;14:232.
103. Mondal P, Abu-Hasan M, Saha A, Pitts T, Rose M, Bolser DC, Davenport PW. Effect of laparotomy on respiratory muscle activation pattern. Physiol Rep. 2016;4:e12668.
104. Taveras LR, Imran JB, Cunningham HB, Madni TD, Taarea R, Tompeck A, Clark AT, Provenzale N, Adeyemi FM, Minshall CT, Eastman AL, Cripps MW. Trauma and emergency general surgery patients should be extubated with an open abdomen. J Trauma Acute Care Surg. 2018;85:1043–7.
105. Bellani G, Laffey JG, Pham T, Fan E, Brochard L, Esteban A, Gattinoni L, van Haren F, Larsson A, McAuley DF, Ranieri M, Rubenfeld G, Thompson BT, Wrigge H, Slutsky AS, Pesenti A, LUNG SAFE Investigators, ESICM Trials Group. Epidemiology, patterns of care, and mortality for patients with acute respiratory distress syndrome in intensive care units in 50 countries. JAMA. 2016;315:788–800.
106. Shah CV, Localio AR, Lanken PN, Kahn JM, Bellamy S, Gallop R, Finkel B, Gracias VH, Fuchs BD, Christie JD. The impact of development of acute lung injury on hospital mortality in critically ill trauma patients. Crit Care Med. 2008;36:2309–15.
107. Chiumello D, Coppola S, Froio S, Gregoretti C, Consonni D. Noninvasive ventilation in chest trauma:

108. Bouzat P, Raux M, David JS, Tazarourte K, Galinski M, Desmettre T, Garrigue D, Ducros L, Michelet P, Expert's Group, Freysz M, Savary D, Rayeh-Pelardy F, Laplace C, Duponq R, Monnin Bares V, D'Journo XB, Boddaert G, Boutonnet M, Pierre S, Léone M, Honnart D, Biais M, Vardon F. Chest trauma: first 48 hours management. Anaesth Crit Care Pain Med. 2017;36:135–45.
109. Wutzler S, Wafaisade A, Maegele M, Laurer H, Geiger EV, Walcher F, Barker J, Lefering R, Marzi I, Trauma Registry of DGU. Lung Organ Failure Score (LOFS): probability of severe pulmonary organ failure after multiple injuries including chest trauma. Injury. 2012;43:1507–12.
110. Pape HC, Remmers D, Rice J, Ebisch M, Krettek C, Tscherne H. Appraisal of early evaluation of blunt chest trauma: development of a standardized scoring system for initial clinical decision making. J Trauma. 2000;49:496–504.
111. Daurat A, Millet I, Roustan J-P, Maury C, Taourel P, Jaber S, Capdevila X, Charbit J. Thoracic Trauma Severity score on admission allows to determine the risk of delayed ARDS in trauma patients with pulmonary contusion. Injury. 2016;47:147–53.
112. Ramin S, Charbit J, Jaber S, Capdevila X. Acute respiratory distress syndrome after chest trauma: epidemiology, specific physiopathology and ventilation strategies. Anaesth Crit Care Pain Med. 2019;38:265–76.
113. Miller PR, Croce MA, Bee TK, Qaisi WG, Smith CP, Collins GL, Fabian TC. ARDS after pulmonary contusion: accurate measurement of contusion volume identifies high-risk patients. J Trauma. 2001;51:223–8; discussion 229–230.
114. Acute Respiratory Distress Syndrome Network, Brower RG, Matthay MA, Morris A, Schoenfeld D, Thompson BT, Wheeler A. Ventilation with lower tidal volumes as compared with traditional tidal volumes for acute lung injury and the acute respiratory distress syndrome. N Engl J Med. 2000;342:1301–8.
115. Mercat A, Richard J-CM, Vielle B, Jaber S, Osman D, Diehl J-L, Lefrant J-Y, Prat G, Richecoeur J, Nieszkowska A, Gervais C, Baudot J, Bouadma L, Brochard L, Expiratory Pressure (Express) Study Group. Positive end-expiratory pressure setting in adults with acute lung injury and acute respiratory distress syndrome: a randomized controlled trial. JAMA. 2008;299:646–55.
116. Meade MO, Cook DJ, Guyatt GH, Slutsky AS, Arabi YM, Cooper DJ, Davies AR, Hand LE, Zhou Q, Thabane L, Austin P, Lapinsky S, Baxter A, Russell J, Skrobik Y, Ronco JJ, Stewart TE, Lung Open Ventilation Study Investigators. Ventilation strategy using low tidal volumes, recruitment maneuvers, and high positive end-expiratory pressure for acute lung injury and acute respiratory distress syndrome: a randomized controlled trial. JAMA. 2008;299:637–45.
117. Ferguson ND, Cook DJ, Guyatt GH, Mehta S, Hand L, Austin P, Zhou Q, Matte A, Walter SD, Lamontagne F, Granton JT, Arabi YM, Arroliga AC, Stewart TE, Slutsky AS, Meade MO, OSCILLATE Trial Investigators, Canadian Critical Care Trials Group. High-frequency oscillation in early acute respiratory distress syndrome. N Engl J Med. 2013;368:795–805.
118. Papazian L, Forel J-M, Gacouin A, Penot-Ragon C, Perrin G, Loundou A, Jaber S, Arnal J-M, Perez D, Seghboyan J-M, Constantin J-M, Courant P, Lefrant J-Y, Guérin C, Prat G, Morange S, Roch A, ACURASYS Study Investigators. Neuromuscular blockers in early acute respiratory distress syndrome. N Engl J Med. 2010;363:1107–16.
119. Brower RG, Lanken PN, MacIntyre N, Matthay MA, Morris A, Ancukiewicz M, Schoenfeld D, Thompson BT, National Heart, Lung, and Blood Institute ARDS Clinical Trials Network. Higher versus lower positive end-expiratory pressures in patients with the acute respiratory distress syndrome. N Engl J Med. 2004;351:327–36.
120. Zochios V, Chandan JS, Dunne É, Sherwin J, Torlinski T. Adherence to least injurious tidal volume ventilation in thoracic trauma: a tertiary trauma centre retrospective cohort analysis. J Intensive Care Soc. 2019;20:NP10–3.
121. Plurad D, Martin M, Green D, Salim A, Inaba K, Belzberg H, Demetriades D, Rhee P. The decreasing incidence of late posttraumatic acute respiratory distress syndrome: the potential role of lung protective ventilation and conservative transfusion practice. J Trauma. 2007;63:1–7; discussion 8.
122. Guérin C, Reignier J, Richard J-C, Beuret P, Gacouin A, Boulain T, Mercier E, Badet M, Mercat A, Baudin O, Clavel M, Chatellier D, Jaber S, Rosselli S, Mancebo J, Sirodot M, Hilbert G, Bengler C, Richecoeur J, Gainnier M, Bayle F, Bourdin G, Leray V, Girard R, Baboi L, Ayzac L, PROSEVA Study Group. Prone positioning in severe acute respiratory distress syndrome. N Engl J Med. 2013;368:2159–68. https://doi.org/10.1056/NEJMoa1214103. Epub 2013 May 20. PMID: 23688302.
123. Dart BW, Maxwell RA, Richart CM, Brooks DK, Ciraulo DL, Barker DE, Burns RP. Preliminary experience with airway pressure release ventilation in a trauma/surgical intensive care unit. J Trauma. 2005;59:71–6.
124. Andrews PL, Shiber JR, Jaruga-Killeen E, Roy S, Sadowitz B, O'Toole RV, Gatto LA, Nieman GF, Scalea T, Habashi NM. Early application of airway pressure release ventilation may reduce mortality in high-risk trauma patients: a systematic review of observational trauma ARDS literature. J Trauma Acute Care Surg. 2013;75:635–41.
125. Maung AA, Schuster KM, Kaplan LJ, Ditillo MF, Piper GL, Maerz LL, Lui FY, Johnson DC, Davis KA. Compared to conventional ventilation, airway pressure release ventilation may increase ventilator

days in trauma patients. J Trauma Acute Care Surg. 2012;73:507–10.
126. Cinnella G, Dambrosio M, Brienza N, Giuliani R, Bruno F, Fiore T, Brienza A. Independent lung ventilation in patients with unilateral pulmonary contusion. Monitoring with compliance and EtCO(2). Intensive Care Med. 2001;27:1860–7.
127. Guirand DM, Okoye OT, Schmidt BS, Mansfield NJ, Aden JK, Martin RS, Cestero RF, Hines MH, Pranikoff T, Inaba K, Cannon JW. Venovenous extracorporeal life support improves survival in adult trauma patients with acute hypoxemic respiratory failure: a multicenter retrospective cohort study. J Trauma Acute Care Surg. 2014;76: 1275–81.
128. Robba C, Ortu A, Bilotta F, Lombardo A, Sekhon MS, Gallo F, Matta BF. Extracorporeal membrane oxygenation for adult respiratory distress syndrome in trauma patients: a case series and systematic literature review. J Trauma Acute Care Surg. 2017;82:165–73.
129. Bakowitz M, Bruns B, McCunn M. Acute lung injury and the acute respiratory distress syndrome in the injured patient. Scand J Trauma Resusc Emerg Med. 2012;20:54.
130. Mascia L, Zavala E, Bosma K, Pasero D, Decaroli D, Andrews P, Isnardi D, Davi A, Arguis MJ, Berardino M, Ducati A, Brain IT Group. High tidal volume is associated with the development of acute lung injury after severe brain injury: an international observational study. Crit Care Med. 2007;35:1815–20.
131. Robba C, Poole D, McNett M, Asehnoune K, Bösel J, Bruder N, Chieregato A, Cinotti R, Duranteau J, Einav S, Ercole A, Ferguson N, Guerin C, Siempos II, Kurtz P, Juffermans NP, Mancebo J, Mascia L, McCredie V, Nin N, Oddo M, Pelosi P, Rabinstein AA, Neto AS, Seder DB, Skrifvars MB, Suarez JI, Taccone FS, van der Jagt M, Citerio G, et al. Mechanical ventilation in patients with acute brain injury: recommendations of the European Society of Intensive Care Medicine consensus. Intensive Care Med. 2020;46:2397–410.

14

Fluid and Blood Management in Traumatic and Non-traumatic Surgical Emergencies

Domien Vanhonacker, Michaël Mekeirele, and Manu L. N. G. Malbrain

Learning Objectives

The readers of this chapter on fluid and blood management in traumatic and non-traumatic surgical emergencies will learn more about:
- The 4 Ds of fluid therapy and the ROSE principle
- Different types of resuscitation fluids and when to use them
- Assessing whether or not a patient will benefit from fluid administration

14.1 Introduction

The first administration of intravenous (IV) fluids was performed almost two centuries ago and has been one of the most frequent medical interventions ever since. The majority of patients undergoing emergency surgery require fluid therapy to correct a state of absolute or relative intravascular volume depletion caused by absolute (e.g. bleeding that needs to be corrected with resuscitation fluids or blood products or insensible losses during open abdomen surgery that need to be corrected with replacement fluids) or relative (e.g. third spacing) fluid losses. Early adequate fluid therapy to restore cardiac output and oxygen

D. Vanhonacker
Department of Critical Care, Vrije Universiteit Brussel (VUB), Universitair ziekenhuis Brussel (UZB), Jette, Belgium

Department of Anesthesiology, Vrije Universiteit Brussel (VUB), Universitair ziekenhuis Brussel (UZB), Jette, Belgium
e-mail: domien.vanhonacker@uzbrussel.be

M. Mekeirele
Department of Critical Care, Vrije Universiteit Brussel (VUB), Universitair ziekenhuis Brussel (UZB), Jette, Belgium
e-mail: michael.mekeirele@uzbrussel.be

M. L. N. G. Malbrain (✉)
International Fluid Academy, Lovenjoel, Belgium

Department of Anaesthesiology and Intensive Care Medicine, Faculty of Medicine, Medical University of Lublin, Lublin, Poland

Medical Department, Medaman, Geel, Belgium

delivery is one of the cornerstones for treating shocked patients [1]. Even though fluids can be lifesaving, recently, more and more evidence shows that positive daily and cumulative fluid balances, as well as inappropriate use of IV fluids, might compromise patient outcomes and survival [2–5].

Every clinician should keep the following two principles in mind whenever considering administering IV fluids: the first is aptly named "the **4 Ds of fluid therapy**", referring to **D**rug, **D**ose, **D**uration, and **D**e-escalation [6]. Like antibiotics, the right resuscitation fluid should be administered at the proper dose for a limited period and treatment is to be stopped as soon as the signs and symptoms of shock have resolved.

The second principle is generally referred to as the **ROSE model** and states that fluid therapy should be tailored to the different phases of critical illness. Four dynamic phases have been described. The first phase is the **R**esuscitation phase, during which the patient's life is saved by aggressively administering fluid therapy. The second phase is characterized by a more calculated approach to **O**ptimize organ perfusion, while the third phase aims at achieving **S**tabilization through neutral daily fluid balances. Finally, during the fourth phase, excess fluids that might have accumulated during previous phases are **E**vacuated [6]. This is illustrated in Fig. 14.1 and Table 14.1.

In this chapter, we will review the current literature on fluid and blood management for patients undergoing emergency surgery and try to shed a light on a topic that has been hotly debated for many years. A lot of questions still remain unanswered, but by using the two above mentioned principles as a conceptual framework, we hope you will be able to see the wood for the trees.

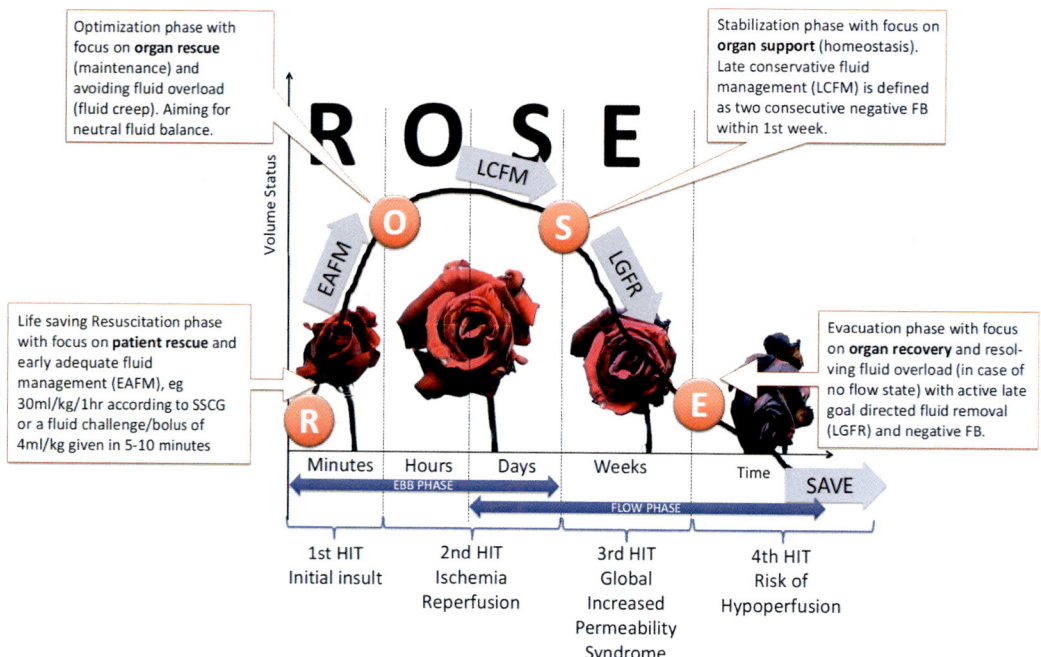

Fig. 14.1 Visualization of the ROSE conceptual model. Graph showing the four-hit model of shock with evolution of patients' cumulative fluid volume status over time during the four distinct phases of resuscitation: Resuscitation (R), Optimization (O), Stabilization (S), and Evacuation (E) (ROSE). (Adapted according to the Open Access CC BY Licence 4.0 with permission from Malbrain et al. [6])

Table 14.1 The ROSE conceptual model avoiding fluid overload (adapted from Malbrain et al. with permission) [7]

	Resuscitation	Optimization	Stabilization	Evacuation
Hit sequence	First hit	Second hit	Second hit	Third hit
Time frame	Minutes	Hours	Days	Days to weeks
Underlying mechanism	Inflammatory insult	Ischaemia and reperfusion	Ischaemia and reperfusion	Global increased permeability syndrome
Clinical presentation	Severe shock	Unstable shock	Absence of shock or threat of shock	Recovery from shock, possible Global Increased Permeability Syndrome
Goal	Early adequate goal-directed fluid management	Focus on organ support and maintaining tissue perfusion	Late conservative fluid management	Late goal-directed fluid removal (de-resuscitation)
Fluid therapy	Early administration with fluid boluses, guided by indices of fluid responsiveness	Fluid boluses guided by fluid responsiveness indices and indices of the risk of fluid administration	Only for normal maintenance and replacement	Reversal of the positive fluid balance, either spontaneous or active
Fluid balance	Positive	Neutral	Neutral to negative	Negative
Primary result of treatment	Salvage or patient rescue	Organ rescue	Organ support (homeostasis)	Organ recovery
Main risk	Insufficient resuscitation	Insufficient resuscitation and fluid overload (e.g. pulmonary edema, intra-abdominal hypertension)	Fluid overload (e.g. pulmonary edema, intra-abdominal hypertension)	Excessive fluid removal, possibly inducing hypotension, hypoperfusion, and a "fourth hit"

14.2 Diagnosis: When to Administer Fluids?

Deciding whether or not fluids should be administered is obvious in some cases (e.g. the septic/haemorrhagic shock patient with a low mean arterial pressure (MAP) and high lactate), but less clear-cut in others. A good clinical exam as well as gathering all of the available hemodynamic information are essential in making a well-considered decision. Advanced hemodynamic monitoring devices measuring cardiac output (CO), stroke volume (SV) and stroke volume variation (SVV) are available, but the clinical exam remains indispensable to evaluate whether a patient's circulation is sufficient to fulfill organ needs. A mottled skin, cold limbs, and a prolonged capillary refill time (>2 s) should always trigger further investigation.

Fluid responsiveness is a concept based on the Frank-Starling mechanism; a patient is dubbed a "fluid responder" when an increase in SV and/or CO of at least 10–15% is seen after the administration of a fluid challenge. Often an increase in MAP of 10% is used as a surrogate marker for fluid responsiveness in the absence of a cardiac output monitoring device. For patients not responding to a fluid challenge, the term "non-responders" is used. A fluid challenge can be performed by administering a fixed amount of fluid over a short period of time (e.g. 250 mL or 4 mL/kg over 2–5 min). An alternative method of testing fluid responsiveness without actually administering a single drop of fluid is increasing venous return by performing a passive leg raise (PLR) test. It is very important to be aware that a fluid-responsive patient will not necessarily benefit from fluid administration. Being fluid-responsive simply tells us the patient's intravascular volume status is situated on the steep part of the Frank-Starling curve [8].

Clinicians confronted with a hemodynamically unstable patient basically have 3 therapeutic options: administer fluids, start vasopressors or inotropes, or do nothing. If an intervention is warranted, then assessing fluid responsiveness is the first step towards making an informed decision. To determine in complex cases whether a fluid responder will truly benefit from extra fluids requires knowledge of the patient's current SV and CO. If a patient's SV or CO are sufficient then they are not likely to benefit from administering more fluids. The golden standard for CO monitoring is invasive thermodilution by means of pulmonary artery (PA) catheterization (Swan-Ganz catheter) or via transpulmonary thermodilution. Because there is no evidence that CO measurement by means of a PA catheter leads to improved outcomes, the invasiveness, and the risk of serious complications, it is no longer routinely used but rather reserved for patients suffering from severe cardiogenic shock, pulmonary hypertension, and those undergoing high-risk cardiac surgery [9]. Echocardiography and pulse contour analysis are less invasive techniques, allowing clinicians to estimate SV/CO [10].

The passive leg raise test requires the patient to sit up in a semi-recumbent position at 45°, the upper body of the patient is then lowered to supine, and the legs are passively raised to 45°; 30–60 s later the SV/CO of fluid-responsive patients should increase by at least 10% [11]. Once again in the absence of cardiac output monitoring device, the MAP is an often-used surrogate. For trauma patients, a physician should always assess whether it is feasible and safe to perform the PLR maneuver. PLR testing could increase ICP; patients at risk of or suffering from intracranial hypertension might not be appropriate candidates. More research is needed to confirm whether the PLR test can be safely used for this specific subpopulation. An alternative for SV/CO is the use of pulse pressure (PP) and pulse pressure variation (PPV). PP is the difference between systolic and diastolic blood pressure, whereas PPV quantifies PP changes during mechanical ventilation. PPV is a dynamic variable allowing us to predict fluid responsiveness.

Monitoring cumulative fluid balances with in- and output also provides valuable information on whether a patient might benefit from additional fluid administration or not. Often forgotten but significant sources of fluid are the volumes used to administer drugs, electrolytes, and nutrition. This so-called fluid creep should always be taken into account when calculating fluid balances.

Another simple but robust method to follow up on volume status is to keep a daily record of patient weight. Increased fluid losses, especially during the acute phase, need to be compensated, whereas the edematous patient with high positive fluid balances might still, but is less likely to, benefit from administering more fluids.

The practice of using central venous pressure (CVP) measurements to guide fluid resuscitation has been abandoned because of the following reasons:

- CVP is the equilibrium of the cardiac function and the central venous return function, it is not a predictor of the intravascular volume
- CVP does not accurately predict fluid responsiveness because right heart function, PEEP, and intra-abdominal pressure have a major impact on CVP

If the clinician decides a patient is likely to benefit from fluid administration, a fixed amount bolus (250 mL or 4 mL/kg) should be given over a short period of time and the patient is to be reassessed on a regular basis. Assessing the patient's hemodynamic response as well as monitoring for signs of adverse effects (e.g. deteriorating respiratory function, electrolyte disturbances, edema) will guide further decision-making.

Even though optimization of tissue perfusion should always be the goal of resuscitation, blood pressure is often used as a surrogate for perfusion. Numerous trials have shown that a MAP lower than 60–65 mmHg leads to increased organ failure rates. Higher MAP levels might be warranted to maintain organ perfusion in the elderly and hypertensive patient populations, whereas younger patients could well tolerate lower MAPs. Some trials even suggest that different types of trauma require varying blood pressure targets [12]. One size obviously does not fit all, and personalized blood pressure management is needed for every patient [13, 14].

In the trauma setting, permissive hypotension (e.g. a systolic blood pressure between 80 and 90 mmHg) is acceptable in certain situations, if rapid transport to the nearest emergency center can be arranged to obtain haemorrhagic control in theatre [15]. Several trials have shown permissive hypotension results in lower transfusion needs without worsening outcome [16]. Accepting a lower blood pressure allows the body to achieve hemostasis with minimal clot disruption. For traumatic brain injury, higher, rather than lower, blood pressure targets should be aimed for since hypotension is likely to worsen brain injury [17].

14.3 Treatment: Choosing the Right Type of Fluid

When picking the "right fluid for the job", the characteristics of different fluids (e.g. osmolality, tonicity, pH, electrolyte composition, and the presence of metabolically active compounds), as well as the reason for fluid administration (e.g. resuscitation, maintenance, or replacement) need to be taken into account. Balanced and unbalanced isotonic crystalloids, synthetic and blood-derived colloids (e.g. albumin), and blood products (e.g. packed red blood cells and plasma) can all be used as resuscitation fluids to restore an intravascular volume deficit. However, as we will discuss further, this does not imply that they are all equal.

14.3.1 Crystalloids

Crystalloids are a diverse group of fluids with very different properties. They are inexpensive, widely available, and form the backbone of fluid therapy.

Hypotonic crystalloids have no place in fluid resuscitation, they can be used as maintenance fluids, but only in the absence of traumatic brain injury or stroke.

Theoretically, **hypertonic** crystalloids should have a bigger impact on volume expansion of the intravascular compartment than isotonic fluids since their hypertonicity draws water from the other compartments into the bloodstream. A number of trials have shown that hypertonic saline (HTS) can be safely used for trauma patients under permissive hypotension during damage control surgery in order to avoid excessive fluid loading [18, 19]. However, two recent trials, HYPER2S and HERACLES, looking at the use of HTS as a resuscitation fluid in septic shock and cardiac surgery patients were unable to show any benefit of using HTS over normal saline [20, 21]. Patients treated with HTS initially received less fluids, but after correcting substantial variations in electrolyte and acid-base homeostasis, fluid balances of both groups no longer differed significantly.

In 2017, De Crescenzo et al. published a systematic review and meta-analysis on the prehospital use of hypertonic fluid resuscitation for trauma patients; 9 trials were used for the systematic review, of which 6 were included in the meta-analysis. The meta-analysis showed no beneficial effects of the use of hypertonic crystalloids when compared to isotonic crystalloids in the general trauma population [22]. HTS can be used to reduce intracranial pressure (ICP) in traumatic brain injury (TBI). However, it is important to note that the out-of-hospital use of HTS in trauma patients might delay the recognition and treatment of haemorrhagic shock, possibly delaying transfusion and increasing overall mortality [23].

Isotonic crystalloids are the most commonly used intravenous fluids. They can be divided into two subcategories: unbalanced (e.g. normal saline) and balanced isotonic crystalloids (e.g. Hartmann's solution or Ringer's lactate, Plasma-Lyte, and Ringer's acetate). Balanced solutions were developed to more closely resemble the composition of human plasma.

Balanced crystalloids generally contain reduced levels of sodium and chloride, the latter anion usually being replaced with lactate, acetate, malate, or gluconate. The accumulation of lactate caused by resuscitation with Hartmann's or lactated Ringer's solution is rarely seen in the absence of liver failure and does not appear to have any clinical consequences unless it is given in extremely large amounts as seen in severe burn injury. Since lactate substitutes glucose as fuel for the brain in the setting of TBI and hypertonic lactate solutions have shown to be effective at reducing ICP, these solutions might prove to be valuable to manage intracranial pressure [24, 25].

However, more data are needed to confirm these findings. Acetate is known to predispose to hypotension when used as a buffer for patients undergoing hemodialysis, but there is no evidence suggesting a similar effect when resuscitating patients with an acetate-containing balanced crystalloid [26]. Because acetate is a very efficient bicarbonate precursor and is metabolized regardless of liver function, balanced fluids containing acetate have superior buffering effects when compared to Ringer's lactate and saline even in patients with a reduced liver function [27]. Very little is known about the metabolism of malate and gluconate.

Normal saline (NaCl 0.9%) is still the most widely used IV crystalloid, despite evidence suggesting its administration is associated with hyperchloremic metabolic acidosis, acute kidney injury, and aggravating the trauma triad of death by inducing acidosis and coagulopathy [28–35]. Normal saline is far from normal or physiological; its use is based on old habits and low cost rather than scientific rationale.

The strong ion difference (SID) is a concept stemming from the Stewart approach for interpreting acid-base disturbances and expresses the influence of so-called strong ions on pH. Strong ions include Na, Ca, Mg, Cl, and organic acids; at a normal pH they are fully dissociated and exert no buffering effect. The SID of a fluid is the difference between the strong cations and anions. An increased SID leads to alkalosis, whereas a decreased SID induces acidosis (normal SID of human plasma = 42 mEq/L). Since Na and Cl are the most abundant strong ions, an abbreviated SID can be calculated as follows: [Na] − [Cl]. The SID of balanced crystalloids is higher and approaches the SID of plasma, therefore these solutions are less acidic than normal saline which has a SID of 0 mEq/L. The volume expanding effects of balanced crystalloids are very similar to those of normal saline. Approximately 25–30% of an infused crystalloid volume will remain in the intravascular space 60 min after administration due to redistribution within the extracellular (interstitial) fluid compartment [34, 35].

In 2015, the SPLIT trial was the first large randomized controlled clinical trial (RCT) comparing the effects of (ab)normal saline vs Plasma-Lyte administration in ICU patients requiring fluid therapy. A total of 2278 patients were enrolled in the trial that took place in the ICU's of 4 New Zealand hospitals. It is noteworthy that only 125 of the 2278 patients included were trauma patients. The primary outcome of the trial was the incidence of AKI during the first 90 days after enrolment. In both groups, a nearly identical proportion of patients developed AKI (9.6% vs 9.2%; $p = 0.77$). No statistical differences were shown for any of the secondary outcomes (need for renal replacement therapy or mechanical ventilation, length of stay, and mortality). The authors concluded that the use of a balanced crystalloid does not reduce the risk of AKI. Although the methodology of the trial was good, a number of important limitations make it difficult to generalize its results: the vast majority of the included patients were elective postoperative patients with few comorbidities and a relatively low APACHE II score. Furthermore, over 90% of the patients had received a balanced crystalloid before enrolment and the median volume of fluid administered was merely 2 L per ICU stay. Finally, the authors failed to monitor the most important adverse effect related to (ab)normal saline, namely hyperchloremia and the presence of metabolic acidosis. With these limitations in mind, we would like to suggest a more balanced conclusion: administering up to 2 L of normal saline in patients undergoing elective surgery or moderately ill critical care patients does not result in an increased risk of developing AKI compared with Plasma-Lyte [36].

In 2018, the New England Journal of Medicine (NEJM) published two large RCT's on the matter, the SMART and the SALT-ED trials [37, 38]. Investigators of the SMART trial examined whether the administration of balanced crystalloids compared with normal saline would reduce a composite 30-day outcome of death, new renal replacement therapy, or persistent renal dysfunction in critically ill patients. Between June 2015 and April 2017, in total 15,802 patients were randomized to receive a balanced crystalloid or normal saline in the 4 ICU's of a single US academic center. The occurrence of the composite 30-day outcome was significantly higher for patients treated with normal saline (15.4% vs 14.3%; $p = 0.04$). Therefore, the authors concluded that balanced crystalloids should be picked over normal saline for treating critically ill patients. Even though the use of a composite endpoint makes interpreting the results more complex, this large and strong methodological study casts more doubt on the safety profile of normal saline, especially when used in critically ill patients [37].

The SALT-ED trial looked at non-critically ill patients to see whether the administration of a balanced crystalloid could reduce hospital-free days (a composite of in-hospital death and length of stay, LOS) up to day 28 compared with normal saline. Upon arrival at the emergency department of a single US academic center, 13,347 patients were enrolled into the normal saline or balanced crystalloid group. There was no difference in hospital-free days between the groups; however, a significantly lower incidence of major adverse kidney events within 30 days was reported for the group treated with balanced crystalloids (4.7% vs 5.6%; $p = 0.01$). The SALT-ED trial, like the SMART trial, is a large and well-designed study suggesting that normal saline might also affect the outcomes of non-critically ill patients in a negative way [38].

Enrolment for the PLUS trial is expected to finish in June 2021. This multi-centered, blinded RCT will compare 90-day mortality in critically ill patients treated with normal saline vs balanced crystalloids. Hopefully the first primary results will be published in 2022, shedding more light on this never-ending story [39].

While waiting for more data and studies to identify the best crystalloid for resuscitating our patients, we suggest avoiding (ab)normal saline as a resuscitation fluid. Balanced crystalloids are widely available and are a good first choice; they are the most sensible option from a physiological point of view; current data are robust enough to pick them over unbalanced solutions and their potential benefits outweigh the added cost, especially when large volumes are administered to the critically ill.

14.3.2 Colloids

Colloids are high molecular weight substances that are ought to largely remain in the intravascular compartment and thereby generate an oncotic pressure, thus drawing in water from the other compartments [34, 35]. Two categories can be differentiated: natural colloids (e.g. human albumin, fresh frozen plasma) and synthetic colloids (e.g. gelatins, dextrans, and hydroxyethyl starches). Traditionally, synthetic colloids were frequently used as resuscitation fluids since data suggested that to obtain the same increase in intravascular volume, one would need to administer double the volume of crystalloids compared to colloids. More recent research has busted this myth, and in reality, the ratio appears closer to 1.3:1 or even 1:1 for patients in shock and as well as patients undergoing surgery [40, 41]. In most countries, human albumin, hydroxy-ethyl starches (HES), and gelatins are the only colloid solutions still being used in the clinical setting.

Human albumin is a plasma protein and exerts approximately 80% of the colloid osmotic pressure (COP) on the interstitial tissues. It therefore plays an essential role in the distribution of fluids between the different compartments. Albumin has been used in trauma and burn patients since the 1940s. Even though large multicenter RCT's have provided us with information on which patient groups are likely to benefit from its use, a lot of questions still remain.

In 2003, a meta-analysis by Vincent et al. of 90 cohort studies concluded that hypoalbuminemia is a powerful and independent risk factor for poor outcome in the acutely ill. Both morbidity and mortality increased as serum albumin levels decreased. The authors advocated monitoring albumin levels as a monitoring tool to identify high-risk patients [42].

The multicentric Saline versus Albumin Fluid Evaluation (SAFE) trial published in 2004 showed that a 4% Albumin solution is as safe as normal saline when used as a resuscitation fluid in critically ill patients [43]. Albumin should not be used in the treatment of patients with TBI since a subgroup analysis of the SAFE trial showed that TBI patients receiving albumin had worse outcomes than those treated with normal saline [44]. Cooper et al. later confirmed that the use of albumin in patients with severe TBI is associated with increased ICP and is most likely the mechanism of increased mortality in these patients [45]. However, in a subgroup of patients with severe sepsis and septic shock, albumin had a beneficial effect with an adjusted odds ratio for death = 0.71 (95% CI: 0.52–0.97; $p = 0.03$) [46].

Another large RCT, the ALBIOS trial, compared the outcome of severe sepsis and septic shock patients treated with crystalloids versus those receiving crystalloids as well as a 20% albumin solution to maintain a target serum albumin concentration of 30 g/L. Those treated with albumin had better hemodynamic indices, but the use of albumin did not impact 28- or 90-day mortality [47].

Burn patients who are generally resuscitated using the Parkland formula often have significant crystalloid requirements. Lawrence et al. administered a combination of albumin and balanced crystalloids to patients with progressively increasing requirements [48]. They concluded that the addition of albumin to Parkland resuscitation reduced hourly fluid requirements, the occurrence of compartment syndrome, and fluid overload.

Since synthetic colloids have fallen out of grace due to the debate concerning potential side effects (as discussed below), albumin received increased interest as a resuscitation fluid. However, not a single RCT has been able to show a significant benefit of using albumin over other fluids. Furthermore, the significant cost of albumin and the availability of balanced crystalloids which are cheap and equally effective have not contributed to its already controversial case. More research is needed to determine whether albumin is superior to balanced crystalloids for certain patient populations.

Gelatin is the name given to the large molecular weight proteins formed by the hydrolysis of collagen when cooking the connective tissues of animals; these proteins dissolve in hot water and form a jelly when cooled. Gelatins have the advantages of being inexpensive compared to other colloids and the fact that the gel-like matrix is negatively charged making them by definition "balanced" with a larger SID. However, they are rapidly excreted by the kidney (2–3 h) and there is evidence suggesting their use is associated with an increased risk of anaphylactic reactions, renal failure, coagulation disturbances, and possibly even mortality [49]. A large prospective RCT, the GENIUS trial is currently enrolling patients and will hopefully provide us with more robust data on the usefulness and safety profile of gelatins [50]. Until then we would not recommend using gelatins as resuscitation fluids.

Dextrans are highly branched polysaccharide molecules; their volume expanding effect is more pronounced than that of HES and albumin and lasts for approximately 6–12 h. They cause more anaphylactic reactions than gelatins and starches. Administering large doses of dextrans is associated with significant bleeding and an increased need for transfusion caused by decreasing blood viscosity and inhibition of coagulation pathways [51]. In most countries, dextrans are no longer available on the market and we would not recommend using them as resuscitation fluids.

Hydroxy-ethyl starches (HES) are derivatives of amylopectin, a highly branched compound of starch resembling glycogen. Following a number of RCTs pointing out the potential negative effects of synthetic colloids, the Pharmacovigilance Risk Assessment Committee (PRAC) of the European Medicines Agency (EMA) took matters into hand and prohibited the use of HES for patients with sepsis, burn injuries, renal impairment or RRT, intracranial or cerebral haemorrhage, impaired liver function, severe coagulopathy, and the critically ill. They can, however, still be used in the perioperative setting to treat hypovolemic shock in surgical patients with acute bleeding and victims of major trauma when crystalloids alone are not sufficient albeit at the lowest effective dose for the shortest period of time. In the US, HES can no longer be used for the critically ill and those with renal dysfunction.

The VISEP, 6S, and CHEST trials were the first RCTs ringing the alarm [3–5]. All three trials looked at the development of new organ failure and overall mortality in patients receiving HES or crystalloids. The VISEP researchers saw significantly higher rates of AKI and need for RRT in the group treated with HES (34.9% vs 22.8%; $p = 0.002$) [4]. The 6S trial not only showed that the administration of HES, compared to Ringer's lactate, is associated with an increased need for RRT, but also significantly increases mortality [3]. The CHEST trial is the largest RCT comparing HES to normal saline in the critically ill. Its authors concluded there was no significant difference in the primary endpoint, 90-day mortality. The use of HES was associated with an increase in RRT, hepatic failure, and some minor adverse events such as pruritus and rash. The CHEST trial received a lot of skepticism due to issues with patient randomization and the refusal of the authors to share the raw data [5].

The CRYSTMAS and CRISTAL trials were published during the same period and questioned the conclusions of the trials mentioned above, sparking hope with the HES supporters and adding fuel to an already heated debate [52, 53]. Patients in the CRYSTMAS study were randomly assigned to receive either HES or normal saline. A lower amount of fluids was used to resuscitate the HES group and no difference in adverse advents was seen. Shortly after publication, the authors of the trial received criticism and when the data were reassessed, both groups appeared to have received equal amounts of fluids. Furthermore, the study was underpowered. If anything, it showed a non-significant trend towards a higher need for RRT and mortality in the HES group [54]. The CRISTAL trial reported similar results as the CRYSTMAS trial, but power calculations showed it was underpowered to detect significant differences in renal failure or mortality [53].

HES, like gelatins and dextrans, impair platelet reactivity and decrease circulating plasma concentrations of coagulation factor VII and von Willebrand factor. There is evidence suggesting that the administration of starches results in weakened clot formation, increased bleeding, and a higher incidence of transfusion compared to those receiving crystalloids [51].

Up to this day, we lack a large-scale clinical trial investigating whether HES can be safely used to treat haemorrhagic shock in trauma patients. A number of retrospective trials and small RCTs suggest the use of HES might be acceptable for trauma patients, but we need a more robust and elaborate trial to confirm these findings, especially given the strong evidence against HES for other indications [55, 56].

A recent systematic review from the Cochrane collaboration concluded that the use of HES in critically ill patients probably makes little or no difference on mortality (moderate-certainty evidence), but slightly increases the need for blood transfusion and RRT. Therefore, we would err on the side of caution and refrain from using HES until more compelling evidence confirms it can be safely used in certain patient groups [57].

Packed red blood cells (PRC) can be used as resuscitation fluids in haemorrhagic resuscitation or anaemic patients. Haemoglobin improves the blood's oxygen-carrying capacity which is essential to provide tissues with the oxygen needed to maintain their aerobic metabolism. Blood transfusion is not without risk and has been shown to be an independent predictor of mortality. Fever, fluid overload, hypotension, infection, and ARDS were the most common side effects reported in the CRIT trial, a multicenter observational study among ICU patients [58].

For many years, a blood haemoglobin concentration above 10 g/dL and a haematocrit higher than 30% were targeted. Over the past few years, the paradigm has shifted from a liberal towards a more restrictive transfusion threshold [59, 60].

The TRICC trial by Hébert et al. was the first large RCT suggesting similar outcomes when aiming for a haemoglobin level between 7 and 9 g/dL rather than a level between 10 and 12 g/dL. Furthermore, a significantly lower in-hospital mortality was seen in the restrictive strategy group as well as a trend favouring general survival [60].

In 2014, the TRISS trial, one of the many trials comparing a "low" haemoglobin transfusion threshold of 7 g/dL with a "high" threshold of 9 g/dL, was published. The authors concluded both groups had similar outcomes, irrespective of patient age, (cardiovascular) comorbidities, and SAPS II score. Acute coronary syndrome, burn, and actively bleeding patients were not included in this trial [61].

In 2016, the Cochrane Collaboration published a systematic review concluding that transfusing at a restrictive haemoglobin concentration (7–8 g/dL) decreases transfusion need and has no impact on 30-day mortality or morbidity. Insufficient data were available to verify these findings in clinical subgroups [62].

Concerning patients requiring massive transfusion (>10 units of PRC in 24 h), the guidelines of the American College of Surgeons Trauma Quality Improvement Program (ACS TQIP) state the following [63]:

- Universal blood product infusion is preferred over crystalloid or colloid solutions
- PRC and FFP should be transfused at a ratio between 1:1 and 2:1
- 1 pool of platelets should be administered for each 6 units of PRC

Fresh frozen plasma (FFP) contains clotting factors, albumin, and other serum proteins as well as plasma protease inhibitors. FFP is indicated for patients who are actively bleeding or undergoing invasive procedures with multiple coagulation factor deficiencies. The recommended dose is 15–20 mL/kg. If bleeding or coagulopathy persists and further FFP administration is warranted, the PRC:FFP ratio should be at least 2:1 [64].

A number of clotting factor concentrates are available on the market; these products can be used for the emergency reversal of vitamin K-dependant anticoagulants [65]. A lot of questions still remain on the efficacy of these concentrates for massive bleeding, especially since none of the concentrates contain all of the clotting factors, whereas FPP does. However, correcting coagulation disorders with clotting factor concentrates requires less fluid administration compared to FFP.

The administration of tranexamic acid, an antifibrinolytic agent, to trauma patients within the first 3 h after injury significantly reduced mortality due to bleeding [66]. When tranexamic acid was started more than 3 h after injury, overall mortality increased. All trauma patients should receive a 1 g loading dose of tranexamic acid over 10 min, followed by an intravenous infusion of 1 g over 8 h during the first 3 h after injury since limiting blood loss early on will reduce the need for resuscitation later.

FFP should not be used as a resuscitation fluid in non-bleeding patients since blood products are of limited supply, less expensive alternatives are available, and transfusion is not without risk.

> **Do and Dont's**
> - Always prevent fluid overload and accumulation
> - Apply ROSE concept to all critical patients
> - Don't underestimate the effect of fluid as drugs to be administered cautiously
> - Don't forget to assess fluid state in all critical patients

> **Take-Home Messages**
>
> Fluid resuscitation has been one of the most common medical interventions for a long time. Fluids are drugs and should only be administered when their benefit outweighs the risk of potential side effects. The 4 D's of fluid resuscitation (**D**rug, **D**ose, **D**uration, and **D**e-escalation) should be taken into account whenever prescribing/administering fluids [6]. Fluid accumulation impacts patient outcomes and mortality and should be avoided at all costs.
>
> Shocked patients, requiring emergency surgery, should be treated in accordance with the ROSE principle (Fig. 14.1 and Table 14.1): during the **R**esuscitation phase, volume status and fluid responsiveness should be monitored regularly while administering aggressive therapy. Advanced hemodynamic monitoring can help **O**ptimizing organ perfusion. Once the shock state has resolved, the **S**tabilization phase begins and neutral to negative fluid balances should be aimed for. During the **E**vacuation phase, excess fluids should be mobilized and removed from the body since they will hinder the diffusion and absorption of oxygen and nutrients [6].
>
> The frequent assessment of both clinical and hemodynamic parameters as well as monitoring for the occurrence of adverse events will help guide the clinician's decision-making on whether the surgical patient is likely to benefit from fluid therapy or not.

Multiple Choice Questions

1. The 4 D's of fluid therapy stand for:
   A. **D**rug, **D**rug interaction, **D**uration, and **D**e-escalation
   B. **Drug, Dose, Duration, and De-escalation**
   C. **D**ose, **D**ynamics, **D**uration, and **D**e-escalation
   D. **D**rug, **D**ose, **D**elivery, and **D**uration

2. Which of the 4 statements below does **not** correctly describe a phase of the ROSE model?
   A. **R**esuscitation phase: the patient's life is saved by aggressively administering fluids
   B. **O**ptimization phase: organ perfusion is optimized through a more calculated approach
   C. **Stabilization phase: the patient is stable, positive daily fluid balances are needed to maintain stability**
   D. **E**vacuation phase: excess fluids are removed from the body compartments

3. Administering fluids is **not** a good idea in the following situations:
   A. A low MAP and a high lactate
   B. **A high CVP**
   C. A SVV > 15% after a fluid bolus was administered
   D. A mottled skin, cold limbs, and a prolonged capillary refill time (>2 s)

4. Concerning mean arterial pressure (MAP):
   A. MAP should never be used as a surrogate for perfusion
   B. A low MAP will not lead to increased organ failure rates
   C. **A normal MAP can be seen in patients with inadequate tissue perfusion**
   D. Targeting a MAP of 65 mmHg will ensure adequate tissue perfusion for every patient

5. The administration of normal saline (NaCl 0.9%)
   A. Is associated with metabolic alkalosis
   B. Is a balanced crystalloid solution
   C. Is useful for the treatment of acute kidney injury
   D. **Can induce coagulopathy and therefore aggravate bleeding in trauma patients**

6. Human albumin
   A. Exerts approximately 50% of the colloid osmotic pressure
   B. Can be safely used in the treatment of patients with TBI
   C. Has significant benefits over crystalloids when used to resuscitate patients
   D. **Is frequently used in the resuscitation of burn patients**

7. Balanced crystalloids
   A. Generally contain higher levels of sodium and chloride compared to Normal Saline (NaCl 0.9%)
   B. Have a lower strong ion difference (SID) than Normal Saline (NaCl 0.9%)
   C. **Often contain lactate, acetate, malate, or gluconate to replace chloride**
   D. More frequently cause acid-base disorders compared to Normal Saline (NaCl 0.9%)

8. Which of the following statements concerning synthetic colloids is true?
   A. Hydroxy-ethyl starches (HES) should, under no circumstances, be used to resuscitate trauma patients
   B. **The use of gelatins is associated with an increased risk of anaphylactic reactions, renal failure, and coagulation disturbances**
   C. Dextrans are cheap colloids, available in many countries worldwide
   D. Hydroxy-ethyl starches (HES) can be safely used to resuscitate septic shock patients

9. Transfusion of packed red blood cells (PRC)
   A. **Is associated with side effects (e.g. fever, fluid overload, infection, ARDS)**

B. Be performed whenever a patient's haemoglobin drops below 9 g/dL
C. And FFP should be done at a ratio between 1:2 and 1:2 for patients requiring massive transfusion
D. Has no impact on patient mortality when a liberal regimen is followed

10. Fresh frozen plasma (FFP) does **not** contain
A. Clotting factors
B. Albumin
C. Serum proteins
D. **Plasma proteinase activators**

References

1. Rivers E, Nguyen B, Havstad S, Ressler J, Muzzin A, Knoblich B, et al. Early goal-directed therapy in the treatment of severe sepsis and septic shock. N Engl J Med. 2001;345(19):1368–77.
2. Vincent JL, Sakr Y, Sprung CL, Ranieri VM, Reinhart K, Gerlach H, et al. Sepsis in European intensive care units: results of the SOAP study. Crit Care Med. 2006;34(2):344–53.
3. Perner A, Haase N, Guttormsen AB, Tenhunen J, Klemenzson G, Åneman A, et al. Hydroxyethyl starch 130/0.42 versus Ringer's acetate in severe sepsis. N Engl J Med. 2012;367(2):124–34.
4. Brunkhorst FM, Engel C, Bloos F, Meier-Hellmann A, Ragaller M, Weiler N, et al. Intensive insulin therapy and pentastarch resuscitation in severe sepsis. N Engl J Med. 2008;358(2):125–39.
5. Myburgh JA, Finfer S, Bellomo R, Billot L, Cass A, Gattas D, et al. Hydroxyethyl starch or saline for fluid resuscitation in intensive care. N Engl J Med. 2012;367(20):1901–11.
6. Malbrain MLNG, Van Regenmortel N, Saugel B, De Tavernier B, Van Gaal PJ, Joannes-Boyau O, et al. Principles of fluid management and stewardship in septic shock: it is time to consider the four D's and the four phases of fluid therapy. Ann Intensive Care. 2018;8(1):66.
7. Malbrain ML, Marik PE, Witters I, Cordemans C, Kirkpatrick AW, Roberts DJ, et al. Fluid overload, de-resuscitation, and outcomes in critically ill or injured patients: a systematic review with suggestions for clinical practice. Anaesthesiol Intensive Ther. 2014;46(5):361–80.
8. Cherpanath TGV, Aarts LPHJ, Groeneveld JAB, Geerts BF. Defining fluid responsiveness: a guide to patient-tailored volume titration. J Cardiothorac Vasc Anesth. 2014;28(3):745–54.
9. Rajaram SS, Desai NK, Kalra A, Gajera M, Cavanaugh SK, Brampton W, et al. Pulmonary artery catheters for adult patients in intensive care. Cochrane Database Syst Rev. 2013;2013(2):CD003408.
10. Pour-Ghaz I, Manolukas T, Foray N, Raja J, Rawal A, Ibeuogu UN, et al. Accuracy of non-invasive and minimally invasive hemodynamic monitoring: where do we stand? Ann Transl Med. 2019;7(17):421.
11. Assadi F. Passive leg raising: simple and reliable technique to prevent fluid overload in critically ill patients. Int J Prev Med. 2017;8(1):48.
12. Wise R, Faurie M, Malbrain MLNG, Hodgson E. Strategies for intravenous fluid resuscitation in trauma patients. World J Surg. 2017;41(5):1170–83.
13. Saugel B, Sessler DI. Perioperative blood pressure management. Anesthesiology. 2021;134(2):250–61.
14. Asfar P, Meziani F, Hamel J-F, Grelon F, Megarbane B, Anguel N, et al. High versus low blood-pressure target in patients with septic shock. N Engl J Med. 2014;370(17):1583–93.
15. Bickell WH, Wall MJ, Pepe PE, Martin RR, Ginger VF, Allen MK, et al. Immediate versus delayed fluid resuscitation for hypotensive patients with penetrating torso injuries. N Engl J Med. 1994;331(17):1105–9.
16. Nevin DG, Brohi K. Permissive hypotension for active haemorrhage in trauma. Anaesthesia. 2017;72(12):1443–8.
17. Carney N, Totten AM, O'Reilly C, et al. Guidelines for the management of severe traumatic brain injury, fourth edition. Neurosurgery. 2017;80:6–15.
18. Duchesne JC, Simms E, Guidry C, Duke M, Beeson E, McSwain NE, et al. Damage control immunoregulation: is there a role for low-volume hypertonic saline resuscitation in patients managed with damage control surgery? Am Surg. 2012;78(9):962–8.
19. Duchesne JC, Kaplan LJ, Balogh ZJ, Malbrain MLNG. Role of permissive hypotension, hypertonic resuscitation and the global increased permeability syndrome in patients with severe hemorrhage: adjuncts to damage control resuscitation to prevent intra-abdominal hypertension. Anaesthesiol Intensive Ther. 2015;47(2):143–55.
20. Asfar P, Schortgen F, Boisramé-Helms J, Charpentier J, Guérot E, Megarbane B, et al. Hyperoxia and hypertonic saline in patients with septic shock (HYPERS2S): a two-by-two factorial, multicentre, randomised, clinical trial. Lancet Respir Med. 2017;5(3):180–90.
21. Pfortmueller CA, Kindler M, Schenk N, Messmer AS, Hess B, Jakob L, et al. Hypertonic saline for fluid resuscitation in ICU patients post-cardiac surgery (HERACLES): a double-blind randomized controlled clinical trial. Intensive Care Med. 2020;46(9):1683–95.
22. de Crescenzo C, Gorouhi F, Salcedo ES, Galante JM. Prehospital hypertonic fluid resuscitation for trauma patients: a systematic review and meta-analysis. J Trauma Acute Care Surg. 2017;82(5):956–62.
23. Bulger EM, May S, Kerby JD, Emerson S, Stiell IG, Schreiber MA, et al. Out-of-hospital hypertonic

23. resuscitation after traumatic hypovolemic shock: a randomized, placebo controlled trial. Ann Surg. 2011;253(3):431–41.
24. Arifianto MR, Ma'ruf AZ, Ibrahim A, Bajamal AH. Role of hypertonic sodium lactate in traumatic brain injury management. Asian J Neurosurg. 2018;13(4):971–5.
25. Ichai C, Armando G, Orban J-C, Berthier F, Rami L, Samat-Long C, et al. Sodium lactate versus mannitol in the treatment of intracranial hypertensive episodes in severe traumatic brain-injured patients. Intensive Care Med. 2009;35(3):471–9.
26. Tessitore N, Santoro A, Panzetta GO, Wizemann V, Perez-Garcia R, Martinez Ara J, et al. Acetate-free biofiltration reduces intradialytic hypotension: a European multicenter randomized controlled trial. Blood Purif. 2012;34(3–4):354–63.
27. Ergin B, Kapucu A, Guerci P, Ince C. The role of bicarbonate precursors in balanced fluids during haemorrhagic shock with and without compromised liver function. Br J Anaesth. 2016;117(4):521–8.
28. Chowdhury AH, Cox EF, Francis ST, Lobo DN. A randomized, controlled, double-blind crossover study on the effects of 2-L infusions of 0.9% saline and plasma-lyte® 148 on renal blood flow velocity and renal cortical tissue perfusion in healthy volunteers. Ann Surg. 2012;256(1):18–24.
29. Hasman H, Cinar O, Uzun A, Cevik E, Jay L, Comert B. A randomized clinical trial comparing the effect of rapidly infused crystalloids on acid-base status in dehydrated patients in the emergency department. Int J Med Sci. 2012;9(1):59–64.
30. Kellum JA. Fluid resuscitation and hyperchloremic acidosis in experimental sepsis: improved short-term survival and acid-base balance with Hextend compared with saline. Crit Care Med. 2002;30(2):300–5.
31. Orbegozo D, Su F, Santacruz C, He X, Hosokawa K, Creteur J, et al. Effects of different crystalloid solutions on hemodynamics, peripheral perfusion, and the microcirculation in experimental abdominal sepsis. Anesthesiology. 2016;125(4):744–54.
32. Potura E, Lindner G, Biesenbach P, Funk GC, Reiterer C, Kabon B, et al. An acetate-buffered balanced crystalloid versus 0.9% saline in patients with end-stage renal disease undergoing cadaveric renal transplantation: a prospective randomized controlled trial. Anesth Analg. 2015;120(1):123–9.
33. White NJ, Ward KR, Pati S, et al. Hemorrhagic blood failure: oxygen debt, coagulopathy, and endothelial damage. J Trauma Acute Care Surg. 2017;82(6S Suppl 1):S41–9.
34. Jaynes MP, Murphy CV, Ali N, Krautwater A, Lehman A, Doepker BA. Association between chloride content of intravenous fluids and acute kidney injury in critically ill medical patients with sepsis. J Crit Care. 2018;44:363–7.
35. Langer T, Santini A, Scotti E, Van Regenmortel N, Malbrain ML, Caironi P. Intravenous balanced solutions: from physiology to clinical evidence. Anaesthesiol Intensive Ther. 2015;47 Spec No:s78–88.
36. Young P, Bailey M, Beasley R, Henderson S, Mackle D, McArthur C, et al. Effect of a buffered crystalloid solution vs saline on acute kidney injury among patients in the intensive care unit: the SPLIT randomized clinical trial. JAMA. 2015;314(16):1701–10.
37. Semler MW, Self WH, Rice TW. Balanced crystalloids versus saline in critically ill adults. N Engl J Med. 2018;378(20):1951.
38. Self WH, Semler MW, Wanderer JP, Wang L, Byrne DW, Collins SP, et al. Balanced crystalloids versus saline in noncritically ill adults. N Engl J Med. 2018;378(9):819–28.
39. Plasma-Lyte 148® versUs Saline Study—Full Text View—ClinicalTrials.Gov [Internet]. Clinicaltrials.gov. [cited 2021 Apr 27]. https://clinicaltrials.gov/ct2/show/NCT02721654.
40. Hahn RG. Volume kinetics for infusion fluids. Anesthesiology. 2010;113(2):470–81.
41. Hahn RG, Lyons G. The half-life of infusion fluids: an educational review. Eur J Anaesthesiol. 2016;33(7):475–82.
42. Vincent J-L, Dubois M-J, Navickis RJ, Wilkes MM. Hypoalbuminemia in acute illness: is there a rationale for intervention? A meta-analysis of cohort studies and controlled trials. Ann Surg. 2003;237(3):319–34.
43. Finfer S, Bellomo R, Boyce N, French J, Myburgh J, Norton R, et al. A comparison of albumin and saline for fluid resuscitation in the intensive care unit. N Engl J Med. 2004;350(22):2247–56.
44. SAFE Study Investigators, Finfer S, McEvoy S, Bellomo R, McArthur C, Myburgh J, et al. Impact of albumin compared to saline on organ function and mortality of patients with severe sepsis. Intensive Care Med. 2011;37(1):86–96.
45. Cooper DJ, Myburgh J, Heritier S, Finfer S, Bellomo R, Billot L, et al. Albumin resuscitation for traumatic brain injury: is intracranial hypertension the cause of increased mortality? J Neurotrauma. 2013;30(7):512–8.
46. Finfer S, McEvoy S, Bellomo R, McArthur C, Myburgh J, Norton R, et al. Impact of albumin compared to saline on organ function and mortality of patients with severe sepsis. Intensive Care Med. 2011;37(1):86–96.
47. Caironi P, Tognoni G, Masson S, Fumagalli R, Pesenti A, Romero M, et al. Albumin replacement in patients with severe sepsis or septic shock. N Engl J Med. 2014;370(15):1412–21.
48. Lawrence A, Faraklas I, Watkins H, Allen A, Cochran A, Morris S, et al. Colloid administration normalizes resuscitation ratio and ameliorates "fluid creep". J Burn Care Res. 2010;31(1):40–7.
49. Moeller C, Fleischmann C, Thomas-Rueddel D, Vlasakov V, Rochwerg B, Theurer P, et al. How safe is gelatin? A systematic review and meta-analysis of gelatin-containing plasma expanders vs crystalloids and albumin. J Crit Care. 2016;35:75–83.

50. Gelatin in ICU and sepsis—Full text view—ClinicalTrials.Gov [Internet]. Clinicaltrials.gov. [cited 2021 Apr 27]. https://clinicaltrials.gov/ct2/show/NCT02715466.
51. Mitra S, Khandelwal P. Are all colloids same? How to select the right colloid? Indian J Anaesth. 2009;53(5):592–607.
52. Guidet B, Martinet O, Boulain T, Philippart F, Poussel JF, Maizel J, et al. Assessment of hemodynamic efficacy and safety of 6% hydroxyethylstarch 130/0.4 vs. 0.9% NaCl fluid replacement in patients with severe sepsis: the CRYSTMAS study. Crit Care. 2012;16(3):R94.
53. Annane D, Siami S, Jaber S, Martin C, Elatrous S, Declère AD, et al. Effects of fluid resuscitation with colloids vs crystalloids on mortality in critically ill patients presenting with hypovolemic shock: the CRISTAL randomized trial. JAMA. 2013;310(17):1809–17.
54. Hartog CS, Reinhart K. CRYSTMAS study adds to concerns about renal safety and increased mortality in sepsis patients. Crit Care. 2012;16(6):454; author reply.
55. Allen CJ, Ruiz XD, Meizoso JP, Ray JJ, Livingstone AS, Schulman CI, et al. Is hydroxyethyl starch safe in penetrating trauma patients? Mil Med. 2016;181(5 Suppl):152–5.
56. Leberle R, Ernstberger A, Loibl M, Merkl J, Bunz M, Creutzenberg M, et al. Association of high volumes of hydroxyethyl starch with acute kidney injury in elderly trauma patients. Injury. 2015;46(1):105–9.
57. Lewis SR, Pritchard MW, Evans DJ, Butler AR, Alderson P, Smith AF, et al. Colloids versus crystalloids for fluid resuscitation in critically ill people. Cochrane Database Syst Rev. 2018;8:CD000567.
58. Corwin HL, Gettinger A, Pearl RG, Fink MP, Levy MM, Abraham E, et al. The CRIT study: anemia and blood transfusion in the critically ill—current clinical practice in the United States. Crit Care Med. 2004;32(1):39–52.
59. Villanueva C, Colomo A, Bosch A, Concepción M, Hernandez-Gea V, Aracil C, et al. Transfusion strategies for acute upper gastrointestinal bleeding. N Engl J Med. 2013;368(1):11–21.
60. Hebert PC, Wells G, Blajchman MA, Marshall J, Martin C, Pagliarello G, et al. A multicenter, randomized, controlled clinical trial of transfusion requirements in critical care. Transfusion Requirements in Critical Care Investigators, Canadian Critical Care Trials Group. N Engl J Med. 1999;340(6):409–17.
61. Holst LB, Haase N, Wetterslev J, Wernerman J, Guttormsen AB, Karlsson S, et al. Lower versus higher hemoglobin threshold for transfusion in septic shock. N Engl J Med. 2014;371(15):1381–91.
62. Carson JL, Stanworth SJ, Roubinian N, Fergusson DA, Triulzi D, Doree C, et al. Transfusion thresholds and other strategies for guiding allogeneic red blood cell transfusion. Cochrane Database Syst Rev. 2016;10:CD002042.
63. Facs.org. [cited 2021 Apr 27]. https://www.facs.org/-/media/files/quality-programs/trauma/tqip/transfusion_guildelines.ashx.
64. Spahn DR, Bouillon B, Cerny V, Coats TJ, Duranteau J, Fernández-Mondéjar E, et al. Management of bleeding and coagulopathy following major trauma: an updated European guideline. Crit Care. 2013;17(2):R76.
65. Leissinger CA, Blatt PM, Hoots WK, Ewenstein B. Role of prothrombin complex concentrates in reversing warfarin anticoagulation: a review of the literature. Am J Hematol. 2008;83(2):137–43.
66. CRASH-2 Trial Collaborators, et al. Effects of tranexamic acid on death, vascular occlusive events, and blood transfusion in trauma patients with significant haemorrhage (CRASH-2): a randomised, placebo-controlled trial. Lancet. 2010;376(9734):23–32.

Compartment Syndrome

15

Rao R. Ivatury

Learning Goals
- Recognize the various compartments in the body
- Understand the relationship between pressure and perfusion
- Learn about the various options to diagnose critical compartment pressure requiring treatment
- Understand the importance of prompt treatment methods of carrying them.

15.1 Introduction

The intricate relationships of pressure and perfusion occur on a regular basis in the many compartments ubiquitous in the human body and have tremendous implications in terms of organ failures, limb loss, and death [1]. This chapter will cover the principal compartment syndromes and briefly sketch the others in smaller compartments.

15.2 Intracranial Compartment Syndrome

The rigid intracranial compartment and the effects of intracranial pressure [IC] elevation are familiar to the emergency surgeon. The outcomes, both short and long term, are poor when the ICP is elevated. In a study of 429 patients with head injury, mortality was significantly higher with ICP greater than 20 mmHg and cerebral perfusion pressure [CPP] lower than 55 mmHg. Of note, even with an elevated CPP of greater than 95 mmHg, disability increased [2]. More recent studies [3–5] are questioning whether the prognosis of traumatic brain injury is totally dependent on ICP and CPP. One study concluded that there are pathologic processes in the injured brain that do not directly involve increases in ICP and decreases in CPP [4]. These authors, in a previous study [3], investigated the relationship between perfusion and focal cerebral blood flow (fCBF) in 23 patients. They noted that CPP did not have a linear relationship with fCBF over a range of 50–150 mmHg in patients who survived. In those who died, four of seven showed some indication of linearity. They concluded that in a normal brain, autoregulation of cerebral blood flow predominates. The onset of a pressure-flow correlation may be an early warning of a clinical deterioration since the metabolic regulation is robust and preserved over a wide range of brain injury. A similar concept of looking beyond

R. R. Ivatury (✉)
Department of Surgery, Virginia Commonwealth University, Richmond, VA, USA

ICP and CPP was proposed by a Swiss group of investigators [5]. They suggested that secondary brain injury may be better managed by multimodal brain monitoring, brain tissue oxygen [$PbtO_2$], cerebral microdialysis, and transcranial Doppler, to optimize cerebral blood flow and the delivery of oxygen/energy substrate [5]. There, evidently, is much more to be discovered in the pressure-perfusion tale of the injured brain. The timing of decompressive craniotomy is also not well-defined, as summarized by the recent review by Coccolini et al. [6].

Diagnosis: ICP monitoring, multimodal brain monitoring

Treatment: Decompressive craniotomy

> **Dos of Treatment**
> - Always consider ICP monitoring in high-risk patients
> - Consult neurosurgeons early
> - Consider decompressive craniotomy if medical measures fail

> **Don'ts of Treatment**
> - Don't forget to elevate head of bed, keep the patient quiet and sedated
> - Don't forget antiepileptic therapy and mannitol (in consultation with neurosurgeons)

15.3 Orbital Compartment Syndrome

The orbit is another closed compartment, bound anteriorly by the eyelids and orbital septum and posteriorly by the bony orbital walls. "Orbital compartment syndrome" [OCS] with the characteristic protrusion of the eye and the limitation of lateral gaze can have disastrous consequences in a short time. The exact mechanism by which OCS causes visual loss has not been fully established, but likely is a result of damage to the optic nerve from prolonged ischemia [7–10]. An excellent collective review was published by McCallum et al. in 2019 [10].

The most common precipitating event of OCS is hemorrhage secondary to trauma which may be subperiosteal or inside the orbit. This is frequently seen in the presence of orbital and facial fractures, surgical trauma from orbital, eyelid and lacrimal surgery, peribulbar or retrobulbar injections, sinus surgery, craniofacial surgery, and neurosurgery [10]. OCS can occur in certain situations of fluid accumulation. Examples include prolonged prone position and facial/periocular chemical burns [10].

Massive fluid resuscitation following extensive thermal burns may cause OCS. Of 13 patients with burns greater than 25% body surface area in one burn center, 5 had intraocular pressures greater than 30 mm Hg and required lateral canthotomy for decompression [8]. Singh et al. [9] reported similar results in a group of 29 patients with burns. In such patients, it is imperative that ocular pressure be monitored.

Symptoms and signs: The patient will typically complain of reduced vision, pain, and increased prominence of the eye or eyelids, with or without double vision. Marked eyelid swelling or ecchymosis with a combination of proptosis, chemosis, and in some cases, extensive subconjunctival hemorrhage may be noted. The vision is often significantly reduced, with no perception of light. Even if there is moderately good vision, color vision can be a sensitive marker of disease severity. Digital ocular palpation often demonstrates resistance to retropulsion and a firm globe indicating an elevated intraocular pressure. Sensation may also be diminished in the distribution of the supra- and infraorbital nerves. Examination of eye movements may demonstrate significant or even complete external ophthalmoplegia [10].

Diagnosis: Ancillary Tests: Computed tomography may be helpful in establishing the diagnosis in milder cases, but is not recommended when the diagnosis of OCS is clear, not to delay treatment. Imaging may help after initial treatment to guide decompression of the orbit. MR with an angiography/venography protocol may assist in finding venous or arterial malformations, lymphangiomatosis of the orbit, or carotid artery pathology [10].

Treatment: Surgical Management. If OCS is suspected and there is evidence of optic nerve compromise, then urgent surgical decompression by a lateral canthotomy and cantholysis (LC/C) is indicated. This can be done expediently at the bedside under local anesthesia. Bony orbital decompression can be considered if adequate response is not achieved after LC/C. Surgery should also target the primary cause of OCS [7–10].

Medical Therapy [10]: Pharmacological agents can be used as an adjunct to surgery or in very mild cases where vision is preserved. The most commonly used agents are corticosteroids, carbonic anhydrase inhibitors, osmotic agents, and aqueous suppressants. All are used with the intention of reducing pressure within the orbital compartment, though their effectiveness in OCS has not been established.

Results [10]: Most patients treated within 2 h will achieve a final Snellen visual acuity better than 6/12. There are reports of mild visual recovery after delayed compression at 5 days and even with no decompression at all. It is therefore still worth considering orbital decompression in cases with delayed presentation. The results of orbital decompression in terms of residual visual acuity or vision loss were recently summarized by Coccolini and associates [6] from the World Society of Emergency Surgery (WSES).

Dos
- Make a clinical diagnosis and institute treatment early

Don'ts
- Waste precious time doing CT scans and other tests

15.4 Thoracic and Mediastinal Compartment Syndrome [11–16]

The syndrome is well known after prolonged cardiac surgery, the effects of excessive volume infusion, leading to cardiac dilatation. The resulting reduction in cardiac output and subendocardial ischemia causes further reduction in cardiac output, and the vicious cycle continues [11]. The phenomenon has also been called "mediastinal tightness". Any attempts at sternal closure cause a reduction of cardiac output and the systolic blood pressure drops. In these cases, leaving the sternum unclosed for a delayed closure after a few days is the recommended approach. On some occasions, the syndrome may manifest itself a few days after the primary sternal closure. Increasing peak airway pressures and increasing hemodynamic instability should suggest the diagnosis [11, 12].

This phenomenon is also seen after trauma [13–15]. In the author's experience, this was illustrated by a young patient who had a gunshot wound of the chest causing a tangential laceration of the heart with cardiac tamponade. He had a prompt thoracotomy, relief of tamponade, and a suture of the laceration. The resuscitation should have ended then. Overzealous fluid administration, however, contributed to a tremendous cardiac dilatation so that the pericardium and the chest could not be closed without compressing the heart and causing hypotension. The chest incision had to be left open with a temporary closure, using an Esmarch bandage sutured to the skin edges. It was closed subsequently, after a few days of diuresis. Three other cases were reported in the literature after chest trauma [13–15]. Kaplan et al. [12] presented a case of a patient with gunshot wounds through the heart and descending thoracic aorta who developed TCS upon clamshell thoracotomy closure. In that case, closure of the chest precipitated an immediate elevation in airway pressure and rapid hemodynamic collapse. Wandling and An [13] described a case of TCS following a chest injury. They identified some risk factors in their patient that precipitated the TCS: intrathoracic hemostatic packing and a trap-door incision causing substantial tissue injury and the need for greater resuscitation fluids. Amos et al. [14] reported a patient with severe blunt chest trauma that developed TCC and was managed with an early implementation of VV-ECMO. This allowed primary closure of the thoracotomy.

Diagnosis and treatment: These cases illustrate the prevention of the complication, prompt diagnosis, and timely intervention by chest decompression when it occurs [15].

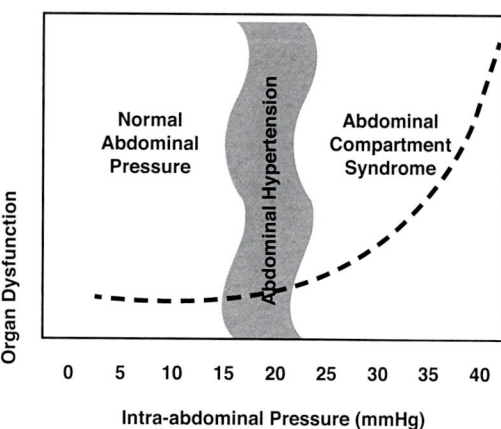

Fig. 15.1 Progression of IAP (intra-abdominal pressure) from normal to IAH (intra-abdominal hypertension) to abdominal compartment syndrome with organ failures

> **Dos**
> - Keep thoracic compartment syndrome (TCS) in mind and try to prevent it

> **Don'ts**
> - Close chest incisions by force and precipitate TCS.

15.5 Abdominal Compartment Syndrome [ACS]

Abdominal compartment syndrome [ACS] has tremendous relevance in the care of critically ill or injured patients., because of the effects of elevated pressure within the confined space of the abdomen on multiple organ systems. We now recognize that ACS should be viewed as the end-result of a progressive, unchecked rise in IAP, called intra-abdominal hypertension, (IAH), as illustrated in Fig. 15.1. We also have learnt that the adverse effects of elevated IAP occur at lower levels than previously thought [16].

15.5.1 Historical Background

The pathophysiology of IAH has been known since late 1800s and is well reviewed in the monograph [16]. Fietsam et al., From William Beaumont Hospital, Royal Oak, Michigan, were the architects of the term intra-abdominal compartment syndrome [17]. As with many advances in medicine, this precious knowledge was forgotten, rediscovered, and forgotten again. Many proponents of the syndrome faced skepticism and ridicule till the clinical syndrome was rediscovered in patients with life-threatening abdominal injuries undergoing 'abbreviated laparotomy' [16, 18–22].

Our knowledge of IAH and ACS was due to the experience of trauma centers dealing with the nightly horrors of "America's uncivil war", as dubbed by Schwab [22]. The phenomena were popularized by the clinical practice of such advances as IAP monitoring by bladder pressure and non-closure of fascia after laparotomy ("open abdomen") [18–21]. Further advances were also realized through the efforts World Society of Abdominal Compartment Syndrome (WSACS). Established in 2004 in Noosa, Australia, the Society redefined the current concepts of IAH and ACS through multinational clinical trials, literature review and analyses, multiple publications, a monograph on the subject [16], and guideline and consensus development [23–25].

WSACS consensus definitions of IAH and ACS [23–25] are summarized:

IAP: Intra-abdominal pressure [IAP] is the pressure concealed within the abdominal cavity. IAP should be measured at end-expiration in the complete supine position after ensuring that abdominal muscle contractions are absent and with the transducer zeroed at the level of the mid-axillary line. The reference standard for intermittent IAP measurement is via the bladder with a maximal instillation volume of 25 mL of sterile saline. Normal IAP is approximately 5–7 mmHg in critically ill adults.

IAH is defined by **a sustained or repeated** pathologic elevation of IAP ≥ 12 mmHg. It is graded as follows: Grade I: IAP 12–15 mmHg, Grade II: IAP 16–20 mmHg, Grade III: IAP 21–25 mmHg, Grade IV: IAP > 25 mmHg.

ACS: Abdominal compartment syndrome [ACS] is defined as a sustained IAP > 20 mmHg with or without an Abdominal Perfusion Pressure (APP = Mean Arterial Pressure, MAP-IAP) < 60 mmHg that is associated with new organ dysfunction/failure. It should be noted that this definition *moves ACS to a much earlier point in the trajectory of clinical course than the traditional fully manifested syndrome with multi-organ failure.*

Primary ACS is a condition associated with injury or disease in the abdomino-pelvic region that frequently requires early surgical or interventional radiological intervention.

Secondary ACS refers to conditions that do not originate from the abdomino-pelvic region. Recurrent ACS refers to the condition in which ACS redevelops following previous surgical or medical treatment of primary or secondary ACS.

Risk Factors for IAH/ACS [16, 26–30]: ACS can develop in both nonsurgical and surgical patients. These factors include: Diminished abdominal wall compliance (abdominal surgery, major trauma, major burns, prone positioning); increased intraluminal contents (e.g., acute pancreatitis, hemoperitoneum/pneumoperitoneum or intraperitoneal fluid collections, intra-abdominal infection/abscess, intra-abdominal or retroperitoneal tumors, liver dysfunction/cirrhosis with ascites, capillary leak/fluid resuscitation from massive fluid resuscitation or positive fluid balance); damage control laparotomy. Other miscellaneous causes include bacteremia, coagulopathy, massive incisional hernia repair, obesity or increased body mass index, PEEP, peritonitis, and sepsis.

15.5.2 Pathophysiology of ACS [16, 26–30]

IAH affects multiple organ systems.

15.5.2.1 Cardiovascular Effects

Elevation in IAP leads to a reduction in cardiac output, most consistently seen at an IAP > 20 mmHg, due to a combination of decreased inferior vena caval flow and an increased thoracic pressure (which decreases both inferior and superior vena caval flow). Other contributory factors include cardiac compression, decreased ventricular end-diastolic volumes, and marked increase in systemic afterload. This may lead to spuriously elevated central venous pressure, pulmonary artery pressure, and pulmonary artery occlusion (wedge) pressure. Combined with a reduced CO, this may erroneously suggest a state of hypervolemia or biventricular failure. Improvement in CO after a saline fluid bolus may be therapeutic and clarify the diagnostic conundrum.

15.5.2.2 Pulmonary Dysfunction

With an acute elevation in IAP, respiratory failure characterized by high ventilatory pressures, hypoxia, and hypercarbia eventually develops. Diaphragmatic elevation leads to a reduction in static and dynamic pulmonary compliance. The increase in IAP also reduces total lung capacity, functional residual capacity, and residual volume. These lead to ventilation-perfusion abnormalities and hypoventilation producing hypoxia and hypercarbia, respectively. Chronic elevation of IAP, as in central obesity, also produces these derangements in the form of obesity hypoventilation syndrome [28]. Abdominal decompression improves the acute respiratory failure almost immediately. A porcine model by Simon et al. demonstrated that prior hemorrhage and resuscitation (ischemia-reperfusion injury) exacerbate the cardiopulmonary sequelae of IAH [31].

15.5.2.3 Renal Sequelae

Oliguria progressing to anuria, and prerenal azotemia unresponsive to volume expansion, characterize the renal dysfunction of ACS. Oliguria can be seen at IAP of 15–20 mmHg, while increases to 30 mmHg or above lead to anuria. Volume expansion and the use of dopaminergic agonists or loop diuretics may be ineffective in these patients. However, decompression and reduction in IAP promptly reverse oliguria, usually inducing a vigorous diuresis. The mechanisms of renal derangements with IAH involve reduced absolute and proportional renal arterial flow, increased renal vascular resistance with changes in intrarenal regional blood flow, reduced glomerular filtration, and increased tubular sodium and water retention [16, 26–29].

15.5.2.4 Abdominal Visceral Abnormalities

Mesenteric arterial, hepatic arterial, intestinal mucosal, hepatic microcirculatory, and portal venous blood flow all have been shown to be reduced with IAH in animal models [16, 26, 31, 32]. Clinically, many investigators demonstrated that gut mucosal acidosis, demonstrable by intramucosal pH (pHi) measured with gastric tonometery, is a sensitive change after ACS [16, 18, 26]. Further increases in IAP may lead to intestinal infarction, often present in the ileum and right colon without arterial thrombosis. Prolonged low-grade elevation of IAP may be associated with bacterial translocation in rat and murine models [33]. Thus, despite normal systemic hemodynamics, profound splanchnic ischemia can be ongoing with IAH. It has been suggested that such ischemia is associated with an increased incidence of multisystem organ failure, sepsis, and increased mortality [16]. Furthermore, laboratory evidence suggests that prior hemorrhage and resuscitation actually lower the critical levels of IAP at which mesenteric ischemia begins [31, 32]. Many investigators note a relationship between IAH, sepsis, multisystem organ failure, and the need for reoperation and mortality [26–33]. *These are some of the strongest arguments for the routine measurement of IAP in critically ill patients.*

15.5.2.5 Abdominal Wall Abnormalities

Increased IAP has been shown to reduce abdominal wall blood flow by the direct, compressive effects of IAH under conditions of stable systemic perfusion, leading to local ischemia and edema [26, 27]. This can decrease abdominal compliance (defined as a measure of the ease of abdominal expansion, which is determined by the elasticity of the abdominal wall and diaphragm and expressed as the change in intra-abdominal volume per change in IAP) and exacerbate IAH. Abdominal wall muscle and fascial ischemia may contribute to such wound complications as dehiscence, herniation, and necrotizing fasciitis.

15.5.2.6 Intracranial Derangements

Elevated intracranial pressure (ICP) and reduced cerebral perfusion pressure (CPP) have been described with acute changes in IAP in animal models and in human studies [34]. In animal models the changes in ICP and CPP are independent of changes in pulmonary or cardiovascular function and appear to be the direct result of elevated intrathoracic and central venous pressures with impairment of cerebral venous outflow. Reduction in IAP by surgical decompression reverses this derangement. Furthermore, chronic elevation in IAP has been implicated as an important etiologic factor in the development of benign intracranial hypertension, or pseudotumor cerebri, in the morbidly obese [26–28].

15.5.3 Poly-compartment Syndrome [34, 35]

A poly-compartment syndrome, where two or more anatomical compartments have elevated compartmental pressures, is a potential companion of IAH, e.g., intra-abdominal leading to intra-thoracic and consequent intracranial hypertension. IAH helps to explain the severe pathophysiological condition occurring in patients with cardiorenal, hepatopulmonary, and hepatorenal syndromes. When more than one compartment is affected, an exponential detrimental effect on end-organ function in both immediate and distant organs may occur. The compliance of each compartment is the key to determining the transmission of a given compartmental pressure from one compartment to another. In high-risk patients, these interactions must be considered for optimal management [35]. All the compartments, namely, intracranial, intrathoracic, and intra-abdominal, have an interplay. Scalea et al. [34] noted that our therapeutic efforts to increase CPP in patients with concomitant head and multisystem injury may have adverse effects on pulmonary function. This will necessitate efforts to improve lung function by increasing ventilator support. The result may be a further increase in IAP and ICP. In some patients, this intracranial hypertension may be resistant to all conventional interventions, until abdominal decompression is performed to reduce IAP and, secondarily, the ICP. This clinical scenario has been dubbed the poly-compartment syndrome [35].

15.5.4 Recommendations in Management [23–25]

The most effective approach in the medical and surgical management of IAH and ACS is best summarized by the algorithms recommended by WSACS (Figs. 15.2 and 15.3) based on the GRADE methodology [Grading, Assessment, Development, and Evaluation]. Quality of evidence is graded from high [A] to very low [D]. Recommendations range from strong recommendations to weaker suggestions.

Results of management: As noted earlier, the efforts of WSACS made a profound impact on our understanding of the disease and our clinical approach. Anticipation of the complication, measures of prophylaxis, earlier recognition, and intervention: all of these translated into fewer organ failures and better survival.

Effect of decompressive laparotomy in IAH and ACS: In 2018, Van Damme and De Waele [36] published a meta-analysis of 15 articles, including three in children only [aged 18 years or younger]. Of 286 patients, 49.7% had primary ACS. The baseline mean IAP in adults decreased with an average of 18.2 ± 6.5 mmHg following decompression, from 31.7 ± 6.4 mmHg to 13.5 ± 3.0 mmHg. There was a decrease in HR [12.2 ± 9.5 beats/min; $p = 0.04$], CVP [4.6 ± 2.3 mmHg; $p = 0.022$], PCWP [5.8 ± 2.3 mmHg; $p = 0.029$], and PIP [10.1 ± 3.9 cmH$_2$O; $p < 0.001$] and a mean increase in P/F ratio [70.4 ± 49.4; $p < 0.001$] and UO [95.3 ± 105.3 mL/h; $p < 0.001$]. In children, there was a significant increase in MAP [20.0 ± 2.3 mmHg; $p = 0.006$], P/F ratio [238.2; $p < 0.001$], and UO [2.88 ± 0.64 mL/kg/h; $p < 0.001$] and a decrease in CVP [7 mmHg; $p = 0.016$] and PIP [9.9 cmH$_2$O; $p = 0.002$]. The overall mortality rate was higher in children following decompressive laparotomy. The authors confirmed that decompressive laparotomy resulted in a significantly lower IAP and had beneficial effects on hemodynamic, respiratory, and renal parameters, even though mortality remained significant, 49.7% in adults and 60.8% in children.

Impact of IAH monitoring and intervention: In a prospective, observational study, Cheatham and Safcsak [37] studied 478 consecutive patients who were treated with open abdomen for IAH and ACS according to a "a continually revised management algorithm" and noted a significantly increased patient survival to hospital discharge from 50 to 72% and an increase in same-admission primary fascial closure from 59 to 81% over the period of the study. This was one of the first clinical series showing better outcomes with a management focus on IAP. Balogh and associates [38] prospectively analyzed 81 consecutive severely injured shock/trauma patients (mean ISS 29) admitted to the intensive care unit with a protocol of two hourly intra-abdominal pressure (IAP) monitoring. No patient developed ACS, even though 61 (75%) had IAH. One patient with IAH and one without died. Multiorgan failure occurred in 1 patient without IAH [5%] vs 4 with IAH [7%]. The authors considered that monitoring and intervening for a less serious IAH avoided the deadly ACS.

As optimistic as these paradigms have been, many institutions around the world have not utilized them and benefited from them. In 2013,

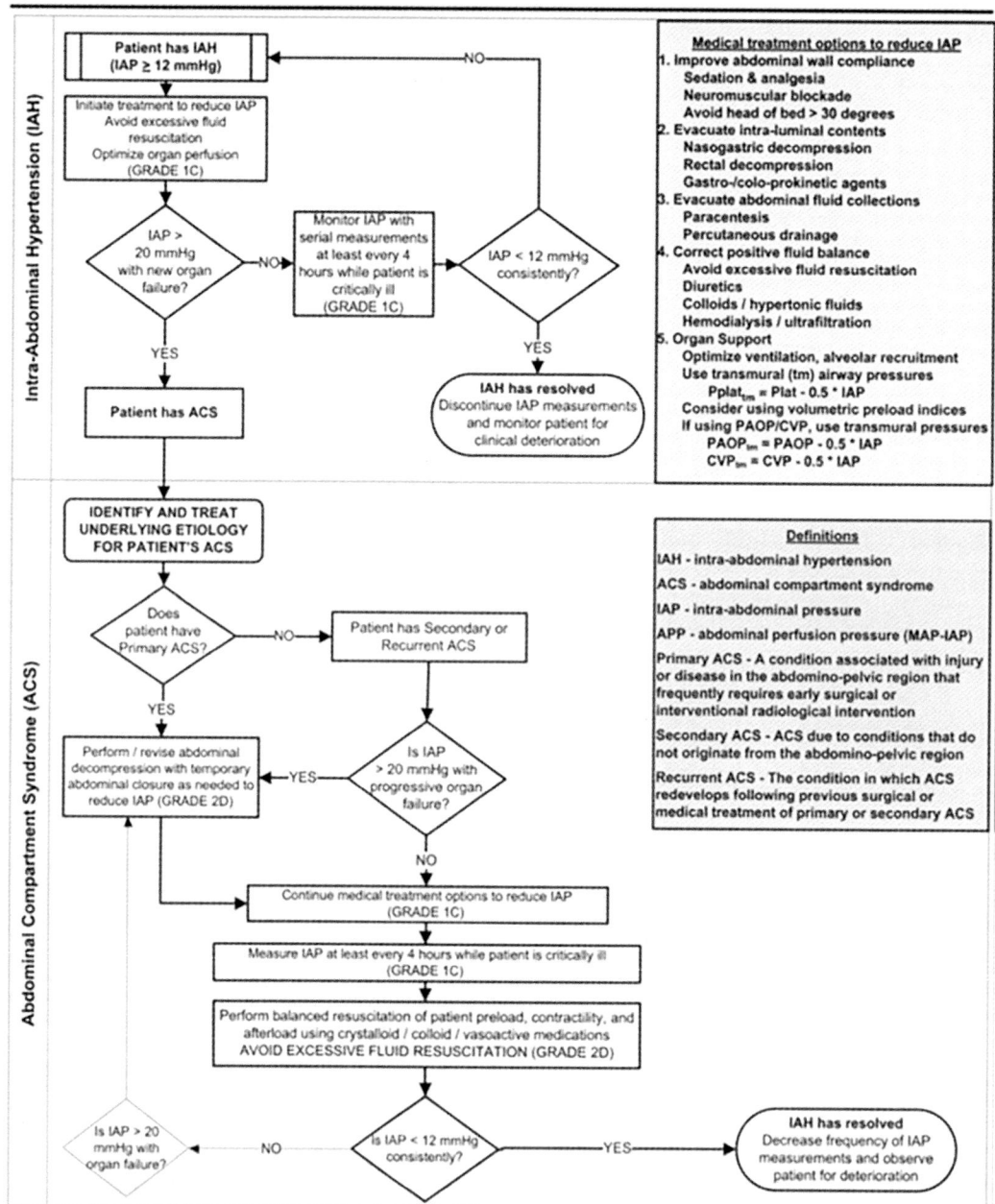

Fig. 15.2 Management algorithm for IAH and ACS (Reproduced from Kirkpatrick AW et al.: Intra-abdominal hypertension and the abdominal compartment syndrome: updated consensus definitions and clinical practice guidelines from the World Society of the Abdominal Compartment Syndrome. Intensive Care Med. 2013;39(7):1190-206)

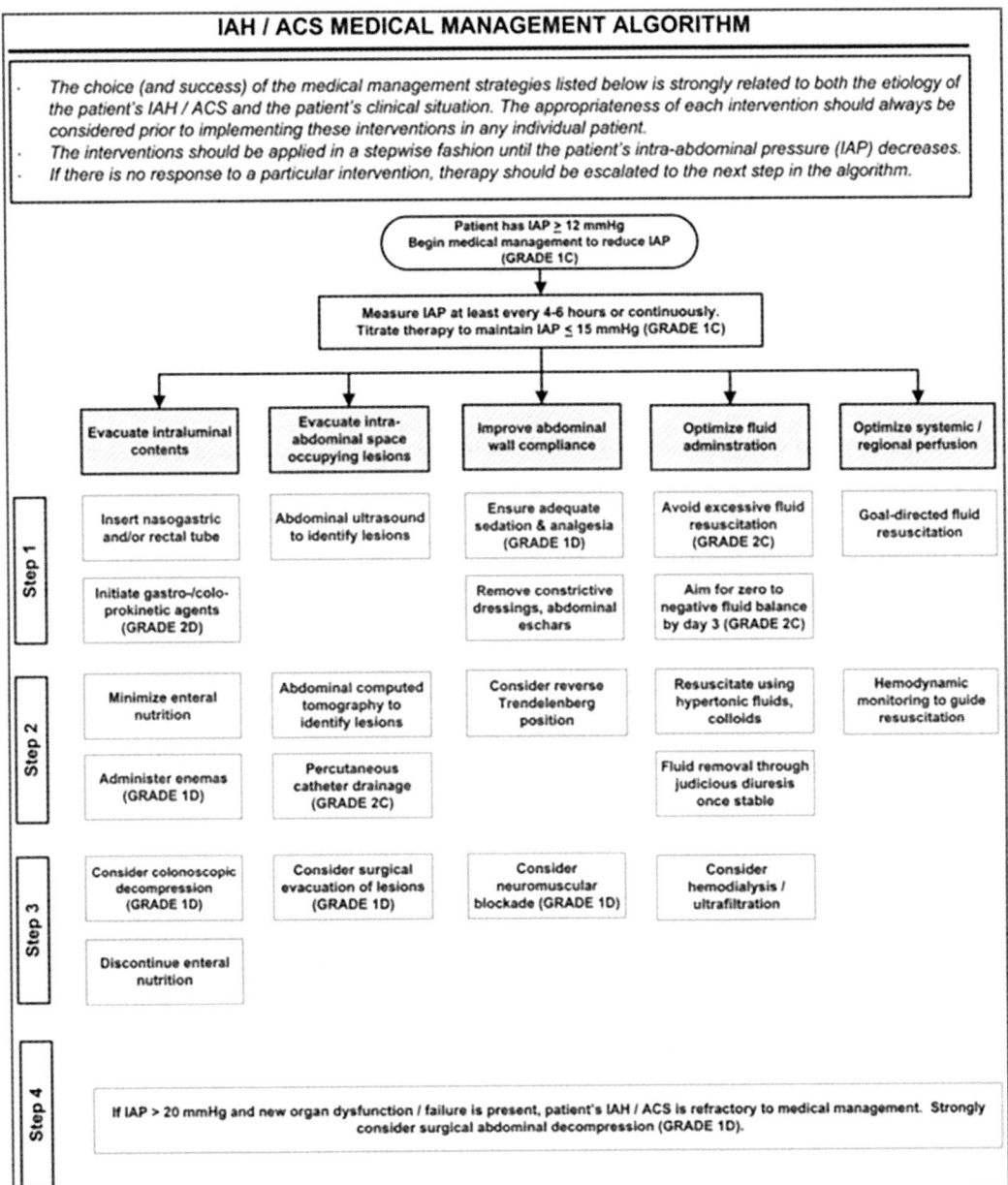

Fig. 15.3 Medical management of IAH and ACS. (Reproduced from Kirkpatrick AW et al.: Intra-abdominal hypertension and the abdominal compartment syndrome: updated consensus definitions and clinical practice guidelines from the World Society of the Abdominal Compartment Syndrome. Intensive Care Med. 2013;39(7):1190-206)

the WSACS distributed a survey of 13 questions to 10,000 members of the WSACS, the European Society of Intensive Care Medicine [ESICM], and the Society of Critical Care Medicine [SCCM]. A total of 2244 clinicians responded [response rate, 22.4%], mostly from North America. The majority of responders [85%] were familiar with IAP/IAH/ACS, but only 28% were aware of the WSACS consensus definitions. Overall knowledge scores were low (43 ± 15%), suggesting ignorance of established consensus definitions and guidelines [39]. A Dutch survey documented that many of their surgeons exhibited a good knowledge of IAH and ACS, but only 27% used this in their daily practice [40]. A similar lack of practice of definitions and guidelines was reported among German pediatric intensivists [41] and Australian critical care nurses [42]. In 2019, the WSACS, now with the new name of World Society of Abdominal Compartment, conducted a revisit of its international survey. They did note an improvement in general awareness and knowledge regarding IAP, IAH, and ACS. The level of understanding and awareness of WSACS guidelines, however, remained low [43]. The editorials of the members of WSACS [44, 45] reflect their continuing frustration with the underappreciation of the critical phenomena of IAH and ACS.

15.5.5 Quaternary ACS [46, 47]

Kirkpatrick et al. [46] recently brought attention to elevated intra-abdominal pressure following abdominal wall reconstruction (AWR) in patients with massive ventral hernia. They reviewed the pathophysiology and warned that surgeons should carefully measure intra-abdominal pressure and its resultant effects on respiratory parameters and function during the reconstruction. They reasserted that IAP is especially at risk of dangerous elevation in instances of "loss of domain" patients with massive ventral hernia in whom the bowel has been outside the peritoneal cavity for a long time. The authors then reviewed potential strategies for surgeons to battle this complication preoperatively: muscular paralysis either temporarily or semi-permanently (Botox induced paralysis, etc.), progressive pneumoperitoneum (PPP), and permanently removing hernial contents by bowel resection. This is an important report for all undertaking abdominal wall reconstruction.

These theoretical considerations got further support from a recent series from Porto by Quintela et al. [47]. Five of 115 patients were diagnosed with QACS, all being hernias with loss of domain (LOD) ≥20% and showing major renal and pulmonary impairment. Four patients had predictable transitory QACS, yet one patient died despite damage control surgery. A total of 19 patients had LOD ≥20%, 14 without QACS development and 5 with this entity. The most important difference between the groups was a significantly higher variation in peak respiratory pressure (PRP) measured before incision and intraoperatively. An LOD ≥20% was an important risk factor. PRP variations between 6 and 10 mmHg during fascial closure was a significant marker for adverse endpoints in AWR.

In summary, IAH and ACS are common complications in the care of the critically ill or injured patients, medical or surgical, young or old. They can cause profound morbidity and mortality, if unanticipated, unrecognized, and uncontrolled. Appropriate monitoring and early intervention, based on the precepts of WSACS, can minimize organ failures, morbidity, and mortality.

Diagnosis: Anticipate, measure IAP

Treatment: Medical management and surgical decompressive laparotomy for recalcitrant cases

> **Dos: Preventive Measures to Be Kept in Mind**
> - In all high-risk situations, institute IAP monitoring q4.
> - Institute medical measures for persistent elevation of IAP and if this is not successful, strongly consider abdominal decompression by laparotomy with open abdomen approach
> - Employ negative pressure vac systems for management of open abdomen
> - Try to close the open abdomen as early as possible to avoid complications.

> **Don'ts**
> - Neglect IAP measurement in ALL critically ill patients.
> - "Hyper resuscitate critically ill patients

15.6 Extremity Compartment Syndrome

Compartment syndrome in the extremities is a particularly frequent and complex clinical entity. It can result from an increase in the contents of rigid compartments. Examples include fractures, hematoma, soft tissue injury, crush syndrome, revascularization, exercise, fluid infusion, snake bite, nephrotic syndrome, myositis, and osteomyelitis. It is also caused by reduced compartmental volume such as after burns. This review will summarize general pathophysiology and controversies in diagnosis and treatment of leg compartment syndrome and then briefly outline other areas.

15.6.1 Pathophysiology

Several theories have been proposed to explain the compartment syndrome [48–51]. One points to an increase in volume and its profound effect on the intra-compartmental pressure. This increase in interstitial tissue pressure, exceeding the perfusion pressure, results in a narrowed A–V gradient, capillary collapse, as well as muscle and tissue ischemia. Ischemic skeletal muscle responds by the secretion of histamine-like substances. The resultant increased vascular permeability leads to leakage of plasma, sludging of capillary flow, and worsening of muscle ischemia. Myocytes undergo lysis; myofibrillar proteins escape into the interstitium, osmotically extract fluid, increasing the compartmental pressure further. Muscle ischemia worsens and perpetuates this vicious cycle.

Other theories postulate the presence of a critical closing pressure [termed the P crit], approximately 30 mmHg, within the muscle compartments, which determines the level at which muscle blood flow decreases. Arterioles allegedly require high arteriole-tissue gradient to maintain patency. Conditions causing extremity compartment syndrome (ECS) cause a reduction or removal of this gradient and lead to arteriolar collapse [49–51].

Regardless of the mechanism, the effect is ischemia-induced cellular destruction and alterations in muscle cell membrane, leading to the release of myoglobin into the circulation. This rhabdomyolysis results in renal injury. The pathophysiology of ECS following vascular occlusion may differ slightly, ischemia-reperfusion injury playing a dominant role and is discussed in detail below.

15.6.1.1 Prevalence

Tibial fracture accounts for approximately 10% of all cases of ECS and seems to be more common in open fractures. According to Schmidt [51], the fracture may be segmental in 48%, a bicondylar tibial plateau fracture in 18%, a medial knee fracture dislocation in 53%. Vascular injury is the other frequent mechanism. Feliciano et al. [52] reported that 19% of patients with vascular injury required fasciotomy for ECS. Secondary ECS describes the syndrome developing without significant injury to the extremity itself and is an iatrogenic phenomenon occurring in massively injured patients receiving large-volume resuscitation. In the first series from Grady reported by Tremblay et al. [53], 10 of 11,996 patients and a mean of 3.1 extremities developed this complication. Mortality in the group was 70%. In their follow-up series [54], these authors presented a similar group of very severely injured patients who had received massive resuscitation, but who were carefully monitored for compartment syndrome. The incidence of renal failure and death was reduced but was still substantial at 35%. Of the 46 extremities with ECS, 7 required amputation.

15.6.1.2 Diagnosis

There are cardinal p's of ECS, namely, pallor, pulselessness, paraesthesia, pressure, poikilothermia, and paralysis. They are, however, more specific than sensitive. Conventional radiographs, computed tomographic scans, and magnetic resonance imaging studies may be indicated in selected patients with compartment syndrome of the pelvis, thigh, and so on [48–51, 55, 56].

Serum biomarkers of inflammation [57, 58]: White cell count (WCC), erythrocyte sedimentation rate (ESR) and C-reactive protein (CRP), creatine kinase, and lactate levels rise, due to muscle breakdown and anaerobic metabolism. Creatinine kinase levels of >2000 units/L can be a warning sign of compartment syndrome in a sedated and ventilated patient. Ischemia-modified albumin [IMA] has been shown to rise with reasonable sensitivity and specificity in the presence of critical limb ischemia. However, no serum marker has been shown to have adequate sensitivity and specificity to quantify the level of skeletal muscle ischemia.

The testing of regional or local biomarker levels such as intramuscular glucose and pH offer had greater potential, in animal experiments. Doro et al. measured intramuscular glucose in 12 canine models and found that an intramuscular glucose concentration of less than 97 mg/dL was 100% sensitive [95% CI 73–100%] and 75% specific [95% CI 40–94%]. These changes could be detected as soon as 15 min after induction of compartment syndrome [57, 58].

The surface pH of skeletal muscle has been confirmed to be a sensitive indicator of peripheral muscle blood flow. The development of probes to measure intramuscular pH is a more recent concept. In an initial study of 62 patients, its sensitivity and specificity were found to be significantly higher than intra-compartmental pressure monitoring. Invasive pH monitoring continues to be investigated, but is not yet a clinical reality [57].

Compartment pressure (CP) monitoring is the most useful test for diagnosis but is fraught with problems [55–63]. This can be performed bedside by several techniques, including the Stryker Quick Pressure Monitor Instrument, manometric IV pump method, and the slit catheter technique. The Stryker instrument has the advantage of simplicity. After being zeroed, the needle is inserted perpendicular to the skin, then into the muscle compartment in question. A total of 0.3 mL of sterile saline is injected through the needle into the compartment. Equilibrium is reached in a few seconds, and the compartmental pressure is then read on a digital screen. If the Stryker system is not available, a pressure transducing system, like that used for an arterial line and similar to Whitesides' original description, can be used. Normal resting CP is approximately 8 mmHg in adults and slightly higher (13–16 mmHg) in children.

There are several issues both in the measurement of the CP and in interpreting the results. The threshold pressure at which a surgeon should intervene is an area that remains unresolved. This difficulty is highlighted by Prayson et al. [63] who carefully followed blood pressure and compartment pressure in 19 patients with isolated lower extremity fractures who did not have compartment syndrome by clinical criteria, or at follow-up. Eighty four percent of the patients had at least one measurement in which their perfusion pressure was less than 30 mmHg, and 58% with less than 20 mmHg.

The most common threshold used by clinicians when assessing compartment pressures remains the delta pressure (ΔP), which is the diastolic blood pressure minus the intracompartmental pressure. ΔP less than or equal to 30 mmHg is defined as ECS. Again, difficulties arise. First, there is spatial variation in the pressure within a given compartment, with pressures being highest within 5 cm of the fracture and more centrally in the muscle. It has never been established whether one should obtain pressures near the fracture to obtain the highest pressure, or measure further away [outside the zone of injury] to obtain a pressure that may be more representative of the majority of the compartment. Second, there may be uncertainty and/or variability in measured values of the pressure. Another potential source of uncertainty when calculating perfusion pressure is what blood pressure value to use, especially if the patient is under general anesthesia. It is recommended to use preoperative blood pressure values when calculating perfusion pressure in a patient under general anesthesia, except when the patient is going to remain under anesthesia for several more hours [49, 55–60].

Continuous CP monitoring with a slit catheter inserted into the compartment and connected to a continuous pressure transducer and trends in CP over time has been suggested to be a more useful than a single pressure. McQueen et al. [61] found the sensitivity and specificity of continuous intracompartmental pressure monitoring to be high, with estimated positive and negative predictive values of 93% and 99%, respectively.

Determination of tissue oxygenation spectroscopy [49, 64–70]: *NIRS* is a noninvasive method for assessing levels of oxygenated muscle hemoglobin and myoglobin. When blood flow is decreased, a reduction in local oxygen saturation and muscle oxygen tension can be seen. An inverse correlation between CP and oxygenation and a correlation between perfusion pressure and oxygenation were demonstrated in an animal model. A human model of compartment syndrome showed that both tissue oxygenation and CP significantly correlated with a decrease in deep peroneal conduction, cutaneous peroneal sensitivity, and pain. Multiple case reports have been published detailing the use of NIRS as an adjunct for continuous monitoring of lower extremity perfusion [69, 70]. Shuler et al. [70] published a series of patients who underwent fasciotomies based on CP monitoring with simultaneous NIRS monitoring. All compartments showed decreasing tissue oxygenation with decreasing perfusion pressure. NIRS has also been used to characterize changes in perfusion following tibial fracture in patients without compartment syndrome, as compared with subjects' contralateral extremity and uninjured extremities in other controls. Of note, a lack of posttraumatic hyperemia (15% increase in tissue oxygenation seen in injured extremities) was felt to actually represent a compartment syndrome even if oxygenation in the injured leg is equivalent to that in the uninjured extremity.

Tissue oxygenation, as determined by NIRS, may help avoid fasciotomy. In a study of patients with clinical signs of compartment syndrome after revascularization surgery for lower limb ischemia, Arató et al. [71] reported that measurement of compartmental pressure and NIRS-measured tissue oxygenation could be used to determine whether fasciotomy was needed. Patients with pressure less than 40 mmHg and normal tissue oxygen saturation were treated conservatively.

While NIRS has the potential to offer the ability to objectively measure tissue perfusion in a noninvasive and continuous manner, it has many limitations, including limited depth of tissue penetration and the tendency for skin color and subcutaneous bruising hematomas to adversely affect readings.

Recently, Resonance Raman spectroscopy (RRS), using excitation by a Krypton ion laser, was tested in animal models of hemorrhagic shock and resuscitation [72] in our laboratory. Raman spectroscopy-derived sublingual oxygen tension [Smo_2] was calculated as the ratio of the oxygenated heme spectral peak height to the sum of the oxyhemoglobin and deoxyhemoglobin spectral peak heights. Measurements were compared with central venous oxygen tension [$Scvo_2$] as well as with other indicators of oxygenation. Smo_2 was significantly [$p < 0.0001$] correlated with $Scvo_2$ [$r = 0.80$], lactate [$r = j0.78$], base excess [$r = 0.80$], and shed blood volume [$r = j0.75$]. The technique was thought to show promise as a method to noninvasively monitor tissue oxygenation. In a subsequent study [73], the ability of resonance Raman spectroscopy to monitor tissue hemoglobin oxygenation [$RRS-StO_2$] during hemorrhage was confirmed to be superior to NIRS tissue hemoglobin oxygenation [$NIRS-StO_2$]. Future investigations, hopefully, will focus on the ability of $RRC-StO_2$ to diagnose critical muscle ischemia from evolving ECS and facilitate an early diagnosis of ECS.

An ultrasound-based measurement [74]: In a prospective study, an ultrasound-based measurement was used to determine the relative elasticity [RE] of the affected and unaffected limb. The difference in the compartment depth with a probe pressure of 80 mmHg (P 80) on the limb minus (P 0 = the compartment depth without compression corresponding to 100%) resulted in a value of relative elasticity (%). These values were compared with the invasive needle measurement [mmHg] regarding their intraindividual difference and correlation of the compartmental pressure. In six trauma patients, the relative elasticity in their paired limbs showed a significant difference. The average values of the repetitively measured RE and the ICP showed a high level of correlation (spearman correlation coefficient: $r = 0.929$). The RE less than 10.5% of the anterior tibial compartment had a sensitivity of 95.8% and a specificity of 87.5% to an appropriate diagnosis of ACS. Obviously, this needs confirmation in lager groups to prove its clinical applicability.

15.6.2 Problems in Treatment

The only effective treatment for ECS is immediate surgical fasciotomy, releasing the skin and muscle fascia in order to reduce compartment pressure. Unfortunately, none of the methods described above tell us what the critical CP is, even though all agree that early diagnosis and the timeliness of fasciotomy obviously are terribly important. Matsen and Krugmire [48] suggest 2–4 h of ischemia as causing functional impairment of muscles and 4–12 h for irreversibility. For nerve tissue, the critical times were 30–45 min and 12–24 h. Awareness of high-risk groups of patients and high-risk situations, when critical muscle ischemia either goes undetected or occurs very early, must be kept in mind. These include tissue previously subjected to intervals of ischemia, patients under general anesthesia, sedated, or obtunded, and those receiving postoperative epidurals after tibial fracture fixation [75–77].

The importance of timeliness of fasciotomy in vascular injuries was investigated by Farber et al. [78], analyzing National Trauma Data Bank data of 612 patients who underwent fasciotomies, 543 early and 69 late (before 8 h and after 8 h of vascular repair). Patients in the early fasciotomy group had lower amputation rate and shorter total hospital stay compared with those in the late fasciotomy group. Early fasciotomy was associated with a fourfold lower risk of amputation and 23% shorter hospital stay, on multivariable analysis.

The role of timely fasciotomy in extremity crush injuries was addressed by two recent articles from the Middle East wars. In the first series [79] of 336 patients, the majority of the fasciotomies were to the lower leg (49%) and forearm (23%). Patients who underwent fasciotomy after evacuation had higher rates of muscle excision (25% vs. 11%), amputation (31% vs. 15%), and mortality (19% vs. 5%) compared with patients who received their fasciotomies in the combat theater, suggesting the poor outcomes of delayed fasciotomies. In a subsequent study, the army confirmed correction of these unfavorable results by an education program designed to improve surgeon knowledge [80].

Surprisingly, timely fasciotomy in the civilian setting was noted to be an exception rather than the rule. Examples include several series from civilian trauma centers. Feliciano et al. [52] reported on 25 fasciotomies (25 upper and 100 lower) and that delayed or incomplete fasciotomies resulted in 75% of amputations. In a review of 81 popliteal artery injuries (39 arterial and 42 combined), Fainzilber et al. [81] noted that 6 of the 35 patients who did not have a primary fasciotomy required an amputation. The current author and his former group [82] noted two amputations for extensive popliteal vascular injury despite primary fasciotomy. One amputation was the result of a delayed fasciotomy and failure of vascular repair. They also observed that four of nine patients who had neurologic deficit in the extremity also had failure of vascular repair and delayed fasciotomy. Another multicenter series from Canada [83] documented significant delays in diagnosis and treatment in both traumatic and nontraumatic cases of ECS.

Kashuk et al. [84] analyzed 83 cases of compartment syndrome over 7 years at a distinguished trauma center. Eight percent died after predominantly orthopedic injuries. Six percent had amputations. Repeated debridement of dead muscle was needed due to delayed fasciotomy in 8%. Of note, CP monitoring was not used in any of them. Another 7% had iatrogenic transection of superficial peroneal nerve during the performance of fasciotomy. The authors concluded that compartment syndrome remained a significant diagnostic and management challenge with great morbidity in terms of limb loss and neurologic outcome. They proposed a key pathway with a multidisciplinary approach for optimal outcome in these patients [84].

An early fasciotomy is recommended before arterial exploration for vascular injuries in high-risk patients [those with prolonged ischemia time, significant preoperative hypotension, associated crush injury, combined arterial and venous injury, or the need for a major venous ligation in the lower limb] [85].

The role of fasciotomy in ECS caused by vascular occlusion is still imperfect [86–88]. If ECS is diagnosed late, fasciotomy is of no benefit and may lead to adverse effects such as severe infection in the necrotic muscle. A compartment with necrotic muscle unopened by fasciotomy may heal with scar tissue and may result in a more functional extremity with fewer complications [89]. This notion of delayed fasciotomy causing more harm than good was supported by this 1989 editorial from the distinguished Blaisdell [87, 88], who was called the father of modern trauma care: "The question is, what factor is responsible for the increased compartmental pressure?— When a limb has been revascularized after many hours of ischemia, the reason for the swelling is not quite so clear. I contend that we still do not have a clear understanding of the reason for the high compartment pressures, nor do we have the precise point at which fasciotomy will be more beneficial than harmful."

The ill effects of delayed fasciotomy were emphasized by other authors. A series of mostly adult patients by Sheridan and Matsen [89] found as early as in 1976 that outcomes were significantly worse for patients who underwent fasciotomy later than 12 h after the onset of compartment syndrome, with only 8% of patients achieving normal function versus 68% of patients who underwent early fasciotomy. Even in crush injuries, patients with closed crush injuries treated by late fasciotomy [≥24 h] had worse outcomes than those treated nonoperatively, as noted by Reis and Michaelson [79], since skin served an important role as a barrier to infection. Likewise, Finkelstein et al. [86] contend that infection secondary to delayed fasciotomy for a crush injury has greater morbidity than the muscle contractures that will occur from myonecrosis.

15.6.2.1 Important Technical Aspects of Fasciotomy [90]

The lower leg has four fascial compartments: anterior, lateral, superficial posterior, and deep posterior. Fasciotomies for CS should decompress all four compartments and may be done with a dual or single incision approach. The dual incision technique is the preferred approach through anterolateral and posteromedial incisions. The anterolateral incision extends from the level of the proximal tibiofibular joint to the level of the distal tibiofibular about 2–5 cm anterior to the fibular shaft or midway between the tibial crest and fibular shaft. It provides access to the anterior and lateral compartments.

The anterior compartment is released along the entire length of the compartment halfway between the intermuscular septum and the tibial crest. The lateral compartment is incised posterior to the septum in line with the fibular shaft and should continue distally until the tendinous portion of the peroneal muscles is visualized. Here, the superficial peroneal nerve must be protected as it exits the fascia in the middle or distal third of the exposure. The posteromedial incision is conducted approximately 2 cm posterior to the posteromedial border of the tibia. The superficial posterior compartment is released initially, with exception of the lateral head of the gastrocnemius muscle.

The soleal bridge, located near proximal metadiaphyseal junction of the tibia, must be completely released to adequately expose and decompress the deep posterior compartment. The deep posterior compartment is then released from the back of the tibia and is the most commonly "missed" compartment when fasciotomies are performed.

Wound closure is typically performed with delayed primary closure or skin graft coverage 3–7 days after fasciotomy. A vessel loop technique and negative pressure wound therapy are useful techniques in managing the fasciotomy wounds.

15.7 Miscellaneous Considerations [90]

15.7.1 Nonsurgical Treatment of ECS

With the morbidity and expense of fasciotomy, investigations are focusing on identifying less invasive approaches to treating ECS. Odland et al. [91] have reported on the potential use of tissue ultrafiltration for both diagnosing ECS by a biomarker measurement and decreasing CP by removal of interstitial fluid. Lawendy and colleagues have shown that the inflammatory response to injury may play a significant role in the pathophysiology [92]. Attenuation of the inflammatory response by indomethacin reduced tissue injury and compartment pressures in an animal model [93].

15.7.2 Pediatric Acute Compartment Syndrome

A recent systematic review of 12 studies of ECS in pediatric patients analyzed the data on 233 children [94]. The average age was 9.7 years. The most common causes were trauma of the lower leg [60%] and forearm [27%]. Pain was the most common presenting symptom [88%] followed by paresthesias [32%]. Compartment pressures were measured in 68% of patients to aid diagnosis. The mean time from injury to fasciotomy was 25.4 h. Patients had good outcomes, with 85% achieving full functional recovery, even when presenting in delayed fashion and undergoing fasciotomies delayed for at least 24 h. The authors, therefore, recommend considering decompressive fasciotomy in children even if there is prolonged time from injury to diagnosis.

15.7.3 Upper Extremity Compartment Syndrome [UECS]

CS of the forearm is the second most common after leg CS. A high level of suspicion with clinical symptoms such as pain to passive stretch and increasing pain or analgesic requirements are the key to diagnosis. The etiologic factors are similar to those of the lower extremity: reduction of compartment size such as external pressure from casts and dressings, or increase in compartmental contents as seen in bleeding, fracture displacement, ischemia, burns, envenomation, iatrogenic extravasations of intravenous fluids, and electrical trauma.

UECS is most commonly encountered in the forearm, which has three designated compartments and the ten designated hand compartments. When performing fasciotomies for UECS, care should be taken to decompress the muscles of the deep flexor compartment. Fasciotomies must be performed protecting key functional structures (e.g., neuro-vascular bundles, tendons, and joints). Early functional rehabilitation including splinting and compression therapy is crucial. The reader is referred to an excellent review of the topic by Prasarn and Ouellette [95].

15.7.4 Gluteal Compartment Syndrome

The gluteal region is a rare location for the development of a compartment syndrome and may result from prolonged immobilization from an obtunded state or prolonged surgeries in the lateral decubitus or lithotomy position. Additional causes may include vascular injury, epidural analgesia after total hip arthroplasty, anticoagulation, and necrotizing fasciitis infections.

The symptoms are severe pain in the gluteal region or lower extremity paresthesias. Physical examination will reveal tense and painful buttocks to touch and possibly ecchymoses. Passive motion of adduction and flexion of the hip would exacerbate pain in the alert patient. Diagnosis is based on either clinical presentation or measurement of compartmental pressures. Henson et al. in 2009 [96] published a systematic review of gluteal compartment syndrome with seven papers and 28 cases. The most common method of treating gluteal compartment syndrome was surgical fasciotomy [71.4%].

15.7.5 Thigh Compartment Syndrome

Thigh compartment syndrome is typically the result of blunt trauma with motor vehicle and motorcycle collisions. In a 2010 review [97],

90% of cases were attributed to blunt injury with 44% having associated femur fractures. Other causes include gunshot wounds, arterial injuries, coagulopathies or anticoagulant therapy, burns, overexertion, reperfusion swelling, or external compression.

The thigh has three anatomical compartments: anterior, posterior, and medial. The anterior compartment includes the sartorius and quadriceps, innervated by the femoral nerve and the proximal portions of the femoral artery and vein pass through this compartment, deep to the sartorius muscle. The posterior compartment hosts biceps femoris, semimembranosus, semitendinosus, and the sciatic nerve. The popliteal vascular bundle crosses from medial to posterior in the distal third of the thigh. The medial compartment is composed of adductors longus, magnus, and brevis as well as the gracilis muscle and the obturator neurovascular bundle.

Diagnosis of compartment syndrome in alert patients is by physical findings of pain out of proportion to neurovascular changes and exacerbated by passive movement of muscles. Some surgeons may choose to use compartment pressure measurements to confirm the diagnosis in an alert patient or to make the diagnosis in an obtunded patient. Treatment of a thigh compartment syndrome is a fasciotomy of the compartments. A single lateral incision allows access for the anterior and posterior compartments.

Significant mortality and morbidity may be associated with thigh compartment syndrome, as also a high association with the development of renal failure due to crush syndrome. Decompression within 8 h leads to significantly better outcomes. A systematic review of thigh compartment syndrome is recommended for further details [97].

15.7.6 Foot Compartment Syndrome

Foot compartment syndrome is a rare but debilitating condition. Clinical presentation and evaluation can differ with classically reported signs and symptoms of compartment syndrome in other areas. Controversy exists in the amount of existing myofascial compartments of the foot, as well as acute versus delayed management of foot compartment syndrome. Multiple surgical approaches have been described for myofascial decompression and are summarized in a recent review [98].

15.8 Summary and Conclusions

Despite many hazy areas, compartment syndromes also have some clarity. At a critical pressure, perfusion goes down and this is worsened by prior shock and resuscitation. A vicious cycle of ischemia and end-organ damage is set in motion. Clinical signs are late, and diagnostic tests are useful but not specific. The result is a delayed diagnosis and treatment, inevitably leading to poor outcomes.

Prevention holds the greatest promise in saving the unfortunate patient from a disastrous functional and financial adversity. Circumventing secondary compartment syndrome by eschewing aggressive crystalloid overloading or "fluid-creep" [99, 100], pursuing the diagnosis in high-risk situations right from the onset, and erring on the side of a timely and technically exquisite compartmental decompression are the keys to success.

It is, indeed, time to pay attention [1].

Treatment Dos and Don'ts
- Do diagnose promptly with a high index of suspicion
- Do a complete decompression (four compartment decompression in legs, two compartment decompression for thigh)
- Don't be fooled by distal pulses
- Don't miss the diagnosis in patients who are intubated and sedated or under anesthesia (general or epidural)
- Don't cause secondary compartment syndrome by overzealous resuscitation with crystalloids

Self Assessment Questions

1. Risk factors for orbital compartment syndrome include:
   A. Massive fluid resuscitation
   B. Local trauma
   C. Chemical burns of the eye
   D. All of the above
   Correct Answer: D

2. A patient with severe thoracic trauma received massive fluid resuscitation. Attempts at closure of chest incision cause hypotension. A provisional diagnosis of thoracic compartment syndrome is made. Treatment approaches should include all except
   A. Tight closure of incision with retention sutures
   B. Open chest management
   C. Diuresis
   D. Closure of chest incision temporarily with prosthetic material
   Correct Answer: A

3. When taking a measurement of intra-abdominal pressure via the intravesical route, one should:
   A. Zero the transducer at the level of the pubic symphysis.
   B. Ensure the head of the bed is elevated to 30°.
   C. Instill 250 mL of saline into the bladder.
   D. After instilling the saline, wait 30–60 s before taking readings.
   Correct Answer: A

4. A patient with abdominal compartment syndrome has reduced cardiac output, but elevated central venous pressure, pulmonary artery pressure, and pulmonary artery occlusion (wedge) pressure. The low cardiac output is most likely a result of:
   A. Biventricular failure
   B. Increased afterload.
   C. Hypervolemia
   D. Hypovolemia
   Correct Answer: D

5. Appropriate statements concerning surgical treatment of abdominal compartment syndrome include:
   A. After laparostomy, the laparostomy wound should be closed provided there are no signs of infection and the risk of abdominal hypertension has decreased.
   B. After laparostomy, abdominal pressure will not rise when the Bogota bag is used.
   C. Subcutaneous release of the linea alba is most unlikely to be effective in reducing intra-abdominal pressure.
   D. Temporary abdominal closure with negative pressure systems is the most effective contemporary management.
   Correct Answer: D

6. A patient with a leg cast for fracture of both bones is complaining of severe pain in the extremity. Management strategy should include
   A. Check to make sure distal pulses are OK
   B. Bivalve the cast to reduce compartment pressure
   C. Reassure the patient the pain will subside
   D. Analgesia and sedation
   Correct Answer: B

7. The most accurate test for extremity compartment syndrome is:
   A. Compartment pressure
   B. NIRS-derived muscle oxygenation
   C. Ps of compartment syndrome
   D. None of the above.
   Correct Answer: D

8. The critical periods of ischemia for functional impairment:
   A. 2–4 h of ischemia for muscles
   B. May go undetected in patients under general anesthesia, sedated, or obtunded, and those receiving postoperative epidurals after tibial fracture fixation

C. May be modified in those receiving postoperative epidurals after tibial fracture fixation
   D. All of the above
   Correct Answer: D
9. Key principles to avoid morbidity from extremity compartment syndrome include:
   A. Judicious use of prophylactic fasciotomy
   B. Avoidance of overzealous crystalloid resuscitation
   C. Compartment pressure monitoring in high-risk patients
   D. All of the above
   Correct Answer: D
10. About extremity compartment syndrome caused by vascular occlusion:
    A. Fasciotomy is of no benefit
    B. Fasciotomy may lead to severe infection in the necrotic muscle.
    C. Primary amputation is the optimal treatment
    D. Necrotic muscle must always be debrided
    Correct Answer: B

References

1. Ivatury R. Pressure, perfusion, and compartments: challenges for the acute care surgeon. J Trauma Acute Care Surg. 2014;76(6):1341–8.
2. Balestreri M, Czosnyka M, Hutchinson P, Steiner LA, Hiler M, Smielewski P, Pickard JD. Impact of intracranial pressure and cerebral perfusion pressure on severe disability and mortality after head injury. Neurocrit Care. 2006;4(1):8–13.
3. Chovanes G, Richards RM. Pressure is only part of the story in traumatic brain injured patients; focal cerebral blood flow goes to zero in some patients with adequate cerebral perfusion pressure. Surg Neurol Int. 2012;3:12. https://doi.org/10.4103/2152-7806.92185.
4. Chovanes GI, Richards RM. The predominance of metabolic regulation of cerebral blood flow and the lack of "Classic" autoregulation curves in the viable brain. J Emerg Med. 2013;44(5):1039–44.
5. Jan Bouzat P, Sala N, Payen JF, Oddo M. Beyond intracranial pressure: optimization of cerebral blood flow, oxygen, and substrate delivery after traumatic brain injury. Ann Intensive Care. 2013;3(1):23.
6. Coccolini F, Improta M, Picetti E, Vergano LB, Catena F, de 'Angelis N, Bertolucci A, Kirkpatrick AW, Sartelli M, Fugazzola P, Tartaglia D, Chiarugi M. Timing of surgical intervention for compartment syndrome in different body region: systematic review of the literature. World J Emerg Surg. 2020;15:60.
7. Sullivan SR, Ahmadi AJ, Singh CN, Sires BS, Engrav LH, Gibran NS, Heimbach DM, Klein MB. Elevated orbital pressure: another untoward effect of massive resuscitation after burn injury. J Trauma. 2006;60:72–6.
8. Singh CN, Klein MB, Sullivan SR, Sires BS, Hutter CM, Rice K, Jian-Amadi A. Orbital compartment syndrome in burn patients. Ophthal Plast Reconstr Surg. 2008;24(2):102–6.
9. Lima V, Burt B, Leibovitch I, Prabhakaran V, Goldberg RA, Selva D. Orbital compartment syndrome: the ophthalmic surgical emergency. Surv Ophthalmol. 2009;54(4):441–9.
10. McCallum E, Keren S, Lapira M, Norris JH. Orbital compartment syndrome: an update with review of the literature. Clin Ophthalmol. 2019;13:2189–94.
11. Riahi M, Tomatis LA, Schlosser RJ, Bertolozzi E, Johnston DW. Cardiac compression due to closure of the median sternotomy in open heart surgery. Chest. 1975;67(1):113–4.
12. Kaplan LJ, Trooskin SZ, Santora TA. Thoracic compartment syndrome. J Trauma. 1996;40(2):291–3.
13. Rizzio AG, Sample GA. Thoracic compartment syndrome secondary to a thoracic procedure. A case report. Chest. 2003;124:1164–8.
14. Amos T, Yeunga M, Gooie J, Fitzgerald M. Survival following traumatic thoracic compartment syndrome managed with VV-ECMO. Trauma Case Rep. 2019;24:100249.
15. Wandling MW, An GC. A case report of thoracic compartment syndrome in the setting of penetrating chest trauma and review of the literature. World J Emerg Surg. 2010;5:22.
16. Ivatury R, Cheatham M, Malbrain M, Sugrue M, editors. Abdominal compartment syndrome. Landes Bioscience: Georgetown; 2006.
17. Fietsam R, Billalba M, Glover JL, Clark K. Intra-abdominal compartment syndrome as a complication of ruptured abdominal aortic aneurysms. Am Surg. 1989;55(6):396–402.
18. Roberts DJ, Ball CG, Feliciano DV, Moore EE, Ivatury RR, Lucas CE, Fabian TC, Zygun DA, Kirkpatrick AW, Stelfox HT. History of the innovation of damage control for management of trauma patients: 1902–2016. Ann Surg. 2017;265(5):1034–44.
19. Rotondo MF, Schwab CW, McGonigal MD, , Phillips GR 3rd, Fruchterman TM, Kauder DR, Latenser BA, Angood PA: "Damage control": an approach for improved survival in exsanguinating penetrating abdominal injury. J Trauma, 1993; 35(3): 375–382.

20. Morris JA Jr, Eddy VA, Blinman TA, Rutherford EJ, Sharp KW. The staged celiotomy for trauma. Issues in unpacking and reconstruction. Ann Surg. 1993;217(5):576–84.
21. Ivatury RR, Porter JM, Simon RJ, Islam S, John R, Stahl WM. Intra-abdominal hypertension after life-threatening penetrating abdominal trauma: prophylaxis, incidence, and clinical relevance to gastric mucosal pH and abdominal compartment syndrome. J Trauma. 1998;44(6):1016–21.
22. Schwab CW. Master surgeon lecture: damage control: 20 years of experience. aast.org. Accessed 15 June 2021
23. Malbrain ML, Cheatham ML, Kirkpatrick A, Sugrue M, Parr M, DeWaele J, Balogh Z, Leppaniemi A, Olvera C, Ivatury R, et al. Results from the international conference of experts on intra-abdominal hypertension and abdominal compartment syndrome. I. Definitions. Intensive Care Med. 2006;32(11):1722–32.
24. Cheatham ML, Malbrain ML, Kirkpatrick A, Sugrue M, Parr M, De Waele J, Balogh Z, Leppäniemi A, Olvera C, Ivatury R, et al. Results from the international conference of experts on intra-abdominal hypertension and abdominal compartment syndrome. II. Recommendations. Intensive Care Med. 2007;33(6):951–62.
25. Kirkpatrick AW, Roberts DJ, De Waele J, Jaeschke R, Malbrain ML, De Keulenaer B, Duchesne J, Bjorck M, Leppaniemi A, Ejike JC, et al. Intra-abdominal hypertension and the abdominal compartment syndrome: updated consensus definitions and clinical practice guidelines from the World Society of the Abdominal Compartment Syndrome. Intensive Care Med. 2013;39(7):1190–206.
26. Ivatury RR, Diebel L, Porter JM, Simon RJ. Intra-abdominal hypertension and the abdominal compartment syndrome. Surg Clin North Am. 1997;77(4):783–800.
27. Ivatury RR, Sugerman HJ, Peitzman AB. Abdominal compartment syndrome: recognition and management. Adv Surg. 2001;35:251–69.
28. Saggi BH, Sugerman HJ, Ivatury RR, Bloomfield GL. Abdominal compartment syndrome. J Trauma. 1998;45(3):597–609.
29. Meldrum DR, Moore FA, Moore E, Franciose RJ, Sauaia A, Burch JM. Prospective characterization and selective management of the abdominal compartment syndrome. Am J Surg. 1997;174:667–72.
30. Mayberry JC, Mullins RJ, Crass RA, Trumkey DD. Prevention of abdominal compartment syndrome by absorbable mesh prosthesis closure. Arch Surg. 1997;132(9):957–61.
31. Simon RJ, Friedlander MH, Ivatury RR, et al. Hemorrhage lowers the threshold for intra-abdominal hypertension-induced pulmonary dysfunction. J Trauma. 1997;42(3):398–403.
32. Friedlander MH, Simon RJ, Ivatury R, et al. Effect of hemorrhage on superior mesenteric artery flow during increased intra-abdominal pressures. J Trauma. 1998;45(3):433–89.
33. Doty JM, Oda J, Ivatury RR, et al. The effects of hemodynamic shock and increased intra-abdominal pressure on bacterial translocation. J Trauma. 2002;52(1):13–7.
34. Scalea TM, Bochicchio GV, Habashi N, et al. Increased intra-abdominal, intrathoracic, and intracranial pressure after severe brain injury: multiple compartment syndrome. J Trauma. 2007;62(3):647–56.
35. Malbrain ML, Roberts DJ, Sugrue M, et al. The polycompartment syndrome: a concise state-of-the-art review. Anaesthesiol Intensive Ther. 2014;46(5):433–50.
36. Van Damme L, De Waele JJ. Effect of decompressive laparotomy on organ function in patients with abdominal compartment syndrome: a systematic review and meta-analysis. Crit Care. 2018;22:179. https://doi.org/10.1186/s13054-018-2103-0.
37. Cheatham ML, Safcsak K. Is the evolving management of intra-abdominal hypertension and abdominal compartment syndrome improving survival? Crit Care Med. 2010;38(2):402–7.
38. Balogh ZJ, Martin A, van Wessem KP, et al. Mission to eliminate postinjury abdominal compartment syndrome. Arch Surg. 2011;146(8):938–43.
39. Wise R, Roberts DJ, Vandervelden S, et al. Awareness and knowledge of intra-abdominal hypertension and abdominal compartment syndrome: results of an international survey. Anaesthesiol Intensive Ther. 2015;47(1):14–29. https://doi.org/10.5603/AIT.2014.0051.
40. Strang SG, Van Lieshout EM, Verhoeven RA, et al. Recognition and management of intra-abdominal hypertension and abdominal compartment syndrome; a survey among Dutch surgeons. Eur J Trauma Emerg Surg. 2017;43(1):85–98. https://doi.org/10.1007/s00068-016-0637.
41. Kaussen T, Steinau G, Srinivasan PK, et al. Recognition and management of abdominal compartment syndrome among German pediatric intensivists: results of a national survey. Ann Intensive Care. 2012;2 Suppl 1(Suppl 1):S8. https://doi.org/10.1186/2110-5820-2-S1-S8.
42. Hunt L, Frost SA, Newton PJ, et al. A survey of critical care nurses' knowledge of intra-abdominal hypertension and abdominal compartment syndrome. Aust Crit Care. 2017;30(1):21–7 . pii: S1036-7314(16)00030-8. https://doi.org/10.1016/j.aucc.2016.02.001.
43. Wise R, Rodseth R, Blaser AR, Roberts DJ, De Waele JJ, Kirkpatrick AW, De Keulenaer BL, Malbrain MLG, et al. Awareness and knowledge of intra-abdominal hypertension and abdominal compartment syndrome: results of a repeat, international, cross-sectional survey. Anaesthesiol Intensive Ther. 2019;51(3):186–99. https://doi.org/10.5114/ait.2019.87648.

44. Ivatury RR. Abdominal compartment syndrome: a century later, isn't it time to accept and promulgate? Crit Care Med. 2006;34(9):2494–5.
45. Malbrain ML, Cheatham ML, Kirkpatrick A, Sugrue M, De Waele J, Ivatury R. Abdominal compartment syndrome: it's time to pay attention! Intensive Care Med. 2006;32(11):1912–4.
46. Kirkpatrick AW, Nickerson D, Roberts DJ, Rosen MJ, McBeth PB, Petro CC, Berrevoet F, Sugrue M, Xiao J, Ball CG. Intra-abdominal hypertension and abdominal compartment syndrome after abdominal wall reconstruction: quaternary syndromes? Scand J Surg. 2017;106(2):97–106.
47. Quintela C, Freire L, Marrana F, Barbosa E, Guerreiro G, Ferreira FC. Quaternary abdominal compartment syndrome in complex ventral hernias. Int J Abdom Wall Hernia Surg. 2021;4:39–44.
48. Matsen FR, Krugmire RB. Compartmental syndromes. Surg Gynecol Obstet. 1978;147:943–9.
49. Shadgan B, Menon M, Sanders D, Berry G, Martin C Jr, Duffy P, Stephen D, O'Brien PJ. Current thinking about acute compartment syndrome of the lower extremity. Can J Surg. 2010;53(5):329–34.
50. McQueen MM, Gaston P, Court-Brown CM. Acute compartment syndrome. Who is at risk? J Bone Joint Surg Br. 2000;82(2):200–3.
51. Schmidt AH. Acute compartment syndrome. Injury. 2017;48 Suppl 1:S22–5.
52. Feliciano DV, Cruse PA, Spjut-Patrinely V, Burch JM, Mattox KL. Fasciotomy after trauma to the extremities. Am J Surg. 1988;156(6):533–6.
53. Tremblay LN, Feliciano DV, Rozycki GS. Secondary extremity compartment syndrome. J Trauma. 2002;53(5):833–7.
54. Goaley TJ Jr, Wyrzykowski AD, MacLeod JB, Wise KB, Dente CJ, Salomone JP, Nicholas JM, Vercruysse GA, Ingram WL, Rozycki GS, et al. Can secondary extremity compartment syndrome be diagnosed earlier? Am J Surg. 2007;194(6):724–6.
55. Shadgan B, Menon M, O'Brien PJ, Reid WD. Diagnostic techniques in acute compartment syndrome of the leg. J Orthop Trauma. 2008;22(8):581–7.
56. Elliott KG, Johnstone AJ. Diagnosing acute compartment syndrome. J Bone Joint Surg Br. 2003;85(5):625–32.
57. Ulmer T. The clinical diagnosis of compartment syndrome of the lower leg: are clinical findings predictive of the disorder? J Orthop Trauma. 2002;16(8):572–7.
58. Tristan E, McMillan TE, Gardner WT, Schmidt AH, Johnstone AJ. Diagnosing acute compartment syndrome—where have we got to? Int Orthop. 2019;43:2429–35.
59. Mubarak SJ, Hargens AR, Owen CA, Garetto LP, Akeson WH. The wick catheter technique for measurement of intramuscular pressure. A new research and clinical tool. J Bone Joint Surg Am. 1976;58(7):1016–20.
60. Whitesides TE, Haney TC, Morimoto K, Harada H. Tissue pressure measurements as a determinant for the need of fasciotomy. Clin Orthop Relat Res. 1975;113:43–51.
61. McQueen MM, Court-Brown CM. Compartment monitoring in tibial fractures. The pressure threshold for decompression. J Bone Joint Surg Br. 1996;78(1):99–104.
62. Nelson JA. Compartment pressure measurements have poor specificity for compartment syndrome in the traumatized limb. J Emerg Med. 2013;44(5):1039–44.
63. Prayson MJ, Chen JL, Hampers D, Vogt M, Fenwick J, Meredick R. Baseline compartment pressure measurements in isolated lower extremity fractures without clinical compartment syndrome. J Trauma. 2006;60:1037–40.
64. Bariteau JT, Beutel BG, Kamal R, Hayda R, Born C. The use of near infrared spectrometry for the diagnosis of lower-extremity compartment syndrome. Orthopedics. 2011;34(3):178.
65. Arbabi S, Brundate SI, Gentilello LM. Near-infrared spectroscopy: a potential method for continuous, transcutaneous monitoring for compartmental syndrome in critically injured patients. J Trauma. 1999;47:829–33.
66. Mancini DM, La Manca J, Donchez L, Henson D, Levine S. Validation of near-infrared spectroscopy in humans. J Appl Physiol. 1994;77:2740–7.
67. Giannotti G, Cohn SM, Brown M, et al. Utility of near-infrared spectroscopy in the diagnosis of lower extremity compartment syndrome. J Trauma. 2000;48:396–9.
68. Gentilello LM, Sanzone A, Wang L, Liu PY, Robinson L. Near-infrared spectroscopy versus compartment pressure for the diagnosis of lower extremity compartmental syndrome using electromyography-determined measurements of neuromuscular function. J Trauma. 2001;51:1–8.
69. Shuler MS, Reisman WM, Whitesides TE, et al. Near-infrared spectroscopy in lower extremity trauma. J Bone Joint Surg Am. 2009;91:1360–8.
70. Shuler MS, Reisman WM, Kinsey TL, Whitesides TE Jr, Hammerberg EM, Davila MG, Moore TJ. Correlation between muscle oxygenation and compartment pressures in acute compartment syndrome of the leg. J Bone Joint Surg Am. 2010;92:863–70.
71. Arató E, Kürthy M, Sínay L, Kasza G, Menyhei G, Masoud S, Bertalan A, Verzár Z, Kollár L, Roth E, et al. Pathology and diagnostic options of lower limb compartment syndrome. Clin Hemorheol Microcirc. 2009;41(1):1–8.
72. Ward KR, Torres Filho I, Barbee RW, Torres L, Tiba MH, Reynolds PS, Pittman RN, Ivatury RR, Terner J. Resonance Raman spectroscopy: a new technology for tissue oxygenation monitoring. Crit Care Med. 2006;34(3):792–9.
73. Tiba MH, Draucker GT, Barbee RW, Terner J, Filho IT, Romfh P, Vakhshoori D, Ward KR. Tissue oxy-

genation monitoring using resonance Raman spectroscopy during hemorrhage. J Trauma Acute Care Surg. 2014;76(2):402–8.
74. Sellei RM, Wollnitz J, Reinhardt N, de la Fuente M, Radermacher K, Weber C, Kobbe P, Hildebrand F. Non-invasive measurement of muscle compartment elasticity in lower limbs to determine acute compartment syndrome: clinical results with pressure related ultrasound. Injury. 2020;51:301–6.
75. Mubarak SJ, Hargens AR. Acute compartment syndromes. Surg Clin North Am. 1983;63(3):539–65.
76. Taylor RM, Sullivan MP, Mehta S. Acute compartment syndrome: obtaining diagnosis, providing treatment, and minimizing medicolegal risk. Curr Rev Musculoskelet Med. 2012;5(3):206–13.
77. Mabvuure NT, Malahias M, Hindocha S, Khan W, Juma A. Acute compartment syndrome of the limbs: current concepts and management. Open Orthop J. 2012;6:535–43.
78. Farber A, Tan TW, Hamburg NM, Kalish JA, Joglar F, Onigman T, Rybin D, Doros G, Eberhardt RT. Early fasciotomy in patients with extremity vascular injury is associated with decreased risk of adverse limb outcomes: a review of the National Trauma Data Bank. Injury. 2012;43(9):1486–91.
79. Ritenour AE, Dorlac WC, Fang R, Woods T, Jenkins DH, Flaherty SF, Wade CE, Holcomb JB. Complications after fasciotomy revision and delayed compartment release in combat patients. J Trauma. 2008;64(Suppl 2):S153–61.
80. Kragh JF Jr, San Antonio J, Simmons JW, Mace JE, Stinner DJ, White CE, Fang R, Aden JK, Hsu JR, Eastridge BJ, et al. Compartment syndrome performance improvement project is associated with increased combat casualty survival. J Trauma Acute Care Surg. 2013;74(1):259–63.
81. Fainzilber T, Roy-Shapira G, Wall MJ Jr, Mattox KL. Predictors of amputation for popliteal artery injuries. Am J Surg. 1995;170:568–71.
82. Abouezzi Z, Nassoura Z, Ivatury RR, Porter JM, Stahl WM. A critical reappraisal of indications for fasciotomy after extremity vascular trauma. Arch Surg. 1998;133(5):547–5515.
83. Vaillancourt C, Shrier I, Falk M, Rossignol M, Vernec A, Somogyi D. Quantifying delays in the recognition and management of acute compartment syndrome. CJEM. 2001;3:26–30.
84. Kashuk JL, Moore EE, Pinski S, Johnson JL, Moore JB, Morgan S, Cothren CC, Smith W. Lower extremity compartment syndrome in the acute care surgery paradigm: safety lessons learned. Patient Saf Surg. 2009;3(1):11.
85. Percival TJ, White JM, Ricci MA. Compartment syndrome in the setting of vascular injury. Perspect Vasc Surg Endovasc Ther. 2011;23(2):119–24.
86. Finkelstein JA, Hunter GA, Hu RW. Lower limb compartment syndrome: course after delayed fasciotomy. J Trauma. 1996;40(3):342–4.
87. Blaisdell FW. Is there a reason for controversy regarding fasciotomy? J Vasc Surg. 1989;9(6):828.
88. Blaisdell FW. The pathophysiology of skeletal muscle ischemia and the reperfusion syndrome: a review. Cardiovasc Surg. 2002;10:620–30.
89. Sheridan GW, Matsen FA 3rd. Fasciotomy in the treatment of the acute compartment syndrome. J Bone Joint Surg Am. 1976;58(1):112–5.
90. Mauffrey C, Hak DJ, Martin MP III, editors. Compartment syndrome: a guide to diagnosis and management. 2019.
91. Odland RM, Schmidt AH. Compartment syndrome ultrafiltration catheters: report of a clinical pilot study of a novel method for managing patients at risk of compartment syndrome. J Orthop Trauma. 2011;25:358–65.
92. Lawendy A-R, Bihari A, Sanders DW, McGarr G, Badhwar A, Cepinskas G. Contribution of inflammation to cellular injury in compartment syndrome in an experimental rodent model. Bone Joint J. 2015;97-B:539–43.
93. Manjoo A, Sanders D, Lawendy A, Gladwell M, Gray D, Parry N, et al. Indomethacin reduces cell damage: shedding new light on compartment syndrome. J Orthop Trauma. 2010;24:526–9.
94. Lina JS, Samoraa JB. Pediatric acute compartment syndrome: a systematic review and meta-analysis. J Pediatr Orthop B. 2020;29:90–6.
95. Prasarn ML, Ouellette EA. Acute compartment syndrome of the upper extremity. J Am Acad Orthop Surg. 2011;19:49–58.
96. Henson J, Roberts C, Giannoudis P. Gluteal compartment syndrome. Acta Orthop Belg. 2009;75(2):147–52.
97. Ojike NI, Roberts CS, Giannoudis PV. Compartment syndrome of the thigh: a systematic review. Injury. 2010;41(2):133–6.
98. Dodd A, Le I. Foot compartment syndrome: diagnosis and management. J Am Acad Orthop Surg. 2013;21(11):657–64.
99. Pruitt BA Jr. Protection from excessive resuscitation: "pushing the pendulum back". J Trauma. 2000;49:567–8.
100. Ball CG. Damage control resuscitation: history, theory and technique. Can J Surg. 2014;57(1):55–60.

Antibiotic and Antimicotic Therapy

Marcelo A. F. Ribeiro Junior, Gabriela Tebar, and José Lucas Rodrigues Salgueiro

Learning Goals
- Identifying the main surgical-related infections
- Understanding the main antibiotics to be used depending on the infection site
- Enabling prompt sepsis identification and starting the protocols

16.1 Introduction

Antimicrobial standardization programs have been promoted to optimize antibiotics using, improve patients' outcome, and reduce antimicrobial resistance. However, the best strategies are not fully established and depend on aspects such as local culture, clinical routine, and limited resources [1].

Sepsis is a potentially life-threatening clinical condition and the most common cause of death in hospitalized patients. In addition, it generates annual costs higher than US $ 20 billion in the USA. Studies have associated increase by 6–7% in mortality rates for every hour taken to start the infusion of antibiotics and intravenous fluids in septic patients [2].

Infections are often hard to be diagnosed, mainly in critically ill surgical patients, since fever is actually attributed to surgical infections in only 1/3 of cases. Increased body temperature is the most common and easily detectable sign of infection; it affects from 44 to 70% of all patients hospitalized in surgical intensive care units [3].

Critically ill patients with complicated medical and surgical history are often subjected to a variety of invasive support devices such as endotracheal tubes and/or nasogastric tubes, central venous or arterial catheters, and urinary catheters, which enable a wide range of potential infectious sites.

Thus, it is necessary conducting a thorough investigation in such cases. Objective data collection based on images and on standardized analyses comprising blood, urine, or bronchial cultures must be performed to help providing proper treat-

M. A. F. Ribeiro Junior (✉)
General and Trauma Surgery Division, Catholic University of São Paulo PUCSP-Sorocaba, São Paulo, Brazil

Chair Division of Trauma, Burns, Critical Care and Acute Care Surgery, Sheikh Shakhbout Medical City - Mayo Clinic Abu Dhabi, Abu Dhabi, United Arab Emirates

Khalifa University and Gulf Medical University, Abu Dhabi, United Arab Emirates

Education Committee of the Panamerican Trauma Society, São Paulo, Brazil

Brazilian Trauma Society, São Paulo, Brazil

American College of Surgeons, Chicago, United States of America
e-mail: mjunior@ssmc.ae

G. Tebar · J. L. R. Salgueiro
Catholic University of São Paulo PUCSP-Sorocaba, São Paulo, Brazil

ment to critically ill patients in order to preserve their lives and to avoid subsequent consequences of incorrect or delayed therapy application. Several studies, such as the Surviving Sepsis Campaign, have shown that early antibiotic administration is associated with better outcomes such as reduced hospital mortality rates.

Prophylactic antibiotics should be infused in all patients subjected to major emergency surgeries. Delayed antibiotic infusion applications are associated with increased complications, reoperation, and mortality rates within 30 days, as well as with longer hospitalization time [2].

On the other hand, besides leading to high mortality rates, excessive antibiotic using is associated with resistant infections such as the one caused by methicillin-resistant *Staphylococcus aureus*, as well as with opportunistic infections such as the one caused by *Clostridioides difficile* [3].

16.2 Surgical Site Infection and Antibiotic Prophylaxis

Appropriate preoperative antibiotic prophylaxis (PAP) application, in compliance with the established principles, can safely circumvent the development of surgical site infections (SSI) in several patients. This prophylaxis comprises timely antibiotic administration to enable high levels of it in patients' tissues at surgical incision time, the use of effective narrower-spectrum agents against the pathogens most likely to cause SSI in a given procedure, and the discontinuity of these antibiotics once the surgery is finished, according to guidelines published by the American College of Surgeons and by the Surgical Infection Society [4, 5] Table 16.1.

Surgical site infection (SSI) is the most common postoperative complication presenting significant morbidity and mortality rates - SSI corresponds to 17% of healthcare-related infections. It is featured by infections developed 30 days after surgical procedures, or 90 days after procedures involving implants or prostheses. The most common causative organisms are those overall endogenous to patients, i.e., organisms deriving from cutaneous tissues or from any viscera that has been opened [5]. Patients who developed this infection were five times more likely to be hospitalized again within 3 days and two times more likely to die.

The risk of SSI development in surgical patients has been affected by several factors in recent decades, namely: microbial resistance has worsened due to multiple-resistant *Staphylococcus aureus* (MRSA) outspread in the community, surgical patients have become older and present more comorbidities, and minimally invasive approaches have increasingly replaced open surgeries.

16.2.1 Antibiotic Prophylaxis

Antibiotic prophylaxis is recommended for clean procedures involving prostheses or implant placement, as well as for clean-contaminated and contaminated operation cases. This prophylaxis is not indicated for infected operation cases, which should be subjected to antibiotic therapy.

Table 16.1 Classification of surgical wounds and risk of surgical site infection (SSI) [4]

Class	Potential for contamination	Features	Example	SSI-incidence estimates
I	Clean	No signs of inflammation, no opening of the respiratory, digestive, or genitourinary tracts	Umbilical herniorrhaphy	<2%
II	Potentially contaminated	Opening of the respiratory, digestive, or genitourinary tracts without significant contamination	Cholecystectomy (without bile leakage)	<10%
III	Contaminated	Inflammatory process or opening of respiratory, digestive, or genitourinary tracts with significant contamination	Appendectomy, colectomies	20%
IV	Infected	Gross contamination secondary to pus or perforation	Cholecystectomy due to suppurative cholecystitis	>40%

Antimicrobial drug selection is based on the microorganisms most often observed in patients' skin and manipulated sites, such as gram-positive *S. aureus* and gram-negative *S. coagulase*, (for clean surgeries), as well as gram-negative and anaerobic bacteria, after contaminated or potentially contaminated procedures. The ideal antimicrobial dose should reach serum and tissue levels that exceed the minimum inhibitory concentration for likely pathogens. Single-dose prophylaxis should be encouraged whenever possible, since prolonged antibiotic using increases the risk of adverse effects - the ideal administration time ranges from 30 to 60 min before skin incision, except for Vancomycin, which should be infused 1–2 h before the incision. Additional doses are only necessary in case of surgeries longer than 4 h or in patients presenting intraoperative blood loss higher than 1500 mL.

Antimicrobial prophylaxis should always be shorter than 24 h, since longer prophylaxis can increase the incidence of acute kidney injury and infection caused by *Clostridium difficile*, without increasing local protection [Branch-Elliman et al.].

Patients colonized with methicillin-resistant *Staphylococcus aureus* (MRSA) must undergo topical 2% mupirocin-based decolonization 3 times a day (intranasal (IN) route) and 2% chlorhexidine baths on a daily basis, for 5 days before elective surgeries.

16.2.1.1 Antibiotic Treatments

Head and Neck

Head and neck infections can lead to high morbidity and mortality rates since they are close to the orbit region and brain, as well as associated with the upper airways and the mediastinum [6].

Old age and its associated comorbidities such as diabetes mellitus, anemia and peripheral vascular disease, as well as nutritional factors, tobacco smoking, and alcohol intake are linked to surgical site infection in the context of head and neck surgery [7].

Infections in the oral cavity, oropharynx, and salivary glands are quite common; approximately 30% of infections affecting the deep cervical planes derive from odontogenic processes; 30% of them derive from pharyngitis; and 10%, from sialadenitis. Lesser common sources of infectious processes affecting the deep cervical planes derive from other pathologies, such as suppurative lymphadenitis, congenital cyst infection, ear infections, and injecting-drug using [6].

Infections can reach deep spaces due to their rapid progression through the fascial planes, which most often include the submandibular triangle, as well as the retropharyngeal, parapharyngeal, and masticatory spaces. Such conditions require urgent treatment, otherwise they can reach the mediastinal, pulmonary, or cardiac planes and lead to mediastinitis, empyema, and pericardial effusion [6].

Dental infections and sialadenitis are often observed in head and neck infection patients. In addition, they can progress to Ludwig's angina, which compromises mylohyoid muscles and leads to inflammation featured by edema at the level of the lower incisors, macroglossia, and posterior ptosis of the tongue. Accessing the airway of these patients is a challenging task given the obstructive pattern presented by this condition, which sometimes require fibroscopy- or tracheostomy-based intubation in conscious patients [6]. Sialadenitis is most often associated with sialolithiasis; it causes further inflammation, although other pathologies related to it also comprise infections caused by the HIV, coxsackie, or influenza viruses [8].

Untreated tonsillitis in the oropharyngeal region can develop into periamygdalic abscess, which is followed by odynophagia for 3–5 days and progresses to worsened pain and ipsilateral otalgia, and may even lead to fever, dysphagia, and vocal changes (hot potato voice). It must be clinically diagnosed and treated with abscess drainage and antibiotic therapy [6].

Mastoiditis is the most common complication of suppurative otitis media in children; it is diagnosed based on patients' clinical history, in association with image showing mastoid bone destruction and collection. Treatment applied to mastoiditis patients is based on targeted antibiotic therapy (*Streptococcus pneumoniae*, *Pseudomonas aeruginosa*, and *Staphylococcus aureus*), which can be associated with surgical treatment (tympanic tube or mastoidectomy), or not. Subperiosteal abscess, with pinna proptosis or protrusion, is the most common complication of mastoiditis. Another complication lies on mastoiditis' extension through digastric and sternocleidomastoid muscles, which leads to infection in deep cervical tissues. It can rarely reach the anterior zygomatic region and take the abscess to the temporal region [6].

Fortunately, intracranial complications resulting from ear infections are not common - meningitis is the main intracranial complication and *Streptococcus pneumoniae* is the main pathogen causing it. In general, *Hemophilus influenzae type B* was the most common pathogen before mass vaccination. *Proteus mirabilis* and *Klebsiella* are often associated with chronic otitis and meningitis cases [6].

Rhinological infections are often associated with viruses; they may spontaneously heal or evolve to sinusitis, which can lead to orbital complications such as preseptal cellulitis, orbital cellulitis, subperiosteal orbital abscess, orbital abscess, and cavernous sinusoid thrombosis [6].

Preseptal cellulitis presents the clinical picture of cellulite associated with inflammatory signs in the lower and upper eyelids; its treatment comprises antibiotic therapy with ampicillin and sulbactam, or with clindamycin for penicillin-allergic patients [6].

Subperiosteal orbital abscess is the second most common complication of sinusitis. It leads to sinusoidal and orbital pain, eyeball proptosis, and conjunctival ecchymosis, and its treatment comprises intravenous antibiotic therapy, in association (or not) with surgical drainage [6].

Orbital cellulitis and cavernous sinusoid thrombosis are ophthalmic emergencies due to high risk of blindness, as well as of intracranial dissemination through orbital fissures. Ocular proptosis and ecchymosis, as well as decreased visual acuity and pupillary response, are observed in many cases. Ophthalmoplegia is a concern in cavernous sinusoid thrombosis cases [6].

Intracranial complications deriving from sinusitis comprise meningitis, epidural and subdural abscesses, encephalitis, and brain abscess. Risk factors for such conditions are observed in patients with history of head trauma or skull fractures, encephalocele, immunosuppression, and skull base defects. Patients with meningeal signs, sensory changes, and headaches (with compatible history) should undergo cranial tomography for clarification purposes [6].

Sinusitis resulting from fungal invasion is a rare, although devastating, disease. *Aspergillus* or *Mucorales* species stand out among its pathogens, which can lead to the fulminant form of the disease. Treatment should be based on antifungal drugs and abscess drainage [6]. Species such as *Candida, Histoplasma, Cryptococcus,* and *Coccidioides* can also be found in these cases [8].

Several strategies are used to reduce the risks of infection in surgical sites. Among them, one finds control of comorbidities and of the surgical environment, as well as proper asepsis and antisepsis of the surgical regions (with adequate trichotomy), correct antibiotic prophylaxis, as well as correct antibiotic administration time in the perioperative period [7].

Antibiotic prophylaxis/therapy implementation changes depending on each service. A retrospective study has used clindamycin, cefazoline in association with metronidazole, cefazolin alone, or ampicillin in association with sulbactam. Clindamycin is the least routinely recommended among them [7].

Staphylococci, Streptococci viridans, Group C *Streptococci,* and Prevotella are the bacterial species most often isolated in odontogenic disorders, which are major causes of infection in the deep cervical planes. Antibiotics such as ampicillin (associated with sulbactam, or not), cefazolin, levofloxacin, gentamicin, penicillin, and piperacillin/tazobactam were effective in treating these disorders. Clindamycin was also used for this purpose, but it did not show the evident success recorded for the aforementioned antibiotics (Table 16.2) [9].

Thorax

Pleural infection corresponds to bacterial invasion of the pleura, mainly after microorganism translocation from the infected lung to the pleural space of pneumonia patients. It is a frequent clinical issue with high annual incidence, as well as morbidity and mortality rates worldwide. Approximately 50% of patients with

Table 16.2 Empirical antimicrobial use in urgent and emergency surgery for head and neck infections

Cephalic pole	Urgency and emergency	Streptococcus pneumoniae, Pseudomonas aeruginosa, Staphylococcus aureus, Hemophilus influenzae type B, Proteus mirabilis and Klebsiella	Ampicillin + sulbactam Cefazolin + metronidazole	Clindamycin Penicillin
Neck	Urgency and emergency	Staphylococci, Streptococci viridans, Streptococci belonging to group C and Prevotella	Ampicillin ± sulbactam Cefazolin in separate Levofloxacin	Gentamycin Penicillin Piperacillin/Tazobactam

community-acquired pneumonia develop parapneumonic effusion and 10% of these effusions get infected [10]. Pleural infection management process comprises proper antibiotic administration in association with infected pleural fluid drainage.

The introduction of antibiotics has reduced the incidence of empyema and changed its bacteriology. Before them, 60–70% of cases were derived from *Streptococcus pneumoniae*, which nowadays only represent approximately 10% of positive culture cases. The prevalence of *Staphylococcus aureus* has increased and the development of staphylococcal resistance in the 1950s has increased complication and mortality rates [11].

Although most patients with community-acquired pleural infection often recover after treatment with antibiotics and pleural drainage, 20% of them require surgical intervention [10]. Inappropriate antibiotic using is a common cause of treatment failure. It is essential to understand the common causative bacteria, as well as their resistance patterns to these drugs, at the time to select the treatment to be applied to these patients.

It is known that pleural infection mostly affects extreme-age groups, i.e., the pediatric and elderly populations. Risk factors for this disease are similar to those of pneumonia, although empyema development is more associated with patients with diabetes mellitus, immunosuppressive patients using corticosteroids, as well as with individuals presenting gastroesophageal reflux, excessive alcohol intake, and intravenous drug abuse.

Most pleural infection forms represent a progressive process that turns a "simple" parapneumonic effusion with spontaneous resolution into a "complicated" multiloculated fibrinopurulent collection associated with clinical and/or biochemical sepsis features.

Based on changes in the bacteriological profile of pulmonary infections, knowledge about the most prevalent bacteria should help implementing empirical antibiotic therapy, which can change disease prognosis, when it is early and properly adopted.

Nowadays, it is known that gram-positive aerobic organisms prevail in community-acquired infections. *Streptococci*, including groups of organisms such as *S. milleri* and *S. aureus*, account for approximately 65% of cases. Gram-negative organisms such as *Enterobacteriaceae*, *Escherichia coli*, and *Haemophilus influenzae* are less often grown and most often seen in patients with comorbidities [10, 11]. On the other hand, hospital-acquired pleural infections are mostly associated with *S. aureus*.

- Methicillin-resistant *S. aureus* (MRSA) may account for up to two-thirds of cases [1]
- Gram-negative organisms - mostly *E. coli*, *Enterobacter* spp. and *Pseudomonas* spp. - account for most of the remainder cases; significantly higher rates of Gram-negative aerobic organisms have been reported in patients requiring hospitalization in intensive care unit [10, 11]
- Polymicrobial infection is often caused by Gram-negative and anaerobic organisms that rarely happen in isolation; this infection mostly affects elderly patients and individuals with comorbidities [10]

Thus, all patients with suspected pleural infection should undergo blood cultures for aerobic and anaerobic bacteria. These cultures are often positive in approximately 14% of patients; moreover, they are the only microbiological source used to guide antibiotic selection [11].

The initial treatment of these patients is mainly based on antibiotic therapy, which must focus on the most common bacterial profile of pleural infection and comply with local policies about local antibiotics and resistance patterns. Its inadequate use, together with misdiagnosis, delayed drainage, and poor positioning of the chest drain are the most common causes of initial treatment failure.

The bacteriology of pleural infections significantly differs from that of pneumonia. In addition, low sensitivity (40–60%) of pleural fluid cultures and lack of culture results at diagnosis time require the implementation of antibiotic treatment without microbiological guidance in most cases [10].

Antibiotics capable of covering anaerobic infections should be used in all patients, except in the ones with culture-proven pneumococcal infection. In addition, antibiotic therapy selection should be guided by bacterial culture results, whenever possible. The selected antibiotic therapy should cover the most common pathogens and anaerobic organisms in case of negative results. Macrolides are not recommended, unless there is objective evidence or high clinical index of suspected "atypical" pathogens.

Aminopenicillin-based treatment (e.g., amoxicillin) application to community-acquired infection patients must cover organisms such as *S. pneumoniae* and *H. influenzae*. In addition, b-lactamase inhibitors such as amoxicillin + clavulanate or metronidazole should also be administered due to frequent coexistence of penicillin-resistant aerobes, such as *S. aureus* and anaerobic bacteria [11].

Clindamycin has good penetration into the infected pleural space and provides adequate antimicrobial coverage. Therefore, penicillin-allergic patients can be treated with clindamycin, either alone or in combination with ciprofloxacin or cephalosporin. Chloramphenicol, carbapenems such as meropenem, third-generation cephalosporins, and broad-spectrum penicillin types, such as piperacillin, are alternative agents.

According to the study conducted by Marianthi Iliopoulou about bacterial resistance, susceptibility test conducted with combinations of these antibiotics has shown that the lowest (56%) and highest (94%) prevalence of sensitivity was observed for penicillin G and meropenem, respectively. With respect to antibiotic combinations, the highest (94%) prevalence of sensitivity was observed for the meropenem/linezolid combination, whereas similar results were observed for combinations comprising aminopenicillin/lactamase inhibitor and respiratory fluoroquinolone (93%), as well as ceftriaxone and respiratory fluoroquinolone (89%) [10].

Thus, it is possible concluding that Gram-positive cocci, mainly non-pneumococcal streptococci, are most often found in patients with community-acquired infections. Most isolates are sensitive to the combination of respiratory fluoroquinolone to ceftriaxone or aminopenicillin/lactamase inhibitor. Therefore, common antibiotic regimens based on local antibiotic policies are highly effective in treating this infection when they are early and properly implemented (Table 16.3).

Table 16.3 Empirical antimicrobial use in urgent and emergency surgery for thorax infections

Community-acquired infection	Urgency and emergency	*Streptococcus spp, Staphylococcus aureus*, gram-negative (*E. coli* and Enterobacteriaceae)	Amoxicillin (preferably in association with clavulanate) + Levofloxacin Ceftriaxone + Levofloxacin	Amoxicillin (preferably in association with clavulanate) + Clindamycin Clindamycin
Hospital infection	Urgency and emergency	Staphylococci, *E. coli*, *Pseudomonas aeruginosa*, *Klebsiella* spp.	Piperacillin/Tazobactam + Clindamycin	Meropenem + Linezolid

Intra-abdominal Region

It is necessary establishing whether the infection is of the community-acquired or healthcare-associated type to enable the proper management of the infectious site, as well as to list the likely pathogens and their potential resistance patterns. Antibiotic therapy application to community-acquired infections should focus on bacteria deriving from the gastrointestinal flora. On the other hand, broader antibiotic therapy application is preferable in healthcare-associated infections. The World Society of Emergency Surgery always recommends implementing short-term antibiotic therapy (3–5 days) after satisfactory infectious source control in complicated cases. On the other hand, etiological investigation should be performed after 5–7 days, in patients with peritonitis or persistent systemic disease.

The antimicrobial option should be based on patients' clinical condition, individual risk of infection by resistant pathogens, and local epidemiological antimicrobial resistance. Culture collections during the intraoperative period are recommended for patients with community-acquired and healthcare-associated infections. They enable the initial expansion of antimicrobial spectrum in critically ill patients, and subsequent therapy focused on the post-culture agent. Empirical antifungal therapy is recommended by the World Society of Emergency Surgery for patients with healthcare-associated infection, mainly for those who were recently subjected to abdominal surgery or who present anastomotic fistula. Thus, recommendations should be made as follows:

Empirical antimicrobial using in patients with early-stage retroperitoneal infections should be based on etiological analysis and on the epidemiology of the pathogen (Table 16.4). Guidelines, such as the Chinese guideline for the diagnosis and management of intra-abdominal infection, have suggested that moxifloxacin, cefoperazone-sulbactam, or ertapenem (alone) are recommended for non-severe retroperitoneal infections. Carbapenems such as imipenem-cilastatin or meropenem, or broad-spectrum antibiotics such as piperacillin-tazobactam, are prescribed, right away, to cover all likely pathogens and to control the infection in critically ill patients [12]. They can have their antimicrobial spectrum narrowed based on culture results (Table 16.4) [13].

Table 16.4 Empirical antimicrobial use in urgent and emergency surgery for intra-abdominal infections

Overall community-acquired infection	Noncritical condition	E. coli, Klebsiella pneumonieae, Pseudomonas aeruginosa, Streptococci, Staphylococcus aureus, Proteus mirabilis, anaerobes	Amoxicillin + clavulanate Ceftriaxone + metronidazole Cefotaxime + metronidazole	Ciprofloxacin + metronidazole Ertapenem Tigecycline
	Critical condition		Piperacillin + tazobactam Cefepime + metronidazole	Meropenem Doripenem or Imipenem/Cilastatin Ampicillin (enterococcus)
Overall hospital infection	Noncritical condition	E. coli, Klebsiella pneumonieae, Pseudomonas aeruginosa, Streptococci, Staphylococcus aureus, Proteus mirabilis, anaerobes	Piperacillin + tazobactam	Meropenem + ampicillin Doripenem + ampicillin Piperacillin/Tazobactam + tigecycline
			High risk of candida infection	(+) Fluconazole
	Critical condition		Meropenem	Ceftolozane/Tazobactam + metronidazole (non-metallo-lactamase-producing pseudomonas)
			Doripenem	Ceftazidime/Avibactam + metronidazole + vancomycin or teicoplanin
			Imipenem/Cilastatin	Linezolid (vancomycin-resistant enterococcus)
			Risk of fungal infection	Caspofungin, micafungin or Liposomal Amphotericin B

Appendix

Perforation is one of the main complications of acute appendicitis since it is correlated to increased morbidity and mortality rates. The risk of perforation increases in younger age groups and in patients in the age group 50 years or older. Appendectomy has been the suggested therapy in most cases since it was first described in the nineteenth century. Appendicitis is diagnosed based on clinical, laboratory, and imaging findings. Surgical site infection, intra-abdominal abscess, and paralytic ileus stand out among its postoperative complications [13].

Antibiotic prophylaxis is recommended for uncomplicated appendectomy cases; it is administered up to 60 min before skin incision. On the other hand, its therapeutic use is adopted for 3–5 days, or for longer, in complicated appendicitis cases (perforating appendicitis presenting abscess or diffuse peritonitis) [13].

Gram-negative and anaerobic bacteria, mainly *E. coli* and *Bacteroides* spp., are the most common pathogens. Both the prophylactic and therapeutic use of antibiotics are adopted to enable this coverage. The most common combination comprises ceftriaxone + metronidazole, whereas the pediatric population can be treated with gentamicin, ampicillin, and metronidazole combination; the most aggressive cases can be treated with piperacillin/tazobactam, in separate [13].

Other antibiotic formulations can be used by taking into consideration Gram-negative pathogens. Some alternatives comprise quinolones (ciprofloxacin or ofloxacin), tinidazole using rather than the mostly used metronidazole, and cefotaxime using as alternative cephalosporin, whose use depends on the profile of each healthcare service (Table 16.5) [14].

Pancreas

Acute pancreatitis (AP) is an inflammatory condition of the pancreas that is most often caused by gallstones or excessive alcohol intake. The disease has mild course in most patients, who present fast clinical improvement after undergoing moderate fluid resuscitation, pain and nausea treatment, and early oral feeding.

Most patients (80–85%) develop mild illness (self-limited, mortality rate < 1–3%), but approximately 20% of them have moderate or severe AP episodes [15] The severe form of the disease results from infected pancreatic and peripancreatic necrosis, which affects approximately 20–40% of patients with severe acute pancreatitis and is associated with worsened organic dysfunctions. Mortality rate in patients with infected necrosis and organ failure reached 35.2%, whereas concomitant sterile necrosis and organ failure were associated with mortality rate of 19.8% [15].

Review conducted by Johnson et al. (2004) has reported that persistent organ failure (POF) for more than 48 h in the first week is strongly associated with the risk of death or local complications.

According to the updated 2012 Atlanta classification, acute necrotic collections (ANC) and Walled-off necrosis (WON) are peripancreatic collections associated with necrosis. ANCs are observed during the first 4 weeks and present varying number of fluids and necrotic tissues involving the pancreatic parenchyma and/or peripancreatic tissues. WON is a mature encapsulated collection of pancreatic and/or peripancreatic necrosis with well-defined and intensified inflammatory wall.

Nowadays, two new studies were performed to review the 2012 Atlanta classifications for pan-

Table 16.5 Empirical antimicrobial use in urgent and emergency surgery for cecal appendix infections

Noncomplicated	*E.coli, Bacteroides spp*	Antibiotic prophylaxis: Cefazolin	
Complicated		Amoxicillin + clavulanate	Ciprofloxacin + metronidazole
		Ceftriaxone + metronidazole	Moxifloxacin
		Cefotaxime + metronidazole	Ertapenem (risk of ESBL enterobacteria)

creatitis prognosis, namely: Revised Atlanta Classification 2012 (RAC)—in addition to AP severity classification, it provides a clear definition of its diagnosis, highlights pain onset as important point of reference, and defines individual local complications, as well as interstitial and necrotizing pancreatitis. RAC comprises three categories: mild, moderately severe, and severe, based on organ failure and on local or systemic complications. The Determinant-Based Classification of Acute Pancreatitis Severity (DBC) has added a fourth (critical) category, which is based on the two main mortality determinants: (peri)pancreatic necrosis and organ failure.

All patients with severe acute pancreatitis should be subjected to contrast computed tomography (CE-CT) or magnetic resonance imaging (MRI) to assess the extent to which the gland is compromised. The ideal time for the first CE-CT assessment is 72–96 h after the onset of symptoms.

Magnetic resonance cholangiopancreatography (MRCP) or endoscopic ultrasound should be taken into consideration for screening hidden common bile ducts in patients with unknown etiology.

C-reactive protein level ≥150 mg/L on the third day can be used as prognostic factor for severe acute pancreatitis. According to the American College of Gastroenterology guideline, C-reactive protein (CRP) is the gold standard used to assess pancreatitis severity. Based on cutoff point ranging from 110 to 150 mg/L, sensitivity and specificity ranged from 38% to 61%, and from 89% to 90%, respectively, at hospitalization time [16, 17].

Other tests such as hematocrit >44% represent independent risk factor for pancreatic necrosis, whereas urea >20 mg/dL is an independent predictor of mortality. Procalcitonin is the most sensitive laboratory test used to detect pancreatic infection—low serum values appear to be strong negative predictors of infected necrosis.

The pathogenesis of secondary bacterial pancreatic infections remains unknown. Pathogens can reach the pancreas via the hematogenous pathway, through the biliary system, and ascend from the duodenum through the main pancreatic duct, or through transmural colonic migration from the colonic bacteria translocation.

The main bacterial agents involved in the infection—gram-negative bacteria such as *Escherichia coli*, *Proteus*, *Klebsiella pneumonia*—emerge through the translocation of the intestinal flora and through damage to the intestinal mucosa. Compromised bodily defenses predispose individuals to the translocation of gastrointestinal organisms and toxins, with subsequent secondary pancreatic infection. However, Gram-positive bacteria (*Staphylococcus aureus*, *Streptococcus faecalis*, *Enterococcus*), anaerobes and, occasionally, fungi are also found [18].

Nowadays, prophylactic antibiotic therapy is not associated with significant decrease in mortality or morbidity rates. Thus, routine prophylactic antibiotics are no longer recommended for all patients with acute pancreatitis [15].

However, antibiotics are always recommended for severe and infected AP, although it is hard to be diagnosed. These patients should receive broad-spectrum empirical antibiotics capable of covering aerobic and anaerobic Gram-negative and Gram-positive microorganisms [19].

Third-generation cephalosporins, such as piperacillin, have intermediate penetration into the pancreatic tissue, are effective against gram-negative organisms, and can cover the minimum inhibitory concentration for most gram-negative organisms found in pancreatic infections [15]. Among these antibiotics, only piperacillin/tazobactam are effective against gram-positive and anaerobic bacteria.

Quinolones (ciprofloxacin and moxifloxacin) and carbapenems show satisfactory penetration into the pancreatic tissue with the additional benefit of anaerobic coverage [15]. However, given the high rate of resistance to quinolones worldwide, they should only be used in patients with allergies to beta-lactam agents.

Carbapenems should always be optimized and only used in very critically ill patients due to the outspread of carbapenem-resistant *Klebsiella pneumoniae*.

Table 16.6 Empirical antimicrobial use in urgent and emergency surgery for pancreas infections

Urgency and emergency	E, coli, Proteus, Klebsiella pneumonieae (the most common ones) Staphylococcus aureus, Streptococcusfaecalis, Enterococcus (also found)	Piperacillin + tazobactam	Quinolones (allergy to beta lactam)
			Meropenem/ Imipenem/ Ertapenem

Metronidazole also shows satisfactory penetration into the pancreas given its bactericidal spectrum, which almost exclusively focuses on anaerobes (Table 16.6).

16.2.1.2 Gallbladder and Bile Ducts

The estimated prevalence of gallstones reaches 10–15% in the overall population, with some differences between countries. From 20 to 40% of patients with gallstones develop complications such as choledocholithiasis, cholecystitis, and pancreatitis—incidence of 1–3% a year [20].

Acute cholecystitis (AC) is the first clinical presentation in 10–15% of cases; cholecystectomy is the gold standard therapeutic approach for these cases, with two exceptions: patients who refuse surgery and patients for whom surgery would be considered a "very high risk", although there is no clear consensus on this second issue.

Choledocholithiasis—i.e., the incidence of common bile duct stone (CBDS)—happens in 10–20% of gallstone cases. It has lower incidence (from 5 to 15%) in the case of acute calculous cholecystitis (ACC) [21, 22].

According to Tokyo Guidelines (2018), Gram-negative (*E. coli*, *Klebsiella* spp., and *Pseudomonas* spp.) and Gram-positive bacteria (Enterococcus spp. and Streptococcus spp.), as well as anaerobes, are the main microorganisms isolated from bile culture in acute cholecystitis and acute cholangitis cases. According to the same guideline, empirical antimicrobial therapy is divided into community-acquired and healthcare-associated bile infections [23].

Cases of community-acquired noncritical infections can be treated with ampicillin/sulbactam, with metronidazole in combination to cefazolin, cefuroxime, ceftriaxone or cefotaxime, ertapenem, or with quinolones such as ciprofloxacin or levofloxacin, in association with metronidazole [23].

Moderate cases of community-acquired biliary infections can be treated with piperacillin/tazobactam, with metronidazole in combination to ceftriaxone, cefepime, ceftazidime, cefozopran or cefotaxime, ertapenem, or with metronidazole combination to ciprofloxacin, levofloxacin, pazufloxacin, or levofloxacin [23].

Critical or healthcare-associated cases can be treated with piperacillin/tazobactam, as well as with metronidazole in association with cefepime, ceftazidime, or cefozopran. They can also be treated with therapy based on carbapenems such as imipenem/cilastatin, meropenem, doripenem, or ertapenem. Another option lies on using Aztreonam, either alone or in combination with metronidazole [23].

Nowadays, laparoscopic cholecystectomy is the gold standard treatment for acute calculous cholecystitis. On the other hand, antibiotic therapy administration in the postoperative period is not recommended for noncomplicated cases. However, there are patients who present biliary sepsis, such as those with cholangitis, who require surgical treatment in association with antimicrobial therapy.

Early administration of correct empirical antimicrobial therapy has significant impact on the outcome of patients with sepsis of abdominal origin. International guidelines focused on managing severe sepsis and septic shock (Surviving Sepsis Campaign) recommend the administration of broad-spectrum intravenous antibiotics with good penetration into the infection site within the first hour. The pharmacokinetics of selected drugs may significantly change in biliary sepsis cases; therefore, antibiotic selection should be reassessed on a daily basis by taking into consideration patients' pathophysiological state and pharmacokinetic properties of specific drugs.

However, complicated acute calculous cholecystitis presents different clinical picture and management approach. It is recommended to adopt treatment with empirical antibiotics based on the most often isolated pathogens, by taking into account local resistance trends, drug availability, and risk factors for the main resistance patterns. Extended-spectrum beta-lactamase production by *Enterobacteriae* remains the main issue associated with resistance to antibiotics in biliary tract infection cases; it is often found in community-acquired infections affecting patients who had been previously exposed to antibiotics [24, 25].

The proper use of broad-spectrum empirical therapy appears to be a crucial factor in reducing postoperative complications and death cases, mainly in critically ill patients. The effectiveness of antibiotics in treating biliary infections may be associated with their bile concentration. However, bile penetration of antibiotics administered to patients hospitalized due to choledocholithiasis may be poor and real bile concentrations are only achieved in a small percentage of patients.

Gram-negative aerobes such as *Escherichiacolia* and *Klebsiella*, as well as anaerobes, mainly *Bacteroides fragilis*, are the most isolated bacteria in biliary infection cases [24, 25].

The potential pathogenicity of bacteria belonging to genus *Enterococci* in biliary sepsis cases remains unclear. Specific coverage against these microorganisms is not often suggested for community-acquired biliary infections, only in immunosuppression cases, i.e., in transplant patients.

Identifying the causative organism(s) is an essential step to manage ACC, mainly in patients at high risk of antimicrobial resistance, such as immunocompromised patients. The positive bile culture rate (of gallbladder culture or bile samples from the common bile duct) ranges from 29 to 54% [26, 27].

Thus, the 2020 WSES about acute calculous cholecystitis, based on updated evidences, reinforces the key role played by laparoscopic cholecystectomy as the main treatment for ACC, even in high-risk patients. The use, or not, of antimicrobial therapy must be based on the physiological status of these patients at hospitalization time (Table 16.7).

16.2.1.3 Small Intestine and Colon

Abdominal issues involving hollow viscera—which require antibiotic using—can be found in traumatic and nontraumatic emergencies; obstructions and perforations are the most common ones.

Prophylactic antibiotic therapy capable of covering gram-negative and anaerobic bacilli is

Table 16.7 Empirical antimicrobial use in urgent and emergency surgery for gallbladder and bile ducts infections

Community-acquired Infection noncritical condition	*Gram-negative (E. coli, Klebsiella* spp. *and Pseudomonas* spp.*)* *Gram-positive (Enterococcus* spp. *and Streptococcus* spp.*)* *Anaerobes*	Ampicillin + sulbactam Cefazolin or Cefotiam or Cefuroxime or Ceftriaxone or Cefotaxime +Metronidazole	Ertapenem Ciprofloxacin, Levofloxacin, Pazufloxacin + Metronidazole
Community-acquired infection moderate condition	*Gram-negative (E. coli, Klebsiella* spp. *and Pseudomonas* spp.*)* *Gram-positive (Enterococcus* spp. *and Streptococcus* spp.*)* *Anaerobes*	Piperacillin + tazobactam Ceftriaxone or Cefotaxime or Cefepime or Cefozopran or Ceftazidime + Metronidazole	Ertapenem Ciprofloxacin, Levofloxacin, Pazufloxacin + Metronidazole
Community-acquired infection critical condition	*Gram-negative (E. coli, Klebsiella* spp. *and Pseudomonas* spp.*)*	Piperacillin + tazobactam	Aztreonam +/= metronidazole
Hospital infection	*Gram-positive (Enterococcus* spp. *and Streptococcus* spp.*)* *Anaerobes*	Cefepime or Ceftazidime or Cefozopran + Metronidazole	Imipenem/Cisplatin or Meropenem or Doripenem or Ertapenem

recommended for patients with obstruction issues, given the likelihood of bacterial translocation. This antibiotic prophylaxis should be discontinued after 24 h or 3 doses, if patients do not present other indication for antibiotic therapy. Antibiotic prophylaxis can be based on third-generation cephalosporin, in association (or not) with metronidazole [28].

The most distal portion of the gastrointestinal tract is more densely populated by aerobes such as *Escherichia coli* and *Pseudomonas* sp., as well as by anaerobes such as *Peptostreptococcus* sp., *Bacteroides oralis*, *B. melaninogenicus*, *B. fragilis,* and *Clostridia* sp. [29].

Antibiotic therapy capable of covering gram-negative and anaerobic bacilli is always recommended for perforation cases. *B. fragilis* and other mandatory anaerobes, as well as *Enterobacteriaceae* such as *E. coli*, stand out among the most common pathogens [28].

Broad-spectrum antibiotics should be empirically used in these cases, mainly in septicemia cases, based on culture of ESBL-producing Enterobacteria strains. Treatment time ranges from 4 to 7 days, on average, depending on clinical parameters such as source, fever, leukocytosis, C-reactive protein, and procalcitonin control [28].

Third-generation cephalosporins are highly effective against gram-negative colonies, whereas ceftriaxone is a good prophylactic option due to its high effectiveness and duration. Ceftriaxone was more effective than other antibiotics, such as the beta-lactam ones (cephalosporins and penicillin); thus, it can be used alone, or in combination with metronidazole, with good therapeutic outcomes (Table 16.8) [30].

Stomach

Patients with perforated peptic ulcers should be treated with broad-spectrum antibiotic therapy, without the need for associated antifungals. Intraoperative culture is recommended for subsequent antibiotic adjustment [31].

Associated pathogens can be of the gram-positive, gram-negative, and anaerobic types. Antibiotic therapy should be initially guided based on infection type (domiciliary or nosocomial), as well as on patients' critical condition and, later, on culture (Table 16.9) [31].

Table 16.8 Empirical antimicrobial use in urgent and emergency surgery for small intestine and colon infections

Obstruction	*E. coli, pseudomonas sp, anaerobes (Peptostreptococcus* sp., *Bacteroides oralis, B. melaninogenicus, B. fragilis,* and *Clostridia sp)*	Ceftriaxone ± metronidazole
Perforation	Anaerobes (*Peptostreptococcus* sp., *Bacteroides oralis, B. melaninogenicus, B. fragilis,* and *Clostridia* sp.) *E. coli*	Ceftriaxone ± metronidazole

Table 16.9 Empirical antimicrobial use in urgent and emergency surgery for stomach infections

Community-acquired infection noncritical condition		Amoxicillin + clavulanate	Ciprofloxacin + metronidazole
		Ceftriaxone + metronidazole	Ertapenem or tigecycline (risk of ESBL)
		Cefotaxime + metronidazole	
Community-acquired infection critical condition		Piperacillin + tazobactam	Meropenem or doripenem
		Cefepime + metronidazole	Imipenem/Cisplatin
Hospital infection noncritical condition		Piperacillin + tazobactam associated with:	Piperacillin + tazobactam associated with:
		Meropenem ± ampicillin Doripenem ± ampicillin Imipenem/cisplatin	Tigecycline
Hospital infection critical condition		Meropenem Imipenem/cisplatin Doripenem associated, or not, with: Vancomycin or Teicoplanin	
Bleeding ulcer	Eradicate *H. pylori*, if positive	Clarithromycin + Amoxicillin + Metronidazole	

Orthopedics and Soft Tissue Infection

Gustilo-Anderson Classification is recommended to classify orthopedic traumas involving open fractures. Pulsating washing at high pressure is recommended, regardless of this classification, because it is effective in removing microbial organisms and contaminants from fractures. On the other hand, it damages soft tissues and can lead to loss of strength mechanisms due to muscle loss. Moreover, antibiotic prophylaxis must be maintained for 72 h, after the trauma, or for 24 h, after the wound was covered [32].

Recommendations for Gustilo-Anderson open-fracture types 1 and 2 comprise early administration of antibiotics with Gram-positive coverage. Cephalosporins, either alone or in association with macrolides, were effective in these cases, as well as high penicillin doses in cases of high risk of fecal or *Clostridium* contamination. Fluoroquinolones using as alternative therapy has shown satisfactory antimicrobial coverage, although they had deleterious effect on fracture healing. With respect to type 3 fractures, in addition to the aforementioned recommendations, it is necessary covering Gram-negative germs, which should be preferably treated based on the association between cephalosporins and aminoglycosides. There is also the alternative option of association with macrolides [32]. A series of previous studies have concluded that the 3-h antimicrobial onset is the gold standard. However, 66 min is the independent predictor of infection in cases of Gustilo-Anderson open fracture III [33].

Approximately 40% of patients subjected to high-energy trauma and soft tissue loss presented monobacterial growth, whereas 35% of them presented polymicrobial growth, although approximately 25% of patients presented negative cultures. Methicillin-sensitive *Staphylococcus aureus* (MSSA) and methicillin-resistant *Staphylococcys aureus* (MRSA) stood out among the main bacteria isolated in these patients [34]. Complex soft tissue injuries caused by high-energy trauma are susceptible to fungal infections. Thus, systemic antifungal therapy with voriconazole or liposomal amphotericin B should be administered. Topical therapy with liposomal amphotericin B (500 mg), voriconazole (200 mg), tobramycin (1.2 g), and vancomycin (1 g) is also recommended [33].

Several studies have shown that burnt patients' hospitalization duration is associated with the isolated bacterium found in them. *Psudomonas aeruginosa* was rarely found in the first 7 days of hospitalization (8% of isolated gram-negative bacteria), but its incidence has increased within 28-day hospitalization (55% of isolated gram-negative bacteria). On the other hand, *Haemophilus influezae* recorded 36% incidence in the first 7 days of hospitalization and it was virtually absent after 7 days. Median time recorded for positive culture of *Staphylococcus aureus* was 3 days (2–8), whereas that of *pseudomonas* was 18 days (9–36) (Table 16.10) [35].

Table 16.10 Empirical antimicrobial use in urgent and emergency surgery for orthopedics and soft tissue infections

Open fractures	Gustilo Anderson I and II	*Staphylococcus aureus, Streptococcus epidermidis*	Cefazolin ± Clindamycin	Vancomycin
	Gustilo Anderson III	*Staphylococcus aureus, Streptococcus epidermidis*	Ceftriaxone + Amikacin / Ceftriaxone + Clindamycin	Vancomycin
High-energy traumas	Soft tissue loss	Associating antifungal coverage	Voriconazole and liposomal Amphotericin B	
Burnt patients		Risk of infection by *pseudomonas aeruginosa, haemophilus influenzae* and *Staphylococcus aureus*	No indication of initial antibiotic therapy	

16.3 Antifungal Drugs

There has been increase in the number of fungal infection cases in hospital environments in the last 25 years. Physicians often associate fungal infections with neutropenic patients; but nowadays, at least half of all nosocomial fungal infections, such as deep and bloodstream infections, affect critically ill surgical patients [36].

Pathogens belonging to genus *Candida*—*Candida albicans* is the prevalent species and it is followed by *C. glabrata*, *C. tropicalis*, *C. parapsilosis*, *C. krusei* and *C. lusitaniae*—are the ones most often involved in fungal infections affecting surgical patients. Species such as *Aspergillus*, *Fusarium*, and *Rhizopus* are less common (10%); they are found in patients with higher immunosuppression degree, such as transplant recipients or individuals subjected to chemotherapy [36].

Amphotericin B, fluconazole, itraconazole, voriconazole, flucytosine, amphotericin lipid products, and echinocandins (caspofungin, micfungin, and anidulafungin) stand out among a wide range of antifungals. Antifungal agent selection depends on the selected fungus, preferential drug administration route (oral or intravenous), agent toxicity, as well as on drug interactions and cost [36].

Species *C. albicans* is often extremely sensitive to fluconazole—sensitivity ranges from 0.125 to 0.250 µg/mL. With respect to *C. glabrata*, fluconazole dose dependence is typically observed at minimum inhibitory concentration of 16 µg/mL, whereas resistance is observed when the minimum inhibitory concentration is higher than, or equal, to 32 µg/mL. *C. glabrata* can be sensitive, dose-dependent, or resistant to fluconazole and itraconazole, depending on its institution; besides, it may show varying sensitivity to amphotericin. Since *C. glabrata* can account for 20–25% of all infections and sensitivity patterns can dictate the therapy to be adopted, physicians must be aware of this pathogen and of the frequency of its institution. Unlike *C. albillicas* and *C. glabrata*, *C. krusei* is always resistant to fluconazole, dose-dependent or resistant to itraconazole, often resistant to flucytosine and presents varying sensitivity to amphotericin. *C. lusitaniae* also has varying sensitivity to amphotericin [36] (Table 16.3).

Initially, treatment with fluconazole is relevant for candidemia cases. There is also the option of using another antifungal drug if patients had previously used any azole component or if they are in critical condition due to unknown pathogen [36].

Peritoneal fluid cultures show high incidence of fungal species, mainly of *Candida albicans*, at perforated peptic ulcer surgery time. Fungal growth in peritoneal fluid is a risk factor for worsened outcomes. Interestingly, there is no evidence of the clinical benefits of empirical antifungal treatment in these patients. On the other hand, delay in treating yeast infections in the bloodstream is an independent predictor of death. If one takes into consideration that *Candida* spp. is often found in the gastrointestinal flora, fungal growth in peritoneal fluid may correspond to colonization rather than to true infection, and it may explain the poor correlation between treatment and outcome [3] (Table 16.11).

Therefore, early empirical antifungal therapy should be taken into consideration since it is significantly associated with lower 30-day mortality rate. Thus, empirical antifungal treatments should be applied to patients at higher risk of invasive candidiasis since the benefit of the treatment outweighs its risk (Table 16.12) [3].

Table 16.11 Empirical antimicrobial use in overall urgent and emergency surgery

Antimicrobial use in urgent and emergency surgery

Surgical site		Clinical condition	Main infectious agents	Antibiotic therapy of choice	Alternative antibiotic therapy
Head and neck	Cephalic pole	Urgency and emergency	Streptococcus pneumoniae, Pseudomonas aeruginosa, Staphylococcus aureus, Hemophilus influenzae type B, Proteus mirabilis and Klebsiella	Ampicillin + sulbactam	Clindamycin
				Cefazolin + metronidazole	Penicillin
	Neck	Urgency and emergency	Staphylococci, Streptococci viridans, Streptococci belonging to group C and Prevotella	Ampicillin ± sulbactam	Gentamycin
				Cefazolin in separate	Penicillin
				Levofloxacin	Piperacillin/Tazobactam
Thorax	Community-acquired infection	Urgency and emergency	Streptococcus spp, Staphylococcus aureus, gram-negative (E. coli and Enterobacteriaceae)	Amoxicillin (preferably in association with clavulanate) + Levofloxacin	Amoxicillin (preferably in association with clavulanate) + Clindamycin
				Ceftriaxone + Levofloxacin	Clindamycin
	Hospital infection	Urgency and emergency	Staphylococci, E. coli, Pseudomonas aeruginosa, Klebsiella spp.	Piperacillin/Tazobactam + Clindamycin	Meropenem + Linezolid
				Piperacillin/Tazobactam + Levofloxacin	
Abdomen	Overall community-acquired infection	Noncritical condition	E. coli, Klebsiella pneumoniae, Pseudomonas aeruginosa, Streptococci, Staphylococcus aureus, Proteus mirabilis, anaerobes	Amoxicillin + clavulanate	Ciprofloxacin + metronidazole
				Ceftriaxone + metronidazole	Ertapenem
				Cefotaxime + metronidazole	Tigecycline
		Critical condition		Piperacillin + tazobactam	Meropenem
					Doripenem or Imipenem/Cilastatin
				Cefepime + metronidazole	Ampicillin (enterococcus)
	Overall hospital infection	Noncritical condition	E. coli, Klebsiella pneumoniae, Pseudomonas aeruginosa, Streptococci, Staphylococcus aureus, Proteus mirabilis, anaerobes	Piperacillin + tazobactam	Meropenem + ampicillin
					Doripenem + ampicillin
					Piperacillin/Tazobactam + tigecycline
				High risk of candida infection	(+) Fluconazole
		Critical condition		Meropenem	Ceftolozane/Tazobactam + metronidazole (non-metallo-lactamase-producing pseudomonas)
				Doripenem	Ceftazidime/Avibactam + metronidazole + vancomycin or teicoplanin
				Imipenem/Cilastatin	Linezolid (vancomycin-resistant enterococcus)
				Risk of fungal infection	Caspofungin, micafungin or Liposomal Amphotericin B

(continued)

Table 16.11 (continued)

Antimicrobial use in urgent and emergency surgery

Surgical site	Clinical condition	Main infectious agents	Antibiotic therapy of choice	Alternative antibiotic therapy
Retroperitoneum	Noncritical condition	E. coli, Klebsiella pneumoniae, Pseudomonas aeruginosa, Streptococci, Staphylococcus aureus, Proteus mirabilis, anaerobes	Moxifloxacin	Ertapenem
	Critical condition		Cefoperazone/Sulbactam	
			Imipenem/Cilastatin or meropenem	
			Piperacillin/Tazobactam	
Stomach	Community-acquired infection noncritical condition		Amoxicillin + clavulanate	Ciprofloxacin + metronidazole
			Ceftriaxone + metronidazole	Ertapenem or tigecycline (risk of ESBL)
			Cefotaxime + metronidazole	
	Community-acquired infection critical condition		Piperacillin + tazobactam	Meropenem or doripenem
			Cefepime + metronidazole	Imipenem/Cisplatin
	Hospital infection noncritical condition		Piperacillin + tazobactam associated with:	Piperacillin + tazobactam associated with:
				Tigecycline
	Hospital infection critical condition		Meropenem ± ampicillin Doripenem ± ampicillin Imipenem/Cisplatin	
			Meropenem Imipenem/Cisplatin Doripenem associated, or not, with:	
			Vancomycin or Teicoplanin	
	Bleeding ulcer	Eradicate H. pylori, if positive	Clarithromycin + Amoxicillin + Metronidazole	
Small intestine and colon	Obstruction	E. coli, pseudomonas sp, anaerobes (Peptostreptococcus sp., Bacteroides oralis, B. melaninogenicus, B. fragilis, and Clostridia sp)	Ceftriaxone ± metronidazole	
	Perforation	Anaerobes (Peptostreptococcus sp., Bacteroides oralis, B. melaninogenicus, B. fragilis, and Clostridia sp.) E. coli	Ceftriaxone ± metronidazole	
Cecal appendix	Noncomplicated	E.coli, Bacteroides spp	Antibiotic prophylaxis: Cefazolin	
	Complicated		Amoxicillin + clavulanate	Ciprofloxacin + metronidazole
			Ceftriaxone + metronidazole	Moxifloxacin
			Cefotaxime + metronidazole	Ertapenem (risk of ESBL enterobacteria)
Pancreas	Urgency and emergency	E. coli, Proteus, Klebsiella pneumoniae (the most common ones) Staphylococcus aureus, Streptococcus faecalis, Enterococcus (also found)	Piperacillin + tazobactam	Quinolones (allergy to beta lactam)
				Meropenem/Imipenem/Ertapenem

Gallbladder cholecystitis and cholangitis	Community-acquired infection noncritical condition	Gram-negative (E. coli, Klebsiella spp. and Pseudomonas spp.) Gram-positive (Enterococcus spp. and Streptococcus spp.) Anaerobes	Ampicillin + sulbactam Cefazolin or Cefotiam or Cefuroxime or Ceftriaxone or Cefotaxime + Metronidazole	Ertapenem Ciprofloxacin, Levofloxacin, Pazufloxacin + Metronidazole
	Community-acquired infection moderate condition	Gram-negative (E. coli, Klebsiella spp. and Pseudomonas spp.) Gram-positive (Enterococcus spp. and Streptococcus spp.) Anaerobes	Piperacillin + tazobactam Ceftriaxone or Cefotaxime or Cefepime or Cefozopran or Ceftazidime + Metronidazole	Ertapenem Ciprofloxacin, Levofloxacin, Pazufloxacin + Metronidazole
	Community-acquired infection critical condition	Gram-negative (E. coli, Klebsiella spp. and Pseudomonas spp.) Gram-positive (Enterococcus spp. and Streptococcus spp.) Anaerobes	Piperacillin + tazobactam	Aztreonam +/= metronidazole
	Hospital infection		Cefepime or Ceftazidime or Cefozopran + Metronidazole	Imipenem/Cisplatin or Meropenem or Doripenem or Ertapenem
Open fractures	Gustilo Anderson I and II	Staphylococcus aureus, Streptococcus epidermidis	Cefazolin ± Clindamycin	Vancomycin
	Gustilo Anderson III	Staphylococcus aureus, Streptococcus epidermidis	Ceftriaxone + Amikacin Ceftriaxone + Clindamycin	Vancomycin
High-energy traumas	Soft tissue loss	Associating antifungal coverage	Voriconazole and liposomal Amphotericin B	
Burnt patients		Risk of infection by Pseudomonas aeruginosa, Haemophilus influenzae and Staphylococcus aureus	No indication of initial antibiotic therapy	

Row group label: Limbs and soft tissues (Open fractures, High-energy traumas, Burnt patients)

Table 16.12 Candida species' sensitivity to drugs

Candida species	Fluconazole	Itraconazole	Flucytosinex	Amphotericin B
C. albicans	Susceptible	Susceptible	Susceptible	Susceptible
C. glabrata	Susceptible to high doses	Susceptible to high doses	Susceptible	Intermediary
C. tropicalis	Susceptible	Susceptible	Susceptible	Susceptible
C. parapsilosis	Susceptible	Susceptible	Susceptible	Susceptible
C. krusei	Resistant	Susceptible to high doses	Intermediary	Intermediary
C. lusitaniae	Susceptible	Susceptible	Susceptible	Intermediary

16.4 Diagnosis

Inappropriate treatment or delay in starting adequate treatment can increase the morbidity and mortality of patients. The ability to discern between infectious and noninfectious sources based on clinical analysis is effective only in 61.5% of cases where the patient effectively presents with infection. Obtaining objective infection data in surgical and critically ill patients is an essential component of good patient outcome. The clinical picture usually progresses with symptoms such as a systemic inflammatory response without necessarily having an infectious cause (pancreatitis, burns, venous thrombosis, aspiration, transfusion, ischemia, neurological damage). Critically ill patients with fever and an infectious origin are most commonly related to intra-abdominal infection, pneumonia, or skin and soft tissue infection [3].

Additionally, the use of clinical scores such as APACHE and serum procalcitonin dosage are poor predictors of infectious etiology in surgical patients due to the presence of several invasive support devices such as endotracheal tube, nasogastric tube, central venous access, arterial catheters, and urinary catheter delays, which include a broad source of infectious and noninfectious sources of fever [3].

Although infectious diagnosis is difficult, identifying the source can be even more challenging. Site-focused diagnostic management (no general cultures) based solely on clinical suspicion may result in delayed diagnosis or even misdiagnosis. Often times, even objective laboratory data such as different sites cultures may fail to reveal the infectious site, but a clinically guided approach alone may prove impossible to diagnose [3].

In a scenario in which the origin of a febrile condition is difficult to identify, it is a consensus to start empirical antibiotics to avoid delays in antimicrobial administration. The more conservative start of antibiotic therapy in stable patients has shown a reduction in mortality, but in critically ill patients it has already been proven, as demonstrated by the Surviving Sepsis Campaign [37], as the best outcome in the early and aggressive start of antibiotic therapy, including reducing hospital mortality [3].

16.5 Sepsis

Sepsis is defined as a life-threatening organ dysfunction caused by an unregulated host response to an infection [38] Its appearance is related to characteristics of pathogens and hosts (examples: sex, ethnicity, and other genetic determinants, age, comorbidities, environment) [38].

The sepsis diagnostic algorithm is based on prognostic scores that assess organ dysfunction. Organ dysfunction can be identified as an acute change in the SOFA (Sequential [Sepsis-related] Organ Failure Assessment) score greater than or equal to two points [38] (Table 16.13).

Although the SOFA score change is a robust mortality stratification tool, it is difficult to calculate and requires laboratory values that are not readily available for rapid screening of patients outside the intensive care unit [39]. The task force began to readily identify accessible screening measures and arrived at 3 criteria, called the qSOFA (quick Sequential Organ Failure Assessment) [39] (Table 16.14).

Table 16.13 SOFA (Sequential [Sepsis-related] Organ Failure Assessment) score

	Escore				
	0	1	2	3	4
Respiratory system - PaO$_2$/FiO$_2$, mmHg (kPa)	≥400	<400	<300	<200 w/ventilatory support	<100 w/ventilatory support
Coagulation - Platelets, × 10^3/μL	≥150	<150	<100	<50	<20
Liver - Bilirrubins, mg/dL (μmol/L)	<1.2	1.2–1.9	2.0–5.9	6.0–11.9	>12
Cardiovascular	MAP ≥70 mmHg	MA < 70 mmHg	Dopamine <5 or dobutamine (any dosage)[a]	Dopamine 5.1–15 ou epinefrine ≤0.1 ou noradrenaline ≤0.1[a]	Dopamine >15 ou epinefrine >0.1 ou noradrenaline >0.1[a]
Central nervous system - Glasgow coma scale	15	13–14	10–12	6–9	<6
Renal - Creatinine, mg/dL (μmol/L) - Urinary output	<1.2	1.2–1.9	2.0–3.4	3.5–4.9 <500	>5.0 <200

FiO fraction of inspired oxygen, *MAP* mean arterial pressure, *PaO2* partial pressure of oxygen
[a] Dosage of catecholamines is μg/kg/min for at least one hour

Table 16.14 qSOFA (quick Sequential Organ Failure Assessment)

qSOFA	
Parameter evaluated	Reference value
Respiratory rate	>22 ipm
Glasgow coma scale	<13
Systolic blood pressure	≤100 mmHg

For patients outside the intensive care unit, with a score greater than or equal to two points by the qSOFA score, mortality was similar to those who were assessed by the full SOFA [39].

After the diagnostic suspicion of a septic condition, the start of therapy should be instituted within the first hour. Defined as "hour-1 bundle", with the explicit intent to begin resuscitation and management immediately [40].

Among this approach, we can cite the measures below [40]:

- Measure serum lactate level. Collect if initially >2 mmol/L;
- Obtain blood cultures before starting antibiotics;
- Administer broad-spectrum antibiotics;
- Start rapid administration of crystalloid solution at a dose of 30 mL/kg, if hypotension or serum lactate ≥4 mmol/L;
- Initiate vasopressors during or after fluid resuscitation to maintain mean arterial pressure ≥ 65 mmHg.

Thinking specifically about the surgical patient, this is subject to evolution to a septic condition and the surgical procedure itself can be the source of infection (in case of emergency surgery, for example).

Many other factors related to hospitalization can contribute to the development of postoperative infections and sepsis. Preoperative identification of patients who are at increased risk for sepsis after surgery can help clinicians predict patients who should be more intensively monitored for sepsis after surgery, which, in turn, can facilitate early detection and the start of therapy [41].

Patient-related risk factors for postoperative sepsis [41]:

1. Male gender;
2. Older patients (age group ≥75 years);
3. Underweight was associated with a higher incidence of sepsis during the first 30 days after surgery.

Preexisting conditions [6]:

1. Chronic obstructive pulmonary disease;
2. Diabetes;
3. Hypertension;
4. Chronic heart failure;
5. Anemia;
6. Chronic kidney disease.

Late recognition of sepsis and late treatment initiation are prognostic indicators of poor outcome and high mortality. Current guidelines recommend the implementation of routine sepsis screening for high-risk patients and advise starting treatment as soon as possible to reduce mortality [41, 42].

16.6 Conclusion

Prevention protocols are cost-effective and can be implemented everywhere, including in places with limited resources. Patients subjected to central and urinary catheters, as well as to ventilators are at high risk of developing hospital infections. Surgical site infection is the most common type observed in surgical patients. Surgeons must identify surgical infections and provide feedback to hospital control sectors by directly interacting with antimicrobial standardization teams and with infection control committees.

Dos and Don'ts
- Sepsis protocol must be implemented as soon as patients present clinical signs of systemic infection.
- Remember to collect fluid samples of all drained collections.
- Interventions, either surgical or by interventional radiology, are often necessary for surgical patients.
- Do not delay surgical procedure recommendation to reduce infection.
- Do not expect surgical infections to be resolved with antibiotics alone.
- Do not forget to offer proper nutritional support during the hypermetabolic phase.

Take-Home Messages
- Surgical patients often develop infectious complications.
- Be aware of clinical signs of sepsis.
- Be effective in treating surgical infections, otherwise it can be devastating for your patients.
- Follow institutional protocols set for infections, according to the local environment.
- Fungal infections may be in progress and they can be devastating for these patients.

Questions
1. A 25-year-old male patient undergoing elective surgical planning for inguinal hernioplasty. How can we classify the surgical wound for such a patient?
   A. **Clean**
   B. Potentially contaminated
   C. Contaminated
   D. Infected
2. What is the recommended time to perform antibiotic prophylaxis?
   A. 24 h before the surgical procedure
   B. **30–60 min before skin incision**
   C. 1 h after the end of the procedure
   D. At the time of skin incision

3. Which bacteria are most found in cervical affections derived from odontogenic processes?
   A. Gram-negative Streptococcus spp., Staphylococcus aureus (E. coli and Enterobacteriaceae),
   B. Escherichia coli, Bacteroides spp.
   C. Escherichia coli, Proteus, Klebsiella pneumonia
   D. **Staphylococci, Streptococci viridans, Group C Streptococci, and Prevotella**

4. What etiologic agent is most commonly found in a patient diagnosed with uncomplicated acute appendicitis?
   A. Klebsiella pneumoniae
   B. Staphylococcus aureus
   C. **Escherichia coli**
   D. Streptococci viridans

5. In case of antibiotic prophylaxis for a patient diagnosed with uncomplicated appendicitis, which of the following is the most suitable?
   A. Gentamicin
   B. **Cefazolin**
   C. Benzathine Penicillin
   D. Amikacin

6. Which patient would benefit from starting antibiotic therapy in the context of acute pancreatitis?
   A. Patient with acute biliary pancreatitis, Ranson 1
   B. Alcoholic patient, with ultrasonography showing focal enlargement of the pancreas
   C. **Patient in intensive care bed, using vasoactive drugs and tomography with the presence of pancreatic necrosis with the presence of gas inside**
   D. Patient with immunosuppression, with tomography showing densification of the peripancreatic planes

7. Patient undergoes rectosigmoidectomy for acute diverticulitis; intraoperatively, colonic perforation was evidenced, with extravasation of feces into the cavity. According to the classification of surgical wounds and the risk of surgical site infection, how could this surgery be classified?
   A. Clean
   B. Potentially contaminated
   C. Contaminated
   D. **Infected**

8. Taking lung pathogens into account, what would be the first line of treatment for community-acquired pneumonia?
   A. **Amoxicillin associated or not with clavulanate + Levofloxacin**
   B. Ciprofloxacin + metronidazole
   C. Gentamicin + amikacin
   D. Ceftriaxone

9. Patient victim of car trauma, with open fracture in the right lower limb, other systems without significant alterations. What would be the first approach with a view to reducing the risk of contamination of the raw area?
   A. Broad spectrum antibiotic therapy
   B. Suture of the bloody area
   C. **Pulsatile washing with high pressure as it is effective in removing microbial organisms and contaminants, in addition to antibiotic prophylaxis**
   D. Call on orthopedic specialist on duty

10. 42-year-old male with previous diagnosis of choledocholithiasis, performed ERCP for treatment of choledocholithiasis and subsequent laparoscopic video cholecystectomy. Returns to the service after a week with fever, leukocytosis, and hemodynamic instability, diagnosed with acute pancreatitis. He was submitted to a computed tomography scan of the total abdomen which showed a single, extensive peripancreatic collection,

with interspersed gas, without other commemoratives. In this scenario, the most appropriate conduct is:
A. Laparotomy with necrosectomy + cavity drainage
B. New ERCP with calculus removal + biliary drainage
C. Initial antibiotic therapy, with ciprofloxacin and metronidazole and subsequent percutaneous drainage if there is no improvement
D. **Nonoperative treatment with exclusive antibiotic therapy**
E. Partial pancreatectomy + cavity drainage

References

1. Sartelli M, Labricciosa FM, Barbadoro P, Pagani L, Ansaloni L, Brink AJ, et al. The *Global Alliance for Infections in Surgery:* defining a model for antimicrobial stewardship-results from an international cross-sectional survey. World J Emerg Surg. 2017;12:34. https://doi.org/10.1186/s13017-017-0145-2. PMID: 28775763; PMCID: PMC5540347.
2. Harmankaya M, Oreskov JO, Burcharth J, Gögenur I. The impact of timing of antibiotics on in-hospital outcomes after major emergency abdominal surgery. Eur J Trauma Emerg Surg. 2020;46(1):221–7. https://doi.org/10.1007/s00068-018-1026-4. Epub 2018 Oct 11. PMID: 30310958.
3. Subramanian M, Hirschkorn C, Eyerly-Webb SA, Solomon RJ, Hodgman EI, Sanchez RE, Davare DL, Pigneri DA, Kiffin C, Rosenthal AA, Pedraza Taborda FE, Arenas JD, Hennessy SA, Minei JP, Minshall CT, Hranjec T. Clinical diagnosis of infection in surgical intensive care unit: you're not as good as you think! Surg Infect (Larchmt). 2020;21(2):122–9. https://doi.org/10.1089/sur.2019.037. Epub 2019 Sep 25. PMID: 31553271.
4. Costa AC, Santa-Cruz F, Ferraz AAB. What's new in infection on surgical site and antibioticoprophylaxis in surgery? Arq Bras Cir Dig. 2020;33(4) https://doi.org/10.1590/0102-672020200004e1558.
5. Mazuski JE. Perioperative antibiotic prophylaxis: can we do better? J Am Coll Surg. 2020;231(6):768–9. https://doi.org/10.1016/j.jamcollsurg.2020.09.012. PMID: 33243403.
6. Russell MD, Russell MS. Urgent infections of the head and neck. Med Clin North Am. 2018;102(6):1109–20. https://doi.org/10.1016/j.mcna.2018.06.015.
7. Chiesa-Estomba CM, Calvo-Henriquez C, Siga Diom E, Martinez F. Head and neck surgical antibiotic prophylaxis in resource-constrained settings. Curr Opin Otolaryngol Head Neck Surg. 2020;28(3):188–93. https://doi.org/10.1097/moo.0000000000000626.
8. Rana RS, Moonis G. Head and neck infection and inflammation. Radiol Clin North Am. 2011;49:165–82. https://doi.org/10.1016/j.rcl.2010.07.013.
9. Heim N, Faron A, Wiedemeyer V, Reich R, Martini M. Microbiology and antibiotic sensitivity of head and neck space infections of odontogenic origin. Differences in inpatient and outpatient management. J Craniomaxillofac Surg. 2017;45(10):1731–5. https://doi.org/10.1016/j.jcms.2017.07.013.
10. Iliopoulou M, Skouras V, Psaroudaki Z, Makarona M, Vogiatzakis E, Tsorlini E, et al. Bacteriology, antibiotic resistance and risk stratification of patients with culture-positive, community-acquired pleural infection. J Thorac Dis. 2021;13(2):521–32. https://doi.org/10.21037/jtd-20-2786.
11. Ali Raza M. Management of pleural infection in adults: British Thoracic Society pleural disease guideline 2010. Yearbook of Pulmonary Disease, 2011, 111–113. https://doi.org/10.1016/j.ypdi.2011.03.019.
12. Li Z, Tang Y, Wang P, Ren J. Diagnosis and treatment of retroperitoneal infection. Surg Infect (Larchmt). 2021;22(5):477–84. https://doi.org/10.1089/sur.2020.126. Epub ahead of print. PMID: 33146587.
13. Di Saverio S, Podda M, De Simone B, et al. Diagnosis and treatment of acute appendicitis: 2020 update of the WSES Jerusalem guidelines. World J Emerg Surg. 2020;15:27. https://doi.org/10.1186/s13017-020-00306-3.
14. Coccolini F, Fugazzola P, Sartelli M, et al. Conservative treatment of acute appendicitis. Acta Biomed. 2018;89(9-S):119–34. https://doi.org/10.23750/abm.v89i9-S.7905.
15. Leppäniemi A, Tolonen M, Tarasconi A, et al. 2019 WSES guidelines for the management of severe acute pancreatitis. World J Emerg Surg. 2019;14:27. https://doi.org/10.1186/s13017-019-0247-0.
16. Lippi G, Valentino M, Cervellin G. Laboratory diagnosis of acute pancreatitis: in search of the holy grail. Crit Rev Clin Lab Sci. 2012;49:18–31.
17. Rompianesi G, Hann A, Komolafe O, Pereira SP, Davidson BR, Gurusamy KS. Serum amylase and lipase and urinary trypsinogen and amylase for diagnosis of acute pancreatitis. Cochrane Database Syst Rev. 2017;4:CD012010.
18. Reuken PA, Albig H, Rödel J, Hocke M, Will U, Stallmach A, et al. Fungal infections in patients with infected pancreatic necrosis and pseudocysts: risk factors and outcome. Pancreas. 2018;47:92–8.
19. Tenner S, Baillie J, DeWitt J, Vege SS, American College of Gastroenterology. American College of Gastroenterology guideline: management of acute pancreatitis. Am J Gastroenterol. 2013;108:1400–15; 1416.
20. Pisano M, Allievi N, Gurusamy K, et al. 2020 World Society of Emergency Surgery updated guidelines for

the diagnosis and treatment of acute calculus cholecystitis. World J Emerg Surg. 2020;15:61. https://doi.org/10.1186/s13017-020-00336-x.
21. Peng WK, Sheikh Z, Paterson-Brown S, et al. Role of liver function tests in predicting common bile duct stones in acute calculous cholecystitis. Br J Surg. 2005;92(10):1241–7.
22. Maple JT, Ben-Menachem T, Anderson MA, et al. The role of endoscopy in the evaluation of suspected choledocholithiasis. Gastrointest Endosc. 2010;71(1):1–9.
23. Gomi H, Solomkin JS, Schlossberg D, Okamoto K, Takada T, Strasberg SM, et al. Tokyo guidelines 2018: antimicrobial therapy for acute cholangitis and cholecystitis. J Hepatobiliary Pancreat Sci. 2018;25(1):3–16. https://doi.org/10.1002/jhbp.518. Epub 2018 Jan 9. PMID: 29090866.
24. Sartelli M, Catena F, Ansaloni L, et al. Complicated intra-abdominal infections worldwide : the definitive data of the CIAOW study. World J Emerg Surg. 2014;9:37.
25. Sartelli M, Catena F, Ansaloni L, et al. Complicated intra-abdominal infections in Europe : a comprehensive review of the CIAO study. World J Emerg Surg. 2012;7(1):36.
26. Csendes A, Becerra M, Burdiles P, et al. Bacteriological studies of bile from the gallbladder in patients with carcinoma of the gallbladder, cholelithiasis, common bile duct stones and no gallstones disease. Eur J Surg. 1994;160:363–7.
27. Salvador V, Lozada MCR. Microbiology and antibiotic susceptibility of organisms in bile cultures from patients with and without cholangitis at an Asian Academic Medical Center. Surg Infect (Larchmt). 2011;12:105–11.
28. Pisano M, et al. 2017 WSES guidelines on colon and rectal cancer emergencies: obstruction and perforation. World J Emerg Surg. 2018;13:36. https://doi.org/10.1186/s13017-018-0192-3.
29. Danziger L, Hassan E. Antimicrobial prophylaxis of gastrointestinal surgical procedures and treatment of intra-abdominal infections. Drug Intell Clin Pharm. 1987;21(5):406–16. https://doi.org/10.1177/106002808702100502.
30. Raua HG, Mittelkötterb U, Zimmermanna A, Lachmannc A, Köhlerd L, Kullmanne KH. Perioperative infection prophylaxis and risk factor impact in colon surgery. Chemotherapy. 2000;46:353–63.
31. Tarasconi A, Coccolini F, Biffl WL, et al. Perforated and bleeding peptic ulcer: WSES guidelines. World J Emerg Surg. 2020;15:3. https://doi.org/10.1186/s13017-019-0283-9.
32. Gümbel D, Matthes G, Napp M, Lange J, Hinz P, Spitzmüller R, Ekkernkamp A. Current management of open fractures: results from an online survey. Arch Orthop Trauma Surg. 2016;136(12):1663–72. https://doi.org/10.1007/s00402-016-2566-x. Epub 2016 Sep 15. PMID: 27628620.
33. Sheean AJ, Tintle SM, Rhee PC. Soft tissue and wound management of blast injuries. Curr Rev Musculoskelet Med. 2015;8(3):265–71. https://doi.org/10.1007/s12178-015-9275-x. PMID: 26002232; PMCID: PMC4596198.
34. Ray-Zack MD, Hernandez MC, Younis M, Hoch WB, Soukup DS, Haddad NN, Zielinski MD. Validation of the American Association for the Surgery of trauma emergency general surgery grade for skin and soft tissue infection. J Trauma Acute Care Surg. 2018;84(6):939–45. https://doi.org/10.1097/TA.0000000000001860. PMID: 29794690.
35. Lachiewicz AM, Hauck CG, Weber DJ, Cairns BA, van Duin D. Bacterial infections after burn injuries: impact of multidrug resistance. Clin Infect Dis. 2017;65(12):2130–6. https://doi.org/10.1093/cid/cix682. PMID: 29194526; PMCID: PMC5850038.
36. Lipsett PA. Surgical critical care: fungal infections in surgical patients. Crit Care Med. 2006;34(9 Suppl):S215–24. https://doi.org/10.1097/01.CCM.0000231883.93001.E0.
37. Dellinger RP, Levy MM, Rhodes A, et al. Surviving sepsis campaign: international guidelines for management of severe sepsis and septic shock, 2012. Intensive Care Med. 2013;39:165–228.
38. Singer M, Deutschman CS, Seymour CW, Shankar-Hari M, Annane D, Bauer M, et al. The third international consensus definitions for sepsis and septic shock (Sepsis-3). JAMA. 2016;315(8):801. https://doi.org/10.1001/jama.2016.0287.
39. Font MD, Thyagarajan B, Khanna AK. Sepsis and septic shock—basics of diagnosis, pathophysiology and clinical decision making. Med Clin North Am. 2020;104(4):573–85. https://doi.org/10.1016/j.mcna.2020.02.011.
40. Levy MM, Evans LE, Rhodes A. The surviving sepsis campaign bundle: 2018 update. Intensive Care Med. 2018;44(6):925–8. https://doi.org/10.1007/s00134-018-5085-0.
41. Plaeke P, De Man JG, Coenen S, Jorens PG, De Winter BY, Hubens G. Clinical- and surgery-specific risk factors for post-operative sepsis: a systematic review and meta-analysis of over 30 million patients. Surg Today. 2020;50(5):427–39. https://doi.org/10.1007/s00595-019-01827-4.
42. Sartelli M, Coccolini F, Abu-Zidan FM, Ansaloni L, Bartoli S, Biffl W, et al. Hey surgeons! It is time to lead and be a champion in preventing and managing surgical infections! World J Emerg Surg. 2020;15(1):28. https://doi.org/10.1186/s13017-020-00308-1. PMID: 32306979; PMCID: PMC7168830.

Pain Management 17

Etrusca Brogi and Francesco Forfori

17.1 Introduction

> **Learning Goals**
> - Assessment of pain: Pain should be considered as a vital parameter. Pain has to be measured periodically, reassessed after therapeutic intervention and recorded on the medical records. It is important to choose pain assessment methods that fit patients' characteristics. Specific assessment tools are available for specific type of population (i.e., pediatric patients, cognitive impairment, heavily sedated patients, geriatrics).
> - Multimodal approach to pain management: A multidisciplinary approach strategy including pharmacological as well as non-pharmacological interventions has to be followed in order to achieve an optimum pain relief, to obtain patient comfort, and to reduce drugs administration (especially opioids consumption).
> - Tailored medicine that fit patients' characteristics (i.e., cognitive impairment, elderly, pediatrics, obese, chronic pain syndrome, opioid misuse) and clinical settings (from prehospital to discharge).

17.1.1 Introduction

Pain is defined by the International Association for the study of Pain (IASP) as "an unpleasant sensory and emotional experience associated with, or resembling that associated with, actual or potential tissue damage" [1]. In 1986, WHO published a first general guide to pain management, followed by several updates [2]. Acute pain, highly prevalent in emergency situations, is typical of sudden onset and variable duration and is provoked by a specific injury or disease. Pain represents the most common symptom reported by the patients in the Emergency Department (ED), and pain management represents a quality-of-care indicator [3, 4].

An appropriate assessment of pain is crucial in order to reach the diagnosis of the source of pain, to allow effective and individualized pain management, to select an appropriate analgesic strat-

E. Brogi (✉)
Department of Anesthesia and Intensive Care,
Azienda Ospedaliero-Universitaria Pisana, Pisa, Italy

F. Forfori
Department of Anesthesia and Intensive Care,
University of Pisa, Pisa, Italy
e-mail: francesco.forfori@unipi.it

egy, and for the evaluation of the response to therapy. It is vital to select a proper and specific assessment tool for pain measurement that fits specific situation and patient's characteristics (e.g., cognitive developmental, unable to communicate verbally, sedated patients, ventilated patients) [5]. Unfortunately, several barriers still exist for a proper pain assessment and consequent adequate pain management, especially in prehospital and emergency settings [6]. Barriers to adequate pain management are multifactorial and include: limited availability of drugs (prehospital setting), fear of opioids' dependence or abuse, overcrowding in ED, lack of knowledge and training (e.g., regional anesthesia), lack of resource (especially in prehospital setting), and lack of local guidelines.

A comprehensive pain management strategy aims to relieve pain, with minimal side effects and interaction with other drugs. A good pain management strategy should also be able to not interfere with general clinical valuation of the patients (e.g., excessive sedation) and to prevent chronification of pain [7]. Pain control should not be delayed, should begin as early as possible and reassess within fixed periods (depending on the pharmacokinetics of the drugs administered and intensity of pain) and after each intervention [8]. Drugs can be administered by the clock to maintain a constant serum level and on demand, depending on the type of pain and patients' characteristics; however, what is important is to provide analgesia before recurrence of pain. Pain management follows all the phase of patient care, from the prehospital setting to discharge. Consequently, patients should be discharged by the hospital with a clear and proper prescribed pain management strategy with a scheduled follow-up evaluation by healthcare personnel [9]. Acute pain service plays a vital role in all these phases [10].

A complete pain treatment represents a fundamental right of the patients and a fundamental ethical aspect of medicine practice, with several beneficial effects. Pain relief facilitates patient care and management; from physical examination, clinical history evaluation, imaging scan acquisition, invasive procedure, and nursing care.

Not to be underestimated, pain relief prevents the negative consequence for untreated pain with important impact on outcome: sleep disorders, impaired immunity, pro-inflammatory effects, post-traumatic stress disorders, hypertension, increased myocardial oxygen demand, insulin resistance changes in protein metabolism, and coagulopathies [11, 12]. In fact, inadequate pain control is associated with delayed recovery time, increased hospital readmission rates, psychological impacts, chronification of pain, increased morbidity, mortality, and higher health-care costs [13].

From this point of view, a multidisciplinary approach to pain management should include both pharmacological and non-pharmacological pain control methods [14]. It is extremely important to reassure patients that their pain will be taken seriously. Establish realistic expectation with the patients and reassure that the risks and benefits of each component of the pain management are understood. De-escalation regimen has to begin as soon as possible. Even more, during clinical examination, it is important not only to analyze the characteristics of pain (localization of pain, temporal characteristics, intensity of pain, associated symptoms, aggravating and alleviating factors), but it is also important to evaluate the impact of pain on quality of life (on daily activities and sleep) and patients' expectation and willing [15].

17.1.2 Pathophysiology of Pain

From a pathophysiologic point of view, pain originates from a noxious stimulus (i.e., invasive procedures, surgeries, trauma, inflammation) arising from damaged tissues. There are three categories of noxious stimuli: mechanical (e.g., invasive procedures, surgeries, trauma), thermal, (e.g., burn) and chemical (e.g., ischemia, sepsis). The noxious stimulus is responsible for the release of local inflammatory mediators (e.g., histamine, prostaglandins, bradykinin, substance P), the activation of the nociceptors, and a consequent electrical pain signal. Nociceptors are distributed in the somatic and visceral organs. Aδ and C fibers represented the pain circuitry in peripheral nervous systems and transmitted pain impulses from the site of transduction to the dorsal horn in the spinal cord [16]. Then, pain signal is transmitted towards the brain stem, the thalamus to the cerebral cortex through nociceptive afferent pathways. During the transmission of pain stimulus through the brain stem and thalamus, several central nervous pathways are activated with the consequent important response. The activation of reticular system is responsible for the automatic and motor response to pain. The activation of the somatosensory cortex is responsible for the perception and interpretation of pain. Then, the activation of limbic system is responsible for the emotional and behavioral response to pain [17]. Even more, pain transmission is influenced by a second circuitry in the spinal cord through descending inhibitory fibers, responsible for the modulation of pain signal [18]. The descending modulatory pain pathways can lead to a modulation of pain transmission through the release of inhibitory neurotransmitters (e.g., serotonin 5-HT, norepinephrine, gamma -aminobutyric acid).

It is important to highlight that pain is a personal experience and the perception of pain to a noxious stimulus is highly variable on the basis of patient's characteristics and socio-cultural aspects. Even more, patients with preexisting chronic pain syndrome, neuropathy, and myopathy are at higher risk of opioid tolerance, central sensitization, hyperalgesia, and allodynia [19]. The incidence of chronic pain syndromes is high in this group of patients, often due to ineffectively treated or recurrent pain experience, leading to higher drugs consumption with a long-term functional impairment and a lower quality of life [20]. The persistence of pain can be responsible for an upregulation of receptors and an amplified response to the stimuli.

The general stress response to pain leads to the activation of neurohormonal systems and to the release of catecholamine and inflammatory mediators with consequent increased catabolism and increased myocardial oxygen consumption/demand and potential negative impact on the cardiovascular and renal system [21]. The immune system and coagulation cascade are also activated resulting in potential immune system dysfunction, hypercoagulable state, and altered metabolic control. Noteworthy, pain can negatively influence the respiratory system. Patients with chest trauma, thoracotomy, and abdominal injuries are at high risk of the development of atelectasis, consolidation, and respiratory failure [22]. An adequate pain control diminishes the pain associated with breathing and coughing and improves ventilator synchrony with a potential positive effect on ventilator weaning. Therefore, it is fundamental to achieve adequate pain control.

17.1.3 Special Patients Group

17.1.3.1 The Elderly Patient

Elderly patients represent a fastest growing part of the population and a large proportion of the overall trauma and emergency surgical population [23, 24]. Pain management is particularly challenging for the presence of several factors [25]:

- Coexisting medical diseases.
- Concomitant medication with possible risk of harmful interaction.
- Difficult pain assessment due to alteration in sensory perception, cognitive impairment, impaired verbal communication, and the possible presence of mood disorders (e.g., fear, depression, and anxiety) choose appropriate behavior assessment scale tools (as shown in Table 17.3).
- Altered pain threshold and pain tolerance with consequent persistent pain, poor rehabilitation, and a late functional recovery.
- Alterations in pharmacokinetics and pharmacodynamics of drugs due to the steady decline of homeostatic mechanism associating with aging. Decline in hepatic function, decrease in albumin concentration (reduce protein binding) and increase in free concentration of drugs requiring a dose adjustment of drugs in order to avoid side effects. Changes in body composition: decreased body water and

increase in adipose tissue with consequent alteration in drug distribution and clearance.
- Risks of respiratory depressant effects of opioids and benzodiazepines due to the diminished response of central nervous systems to hypercapnia, combined with reduced pulmonary reserve. Titrate accurately drug dose and choose a multimodal approach to pain control especially in this kind of population.
- Increased risk of renal impairment, platelet dysfunction, and gastrointestinal bleeding with the use of NSAIDs.

17.1.3.2 The Pediatric Patient

The development of the nervous system is characterized by a great plasticity of the fibers and the complete development of the nociceptive system is completed in the first month of life. Inadequate pain control can lead to the establishment of long-term consequences.

Specific pain assessment has to be chosen for pediatric pain management, taking into account age, cognitive impairment, and communication (as shown in Table 17.2) [26]. The role of the family member is pivotal, and the presence of family members should be encouraged. Both pharmacologic and non-pharmacologic methods have to be implemented. Cognitive-behavioral techniques reduce the stress associated with the procedure [27]. Pain control strategies have to be chosen in accordance with the patient's age (e.g., neonates, infants, pediatrics), the type of procedure performed, previous experience, and the availability of drugs/equipment (e.g., regional analgesia). Analgesics can be administered through different routes of administration. Intranasal and nebulized short acting analgesics (e.g., ketamine and fentanyl) could represent a good option, especially in non-collaborative patients to avoid intravenous drugs.

Paracetamol and NSAIDs are effective for moderate pain and reduce opioids consumption after major surgery [28]. For major procedures, regional anesthesia can be employed with local anesthetic in addition to general anesthesia. Whatever the technique used, the accurate monitoring of possible side effects and the collaboration of an expert team with specific expertise in child are very important.

17.1.3.3 The Obese Patient

Obese-induced pharmacokinetic alterations can severely alter response to medications. Changes in gastric pH, cardiac output, and intestinal motility may alter oral analgesic absorption and efficacy. Due to changes in total body water, plasma concentration of drugs may decrease as distribution volume increases. Decreased plasma protein binding increases free drug concentrations and further increases drug distribution into tissue. The altered drug metabolism may increase risks of toxicity or decrease efficacy [29]. Even more, coexisting medical disease and concomitant medication may increase the possible risk of harmful drug interaction. It is necessary to reduce the dosage of opioids since the volume of distribution is small compared to the total body weight. Central and regional techniques are recommended, although the local regional techniques present greater technical difficulties and higher incidence of complications [30].

Obese patients are at higher risk of obstructive sleep apnea and it is recommended to prefer an opioid-sparing analgesia technique and monitor the level of sedation, as well as the respiratory rate.

17.1.3.4 Chronic Opiod Therapy: An Opiod Disorder

Patients with preexisting chronic pain syndrome are at higher risk of opioid tolerance, central sensitization, hyperalgesia, and allodynia [31]. It is important to identify patients with chronic opioid therapy or opioids abuse and rapidly activate specific local referral services specialized in substance abuse or chronic pain syndrome treatment [32].

However, the use of routine use of drug testing in patients with trauma or in emergency setting is variable and depends on local rules. It is important to not reduce the usual daily doses of opiates, to use short acting oral opioids, titrate the dose, and use adjuvants in combination (e.g., alpha-2-agonists, ketamine, gabapentin). Evaluate the possible recourse to the rotation of opioids to methadone or buprenorphine. Patients should continue their treatment (e.g., methadone, buprenorphine, naloxone) throughout the period of acute pain with confirmation of the health care provider of reference (e.g., methadone dosage). This aspect represents a strategy to prevent withdrawal syndrome, but it is not enough to treat acute pain [33]. In this case, patients may require further opioid analgesics. It is important to avoid both analgesic holes and oversedation phases and plan the transition to the oral route for the following days. Finally, a proper discharged plan has to be organized in accordance with the referral pain specialist. The coordination between trauma center and chronic opioid prescribers is a vital aspect to implement.

Patients on chronic opioid therapy or opioid use disorders present special challenge for the presence of several factors:

- higher incidence of pain in the perioperative period
- rapid development of tolerance
- treatment for withdrawal syndrome as well as acute pain due to trauma
- higher dose of drugs requirement for a longer period
- high incidence of behavioral factors: anxiety, psychosis, depression, personality disorders
- opioid-induced hyperalgesia, also triggered by withdrawal syndromes and / or by reduction of daily doses.
- Increase length of hospital stay, more likely to be admitted to ICU, higher rate if complication and hospital readmission after discharge.

17.1.3.5 End of Life

Pain management represents an essential part of end-of-life care [34]. The coordination between the withdrawing of life sustaining treatment and to prevent discomfort, dyspnea, and pain for the patient is a crucial aspect and requires specific knowledge on pharmacologic treatment and organ failure. Not to be underestimated, another crucial aspect is represented by the communication with the family and their presence during the end-of-life care of the patient. This requires the creation of a peaceful environment. Caregivers have to silence the alarm and remove all the unnecessary equipment or treatment. Provide the family with a confront environment (e.g., provide chairs, tissue, water) and discuss with the family about the process.

17.2 Diagnosis: Assessment of Pain

In prehospital and emergency settings, pain is often poorly assessed due to the presence of several confounding factors. The clinical condition of the patients and their level of alertness influence the possibility to take a reliable pain history by clinicians. Even more, restricted access of the patient on the field or the overcrowding in the ED represents barrier to carry out a reliable pain assessment [6].

During clinical evaluation, it is important to assess several pain characteristics such as the location of pain, aggravating and alleviating factors, impact of pain on function, duration of pain, medications, and patient's expectation [35]. Then, the intensity of pain has to be clearly evaluated and reported [5]. It is important to report on clinical diary the intensity of pain in order to reassess the effectiveness of therapeutic regimen and to evaluate pain over time.

Pain should be considered a vital parameter [36]. Consequently, pain, as well as heart rate, blood pressure, blood oxygen saturation, and temperature, has to be measured, periodically evaluated with reliable tools. Considering the multidimensional characteristics of pain and the wide variability of the perception of pain among patients, consequently, it is important to choose pain assessment methods that fit patients' characteristics. In particular, it is important to take into account the capability to communicate and the cognitive level [37]. Specific assessment tools are available for specific types of population (i.e., pediatric patients, cognitive impairment, heavily sedated patients, geriatrics). Self-report is the most valid and reliable indicator of pain; however, in the elderly, pain assessment may be complicated by dementia and cognitive and sensory impairments, then, alternative assessment tools are available to guide pain management [25]. As an example, behavior scale incorporates behavioral components (facial expression, upper limb movement, compliance with ventilation) for pain scoring [38]. These scales can be used in patients with difficulty or impossibility to self-reported and evaluate pain (e.g., dementia, sedated, or unconscious patients). Even more, several pediatric pain rating scales have been developed since pediatric patients are unable to communicate or communicate properly verbally. These scales rely on observation of the presence or absence of crying, facial expression, heart rate, and vital signs [26, 39]. Other special circumstances that pose significant challenge are represented by breakthrough pain (transient exacerbation of pain) in cancer patients or in patient suffering from chronic pain and patients with active or previous drug misuse (genuine pain vs. seeking for medications in ED). Finally, it is also important to evaluate the degree of consciousness and level of agitation, possible factors that can increment the level of analgesic requirement.

Several pain assessment tools are available for rating pain [26, 38–43]:

- Categorial pain scales: self-reported scores, verbal rating scale. Pain is evaluated using a verbal descriptor scale. Generally, categorial pain scales use 4–5 descriptors from "no pain" to "intense pain" (as shown in Table 17.1). Not suitable for patients with language barriers.
- Numeric rating scales (NRS): unidimensional measure of pain intensity in adults, self-reported scores. Patients are scored on a scale from 0 (no pain) to 10 (worst imaginable pain). A pain score of 1–3 is considered as a mild pain, a score of 4–7 a moderate pain, and a score of above 7 a severe pain (as shown in Table 17.1).
- Visual analogue scale (VAS): self-reported scores. A measurement tool represented as a 100 mm/10 cm horizontal line. The patients mark their pain level on the scale with the left side representing no pain and the right side worst pain imaginable (as shown in Table 17.1).
- Color analog scale: use color for representing pain, from blue (mild), yellow (moderate) to red (severe).
- Functional activity scale (FAS): a 3-level categorical score used to assess the incapability of the patients to perform specific activities due to the occurrence of pain; from level A (no limitation) to C (significant limitation due to the presence of pain).
- Clinically aligned pain assessment (CAPA): healthcare providers evaluate pain intensity, the effect of pain on function and sleep, the efficacy of treatment, and the progress towards relief. Do not provide a score but an assessment of the effect of pain on their functional status.
- Functional pain scale (FPS): healthcare provider evaluates the presence of the pain, its tolerability, and eventual interference with activities of daily living.
- McGill Pain Scale: The McGill Pain Questionnaire consists of 78 words that describe pain, especially useful for rehabilitation program.
- Wong-Baker FACES pain rating scale: combines picture (faces) and number for rating pain. It can be used in children>3 years old. The faces depict several expressions, from smiling to crying. The patients can choose the picture that best represents the intensity of pain.

Table 17.1 Numeric rating scale (NRS), Verbal rating scale (VRS), and visual analogue (VAS) scale

NRS										
No pain	Mild pain			Moderate pain			Severe pain			
0	1	2	3	4	5	6	7	8	9	10
VRS										
No pain		Mild pain		Moderate pain		Severe pain	Very severe pain		Worst imaginable pain	
VAS										
No pain	Mild pain			Moderate pain			Severe pain			
0	10	20	30	40	50	60	70	80	90	100

- FLACC Scale (Face, legs, activity, crying, and consolability): 2 months to 7 years. The assessment of the level of pain in children who are too young to cooperate verbally is based on the observations of 5 criteria (facial expression, position/movement of the legs, overall activity, presence/degree of crying, ability to be consoled or comforted).
- FLACC -Revised Scale: assessment of pain evaluating the five aforementioned categories of FLACC Scale, validated for children with cognitive impairment. The central role of parents/caregivers for additional indicators of pain (as shown in Table 17.2).
- CRIES (C-crying, R-requires oxygen administration, I-increased vital signs, E-expression, S-sleeplessness) Scale: for neonates. It consists of the assessment of crying, oxygenation, vital signs, facial expression, and sleeplessness (0 point for no pain, 2 point for signs of maximal pain, as shown in Table 17.2).
- Premature Infant Pain Profile (PIPP): for Neonates and preterm. The behavioral state is scored by observing the infant before and after

Table 17.2 Revised Face Legs Activity Cry and Consolability (r-FLACC) Scale behavioral pain assessment tool and Children's Revised Impact of Event Scale (CRIES)

r-FLACC Scale				
Face	**Legs**	**Activity**	**Cry**	**Consolability**
0 No expression or smile	0 Normal position or relaxed	0 Lying quietly, normal position, moves easily; regular rhythmic breaths	0 No cry (awake or asleep)	0 Content, relaxed
1 Occasional grimace or frown, withdrawn, disinterested; appears sad or worried	1 Uneasy, restless, tense; occasional tremors	1 Squirming, shifting back and forth, tense or guarded movements; mildly agitated, shallow, splinting breaths	1 Moans or whimpers, occasional complaint; occasional verbal outburst or grunt	1 Reassured by occasional touching, hugging, Can be distracted
2 Distressed looking face; expression of fright or panic Individualized behavior described by family	2 Kicking, or legs drawn up; increase in spasticity; constant tremors or jerking Individualized behavior described by family	2 Arches, rigid, or jerking; severe agitation; shivering, breath holding, sharp intake of breaths Individualized behavior described by family	2 Crying steadily, screams, frequent complaints; constant grunting Individualized behavior described by family	2 Difficult to console or comfort; pushing away caregiver; resisting comfort measures Individualized behavior described by family
Total score				_____ of 10
CRIES Scale				
Crying	**Requires O$_2$ for SaO$_2$ < 95%**	**Increased vital signs**	**Expression**	**Sleepless**
0 No cry	0 No oxygen required	0 Heart rate and mean blood pressure equal to baseline	0 No grimace	0 Continuously asleep
1 Cry high pitched but consolable	1 <30% supplemental oxygen required (target SaO$_2$ > 95%)	1 Heart rate or mean blood pressure increased <= 20% from baseline	1 Grimace	1 Awakened at frequent intervals
2 Cry high pitched, inconsolable	2 >30% supplemental oxygen required (target SaO$_2$ > 95%)	2 Heart rate or mean blood pressure increased >20% from baseline	2 Grimace with grunting	2 Constantly awake
Total score				_____ of 10

a painful event and pain medication administration. The following categories are evaluated: behavioral state, maximum heart rate, minimum oxygen saturation, brow bulge eye squeeze, nasolabial furrow.
- NFCS Scale (neonatal facial coding scale). Evaluation of different facial expressions specifically coded in premature neonates, term-born neonates, and infants up to 18 months of age.
- The behavioral pain scale (BPS): three domain tools (facial expression, upper limb movements, and compliance with mechanical ventilator), validated in critically ill patients, sedated and mechanically ventilated patients with a score ranging from 1 to 4. Scores above 6 indicate an unacceptable level of pain (as shown in Table 17.3).

Table 17.3 Behavioral Pain Scale (BPS) and Richmond Agitation Sedation Scale (RASS)

Behavioral Pain Scale (BPS)					
Facial expression		Upper limbs		Compliance with ventilation	
1	Relaxed	1	No movement	1	Tolerating movement
2	Partially tightened	2	Partially bent	2	Coughing but tolerating ventilation most of the time
3	Fully tightened	3	Fully bent with finger extension	3	Fighting ventilator
4	Grimacing	4	Permanently retracted	4	Unable to control ventilation
Total score					___of 12
RASS Score					
Combative; danger to staff					+4
Very agitated, Aggressive behavior, removes tubes or devices					+3
Agitated, Non purposeful movement, fight ventilator, ventilator dyssynchrony					+2
Restless, Anxious, not aggressive					+1
Alert and calm					0
Drowsy, Awakens to voice, eye contact					−1
Light sedation, Awakens to voice, eye contact					−2
Moderate sedation, movement to voice, no eye contact					−3
Deep sedation, no response to voice, open eye to physical stimulation					−4
Unarousable, no response to voice or to physical stimuli					−5

- Critical Care Pain Observation Tool (CPOT): assessment of pain based on the evaluation of facial expression, body movement, ventilator compliance (ventilated patients) and vocalization (extubated patients), and passive muscle tension either at rest (baseline evaluation) and after procedures that may cause discomfort.
- COMFORT Scale: for patients who are unable to rate or communicate the pain (e.g., Children, cognitively impaired, sedated). This scale evaluates nine different parameters, each rated from one to five: Alertness, Calmness, Respiratory distress, Crying, Physical movement, Muscle tone, Facial tension, Blood pressure, and heart rate.
- Pain assessment in advanced dementia (PAINAD): a 0–10 scale evaluating five domains (breathing, negative vocalization, facial expression, body language, consolability).
- DOLOPLUS-2: evaluation of three domains: somatic, psychomotor, and psychosocial in patient with cognitive impairment severity.
- Ramsay SCORE: defines the level of sedation in 6 categories. Patients are scored according to the level of alertness and agitation from level 1 to 6.
- Richmond agitation sedation scale (RASS): assess the level of vigilance and distressed behavior in critically ill patients. It is a 10-point scale from −5 to +4. From −5 to −1, describe the level of sedation (from unarousable to awakens to voice), from +1 to +4 describe an increasing level of agitation (from anxiety to combative, as shown in Table 17.3).

17.3 Special Settings

17.3.1 Pain Management in the Prehospital Setting and in the Emergency Department

A fundamental aspect of emergency care is represented by pain management. However, on the field, pain assessment and treatment can be difficult. The availability of analgesic drugs is often limited, and the limited prescribing rights of the emergency services represent important obstacles. In case of localized injury, regional anesthesia has to be considered; however, it is often difficult to perform due to special environment issues, lack of resources, and highly depending on skills' retention of healthcare personal [6]. To overcome these barriers, it is important to create specific protocols that fit local characteristic. Especially in prehospital and emergency settings, patients required close monitoring of vital parameters, not only for the evaluation of pain management, but also for a quick recognition of side effects and deterioration. It is preferable to choose short-acting analgesics with the least hemodynamics and respiratory impact (e.g., ketamine IV). Analgesic dose of Ketamine plays a central role with a safe hemodynamic and respiratory profile, avoiding exacerbation of hypoxia, respiratory depression, apnea, and hypotension [44]. Among opioids, fentanyl has a safer hemodynamic and respiratory profile, and it is widely used in emergency settings for these advantages [45].

The intravenous route represents the most common route of administration with faster onset and not influenced by absorption as for the oral route. Intramuscular or intranasal route can be chosen in case of difficult venous access or in extremely uncollaborative patients. Even more, intraosseous access is an effective route for drug administration without the need of dose adjustment in comparison to intravenous route [46]. Nonpharmacologic strategies, such as positioning, splinting, and heat/cold therapy are commonly used, especially for fracture and injury to the extremity.

It is worth remembering that compartment syndromes require urgent treatment and should always be evaluated, especially in patients with fractures or crush injuries and increasing pain scores or analgesic requirements.

17.3.2 Acute Pain Service

The Acute Pain Service is a multidisciplinary service that involves several different kinds of health care specialists (i.e., anesthetists, surgeons, nurses, physiotherapists) [10]. The general organization has to be adapted to the local reality and possibilities. It is important to identify a referring physician, to draft therapeutic protocols and to collect the efficacy and adverse effects of the protocols used. An accurate medical history of the patient's algological history should be conducted to plan a personalized treatment strategy on the basis of planned invasive procedures, expected subsequent pain, and the possibility of chronicity. A fundamental aspect is to inform the patient about the advantages and risks related to drugs and techniques that can be used to obtain the maximum benefit from the treatments.

The implementation of this kind of service within the hospital leads to better management of acute pain and a reduction of side effects (e.g., postoperative nausea and vomiting) and of the incidence of chronic pain [47]. In fact, this multimodal approach allows for a rapid individualization of high-risk patients and to quickly integrate strategies and multimodal intensive rehabilitation paths. Furthermore, this kind of organization allows for the implementation of the most advanced analgesic techniques (e.g., PCA and epidural analgesia, regional analgesia).

17.3.3 Pain Management in Perioperative Care and in the Intensive Care Unit

Inadequate postoperative pain is associated with decreases in patient satisfaction, delayed ambulation, and increased complications, morbidity, and mortality. Postoperative pain is caused not only by the surgical procedure (including drains, tubes), but can be exacerbated by the pre-existing disease and by possible complications. Preexisting psychosocial factors and chronic opioid use have an important impact on postoperative pain.

Consequently, the treatment of the postoperative pain represents a priority institutional objective being an integral part of the therapeutic plan for the perioperative care. In this view, specific protocols for postoperative pain management characterized by multimodal and interdisciplinary perioperative analgesia programs have to be present in each hospital in order to increase the safety and effectiveness of postoperative management and improve the patient's quality of life, reducing all the adverse effects related to inadequate management of the pain as well as the costs associated with prolonging the hospital stay and altering the patient's quality of life for the development of chronic pain [48].

Personalized pain treatment plan requires:

- The evaluation, during the preoperative visit when possible, of the medical history and medication.
- Patients' characteristics: elderly, pediatric, neurocognitive disorders, obese, obstructive sleep apnea, ischemic cardiac disease.
- Identify patient at risk of pain chronification or opioid misuse.
- Route of drugs administration: impossible to use oral route in surgical abdominal patient, soporous or not collaborative patients.
- Dose adjustment in case of organ failure.
- Evaluation of coagulation disorder in case of regional or neuraxial anesthetic technique.
- Type of surgery/invasive procedure and the expected subsequent pain and duration of pain.
- The possibility of chronicity.
- Evaluation of the risk/benefit ratio of all the planned procedures.
- Local resources, healthcare skills.

17.3.4 Pain Management at Hospital Discharge

Patients should be discharged by the hospital with a clear and proper prescribed pain management strategy with a scheduled follow-up evaluation by healthcare personnel [9]. It is recommended to provide clear and comprehensive information to the patients about drug administration (route, time), possible side effects, therapeutic expectation as well as emergency telephone number, both orally and in writing. It is also recommended to evaluate the level of acceptance of patients in the face of the prospect of discharge with mild pain still present. The analgesic therapy regimen and the contact number have to be reported on the discharge letter.

Even more, in case of opioid prescription, healthcare personnel have to explain clearly the possible side effects of opioid abuse/misuse and plan a clear anticipated scheme for weaning from opioids at home. It is recommended to prescribe the lowest dosage and duration of prescription opioids.

17.4 Treatment

17.4.1 Multimodal Pain Management

A multimodal approach to pain management includes both pharmacological and non-pharmacological pain control methods that may be applied across the continuum of care [49].

Fundamental steps for the creation of a multidisciplinary management approach are represented by the evaluation of local resources, the identification and training of the personnel involved, and the implementation of active physiotherapy and nursing care. Each hospital facility should create a clear pain management pathway and draft pain treatment algorithm specific for different clinical settings (e.g., ED, perioperative, at discharge). Acute Pain Service is the organization of different kinds of health care specialists (i.e., anesthetists, surgeons, nurses, physiotherapists), focusing on the diagnosis and treatment of pain. These kinds of facilities play a central role in all the phases of clinical care [10].

A multimodal analgesia is characterized by the prescription of different analgesic drugs with different mechanisms of action with the aim of achieving effective pain control and of reducing doses, especially opioids [14]. In fact, one of the main goals of multimodal treatment is the reduction of opioid consumption and drugs' side effects (i.e., nausea, vomiting, respiratory depression, and sedation). Nonsteroidal anti-inflammatory drugs (NSAIDs), Paracetamol, Ketamine, Clonidine, and Gabapentin have already shown evidence of opioid-sparing effect [50]. In fact,

NSAIDs, cyclooxygenase inhibitors, or Paracetamol in combination with Morphine determine "opioid-sparing effect" with a reduction of the consumption of morphine, pain score, the incidence of sedation, and post-operative nausea and vomiting [51]. The combination of different classes of drugs may increase the synergistic pain control effect of the different pain strategies with a reduction of the risk profile of each drug. In addition, central neuraxial blocks and regional anesthetic techniques with the administration of local anesthetic and adjuvants improve analgesia management after different types of injuries.

17.4.2 Non-pharmacological Pain Management

The evidence of non-pharmacological interventions on trauma patients and emergency setting available in the literature is scarce. However, non-pharmacological measures should be implemented as part of multimodal approach and considered as adjuvants especially for anxiety and distress management. One vital aspect is represented by psychological interventions [52]. It is important to provide patient with information and use relaxation techniques (e.g., breathing patterns, attention control methods, cognitive behavioral intervention) and to educate patients about expectation for pain management. It is important to communicate clearly with the patient and explain the plan for managing the pain and the effect expected. The reassessment of the pain is extremely important in order to evaluate the therapeutic effect and for physiological aspect (reassurance).

Non-pharmacological interventions include but are not limited to:

- cognitive behavioral therapy: consists of a series of techniques performed by trained social workers with the aim of making patients control over their perception of pain, (e.g., relaxation technique, active distraction technique, meditation, diversion, attention control methods) [53, 54];
- acupressure and acupuncture: different body part is stimulated in order to relieve pain in specific body area. No studies are available for the use of acupuncture and acupressure in pre-hospital setting. Acupressure showed a reduction of pain score and anxiety in ED [55];
- iontophoresis: medication delivered to tissue with low-voltage electrical current (i.e., anesthetics and corticosteroids) [56];
- transcutaneous electrical nerve stimulation (TENS): low-voltage electrical currents over the skin with a portable device in order to stimulate peripheral nerve fibers [57];
- patient positioning and immobilization: stabilize the injured region (pelvic, extremity) prior to surgical repair with an important beneficial effect on hemorrhage reduction, fracture healing, and pain management [58];
- temperature therapy: cryotherapy reduces tissue edema, local inflammatory, vascular permeability, generally used in orthopedic injuries [59];
- ultrasound: the usage of ultrasound waves to generate heat in the soft tissue (tendinitis, chronic joint swelling, muscle spasm) [60].

17.4.3 Pharmacological Analgesia

Different classes of drugs can be used in the treatment of acute pain, individually or in combination with each other [14]. The choice for using one drug over the other is influenced by the intensity of the pain, routes of administration, allergy, comorbidities, and availabilities of the drugs in specific setting. When used in combination, prescription has to take into account the pharmacokinetics and pharmacodynamics of the different classes of drugs in order to maximize the pain relief and reduce the possible side effects. It is extremely important to record pain intensity and to monitor for possible side effects and reassess periodically, with fixed time, the effectiveness of analgesia [8]. In case of exacerbation of pain, it is important to promptly investigate the possible cause of increasing pain rather than increase the administration of the drugs.

In the ED and prehospital setting and critical patients, drugs are generally administered through intravenous route [46]. In fact, it is not possible to use the oral route in several kinds of patient with acute pain (e.g., surgical abdominal patient, soporous or not collaborative patients). Even more, depending on the expertise of the physician, local anesthetics with or without adjuvants can be used to provide pain relief in specific anatomic areas.

17.4.3.1 Paracetamol

Paracetamol inhibits prostaglandin endoperoxide H2 synthase and cyclooxygenase activity with pain relieving and antipyretic properties, generally used for the treatment of mild to moderate acute pain [61]. However, paracetamol has no anti-inflammatory effects. Paracetamol can be administered in combination with opioids or NSAIDs in order to increase the analgesic efficacy, through oral, rectum, or intravenous routes. Paracetamol does not present effects on gastrointestinal tract or kidney. In case of overdose (≥ 100 mg/kg/day), paracetamol can cause acute liver toxicity; specific antidote is available (i.e., n-acetyl-cysteine) [37]. Paracetamol presents a dose-dependent effect on platelet aggregation and can enhance the antiplatelet effect of NSAIDs and the anticoagulant effect of vitamin K inhibitors. Paracetamol does not require dosage adjustments in patients with mild liver disease, whereas, in the hepatopathy patient, physician should take into account the narrow therapeutic window [62]. Consequently, paracetamol has to be used with caution in alcoholics, hepatic impairment, and cirrhosis. In this case, physicians have to reduce doses, lengthening the intervals of administration and monitoring of liver function. Allergic reactions to acetaminophen are also described with a low incidence in the general population.

Paracetamol produces comparable analgesic effects to that of NSAIDs. Furthermore, the association of paracetamol and morphine reduces the daily consumption of opioids [63]. It is also observed that the use of paracetamol leads to a reduction of rescue pain medications, such as opioids. One of the major advantages of using paracetamol is the wide availability of this drug in different clinical settings.

17.4.3.2 NSAIDs

Nonsteroidal anti-inflammatory drugs (NSAIDs) represented the most widely painkiller prescribed for the management of mild to moderate acute pain [3]. NSAIDs inhibit the cyclooxygenase 1 (COX-1) and the cyclooxygenase 2 (COX-2) enzymes with consequent anti-inflammatory, analgesic, and antipyretic effects. NSAIDs can be administered in combination with opioids or with paracetamol in order to increases the analgesic efficacy, through oral, sublingual, topical, or intravenous routes [63].

NSAIDs presents several important side effects to take into account; gastritis, bleeding, renal impairment, and antiplatelet activities. Consequently, NSAIDs are contraindicated in patients with active peptic ulceration, stomach bleeding, renal impairment, inflammatory bowel disease, and ulcerative colitis.

NSAIDs are extensively used in ED, especially for its analgesic efficacy for musculoskeletal pain, osteopathic manipulation, fracture, and acute low back pain [64]. Furthermore, the association of NSAIDs and morphine reduces the daily consumption of opioids [50]. It is also observed that the use of NSAIDs leads to a reduction of rescue pain medications, such as opioids. One of the major advantages of using NSAIDs is the wide availability of this drug in different clinical settings.

COXIBs, selective blockers of COX-2 isoforms, is mainly used in arthritis and ankylosing spondylitis. Few evidences are available for their use in acute pain and ED setting. Parecoxib is the only COXIBs available for intravenous administration and licensed for postoperative acute pain [65]. Contraindications are represented by ischemic heart disease and/or overt cerebrovascular disease, congestive heart failure, and postoperative aorto-coronary bypass surgery.

17.4.3.3 Ketamine

Ketamine is one of the most used drugs in anesthesia with several pharmacological effects (e.g., dissociation, analgesia, sedation, and bronchodilation). Even if ketamine is known most widely for its anesthetic properties (including utility for anesthesia induction in hemodynamically unstable patients), recent research has uncovered multiple novels uses (e.g., neuroprotection, seizures, chronic pain, and headache) [66]. As a nonselective NMDA receptor antagonist, it has equal affinity for different NMDA receptor types [67]. Even more, ketamine can be used in ethanol withdrawal syndrome. Like ethanol, ketamine is an N-methyl-d-aspartate receptor antagonist and treats ethanol withdrawal at a receptor infrequently addressed by traditional therapy [68].

Ketamine can be administered in combination with other analgesic drugs as adjuvants in order to increase the analgesic efficacy, through intravenous routes either as a continuous infusion or in repeated boluses. Ketamine can also be administered through intramuscular or intranasal routes.

The use of ketamine reduces the intensity of postoperative pain and/or the need for analgesics to reduce the consumption of morphine [3]. Not to be underestimated, ketamine is able to prevent the development of hyperalgesia following surgery. Ketamine is extensively used in prehospital setting and in critical patients for its wide therapeutic index, hemodynamics stability, and no respiratory depression [44]. Even more, its safe hemodynamic profile allows the usage of ketamine in prehospital settings and a good drug during rapid sequence intubation.

17.4.3.4 Opiods

Opioids have always been the cornerstone of the treatment of moderate to severe acute postoperative pain [3]. Opioids act on membrane receptors (μ, δ, κ, N) distributed in the central nervous system in a nonuniform way. This class of drugs presents a direct inhibition of the ascending nociceptive system (k, μ) and a peripheral inhibition of the release of inflammatory mediators of the cells of the immune system (μ). Furthermore, opioids activate the descending pain control system (k, μ) and inhibit pain transmission at the thalamic level (μ). Opioids present several side effects to take into account (i.e., sedation, potential respiratory depression, nausea, vomiting, itch anaphylaxis, and paralytic ileus) [61]. The main adverse effects are dose-dependent, thus avoidable with dose titration. Opioids can be used in combination with other classes of drugs, as described above, in order to reduce opioid needs through intravenous routes. When used in epidural or spinal anesthesia, the association between low doses of local anesthetic and lipophilic opioids enhances post-operative pain control and reduced incidence of side effects [69].

Opioids can be administered through intramuscular, intranasal, oral, and intravenous routes, depending on the intensity of the pain and patients' characteristics. Intravenous PCA (patient control anesthesia) device represents another interesting administration route [70]. PCA is a method for treating postoperative pain that allows the patient to self-administer predetermined doses of analgesic as needed. The PCA can be programmed on demand administration (a fixed dose is self-administered intermittently) or with continuous basal infusion plus administration on demand. Finally, transdermal PCA is a new noninvasive method based on the iontophoresis technique that uses a low intensity current to carry ionized substances through the skin to the bloodstream [70].

Morphine

Morphine is a strong opioid and a pure agonist for opioid receptors, without a ceiling effect. The excretion of metabolites is dependent on renal function. In case of hepatic or renal insufficiency or in other situations that alter the metabolism or kinetics of drugs, doses should be reduced.

Titration should be carried out gradually by administering boluses and reassessing pain relief by the patient and evaluated through a numerical or verbal scale. In the post-operative period, PCA administration represents an useful and effective pain control method with low sedation and low incidence of complications [70].

Fentanyl-Sufentanil-Remifentanil

Fentanyl is used intravenously and in epidural (off label) in combination with local anesthetics. Its analgesic efficacy is 100 times more potent than morphine. Fentanyl is commonly administered as intranasal, intramuscular, and intravenous formulation. Fentanyl is widely used in the control of acute pain due to its lack of active metabolites and its rapid onset [3]. Even more, its safe hemodynamic profile allows the usage of fentanyl in prehospital setting and for rapid sequence intubation [45]. A transdermal patch formulation is available with similar results to analgesic relief in comparison to morphine in PCA [70]. Intranasal formulation provides a fast onset of action, particularly useful in children.

Sufentanil is a highly selective opioid for μ receptors, much more potent than morphine. Unlike morphine, it is highly liposoluble and has a very high protein bond. Its analgesic efficacy is 100 times more potent than morphine. Sufentanil guarantees excellent hemodynamic stability [71]. It can be used both intravenously and peridural in association with local anesthetics.

Remifentanil is the opioid of choice in renal and hepatopathy patients and newborns. It is characterized by a rapid onset of action and by the absence of an analgesic tail.

Oxycodone-Buprenorphine-Tramadol

Oxycodone is a semisynthetic opioid, a pure agonist of opioid receptors characterized by a high oral bioavailability (60%). It is metabolized in the liver to noroxycodone and oxymorphone which are weakly active. Oxycodone is a strong opioid for the treatment of severe pain. Oxycodone is indicated for the treatment of chronic pain and for the control of acute pain and post-operative pain [72].

Buprenorphine is a partial agonist (mu opioid receptor) and an antagonist (kappa receptor). It has depressant effects on the respiratory system similar to morphine [73]. There are currently no controlled clinical studies on its use in the treatment of postoperative pain.

Tramadol is typically used for moderate to severe acute pain, through oral, intramuscular, and intravenous routes [74]. Tramadol is a central synthetic analgesic. Its action is expressed through the inhibition of the reuptake of biogenic amines (noradrenaline and serotonin) and as a weak activation of the μ receptors for opioids (via the metabolite M 1). Tramadol causes less respiratory depression than other major opioids with inferior impact on intestinal motility and gastric emptying. However, nausea and vomiting are the most common side effects and have a similar incidence to that of other opioids. Tramadol can be administered in combination with NSAIDs, Ketorolac, and Paracetamol.

Local Anesthetics

Local anesthetics (AL) are a heterogeneous pharmacological class sharing a similar mechanism of action based on the transient and reversible interruption of nerve conduction at the site where they are injected. Their main use is to allow the execution of surgical/diagnostic interventions and in the management of post-operative pain or chronic pain. The greatest advantage of using ALs is the maintenance of the patient's consciousness and spontaneous breathing during the execution of these procedures. These drugs can be administered intrathecally, perineurally, topically, intravenously (Bier block), and by infiltration.

Several factors influence the mechanism of action, the onset, and the duration of ALs [73, 75, 76]:

- percentage of protein binding.
- the influence of pH: poor effectiveness of ALs in the event of infection or acidosis and sepsis.
- stereoisomerism of ALs: R isomers have a capacity to block the membrane channels with higher affinity in comparison to the S isomers. Bupivacaine has a lower safety margin than Ropivacaine and Levobupivacaine.
- dose administered.
- the injection site: depending on the different local blood flow that influences the absorption rate and therefore the achievement of the plasma peak.
- use of adjuvants: Clonidine and magnesium are adjuvants widely recognized, increasing the analgesic effect of ALs.
- use of AL formulations: combination of a local anesthetic with a short duration of action and rapid onset with a longer lasting AL and a later onset has the goal of obtaining a block that sets in quickly and with a longer duration. It should be remembered that for AL mixtures, it is not possible to reach maximum doses of the respective ALs.
- use of a vasoconstrictor: reduces the systemic absorption of local anesthetic and will consequently reduce plasma absorption. The association with adrenaline prolongs the duration of the anesthetic block and reduces the systemic absorption of the anesthetic.

- Alkalinization of the local anesthetic solutions: reduce the time required for the anesthetic block to establish. The addition of sodium bicarbonate increases the pH and increases the amount of non-ionized bases, causing a greater diffusion of the drug and a faster onset of the neural block.
- The association with opioids increases the analgesic effect.

Adverse reactions may occur if toxic blood concentrations of AL are reached. Therefore, the factors that influence the rate of reabsorption of ALs will be the same ones that will influence the achievement of toxic blood concentrations and therefore the probability of observing adverse reactions.

17.4.4 Regional Analgesia

Regional anesthesia can provide pain relief for the management of trauma-related issues and during surgical or invasive procedures confined to specific anatomic regions (i.e., thoracotomy, rib fractures, upper or lower extremity procedures) [77]. The major limitations of the implementation of regional anesthesia in prehospital setting are represented by the availability of specific equipment and by operator skill acquisition and retention.

It is worth highlighting that the implementation of regional anesthesia in the management of pain allows achieving a good and reliable analgesic effect with a consequent reduction of opioid use. An important advantage of performing regional anesthesia is the maintenance of the patient's consciousness and spontaneous breathing with consequent reliable neurological evaluation and without respiratory depression. Even more, in the literature are described numerous potential systemic benefits of regional anesthetic technique: anti-inflammatory and antithrombotic effects, improvement of gastrointestinal microcirculation, and enhancement in respiratory function [78].

Central neuraxial anesthesia and regional anesthesia allow the administration of local anesthetics or adjuvant drugs (i.e., clonidine) around peripheral nerves/plexus, or directly into spinal fluid. A summary of the regional anesthesia techniques is provided in Table 17.4. The choice of one technique over the other is influenced by the location of a planned intervention and of the anticipated or actual severity of the pain.

Table 17.4 A summary of the major type of regional anesthesia

	Indications
Endotracheal intubation	Awake fiberoptic intubation in patients with cervical spine fractures or with suspected difficult intubation
NEURAXIAL techniques	Chest trauma, thoracic and abdominal surgery, major orthopedic surgery, acute pancreatitis, cardiac surgery
Paravertebral block	Thoracic surgery, rib fractures, treatment of chronic pain
Intercostal block	Thoracic or upper abdominal surgery, rib fractures, breast surgery
Intrapleural analgesia	Rib fractures, pain treatment for chest and upper abdomen, herpes zoster, complex regional pain syndromes, and pancreatitis
TAP block	Postoperative analgesia for laparotomy, appendectomy, laparoscopic surgery, abdominoplasty, gynecological procedures, and caesarean delivery
Iliohypogastric and ilioinguinal nerve blocks	Somatic procedure for lower abdominal wall/inguinal region
Interscalene block	Shoulder, upper arm surgery
Supraclavicular block	Arm, elbow, forearm, and hand surgery
Infraclavicular block	Arm, elbow, forearm, hand surgery
Axillary block	Elbow, forearm, and hand surgery
Femoral block	Anterior thigh, femur, and knee surgery. Proximal femur fracture
Sciatic block	Foot and ankle surgery; analgesia after knee surgery/trauma
Lumbar plexus block	Abdominal, lower extremity procedures
Erector spinae blocks	Anterior and posterior chest wall trauma
PECS AND Serratus anterior plane block	Breast surgery, lateral thoracic surgery, and chest wall trauma
Fascia iliaca block	Anterior thigh and knee surgery, proximal femur fracture

Central neuraxial anesthesia (i.e., spinal, epidural analgesia) provides effective and stable pain control; however, these techniques face special challenges in critically ill patients (e.g., coagulopathies, infections, sedation) and cannot be performed on the field. The most common indications for neuraxial blocks are multiple rib fractures and acute postoperative pain following laparotomy or thoracotomy. In thoracic trauma and rib fractures, the placement of thoracic epidural catheters or the administration of local analgesia through paravertebral block or intercostal nerve blocks are effective in the alleviation of pain with associated improvement in respiratory function, consequent shorten of mechanical ventilation days, and enhancement of ventilator weaning process [79]. However, the placement of epidural catheters is contraindicated in case of coagulopathies and in patients receiving anticoagulants [80]. In these cases, fascial plane blocks (with the exception of the quadratus lumborum block) may be considered an acceptable alternative.

On the other hand, single-shot peripheral nerve block technique, topical local anesthesia, and skin infiltration can be utilized for pain management during invasive procedures also in the prehospital setting (e.g., placement of chest tube or central venous catheter, fracture repositioning). Current evidence showed that the implementation of ultrasound guidance has an important impact in increasing success rate and reducing the incidence of complications [81]. Ultrasound guidance provides the direct visualization of the needle, the localization of the nerve, and the effective identification of the LA spread around the nerve.

Not to be underestimated, topical local analgesia (i.e., spray nebulizer, direct cotton swabs, inhaling aerosolized local aesthetic) or nerve block (i.e., glossopharyngeal and superior laryngeal nerves block) can represent important ads during endotracheal intubation (i.e., awake fiberoptic intubation, anticipated difficult airway management) [82].

Dos and Don'ts
- Plan pain treatment algorithm in different settings. Implement a clear pathway (acute pain service) for comprehensive pain management and safe de-escalation with the collaboration of different specialists.
- Reassure patient that their pain will be taken seriously. Establish realistic expectation with the patients. Evaluate the impact of pain on quality of life and patient's expectations and willing.
- Pain has to be measured, reassessed after therapeutic intervention, and recorded on the medical record with the side effects. Pain control should not be delayed. Provide analgesia before recurrence of pain.
- Choose specific assessment tools for specific types of population (i.e., pediatric patients, cognitive impairment, heavily sedated patients, geriatrics).
- Evaluate the degree of consciousness and level of agitation.
- Follow a multimodal approach to pain management including both pharmacological and non-pharmacological pain control methods.
- Use different classes of analgesic drugs in combination with the aim of reducing opioids consumption.
- Provide a proper prescribed pain management strategy with a scheduled follow-up at discharged.

Take-Home Messages

- The implementation of "Acute Pain Service" within the hospital leads to better management of acute pain and a reduction of side effects. A multidisciplinary service involves several different kinds of health care specialists with the goal to draft therapeutic protocols and to collect efficacy and adverse effects of the protocols use. This multimodal approach allows for a rapid individualization of high-risk patients and to quickly integrate strategies and multimodal intensive rehabilitation paths.
- Assessment of pain with specific assessment tools. It is important to choose pain assessment methods that fit patients' characteristics. Specific assessment tools are available for specific types of population (i.e., pediatric patients, cognitive impairment, heavily sedated patients, geriatrics).
- Multimodal approach to pain management: A multidisciplinary approach strategy including pharmacological as well as non-pharmacological interventions has to be followed in order to achieve an optimum pain relief, to obtain patient comfort and to reduce drug administration (especially opioids consumption).
- Tailored medicine that fits patients' characteristics (i.e., cognitive impairment, elderly, pediatrics, obese, chronic pain syndrome, opioid misuse) and clinical settings (from prehospital to discharge).

Multiple Choice Questions (Only 1 Right Answer)

1. Possible barriers to inadequate pain management include:
   A. limited availability of drugs
   B. fear of opioids dependence or abuse
   C. lack of resource and lack of local guidelines
   D. all the above
2. Inadequate pain control is associated with:
   A. delayed recovery time
   B. hospital readmission rates, increased morbidity, mortality, and higher health-care costs
   C. chronification of pain
   D. all of the above
3. A multidisciplinary approach to pain management should include:
   A. both pharmacological and non-pharmacological pain control methods
   B. pharmacological methods
   C. non-pharmacological pain control methods
   D. None of the above
4. A proper and specific assessment tool for pain measurement:
   A. fit specific situation and patient's characteristics
   B. takes into account the capability to communicate, and the cognitive level of the patients
   C. takes into account the multidimensional characteristics of pain and the wide variability of the perception of pain among patients
   D. All of the above

5. Categorial pain scales:
   A. rate pain using verbal or visual descriptor of pain
   B. for children, faces or images are commonly used
   C. generally, use 4–5 descriptors from "no pain" to "intense pain"
   D. all the above
6. FLACC Scale:
   A. assessment of the level of pain in children who are too young to cooperate verbally
   B. is based on the observations of 5 criteria (facial expression, position/movement of the legs, overall activity, presence /degree of crying, ability to be consoled or comforted)
   C. the revised form of the FLACC Scale (FLACC -Revised Scale) is validated for children with cognitive impairment
   D. all the above
7. RASS:
   A. Is the acronym of the Richmond agitation sedation scale
   B. assesses the level of vigilance and distressed behavior in critically ill patients
   C. it is a 10-point scale from −5 to+4
   D. all of the above
8. Acute pain service:
   A. is a multidisciplinary service that involves several different kinds of health care specialists with the aim of a better management of acute pain and of reducing the side effects and the incidence of chronic pain
   B. allows for a rapid individualization of high-risk patients
   C. allows for the implementation of the most advanced analgesic techniques
   D. all of the above
9. Fentanyl:
   A. is commonly administered as intranasal, intramuscular, and intravenous formulation.
   B. presents a safe hemodynamic profile
   C. is highly used in prehospital setting and for rapid sequence intubation
   D. all of the above
10. Regional anesthesia:
    A. can provide pain relief for the management of trauma-related issues and during surgical or invasive procedures confined to specific anatomic regions
    B. allow the administration of local anesthetics or adjuvant drugs around peripheral nerves/plexus, or directly into spinal fluid
    C. major limitations of the implementation of regional anesthesia in prehospital setting are represented by the availability of specific equipment and by operator skill acquisition and retention
    D. All of the above

Answers
1. D, 2. D, 3. A, 4. D, 5. D, 6. D, 7. D, 8. D, 9. D, 10. D

References

1. Raja SN, Carr DB, Cohen M, Finnerup NB, Flor H, Gibson S, et al. The revised International Association for the Study of Pain definition of pain: concepts, challenges, and compromises. Pain. 2020;161(9):1976–82.
2. McGuire LS, Slavin K. Revisiting the WHO analgesic ladder for surgical management of pain. AMA J Ethics. 2020;22(1):E695–701.
3. Abdolrazaghnejad A, Banaie M, Tavakoli N, Safdari M, Rajabpour-Sanati A. Pain management in the emergency department: a review article on options and methods. Adv J Emerg Med. 2018;2(4):e45.
4. Carr EC, Meredith P, Chumbley G, Killen R, Prytherch DR, Smith GB. Pain: a quality of care issue during patients' admission to hospital. J Adv Nurs. 2014;70(6):1391–403.
5. Gordon DB. Acute pain assessment tools: let us move beyond simple pain ratings. Curr Opin Anaesthesiol. 2015;28(5):565–9.

6. Al-Mahrezi A. Towards effective pain management: breaking the barriers. Oman Med J. 2017;32:357–8.
7. Morlion B, Coluzzi F, Aldington D, Kocot-Kepska M, Pergolizzi J, Mangas AC, et al. Pain chronification: what should a non-pain medicine specialist know? Curr Med Res Opin. 2018;34(7):1169–78.
8. Ahmadi A, Bazargan-Hejazi S, Heidari Zadie Z, Euasobhon P, Ketumarn P, Karbasfrushan A, et al. Pain management in trauma: a review study. J Inj Violence Res. 2016;8(2):89–98.
9. McIntosh SE, Leffler S. Pain management after discharge from the ED. Am J Emerg Med. 2004;22:98–100.
10. Frenette L. The acute pain service. Crit Care Clin. 1999;15(1):143–50.
11. Finan PH, Goodin BR, Smith MT. The association of sleep and pain: an update and a path forward. J Pain. 2013;14(12):1539–52.
12. Liang X, Liu R, Chen C, Ji F, Li T. Opioid system modulates the immune function: a review. Transl Perioper Pain Med. 2016;1(1):5–13.
13. Gan TJ. Poorly controlled postoperative pain: prevalence, consequences, and prevention. J Pain Res. 2017;10:2287–98.
14. Helander EM, Menard BL, Harmon CM, Homra BK, Allain AV, Bordelon GJ, et al. Multimodal analgesia, current concepts, and acute pain considerations. Curr Pain Headache Rep. 2017;21(1):3.
15. McCarberg BH, Nicholson BD, Todd KH, Palmer T, Penles L. The impact of pain on quality of life and the unmet needs of pain management: results from pain sufferers and physicians participating in an Internet survey. Am J Ther. 2008;15(4):312–20.
16. Loeser JD, Melzack R. Pain: an overview. Lancet. 1999;353(9164):1607–9.
17. Rolls ET. Limbic systems for emotion and for memory, but no single limbic system. Cortex. 2015;62:119–57.
18. Ossipov MH. The perception and endogenous modulation of pain. Scientifica (Cairo). 2012;2012:561761.
19. Baron MJ, McDonald PW. Significant pain reduction in chronic pain patients after detoxification from high-dose opioids. J Opioid Manag. 2006;2(5):277–82.
20. Clark F, Gilbert HC. Regional analgesia in the intensive care unit. Principles and practice. Crit Care Clin. 2001;17(4):943–66.
21. Hannibal KE, Bishop MD. Chronic stress, cortisol dysfunction, and pain: a psychoneuroendocrine rationale for stress management in pain rehabilitation. Phys Ther. 2014;94(12):1816–25.
22. Richardson J, Sabanathan S, Shah R. Post-thoracotomy spirometric lung function: the effect of analgesia. A review. J Cardiovasc Surg. 1999;40(3):445–56.
23. Jiang L, Zheng Z, Zhang M. The incidence of geriatric trauma is increasing and comparison of different scoring tools for the prediction of in-hospital mortality in geriatric trauma patients. World J Emerg Surg. 2020;15(1):59.
24. Deiner S, Westlake B, Dutton RP. Patterns of surgical care and complications in the elderly. J Am Geriatr Soc. 2014;62(5):829–35.
25. Lindenbaum L, Milia DJ. Pain management in the ICU. Surg Clin North Am. 2012;92(6):1621–36.
26. Johansson M, Kokinsky E. The COMFORT behavioural scale and the modified FLACC scale in paediatric intensive care. Nurs Crit Care. 2009;14(3):122–30.
27. Schmitt YS, Hoffman HG, Blough DK, Patterson DR, Jensen MP, Soltani M, et al. A randomized, controlled trial of immersive virtual reality analgesia, during physical therapy for pediatric burns. Burns. 2011;37(1):61–8.
28. Benini F, Corsini I, Castagno E, Silvagni D, Lucarelli A, Giacomelli L, et al. COnsensus on Pediatric Pain in the Emergency Room: the COPPER project, issued by 17 Italian scientific societies. Ital J Pediatr. 2020;46:101.
29. Brill MJ, Diepstraten J, van Rongen A, van Kralingen S, van den Anker JN, Knibbe CA. Impact of obesity on drug metabolism and elimination in adults and children. Clin Pharmacokinet. 2012;51(5):277–304.
30. Ingrande J, Brodsky JB, Lemmens HJ. Regional anesthesia and obesity. Curr Opin Anaesthesiol. 2009;22(5):683–6.
31. White JM. Pleasure into pain: the consequences of long-term opioid use. Addict Behav. 2004;29(7):1311–24.
32. Shanahan CW, Beers D, Alford DP, Brigandi E, Samet JH. A transitional opioid program to engage hospitalized drug users. J Gen Intern Med. 2010;25(8):803–8.
33. Rehni AK, Jaggi AS, Singh N. Opioid withdrawal syndrome: emerging concepts and novel therapeutic targets. CNS Neurol Disord Drug Targets. 2013;12(1):112–25.
34. Mularski RA, Puntillo K, Varkey B, Erstad BL, Grap MJ, Gilbert HC, et al. Pain management within the palliative and end-of-life care experience in the ICU. Chest. 2009;135(5):1360–9.
35. Levy N, Sturgess J, Mills P. "Pain as the fifth vital sign" and dependence on the "numerical pain scale" is being abandoned in the US: why? Br J Anaesth. 2018;120(3):435–8.
36. Morone NE, Weiner DK. Pain as the fifth vital sign: exposing the vital need for pain education. Clin Ther. 2013;35(11):1728–32.
37. Kim EB, Han HS, Chung JH, Park BR, Lim S, Yim KH, et al. The effectiveness of a self-reporting bedside pain assessment tool for oncology inpatients. J Palliat Med. 2012;15(11):1222–33.
38. Rose L, Haslam L, Dale C, Knechtel L, McGillion M. Behavioral pain assessment tool for critically ill adults unable to self-report pain. Am J Crit Care. 2013;22(3):246–55.
39. Merkel SI, Voepel-Lewis T, Shayevitz JR, Malviya S. The FLACC: a behavioral scale for scoring postoperative pain in young children. Pediatr Nurs. 1997;23(3):293–7.
40. Williamson A, Hoggart B. Pain: a review of three commonly used pain rating scales. J Clin Nurs. 2005;14(7):798–804.

41. Stevens B, Johnston C, Petryshen P, Taddio A. Premature infant pain profile: development and initial validation. Clin J Pain. 1996;12(1):13–22.
42. Peters JW, Koot HM, Grunau RE, de Boer J, van Druenen MJ, Tibboel D, et al. Neonatal facial coding system for assessing postoperative pain in infants: item reduction is valid and feasible. Clin J Pain. 2003;19(6):353–63.
43. Rostad HM, Utne I, Grov EK, Puts M, Halvorsrud L. Measurement properties, feasibility and clinical utility of the Doloplus-2 pain scale in older adults with cognitive impairment: a systematic review. BMC Geriatr. 2017;17(1):257.
44. Petz LN, Tyner S, Barnard E, Ervin A, Mora A, Clifford J, et al. Prehospital and en route analgesic use in the combat setting: a prospectively designed, multicenter, observational study. Mil Med. 2015;180(3 Suppl):14–8.
45. Garrick JF, Kidane S, Pointer JE, Sugiyama W, Van Luen C, Clark R. Analysis of the paramedic administration of fentanyl. J Opioid Manag. 2011;7(3):229–34.
46. Bennett JD. Emergency drug therapy. Drugs and routes of administration. Dent Clin North Am. 1995;39(3):501–21.
47. Low SJ, Wong SSC, Qiu Q, Lee Y, Chan TCW, Irwin MG, et al. An audit of changes in outcomes of acute pain service: evolution over the last 2 decades. Medicine (Baltimore). 2015;94(40):e1673.
48. Elsamadicy AA, Adogwa O, Fialkoff J, Vuong VD, Mehta AI, Vasquez RA, et al. Effects of immediate post-operative pain medication on length of hospital stay: does it make a difference? J Spine Surg. 2017;3(2):155–62.
49. Hyland SJ, Brockhaus KK, Vincent WR, Spence NZ, Lucki MM, Howkins MJ, et al. Perioperative pain management and opioid stewardship: a practical guide. Healthcare (Basel). 2021;9(3):333.
50. Chen JY, Ko TL, Wen YR, Wu SC, Chou YH, Yien HW, et al. Opioid-sparing effects of ketorolac and its correlation with the recovery of postoperative bowel function in colorectal surgery patients: a prospective randomized double-blinded study. Clin J Pain. 2009;25:485–9.
51. Kumar K, Kirksey MA, Duong S, Wu CL. A review of opioid-sparing modalities in perioperative pain management: methods to decrease opioid use postoperatively. Anesth Analg. 2017;125(5):1749–60.
52. Powell R, Scott NW, Manyande A, Bruce J, Vögele C, Byrne-Davis LM, et al. Psychological preparation and postoperative outcomes for adults undergoing surgery under general anaesthesia. Cochrane Database Syst Rev. 2016;2016(5):CD008646.
53. Zatzick D, Jurkovich G, Rivara FP, Russo J, Wagner A, Wang J, et al. A randomized stepped care intervention trial targeting posttraumatic stress disorder for surgically hospitalized injury survivors. Ann Surg. 2013;257(3):390–9.
54. Heutink M, Post MW, Luthart P, Schuitemaker M, Slangen S, Sweers J, et al. Long-term outcomes of a multidisciplinary cognitive behavioural programme for coping with chronic neuropathic spinal cord injury pain. J Rehabil Med. 2014;46(6):540–5.
55. Kober A, Scheck T, Greher M, Lieba F, Fleischhackl R, Fleischhackl S, et al. Prehospital analgesia with acupressure in victims of minor trauma: a prospective, randomized, double-blinded trial. Anesth Analg. 2002;95(3):723–7. table of contents
56. Neeter C, Thomeé R, Silbernagel KG, Thomeé P, Karlsson J. Iontophoresis with or without dexamethazone in the treatment of acute Achilles tendon pain. Scand J Med Sci Sports. 2003;13(6):376–82.
57. Chou R, Gordon DB, de Leon-Casasola OA, Rosenberg JM, Bickler S, Brennan T, et al. Management of postoperative pain: a clinical practice guideline from the American Pain Society, the American Society of Regional Anesthesia and Pain Medicine, and the American Society of Anesthesiologists' Committee on Regional Anesthesia, Executive Committee, and Administrative Council. J Pain. 2016;17(2):131–57.
58. Oakley E, Barnett P, Babl FE. Backslab versus non-backslab for immobilization of undisplaced supracondylar fractures: a randomized trial. Pediatr Emerg Care. 2009;25(7):452–6.
59. Nadler SF, Weingand K, Kruse RJ. The physiologic basis and clinical applications of cryotherapy and thermotherapy for the pain practitioner. Pain Physician. 2004;7(3):395–9.
60. Griffin XL, Smith N, Parsons N, Costa ML. Ultrasound and shockwave therapy for acute fractures in adults. Cochrane Database Syst Rev. 2012(2):CD008579.
61. Oyler DR, Parli SE, Bernard AC, Chang PK, Procter LD, Harned ME. Nonopioid management of acute pain associated with trauma: focus on pharmacologic options. J Trauma Acute Care Surg. 2015;79(3):475–83.
62. Prescott LF. Paracetamol, alcohol and the liver. Br J Clin Pharmacol. 2000;49(4):291–301.
63. Elia N, Lysakowski C, Tramèr MR. Does multimodal analgesia with acetaminophen, nonsteroidal antiinflammatory drugs, or selective cyclooxygenase-2 inhibitors and patient-controlled analgesia morphine offer advantages over morphine alone? Meta-analyses of randomized trials. Anesthesiology. 2005;103(6):1296–304.
64. Atchison JW, Herndon CM, Rusie E. NSAIDs for musculoskeletal pain management: current perspectives and novel strategies to improve safety. J Manag Care Pharm. 2013;19(9 Suppl A):S3–S19.
65. Huang JM, Lv ZT, Zhang YN, Jiang WX, Li HN, Nie MB. Efficacy and safety of postoperative pain relief by parecoxib injection after laparoscopic surgeries: a systematic review and meta-analysis of randomized controlled trials. Pain Pract. 2018;18(5):597–610.
66. Kurdi MS, Theerth KA, Deva RS. Ketamine: current applications in anesthesia, pain, and critical care. Anesth Essays Res. 2014;8(3):283–90.
67. Pribish A, Wood N, Kalava A. A review of non-anesthetic uses of ketamine. Anesthesiol Res Pract. 2020;2020:5798285.

68. Krystal JH, Petrakis IL, Webb E, Cooney NL, Karper LP, Namanworth S, et al. Dose-related ethanol-like effects of the NMDA antagonist, ketamine, in recently detoxified alcoholics. Arch Gen Psychiatry. 1998;55(4):354–60.
69. Bernards CM. Recent insights into the pharmacokinetics of spinal opioids and the relevance to opioid selection. Curr Opin Anaesthesiol. 2004;17(5):441–7.
70. Momeni M, Crucitti M, De Kock M. Patient-controlled analgesia in the management of postoperative pain. Drugs. 2006;66(18):2321–37.
71. Stephen R, Lingenfelter E, Broadwater-Hollifield C, Madsen T. Intranasal sufentanil provides adequate analgesia for emergency department patients with extremity injuries. J Opioid Manag. 2012;8(4):237–41.
72. Cheung CW, Ching Wong SS, Qiu Q, Wang X. Oral oxycodone for acute postoperative pain: a review of clinical trials. Pain Physician. 2017;20(2S):SE33–52.
73. Becker DE, Reed KL. Essentials of local anesthetic pharmacology. Anesth Prog. 2006;53(3):98–109.
74. Lehmann KA. [Tramadol in acute pain]. Drugs. 1997;53 Suppl 2:25–33
75. Vaida GT, Moss P, Capan LM, Turndorf H. Prolongation of lidocaine spinal anesthesia with phenylephrine. Anesth Analg. 1986;65(7):781–5.
76. Pöpping DM, Elia N, Marret E, Wenk M, Tramèr MR. Clonidine as an adjuvant to local anesthetics for peripheral nerve and plexus blocks: a meta-analysis of randomized trials. Anesthesiology. 2009;111(2):406–15.
77. Slade IR, Samet RE. Regional anesthesia and analgesia for acute trauma patients. Anesthesiol Clin. 2018;36(3):431–54.
78. Freise H, Lauer S, Konietzny E, Hinkelmann J, Minin E, Van Aken HK, et al. Hepatic effects of thoracic epidural analgesia in experimental severe acute pancreatitis. Anesthesiology. 2009;111(6):1249–56.
79. Jensen CD, Stark JT, Jacobson LL, Powers JM, Joseph MF, Kinsella-Shaw JM, et al. Improved outcomes associated with the liberal use of thoracic epidural analgesia in patients with rib fractures. Pain Med. 2017;18:1787–94.
80. Regional anaesthesia and patients with abnormalities of coagulation: the Association of Anaesthetists of Great Britain & Ireland the Obstetric Anaesthetists' Association Regional Anaesthesia UK. Anaesthesia. 2013;68(9):966–972.
81. Marhofer P, Greher M, Kapral S. Ultrasound guidance in regional anaesthesia. Br J Anaesth. 2005;94(1):7–17.
82. Saxena KN, Bansal P. Endotracheal intubation under local anesthesia and sedation in an infant with difficult airway. J Anaesthesiol Clin Pharmacol. 2012;28(3):358–60.

Damage Control Surgery

Carlo Vallicelli and Federico Coccolini

18.1 Introduction

Learning Goals
- Damage control surgery (DCS) and open abdomen (OA) are effective surgical strategies in trauma and nontrauma patients presenting with a deranged physiology, in order to prevent intra-abdominal hypertension (IAH) and abdominal compartment syndrome (ACS), conditions that may aggravate the physiological deranging potentially leading to multiorgan failure.
- Abdominal decompression is indicated whenever the abdomen cannot be closed due to visceral edema, the surgeon cannot reach a complete source control of the infection, there is the need to reexplore the abdomen in a second-look operation, due to bowel ischemia or to complete the DCS procedures, and in cases of abdominal wall damage.
- OA is a nonanatomical situation and must be transitory. The abdomen should be closed as soon as possible, and no longer than 7 days from the index operation. DCS and OA are procedures with their own complication risks and should be reserved to accurately selected patients.

The principle of abbreviated laparotomy and OA is to minimize the surgical procedure and perform a damage control in severely deranged patients, stabilize the patient, and plan a second-look exploration of the abdomen. DCS has been historically developed in trauma surgery, with the involvement of some of the notable and iconic names within the field of traumatology. It has subsequently been extended also to nontrauma patients, since the principles of performing the OA are the same in these two surgical scenarios. The aim of DCS is to avoid an IAH in patients with a deranged physiology, regardless of its cause. IAH can potentially evolve to ACS. This

C. Vallicelli (✉)
Department of General, Acute Care and Trauma Surgery, Bufalini Hospital, Cesena, Italy
e-mail: carlo.vallicelli@auslromagna.it

F. Coccolini
General Emergency and Trauma Surgery Department, Pisa University Hospital, Pisa, Italy

can result in a trigger to additionally aggravate the physiologic derangement, leading to a multi-organ failure in a vicious circle that should be interrupted by abdominal decompression. Moreover, in other clinical situations the abdomen cannot be closed due to visceral oedema, the inability to have a complete control of the source of infection, and the need to reexplore or complete a DCS procedure.

However, OA is a nonanatomical situation with potential side effects that must remain temporary. OA consists in intentionally leaving the abdominal fascial edges of the paired rectus abdominis muscles unapproximated. Several temporary abdominal closure techniques have been described in order to protect the abdominal viscera while leaving the fascia open, including negative-pressure wound therapy (NPWT) techniques. The abdomen should be closed as soon as possible, and no longer than 7 days after the index operation, otherwise the risk of side effects is increasing. Although we have guidelines from surgical societies defining the indications for DCS, it is often difficult to clearly define in clinical practice the ideal patients to treat with an OA or with a definitive abdominal closure with drains. There has been a large spread in the indications to OA, but there is an ongoing debate in literature to evaluate the clear effectiveness of all these indications. The surgeon must always keep in mind when leaving the abdomen open that we always start with a Björck IA classification, i.e., clean OA without adherence between bowel and abdominal cavity, but we don't know how far the patient is going to end. The Björck grade IV consists of established entero-atmospheric fistula (EAF) and frozen abdomen, which represent a nightmare for the surgeon and for the patient. Other described side effects of the OA include ventral hernia, abdominal abscesses, bowel resection, and anastomotic leak, even with the most effective temporary abdominal closure techniques. Therefore, there is a strong need to identify the ideal patients for these procedures, in order to avoid unnecessary complications and to clearly define the borders of application of the DCS (Table 18.1).

Table 18.1 Indications to DCS according to WSES guidelines

Trauma patients	Nontrauma patients

• Lethal triad and physiological derangement
• Risk of ACS or established ACS
• Packing and planned reoperation
• No source control of posttraumatic contamination
• Need to reevaluate bowel perfusion
	• Peritonitis and sepsis or septic shock plus:
	  – Severe physiological derangement
	  – Need to defer bowel anastomosis
	  – Bowel ischemia
	  – Failure of peritonitis source control
	  – Visceral edema and risk for ACS
	• Hemorrhagic vascular catastrophies
	• Pancreatitis developing ACS unresponsive to step-up medical treatment

18.2 Diagnosis

18.2.1 Trauma Patients

Indication to DCS can result from many clinical situations eventually presenting to the surgeon. DCS consists in quickly controlling exsanguinating haemorrhage and/or gross contamination using one or more abbreviated interventions. Normally, DCS is indicated whenever the patient is severely injured or physiologically deranged. In trauma patients, the lethal triad of persistent hypotension, acidosis (pH < 7.2), hypothermia (temperature < 34 °C), and coagulopathy are all strong predictors of the need for abbreviated laparotomy and OA. Other predictors of the need of OA in trauma patients are risk factors for ACS, such as injuries requiring packing and a planned reoperation, extreme visceral and retroperitoneal swelling, obesity, elevated bladder pressure when abdominal closure is attempted, abdominal wall tissue loss, and aggressive resuscitation [1]. Moreover, decompressive laparotomy is indicated in ACS, if the medical treatment has failed. ACS is defined according to the World Society of Abdominal Compartment Syndrome as an intra-abdominal pressure greater than 20 mmHg with the onset of a new organ dysfunction or organ failure (Table 18.2) [2]. The inability to obtain a definitive source control of infection or the need

Table 18.2 World Society of Abdominal Compartment Syndrome classification of intra-abdominal hypertension

IAH grade	IAP (mmHg)
Grade I	12–15
Grade II	16–20
Grade III	21–25
Grade IV	>25
ACS	>20 with new organ dysfunction/failure

to reevaluate bowel perfusion is also an indicator to OA in post-traumatic bowel injuries.

A recent systematic review analyzed the appropriateness of indication to DCS in civilian trauma patients. Although widely assumed to reduce mortality in critically injured patients, survivors of DC surgery have been reported to have a high risk of complications (e.g., intra-abdominal sepsis, enteric fistulae, and ventral hernia) and often suffer long lengths of ICU and hospital stay. A huge variation in the indication to DCS across different trauma centers has been described and an overuse has been hypothesized [3–6]. The review included 36 cohort studies and three cross-sectional surveys. The 39 included studies assessed the content, construct, and criterion validity of 116 indications for DCS and 32 indications for temporary abdominal closure (TAC) or OA management. Of the 59 unique indications identified using directed qualitative content analysis, two had moderate or strong evidence of content validity: upper quadrant abdominal gunshot wound with a horizontal shift trajectory (e.g., from the right to the left upper quadrant) and a systolic BP < 105 mmHg or right upper quadrant wound with a bullet retained in the same quadrant and a systolic BP < 90 mmHg. Further, nine had moderate or strong evidence of construct validity (high ISS score, preoperative hypothermia, unstable patients with combined abdominal vascular and pancreas gunshot injuries, and transfusion >10 U PRBCs and ISS score > 25 or lowest temperature < 34 °C in the pre- or intraoperative setting) and six had moderate or strong evidence of criterion validity (pre- or intraoperative hypothermia, increased lactate, or decreased pH). The authors identified only six indications that had evidence to support the use of DCS by improving patient survival. These indications include the finding of hypothermia or acidosis, development of a coagulopathy during operation, or the identification of two injury patterns that preclude expedient definitive repair (combined abdominal vascular and pancreas gunshot injuries and ≥1 major abdominal vascular and ≥2 abdominal visceral injuries in patients who have received >10 U packed red blood cells). The authors conclude that the above data suggest that there exists little evidence to support the high DC surgery utilization rates reported by many level 1 trauma centers [7]. In a recently reported post-hoc analysis of the PROPPR randomized trial, DC was used among 33–83% of patients requiring urgent laparotomy across 12 of the participating institutions. Interestingly, the unadjusted risk of sepsis and ventilator-associated pneumonia was higher among those treated with DCS as compared to definitive surgery with no difference in mortality rates [6]. Therefore, additional studies are strongly required to better understand proper indications to DCS in civilian trauma patients.

18.2.2 Peritonitis

The OA is an option in patients with peritonitis and severe sepsis or septic shock if one of the following circumstances is represented: severe physiological derangement, the need for a deferred anastomosis, a planned second-look for bowel ischemia, a persistent source of peritonitis with the failure of source control, or an extensive visceral edema with the concern for development of ACS [1]. According to Sepsis-3 definition, shock is a condition of hypotension that requires vasopressors to maintain a mean arterial pressure of 65 mmHg and a serum lactate level greater than 2 mmol/L after adequate resuscitation. Other validated scores are the Word Society of emergency Surgery Sepsis Severity Score (WSESSSS) (Table 18.3), the Apache II score, Manheim Peritonitis Index (MPI), and the Calgary Predisposition, Infection, Response, and Organ dysfunction (CPIRO) score. These scores all demonstrated some validity in identifying severe complicated intra-abdominal sepsis patients [8].

Table 18.3 WSES sepsis severity score for patients with complicated intra-abdominal infections (Range: 0–18). (From World Journal of Emergency Surgery, publisher under Creative Commons Attribution License 4.0)

Clinical condition at the admission	
• Severe sepsis (acute organ dysfunction) at the admission	3 score
• Septic shock (acute circulatory failure characterized by persistent arterial hypotension. It always requires vasopressor agents) at the admission	5 score
Setting of acquisition	
• Healthcare associated infection	2 score
Origin of the IAIs	
• Colonic non-diverticular perforation peritonitis	2 score
• Small bowel perforation peritonitis	3 score
• Diverticular diffuse peritonitis	2 score
• Post-operative diffuse peritonitis	2 score
Delay in source control	
• Delayed initial intervention [Preoperative duration of peritonitis (localized or diffuse) >24 h]	3 score
Risk factors	
• Age > 70	2 score
• Immunosuppression (chronic glucocorticoids, immunosuppresant agents, chemotherapy, lymphatic diseases, virus)	3 score

The debate is currently ongoing about the opportunity to leave the patient with an OA in case of peritonitis. The "Closed or Open after source control Laparotomy for severe complicated intra-abdominal sepsis" (the COOL trial) study is currently randomizing patients with a secondary peritonitis and a shock to OA or definitive closure after the source control laparotomy. Patients should present with a complicated secondary peritonitis and a shock defined according to Sepsis-3 or with a CPIRO score 3 or more, or with a WSESSSS 8 or more. Primary outcome of the study is 90-day mortality. Secondary outcomes include logistical, physiological, safety, biological, microbiological, mass citometry, economic, and quality of life outcome [9]. Results of the trial are awaited and will further clarify the proper indication to OA in this subgroup of patients.

18.2.3 Vascular Emergencies

Indication to DCS and OA can be a ruptured abdominal aortic aneurism or the management of acute mesenteric ischemia.

18.2.4 Pancreatitis

Patients with severe acute pancreatitis developing an abdominal compartment syndrome unresponsive to step-up medical therapy are candidates to decompressive laparotomy and OA.

18.3 Treatment

18.3.1 Medical Treatment

Together with DCS, damage control resuscitation (DCR) is the cornerstone of the treatment of severely injured and severely physiologically deranged patients. DCR is fundamental in OA management and influences the outcome of the patient. DCR includes several actions taken in the Intensive care Unit (ICU) setting, such as volume resuscitation, reversal of coagulopathy, and correction of acidosis. In trauma patients, the lethal triad must be interrupted as soon as possible [10–16]. Abdominal pressure should be routinely measured, ideally every 4–6 h once IAH is established [17]. Physiologic optimization of the patient is one of the keys of success and hypothermia must be avoided together with its related hypoperfusion effects. Analgesia should ideally consist in multimodal analgesia, thus reducing the need for opioids. The infusion of vasopressors and inotropic agents should be patient-tailored and fluid infusion accurately balanced. Moreover, early enteral nutrition should be started as soon as possible in presence of viable and functional gastrointestinal tract [18–21].

Multidisciplinary management is of utmost importance in such a complex patient.

18.3.2 Surgical Treatment

OA management consists in intentionally leaving the fascial edges of the paired rectus abdominus muscles unapproximated. In the so-called laparostomy, several methods have been described to temporary close the abdomen. In loose packing, the defect is closed by standard wound dressing. In mesh-mediated techniques, an absorbable or nonabsorbable mesh is temporarily sutured to the fascial edges. The Bogota bag consists of a sterile irrigation bag that is sutured between the fascial edges. In the Wittmann patch, two Velcro pieces are sutured to the fascial edges and facilitate gaining access to the abdominal cavity and

gradual reapproximation of the abdominal wall. Dynamic retention sutures consist of extraperitoneally placed large, nonabsorbable sutures through all layers of the abdominal wall, including the skin.

Sutures can be gradually tightened. The latest two techniques can be combined with NPWT. NPWT technique has progressively emerged and demonstrated its validity as compared to traditional temporary abdominal closure techniques. In the NPWT technique, a plastic sheet is positioned to cover the bowel loops, then a polyurethane sponge is placed on top, between the fascial edges. Then the wound is covered with an airtight seal and is centrally pierced by a suction drain, which is connected to a pump and fluid collection system (Fig. 18.1). Self-made variations of this technique (using towels/gauzes) are commonly referred to as Barkers' "Vacuum Pack". Commercially available systems include VAC Abdominal Dressing (KCI), Renasys NPWT (S&N), Avance (MöInlycke), and ABThera Open Abdomen Negative Pressure Therapy System (KCI). NPWT with continuous fascial traction (CFT) is a modification of NPWT, using a mesh or sutures sutured to the fascial edges, which can be tightened with every NPWT system change.

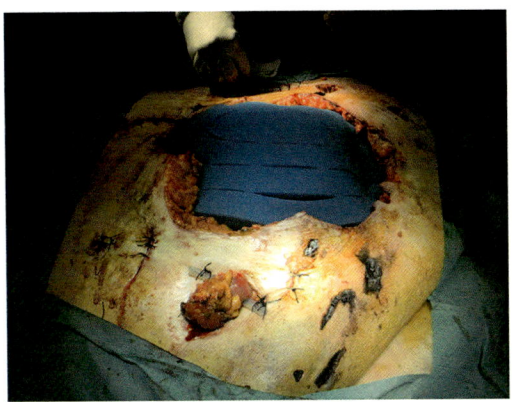

Fig. 18.1 NPWT in an obese trauma patient

Two meta-analyses investigated the effectiveness of all these TAC techniques [22, 23]. The authors systematically reviewed the current literature regarding indications and outcomes after DCS with OA. Globally, the overall quality of the available evidence was poor, and surgical indications were heterogeneous. NPWT was the most frequently described TAC technique. However, the authors found that the highest weighted fascial closure rate was obtained in series describing NPWT with continuous mesh or suture-mediated fascial traction and dynamic retention sutures. Atema et al. analyzed 74 studies with 78 series of patients. Information about the indications for leaving the abdomen open was provided in 59 of 78 series (76%). In 31 series, these indications were multiple, whereas in 28 series only one general indication was described. The most frequent single indication for open abdominal management was a planned relaparotomy strategy. The highest weighted fascial closure rate was seen for NPWT with CFT (73.1%) and dynamic retention sutures. The weighted fistula rate for all included studies was 12.1%. The highest rate was seen after mesh placement (17.2%), whereas NPWT with fascial traction showed the lowest weighted fistula rate (5.7%). NPWT (without fascial traction) had a weighted fistula rate of 14.6%. The authors concluded that published results for NPWT with CFT were superior to those of mere NPWT and other TAC, in terms of achieving delayed fascial closure and risk of enteroatmospheric fistula [10]. However, there was an overall lack of good quality evidence and a substantial heterogeneity existed between the included studies, urging the need of well-conducted prospective studies with clear descriptions of included patients, applied indications for OA, and outcome evaluation.

OA reexploration should be conducted after 24–48 h after the index operation and after any subsequent operation [24, 25]. The duration of the interval shortens if the patient has no physiological improvement and a haemodynamic instability. The abdomen should be maintained open again if the requirements for ongoing resuscitation or the source of contamination persist, if a deferred bowel anastomosis is required, if there is a need for a second-look to evaluate bowel viability, and if there are concerns for the development of an ACS. Ideally, the abdomen should be closed no longer than 7 days after the index operation.

The abdomen should be closed as soon as possible. Early fascial and/or abdominal closure should be the strategy for the management of OA once any requirement for ongoing resuscitation has ceased, there is a definitive source control, there are no concerns on bowel viability, no further surgical reexploration is required, and there are no concerns for ACS. As compared to trauma patients, those affected by peritonitis or abdominal sepsis have a reported lower rate of early fascial closure [26], even though CFT techniques seem to be increasing this rate [27]. Primary fascia closure is the ideal solution to restore the abdominal closure but, if the OA is prolonged, fascia retraction and large abdominal wall defects may require complex abdominal wall reconstructions. Planned ventral hernia represents a valid alternative to cover the viscera and to prevent EAF, when delaying the prosthetic reconstruction is safer, such as in case of persistent contamination, several comorbidities, or in severely ill patients. It consists of skin graft or skin closure only, depending on the wound conditions, the dimension of the skin defect, and the center facilities [28]. When a planned ventral hernia is performed, a staged reconstruction of the abdominal wall should be planned once the patient has recovered. Abdominal component separation is an effective technique in the elective management of the ventral hernia repair, with very good results reported [29].

Mesh-mediated closure techniques have also been reported in the management of abdominal closure after OA. The use of synthetic mesh as fascial bridge should not be recommended due to the risk of local side effects, such as adhesions, erosions, and fistula formation. Biological meshes instead are reliable for definitive abdominal wall reconstruction in presence of large wall defects, bacterial contamination, comorbidities, and difficult wound healing. Not cross-linked biologic meshes are preferable in sublay position when the linea alba can be reconstructed, but have a high rate of recurrent ventral hernia when placed as fascial bridge. Therefore, when the linea alba cannot be closed, cross-linked biologic meshes are recommended in fascial-bridge position. Biologic meshes can also be used in combination with NPWT in order to facilitate granulation and skin closure [30–32].

As previously discussed, all the preemptive measures to avoid an EAF and a frozen abdomen should be accurately followed when performing an OA. Early abdominal wall closure, bowel coverage with plastic sheets, no direct application of synthetic prosthesis over bowel loops, no direct application of NPWT systems on the viscera, and deep burying of bowel anastomoses under bowel loops are all mandatory measures in the management of OA. However, a global fistula rate of 12% has been reported in meta-analyses. The treatment of EAF should be tailored according to patient condition, fistula output and position, and anatomical features. In presence of EAF, the caloric intake and protein demands are increased. Therefore, nutrition should be optimized accordingly. EAF effluent isolation is essential for a proper wound healing. The wound should be separated in different compartments in order to facilitate the collection of the fistula output and to allow granulation tissue formation. NPWT in all its variants is effective and the most accepted technique, allowing EAF isolation, proper wound management, re-epithelization, and converting the EAF in a sort of enterostomy (Fig. 18.2).

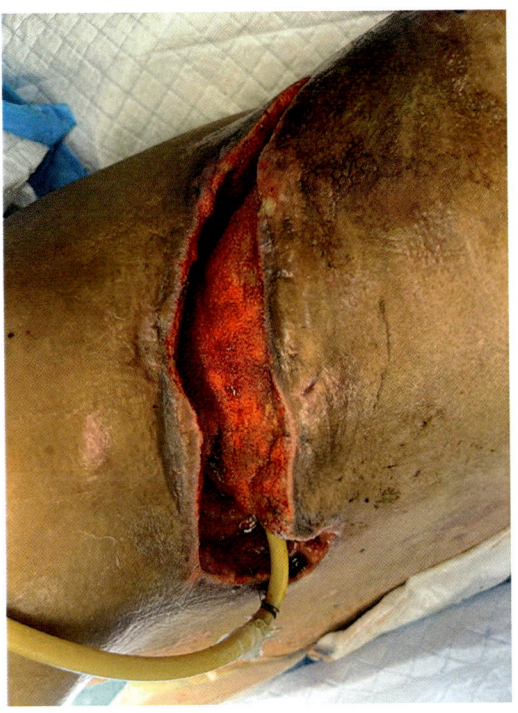

Fig. 18.2 EAF of the right flank in a trauma patient. Foley catheter allows isolation of the fistula output, whereas granulation tissue formation is facilitated by NPWT application

Definitive management of EAF should be postponed at least 6 months to after the patient has completely recovered and the wound has healed.

18.3.3 Prognosis

DCS is a strong arrow in the bow for the surgeon facing trauma and nontrauma patients with a deranged physiology, severe injuries, or critical illness. In these life-threatening situations, OA is dramatically effective. Guidelines clearly report all the indications to perform DCS and OA. However, translating these indications into clinical practice is not always easy due to the variability of the clinical scenarios a surgeon is dealing with. Therefore, its use remains very controversial and is a matter of debate. The lack of definitive data requires a careful tailoring of its use to every single patient and every single situation. An overuse of DCS has been reported, even in level 1 trauma centers. When performing an OA, the surgeons must put in practice all the preemptive measures in order to prevent the development of EAF and frozen abdomen. The globally reported rate of EAF is 12%. Moreover, the abdominal wall should be closed as soon as possible, in order to prevent hernia formation, to reduce ICU and hospital stay, and to facilitate the return to social and working life [33]. Chronic incisional hernia is one of the major complications directly related to OA and often requires a delayed further operation consisting of a complex abdominal reconstruction. The rates of successful abdominal closure have increased with the development of modern TAC techniques, such as NPWT and CFT, with a reported fascial closure rate of 73%. Other reported complications of OA include abscesses (13%), bowel resections (32%), and anastomotic leaks (4.3%). Patients undergoing DCS have a 16% peri-operative mortality. Therefore, the beneficial effect of DCS and OA must be accurately weighted together with its possible complications. The decision, again, should be patient-tailored. Further evidence is required and additional studies are strongly encouraged.

> **Dos and Don'ts**
> - In the DCS management, always apply a DCR: volume resuscitation, reversal of coagulopathy, and correction of acidosis.
> - In trauma patients, stop the lethal triad as soon as possible.
> - Ensure to routinely measure the abdominal pressure.
> - If possible, leave the abdomen open with NPWT and CFT.
> - Reexplore the abdomen every 24–48 h from the index operation and from any subsequent operation.
> - Apply all the prophylactic measures to prevent complications and EAF.
> - Close the abdomen as soon as possible.

Take-Home Messages

- DCS is a strong arrow in the bow for the surgeon facing trauma and nontrauma patients with a deranged physiology, severe injuries, or critical illness. In these life-threatening situations, OA is dramatically effective.
- Several indications to DCS have been reported, but some of those have not reported a clear benefit. Therefore, guidelines should be followed and the indication to DCS and OA should be tailored to every single patient and every single situation.
- DCR is the cornerstone of the treatment of severely injured and severely physiologically deranged patients. Multidisciplinary management is of utmost importance for these patients.
- When performing OA, several TAC techniques have been described. Two meta-analyses report that NPWT with CFT is the most effective in terms of fascial closure.
- OA reexploration should be conducted after 24–48 h after the index operation and after any subsequent operation. The abdominal wall should be closed as soon as possible.
- Preventing measures should be applied to avoid complications, such as chronic hernia, EAF and frozen abdomen, abscesses, bowel resections, and anastomotic leaks. All these measures are mandatory and include early abdominal wall closure, bowel coverage with plastic sheets, no direct application of synthetic prosthesis over bowel loops, no direct application of NPWT systems on the viscera, and deep burying of bowel anastomoses under bowel loops.
- There is a lack of high-quality evidence in literature and further studies are required.

Multiple Choice Questions

1. According to international guidelines, a proper indication to DCS and OA in trauma patients is:
   A. Severely injured patient undergoing laparotomy with the need of bowel resection
   B. Severely injured patient with abdominal pain and grade II IAH
   C. **Severely injured patient undergoing laparotomy with the lethal triad and a severe physiological derangement**
   D. Severely injured patient with haemodynamic instability at admission in the emergency department
2. According to international guidelines, a proper indication to DCS and OA in a peritonitis patient undergoing surgery is:
   A. A massive abdominal contamination
   B. **The inability to reach an effective source control**
   C. The need for bowel resection
   D. The inability to complete a laparoscopic procedure
3. In the damage control resuscitation, how often should intra-abdominal pressure be measured?
   A. According to clinical judgement
   B. Every hour
   C. **Every 4–6 h**
   D. Every 24 h
4. Which is the most effective TAC technique in terms of fascial closure?
   A. Dynamic suture retention
   B. NPWT
   C. **NPWT with continuous fascial traction**
   D. Bogotà bag
5. Which is the average rate of fistula in OA, as reported in meta-analyses?
   A. 3%
   B. **12%**
   C. 18%
   D. 34%

6. When should the OA be reexplored and closed?
   A. OA should be reexplored every day and closed within one week
   B. OA should be reexplored every 24–48 h and closed within 10 days
   C. OA should be reexplored every day and closed as soon as possible
   D. **OA should be reexplored every 24–48 and closed as soon as possible**
7. The definitive management of an established EAF:
   A. Should be obtained as soon as possible
   B. Should be postponed to when the patient has improved, during the index admission
   C. Should be postponed to when the patient has completely recovered and the wound has **completely healed**
   D. Should be postponed at 2 years
8. Mesh-mediated closure techniques of an OA:
   A. Are contraindicated due to the risk of erosions and fistulae
   B. Are allowed as fascial bridges, especially not cross-liked biological meshes
   C. Are allowed as fascial bridges, especially cross-liked biological meshes
   D. Should always be placed in a sublay position
9. DCS in case of secondary peritonitis and shock:
   A. Is always necessary, regardless of the surgery effectiveness
   B. Is never indicated, if surgery reaches an effective source control
   C. **Should be tailored to every single patient, and trials are ongoing to evaluate its effectiveness as compared to definitive abdominal closure**
   D. Is contraindicated
10. In the meta-analyses by Roberts et al.
    A. **Several in**dications to DCS in trauma patients have been reported, but few of them demonstrated a clear validity
    B. Few indications to DCS in trauma patients have been reported, and most of them demonstrated a clear validity
    C. Several indications to DCS in peritonitis patients have been reported, but few of them demonstrated a clear validity
    D. Few indications to DCS in peritonitis patients have been reported, and most of them demonstrated a clear validity

References

1. Coccolini F, Roberts D, Ansaloni L, et al. The open abdomen in trauma and non-trauma patients: WSES guidelines. World J Emerg Surg. 2018;13:7.
2. Kirkpatrick AW, Roberts DJ, De Waele J, et al. Intra-abdominal hypertension and the abdominal compartment syndrome: updated consensus definitions and clinical practice guidelines from the World Society of the Abdominal Compartment Syndrome. Intensive Care Med. 2013;39:1190–206.
3. Higa G, Friese R, O'Keeffe T, et al. Damage control laparotomy: a vital tool once overused. J Trauma. 2010;69(1):53–9.
4. Hatch QM, Osterhout LM, Podbielski J, et al. Impact of closure at the first take back: complication burden and potential overutilization of damage control laparotomy. J Trauma. 2011;71(6):1503–11.
5. Martin MJ, Hatch Q, Cotton B, et al. The use of temporary abdominal closure in low-risk trauma patients: helpful or harmful? J Trauma Acute Care Surg. 2012;72(3):601–8.
6. Watson JJ, Nielsen J, Hart K, et al. Damage control laparotomy utilization rates are highly variable among level I trauma centers: pragmatic, randomized optimal platelet and plasma ratios findings. J Trauma Acute Care Surg. 2017;82(3):481–8.
7. Roberts DJ, Bobrovitz N, Zygun DA, et al. Evidence for use of damage control surgery and damage control interventions in civilian trauma patients: a systematic review. World J Emerg Surg. 2021;16:10.
8. Tolonen M, Coccolini F, Ansaloni L, et al. Getting the invite list right: a discussion of sepsis severity scoring systems in severe complicated intra-abdominal sepsis and randomized trial inclusion criteria. World J Emerg Surg. 2018;6:13–7.

9. Kirkpatrick AW, Coccolini F, Ansaloni L, et al. Closed or Open after Source Control Laparotomy for Severe Complicated Intra-Abdominal Sepsis (the COOL trial): study protocol for a randomized controlled trial. World J Emerg Surg. 2018;13:26.
10. Rotondo MF, Zonies DH. The damage control sequence and underlying logic. Surg Clin North Am. 1997;77:761–77.
11. Sagraves SG, Toschlog EA, Rotondo MF. Damage control surgery—the intensivist's role. J Intensive Care Med. 2006;21:5–16.
12. Chabot E, Nirula R. Open abdomen critical care management principles: resuscitation, fluid balance, nutrition, and ventilator management. Trauma Surg Acute Care Open. 2017;2:e000063.
13. Rohrer MJ, Natale AM. Effect of hypothermia on the coagulation cascade. Crit Care Med. 1992;20:1402–5.
14. Davenport R, Khan S. Management of major trauma haemorrhage: treatment priorities and controversies. Br J Haematol. 2011;155:537–48.
15. Abramson D, Scalea TM, Hitchcock R, Trooskin SZ, Henry SM, Greenspan J. Lactate clearance and survival following injury. J Trauma. 1993;35:584–9.
16. Davenport R. Pathogenesis of acute traumatic coagulopathy. Transfusion. 2013;53:23S–7S.
17. Sugrue M, Bauman A, Jones F, Bishop G, Flabouris A, Parr M, et al. Clinical examination is an inaccurate predictor of intraabdominal pressure. World J Surg. 2002;26:1428–31.
18. Cothren CC, Moore EE, Ciesla DJ, Johnson JL, Moore JB, Haenel JB, et al. Postinjury abdominal compartment syndrome does not preclude early enteral feeding after definitive closure. Am J Surg. 2004;188:653–8.
19. Dissanaike S, Pham T, Shalhub S, Warner K, Hennessy L, Moore EE, et al. Effect of immediate enteral feeding on trauma patients with an open abdomen: protection from nosocomial infections. J Am Coll Surg. 2008;207:690–7.
20. McClave SA, Heyland DK. The physiologic response and associated clinical benefits from provision of early enteral nutrition. Nutr Clin Pract. 2009;24:305–15.
21. Collier B, Guillamondegui O, Cotton B, Donahue R, Conrad A, Groh K, et al. Feeding the open abdomen. JPEN J Parenter Enteral Nutr. 2007;31:410–5.
22. Atema JJ, Gans SL, Boermeester MA. Systematic review and meta-analysis of the open abdomen and temporary abdominal closure techniques in non-trauma patients. World J Surg. 2015;39:912–25.
23. Cristaudo A, Jennings S, Gunnarsson R, et al. Complications and mortality associated with temporary abdominal closure techniques: a systematic review and meta-analysis. Am Surg. 2017;83:191–216.
24. Pommerening MJ, Dubose JJ, Zielinski MD, et al. Time to first take-back operation predicts successful primary fascial closure in patients undergoing damage control laparotomy. Surgery. 2014;156:431–8.
25. Coccolini F, Montori G, Ceresoli M, et al. The role of open abdomen in non-trauma patient: WSES consensus paper. World J Emerg Surg. 2017;12:39.
26. Paul JS, Ridolfi TJ. A case study in intra-abdominal sepsis. Surg Clin North Am. 2012;92:1661–77.
27. Tolonen M, Mentula P, Sallinen V, et al. Open abdomen with vacuum-assisted wound closure and mesh-mediated fascial traction in patients with complicated diffuse secondary peritonitis. J Trauma Acute Care Surg. 2017;82:1100–5.
28. Chiara O, Cimbanassi S, Biffl W, et al. International consensus conference on open abdomen in trauma. J Trauma Acute Care Surg. 2016;80:173–83.
29. Rasilainen SK, Mentula PJ, Leppaniemi AK. Components separation technique is feasible for assisting delayed primary fascial closure of open abdomen. Scand J Surg. 2016;105:17–21.
30. Caviggioli F, Klinger FM, Lisa A, Maione L, Forcellini D, Vinci V, et al. Matching biological mesh and negative pressure wound therapy in reconstructing an open abdomen defect. Case Rep Med. 2014;2014:235930.
31. Dietz UA, Wichelmann C, Wunder C, Kauczok J, Spor L, Strauß A, et al. Early repair of open abdomen with a tailored two-component mesh and conditioning vacuum packing: a safe alternative to the planned giant ventral hernia. Hernia. 2012;16:451–60.
32. Rasilainen SK, Mentula PJ, Leppäniemi AK. Vacuum and mesh-mediated fascial traction for primary closure of the open abdomen in critically ill surgical patients. Br J Surg. 2012;99:1725.
33. Cheatham M, Safcsak K. Longterm impact of abdominal decompression: a prospective comparative analysis. J Am Coll Surg. 2008;207:573–9.

Further Reading

Atema JJ, Gans SL, Boermeester MA. Systematic review and meta-analysis of the open abdomen and temporary abdominal closure techniques in non-trauma patients. World J Surg. 2015;39:912–25.

Coccolini F, Roberts D, Ansaloni L, et al. The open abdomen in trauma and non-trauma patients: WSES guidelines. World J Emerg Surg. 2018;13:7.

Cristaudo A, Jennings S, Gunnarsson R, et al. Complications and mortality associated with temporary abdominal closure techniques: a systematic review and meta-analysis. Am Surg. 2017;83:191–216.

Kirkpatrick AW, Roberts DJ, De Waele J, et al. Intra-abdominal hypertension and the abdominal compartment syndrome: updated consensus definitions and clinical practice guidelines from the World Society of the Abdominal Compartment Syndrome. Intensive Care Med. 2013;39:1190–206.

Roberts DJ, Bobrovitz N, Zygun DA, et al. Evidence for use of damage control surgery and damage control interventions in civilian trauma patients: a systematic review. World J Emerg Surg. 2021;16:10.

Nutritional Support

19

Swathikan Chidambaram, En Lin Goh, and Mansoor Ali Khan

19.1 Introduction

Learning Objectives
- To outline the metabolic response of the body towards trauma, namely the anabolic and catabolic phases.
- To understand the variation in nutritional needs of a trauma patient depending on both patient and trauma-related factors and enable the administration of nutrition in a tailored fashion to optimise outcomes.
- To appreciate that the management of nutrition in a trauma patient requires a multi-disciplinary team and their roles in this process.

The multidisciplinary management of patients who have undergone major trauma involves optimum nutritional support to improve their outcomes. There is well-established guidelines to prove that nutrition is an integral component in minimising the morbidity of patients; however, the specific details of how nutrition is delivered are areas of much debate with conflicting evidence [1, 2]. Historically, given the nature of trauma, there has often been a paucity of high grade evidence, and most guidelines are based on retrospective work with significant heterogeneity that reduces the generalizability of the results. However, over the last decade, there have been several landmark critical care nutrition studies providing new insights into the route, dose, and timing of nutritional support. This chapter aims to review the current evidence base for the different facets of nutritional management that are often the focus of guidelines in managing the trauma patient.

19.2 Physiology of Nutrition in Trauma

The metabolic response to injury has been heavily studied in the literature and was described to go through three different phases, namely, the ebb/shock phase, the flow/catabolic phase, and anabolic phase [3]. The shock phase describes the first 24–48 h after injury and is characterised

---

S. Chidambaram
Faculty of Medicine, Imperial College London, South Kensington, London, UK
e-mail: swathikan.chidambaram12@imperial.ac.uk

E. L. Goh
Oxford Trauma, Nuffield Department of Orthopaedics, Rheumatology and Musculoskeletal Sciences, University of Oxford John Radcliffe Hospital, Oxford, UK
e-mail: enlin.goh@ndorms.ox.ac.uk

M. A. Khan (✉)
University of Brighton, Brighton and Sussex University Hospitals NHS Trust, Royal Sussex County Hospital, Brighton, UK
e-mail: mansoorkhan@nhs.net

by haemodynamic instability due to decreased circulating volume where the body is trying to maintain homeostasis by decreasing the total body energy expenditure and urinary nitrogen excretion [4]. This is where the body mobilises its caloric reserves towards gluconeogenesis to generate up to 75% of glucose needs during illness [5]. The catabolic phase follows the shock phase and is driven by a surge in catecholamines, glucagon, and corticosteroids. These induce a state of insulin resistance and muscle breakdown to generate the precursors necessary for wound healing, although this clinically translates into progressive muscle loss and weakness [5]. The body experiences an increase in metabolic needs, and sources of energy supply need to come from an exogenous energy source rather than endogenous. In the anabolic phase, the body switches to a positive nitrogen balance and increased protein synthesis leading to a progressive increase in muscle gain and strength when combined with exercise [6]. It eventually concludes by restoration of body protein stores and normalisation of nitrogen balance after trauma [7]. There is a high metabolic requirement with an increase in energy and protein needs, especially during rehabilitation. Nutrition support plans should be designed to match the course of critical illness, adjusting for the shock, catabolic, and recovery phases, although clinical criteria for when a patient moves from one phase to another are poorly defined [8].

19.3 Assessment of Malnutrition

The 2015 ESPEN defines malnutrition as a BMI <18.5 kg/m^2; or suffering from an unintentional weight loss >10% irrespective of time; or >5% over the last 3 months combined with either a BMI < 20 if <70 years of age, or BMI < 22 if >70 years of age; or a fat-free mass index <15 and 17 kg/m^2 in women and men, respectively [9, 10]. In response to any injury, the body initiates a series of endocrine, metabolic, and immunological changes that are collectively termed the stress response [3]. This generally results in a hypercatabolic, inflammatory, and pro-coagulant state that results in the breakdown of protein and fat in the body. Coupled with this, patients who undergo trauma are often a group of individuals already predisposed to a significant state of malnutrition. For example, recent epidemiological data show that trauma is increasingly prevalent in the elderly population; people with other major comorbidities; and areas of social deprivation and high violence, including war-torn areas [11–13]. In a recent study of 1055 trauma patients, a higher rate of malnutrition was detected in the geriatric population with up to 29–31% in those aged 65–80 years and 54–60% in those over 80 years. Malnourished patients had a more a prolonged hospital stay (13.7 ± 11.1 vs. 18.2 ± 11.7 days, $p < 0.05$), delayed post-operative mobilisation (2.2 ± 2.9 vs. 4.0 ± 4.9 days, $p < 0.05$), and a significantly higher rate of adverse events (37.2% vs. 21.1%, $p < 0.001$) [14]. Malnutrition in trauma patients is associated with increased mortality and up to 28 days longer in rehabilitation [15]. Hence, the delivery of adequate nutrition necessitates a reliable method to assess malnutrition.

Assessment of nutritional needs should be individualised given the range of patient and disease-related factors, with an approximate target of 20–35 kcal/kg/day depending on the phase of injury. Lower energy provision has been suggested in the resuscitative phase with an increase in energy delivery as the patient enters the rehabilitation phase. Requirements for protein are similar to other ICU patients, but maybe at the higher end of the range at 1.2–2 g/kg/day [16]. This can be tricky given that body weight and body mass index (BMI) are not reliable indicators of nutritional status in the trauma patient who needs critical care support. Often, despite an obese BMI, patients have a high degree of sarcopenia due to loss of lean body muscle [17]. Laboratory tests such as C-reactive protein and albumin are not the best markers of nutritional status as they are increased in pro-inflammatory states such as trauma [18–20]. Tools such as the subjective global assessment (SGA), mini-nutrition assessment (MNA), nutritional risk screening (NRS), MNA-short form (MNA-SF), Clinical Frailty Score (CRF), malnutrition universal screening tool (MUST) score and Nutrition Risk in Critically ill (NUTRIC) score have been evaluated in the critically ill patients, with whom the trauma cohort largely overlaps [10, 21–26]. All of these scoring systems have variable specificities and sensitivities and are yet to be validated in the trauma cohort using higher levels of evidence and calls for a more vigilant approach towards malnutrition. For now, the assessment of these patients should be multi-modal involving clinical status, blood tests, and the aforementioned scores to gain a global appreciation of the nutritional status and make early efforts to optimise it.

19.4 Route of Nutrition: Enteral Vs Parenteral Nutrition

Traditionally, trauma patients received parenteral nutrition (PN) in the initial days of their admission, especially if they had trauma to the abdomen. In fact, it was not until 2003 that the use of enteral nutrition (EN) in the open abdomen was first reported [27]. EN has numerous positive effects including the maintenance of gastrointestinal mucosal integrity, promotion of wound healing, immune function, the response to tissue damage in addition to reducing the rate of nosocomial infections, length of hospital stay, and subsequently, overall health care costs. The landmark CALORIES multicentre randomised controlled trial was published in 2014 and investigated the optimal route of early nutrition support in critically ill patients (EN vs. PN) [28]. Two thousand three hundred and eighty eight adult patients from 33 ICUs in England were included. It demonstrated no mortality benefit for either route and there was also no difference in rate of infection. This finding has been replicated in the recent NUTRIREA-2 trial of 2400 patients on vasopressor support for shock [29]. Both studies challenge old perceptions regarding the safety of PN in critically ill patients and open the door for PN consideration as a viable alternative in cases where EN is not feasible. The CALORIES trial data have been included in the latest systematic review comparing EN and PN, which demonstrated that PN is only associated with more infections when the calories provided by PN were greater than EN, this adding to the argument that it is the dose of nutrition that is more harmful than the route.

Current guidelines recommend the initiation of enteral nutrition as much as possible as it is a more physiological way of feeding the patient with high calorific needs. Oral diet is preferred in patients able to eat, and if that is not possible, then other routes of enteral nutrition including nasogastric feeding, naso-jejunal feeding, and gastrostomy feeding should be considered. If a trauma patient has contraindications to EN, low dose PN should be initiated after carefully considering and balancing against the risks of overfeeding and refeeding, which may outweigh the expected benefits. Contraindications may include uncontrolled shock, uncontrolled hypoxemia and acidosis, uncontrolled upper gastrointestinal bleeding, gastric aspirate >500 mL/h, bowel ischemia, bowel obstruction, abdominal compartment syndrome, and high-output fistula without distal feeding access. A recent meta-analysis of studies comparing EN and PN reported a significant reduction in infections with the former [30]. This is concordant with early work by Moore et al. on trauma patients, who reported a lower rate of septic complications such as pneumonia, intra-abdominal abscess, and line sepsis [31, 32]. Even in patients requiring repeated procedures such as relook laparotomies, enteral feeding has been shown to be safe [33]. Some studies have reported PN to have better outcomes, but this is largely in specific cohorts with head injury, which remains an area needing further research [34–36]. Regardless, nutritional support should not be delayed in favour of EN in cases where EN is not possible, as nutritional deficits during a hypermetabolic state only lead to worse outcomes.

19.5 Timing and Site of Enteral Nutrition

Enteral nutrition can be instituted at an early stage (defined as before 72 h from time of injury) or later than 72 h, termed as delayed EN [37]. The evidence investigating the timing of EN is heterogenous and often there is a variation in the definition of "early" and "late" used. For example, Eyre et al. used 39 h as the cut-off for early in their analysis showing no benefit between early and delayed feeding [38]. Current guidelines state no significant advantage in initiating early EN in severely injured blunt/penetrating trauma patients. However, the European Society for Clinical Nutrition and Metabolism guidelines advocates for early enteral nutrition within 48 h if oral intake is not possible, but this should not, however, delay enteral nutrition [2, 39]. Unlike other facets of nutrition, the timing of nutrition is an area that has never been truly investigated with RCTs. Better prospective work using a widely agreed definition of "early" and "delayed" with clinically relevant outcome measures in specific populations is required as future work.

The provision of enteral nutrition varies depending on the feasibility of access [40]. This is usually done through the nasogastric or nasoenteric tubes; endoscopically or radiologically placed gastric or gastro-jejunal tubes; and lastly surgically placed gastrostomy or jejunostomy tubes if the patient was also undergoing a laparotomy [41]. Usually, feeding into the stomach is convenient as access to the stomach is easier to obtain than the duodenum. However, patients who have delayed gastric emptying (gastric retention) or lower esophageal sphincter dysfunction (severe GORD) are at risk of aspiration and would benefit from post-pyloric feeding methods [42–44]. For example, patients with brain injury failed to meet caloric needs when fed enterally due to delayed gastric emptying and had better outcomes with parenteral nutrition instead. However, other studies have shown that gastric feeding is possible if initiated early on, but this again goes back to the question of correctly timing EN. In patient with abdominal trauma, feeding through naso-jejunal feeding tube, gastro-jejunal feeding tube, or feeding jejunostomy is recommended to gain direct access to the small bowel; however, this requires careful planning and monitoring for complications such as distension, bloating, diarrhea, and intestinal necrosis. Studies comparing jejunal and gastric feeding are limited by their heterogeneity and small sample sizes [45–47]. Taken together, there is no clear evidence to recommend either gastric or jejunal feeding, but it is important to avoid the risk of aspiration. Further work is required to evaluate the safety and efficacy of the different forms of post-pyloric feeding in trauma patients.

19.6 Nutrition in the Open Abdomen

The open abdomen is typically encountered after damage control surgery (DCS) or in patients with abdominal compartment syndrome (ACS) [48, 49]. DCS refers to the surgical strategy of performing only essential interventions during a laparotomy in an unstable patient, with postponement of procedures that do not offer immediate steps toward survival [50–52]. The open abdomen can be classified as either acute (<7 days) or chronic (>7 days) [53]. Patients with a chronic open abdomen tend to have higher nutritional requirements, and hence will benefit from early enteral nutrition [54]. As mentioned earlier, early EN will reduce septic complications [16, 28–30, 55–57]. But, there is a risk of paralytic ileus that can not only worsen any underlying intestinal injury, but also predisposes patients to aspiration risk and further bowel dilation that will delay closure [58]. The recent meta-analysis by Goh et al. showed a statistically significant reduction in the overall mortality and morbidity (infection and fistulae formation) in using EN instead of PN in the management of the open abdomen [59]. However, the analysis also showed that early initiation of EN is associated with increased time to abdominal closure, higher incidence of pneumonia, and longer hospital stay [60–64]. Delayed closure carries a risk of further septic complications. This could be attributed to the inclusion of patients with bowel injury, since subgroup analysis by Burlew et al. excluding such patients showed better outcomes for early EN [60]. Overall, there is insufficient evidence to recommend either approach in the open abdomen, which is an area that requires further prospective work.

19.7 Nutrition Protocols

There is a wide variation in the route, type, and timing of feed. Much work was carried out to establish standardised feeding protocols that delivered enteral nutrition that more closely matches energy and protein requirements, and thus improves the adequacy of enteral nutrition delivery [65–67]. For example, in their study, Barr et al. used feedback from ICU staff to design a feeding protocol for 100 critically ill patients and showed no difference in time to feeding, caloric intake on day 4, and ICU or hospital length of stay [67]. The multicentre, cluster-randomised ACCEPT trial showed that protocols reduced hospital stay and mortality, but delayed EN, though the complications from this were not fully assessed [68]. This contradicted with a larger trial involving 1118 patients where protocols led to more patients receiving EN and within 24 h of admission [68]. Soguel et al. reported that in their study of 572 patients, their 2-step program involving a feeding protocol and a dedicated dietician to implement it led a 31.6% improvement in caloric delivery [65]. Heyland et al. used a bundle of interventions, namely a 24-h volume goal of enteral feeding instead of a rate-based goal, prokinetic agents, a high cutoff for gastric residual volume of 300 mL/h, and protein supplementation [69]. In both the PEPuP study and the FEEDME study, protocols significantly increased the proportion of enteral nutrition volume and calories delivered to patients, resulting in increased protein and body weight [70]. Despite the abundance of evidence, not many units use feeding protocols that are tailored to a patient's demographics and pathology. A limitation of these studies is that while they included critically ill patients, they are not necessarily exposed to major trauma, suggesting a paucity of evidence for feeding protocols specifically in the trauma cohort.

19.8 The Role of the Multidisciplinary Team in Nutritional Support

A major reason for the lack of effectiveness of many nutritional protocols is the lack of a team-based approach in delivering the nutritional support. The most effective protocols employ a multi-disciplinary team approach involving nursing and a dedicated dietician involvement. Inevitably, nurses are at the forefront of caring for the patient and are best placed to both identify patients who need better nutrition and patients at risk of malnutrition [71]. The administration of nutrition requires careful consideration of other issues such as glucose control, infection risks, pain symptoms, aspiration risks, and access issues, all of which require nursing experience [47, 72, 73]. Furthermore, limited knowledge of nutrition support has been identified as a key problem, so the placement of a dedicated dietician to look after trauma patients is essential [74]. Dieticians can provide expert advice with updated knowledge of the evidence tailored to the trauma patient; develop and institute new feeding protocols; monitor the nutritional status of patients; and educate the remainder of team in any nutrition-related issues [65]. In the UK, many hospitals have specific teams looking after the nutrition of these patients, and often also include a senior doctor specialising in clinical biochemistry, chemical pathology, or nutrition [75]. Together, the multi-disciplinary team including doctors, nurses, and auxiliary staff such as dieticians play a vital role in the institution of the correct nutritional support for the trauma patient.

19.9 Areas of Future Work

Nutritional research has been carried for several decades, yet there is much room for further work. There is little work surrounding specific situations, and current evidence only highlights the broad strokes of how to feed the trauma patient. First, there is still no consensus on the timing or route of enteral nutrition. While it is generally agreed that the most physiologically feasible form of feeding is the best mode, this may not always be the case. Furthermore, trials have produced conflicting results on whether EN is truly superior to PN, and we are at a stage where we need to consolidate the lessons from international trials but also smaller work. The feeding requirements for each trauma patient are different, and to match this, further work is needed on feeding protocols that correct nutritional deficiencies and improve non-nutritional outcomes. At present, there is a lack of an agreed method to assess and monitor malnutrition. Better tools incorporating clinical status, laboratory, and imaging information are required. With the advent of artificial intelligence and "big data", there is a potential to overcome the cofounding that is usually present in the heterogeneous nature of previous work. Current guidelines do not incorporate the latest work in this field and often seem outdated, calling for an international collaborative effort to answer these questions and update the consensus statements and current guidance on issues related to nutrition.

19.10 Conclusion

Malnutrition is a common but frequently underestimated problem in patients presenting with traumatic injury. Inadequate nutrition has been significantly linked to increased morbidity, mortality, length of hospital stay, and overall cost of care. Thus, providing adequate nutritional support throughout the critical care and rehabilitation journey should be considered as an integral part of the management of trauma patients. Early EN should be considered in the haemodynamically stable patient in the absence of contraindications, and interruptions to the feed must be kept at a minimum. For this goal to be achieved, it is crucial to raise the awareness about the importance of adequate nutritional support in trauma management, both at the level of healthcare providers and institutions, in addition to adopting evidence-based nutritional guidelines and practical solutions for overcoming the challenges in delivering nutrition support to this group of patients.

> **Dos and Don'ts**
>
> **Do**
> - Evaluate a tailored approach for nutritional planning.
> - Involve a multi-disciplinary team.
>
> **Don't**
> - Underestimate the nutrition needs of your patient.
> - Underestimate trauma's ever-changing physiology.

> **Take-Home Messages**
> - Nutritional needs evolve to match the ever-changing physiology of trauma, and hence must be dynamically monitored and adjusted in the period following injury.
> - There is no overarching accepted protocol for delivering nutrition. Nutritional needs of each patient should be assessed on an individual basis and tailored to meet the caloric needs, depending on both patient and trauma-related factors.
> - The optimum delivery of nutrition should involve a multi-disciplinary team consisting of dieticians, physicians, nurses, and other auxiliary staff that is focused on managing the nutritional needs of a patient.

> **Questions**
> 1. Which of the following describes the correct sequence of the phases of metabolic response to injury?
>   A. **Shock, catabolic, anabolic**
>   B. Catabolic and anabolic only
>   C. Shock and catabolic only
>   D. Shock and anabolic only

2. Which of the following describes the outcomes of the CALORIES trial?
   A. Enteral route resulted in better mortality than parenteral route.
   B. Enteral route resulted in lower infections than parenteral route.
   C. **No difference in mortality or infection rate between enteral and parenteral routes.**
   D. Parenteral route resulted in overall survival than enteral nutrition.

3. Which of the following best describes the recommended type of feeding in patients with an open abdomen?
   A. Enteral only
   B. Parenteral only
   C. Enteral followed by parenteral
   D. **No absolute recommendations made and needs adjusting to the patient**

4. Which of the following time points has traditionally described "late" enteral feeding?
   A. Greater than 24 h
   B. Greater than 48 h
   C. **Greater than 72 h**
   D. Greater than 120 h

5. Which of the following describes the outcomes of the ACCEPT trial?
   A. **Nutrition protocols reduced hospital stay and mortality, but delayed enteral nutrition**
   B. Nutrition protocols increased hospital stay and mortality, but delayed enteral nutrition
   C. Nutrition protocols increased hospital stay, mortality, and allowed earlier enteral nutrition.
   D. Nutrition protocols reduced rate of infection-related complications.

References

1. Jacobs DG, Jacobs DO, Kudsk KA, Moore FA, Oswanski MF, Poole GV, et al. Practice management guidelines for nutritional support of the trauma patient. J Trauma. 2004;57:660–78.
2. Singer P, Blaser AR, Berger MM, Alhazzani W, Calder PC, Casaer MP, et al. ESPEN guideline on clinical nutrition in the intensive care unit. Clin Nutr. 2019;38(1):48–79.
3. Preiser JC, Ichai C, Orban JC, Groeneveld ABJ. Metabolic response to the stress of critical illness. Br J Anaesth. 2014;113(6):945–54.
4. Stahel PF, Flierl MA, Moore EE. "Metabolic staging" after major trauma—a guide for clinical decision making? Scand J Trauma Resusc Emerg Med. 2010;18:34.
5. Wischmeyer PE. Tailoring nutrition therapy to illness and recovery. Crit Care. 2017;21:316.
6. Hasenboehler E, Williams A, Leinhase I, Morgan SJ, Smith WR, Moore EE, et al. Metabolic changes after polytrauma: an imperative for early nutritional support. World J Emerg Surg. 2006;1:29.
7. Heyland DK, Stapleton RD, Mourtzakis M, Hough CL, Morris P, Deutz NE, et al. Combining nutrition and exercise to optimize survival and recovery from critical illness: conceptual and methodological issues. Clin Nutr. 2016;35(5):1196–206.
8. Preiser JC, van Zanten ARH, Berger MM, Biolo G, Casaer MP, Doig GS, et al. Metabolic and nutritional support of critically ill patients: consensus and controversies. Crit Care. 2015;19(1):35.
9. Cederholm T, Barazzoni R, Austin P, Ballmer P, Biolo G, Bischoff SC, et al. ESPEN guidelines on definitions and terminology of clinical nutrition. Clin Nutr. 2017;36(1):49–64.
10. Cederholm T, Jensen GL, Correia MITD, Gonzalez MC, Fukushima R, Higashiguchi T, et al. GLIM criteria for the diagnosis of malnutrition—a consensus report from the global clinical nutrition community. J Cachexia Sarcopenia Muscle. 2019;10(1):207–17.
11. Krug EG, Sharma GK, Lozano R. The global burden of injuries. Am J Public Health. 2000;90:523–6.
12. Alberdi F, García I, Atutxa L, Zabarte M. Epidemiology of severe trauma. Med Intensiva. 2014;38(9):580–8.
13. Müller FS, Meyer OW, Chocano-Bedoya P, Schietzel S, Gagesch M, Freystaetter G, et al. Impaired nutritional status in geriatric trauma patients. Eur J Clin Nutr. 2017;71(5):602–6.
14. Ihle C, Freude T, Bahrs C, Zehendner E, Braunsberger J, Biesalski HK, et al. Malnutrition—an underestimated factor in the inpatient treatment of traumatol-

14. ogy and orthopedic patients: a prospective evaluation of 1055 patients. Injury. 2017;48(3):628–36.
15. Dénes Z. The influence of severe malnutrition on rehabilitation in patients with severe head injury. Disabil Rehabil. 2004;26(19):1163–5.
16. McClave SA, Taylor BE, Martindale RG, Warren MM, Johnson DR, Braunschweig C, et al. Guidelines for the provision and assessment of nutrition support therapy in the adult critically ill patient: Society of Critical Care Medicine (SCCM) and American Society for Parenteral and Enteral Nutrition (A.S.P.E.N.). J Parenter Enter Nutr. 2016;40(2):159–211.
17. Studenski SA, Peters KW, Alley DE, Cawthon PM, McLean RR, Harris TB, et al. The FNIH sarcopenia project: rationale, study description, conference recommendations, and final estimates. J Gerontol A Biol Sci Med Sci. 2014;69(5):547–58.
18. Oh TK, Song IA, Lee JH. Clinical usefulness of C-reactive protein to albumin ratio in predicting 30-day mortality in critically ill patients: a retrospective analysis. Sci Rep. 2018;8(1):14977.
19. Yeh DD, Johnson E, Harrison T, Kaafarani HMA, Lee J, Fagenholz P, et al. Serum levels of albumin and prealbumin do not correlate with nutrient delivery in surgical intensive care unit patients. Nutr Clin Pract. 2018;33(3):419–25.
20. Bharadwaj S, Ginoya S, Tandon P, Gohel TD, Guirguis J, Vallabh H, et al. Malnutrition: laboratory markers vs nutritional assessment. Gastroenterol Rep. 2016;4:272–80.
21. Detsky AS, Baker JP, Mendelson RA, Wolman SL, Wesson DE, Jeejeebhoy KN, et al. Evaluating the accuracy of nutritional assessment techniques applied to hospitalized patients: methodology and comparisons. J Parenter Enter Nutr. 1984;8(2):153–9.
22. Sheean PM, Peterson SJ, Chen Y, Liu D, Lateef O, Braunschweig CA. Utilizing multiple methods to classify malnutrition among elderly patients admitted to the medical and surgical intensive care units (ICU). Clin Nutr. 2013;32(5):752–7.
23. Coltman A, Peterson S, Roehl K, Roosevelt H, Sowa D. Use of 3 tools to assess nutrition risk in the intensive care unit. J Parenter Enter Nutr. 2015;39(1):28–33.
24. Rockwood K, Song X, MacKnight C, Bergman H, Hogan DB, McDowell I, et al. A global clinical measure of fitness and frailty in elderly people. CMAJ. 2005;173(5):489–95.
25. Elia M. THE MUST REPORT—Nutritional screening of adults: a multidisciplinary responsibility. Malnutrition Advis Gr. 2003.
26. Reber E, Gomes F, Vasiloglou MF, Schuetz P, Stanga Z. Nutritional risk screening and assessment. J Clin Med. 2019;8(7):1065.
27. McKibbin B, Cresci G, Hawkins M. Nutrition support for the patient with an open abdomen after major abdominal trauma. Nutrition. 2003;19(6):563–6.
28. Harvey SE, Parrott F, Harrison DA, Bear DE, Segaran E, Beale R, et al. Trial of the route of early nutritional support in critically ill adults. N Engl J Med. 2014;371(18):1673–84.
29. Reignier J, Boisramé-Helms J, Brisard L, Lascarrou JB, Ait Hssain A, Anguel N, et al. Enteral versus parenteral early nutrition in ventilated adults with shock: a randomised, controlled, multicentre, open-label, parallel-group study (NUTRIREA-2). Lancet. 2017;391:133–43.
30. Elke G, van Zanten ARH, Lemieux M, McCall M, Jeejeebhoy KN, Kott M, et al. Enteral versus parenteral nutrition in critically ill patients: an updated systematic review and meta-analysis of randomized controlled trials. Crit Care. 2016;20(1):117.
31. Alverdy JC, Aoys E, Moss GS. Total parenteral nutrition promotes bacterial translocation from the gut. Surgery. 1988;104(2):185–90.
32. Deitch EA, Winterton J, Li M, Berg R. The gut as a portal of entry for bacteremia. Role of protein malnutrition. Ann Surg. 1987;205(6):681–92.
33. Moncure M, Samaha E, Moncure K, Mitchell J, Rehm C, Cypel D, et al. Jejunostomy tube feedings should not be stopped in the perioperative patient. J Parenter Enter Nutr. 1999;23(6 SUPPL):356–9.
34. Borzotta AP, Pennings J, Papasadero B, Paxton J, Mardesic S, Borzotta R, et al. Enteral versus parenteral nutrition after severe closed head injury. J Trauma. 1994;37(3):459–68.
35. Rapp RP, Young DB, Twyman D, Bivins BA, Haack D, Tibbs PA, et al. The favorable effect of early parenteral feeding on survival in head-injured patients. J Neurosurg. 1983;58(6):906–12.
36. Young B, Ott L, Twyman D, Norton J, Rapp R, Tibbs P, et al. The effect of nutritional support on outcome from severe head injury. J Neurosurg. 1987;67(5):668–76.
37. Moore EE, Jones TN. Benefits of immediate jejunostomy feeding after major abdominal trauma—a prospective, randomized study. J Trauma. 1986;26(10):874–81.
38. Eyer SD, Micon LT, Konstantinides FN, Edlund DA, Rooney KA, Luxenberg MG, et al. Early enteral feeding does not attenuate metabolic response after blunt trauma. J Trauma. 1993;34(5):639–43; discussion 643–4.
39. Reintam Blaser A, Deane AM, Starkopf J. Translating the European Society for Clinical Nutrition and Metabolism 2019 guidelines into practice. Curr Opin Crit Care. 2019;25:314–21.
40. Adams S, Dellinger EP, Wertz MJ, Oreskovich MR, Simonowitz D, Johansen K. Enteral versus parenteral nutritional support following laparotomy for trauma: a randomized prospective trial. J Trauma. 1986;26(10):882–91.
41. Burtch GD, Shatney CH. Feeding jejunostomy (versus gastrostomy) passes the test of time. Am Surg. 1987;53(1):54–7.
42. Saxe JM, Ledgerwood AM, Lucas CE, Lucas WF. Lower esophageal sphincter dysfunction precludes safe gastric feeding after head injury. J Trauma. 1994;37(4):581–4; discussion 584–6.
43. Ott L, Young B, Phillips R, McClain C, Adams L, Dempsey R, et al. Altered gastric emptying in the

head-injured patient: relationship to feeding intolerance. J Neurosurg. 1991;74(5):738–42.
44. Kao CH, Changlai SP, Chieng PU, Yen TC. Gastric emptying in head-injured patients. Am J Gastroenterol. 1998;93(7):1108–12.
45. Kortbeek JB, Haigh PI, Doig C. Duodenal versus gastric feeding in ventilated blunt trauma patients: a randomized controlled trial. J Trauma. 1999;46(6):992–6; discussion 996–8.
46. Kadakia SC, Sullivan HO, Starnes E. Percutaneous endoscopic gastrostomy or jejunostomy and the incidence of aspiration in 79 patients. Am J Surg. 1992;164(2):114–8.
47. Spain DA, DeWeese RC, Reynolds MA, Richardson JD. Transpyloric passage of feeding tubes in patients with head injuries does not decrease complications. J Trauma. 1995;39(6):1100–2.
48. Rotondo MF, Schwab CW, McGonigal MD, Phillips GR, Fruchterman TM, Kauder DR, et al. "Damage control": an approach for improved survival in exsanguinating penetrating abdominal injury. J Trauma. 1993;35(3):375–82; discussion 382–3.
49. Waibel BH, Rotondo MF. Damage control in trauma and abdominal sepsis. Crit Care Med. 2010;38(9 Suppl):S421–30.
50. Cheatham ML, Malbrain MLNG, Kirkpatrick A, Sugrue M, Parr M, De Waele J, et al. Results from the international conference of experts on intra-abdominal hypertension and abdominal compartment syndrome. II. Recommendations. Intensive Care Med. 2007;33:951–62.
51. Diaz JJ, Cullinane DC, Dutton WD, Jerome R, Bagdonas R, Bilaniuk JO, et al. The management of the open abdomen in trauma and emergency general surgery: part 1—damage control. J Trauma. 2010;68(6):1425–38.
52. Chidambaram S, Goh EL, Rey VG, Khan MA. Vasopressin vs noradrenaline: have we found the perfect recipe to improve outcome in septic shock? J Crit Care. 2019;49:99–104.
53. Fox N, Crutchfield M, La Chant M, Ross SE, Seamon MJ. Early abdominal closure improves long-term outcomes after damage-control laparotomy. J Trauma Acute Care Surg. 2013;75(5):854–8.
54. Moore SM, Burlew CC. Nutrition support in the open abdomen. Nutr Clin Pract. 2016;31(1):9–13.
55. Kudsk KA, Croce MA, Faian TC, Minard G, Tolley EA, Poret HA, et al. Enteral versus parenteral feeding effects on septic morbidity after blunt and penetrating abdominal trauma. Ann Surg. 1992;215(5):503–13.
56. Reintam Blaser A, Starkopf J, Alhazzani W, Berger MM, Casaer MP, Deane AM, et al. Early enteral nutrition in critically ill patients: ESICM clinical practice guidelines. Intensive Care Med. 2017;43:380–98.
57. Moore FA, Feliciano DV, Andrassy RJ, McArdle AH, Booth FV, Morgenstein-Wagner TB, et al. Early enteral feeding, compared with parenteral, reduces postoperative septic complications the results of a meta-analysis. Ann Surg. 1992;216(2):172–83.
58. Fong Y, Marano MA, Barber A, He W, Moldawer LL, Bushman ED, et al. Total parenteral nutrition and bowel rest modify the metabolic response to endotoxin in humans. Ann Surg. 1989;210(4):449–57.
59. Goh EL, Chidambaram S, Segaran E, Garnelo Rey V, Khan MA. A meta-analysis of the outcomes following enteral vs parenteral nutrition in the open abdomen in trauma patients. J Crit Care. 2020;56:42–8.
60. Burlew CC, Moore EE, Cuschieri J, Jurkovich GJ, Codner P, Nirula R, et al. Who should we feed? A Western Trauma Association multi-institutional study of enteral nutrition in the open abdomen after injury. J Trauma Acute Care Surg. 2012;73(6):1380–7.
61. Byrnes MC, Reicks P, Irwin E. Early enteral nutrition can be successfully implemented in trauma patients with an "open abdomen". Am J Surg. 2010;199(3):359–63.
62. Cothren CC, Moore EE, Ciesla DJ, Johnson JL, Moore JB, Haenel JB, et al. Postinjury abdominal compartment syndrome does not preclude early enteral feeding after definitive closure. Am J Surg. 2004;188(6):653–8.
63. Dissanaike S, Pham T, Shalhub S, Warner K, Hennessy L, Moore EE, et al. Effect of immediate enteral feeding on trauma patients with an open abdomen: protection from nosocomial infections. J Am Coll Surg. 2008;207(5):690–7.
64. Collier B, Guillamondegui O, Cotton B, Donahue R, Conrad A, Groh K, et al. Feeding the open abdomen. J Parenter Enter Nutr. 2007;31(5):410–5.
65. Soguel L, Revelly JP, Schaller MD, Longchamp C, Berger MM. Energy deficit and length of hospital stay can be reduced by a two-step quality improvement of nutrition therapy: the intensive care unit dietitian can make the difference. Crit Care Med. 2012;40(2):412–9.
66. Spain DA, McClave SA, Sexton LK, Adams JL, Blanford BS, Sullins ME, et al. Infusion protocol improves delivery of enteral tube feeding in the critical care unit. J Parenter Enter Nutr. 1999;23(5):288–92.
67. Barr J, Hecht M, Flavin KE, Khorana A, Gould MK. Outcomes in critically Ill patients before and after the implementation of an evidence-based nutritional management protocol. Chest. 2004;125(4):1446–57.
68. Doig GS, Simpson F, Finfer S, Delaney A, Davies AR, Mitchell I, et al. Effect of evidence-based feeding guidelines on mortality of critically ill adults: a cluster randomized controlled trial. JAMA. 2008;300(23):2731–41.
69. Heyland DK, Murch L, Cahill N, McCall M, Muscedere J, Stelfox HT, et al. Enhanced protein-energy provision via the enteral route feeding protocol in critically ill patients: results of a cluster randomized trial. Crit Care Med. 2013;41(12):2743–53.
70. Taylor B, Brody R, Denmark R, Southard R, Byham-Gray L. Improving enteral delivery through the adoption of the feed early enteral diet adequately for maximum effect (FEED ME) protocol in a surgical

71. Metheny NA, Mills AC, Stewart BJ. Monitoring for intolerance to gastric tube feedings: a national survey. Am J Crit Care. 2012;21(2):e33–40.
72. Bell L. Monitoring patients receiving enteral feedings. Am J Crit Care. 2012;21:133.
73. Goh EL, Chidambaram S, Ma D. Complex regional pain syndrome: a recent update. Burns Trauma. 2017;5:2.
74. Racco M. An enteral nutrition protocol to improve efficiency in achieving nutritional goals. Crit Care Nurse. 2012;32(4):72–5.
75. O'Leary-Kelley C, Bawel-Brinkley K. Nutrition support protocols: enhancing delivery of enteral nutrition. Crit Care Nurse. 2017;37(2):e15–23.

Further Reading

McClave SA, Taylor BE, Martindale RG, Warren MM, Johnson DR, Braunschweig C, et al. Guidelines for the provision and assessment of nutrition support therapy in the adult critically ill patient: Society of Critical Care Medicine (SCCM) and American Society for Parenteral and Enteral Nutrition (A.S.P.E.N.). J Parenter Enter Nutr. 2016;40(2):159–211.

McKibbin B, Cresci G, Hawkins M. Nutrition support for the patient with an open abdomen after major abdominal trauma. Nutrition. 2003;19(6):563–6.

Singer P, Blaser AR, Berger MM, Alhazzani W, Calder PC, Casaer MP, et al. ESPEN guideline on clinical nutrition in the intensive care unit. Clin Nutr. 2019;38:48–79.

(Note: Entry starts with "trauma ICU: a quality improvement review. Nutr Clin Pract. 2014;29(5):639–48.")

Palliative Care in the ICU

20

Mayur Narayan and Jeffry Kashuk

Life is a song—sing it. Life is a game—play it. Life is a challenge—meet it.
Life is a dream—realize it. Life is a sacrifice—offer it. Life is love—enjoy it.
—Sathya Sai Baba

> **Learning Goals**
> - Understand the definition of palliative care and palliation and how it differs from hospice care
> - Understand the global need for palliation, including the economic impact
> - Understand the challenges and future directions of palliative care

20.1 Introduction

Death is inevitable for all humans. The manner in which we die, especially when confronted with terminal illness or disease, is an area of healthcare that is greatly contested and debated. The Institute of Medicine (IOM) in the United States has defined a *good death* as "one that is free from avoidable distress and suffering for patients, families, and caregivers, in general accord with patients' families' wishes, and reasonably consistent with clinical, cultural, and ethical standards." It has recommended strategies to improve five vital components of care: (1) the delivery of person-centered, family-oriented end-of-life care; (2) clinician–patient communication and advance care planning; (3) professional education and development; (4) policies and payment systems to support high-quality end-of-life care; and (5) public education and engagement [1].

In 1990, the World Health Organization (WHO) defined *palliative care* as "the active and total care of patients whose disease is not responsive to curative treatment." Key components of the care they described included an emphasis on pain control as well as optimizing the psychological, social, and spiritual concerns of patients. Palliation also includes an understanding of how to achieve the best quality of life for patients *and* their families. Many aspects of palliative care are applicable earlier in the course of illness, especially in patients requiring intensive care unit (ICU) care [2]. A visual representation of the continuum of care, and specifically the role palliative care plays as a bridge to end-of-life care, is shown in Fig. 20.1 [3].

Although the holistic approach to the care of ill patients described above seems ideal, studies

M. Narayan (✉)
Division of Trauma, Burns, Critical and Acute Care, Weill Cornell Medicine/New York-Presbyterian Hospital, New York, NY, USA
e-mail: man9137@med.cornell.edu

J. Kashuk
Department of Surgery, Tel Aviv University Sackler School of Medicine, Tel Aviv, Israel

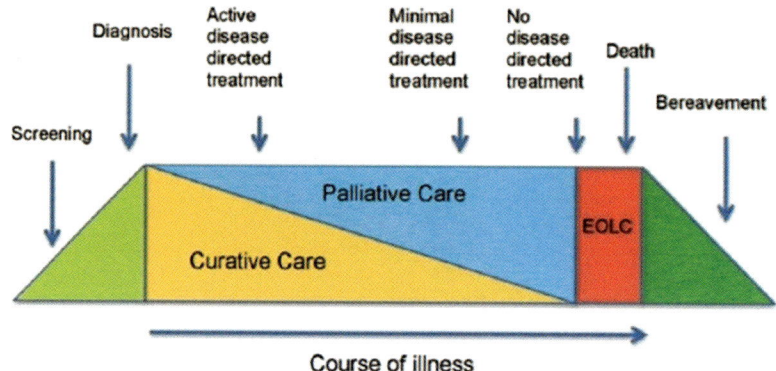

Fig. 20.1 Representing the continuum of palliative care and end-of-life care in an illness trajectory (Modified from Fox, S., FitzGerald, C., Harrison Dening, K. et al. Better palliative care for people with a dementia: summary of interdisciplinary workshop highlighting current gaps and recommendations for future research. BMC Palliat Care 17, 9 (2018). Distributed under the terms of the Creative Commons Attribution 4.0 International License (http://creativecommons.org/licenses/by/4.0/))

have shown that palliative care is underutilized globally. In 2014, the 67th World Health Assembly created a resolution on palliative care that urgently called for all countries to incorporate palliative care provision into their health care systems—a lofty initiative that was intended to ensure access to palliative care for all patients in need but, unfortunately, has not been met [4]. In fact, a report on Palliative Care from the WHO in 2020 estimated that 40 million people are in need of palliative care: 78% of them people living in low- and middle-income countries. An even more concerning statistic is that only an estimated 14% of people who actually need palliative care currently receive it. A lack of a defined public health model for palliative care including poor policies and implementation, limited education on palliative care principles, and a lack of access to medications are universally the main barriers to palliative care development [5].

In addition to the barriers to implementing palliative care, there are also significant differences in resource utilization and costs of end-of-life care globally. In the United States, end-of-life care is considered resource intensive, expensive, and often not aligned with the wishes of the patient and their families [6–8].

For the longest time, the majority of deaths due to terminal illness were reported to occur in the hospital setting. As a result, the last year of life, and specifically the last month, has been found to be the costliest. According to a report published by Arcadia Healthcare Solutions in 2016, people who die in a hospital undergo more intensive tests and procedures than those who die anywhere else. They study also found that spending on people who die in a hospital is about seven times that on people who die at home [9].

Adding to these astonishing numbers is the finding that more than a quarter of the entire Medicare budget, which pays for the health care of Americans aged 65 years or older, is devoted to the care of beneficiaries in the year they die [1, 8, 9].

As the population ages, it is no surprise that elderly patients, many with multiple co-morbidities and sickness, are increasingly visiting emergency departments (ED). These older adults are more likely to present with conditions requiring immediate life-sustaining and/or palliative treatments [10]. In response to the growing numbers of older adults with advanced illnesses cared for in the ED, medical centers have started to develop programs to deliver ED-based palliative care consultation. Implementation and sustaining these programs is especially challenging in this setting given the significant time restraints, lack of a developed rapport in discussing topics such as palliation, and staff shortages [11].

In the United States, there have been significant improvements in the implementation of hospital-based palliative care programs. According to a 2019 report on access to palliative care in US hospitals conducted by the Center to Advance Palliative Care (CAPC), only 7% of hospitals with 50 or more beds had a palliative care program. These hospitals were chosen using 50 beds as a cut-off, as these institutions care for 87% of all hospitalized patients nationwide. With the implementation of policies, education, and incentives, this number rose to 67% in 2015 and up to 72% in 2019 [12].

Even with this progress, there is much more to be done. Yadav et al. found that only one in three US adults completes any type of advanced directive for End of Life Care (EOLC). Much more work needs to be done to educate both the public and healthcare providers on the role of palliative care. This will most definitely need to include a culture shift in how we infuse palliative care into our daily care plans [6].

20.2 Establishing Definitions and A Common Language

The lack of common definitions and language regarding palliative care has unfortunately played a significant role in the widespread utilization if palliative care. The terms "actively dying," "end of life," "terminally ill," "terminal care," "hospice," "transition of care," and "palliative care" are commonly used but rarely and inconsistently defined. The Consensus for Worldwide End-of-Life Practice for Patients in Intensive Care Units (WELPICUS) Study conducted in 2014 aimed to achieve universal consensus on key end-of-life issues and terminology. Responses from 32 countries were recorded, and using a Delphi technique requiring 80% agreement, the consensus was obtained on 35 definitions and 46 statements regarding 22 end-of-life ICU issues [13] (see Appendix 1). It is important to remember that the basic philosophy of palliative care is to relieve symptoms and enable the best possible quality of life for patients and their families when a cure is no longer possible. The importance of a multi-disciplinary approach cannot be over-emphasized [14].

CAPC (defined above) has also defined palliative care as "specialized medical care for people living with serious illnesses, [focused] on providing patients with relief from the symptoms and stress of a serious illness—whatever the diagnosis." They stress that the goal of palliative care is to improve the quality of life for *both* the patient and the family. CAPC also emphasizes that palliative care can be appropriate at any age and any stage in a serious illness and can be provided together with curative treatment [12].

The National Consensus Project for Quality Palliative Care has identified eight key domains of practice for palliative care. Initially developed in 2004, these guidelines illustrate core concepts, structures, and processes necessary for quality palliative care. These domains provide guidance on key areas to improve access to quality palliative care for all people with serious illnesses regardless of setting, diagnosis, prognosis, or age. The guidelines were written to guide healthcare organizations and clinicians across the care continuum to integrate palliative care principles and best practices into their routine assessment and care of all seriously ill patients. It is important to note that palliative care not only incorporates what is happening to the body from a physical standpoint but also addresses psychosocial, spiritual, religious, and family concerns well [15, 16].

Readers are reminded that the concept of palliation, especially in consideration during severe illness or end-of-life care, dovetails with the four cardinal ethical principles initially described by Beauchamp and Childress: respect for autonomy, beneficence, non-maleficence, and justice [17] (see Table 20.1).

These principles help enable healthcare workers from totally disparate moral, spiritual, and religious cultures to share a fairly basic, common moral commitment, common moral language, and common analytical framework for reflecting on problems in healthcare ethics. Beauchamp and Childress espoused that an approach that is neutral between competing for religious, political, cultural, and philosophical theories could be

Table 20.1 The four prima facie principles of medical ethics

Autonomy	Respect for persons; upholding a person's right to make choices about their body
Beneficence	Obligation to contribute to a person's welfare Interventions should provide direct benefit to a patient; not merely avoiding harm
Non-maleficence	Obligation to not inflict harm on persons Harm must be avoided or minimized
Justice	Distribution of resources in a fair and equitable manner

shared by most practitioners regardless of their background [17].

When considering palliative care, it is important to differentiate it from the concept of hospice. Whereas palliative care, as defined by the IOM above, is "care that provides relief from pain and other symptoms, supports quality of life, and is focused on patients with serious advanced illness and their families," hospice is a system of care delivery for patients at the end of life. Of note, hospice is a *philosophy of care* and a system of care delivery, not a place. Complicating this initial definition is the fact that hospice typically includes four levels of care: routine hospice care, general inpatient care, continuous home care, and inpatient respite care [18]. A more detailed breakdown of the key differences between the two is shown in Fig. 20.2 and Table 20.2 [19].

20.2.1 The Need for Palliative Care

The implementation of palliative care has benefits beyond those directly for patient care. There is a growing body of evidence that suggests that integrating palliative care early into the management of ill patients decreases overall healthcare costs and improves quality at the end of life. Benefits of early palliative care for patients with cancer, for example, lead to overall lower costs due to lower rates of emergency department visits, fewer hospital admissions, and ICU stays on admission, fewer in-hospital deaths, improved satisfaction with care, better quality of life, less severe symptoms, improved mood, less aggressive end-of-life care, and longer median survival [8, 20, 21].

Cancer patients are a subset of ill patients that have generated significant interest in the concept of palliative care. Many of these patients present with advanced or incurable diseases leading to difficult decisions and challenges for patients, families, and members of the health care team [21]. A recent Cochrane review aimed to look at the effects of early palliative care on quality of life, survival, depression, and symptom intensity in people with advanced cancer. The results of the meta-analysis based on 1614 participants in seven randomized and cluster-randomized controlled trials showed that in patients with advanced cancer, early palliative care may slightly increase the quality of life. It may also decrease symptom intensity to a small degree. Effects on survival and depression were uncertain [21].

Cauley et al. conducted a retrospective cohort study of 875 disseminated cancer patients undergoing emergency surgery for perforation or obstruction. Among patients who underwent surgery for perforation, 30-day mortality was 34%, 67% had complications, and 52% were discharged to an institution. Renal failure, septic shock, ascites, dyspnea at rest, and dependent functional status were independent preoperative predictors of death at 30 days. When complications were considered, postoperative respiratory complications and age (75–84 years) were also predictors of mortality. The authors concluded that emergency abdominal operations in patients with disseminated cancer are highly morbid, and many patients die soon after surgery. High rates of complications and low rates of pre-existing DNR orders highlight the need for targeted interventions to reduce complications and integrate palliative approaches into the care of these patients [22, 23].

Pancreatic cancer is a particular type of cancer associated with high mortality and morbidity. Several studies have tried to assess the effect of universal palliative care in these patients. Mayer et al. conducted a population study look-

Fig. 20.2 Similarities and differences between hospice and palliative care. (Adopted from Tatum & Mills [18])

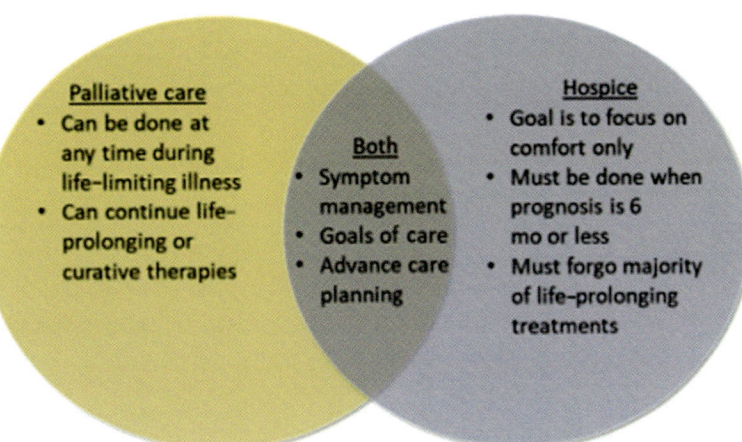

Table 20.2 Palliative care as compared with hospice (*Adopted from Kelley and Morrison. N Engl J Med. 2015; 373*(8): *747–755, with permission*)

Palliative care as compared with hospice		
Characteristic	Palliative care	Hospice
Model of care	Interdisciplinary team, including physicians, nurses, social workers, chaplains, and staff from other disciplines as needed; primary goal is improved quality of life	Interdisciplinary team, including physicians, nurses, social workers, chaplains, and volunteers, as dictated by statute; primary goals are improved quality of life and relief of suffering (physical, emotional, and spiritual)
Eligibility	Patients of all ages and with any diagnosis or stage of illness; patients may continue all life-prolonging and disease-directed treatments	Patients of all ages who have a prognosis of survival of ≤6 months, if the disease follows its usual course; patients must forgo Medicare coverage for curative and other treatments related to terminal illness
Place	Hospitals (most common), hospital clinics, group practices, cancer centers, home care programs, or nursing homes	Home (most common), assisted-living facilities, nursing homes, residential hospice facilities, inpatient hospice units, or hospice-contracted inpatient beds
Payment	Physician and nurse practitioner fees covered by Medicare Part B for inpatient or outpatient care; hospital teams are included within Medicare Part A or commercial insurance payments to hospitals for care episodes; flexible bundled payments under Medicare Advantage, Managed Medicaid, ACOs[a], and other commercial payers	Medicare hospice benefit; standard hospice benefit from commercial payers is usually modeled after Medicare; Medicaid, although coverage varies by state; medication costs are included for illnesses related to the terminal illness

[a] ACO denotes accountable care organization

ing at why patients with cancer visit emergency departments. They found that the most common reason cancer patients seek care in the ER is uncontrolled symptoms which suggests ER visits may be a surrogate measure for poor symptom control [24].

An end-of-life study in 2018 looking at elderly patients with pancreatic cancer found that the rate of palliative care increased between 2000 and 2009. Referral to palliative care was not associated with a reduction in end-of-life ICU care and ED visits. Unfortunately, the study found that referrals for palliative care were placed very late in the disease course and increasingly used for sicker patients. The authors opined that early referral to palliative care might allow patients a greater opportunity to benefit from services targeting symptom control which may reduce potentially futile end-of-life healthcare utilization [25].

Elderly patients presenting to ICUs around the globe are increasing of advanced age, with multiple co-morbidities and more frail. Older adults also make up a large portion of surgical practice in the United States. In 2010, 37% of all inpatient operations performed in the United States were in patients 65 years and older. Frail patients are more likely than their non-frail peers to experience adverse health outcomes, including falls, hospitalizations, and even death [3]. In fact, frail patients (regardless of age) are at increased risk of dying within 6 months to 5 year [26]. They also require palliative care input preoperatively to help define their care goals. Ernst et al. state that a systematic frailty-screening program effectively identifies at-risk surgical patients and is associated with a significant reduction in mortality for patients undergoing palliative care consultation [26]. Value decisions should be grounded in patient-oriented expectations and outcomes and should be discussed before any major operative intervention [27].

Intensivists, acute care surgeons, and many other specialists who deal with sick and dying patients are often left with patients, families, of health care proxies who request that "everything be done." This places a significant burden on health care providers who are often left to decide if doing "everything" is in fact doing things *to the patient* and not necessarily *for the patient*. Cauley et al. conducted a qualitative study on surgeons' perspectives on avoiding non-beneficial treatments in seriously ill older patients with surgical emergencies. The authors found that emergency general surgeons felt responsible for having preoperative discussions about EOL care with seriously ill older patients to avoid non-beneficial surgery. However, the same group of surgeons identified multiple factors that undermine adequate communication, eventually leading to non-beneficial surgery [23] (see Table 20.3).

The term futility remains controversial in medical terminology. Part of the controversy is that the word brings up the notion of rationing of

Table 20.3 Surgeons' perspectives on avoiding nonbeneficial treatments in seriously ill older patients with surgical emergencies [23]

Domain 1	Surgeon responsibility	Participants felt that "discussing EOL decisions is our [surgeons'] responsibility"
Domain 2	Assessing risk	First, they had difficulty formulating the prognosis due to the lack of clear data about postoperative outcomes. Several participants discussed the use of preoperative functional status as crucial to assessing potential outcomes to formulate a prognosis but felt this was imperfect
Domain 3	Appropriateness	Whether an operation could or should be done by discussing the patient's goals and how those goals fit into the burdens and benefits of an intervention
Domain 4	Patient and family	All participants agreed that patients or surrogates who are unprepared for EOL conversations—emotionally or in lack of understanding of their illness—complicate an already difficult situation. These conversations require more time to allow unprepared patients or surrogates to process medical information and identify preference
Domain 5	Palliative care	Views on the role and definition of palliative care ranged from an active role in controlling symptoms, helping families cope, and improving QOL, to "doing nothing" Requesting palliative care consultations was limited by concerns that recommending these consults was not their place, lack of access to palliative care in the emergency department, or beliefs that palliative care would not solve the patient's problem
Domain 6	System factors	Time constraints hinder surgeons' ability to fulfill responsibilities regarding communication with their patients. For example, time to discuss goals and wishes preoperatively must be weighed against the risk of a patient's condition declining and "significantly altering their chances of survival

care. Rationing can be understood under a similar lens of triage in mass casualty. It is the allocation of healthcare resources in the face of limited availability, which necessarily means that beneficial interventions are withheld from some while shifted to others [3]. Although many definitions exist, futility can be thought of as "efforts to achieve a result that is possible but that reasoning or experience suggests is highly improbable and cannot be systematically produced" [28]. A treatment that does not improve a patient's prognosis, comfort, well-being, or general state of health could be considered futile, or as described by Narayan and Kashuk, not appropriate [3]. Decisions about the appropriateness of care can involve moral judgments about right or good care. Multiple studies from around the globe have shown that healthcare workers feel that they have participated in inappropriate for at least part of a patient's overall hospital stay. These findings include inappropriate ICU admissions on elderly frail patients with poor prognosis or limited chance of survival, patients who lack clear advanced directives, or performing CPR on patients regardless of actual benefit [29–32].

Many reasons were given for why healthcare workers went on to provide "futile care" even when they felt it was inappropriate. These include clinical doubt about the diagnosis or outcome, limited decision-making time, assessment error, pressure from superiors, referring clinicians or families, and the perceived threat of legal action [31]. A clearly written advanced directive that states the wishes of the patient can help avoid care that is futile. Although helpful in providing guidance, these documents also have their limitations. Written language is subject to interpretation and can be ambiguous to both healthcare proxies and providers. Further complicating the issue is that many of these documents may not have significance or legal standing in other countries outside the US.

Strategies to manage potentially inappropriate treatments have recently been developed and are shown in Table 20.4.

There is also a need to implement palliative care globally. Jordan et al. conducted a systematic review of 169 studies from 23 countries and found that half of all patients accessing palliative care services are referred less than 19 days before death. Of particular interest, while the median number of days of palliative care prior to death for all US studies was 19 days, for all non-US studies, it was 29 days. This finding illustrates that much more work is needed to promulgate palliative care. The authors concluded that reducing barriers to accessing palliative care and pro-

Table 20.4 Managing potentially inappropriate care

1	Institutions should implement strategies to prevent intractable treatment conflicts, including proactive communication, and early involvement of expert consultation
2	The term "potentially inappropriate" should be used, rather than "futile," to describe treatments that have at least some chance of accomplishing the effect sought by the patient, but clinicians believe that competing ethical considerations justify not providing them. Clinicians should communicate and advocate for the treatment plan they believe is appropriate. Requests for potentially inappropriate treatment that remain intractable despite intensive communication and negotiation should be managed by a fair process of dispute resolution
3a	Requests for strictly futile interventions. The term "futile" should only be used in the rare circumstance that an intervention simply cannot accomplish the intended physiologic goal. Clinicians should not provide futile interventions and should carefully explain the rationale for the refusal. If disagreement persists, clinicians should generally obtain expert consultation to assist in conflict resolution and communication
3b	Requests for legally proscribed or legally discretionary treatments. "Legally proscribed" treatments are those that are prohibited by applicable laws, judicial precedent, or widely accepted public policies (e.g., organ allocation strategies). "Legally discretionary" treatments are those for which there are specific laws, judicial precedent, or policies that give physicians permission to refuse to administer them. In responding to requests for either legally proscribed or legally discretionary treatments, clinicians should carefully explain the rationale for treatment refusal and, if there is uncertainty regarding the interpretation and application of the relevant rule, should generally seek expert consultation to confirm accurate interpretation of the rule
4	The medical profession should lead public engagement efforts and advocate for policies and legislation about when life-prolonging technologies should not be used

Am J Respir Crit Care Med. 2015;191(11):1318–1330

moting earlier integration alongside active treatment would maximize benefits to patients before they die and potentially reduce costs to the wider healthcare service [33].

In many palliative care decisions, emergency high-risk general surgery is considered. Patients facing intra-abdominal catastrophes are faced with options to undergo operation, with its associated pain, morbidity, and potential for mortality or a likely assured death as an alternative. Aggarwal et al. conducted a large retrospective review of 14,000 patients who underwent emergency laparotomy at 28 hospitals in England. Analysis revealed that almost 40% of patients died did so within 3 days of surgery. The authors proposed that death early after surgery could reflect sustained physiological insults from underlying conditions, which for that individual patient, perhaps due to comorbidity and the time course of the intervention, was not survivable. They suggest that multi-disciplinary team involvement from intensive care, care of the elderly physicians, and early involvement of palliative care may help both the communication and the burden of responsibility in deciding on the risk–benefit of operative versus nonoperative approaches to care [34].

Cooper et al. highlighted several other reasons for carrying out surgery that may not have benefits, citing surgeon, patient, surrogate, and structural factors [35]. These structural factors include uncertainty about diagnoses, and fragmented sources of information, such as consent. Although consent is meant to assure understanding of the indications, benefits, risks, and alternatives of a particular intervention, surgeons often interpret it as a form of "surgical buy in." The patient is then presumed to consent to all other post-operative measures and interventions required for a successful outcome. Clearly, that is often not the case. The surgeon may feel everything possible should be done whatever the likelihood of success, especially when the alternative is almost certain death. The surgeon may have limited time for discussion due to the urgency of the case or may feel uncomfortable discussing palliative care [36]. Complicating the issue even further is that patients—or, more often, their advocates—may not fully understand what the patient's best interests actually are [35].

20.2.1.1 Economic Concerns and Impact

Quality of end-of-life care indicators endorses referring individuals to hospice in a timely manner, avoiding unnecessary emergency room visits, intensive care stays, and inpatient admissions, and discontinuing chemotherapy when death is imminent. Decreasing aggressive care at the end of life, by reducing frequent hospital and ICU admissions, can lead to decreased use of cardiac catheterization, dialysis, ventilators, and pulmonary artery monitors, significantly reducing end-of-life cost [37].

In the US, the cost of ICU care in the last months of life is the most expensive in a patient's lifetime. During this time, it is common for ethical dilemmas to arise. Medical care teams are left to balance the advancements of medical capabilities that allow for continued physiologic functioning with realism in cases of no meaningful recovery. Nowhere is this truer than in acute surgical emergencies. Adding to the complexity of the situation is the fact that the majority of the US population still lacks an advanced directive of their own wishes regarding care. Those who have planned ahead and stated their wishes often leave decisions in the hands of a medical decision-maker or surrogate [6, 38, 39].

Resource allocation at the end of life is a hot topic for healthcare delivery systems around the world. In the United States, the Affordable Care Act has expanded provisions for palliative care and hospice. Not gone unrecognized is the fact that nearly 30% (~$133 billion dollars) of the entire Medicare (US social healthcare plan covering the elderly) budget in 2009 was spent on acute care services. The percentage of total Medicare payments for decedents in the last year of life also approximates 30%. [40, 41] Overall, Medicare spending is rising by almost 4% annually, with a significant demographic variation. The slice of the health care pie that drives cost most precipitously is end-of-life care. A more granular look at Medicare expenditures finds that approximately one-quarter of the spending is attributable to the 5% of beneficiaries who die each year, and acute care in the last 30 days of life accounts for almost 80% of costs incurred in the final year of life [42].

The direct economic benefit of palliative care program implementation may be hard to define. May et al. conducted a meta-analysis of 6 studies with nearly 134K patients. Their analysis found that hospital costs were *lower* for patients seen by a palliative care consultation team than for patients who did not receive this care. They highlighted the fact that the estimated association was greater for those with a primary diagnosis of cancer and those with more comorbidities (more ill) compared with those with a non-cancer diagnosis and those with fewer comorbidities (less ill) [8].

Luta et al. tried to identify the evidence of the economic value of end-of-life and palliative care interventions.

The authors found the most compelling evidence on cost-effectiveness related to home-based interventions because they offer substantial savings to the health system, including a decrease in total healthcare costs, resource use, and improvement in patient and caregivers' outcomes [20]. Zhang et al. studied the impact of end-of-life conversations on healthcare costs in the last week of life. They found that addressing end-of-life goals with patients could rationalize and contain costs by reducing undesired, aggressive care without rationing or denying individuals aggressive care they may want. Patient-reported outcomes have shown that if a discussion about end-of-life goals is had at baseline, the cost of care in the last week of life care is reduced by 36% (from $2917 to $1876) [43].

Containing costs is a topic not just specific to the US healthcare delivery system. An important point that must be considered here is that the primary purpose of integrated palliative care is *not* cost. Palliative care focuses on quality of life, symptom management, and psychosocial support, a patient-centered approach through which reduced cost or improved value is a *secondary* byproduct, not a primary concern. Palliative care interventions both in the United States and internationally have been successful in utilizing patient care to improve outcomes for patients. These outcomes include quality of life, pain management, psychosocial health, family assessment of care and bereavement, and even survival [16, 44].

Integration of palliative care leads to lower inpatient costs, and inpatient collaboration with palliative care teams could result in lower pharmacy and laboratory expenses, decreased lengths of stay, and fewer admissions to the ICU. The potential cost savings could be substantial. Outpatient palliative care can further decrease costs by up to 33% in some patients by decreasing acute care services, minimizing hospitalizations, and decreasing emergency room visits. Thus, delivering value-congruent care at the end of life by addressing goals with all patients (but denying care to none) decreases the cost of care and improves the quality of life without reducing its quantity [45–47].

The Institute of Medicine report, Dying in America, recommends that palliative care be made available to all patients with serious illness, and that all clinicians who treat them become skilled in palliative care. Refining these skills will enable clinicians to further hone their communication skills, help ailing patients manage their symptoms, help families and healthcare proxies cope, while also being able to provide a clear vision of a peaceful death as an achievable outcome for patients who are unlikely to benefit from aggressive interventions [48].

20.2.1.2 Barriers and Solutions to the Implementation of Palliative Care

After reviewing the section on the need for palliative care above, the reader is left with a better understanding of its potential impact on the ICU management of sick, elderly, or dying patients. Unfortunately, there are many barriers and challenges that healthcare systems and providers must address in order to move the palliative care concept forward. First, and foremost, are clinicians attitudes toward palliative care. Intensivists, surgeons, and others managing complex acute problems are vested in the care of sick, critically-ill patients. Often healthcare teams grapple with the word "palliation" since it potentially implies a certain level of "defeat"—that they have not been able to meet the medical or surgical challenge a patient presents.

The second barrier relates to effective communication and logistics. Many patient care teams often round very early in the morning, often before the family is present. Providers have complained that difficulties exist with being able to assemble the entire team for important discussions with the family. (ICU doctors, surgeons, nurses). Other support resources that may provide insight into prognosis such as social work, pastoral care, or palliative care may not always be available.

Other issues in the effective communication category are the actual or perceived lack of time to discuss complex care issues such as palliation during meetings with the patient, family, or healthcare proxy. Further complicating the communication problem is the presence of multiple decision-makers in a family, often with discordant views, on how best to proceed in the care of their loved one. The end result is often a family who is confused about what their options are, occasionally feeling that the care team has "given-up," or pressured to make a decision they are not comfortable with [49].

The third barrier to implementing palliative care is the healthcare provider's discomfort with holding complex discussions regarding goals of care, end-of-life, hospice, palliation, or a transition to comfort care measures. Often this is due to a lack of formal training or experience in discussing these topics. Healthcare providers not adept at conducting these meetings may use language or medical jargon that the patient, family, or proxy may not understand. In some instances, depending on cultural/societal norms, questioning the care team may or may not be favorably received. The approach to palliative care in a paternalistic medical environment may, therefore, be even more challenging.

Occasionally, different care teams may have divergent views on how well a patient is doing. This could lead to the third barrier, fear of conflict. This conflict could be within and between care teams or involve other providers such as nurses, social workers, palliative care, ethics, or pastoral care. For example, a 84-year-old patient with multiple co-morbidities including known metastatic colon cancer to the liver, chronic obstructive pulmonary disease, peripheral vascular disease, and known poor ejection fraction undergoes an exploratory laparotomy with small bowel resection with anastomosis for acute small bowel obstruction. The patient survives the initial operation and is subsequently extubated in the ICU. Several days later, the patient develops fever, leukocytosis and is found to have anastomotic disruption. The patient develops tachypnea and requires re-intubation as the family has requested "everything be done." Discussions with the colorectal service and the ICU team find completely differing views on how best to proceed. The ICU team would like to advance palliative care discussions, while the colorectal team would like to hold off and proceed full-steam ahead.

Occasionally, care teams deliver prognoses that are unrealistic and often portray "small victories" instead of overall prognosis, leading to prolonged suffering for patients and their families.

The barriers to the implementation of palliative care listed above highlight the importance of open, regular communication within the multidisciplinary care team framework as well as with the family, healthcare proxy. The reader is reminded that the ICU has the potential of being a very intimidating place for both patients and their families. The presence of multiple care teams, a rounding structure that may differ from week to week, multiple machines that may be providing life-sustaining measures, surrounded by other very sick patients all add to the potential confusing nature of the ICU [3].

A scheduled multi-disciplinary meeting (MDM) held at periodic intervals, especially for those patients who have a prolonged ICU stay (greater than a week) can help offset some of the barriers described above. Decision-making in critical illness involves multiple discussions regarding the potential outcomes and processes of care, across the whole disease trajectory. The greatest conflict appears to be when prescribed measures waver between curative and comfort care. The MDM provides a forum where early communication, especially around values and preferred care outcomes, can help offset anxiety or discomfort experienced by many families. Offering further support, possibly with expert palliative care, communication, and discussion of 'trial of treatment' may be beneficial at this time, rather than waiting until the "end of life" [50].

Cook et al. describe a technique developed by the VITALtalk group using the GUIDE mnemonic shown in Table 20.5.

It is important to note that the GUIDE first meeting has no space reserved for decision-making. This is intentional as the first family meeting is framed as a meeting to deliver news that may be upsetting, for medical updates, gathering information, and building relationships. The emotional toll of this meeting can overwhelm families and/or their surrogates, limiting their ability to make complex decisions. Another framework espoused by VITALTalk is the "REMAP" approach, especially when there has been a change in the clinical status of a sick patient [50].

20.2.1.3 REMAP

- **Reframe**: important to warn the family that a change in a status update is coming and that the clinical scenario duration may have changed from previous updates
- **Expect emotion and empathize**: The NURSE (Name, Understand, Respect, Support, Explore) mnemonic of emotional response can be helpful, as responding to emotions from the family improves information retention
- **MAP the future**: Use an understanding of patient's goals to frame medical recommendations

Given the aging population with increasing co-morbidities, assessment of frailty and geriatrics care in the ICU will become more important than ever. Balancing patient and family requests to "do everything" while at the same time re-emphasizing that the goal is always to do something *for* our patients and not just something *to* them can be much harder in practice than in simply understanding the terminology. The overarching message is to ensure that whatever pain and suffering a patient must endure, the end result is worth the temporary discomfort. If, however, the pain and suffering undertaken will result in no such benefit or begets only more pain and suffering, the care team should pause and re-communicate and discuss goals of care with the patient and or surrogates before proceeding to perform potentially unnecessary interventions. Tools such as the Best Case/Worst Case model developed by Olson et al. is a framework that was specifically designed to support in-the-moment decision-making [51]. This simple yet highly effective tool can help aid communication by shifting the focus of decision-making conversations from an isolated problem to a discussion about treatment alternatives and outcomes. As shown below in the figures, the BC/WC model helps promote shared decision-making and facilitates the development of informed preferences. Patients and their families are encouraged to verbalize their choices and options at the very outset of the decision process, allowing them more control and understanding of the varying treatment options [51]. Todi et al. provide another framework to help practitioners and families in making informed decisions about palliation in the ICU setting [52] (Fig. 20.3 *permission obtained*).

Table 20.5 GUIDE Mnemonic

G	**G**et ready: pre-meet, get the right people, find quiet place, and sit down
U	**U**nderstand: what the patient knows
I	**I**nform: starting with a headline & STOP for questions and emotions
D	**D**emonstrate: empathy & respond to emotion
E	**E**quip: the family to understand the next step in care

20.2.1.4 How and When to Implement Palliative Care

Healthcare providers grapple with how best to integrate palliative care within their respective patient care paradigms.

Bradley and Brasel developed guidelines or triggers for identifying patients in the SICU who would benefit from palliative care services. The top five "triggers" for a palliative care consulta-

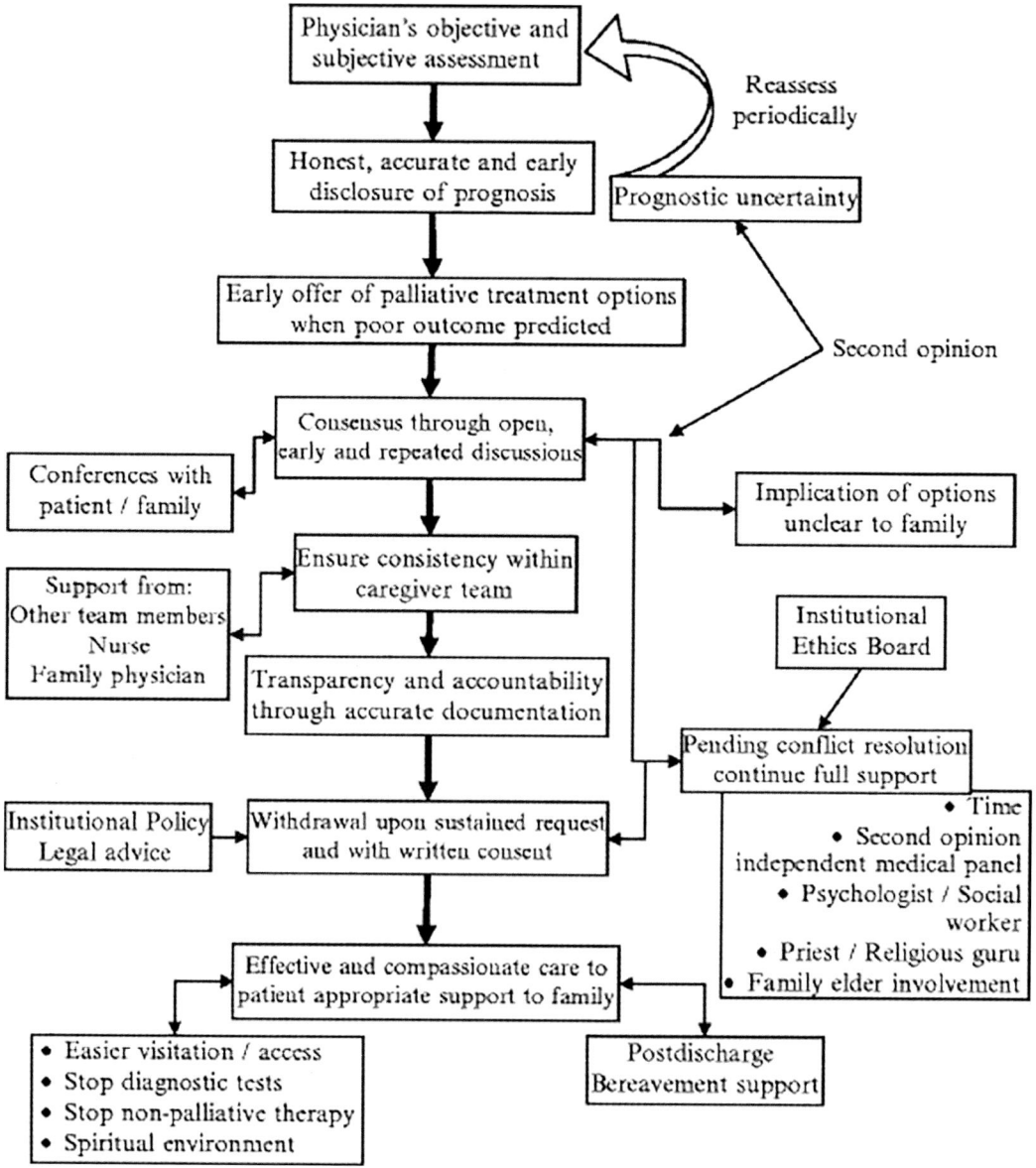

Fig. 20.3 Framework for Integrating Palliative Care in the ICU setting

tion identified were: (1) family request; (2) futility considered or declared by the medical team; (3) family disagreement with the medical team, advance directive, or each other lasting >7 days; (4) death expected during the same SICU stay; or (5) SICU stay greater than 1 month [53].

As previously described, the BC/WC model is one tool that brings to the surface need for palliative care discussions. Additional tool that surgeons can use for discussions with patients and surrogate decision-makers is the American College of Surgeons National Surgical Quality Improvement Program (ACS NSQIP) surgical risk calculator. This tool utilizes outcomes data from the NSQIP database to estimate the chances of an unfavorable outcome such as a complication or death after surgery. The tool enables surgeons to use objective, evidenced-based

Table 20.6 Principles of palliative care

Respect the dignity and autonomy of patients, patients' surrogates, and caregivers
Honor rights of competent patients/surrogates to choose among treatments, including those that may or may not prolong life
Communicate effectively and empathically with patients, their families, and caregivers
Identify the primary goals of care from the patient's perspective, and address how the surgeon's care can achieve the patient's objectives
Strive to alleviate pain and other burdensome physical and nonphysical symptoms
Recognize, assess, discuss, and offer access to services for psychological, social, and spiritual issues
Provide access to therapeutic support, encompassing the spectrum from life-prolonging treatments through hospice care, when they can realistically be expected to improve the quality of life as perceived by the patient
Recognize the physician's responsibility to discourage treatments that are unlikely to achieve the patient's goals, and encourage patients and families to consider hospice care when the prognosis for survival is likely to be less than a half-year
Arrange for continuity of care by the patient's primary and/or specialist physician, alleviating the sense of abandonment patients may feel when "curative" therapies are no longer useful
Maintain a collegial and supportive attitude toward others entrusted with care of the patient

Adopted from the American College of Surgeons Task Force on Surgical Palliative Care and the Committee on Ethics

Table 20.7 8 key domains of palliative care. *Clinical Practice Guidelines for Quality Palliative Care, 4th edition*

Structure & Processes of Care	The composition of an interdisciplinary team is outlined, including the professional qualifications, education, training, and support needed to deliver optimal patient- and family-centered care. Domain 1 also defines the elements of the palliative care assessment and care plan, as well as systems and processes specific to palliative care
Physical Aspects of Care	The palliative care assessment, care planning, and treatment of physical symptoms are described, emphasizing patient- and family-directed holistic care
Psychological & Psychiatric Aspects	The domain focuses on the processes for systematically assessing and addressing the psychological and psychiatric aspects of care in the context of serious illness
Social Aspects of Care	Outlines the palliative care approach to assessing and addressing patient and family social support needs
Spiritual, Religious, & Existential Aspects of Care	The spiritual, religious, and existential aspects of care are described, including the importance of screening for unmet needs
Cultural Aspects of Care	The domain outlines the ways in which culture influences both palliative care delivery and the experience of that care by the patient and family, from the time of diagnosis through death and bereavement
Care of the Patient Nearing the End of Life	This domain focuses on the symptoms and situations that are common in the final days and weeks of life
Ethical and Legal Aspects of Care	Content includes advance care planning, surrogate decision-making, regulatory and legal considerations, and related palliative care issues, focusing on ethical imperatives and processes to support patient autonomy

Adopted from NCP Guidelines, 4th edition

outcomes data to better facilitate discussions with patients [54].

Before mentioning the strategies for implementing palliative care, the reader is encouraged to review the basic principles of palliative care as well as the palliative care domains essential to understanding how palliative care will be integrated into patient care (see Tables 20.6 and 20.7). *Adopted from Kelley and Morrison N Engl J Med. 2015 August 20; 373(8): 747–755. need permission*

The integration of palliative care into healthcare delivery systems is predominantly described as being based on an ***integration strategy*** or a ***consultation strategy***. Primary palliative care (PPC) is defined as palliative care provided by the primary treating service. This approach emphasizes the co-provision of palliative intensive care and may best integrate palliative communication principles into the ICU. This strategy has been shown to promote stronger clinician and patient relationships and reduce the fragmentation of care and can be integrated with other critical care interventions and therapies. One method of the integration strategy is to embed a subspecialty trained palliative care provider who routinely sees all patients within the ICU, either as part of the rounding team or as a scheduled check-in.

Advantages of the integration strategy are that the provider (1) is distinctively aware of all aspects of the patient's current medical problems; (2) understands the potentially differing viewpoints of multiple services providing teams; (3) has been a part of multi-disciplinary meetings to understand goals of care; and (4) can acknowledge other issues from a social, psychosocial, cultural, spiritual or religious context that may influence patient decision making. Disadvantages of the integration strategy are that (1) it requires a designated palliative care provider to be a part of medical rounds and decision-making (this may be seen as exhausting for the palliative care provider as the ICU team goes through problems by systems and may only be given a few moments at the end of each patient presentation to bring up palliative issues) and also be potentially less cost-effectiveness for hospitals as each unit or designated care area may require a provider; (2) primary medical care providers may feel they already do the job of addressing palliative care needs well and may further feel imposed upon by the palliative care specialist.

The other model of addressing palliative care needs in the ICU is to use a consultation strategy. In this model, the palliative care consultant works in a similar manner to any other consultant service in the ICU. The assumption in this model is that there is a baseline degree of comfort from the ICU team with defining goals of care and palliative care issues, providing goal-concordant care and transitioning goals to comfort. The palliative care consultant's services are then requested on an as-needed basis. Advantages of the consultation integration model are that (1) the palliative care provider's services can be used elsewhere in the hospital (in the emergency department, on the floor, or in other ICUs), thus becoming more cost-effective by multiplying their reach and coverage; (2) the consultant's presence and recommendations are given dedicated time since a formal consult has been placed and not just left to provide input at the end of a lengthy systems based ICU presentation. Disadvantages of the consultant model are (1) the consultant does not have the benefit of a longitudinal experience of understanding medical care teams plans that may influence palliative care decisions; (2) the consultant may not have been present for detailed family meetings where goals of care were previously discussed; (3) the consultant may not feel as vested as other members of the team, especially when discussing difficult topics such as hospice, palliative care, or end-of-life care. Another concern about the consultant model is a lack of defined "triggers" to prompt the initial consultation. Hua et al. describe primary and alternative triggers for palliative care consultation below [55, 56] (see Table 20.8).

A summary of the key differences between the two strategies is provided in Table 20.8. Figure 20.4 highlights the indications and key components of each of the three categories of palliative care: primary palliative care, specialty palliative care, and hospice (Table 20.9).

Table 20.8 Clinical triggers for palliative care consultation

Primary triggers[a]	Alternative triggers (Surgical)
ICU admission after hospital stay >10 days Age > 80 with two or more life-threatening comorbidities Diagnosis of active stage IV malignancy (metastatic disease) Status after cardiac arrest Diagnosis of intracerebral hemorrhage requiring mechanical ventilation	Family request Futility considered/declared by the medical team Presence of advanced directive, family disagreement with each other, or family disagreement with medical team >7 days Death expected during same ICU stay ICU stay >1 mo Diagnosis with median survival <6 mo >3 ICU admissions during the same hospitalization GCS < 8 for >1 week in patient >75 year GCS = 3 Multisystem organ failure of >3 systems (PaO/FiO$_2$, <300, platelet count <100,000/mm, acute increase in creatinine >2 mg/dL, acute increase in total bilirubin >2 mg/dL, use of vasopressors, GCS < 13)

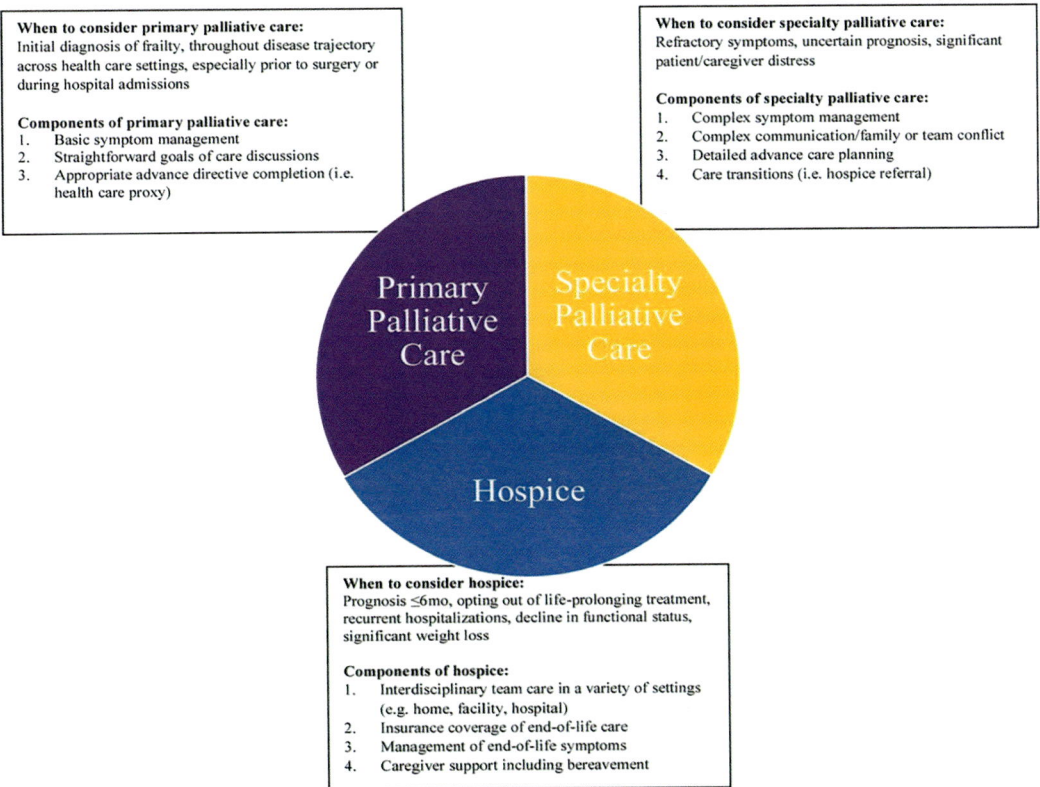

Fig. 20.4 Indications and key components of each of the three categories of palliative care [57] (*adopted from Crooms Anesth Analg. 2020 June*)

Table 20.9 Primary vs specialty palliative care for patients with frailty (*adapted from* [57], with permission)

NHPC-NPC domain		When to use	
		Primary palliative care	Specialty palliative care
Structure and Processes of Care	Interdisciplinary care	• Understand the role of an interdisciplinary team • Refer to ancillary services if indicated and available • **Basic advance care planning**	• Complex psychosocial needs • Spiritual distress
Symptom management [16]	Weight loss	• Encourage liberal diet • Consider high-calorie supplements • Consider nutrition referral	• >10% weight loss over 6 months • Consideration of artificial nutrition
	Weakness	• Consider rehab or physical therapy referral • Encourage strength and balance training	• Decline in functional status, especially loss of independence in ADLs
	Fatigue	• Investigate/treat underlying conditions • Discontinue contributing medications if possible • Encourage physical activity	• Symptoms refractory to primary palliative care interventions
	Falls	• Investigate/treat underlying conditions • Consider rehab or physical therapy referral • Refer for home safety evaluation • Encourage strength and balance training • Review medications for potential contributors	• Ongoing falls despite primary palliative care interventions • Complex decision-making or conflict regarding nursing home placement when indicated
	Pain	• Investigate/treat underlying conditions • Prescribe analgesics including non-opioid medications (acetaminophen, NSAIDs) or single- agent opioid therapy when indicated	• Symptoms refractory to primary palliative care interventions
Psychological and Psychiatric Care		• Screen routinely for depression • Explore patient/caregiver concerns and offer support • Refer for psychotherapy or psychiatry when indicated	• Refractory symptoms (e.g., anxiety, depression, suicidal ideation, and PTSD) • Complex psychiatric issues
Social Support		• Explore the availability of caregivers/social supports • Refer to social work when appropriate	• Complex psychosocial needs • Caregiver burnout
Spiritual, Religious, and Existential Care		• Recognize spiritual care needs and refer to chaplaincy if available	• Significant spiritual distress related to illness • Spiritual history that affects medical decision-making
Culturally Competent Care		• Use interpreter services when necessary • Recognize cultural influences on medical decision-making	• Primary team or patient/caregiver distress related to medical decision- making

Table 20.9 (continued)

NHPC-NPC domain	When to use	
	Primary palliative care	Specialty palliative care
End-of-Life Care	• Recognize hospice eligibility • Discuss code status • Discuss preferences for life-sustaining therapies	• Patients/caregivers with limited understanding of illness/prognosis • Patients unable to verbalize clear preferences • Family or team conflict
Ethical and Legal Concerns	• Assist patient in designating a healthcare agent and completing other advance directives • Identify a legal surrogate decision maker if no designated healthcare agent	• Patient without capacity and no clear surrogate decision maker • Requests for non-beneficial treatments • Requests for physician aid in dying

Table 20.9 describes the eight domains of palliative care identified by the National Coalition for Hospice and Palliative Care-National Consensus Project Clinical Practice Guidelines and provides recommendations for associated primary palliative care interventions and indications for specialty palliative care referral in the frail patient

NCHPC-NCP National Coalition for Hospice and Palliative Care-National Consensus Project, *ADLs* activities of daily living, *NSAIDs* non- steroidal anti-inflammatory drugs, *PTSD* post-traumatic stress disorder

20.3 Integrative, Complementary, and Alternative Medicine

Integrative, complimentary, and alternative medicine are tools available to ICU physicians to help with palliation depending on locale and terms that are often used interchangeably but have distinct and separate meanings. Integrative medicine, as defined by the Academic Consortium for Integrative Medicine and Health, is the practice of medicine that reaffirms the importance of the relationship between practitioner and patient, focusing on the whole person, is informed by evidence, and makes use of all appropriate therapeutic approaches, health care professionals, and disciplines to achieve optimal health and healing. Complementary medicine refers to the use of non-conventional practices *used together with* mainstream medicine treatment. Alternative medicine typically refers to non-conventional practices *in place of* conventional medicine [58].

Complementary or alternative medicines are broadly classified into five major categories of practice: (1) Whole medical systems, (2) mind-body techniques, (3) biologically based practices, (4) manipulative and body-based therapies, and (5) energy therapies. These techniques, shown in detail in Table 20.10, offer an approach to palliative care that addresses the physical environment, relationships, conversations, and behaviors, not only for patients but also for families and for healthcare professionals providing care in acute care settings, and truly integrates the mind, body, and spirit in the work of healing [58–60].

Integrative medicine techniques and hospital-based programs are starting to become more mainstream than in the past but still remain relatively new concepts in modern medicine in the United States. The R Adams Cowley Shock Trauma Center, one of the oldest free-standing such centers in the the United States, was the first trauma center in the country to establish a Center for Integrative Medicine. Interestingly, the University of Maryland Pain Center was the first US academic medical center-based program in integrative medicine.

Table 20.10 Types of complementary and alternative medicine

Types	Description
Whole medical systems	**All-encompassing approaches that include philosophy, diagnosis, and treatment**
Ayurveda	Aims to restore balance within the body Uses diet, massage, herbs, meditation, therapeutic elimination, and yoga
Homeopathy	Based on the law of similars: A substance that causes certain symptoms when given in large doses can cure the same symptoms when it is used in minute doses[a]
Naturopathy	Aims to prevent and treat disease by promoting a healthy lifestyle, treating the whole person, and using the body's natural ability to heal itself Uses a combination of therapies, including acupuncture, counseling, exercise therapy, guided imagery, homeopathy, hydrotherapy, medicinal herbs, natural childbirth, nutrition, physical therapies, and stress management
Traditional Chinese medicine	Aims to restore the proper flow of life force (qi) in the body by balancing the opposing forces of yin and yang within the body Uses acupuncture, massage, medicinal herbs, and meditative exercise (qi gong)
Mind-body medicine	**Use of behavioral, psychologic, social, and spiritual techniques to enhance the mind's capacity to affect the body and thus to preserve health and prevent or cure disease**
Biofeedback	Uses electronic devices to provide people with information about biologic functions (such as heart rate, blood pressure, and muscle tension) and teaches people how to control these functions
Guided imagery	Uses mental images to help people relax or to promote wellness or healing of a particular condition, such as insomnia or psychologic trauma
Hypnotherapy	Puts people into a state of relaxation and heightened attention to help them change their behavior and thus improve their health
Meditation, including mindfulness	Intentionally regulating attention or systematically focusing on particular aspects of experience
Relaxation techniques	Using techniques to slow certain body functions down (for example, by slowing the heart rate) and thus to relieve tension and stress
Biologically based practices	**Use of naturally occurring substances (such as particular foods and micronutrients) to promote wellness**
Botanical medicine and natural products	Uses substances that occur naturally in plants or animals to treat symptoms or disease (such as cartilage used to treat joint pain)
Chelation therapy	Uses a drug to bind with and remove a metal or mineral that is believed to be present in excess or toxic amounts in the body
Diet therapies	Use specialized dietary regimens (such as the macrobiotic, Paleo, low carbohydrate, or Mediterranean diet) to treat or prevent a specific disease, to generally promote wellness, or to detoxify the body
Manipulative and body-based practices	**Manipulation of parts of the body (such as joints and muscles) to treat various conditions and symptoms** **Based on the belief that the body in balance will improve certain symptoms and that its parts are interdependent**
Chiropractic	Involves manipulating the spine (mainly) to restore the normal relationship between the spine and nervous system May involve physical therapy (such as heat and cold therapy and electrical stimulation), massage, acupressure, and/or exercises or lifestyle changes
Cupping	Uses heated cups, inverted and placed on the skin to create vacuum that sucks the skin partway into the cup, which may be left in place for several minutes Considered a form of massage that increases blood flow to targeted regions in an effort to alter inflammation and certain conditions
Massage	Involves manipulating muscles and other tissues to reduce pain and muscle spasm and to reduce stress and enhance relaxation
Moxibustion	Uses dried moxa herb (a mugwort) that is burned usually just above but sometimes directly on the skin over acupuncture points

Table 20.10 (continued)

Types	Description
Reflexology	Involves applying manual pressure to specific areas of the foot, hand, or ear that are believed to correspond to different organs or systems of the body
Scraping (e.g., coining, spooning)	Involves rubbing a dull implement across skin, usually on the back, neck, or extremities. Considered a form of massage, also called gua sha
Energy therapies	**Manipulation of energy fields thought to exist in and around the body (biofields) to maintain or restore health** **Based on the belief that a universal life force or subtle energy resides in and around the body and throughout the universe**
Acupuncture	Stimulates specific points on the body, usually by inserting very thin needles into the skin and underlying tissues to affect the flow of qi along energy pathways (meridians) and thus restore balance in the body
Qi gong	A gentle movement practice in traditional Chinese medicine using postures, breathing, and meditation to improve healing
Magnets	An energy therapy involving placing magnets on the body to reduce pain or enhance healing
Reiki	An energy therapy involving practitioners channeling energy through their hands and transferring it into a person's body to promote healing
Therapeutic touch	An energy therapy using the therapist's healing energy, usually without touching the person, to identify and repair imbalances in the person's biofield

20.4 Spiritual Care

Intensivists around the globe are increasingly acknowledging that the healing of critically ill or injured patients, especially those requiring ICU services, happens best when the mind, the body, and the spirit are aligned. Despite growing empirical evidence for spiritual care as part of palliative care, religious and spiritual concerns remain insufficiently addressed by the medical system [61]. Even more concerning is that less than 50% of physicians believe that it is their role to address such concerns, and only a minority of patients report having their spiritual needs addressed [62]. Various studies highlight the importance of spirituality and religious practice with respect to outcomes in seriously ill patients. An observational study by Winkelman et al. showed that patients with cancer who had unmet spiritual concerns were more likely to have a significantly worse psychological quality of life than those whose spiritual concerns were addressed [63]. Vilalta et al. conducted an observation study on patients with advanced cancer in a palliative care unit. They found that the two specific spiritual needs were most relevant to patients: (1) the need to be recognized as a person until the end of their life (not just a body) and (2) they had a need to know the truth about their illness [64]. Ethnic, religious, and cultural traditions have all been linked with guiding end-of-life healthcare priorities and decision-making and should be considered as possible contributors to overall patient satisfaction. Ratshikana-Moloko et al. studied the religious and spiritual needs of the patient with advanced cancer in South Africa. Patients who received dedicated religious and spiritual care reported less pain, used less morphine, and were more likely to die at home than those who did not [65]. It is not surprising then that patients with serious illnesses have expressed a desire to discuss their spirituality with their physicians [19].

Although patients want to discuss these issues with their treating physicians, time constraints, a lack of confidence in how to speak about such issues, and a fear of imposing one's own spiritual beliefs onto patients are all cited as reasons why physicians don't routinely engage in these discussions. In many parts of the world, chaplains are called upon to lead spiritual discussions as some physicians purposefully keep an arm's length distance on this topic. Unfortunately, there are insufficient numbers of health care chaplains, and very few are certified in palliative care. Thus, most seriously ill patients depend on other members of the health care team to address spiritual concerns.

Balboni et al. conducted a multi-institutional study of 343 patients with advanced cancer to determine whether spiritual care from the medical team impacts medical care received and quality of life at the end of life. They found that patients whose spiritual needs were supported received more hospice care and were less likely to have burdensome non-beneficial interventions near the end of life than those whose needs were not met. Additionally, they found that spiritual support provided by the medical team or chaplain was associated with higher quality-of-life scores [66, 67].

It is interesting to note that in the same cohort of cancer patients, those who relied highly on religious faith to cope with their underlying disease were more likely than those with a low level of religious coping with receiving mechanical intubation and ICU care near the end of life [68]. Healthcare workers and hospital systems looking to start palliative care programs would do well to consider spiritual care training for their staff. This would include an improved understanding of clinicians' appropriate role in spiritual care provision to severely ill patients, which in turn may lead to increased spiritual provision [62]. More research is needed to understand how spirituality and religion affect patient, family, and surrogate decision-making in palliative care.

20.4.1 Palliative Intervention: Is There a Role?

Palliative care does not necessarily mean avoiding any invasive interventions or procedures. As previously defined, the basic premise of palliative care is to alleviate suffering and improve the quality of life for patients with serious underlying diseases. It is important to realize that while palliation helps patients avoid intensive interventions that may not be beneficial to a patient, it does not consider or quantify how intense that palliation should be. For example, patients with malignant small obstruction may opt for palliative surgery in hopes of avoiding death as a result of obstruction, a particularly unpleasant way to die.

In a large systematic review on the role of palliative surgery for malignant bowel obstruction from carcinomatosis, Olson et al. screened 2347 unique articles, selected 108 articles for full-text review, and included a total of 17 studies. Surgery was able to palliate obstructive symptoms for 32–100% of patients, enable resumption of a diet for 45–75% of patients, and facilitate discharge to home in 34–87% of patients. Unfortunately, mortality was noted to be significant (6–32%), and serious complications occurred in up to 45% of patients. Frequent re-obstructions, readmissions to the hospital, and re-operations were additional complications. Median survival was limited (median 26–237 days), and hospitalization for surgery consumed a substantial portion of the patient's remaining life. The authors concluded that although palliative surgery can benefit some patients, it comes at the cost of high mortality and substantial hospitalization relative to the patient's remaining survival time. They emphasized the importance of preoperative discussions to lay out realistic goals and limitations of surgery [69].

Gastric cancer patients are also a subset of cancer patients who typically present with late-stage disease. Progressive tumor growth in this setting can lead to severe complications such as gastric outlet obstruction, perforation, and bleeding. Cowling et al. conducted a systematic review and meta-analysis of the literature for all papers describing palliative resections for gastric cancer and reporting peri-operative or survival outcomes. Their analysis included nearly 60,000 patients from 128 papers. They found that palliative gastrectomy was associated with a *small* improvement in survival at 1 year when compared to non-resectional surgery and chemotherapy. Unfortunately, the benefit seems to occur only at 1 year as survival drops dramatically after that [70].

Colorectal cancer (CRC) is the third most common cancer and the fourth cancer-related cause of death in the world population. CRC education, awareness, and screening campaigns have all helped decrease death rates since the late 80s. Even then, an estimated 20% of patients affected by CRC will present with distant metastasis. Multiple interventions have been described, including open surgery, minimally invasive techniques, or chemotherapy. While emergency situations (perforation) may require surgical intervention or an option for transition to full palliation/comfort care, the role of surgery in the palliative management of asymptomatic patients is being challenged, given advances in chemotherapy. Costi et al. stress that a multi-disciplinary approach to the patient including oncologists, surgeons, and other care-takers should discuss all options with the patient and/or their families or surrogates to help guide which intervention or non-intervention is most aligned with the patient's wishes [71].

Patients with acute malignant colorectal surgery are another example of patients who may opt for a palliative intervention. In this case, patients have an option of choosing a self-expandable metallic stenting either as a definitive procedure or as a bridge to elective surgery rather than undergoing emergency surgery. Li et al. conducted a retrospective review of patients with acute malignant obstruction of the right colon, comparing stent versus emergency surgery. Although the study found no differences in progression-free survival, the patients who underwent stent placement had reduced incidence of post-procedural complications and a shorter post-operative length of stay [72].

Regardless of which intervention a patient ultimately chooses, it is critical to remember that the primary goal is to reduce suffering. The patient-surgeon relationship has evolved from one of paternalistic authority to more of partnering in decision making. Surgeons must express respect for patients' autonomy and practice patient-centered care [73]. The decision making in a patient-centered care approach should be "responsive to individual patient preferences, needs, and values" as defined by the Institute of Medicine [74].

20.4.2 Looking Forward: Changing Culture, Education and Research

A common misconception about palliative care, and supportive care in general, is that it amounts to "doing nothing" or "giving up" on aggressive treatments for patients who are generally the sickest or dying when these decisions are being made [75]. Changing the healthcare culture to infuse palliative care into our daily thinking is difficult. In fact, a change of culture, whether in healthcare or in business, is extremely difficult as it takes years to develop. Entire business school courses have been dedicated to the topic. Torben Rick, for example, writes that the culture of an organization is practically its DNA and that it is what determines how everything else in the organization unfolds. He also emphasizes that organizational culture can evolve over time even though it is deeply linked to its history and development [76]. The implementation of palliative care, either as a primary or consultative service, early in the course of illness will hopefully be a major change in how we manage sick and dying patients. It is not a far-fetched thought then that the culture of integrating palliative care into our everyday healthcare vernacular will include buy-in from primary care physicians, surgeons, spiritual guides, and the public itself. In doing so, the current visceral emotion that occurs by simply uttering the term "palliation" will hopefully give away to acceptance and a more holistic view of life, and inevitably, death.

Education of the healthcare work-force, healthcare organization and delivery systems, patients, their families, and healthcare proxies will be essential to helping change the culture around palliative care.

The WHO has resolved that palliative care is "an ethical responsibility of health systems" and that the integration of palliative care into public health care systems is absolutely essential [77]. The WHO World Health Assembly also has also called to "put people at the center of health care" by providing them "comprehensive primary care services, including health promotion, disease prevention, curative care and palliative care, that are integrated with other levels of care" [77].

Since the patients and their families are the ones who are the most impacted when they are sick and dying, a greater emphasis is being placed on education about palliative care. The WHO recognizes that the greatest majority of people who need palliative care prefer to remain at home so it is critical that that palliative care be provided in the community, as part of primary health care. These specialists are typically primary health care providers with basic training in palliative care and symptom relief. They can appropriately respond to most palliative care needs and arrange for transfer to a higher level of care as needed [77].

Despite the efforts of the WHO, many training programs around the world lack a defined palliative care curriculum or have not achieved consistent and effective implementation of palliative care education. Klaristenfeld et al. conducted a survey of junior and senior surgery residents at a major academic medical center and found that <10% of respondents reported receiving adequate training in palliative care, whereas 100% believed that such training was valuable for surgeons and should be provided during the residency [78]. Bradley et al. discovered that while developing an intervention of implementing a palliative care curriculum for postgraduate year 2 surgical residents at a large, academic center noted that chief surgical residents comprising the control group lacked any formal training in palliative care other than a single, 1-h lecture on general principles of pain management. While training in palliative care is woefully inadequate for our trainees, it is even worse for those in current practice as they have never received any formal training at all [53].

Mosenthal et al. have warned that if surgical faculty themselves lack knowledge of palliative care, they may actually undermine the effectiveness of palliative care education by conveying a "hidden curriculum" in which the educational content of palliative care gets devalued. More worrisome is that this lack of knowledge and skills in palliative care may consciously or subconsciously lead the provider to avoid or delay having discussions regarding palliative care. The importance of dedicated palliative care training remains an important challenge for optimal integration of palliative care in many ICU settings [55].

Bateni et al. conducted a survey on Palliative Care Training and Decision-Making for Patients with Advanced Cancer Surgery. They included practicing surgeons, medical oncologists, intensivists, and palliative care physicians from a large urban city and its surrounding areas. They found "substantial deficiencies in palliative care training" especially among surgeons. These deficiencies in turn led to more aggressive recommendations for treatment. The authors concluded that greater efforts need to be made system-wide in palliative care education among surgeons, including the incorporation of a structured palliative care training curriculum in graduate and continuing surgical education [79].

Simulation-based medical education and simulation-based learning experiences [SBME/SBLE] have been touted as a starting point to train healthcare professionals on how to broach the topic of palliative care. Ann Faulkner, one of the early advocates of the use of simulation in palliative care training, found that SBLE provided a unique opportunity to practice communication skills by immersing learners in a safe and constructive environment without having to deal with the consequences or impact in a real patient scenario where the stakes are much higher [80]. As with any simulations, the fidelity of the simulation is less important than the value of lessons learned during the debriefing and discussion of what was learned. The use of standardized patients to simulate real-world scenarios has made simulation exercises more realistic for the trainee as they can practice on an innumerable amount of scenarios they may have to contend with in a care setting. In fact, SBLE trainees have reported that the addition of human standardized patients to a robotic simulator was what made the experience more realistic, powerful, and moving than with a robotic simulator alone [81].

Another advantage of SBME/SBLE and area that is ripe for additional study is the opportunity to involve learners from multiple specialties involved in the care of seriously ill patients with palliative care needs. Inter-professional training allows trainees to not only understand differing specialty-specific viewpoints but also to play roles they would not normally do given their chosen specialty. This ability to assume different avatars could improve team dynamics and multidisciplinary meetings in the ICU when discussing end-of-life-care, dying, hospice, and palliative care [82, 83].

One example of structured palliative care training is the development of a formalized curriculum to educate clinicians about end-of-life care by the American Medical Association Institute for Ethics' Education for Physicians on End-of-Life Care (EPEC) Project. This is a comprehensive training program, developed jointly by the AMA and the Robert Wood Johnson Foundation, to educate physicians on the clinical competencies required to provide quality, compassionate care to dying patient. The specific goals of EPEC are to define the essential skills required for quality end-of-life care and to use a train-the-trainer approach to educate a cadre of physician trainers, who would, in turn, teach these skills to practicing physicians. The EPEC curriculum consists of four 30-min plenary modules and 12 workshop modules designed to teach fundamental skills in communication, ethical decision-making, palliative care, psychosocial considerations, and symptom management (see Table 20.4) [84, 85].

The American College of Surgeons Division of Education has created a Surgical Palliative Care Task Force to promote the integration of palliative care precepts and techniques into surgical practice and education. They have developed instructional tools such as "Surgical Palliative Care: A Residents' Guide" that help surgical trainees how implement palliative care discussions into their daily practice. Despite the overall enthusiasm and potential benefits of simulation-based curriculums using standardized patients or robots, the costs of developing and maintaining a curriculum need to be weighed.

20.5 Future Research Areas

Healthcare professionals around the globe will need to critically analyze the implementation of palliative care programs in their local environments. It will be imperative to define outcomes that, first and foremost, matter to the patients we are serving. Currently, the scope of most outcome-based surgical research is limited to short-term survival. Few studies have examined other outcomes such as functional quality of life and time spent in ICU, or others that patient's value after surgery or define the benefits and trade-offs of surgery from the patient's perspective. Another key area of study is the area of effective communication and difficult decision-making. Tools such as the Best Case/Worst Case Scenario are a starting point to improve communication. More research is needed to identify strategies that will help patients, families, and healthcare proxies, lead to treatment decisions that are concordant with patients' preferences and that stress quality of life versus simply quantity. Additionally, few studies have examined the feasibility or efficacy of integrating primary palliative care into surgical practice and culture, including strategies for process change and workforce education. The role of simulation and use of standardized scenarios and patients will also need to be evaluated further. On a larger scale, there have been very few studies evaluating models for surgical palliative care that can be scaled to populations in the perioperative setting [86–88].

20.6 Summary

The goal of ICU care is to provide a setting where vital organ function can be maintained and optimized to restore health and reduce mortality and prevent morbidity in patients with severe critical illness. Yet, despite the development of new technologies and the improvement of intensive care treatment, death rates in ICUs around the globe remain high. The purpose of palliative care is to optimize the patient's quality of life by anticipating, preventing, and treating suffering. Ideal programs will realize that treatment is not just limited to the body but should also incorporate the mind and the spirit to achieve optimal results. More training and education are needed to ensure a working knowledge of palliative measures.

Do and Don'ts

- Do relieve patient and family distress
- Do integrate palliative care into the management
- Don't forget to educate health-care work forces
- Don't forget to consider patient provenience and cultural behavior

Take-Home Messages

- Palliative care is care provided to a patient and their family to relieve distress and suffering as a result of disease, illness, or injury while optimizing their psychological, social, and spiritual concerns. It is distinct from hospice care.
- Integrating palliative care early into the management of ill patients decreases overall healthcare costs and improves quality at the end of life.
- Palliative care interventions have been successful in utilizing patient care to improve outcomes for patients. These outcomes include quality of life, pain management, psychosocial health, family assessment of care and bereavement, and even reduced overall healthcare costs.
- Integration of palliative care into healthcare delivery systems is broadly based on an integration strategy or a consultation strategy.
- Education of the healthcare work-force, healthcare organizations and delivery systems, patients, their families, and healthcare proxies will be essential to helping change the culture around palliative care.

Multiple Choice Questions

1. Palliative care
   A. is not possible in acute care surgery
   B. is possible only in trauma surgery
   C. is possible only in oncology
   D. has to be considered whenever indicated

Answer: D

2. Family
   A. must be involved in palliative care management
   B. is not important
   C. is important only the wife
   D. has to drive and decide all the care process

Answer: A

3. Analgesic drugs
   A. are the only real palliative treatment
   B. are part of the palliative treatment
   C. are not useful
   D. are useful only with anxiolytic drugs

Answer: B

References

1. Institute of Medicine Committee on Care at the End of Life. Approaching death: improving care at the end of life. In: Field MJ, Cassel CK, editors. Approaching death: improving care at the end of life. Washington (DC): National Academies Press (US). Copyright 1997 by the National Academy of Sciences. All rights reserved.; 1997.
2. Organization WECoCPRaASCWH. Cancer pain relief and palliative care: report of a who expert committee. 1990.
3. Narayan M, Kashuk JL. Admission/discharge criterion for acute care surgery patients in the ICU: a general review of ICU admission and discharge indications. In: Picetti E, Pereira BM, Razek T, Narayan M, Kashuk JL, editors. Intensive care for emergency surgeons. Cham: Springer International Publishing; 2019. p. 1–21.
4. Strengthening of palliative care as a component of comprehensive care throughout the life course. 2014 2021.
5. Palliative care. 2020.
6. Yadav KN, Gabler NB, Cooney E, Kent S, Kim J, Herbst N, et al. Approximately one in three us adults completes any type of advance directive for

7. Aslakson RA, Curtis JR, Nelson JE. The changing role of palliative care in the ICU. Crit Care Med. 2014;42:2418–28.
8. May P, Normand C, Cassel JB, Del Fabbro E, Fine RL, Menz R, et al. Economics of palliative care for hospitalized adults with serious illness: a meta-analysis. JAMA Intern Med. 2018;178:820–9.
9. Stepro N. The final year: Where and how we die. 2016;2021.
10. Grudzen CR, Richardson LD, Morrison M, Cho E, Morrison RS. Palliative care needs of seriously ill, older adults presenting to the emergency department. Acad Emerg Med. 2010;17:1253–7.
11. Goldonowicz JM, Runyon MS, Bullard MJ. Palliative care in the emergency department: an educational investigation and intervention. BMC Palliat Care. 2018;17:43.
12. Morrison RS, Augustin R, Souvanna P, Meier DE. America's care of serious illness: a state-by-state report card on access to palliative care in our nation's hospitals. 2019.
13. Sprung CL, Truog RD, Curtis JR, Joynt GM, Baras M, Michalsen A, et al. Seeking worldwide professional consensus on the principles of end-of-life care for the critically ill. The consensus for worldwide end-of-life practice for patients in intensive care units (welpicus) study. Am J Respir Crit Care Med. 2014;190:855–66.
14. Hahne P, Lundstrom S, Levealahti H, Winnhed J, Ohlen J. Changes in professionals' beliefs following a palliative care implementation programme at a surgical department: a qualitative evaluation. BMC Palliat Care. 2017;16:77.
15. National Consensus Project for Quality Palliative Care. Clinical practice guidelines for quality palliative care, 4th ed. Richmond: National Coalition for Hospice and Palliative Care; 2018. https://www.nationalcoalitionhpc.org/ncp.2018.
16. Bergman J, Laviana AA. Opportunities to maximize value with integrated palliative care. J Multidiscip Healthc. 2016;9:219–26.
17. Gillon R. Defending the four principles approach as a good basis for good medical practice and therefore for good medical ethics. J Med Ethics. 2015;41:111–6.
18. Tatum PE, Mills SS. Hospice and palliative care: an overview. Med Clin North Am. 2020;104:359–73.
19. Kelley AS, Morrison RS. Palliative care for the seriously ill. N Engl J Med. 2015;373:747–55.
20. Luta X, Ottino B, Hall P, Bowden J, Wee B, Droney J, et al. Evidence on the economic value of end-of-life and palliative care interventions: a narrative review of reviews. BMC Palliat Care. 2021;20:89.
21. Haun MW, Estel S, Rucker G, Friederich HC, Villalobos M, Thomas M, et al. Early palliative care for adults with advanced cancer. Cochrane Database Syst Rev. 2017;6:CD011129.
22. Cauley CE, Panizales MT, Reznor G, Haynes AB, Havens JM, Kelley E, et al. Outcomes after emergency abdominal surgery in patients with advanced cancer: opportunities to reduce complications and improve palliative care. J Trauma Acute Care Surg. 2015;79:399–406.
23. Cauley CE, Block SD, Koritsanszky LA, Gass JD, Frydman JL, Nurudeen SM, et al. Surgeons' perspectives on avoiding nonbeneficial treatments in seriously ill older patients with surgical emergencies: a qualitative study. J Palliat Med. 2016;19:529–37.
24. Mayer DK, Travers D, Wyss A, Leak A, Waller A. Why do patients with cancer visit emergency departments? Results of a 2008 population study in North Carolina. J Clin Oncol. 2011;29:2683–8.
25. Bhulani N, Gupta A, Gao A, Li J, Guenther C, Ahn C, et al. Palliative care and end-of-life health care utilization in elderly patients with pancreatic cancer. J Gastrointest Oncol. 2018;9:495–502.
26. Ernst KF, Hall DE, Schmid KK, Seever G, Lavedan P, Lynch TG, et al. Surgical palliative care consultations over time in relationship to systemwide frailty screening. JAMA Surg. 2014;149:1121–6.
27. Robinson TN, Walston JD, Brummel NE, Deiner S, Brown CH 4th, Kennedy M, et al. Frailty for surgeons: review of a national institute on aging conference on frailty for specialists. J Am Coll Surg. 2015;221:1083–92.
28. Schneiderman LJ, Jecker NS, Jonsen AR. Medical futility: its meaning and ethical implications. Ann Intern Med. 1990;112:949–54.
29. Anstey MH, Adams JL, McGlynn EA. Perceptions of the appropriateness of care in California adult intensive care units. Crit Care. 2015;19:51.
30. Vincent JL. European attitudes towards ethical problems in intensive care medicine: results of an ethical questionnaire. Intensive Care Med. 1990;16:256–64.
31. Giannini A, Consonni D. Physicians' perceptions and attitudes regarding inappropriate admissions and resource allocation in the intensive care setting. Br J Anaesth. 2006;96:57–62.
32. Wunsch H, Linde-Zwirble WT, Harrison DA, Barnato AE, Rowan KM, Angus DC. Use of intensive care services during terminal hospitalizations in England and the United States. Am J Respir Crit Care Med. 2009;180:875–80.
33. Jordan RI, Allsop MJ, ElMokhallalati Y, Jackson CE, Edwards HL, Chapman EJ, et al. Duration of palliative care before death in international routine practice: a systematic review and meta-analysis. BMC Med. 2020;18:368.
34. Aggarwal G, Broughton KJ, Williams LJ, Peden CJ, Quiney N. Early postoperative death in patients undergoing emergency high-risk surgery: towards a better understanding of patients for whom surgery may not be beneficial. J Clin Med. 2020:9, 1288.
35. Cooper Z, Courtwright A, Karlage A, Gawande A, Block S. Pitfalls in communication that lead to nonbeneficial emergency surgery in elderly patients with serious illness: description of the problem and elements of a solution. Ann Surg. 2014;260:949–57.

36. Cooper Z, Scott JW, Rosenthal RA, Mitchell SL. Emergency major abdominal surgical procedures in older adults: a systematic review of mortality and functional outcomes. J Am Geriatr Soc. 2015;63:2563–71.
37. Walling AM, Asch SM, Lorenz KA, Roth CP, Barry T, Kahn KL, et al. The quality of care provided to hospitalized patients at the end of life. Arch Intern Med. 2010;170:1057–63.
38. Rao JK, Anderson LA, Lin FC, Laux JP. Completion of advance directives among US consumers. Am J Prev Med. 2014;46:65–70.
39. Buiar PG, Goldim JR. Barriers to the composition and implementation of advance directives in oncology: a literature review. Ecancermedicalscience. 2019;13:974.
40. Meier DE. Increased access to palliative care and hospice services: opportunities to improve value in health care. Milbank Q. 2011;89:343–80.
41. Lubitz J, Cai L, Kramarow E, Lentzner H. Health, life expectancy, and health care spending among the elderly. N Engl J Med. 2003;349:1048–55.
42. Riley GF, Lubitz JD. Long-term trends in medicare payments in the last year of life. Health Serv Res. 2010;45:565–76.
43. Zhang B, Wright AA, Huskamp HA, Nilsson ME, Maciejewski ML, Earle CC, et al. Health care costs in the last week of life: associations with end-of-life conversations. Arch Intern Med. 2009;169:480–8.
44. Callaway M, Foley KM, De Lima L, Connor SR, Dix O, Lynch T, et al. Funding for palliative care programs in developing countries. J Pain Symptom Manag. 2007;33:509–13.
45. Morrison RS, Penrod JD, Cassel JB, Caust-Ellenbogen M, Litke A, Spragens L, et al. Cost savings associated with us hospital palliative care consultation programs. Arch Intern Med. 2008;168:1783–90.
46. Penrod JD, Deb P, Luhrs C, Dellenbaugh C, Zhu CW, Hochman T, et al. Cost and utilization outcomes of patients receiving hospital-based palliative care consultation. J Palliat Med. 2006;9:855–60.
47. Penrod J, Morrison RS, Meier DE. Studying the effectiveness of palliative care. JAMA. 2008;300:1022–3; author reply 1023–1024.
48. Committee on Approaching Death: Addressing Key End of Life Issues; Institute of Medicine. Improving quality and honoring individual preferences near the end of life. Washington, DC: National Academies Press (US); 2015.
49. Aslakson RA, Wyskiel R, Thornton I, Copley C, Shaffer D, Zyra M, et al. Nurse-perceived barriers to effective communication regarding prognosis and optimal end-of-life care for surgical ICU patients: a qualitative exploration. J Palliat Med. 2012;15:910–5.
50. Cook M, Zonies D, Brasel K. Prioritizing communication in the provision of palliative care for the trauma patient. Curr Trauma Rep. 2020;6(4):183–93.
51. Kruser JM, Nabozny MJ, Steffens NM, Brasel KJ, Campbell TC, Gaines ME, et al. "Best case/worst case": qualitative evaluation of a novel communication tool for difficult in-the-moment surgical decisions. J Am Geriatr Soc. 2015;63:1805–11.
52. . !!! INVALID CITATION !!! {}.
53. Bradley CT, Webb TP, Schmitz CC, Chipman JG, Brasel KJ. Structured teaching versus experiential learning of palliative care for surgical residents. Am J Surg. 2010;200:542–7.
54. Vidri RJ, Blakely AM, Kulkarni SS, Vaghjiani RG, Heffernan DS, Harrington DT, et al. American College of Surgeons national surgical quality improvement program as a quality-measurement tool for advanced cancer patients. Ann Palliat Med. 2015;4:200–6.
55. Mosenthal AC, Weissman DE, Curtis JR, Hays RM, Lustbader DR, Mulkerin C, et al. Integrating palliative care in the surgical and trauma intensive care unit: a report from the improving palliative care in the intensive care unit (IPAL-ICU) project advisory board and the center to advance palliative care. Crit Care Med. 2012;40:1199–206.
56. Hua MS, Li G, Blinderman CD, Wunsch H. Estimates of the need for palliative care consultation across United States intensive care units using a trigger-based model. Am J Respir Crit Care Med. 2014;189:428–36.
57. Crooms RC, Gelfman LP. Palliative care and end-of-life considerations for the frail patient. Anesth Analg. 2020;130:1504–15.
58. Millstine D. Overview of integrative, complementary, and alternative medicine. Merck Manual Consumer Version. 2019.
59. Armstrong M, Flemming K, Kupeli N, Stone P, Wilkinson S, Candy B. Aromatherapy, massage and reflexology: a systematic review and thematic synthesis of the perspectives from people with palliative care needs. Palliat Med. 2019;33:757–69.
60. Estores IM, Frye J. Healing environments: integrative medicine and palliative care in acute care settings. Crit Care Nurs Clin North Am. 2015;27:369–82.
61. El Nawawi NM, Balboni MJ, Balboni TA. Palliative care and spiritual care: the crucial role of spiritual care in the care of patients with advanced illness. Curr Opin Support Palliat Care. 2012;6:269–74.
62. Rodin D, Balboni M, Mitchell C, Smith PT, VanderWeele TJ, Balboni TA. Whose role? Oncology practitioners' perceptions of their role in providing spiritual care to advanced cancer patients. Support Care Cancer. 2015;23:2543–50.
63. Winkelman WD, Lauderdale K, Balboni MJ, Phelps AC, Peteet JR, Block SD, et al. The relationship of spiritual concerns to the quality of life of advanced cancer patients: preliminary findings. J Palliat Med. 2011;14:1022–8.
64. Vilalta A, Valls J, Porta J, Vinas J. Evaluation of spiritual needs of patients with advanced cancer in a palliative care unit. J Palliat Med. 2014;17:592–600.
65. Ratshikana-Moloko M, Ayeni O, Tsitsi JM, Wong ML, Jacobson JS, Neugut AI, et al. Spiritual care, pain reduction, and preferred place of death among advanced cancer patients in soweto, South Africa. J Pain Symptom Manag. 2020;60:37–47.

66. Balboni TA, Paulk ME, Balboni MJ, Phelps AC, Loggers ET, Wright AA, et al. Provision of spiritual care to patients with advanced cancer: associations with medical care and quality of life near death. J Clin Oncol. 2010;28:445–52.
67. Balboni TA, Vanderwerker LC, Block SD, Paulk ME, Lathan CS, Peteet JR, et al. Religiousness and spiritual support among advanced cancer patients and associations with end-of-life treatment preferences and quality of life. J Clin Oncol. 2007;25:555–60.
68. Phelps AC, Maciejewski PK, Nilsson M, Balboni TA, Wright AA, Paulk ME, et al. Religious coping and use of intensive life-prolonging care near death in patients with advanced cancer. JAMA. 2009;301:1140–7.
69. Paul Olson TJ, Pinkerton C, Brasel KJ, Schwarze ML. Palliative surgery for malignant bowel obstruction from carcinomatosis: a systematic review. JAMA Surg. 2014;149:383–92.
70. Cowling J, Gorman B, Riaz A, Bundred JR, Kamarajah SK, Evans RPT, et al. Peri-operative outcomes and survival following palliative gastrectomy for gastric cancer: a systematic review and meta-analysis. J Gastrointest Cancer. 2021;52:41–56.
71. Costi R, Leonardi F, Zanoni D, Violi V, Roncoroni L. Palliative care and end-stage colorectal cancer management: the surgeon meets the oncologist. World J Gastroenterol. 2014;20:7602–21.
72. Li B, Cai SL, Lv ZT, Zhou PH, Yao LQ, Shi Q, et al. Self-expandable metallic stenting as a bridge to elective surgery versus emergency surgery for acute malignant right-sided colorectal obstruction. BMC Surg. 2020;20:326.
73. Barry MJ, Edgman-Levitan S. Shared decision making—pinnacle of patient-centered care. N Engl J Med. 2012;366:780–1.
74. Institute of Medicine (US) Committee on Quality of Health Care in America. Crossing the quality chasm: a new health system for the 21st century. Washington, DC: National Academies Press (US). Copyright 2001 by the National Academy of Sciences. All rights reserved.; 2001.
75. Callahan D. End-of-life care: a philosophical or management problem? J Law Med Ethics. 2011;39:114–20.
76. Rick T. Why is organizational culture change difficult 2015 2021.
77. Integrating palliative care and symptom relief into primary health care: a who guide for planners, implementers and managers. 2018.
78. Klaristenfeld DD, Harrington DT, Miner TJ. Teaching palliative care and end-of-life issues: a core curriculum for surgical residents. Ann Surg Oncol. 2007;14:1801–6.
79. Bateni SB, Canter RJ, Meyers FJ, Galante JM, Bold RJ. Palliative care training and decision-making for patients with advanced cancer: a comparison of surgeons and medical physicians. Surgery. 2018.
80. Faulkner A. Using simulators to aid the teaching of communication skills in cancer and palliative care. Patient Educ Couns. 1994;23:125–9.
81. Choi H, Crump C, Duriez C, Elmquist A, Hager G, Han D, et al. On the use of simulation in robotics: opportunities, challenges, and suggestions for moving forward. Proc Natl Acad Sci U S A. 2021;118:e1907856118.
82. Saylor J, Vernoony S, Selekman J, Cowperthwait A. Interprofessional education using a palliative care simulation. Nurse Educ. 2016;41:125–9.
83. INACSL Standards Committee. INACSL standards of best practice: simulationsm simulation design. Standards of Best Practice: Simulation. 2016;12:S5-S12.
84. Grant M, Elk R, Ferrell B, Morrison RS, von Gunten CF. Current status of palliative care—clinical implementation, education, and research. CA Cancer J Clin. 2009;59:327–35.
85. VanGeest JB. Process evaluation of an educational intervention to improve end-of-life care: the education for physicians on end-of-life care (EPEC) program. Am J Hosp Palliat Care. 2001;18:233–8.
86. Lilley EJ, Cooper Z, Schwarze ML, Mosenthal AC. Palliative care in surgery: defining the research priorities. J Palliat Med. 2017;20:702–9.
87. Kozhevnikov D, Morrison LJ, Ellman MS. Simulation training in palliative care: state of the art and future directions. Adv Med Educ Pract. 2018;9:915–24.
88. Hasson F, Nicholson E, Muldrew D, Bamidele O, Payne S, McIlfatrick S. International palliative care research priorities: a systematic review. BMC Palliat Care. 2020;19:16.

Immunosuppression in Surgical Patients

21

Hannah Groenen and Marja A. Boermeester

21.1 Introduction

> **Learning Goals**
> - To understand the risk of surgery in immunosuppressed patients.
> - To understand how all forms of stress, including illness and surgery, can alter immunocompetence.
> - To understand and recognize the clinical manifestation of some acute surgical diseases in immunosuppressed patients.

Patients with a compromised immune system are a heterogeneous group who do not have a normal response to acute physiologic or psychologic stress such as surgery. So when in need of surgery, immunosuppressed patients have an increased perioperative risk and therefore remain a challenge. Furthermore, clinical manifestations of diseases or postoperative complications can be disguised, causing a delay in treatment and an inferior outcome. It is difficult to stratify immunosuppressed patients because the aetiology and pathophysiology differs. Therefore, this chapter provides an overview of immunosuppressed patients undergoing surgery categorized into six different groups: patients on steroids, after transplantation, with HIV or AIDS, elderly, patients with malnutrition, and with malignancy. We provide different treatment strategies for each of these patient categories.

21.2 Patients on Steroids

21.2.1 Summary

Exogenous steroids can suppress the hypothalamic–pituitary–adrenal axis (HPAA). Consequently, the counterregulatory stress hormone response to illness and tissue injury such as surgery is diminished. Patients on chronic steroid therapy may develop secondary adrenal insufficiency in the perioperative period. Besides immunosuppression, chronic steroid therapy is known to be associated with impaired wound healing, hyperglycaemia, and psychologic disturbances in the postoperative period.

H. Groenen · M. A. Boermeester (✉)
Department of Surgery, Amsterdam UMC Location University of Amsterdam, Amsterdam, The Netherlands

Amsterdam Gastroenterology Endocrinology & Metabolism, Amsterdam, The Netherlands
e-mail: h.groenen@amsterdamumc.nl; m.a.boermeester@amsterdamumc.nl

21.2.2 Secondary Adrenal Insufficiency

The HPAA is activated in response to acute physiologic or psychologic stress (Fig. 21.1). This activation is characterized by the secretion of corticotropin-releasing hormone (CRH) by the hypothalamus, which stimulates the production of adrenocorticotrophic hormone (ACTH) in the anterior pituitary. ACTH causes the adrenal glands to produce cortisol, which stimulates gluconeogenesis, catecholamine production, activates antistress and anti-inflammatory pathways, and is essential for the maintenance of cardiac output and contractility. Negative feedback loops regulate cortisol production leading to decreased secretion of CRH and ACTH. Secondary adrenal insufficiency can occur in patients on chronic steroid therapy due to HPAA suppression. This leads to diminished CRH and ACTH levels that cause atrophy of the adrenal zona fasciculata and lower cortisol production.

21.2.3 Surgical Stress

The adrenal cortex plays an important role in the endocrine response to many forms of stress, including surgery. Cortisol seems to be necessary for survival in critical illness [1].

Periods of stress, such as during surgery, in patients on chronic steroid therapy can lead to adrenal crisis due to their diminished ability to increase a cortisol response. Inadequate cortisol release can cause vasodilatation and hypotension. Nonspecific symptoms of adrenal crisis in patients include nausea, vomiting, abdominal

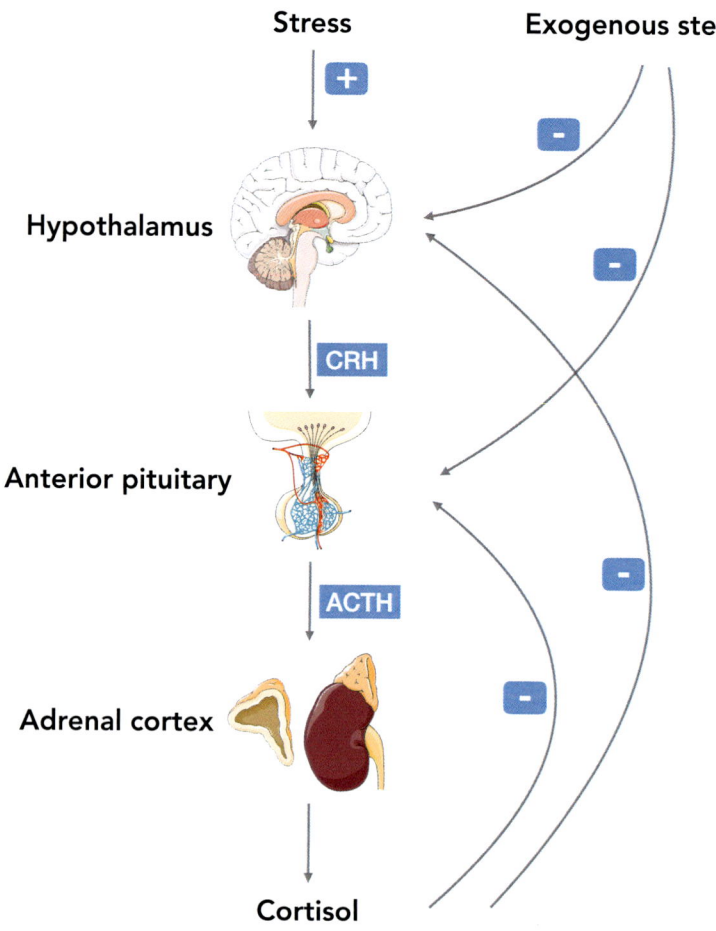

Fig. 21.1 Hypothalamic–pituitary–adrenal axis (HPAA) and exogenous steroids

pain, altered mental status, weakness, hypotension, or coma [2, 3].

There is no agreement on the dose or duration of exogenous steroids required to cause HPAA dysfunction. Generally, prednisone 20 mg/day or its equivalent for more than 3 weeks is considered a threshold [1]. The exact period of recovery from HPAA suppression differs between individuals and is difficult to predict, although HPAA suppression does not continue beyond 1 year after cessation of exogenous steroid therapy [2].

21.2.4 Diagnosis

In patients on steroids who are in need of emergency surgery, there is no time to test for HPAA dysfunction in the preoperative assessment. However, it is important to consider a perioperative adrenal crisis can be the cause of their nonspecific symptoms such as hypotension [2].

21.2.5 Treatment

Administration of perioperative stress-dose steroids in patients on chronic steroids lacks solid data. One of the largest series, published in 1973, has included 73 patients on chronic steroids undergoing surgery. Patients received 5–80 mg/day prednisone or equivalent, withholding all steroids preoperatively for 36 and not restarted until a minimal 24 h postoperatively. Plasma cortisol levels are measured using a fluorometric assay rarely used today, and vitals were registered. Only 3 patients demonstrated unexplained hypotension and low cortisol levels (<15 μg/100 mL) but did not respond to treatment with rescue steroids [4].

A Cochrane review in 2013 concluded supplemental administration of perioperative steroids in patients with adrenal insufficiency was not required. This review was retracted because of comments that debated the eligibility criteria and interpretation of the evidence [5].

Purely based on available evidence, a recommendation for stress-dose steroids for chronic steroid users is weak. A recent systematic review has found two RCTs (a total of 37 patients), five cohort studies (a total of 462 patients), and four systematic reviews. The quality of the evidence is low. Given the significant studies' limitations, it is not possible to conclude that perioperative administration of corticosteroids, compared to placebo, reduces the incidence of adrenal insufficiency [6].

Although the literature is inconsistent, others have concluded that patients who have been on steroid therapy in doses equivalent or above 20 mg/day of prednisone for more than 3 weeks or who have clinical signs of Cushing syndrome are at high risk of HPAA suppression and require perioperative stress-dose steroids. Moreover, patients who have been treated with any dose of glucocorticoid for less than 3 weeks, and a dosage of prednisone of 5 mg/day or less are at low risk of HPAA suppression and may not need perioperative stress-dose steroids [7].

In the event of a perioperative adrenal crisis, it is important to immediately start treatment with stress-dose steroids [7].

Dos and Don'ts
- Do: patients on steroids who need surgery should continue their usual therapy scheme.
- Do: the surgeon should be aware of an increased risk of postoperative complications in patients on steroids.
- Do: in the event of an adrenal crisis, it is important to immediately start treatment with stress-dose steroids.
- Don't: the administration of perioperative stress-dose steroids in patients on chronic steroids because this lacks solid data.

21.3 Transplanted Patients

21.3.1 Summary

Non-transplant surgery in solid organ transplanted patients is accompanied by medical problems unique to the transplant as well as the need to preserve the transplanted organ function during and after surgery. Close attention is paid to considerations of immunosuppressive medication, interaction with anaesthetic drugs, blood product administration, the risk and benefits of invasive monitoring, and risks of infection.

21.3.2 Non-transplant Surgery

When transplant patients need elective or emergency non-transplant surgery, immunocompetence can be altered due to stress of surgery, acute illness such as infectious diseases as an indication for surgery, postoperative infectious complications, or disruption of the regimen by inexperienced health care providers. There are various regimens of immunosuppressive therapy. We need to distinguish induction immunosuppressive therapy starting immediately before organ implantation and, more relevant in the context of this chapter, immunosuppressive maintenance therapy. Maintenance therapy involves one drug from each group: calcineurin inhibitors (e.g., Tacrolimus or Cyclosporine), antimetabolites (e.g., Azathioprine, Cyclophosphamide, Mycophenolate mofetil), and corticosteroids [8].

A fairly recent systematic review has included 71,671 patients presented after a solid organ transplantation (heart, lung, liver, pancreas, or kidney) with graft-unrelated surgical abdominal diseases from 39 case series. Overall, 1761 of these patients (2.5%) underwent emergency abdominal surgery, indicated because of gallbladder diseases (80.3%), gastrointestinal perforations (9.2%), complicated diverticulitis (6.2%), small bowel obstructions (2%), and appendicitis (2%). The immunosuppressive therapy was not modified postoperatively in most patients. The overall mortality rate reported was 5.5% (range 0–17.5%) [9].

In immunosuppressed transplanted patients, the clinical signs and symptoms of gastrointestinal perforation were often absent or nonspecific, with an overall mortality rate of 17.5% [9].

Complicated diverticulitis requiring emergency abdominal surgery has an incidence rate of 0.88–4% in transplant patients (1–4%) [10, 11], which is definitely higher than in the general population (estimated incidence of 0.025–0.053%) [11, 12]. The pooled incidence of acute diverticulitis in post-transplant patients is 1.7% (95% CI 1.0–2.7%). Pooled proportion of complicated diverticulitis among these patients is 40.1% (95% CI 32.2–49.7%) [13].

21.3.3 Diagnosis

Preoperative assessment in transplanted patients who need an emergency surgery is different from the general population because of their chronic immunosuppression. Their atypical or disguised clinical manifestation can lead to misdiagnosis or underestimation of the severity of their disease or complication. Moreover, any stress such as acute illness or surgery can also affect the functional capacity of the transplanted organ [9].

21.3.4 Treatment

In transplant patients, immunosuppression claims for more aggressive treatment of acute abdominal diseases but also the direct impact of immunosuppressive therapies on postoperative complication risk is crucial. Emergency abdominal surgery is associated with enhanced morbidity and mortality rates, respectively, up to 32.7% and 17.5% [9].

> **Dos and Don'ts**
> - Do: continue the immunosuppressive therapy postoperatively in transplanted patients.
> - Do: a more aggressive treatment of acute abdominal diseases in immunosuppressed transplanted patients.
> - Do: be aware of the increased surgical complication risks in transplanted patients.

21.4 Patients with HIV/AIDS

21.4.1 Summary

Human immunodeficiency virus (HIV) or acquired immune deficiency syndrome (AIDS) patients undergo emergency surgery more often nowadays because of longer life expectancy. Recent evidence showed similar postoperative complication and mortality rate in HIV-positive patients with high CD4 cell count compared to HIV-negative patients. Patients with a low CD4 cell count often have AIDS-defining opportunistic infections and are more prone to infectious adverse postoperative outcomes, e.g., surgical site infection, urinary tract infection, and pneumonia.

21.4.2 Immune Function in HIV and AIDS Patients

HIV is a member of the retrovirus family and infects CD4 cells, which normally regulate immune function. After infection, the virus enters the cell by binding to the CD4 protein on the surface and destroys the CD4 cell. Therefore, infection with HIV is characterized by loss of CD4 cell count [14]. The WHO defined AIDS as the most advanced stage of HIV infection with the occurrence of any of the documented AIDS-defining opportunistic infections or AIDS-related cancers [15]. The introduction of Highly Active Antiretroviral Therapies (HAART) has dramatically decreased the incidence of AIDS-defining illnesses and improved the life expectancy of patients with a diagnosis of HIV or AIDS. Most patients receiving HAART achieve viral load (plasma HIV-1 RNA) suppression and regain or maintain immune function [16].

AIDS-defining illnesses occur more often in patients with low CD4 cell counts. The prevalence of opportunistic infections in HIV-infected patients is 25.9%, including shingles (25%), pulmonary tuberculosis (20%), and oral candidiasis (12%). Of the HIV-infected patients with an opportunistic infection, 60.6% have a CD4 cell count <200 cells/mm^3 [17]. A common abdominal opportunistic infection primarily related to HIV or AIDS is abdominal tuberculosis. This co-infection affects the respiratory reserve and leads to the depletion of macronutrients and micronutrients, causing malnutrition [18]. In patients with extrapulmonary tuberculosis, a 60–90% prevalence of HIV infection has been found in Sub-Saharan Africa [19]. Globally, 9.5% of tuberculosis patients are co-infected with HIV [20]. End-stage liver disease can occur in HIV or AIDS patients that suffer a co-infection with Hepatitis B and Hepatitis C viruses. An estimated 4–7% of HIV patients have end-stage renal failure [21]. HIV-infected persons have a 69% increased risk for virus-related cancers than the general population. The most common malignancy types are AIDS-defining non-Hodgkin lymphomas, lung cancer, Kaposi's sarcoma, anal cancer, prostate cancer, liver cancer, and Hodgkin's lymphoma [22]. The correlation between the reported CD4 cell count and the incidence of AIDS-defining cancer varies by cancer type. Kaposi's sarcoma and non-Hodgkin lymphoma are strongly and inversely associated with CD4 cell counts [23].

Several individual AIDS-defining illnesses have been reported at higher CD4 cell counts. Oesophageal candidiasis (13.4%), Kaposi sarcoma (10.9%), and pulmonary tuberculosis (10.4%) are found in more than 200,000 HIV-infected individuals with CD4 cell count of 200 cells/mm^3 or greater. Factors correlated with increased risk of AIDS-defining illness in patients with CD4 cell count over 500 cells/mm^3 are intravenous drug users, viral load greater than 10,000 copies/mL, and older age [24].

21.4.3 Outcomes of Surgery

An estimated 20–25% of the HIV population will undergo an elective or emergency surgical intervention in their life [25]. Literature of the last decade about emergency surgery in HIV or AIDS patients reported high morbidity and mortality rates. The most common adverse outcomes are perioperative infections and impaired wound healing due to the highly compromised immune status, the presence of opportunistic infections, and malnutrition. Most of the literature was published before HAART was introduced in the mid-1990s. Reported results often did not discriminate between HIV-positive patients without AIDS and AIDS patients [26].

More recent evidence showed that CD4 cell count and viral load are important markers in surgical outcomes. Similar operative risk and mortality rates have been found in HIV-positive patients who are AIDS-negative and have high CD4 cell counts (>500 cells/mm^3) compared to HIV-negative patients. *Chicom-Mefire* et al. have compared two groups of HIV-positive patients with different CD4 cell counts (cut-off at 200 cells/mm^3) and HIV-negative patients undergoing major abdominal surgery. HIV-positive patients with low CD4 cell counts have a significantly higher complication rate compared to patients with high CD4 cell counts (62% vs. 19%, $p < 0.01$), while mortality among all subgroups is comparable [27]. Another study has shown an overall complication rate of 55% after major abdominal surgery in HIV and AIDS patients. Significantly lower preoperative CD4 cell counts are found in patients suffering an adverse event (146–156 vs. 288–319, $P = 0.013$) [28].

Sandler et al., in a large series, have compared outcomes after emergency surgery in AIDS patients, HIV-positive patients without AIDS, and HIV-negative patients. AIDS patients were more likely to develop a complication compared to HIV-negative patients (34.6% vs. 17.2%), including pneumonia, respiratory failure, urinary tract infection, septic shock, and admission of a transfusion. HIV-positive patients without AIDS have outcomes comparable to HIV-negative patients. The mortality rate in AIDS patients after emergency surgery was 4.4%, compared to 0.5% in HIV-positive patients without AIDS and 1.6% in HIV-negative patients. However, the HIV-positive patients without AIDS undergoing emergency surgery were of relatively younger age with less comorbidity compared to the HIV-negative patients [26].

21.4.4 Perioperative Admission of HAART

In patients undergoing emergency abdominal surgery oral intake is frequently interrupted. Therefore, also the administration of oral medication including HAART drugs for HIV patients is interrupted. This period is sometimes prolonged after surgery in the case of postoperative ileus. *Yang* et al. have analysed the effect of the interruption of HAART drugs and adding Albuvirtide, a long-acting intravenous fusion inhibitor that inhibits HIV entrance in the cell, in patients undergoing emergency abdominal surgery. In patients on HAART drugs preoperatively, the addition of Albuvirtide revealed no major clinical benefit. In patients not on HAART drugs, adding Albuvirtide reduced the viral load quickly and decreased the postoperative morbidity rate [29].

21.4.5 Diagnosis

In HIV-infected patients who require emergency surgery, it is important to evaluate the clinical stage of the patient's disease by measuring CD4 cell count and viral load preoperatively in order to predict the risk of postoperative complications [18].

21.4.6 Treatment

The level of immunosuppression and the urgency of the surgical procedure are the factors that influence the perioperative morbidity and mortality rate of emergency surgery in HIV or AIDS patients, which is comparable to other immunocompromised patients. However, emergency surgery because of the presence of AIDS-defining illnesses increases morbidity and mortality risk from 15 to 44% [30].

> **Dos and Don'ts**
> - Do: consider CD4 cell count and viral load to be important markers in surgical outcomes in HIV and AIDS patients.
> - Do: it is safe to perform surgery in HIV-positive patients with high CD4 cell count, because of comparable postoperative complication and mortality rate compared to HIV-negative patients.

21.5 Elderly

21.5.1 Summary

The ageing population is increasing and often in need of emergency surgery with a higher complication and mortality rate compared to the general population. One of the main underlying factors is the immune system, which gradually deteriorates with age. In elderly, this leads to a diminished ability to respond to illness and physical stressors such as surgery. By screening for frailty, adverse events can be reduced through the application of perioperative care programs specifically focused on geriatric patients.

21.5.2 Immunosenescence in Elderly

Immunosenescence is characterized by a decrease in the amount of peripheral blood naïve cells and a relative increase in the number of memory cells. In the aged population, this manifests as decreased ability to respond to physical stressors such as surgery, increased onset and progression of autoimmune diseases, and onset of malignancies. Similarly, the level of circulating cytokines and chemokines, particularly pro-inflammatory cytokines, is shifted towards the pro-inflammatory end of the spectrum. Therefore, a constant low-grade inflammatory state is induced, contributing to the progression of chronic diseases such as diabetes, Alzheimer's, atherosclerosis, and osteoporosis [31].

21.5.3 Aging of the Population

Because of the worldwide aging population, the number of geriatric patients undergoing emergency surgery is rapidly expanding. The percentage of trauma patients aged 65 years or above rose from 18 to 30% between 2005 and 2015 according to reports of the National Trauma Database in the United States [32]. In patients undergoing abdominal emergency surgery, the percentage of patients aged 80 years or older significantly increased from 42% (1986–1990) to 53% (1991–1995) [33]. These numbers underscore the importance of specialized perioperative care for this expanding vulnerable population.

21.5.4 Frailty

Advanced age has long been recognised as the most important negative prognostic factor for outcomes after surgery in the geriatric patient. Emerging evidence indicates patients of the same age can be at different risks. Therefore, frailty seems to be a more accurate predictor of postoperative morbidity and mortality. Frailty can be defined as an age-related cumulative decline in multiple physiological systems. Currently, no standardised method to measure frailty is used. A systematic review from *Lin* et al. including 23 studies has identified 21 different instruments to measure frailty [34]. Variations of the Fried Criteria or models based on Comprehensive Geriatric Assessment (CGA), e.g., the Frailty index, have been used in most of the studies. According to the Fried Criteria, patients are described to be frail when they have at least three of the features of slowness, weakness, exhaustion, weight loss, and low physical activity [35] (Fig. 21.2). The Frailty Index quantifies frailty by the number of deficits present in an individual. Deficits include physical and cognitive impairments, co-morbidities, psychosocial risk factors, and common geriatric syndromes [36]. All reviewed studies report a significant association between frailty in patients aged 75 years or greater, postoperative mortality, complications, and longer hospital stays [34].

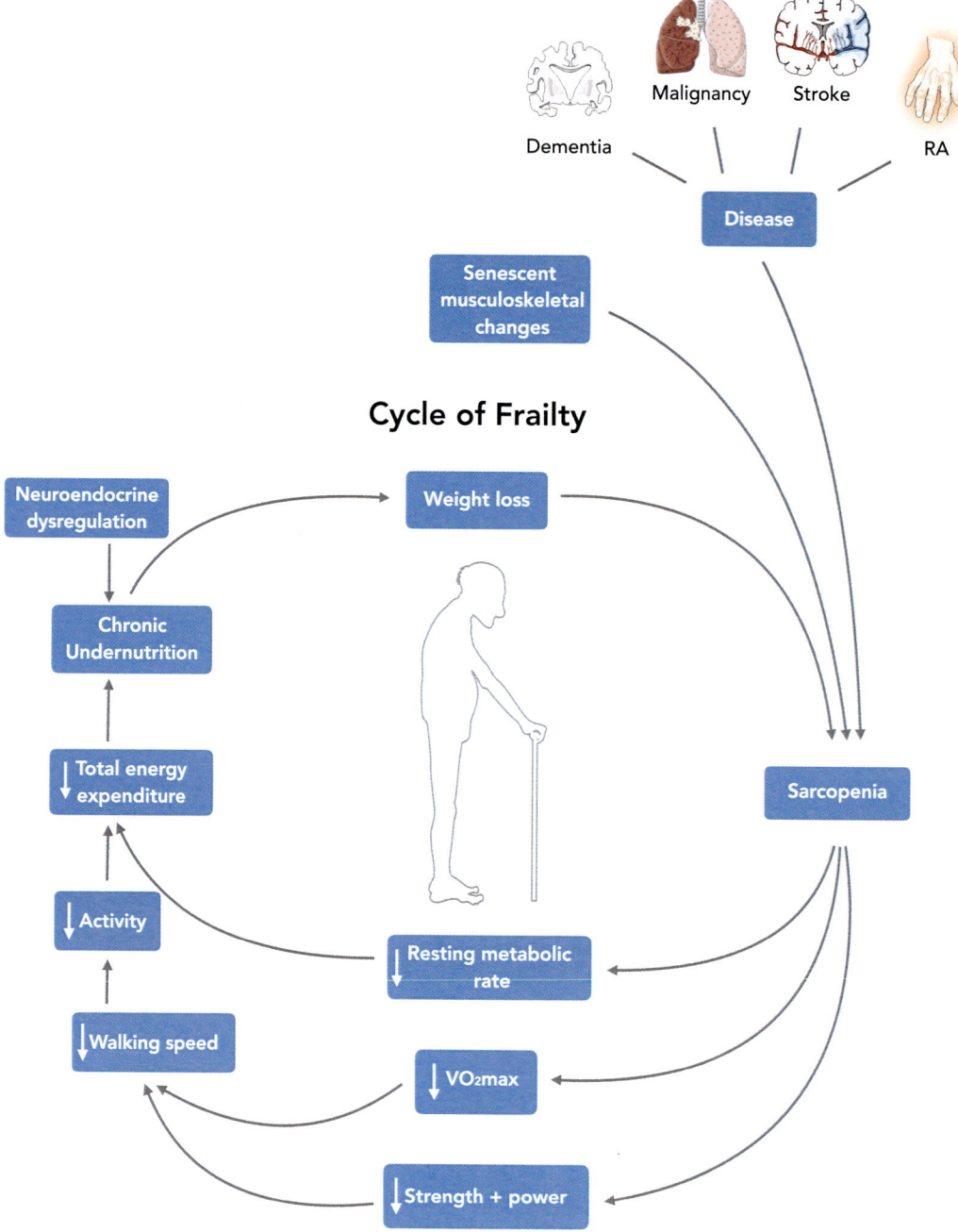

Fig. 21.2 Cycle of frailty in elderly. (Figure inspired by *Fried* et al. [35])

21.5.5 Most Common Emergency Surgeries

Hip fracture surgery is one of the most common procedures performed on geriatric patients. *Mariconda* et al. have shown a 29.4% in-hospital complication rate, including delirium (12%), pressure sores (7.7%), and anaemia (3.9%) [37]. Also, a high readmission rate (15%) within 30 days after discharge has been reported by *Lee* et al., associated with increased morbidity and mortality [38]. A 1-year mortality rate after hip fracture surgery ranging between 15 and 30% has been reported [37–39]. *Panula* et al. have found a three-fold increased risk of mortality after hip fracture compared to the general population during a mean follow-up of 3.7 years [40]. A systematic review from *Smith* et al., including 544,733 patients, has identified 12 significant indicators for risk of mortality, whereof the strongest are pre-fracture mobility, age, the presence of an abnormal ECG, and cognitive impairment [41]. Furthermore, greater time to surgery has been associated with increased postoperative complications such as pneumonia, pressure sores, and mortality (OR 0.74, 95% CI 0.67–0.81; $p < 0.0001$) [42].

Acute abdomen can be a challenging diagnosis in the geriatric patient. *Arenal* et al. found 50% of geriatric patients visited the hospital 48 h after the onset of symptoms, causing a delay in surgery and increased morbidity and mortality [33]. This can be particularly explained by the atypical presentation of abdominal complaints in older individuals, including nonspecific alterations in vital signs and during physical examination. A multicentre study from the UK has reported a 24.4% 30-day mortality rate in patients 80 years of age or greater after emergency laparotomy vs. 14.9% mortality overall [43].

In general, population admitted with acute appendicitis, the incidence of a perforated appendix is estimated to be in the range of 20–30%. This incidence increases with ageing with a reported incidence of 41% in patients over 60 years of age. The pre-hospital delay was the most important negative prognostic factor. Twenty-one percent of the patients suffered postoperative complications and 3% died [44].

Acute cholecystitis in high-risk patients is often treated with percutaneous catheter drainage instead of a laparoscopic cholecystectomy because it is assumed that laparoscopic cholecystectomy is associated with high morbidity and mortality. Recently, a randomized trial, the CHOCOLATE study, compared laparoscopic cholecystectomy with percutaneous catheter drainage in high-risk patients. Mean age in the cholecystectomy cohort was 71.4 (SD 10.6) vs. 74.9 (SD 8.6) in the drainage cohort. Postprocedure complications are significantly higher in the drainage cohort: 65% vs. 12% in the cholecystectomy cohort. The mortality rate is not significantly different between the drainage group and cholecystectomy group (9% vs. 3%, $P = 0.27$) [45].

21.5.6 Diagnosis

Frailty assessment is a valuable tool in the perioperative assessment of the elderly population undergoing emergency surgery to predict postoperative morbidity, mortality, and length of in-hospital stay [34].

21.5.7 Treatment

Delay in treatment of abdominal surgical disease is a common problem in elderly patients, which is the most important prognostic factor for increased postoperative complication and mortality rate [43, 44]. Also, in hip fracture surgery, longer time to surgery is associated with increased complications such as pneumonia, pressure sores, and mortality [42]. The application of perioperative care programs specifically focused on geriatric patients can reduce adverse events postoperatively [34].

> **Dos and Don'ts**
>
> - Do: by screening for frailty in elderly, adverse events can be reduced through the application of perioperative care programs specifically focused on geriatric patients.
> - Don't: do not delay surgery in geriatric patients as longer time to surgery is associated with increased postoperative complications such as pneumonia, pressure sores, and mortality.

21.6 Malnutrition

21.6.1 Summary

Malnutrition is correlated with immune suppression and is a common problem in hospitalized patients causing increased mortality, morbidity, length of stay in hospital, readmissions, and health care costs. Early assessment of nutritional status and introduction of nutritional therapy is important, especially in the emergency surgery population, to reduce major adverse events and increase fast recovery.

21.6.2 Definition of Malnutrition

Malnutrition is a prevalent cause of immunodeficiency worldwide and a common problem in hospitalized patients. Malnutrition can be described as a combination of a negative nutrient balance and increased inflammatory activity. Many definitions for malnutrition and a variety of different screening tools for the assessment of nutrition status have been described. According to The European Society for Clinical Nutrition and Metabolism (ESPEN), malnutrition can be diagnosed in surgical patients if one of the following criteria is present: weight loss >10–15% within 6 months, a body mass index (BMI) <18.5 kg/m^2, a Nutritional Risk Score >5 or a preoperative serum albumin <30 g/L [46]. The Nutritional Risk Score is a validated tool to detect the metabolic risk caused by loss of body cell mass associated with disease-related malnutrition [47]. Dutch hospitals frequently use the SNAQ (short nutritional assessment questionnaire) score, an easy and validated questionnaire, achieved by the nurse at admission, for early detection of hospital malnutrition [48].

21.6.3 Patients at Risk for Malnutrition

The reported prevalence of malnutrition in general hospitalized patients is approximately 30% [49–51]. In a prospective cohort study by *Lim* et al., malnourishment was associated with longer hospital stays (6.9–7.3 days vs. 4.6–5.6 days, $P < 0.001$), more readmissions within 15 days (adjusted relative risk 1.9, 95% CI 1.1–3.2, $P = 0.025$), higher costs of care and increased mortality rate (adjusted hazard ratio 4.4, 95% CI 3.3–6.0, $P < 0.001$) [51].

Several patient groups are at high risk for malnutrition. In an observational study of 1361 patients treated in a single institution ICU after emergency surgery, 60% had nonspecific malnutrition and 8% had protein-energy malnutrition [52]. *Zhenyi Jia* et al. have shown in a cohort of 82,725 patients 65 years or older undergoing emergency surgery in the United States, that 66.74% was malnourished according to the GNRI (The Geriatric Nutritional Risk Index) [53]. The GNRI measures the nutrition status using the serum albumin concentration and the ratio of actual to ideal weight [54]. In six common emergency surgery procedures (appendectomy, cholecystectomy, laparotomy, partial colectomy, surgical management of peptic ulcer disease, and adhesiolysis), malnutrition was strongly associated with higher 30-day morbidity, prolonged hospital length of stay, and mortality rates [53]. Patients with gastrointestinal cancer who require surgery are more prone to malnutrition because of the catabolic effect of cancer, possible insufficient nutrient intake, and nutrient loss. The stress of surgery will aggravate this metabolic response even more. In a cohort of 95 patients admitted for elective upper gastrointestinal or colorectal surgery, 32% were mild-moderately malnourished and 16% severely malnourished. Decreased preoperative albumin is associated with longer hospital stay and longer nil-by-mouth status, 2.0 (2.1) days vs. 3.3 (2.1) days; $P < 0.05$. Also, time taken to achieve adequate nutrition is significantly prolonged in malnourished patients, 6.7 (3.2) days vs. 8.7 (4.4) days, $P < 0.05$ [55].

21.6.4 Effects of Surgery

Any type of injury, including surgery, can be seen as a major stressor causing a metabolic response with an excessive release of stress hormones and cytokines. This induces a breakdown of glycogen, fat, and protein and therefore loss of body cell mass [46]. To rebuild body cell mass and recover from surgery, adequate nutrition and physical activity is required [56]. These aspects are implemented in the Enhanced Recovery After Surgery (ERAS) programmes, which are standard in perioperative management in elective surgery. The goal is to reduce the stress of surgery and therefore minimalizing catabolism and increasing fast recovery. *Zhuang* et al. have shown in a systematic review the efficacy of ERAS programs in elective colorectal surgery in comparison to conventional care. Significantly decreased primary hospital stay (mean difference −2.44 days; $p < 0.000001$), total hospital stay (mean difference −2.39 days; $p = 0.0003$), and total complications rate (relative risk 0.71; $p = 0.0006$) have been found. Readmission rates, surgical complications, and mortality did not differ significantly [57]. Nutritional support is an essential component of the ERAS programmes and includes early oral feeding and avoidance of long periods without any nutritional therapy perioperative. In emergency surgery, malnutrition cannot be prevented preoperatively, but recognition and early assessment of nutritional status are important to start early intervention. A recent systematic review, including 4 cohort studies, has found similar beneficial effects in emergency colorectal surgery using the ERAS program compared to traditional care [58].

Weimann et al. have reviewed 35 controlled trials about the effect of early enteral feeding compared with normal food, administration of crystalloids, and parenteral nutrition in surgical patients. Significant benefits of early enteral feeding were reported in 24 of the 35 trials, especially a decrease in infectious complications, length of in-hospital stay, and health costs. No benefits were reported by 8 of the 35 trials, and some trials reported possible advert outcomes that were probably related to too early administration of enteral feeding [46].

21.6.5 Diagnosis

Early assessment of nutritional status using a validated screening tool is important in all surgical patients, including a preoperative serum albumin to detect possible malnutrition [46–48].

21.6.6 Treatment

In malnourished patients who are in need of emergency surgery, the malnutrition cannot be prevented preoperatively, but the early start of oral feeding and avoidance of days without any nutritional therapy perioperative is associated with a lower overall complication rate and decreased length of in-hospital stay [58].

Dos and Dont's
- Do: early assessment of nutritional status in emergency surgical patients.
- Do: start early feeding to decrease infectious complications, length of in-hospital stay, and health costs. If oral intake is not possible or expected to be inadequate for some time, start enteral or parenteral nutrition without any delay.
- Don't: days without any nutritional therapy perioperative.

21.7 Malignancy

21.7.1 Summary

Emergency surgery in oncological patients is often indicated because of malignancy-related obstruction of the gastrointestinal tract or infectious diseases and can mark the end-stage disease. Increased morbidity and mortality rates have been reported in oncological patients after emergency surgery, especially in patients with severe neutropenia or immunosuppression. These manifestations can be disguised, causing delay in surgery and an inferior outcome.

21.7.2 Immune Status

Oncological patients can suffer from immunosuppression because of the malignant disease or its treatment. Besides that, nutritional impairment in cancer patients is a major problem, with a reported prevalence of 51% at the first oncologist visit, also associated with diminished immune status [59]. All these elements can lead to emergency surgical conditions and can mimic signs of end-stage disease. Pain is the most common reason for oncology-related emergency department consultations (23%), while neutropenic fever is present in 4% [60]. Infections in immune-deficient patients often develop in the gastrointestinal tract, and may be masked.

21.7.3 Abdominal Complications in Malignancy

Malignant obstruction (e.g., colorectal, biliary, small intestine) and infection (e.g., postoperative wound infection, neutropenic enterocolitis, intra-abdominal infections) are the most common reasons for surgical oncological emergency department visits; 42% and 32%, respectively. Patients with a malignant obstruction often suffer from a pre-existent weak medical condition. Still, emergency surgery was performed in 61% of the patients to relieve the obstruction of the gastrointestinal tract [61]. Mortality rates after emergency surgery in patients with acute colonic obstructions range between 12 and 24%, with morbidity rates from 41 to 78%. Fuelled by these high morbidity and mortality rates, the placement of a colonic stent has been adopted from palliative care to serve as a bridge to (curative) surgery. During this time, patients could rehabilitate for definitive surgical resection. A systematic review by *Spannenburg* et al., including 27 studies with 3894 patients, has compared self-expanding metallic stents and emergency surgery for malignant large bowel obstruction. The 3-year and 5-year disease-free and overall survival did not significantly differ. However, placing a stent improved short-term surgical outcomes. The 30-day mortality and overall complication rate were lower in the stent group (respectively RR 0.65, $P = 0.01$, and RR 0.65, $P < 0.001$). Also, shorter in-hospital and ICU stays were observed (respectively mean difference -7.24, $P < 0.0001$ and -2.27, $P = 0.02$) [62].

Acute abdominal pain in neutropenic patients can be caused by neutropenic enterocolitis, a life-threatening condition, characterized by transmural inflammation of the caecum, often ascending colon and ileum, together with neutropenia. It occurs most frequently in patients with leukaemia or after high-dose chemotherapy for solid tumours. High-quality studies on neutropenic enterocolitis are lacking, but estimated incidence has been reported between 0.8 and 26% with a high mortality rate, 50–100% in some reports [63]. Clinical features typically appear 2–3 weeks after administration of chemotherapy, due to mucosal damage. Diagnosis of neutropenic enterocolitis may be delayed because clinical findings are nonspecific: abdominal pain, fever, diarrhoea or bowel wall thickening accompanied by neutropenia [64–66]. Bowel thickening >10 mm diagnosed on ultrasound or CT-scan is associated with an increased mortality rate: 60% vs. 4.2% in patients with a mural thickness of <10 mm [66, 67]. Conservative management is preferred by using broad-spectrum antibiotics and bowel rest. Only in case of bowel perforation, unstoppable haemorrhage or ischemia, emergency surgery is indicated. If possible, surgery should be postponed until recovery from neutropenia, because this is directly associated with the resolution of symptoms [68].

Neutropenic patients diagnosed with acute appendicitis often visit the emergency department with advanced disease because of their atypical presentation. Signs of peritonitis can be masked due to inadequate inflammatory response. Also, ultrasound findings may not be reproduced in some patients due to neutropenia; therefore, abdominal CT is the standard tool for diagnosis. Early appendectomy is preferred and causes no additional adverse outcomes in neutropenic patients [69, 70].

Acute cholecystitis in neutropenic patients can occur secondary to immune deficiency, as complication of locoregional treatment or nonmalignancy related because of cholelithiasis. Late emergency department presentation can result in gangrenous cholecystitis, emphysematous cholecystitis, or gallbladder perforation [71].

21.7.4 Effect of Chemotherapy

Increased morbidity and mortality rates have been reported after emergency surgery in patients on chemotherapy. Emergency surgery within 30 days of chemotherapy is associated with increased morbidity (44% vs. 39.2%, $P = 0.047$) and increased mortality rates (22.4% vs. 10.3%, $P < 0.001$) compared to controls [72]. Emergency surgery in leukaemia patients within 30 days of chemotherapy had a 57% mortality rate, with leukopenia as an important negative prognostic factor [73]. While elective surgery does not cause increased risks in patients within 30 days of chemotherapy [74]. Although leukopenia is associated with elevated morbidity and mortality after emergent abdominal surgery (45.4% vs. 26.9% ($P < 0.001$) and 24.4% vs. 10.8% ($P < 0.001$), respectively), it is not necessarily prohibitive [75]. It is essential to completely assess the risks and inform the patient before surgery.

21.7.5 Diagnosis

The heterogeneity of oncological patients is evident and therefore, the preoperative assessment is different for every patient. Management of oncological emergency patients should be done multidisciplinary, involving the oncological stage and patients' performance state [61].

21.7.6 Treatment

In most of the oncological patients who present to the emergency department with a malignant obstruction or infection, emergency surgery is performed. However, surgery often has an adverse effect on life expectancy and quality of life. Therefore, the best appropriate personalized oncological care has to be performed, preventing overtreatment and to regain clinical benefit [61].

Dos and Dont's
- Do: placement of a colonic stent for malignant large bowel obstruction in a palliative setting or to serve as a bridge to (curative) surgery.
- Do: treat neutropenic enterocolitis with conservative management using broad-spectrum antibiotics and bowel rest.
- Do: abdominal CT is the standard tool for the diagnosis of acute appendicitis in neutropenic patients.

Take-Home Messages
- The administration of perioperative stress-dose steroids in patients on chronic steroids lacks solid data.
- In transplant patients, immunosuppression claims for more aggressive treatment of acute abdominal diseases but also the direct impact of immunosuppressive therapies on postoperative complication risk is crucial.
- Similar operative risk and mortality rates have been found in HIV-positive patients who are AIDS-negative and have high CD4 cell counts (>500 cells/mm^3) compared to HIV-negative patients.
- Frailty seems to be a more accurate predictor of postoperative morbidity and mortality in elderly patients.
- The reported prevalence of malnutrition in general hospitalized patients is approximately 30% and is a common cause of immunodeficiency, causing increased morbidity and mortality.
- If possible, surgery in patients with neutropenic enterocolitis should be postponed until recovery from neutropenia, because this is directly associated with the resolution of symptoms.

Multiple Choice Questions

1. What hormone is produced in the anterior pituitary in the hypothalamic–pituitary–adrenal axis (HPAA)?
   A. Cortisol.
   B. Adrenocorticothrophic hormone (ACTH).
   C. Corticotropin-releasing hormone (CRH).
   D. Adrenaline.
2. Which of the following is not a consequence of chronic steroid therapy?
   A. Hypoglycaemia.
   B. Hyperglycaemia.
   C. Impaired wound healing.
   D. Immunosuppression.
3. What group of drugs are involved in immunosuppressive maintenance therapy when transplanted patients need surgery?
   A. Calcineurin inhibitors, antimetabolites, and corticosteroids.
   B. Corticosteroids and antibiotics.
   C. Calcineurin inhibitors, antimetabolites, antibiotics, and corticosteroids.
   D. Calcineurin inhibitors and corticosteroids.
4. What is the most common abdominal opportunistic infection primarily related to HIV/AIDS?
   A. Clostridium Difficile colitis.
   B. Abdominal tuberculosis.
   C. Neutropenic enterocolitis.
   D. Cytamegalo-Virus colitis.
5. What of the following malignancy types is not associated with HIV/AIDS?
   A. Breast cancer.
   B. Non-Hodgkin's lymphoma.
   C. Anal cancer.
   D. Kaposi's sarcoma.
6. What is the reported prevalence of malnutrition in general hospitalized patients approximately?
   A. 15%
   B. 50%
   C. 40%
   D. 30%
7. What values are used to measure nutrition status according to the GNRI (Geriatric Nutritional Risk Index)?
   A. The BMI, serum albumin concentration, and the Nutritional Risk score.
   B. The BMI, serum albumin concentration, and the ratio of actual to ideal weight.
   C. Serum albumin concentration and the ratio of actual to ideal weight.
   D. Serum albumin concentration and the Nutritional Risk score.
8. What are the most common reasons for surgical oncological emergency department visits?
   A. Anaemia and infection.
   B. Malignant obstruction and infection.
   C. Malignant obstruction and anaemia.
   D. Trauma and infection.
9. What are characteristics of neutropenic enterocolitis and when do they typically appear?
   A. Gastrointestinal perforation, often caecum, together with neutropenia, 4–7 days after administration of chemotherapy.
   B. Gastrointestinal perforation, often caecum, together with neutropenia, 2–3 weeks after administration of chemotherapy.
   C. Transmural inflammation of the caecum, often ascending colon and ileum, together with neutropenia, 4–7 days after administration of chemotherapy.
   D. Transmural inflammation of the caecum, often ascending colon and ileum, together with neutropenia, 2–3 weeks after administration of chemotherapy.
10. What treatment is preferred in neutropenic enterocolitis?
    A. Conservative treatment using broad-spectrum antibiotics and bowel rest.
    B. Emergency surgery and broad-spectrum antibiotics.
    C. Emergency surgery.
    D. Conservative treatment using steroids and bowel rest.

Answers: 1B; 2A; 3A; 4B; 5A; 6D; 7C; 8B; 9D; 10A

References

1. Jabbour SA. Steroids and the surgical patient. Med Clin North Am. 2001;85(5):1311–7.
2. Axelrod L. Perioperative management of patients treated with glucocorticoids. Endocrinol Metab Clin North Am. 2003;32(2):367–83. https://doi.org/10.1016/S0889-8529(03)00008-2.
3. Bornstein SR, Allolio B, Arlt W, Barthel A, Don-Wauchope A, Hammer GD, Husebye ES, Merke DP, Murad MH, Stratakis CA, Torpy DJ. Diagnosis and treatment of primary adrenal insufficiency: an endocrine society clinical practice guideline. J Clin Endocrinol Metab. 2016;101(2):364–89. https://doi.org/10.1210/jc.2015-1710.
4. Kehlet H, Binder C. Adrenocortical function and clinical course during and. Br J Anaesth. 1973;45(10):1043–8. https://doi.org/10.1093/bja/45.10.1043.
5. Yong SL, Coulthard P, Wrzosek A. Supplemental perioperative steroids for surgical patients with adrenal insufficiency. Cochrane Database Syst Rev. 2013;2013(10):CD005367. https://doi.org/10.1002/14651858.CD005367.pub4.
6. Groleau C, Morin SN, Vautour L, Amar-Zifkin A, Bessissow A. Perioperative corticosteroid administration: a systematic review and descriptive analysis. Perioper Med (Lond). 2018;7(1):1–8. https://doi.org/10.1186/s13741-018-0092-9.
7. Liu M, Reidy A, Saatee S, Collard CD. Perioperative steroid management: approaches based on current evidence. Anesthesiology. 2017;127(1):166–72.
8. Shapiro R, Young JB, Milford EL, Trotter JF, Bustami RT, Leichtman AB. Immunosuppression: evolution in practice and trends, 1993–2003. Am J Transplant. 2005;5(4 Pt 2):874–86. https://doi.org/10.1111/j.1600-6135.2005.00833.x.
9. de'Angelis N, Esposito F, Memeo R, Lizzi V, Martìnez-Pérez A, Landi F, Genova P, Catena F, Brunetti F, Azoulay D. Emergency abdominal surgery after solid organ transplantation: a systematic review. World J Emerg Surg. 2016;11(1):1–12. https://doi.org/10.1186/s13017-016-0101-6.
10. Maurer JR. The spectrum of colonic complications in a lung transplant population. Ann Transplant. 2000;5(3):54–7. http://www.ncbi.nlm.nih.gov/pubmed/11147030.
11. Kang JY, Hoare J, Tinto A, Subramanian S, Ellis C, Majeed A, Melville D, Maxwell JD. Diverticular disease of the colon—on the rise: a study of hospital admissions in England between 1989/1990 and 1999/2000. Aliment Pharmacol Ther. 2003;17(9):1189–95. https://doi.org/10.1046/j.1365-2036.2003.01551.x.
12. Hjern F, Johansson C, Mellgren A, Baxter NN, Hjern A. Diverticular disease and migration—the influence of acculturation to a Western lifestyle on diverticular disease. Aliment Pharmacol Ther. 2006;23(6):797–805. https://doi.org/10.1111/j.1365-2036.2006.02805.x.
13. Oor JE, Atema JJ, Boermeester MA, Vrouenraets BC, Ünlü Ç. A systematic review of complicated diverticulitis in post-transplant patients. J Gastrointest Surg. 2014;18(11):2038–46. https://doi.org/10.1007/s11605-014-2593-2.
14. Bender BS, Bender JS. Surgical issues in the management of the HIV-infected patient. Surg Clin North Am. 1993;73(2):373–88. https://doi.org/10.1016/s0039-6109(16)45988-8.
15. World Health Organization. World Health Organization. Interim WHO clinical staging of HIV/AIDS and HIV/AIDS case definitions for surveillance: African region. World Health Organization. 2005. https://doi.org/10.1097/01.nme.0000430823.37826.35.
16. Trickey A, May MT, Vehreschild JJ, Obel N, Gill MJ, Crane HM, Boesecke C, Patterson S, Grabar S, Cazanave C, Cavassini M, Shepherd L, d'Arminio Monforte A, van Sighem A, Saag M, Lampe F, Hernando V, Montero M, Zangerle R, Justice AC, Sterling T, Ingle SM, Sterne JAC. Survival of HIV-positive patients starting antiretroviral therapy between 1996 and 2013: a collaborative analysis of cohort studies. Lancet HIV. 2017;4(8):e349–56. https://doi.org/10.1016/S2352-3018(17)30066-8.
17. Kouanfack OSD, Kouanfack C, Billong SC, Cumber SN, Nkfusai CN, Bede F, Wepngong E, Hubert C, Tsague Georges GNK, Singwe MN. Epidemiology of opportunistic infections in HIV infected patients on treatment in accredited HIV treatment centers in Cameroon. Int J MCH AIDS. 2019;8(2):163–72. https://doi.org/10.21106/ijma.302.
18. Madiba TE, Muckart DJJ, Thomson SR. Human immunodeficiency disease: how should it affect surgical decision making? World J Surg. 2009;33(5):899–909. https://doi.org/10.1007/s00268-009-9969-6.
19. Watters DA. Surgery for tuberculosis before and after human immunodeficiency virus infection: a tropical perspective. Br J Surg. 1997;84(1):8–14. http://www.ncbi.nlm.nih.gov/pubmed/9043439.
20. World Health Organization. Global tuberculosis report 2020; 2020.
21. Ross M, Klotman P, Winston J. HIV-associated nephropathy: case study and review of the literature. AIDS Patient Care STDs. 2000;14(12):637–45.
22. Hernández-Ramírez RU, Shiels MS, Dubrow R, Engels EA. Cancer risk in HIV-infected people in the USA from 1996 to 2012: a population-based, registry-linkage study. Lancet HIV. 2017;4(11):e495–504. https://doi.org/10.1016/S2352-3018(17)30125-X.
23. Biggar RJ, Chaturvedi AK, Goedert JJ, Engels EA. AIDS-related cancer and severity of immunosuppression in persons with AIDS. J Natl Cancer Inst. 2007;99(12):962–72. https://doi.org/10.1093/jnci/djm010.
24. Mocroft A, Furrer HJ, Miro JM, Reiss P, Mussini C, Kirk O, Abgrall S, Ayayi S, Bartmeyer B, Braun D, Castagna A, D'Arminio Monforte A, Gazzard B, Gutierrez F, Hurtado I, Jansen K, Meyer L, Muñoz P, Obel N, Soler-Palacin P, Papadopoulos A, Raffi

F, Ramos JT, Rockstroh JK, Salmon D, Torti C, Warszawski J, De Wit S, Zangerle R, Fabre-Colin C, Kjaer J, Chene G, Grarup J, Lundgren JD. The incidence of AIDS-defining illnesses at a current CD4 count ≥200 cells/μL in the post-combination antiretroviral therapy era. Clin Infect Dis. 2013;57(7):1038–47. https://doi.org/10.1093/cid/cit423.
25. Owotade F, Ogunbodede E, Sowande O. HIV/AIDS pandemic and surgical practice in a Nigerian teaching hospital. Trop Doct. 2003;33:228–31. https://doi.org/10.1258/0049475054036832.
26. Sandler BJ, Davis KA, Schuster KM. Symptomatic human immunodeficiency virus-infected patients have poorer outcomes following emergency general surgery: a study of the nationwide inpatient sample. J Trauma Acute Care Surg. 2019;86(3):479–88. https://doi.org/10.1097/TA.0000000000002161.
27. Chichom-Mefire A, Azabji-Kenfack M, Atashili J. CD4 count is still a valid indicator of outcome in HIV-infected patients undergoing major abdominal surgery in the era of highly active antiretroviral therapy. World J Surg. 2015;39(7):1692–9. https://doi.org/10.1007/s00268-015-2994-8.
28. Deneve JL, Shantha JG, Page AJ, Wyrzykowski AD, Rozycki GS, Feliciano DV. CD4 count is predictive of outcome in HIV-positive patients undergoing abdominal operations. Am J Surg. 2010;200(6):694–700. https://doi.org/10.1016/j.amjsurg.2010.07.030.
29. Yang J, Wei G, He Y, Hua X, Feng S, Zhao Y, Chen T, Wang H, Guo L. Perioperative antiretroviral regimen for HIV/AIDS patients who underwent abdominal surgery. World J Surg. 2020;44(6):1790–7. https://doi.org/10.1007/s00268-020-05402-8.
30. Harris HW, Schecter WP. Surgical risk assessment and management in patients with HIV disease. Gastroenterol Clin North Am. 1997;26(2):377–91. https://doi.org/10.1016/S0889-8553(05)70300-9.
31. Castelo-Branco C, Soveral I. The immune system and aging: a review. Gynecol Endocrinol. 2014;30(1):16–22. https://doi.org/10.3109/09513590.2013.852531.
32. Jiang L, Zheng Z, Zhang M. The incidence of geriatric trauma is increasing and comparison of different scoring tools for the prediction of in-hospital mortality in geriatric trauma patients. World J Emerg Surg. 2020;15(1):1–8. https://doi.org/10.1186/s13017-020-00340-1.
33. Arenal JJ, Bengoechea-Beeby M. Mortality associated with emergency abdominal surgery in the elderly. Can J Surg. 2003;46(2):111–6. http://www.ncbi.nlm.nih.gov/pubmed/12691347.
34. Lin HS, Watts JN, Peel NM, Hubbard RE. Frailty and post-operative outcomes in older surgical patients: a systematic review. BMC Geriatr. 2016;16(1):157. https://doi.org/10.1186/s12877-016-0329-8.
35. Fried LP, Tangen CM, Walston J, Newman AB, Hirsch C, Gottdiener J, Seeman T, Tracy R, Kop WJ, Burke G, McBurnie MA. Frailty in older adults: evidence for a phenotype. J Gerontol A Biol Sci Med Sci. 2001;56(3):146–57. https://doi.org/10.1093/gerona/56.3.m146.
36. Rockwood K, Song X, MacKnight C, Bergman H, Hogan DB, McDowell I, Mitnitski A. A global clinical measure of fitness and frailty in elderly people. CMAJ. 2005;173(5):489–95. https://doi.org/10.1503/cmaj.050051.
37. Mariconda M, Costa GG, Cerbasi S, Recano P, Aitanti E, Gambacorta M, Misasi M. The determinants of mortality and morbidity during the year following fracture of the hip: a prospective study. Bone Joint J. 2015;97-B(3):383–90. https://doi.org/10.1302/0301-620X.97B3.34504.
38. Lee TC, Ho PS, Lin HT, Ho ML, Huang HT, Chang JK. One-year readmission risk and mortality after hip fracture surgery: a national population-based study in Taiwan. Aging Dis. 2017;8(4):402–9. https://doi.org/10.14336/AD.2016.1228.
39. Civinini R, Paoli T, Cianferotti L, Cartei A, Boccaccini A, Peris A, Brandi ML, Rostagno C, Innocenti M. Functional outcomes and mortality in geriatric and fragility hip fractures—results of an integrated, multidisciplinary model experienced by the "Florence hip fracture unit". Int Orthop. 2019;43(1):187–92. https://doi.org/10.1007/s00264-018-4132-3.
40. Panula J, Pihlajamäki H, Mattila VM, Jaatinen P, Vahlberg T, Aarnio P, Kivelä SL. Mortality and cause of death in hip fracture patients aged 65 or older—A population-based study. BMC Musculoskelet Disord. 2011;12:2–7. https://doi.org/10.1186/1471-2474-12-105.
41. Smith T, Pelpola K, Ball M, Ong A, Myint PK. Pre-operative indicators for mortality following hip fracture surgery: a systematic review and meta-analysis. Age Ageing. 2014;43(4):464–71. https://doi.org/10.1093/ageing/afu065.
42. Moja L, Piatti A, Pecoraro V, Ricci C, Virgili G, Salanti G, Germagnoli L, Liberati A, Banfi G. Timing matters in hip fracture surgery: patients operated within 48 hours have better outcomes. A meta-analysis and meta-regression of over 190,000 patients. PLoS One. 2012;7(10):e46175. https://doi.org/10.1371/journal.pone.0046175.
43. Saunders DI, Murray D, Pichel AC, Varley S, Peden CJ. Variations in mortality after emergency laparotomy: the first report of the UK emergency laparotomy network. Br J Anaesth. 2012;109(3):368–75. https://doi.org/10.1093/bja/aes165.
44. Omari AH, Khammash MR, Qasaimeh GR, Shammari AK, Yaseen MKB, Hammori SK. Acute appendicitis in the elderly: risk factors for perforation. World J Emerg Surg. 2014;9(1):1–6. https://doi.org/10.1186/1749-7922-9-6.
45. Loozen CS, Van Santvoort HC, Van Duijvendijk P, Besselink MG, Gouma DJ, Nieuwenhuijzen GA, Kelder JC, Donkervoort SC, Van Geloven AA, Kruyt PM, Roos D, Kortram K, Kornmann VN, Pronk A, Van Der Peet DL, Crolla RM, Van Ramshorst B, Bollen TL, Boerma D. Laparoscopic cholecystectomy versus percutaneous catheter drainage for acute cholecystitis in high risk patients (CHOCOLATE): multicentre randomised clinical trial. BMJ. 2018;363:k3965. https://doi.org/10.1136/bmj.k3965.

46. Weimann A, Braga M, Carli F, Higashiguchi T, Hübner M, Klek S, Laviano A, Ljungqvist O, Lobo DN, Martindale R, Waitzberg DL, Bischoff SC, Singer P. ESPEN guideline: clinical nutrition in surgery. Clin Nutr. 2017;36(3):623–50. https://doi.org/10.1016/j.clnu.2017.02.013.
47. Kondrup J, Allison SP, Elia M, Vellas B, Plauth M. ESPEN guidelines for nutrition screening 2002. Clin Nutr. 2003;22(4):415–21. https://doi.org/10.1016/S0261-5614(03)00098-0.
48. Kruizenga H, Van Keeken S, Weijs P, Bastiaanse L, Beijer S, Huisman-De Waal G, Jager-Wittenaar H, Jonkers-Schuitema C, Klos M, Remijnse-Meester W, Witteman B, Thijs A. Undernutrition screening survey in 564,063 patients: patients with a positive undernutrition screening score stay in hospital 1.4 d longer. Am J Clin Nutr. 2016;103(4):1026–32. https://doi.org/10.3945/ajcn.115.126615.
49. Felder S, Braun N, Stanga Z, Kulkarni P, Faessler L, Kutz A, Steiner D, Laukemann S, Haubitz S, Huber A, Mueller B, Schuetz P. Unraveling the link between malnutrition and adverse clinical outcomes: Association of Acute and Chronic Malnutrition Measures with blood biomarkers from different pathophysiological states. Ann Nutr Metab. 2016;68(3):164–72. https://doi.org/10.1159/000444096.
50. Sorensen J, Kondrup J, Prokopowicz J, Schiesser M, Krähenbühl L, Meier R, Liberda M. EuroOOPS: an international, multicentre study to implement nutritional risk screening and evaluate clinical outcome. Clin Nutr. 2008;27(3):340–9. https://doi.org/10.1016/j.clnu.2008.03.012.
51. Lim SL, Ong KCB, Chan YH, Loke WC, Ferguson M, Daniels L. Malnutrition and its impact on cost of hospitalization, length of stay, readmission and 3-year mortality. Clin Nutr. 2012;31(3):345–50. https://doi.org/10.1016/j.clnu.2011.11.001.
52. Havens JM, Peetz AB, Do WS, Cooper Z, Kelly E, Askari R, Reznor G, Salim A. The excess morbidity and mortality of emergency general surgery. J Trauma Acute Care Surg. 2015;78(2):306–11. https://doi.org/10.1097/TA.0000000000000517.
53. Jia Z, El Moheb M, Nordestgaard A, Lee JM, Meier K, Kongkaewpaisan N, Han K, El Hechi MW, Mendoza A, King D, Fagenholz P, Saillant N, Rosenthal M, Velmahos G, Kaafarani HMA. The geriatric nutritional risk index is a powerful predictor of adverse outcome in the elderly emergency surgery patient. J Trauma Acute Care Surg. 2020;89(2):397–404. https://doi.org/10.1097/TA.0000000000002741.
54. Bouillanne O, Morineau G, Dupant C, Coulombel I, Vincent JP, Nicolis I, Benazeth S, Cynober L, Aussel C. Geriatric nutritional risk index: a new index for evaluating at-risk elderly medical patients. Am J Clin Nutr. 2005;82(4):777–83. https://doi.org/10.1093/ajcn/82.4.777.
55. Garth AK, Newsome CM, Simmance N, Crowe TC. Nutritional status, nutrition practices and postoperative complications in patients with gastrointestinal cancer. J Hum Nutr Diet. 2010;23(4):393–401. https://doi.org/10.1111/j.1365-277X.2010.01058.x.
56. Gillis C, Carli F. Promoting perioperative metabolic and nutritional care. Anesthesiology. 2015;123(6):1455–72. https://doi.org/10.1097/ALN.0000000000000795.
57. Zhuang CL, Ye XZ, Zhang XD, Chen BC, Yu Z. Enhanced recovery after surgery programs versus traditional care for colorectal surgery: a meta-analysis of randomized controlled trials. Dis Colon Rectum. 2013;56(5):667–78. https://doi.org/10.1097/DCR.0b013e3182812842.
58. Lohsiriwat V, Jitmungngan R. Enhanced recovery after surgery in emergency colorectal surgery: review of literature and current practices. World J Gastrointest Surg. 2019;11(2):41–52. https://doi.org/10.4240/wjgs.v11.i2.41.
59. Muscaritoli M, Lucia S, Farcomeni A, Lorusso V, Saracino V, Barone C, Plastino F, Gori S, Magarotto R, Carteni G, Chiurazzi B, Pavese I, Marchetti L, Zagonel V, Bergo E, Tonini G, Imperatori M, Iacono C, Maiorana L, Pinto C, Rubino D, Cavanna L, Di Cicilia R, Gamucci T, Quadrini S, Palazzo S, Minardi S, Merlano M, Colucci G, Marchetti P, Fioretto L, Cipriani G, Barni S, Lonati V, Frassoldati A, Surace GC, Porzio G, Martella F, Altavilla G, Santarpia MC, Pronzato P, Levaggi A, Contu A, Contu M, Adamo V, Berenato R, Marchetti F, Pellegrino A, Violante S, Guida M. Prevalence of malnutrition in patients at first medical oncology visit: the PreMiO study. Oncotarget. 2017;8(45):79884–96. https://doi.org/10.18632/oncotarget.20168.
60. Yucel N, Sukru Erkal H, Sinem Akgun F, Serin M. Characteristics of the admissions of cancer patients to emergency department. J BUON. 2012;17(1):174–9. http://www.ncbi.nlm.nih.gov/pubmed/22517714.
61. Bosscher MRF, Van Leeuwen BL, Hoekstra HJ. Current management of surgical oncologic emergencies. PLoS One. 2015;10(5):1–12. https://doi.org/10.1371/journal.pone.0124641.
62. Spannenburg L, Sanchez Gonzalez M, Brooks A, Wei S, Li X, Liang X, Gao W, Wang H. Surgical outcomes of colonic stents as a bridge to surgery versus emergency surgery for malignant colorectal obstruction: a systematic review and meta-analysis of high quality prospective and randomised controlled trials. Eur J Surg Oncol. 2020;46(8):1404–14. https://doi.org/10.1016/j.ejso.2020.04.052.
63. Snydman DR, Nesher L, Rolston KVI. Neutropenic enterocolitis, a growing concern in the era of widespread use of aggressive chemotherapy. Clin Infect Dis. 2013;56(5):711–7. https://doi.org/10.1093/cid/cis998.
64. Gorschlüter M, Mey U, Strehl J, Ziske C, Schepke M, Schmidt-Wolf IGH, Sauerbruch T, Glasmacher A. Neutropenic enterocolitis in adults: systematic analysis of evidence quality. Eur J Haematol. 2005;75(1):1–13. https://doi.org/10.1111/j.1600-0609.2005.00442.x.
65. Clarenbach R, Ho K, Gorschlu M, Baumgartner S, Hahn C, Ziske C, Mey U, Heller R, Sauerbruch T, Schmidt-Wolf IGH, Eis-Hübinger AM. Abdominal infections in patients with acute leukaemia: a pro-

spective study applying ultrasonography and microbiology. Br J Haematol. 2002;117:351–8.
66. Cartoni C, Dragoni F, Micozzi A, Pescarmona E, Mecarocci S, Chirletti P, Petti MC, Meloni G, Mandelli F. Neutropenic enterocolitis in patients with acute leukemia: prognostic significance of bowel wall thickening detected by ultrasonography. J Clin Oncol. 2001;19(3):756–61. https://doi.org/10.1200/JCO.2001.19.3.756.
67. Davila ML. Neutropenic enterocolitis (Typhlitis). Imaging Gastroenterol 2018:256–257. https://doi.org/10.1016/b978-0-323-55408-4.50127-0.
68. Rodrigues FG, Dasilva G, Wexner SD. Neutropenic enterocolitis. World J Gastroenterol. 2017;23(1):42–7. https://doi.org/10.3748/wjg.v23.i1.42.
69. Kim KU, Kim JK, Won JH, Hong DS, Park HS. Acute appendicitis in patients with acute leukemia. Korean J Intern Med. 1993;8(1):40–5. https://doi.org/10.3904/kjim.1993.8.1.40.
70. Forghieri F, Luppi M, Narni F, Morselli M, Potenza L, Bresciani P, Volzone F, Rossi G, Rossi A, Trenti L, Barozzi P, Torelli G. Acute appendicitis in adult neutropenic patients with hematologic malignancies. Bone Marrow Transplant. 2008;42(10):701–3. https://doi.org/10.1038/bmt.2008.235.
71. Kogut MJ, Bastawrous S, Padia S, Bhargava P. Hepatobiliary oncologic emergencies: imaging appearances and therapeutic options. Curr Probl Diagn Radiol. 2013;42(3):113–26. https://doi.org/10.1067/j.cpradiol.2012.08.003.
72. Sullivan MC, Roman SA, Sosa JA. Does chemotherapy prior to emergency surgery affect patient outcomes? Examination of 1912 patients. Ann Surg Oncol. 2012;19(1):11–8. https://doi.org/10.1245/s10434-011-1844-7.
73. Koretz MJ, Neifeld JP. Emergency surgical treatment for patients with acute leukemia. Surg Gynecol Obstet. 1985;161(2):149–51. http://www.ncbi.nlm.nih.gov/pubmed/3860992.
74. Fahy BN, Aloia TA, Jones SL, Bass BL, Fischer CP. Chemotherapy within 30 days prior to liver resection does not increase postoperative morbidity or mortality. HPB. 2009;11(8):645–55. https://doi.org/10.1111/j.1477-2574.2009.00107.x.
75. Gulack BC, Englum BR, Lo DD, Nussbaum DP, Keenan JE, Scarborough JE, Shapiro ML. Leukopenia is associated with worse but not prohibitive outcomes following emergent abdominal surgery. J Trauma Acute Care Surg. 2015;79(3):437–43. https://doi.org/10.1097/TA.0000000000000757.

Pregnant Women

22

Pintar Tadeja

22.1 Introduction

Learning Objectives
- Assess, resuscitate, and stabilize a surgical emergency patient's condition rapidly and accurately and comprehensive strategy
- Understand the basic pathophysiology of pregnancy and surgical and non-surgical emergency
- Evaluate patients with surgical priority, fetal and maternal urgent surgical/non-surgical clinical situations
- Perform a focused examination in pregnant women with special focus on fetal urgent pathology
- Explain the importance of adequate resuscitation in limiting secondary fetal and maternal morbidity and mortality
- Determine the need for pregnant /obstetrical patient transfer, admission, consultation, or discharge
- Arrange appropriately for a patient's inter-hospital or intra-hospital transfer (what, who, when, how)

Identifying pregnant and obstetric patients at risk for clinical deterioration of baseline or pregnancy-related disease has an important impact to critical illness. Proper and immediate identification is a mandatory comprehensive strategy [1] based on early transfer to high-risk center, and planned and timely proper intervention provides reduced trends in maternal and fetal morbidity and preterm mortality [1–3].

Maternal adaptation to pregnancy corresponds to increased plasma volume (50%) and related red cell mass increase (20%) and this resulting in the pregnancy-related anemia with average hematocrit value of 31–33% [2–4]. Basic physiological adaptations in a healthy pregnancy alter the bleed-

P. Tadeja (✉)
University Medical Center Ljubljana,
Ljubljana, Slovenia

Medical Faculty, University of Ljubljana,
Ljubljana, Slovenia
e-mail: tadeja.pintar@kclj.si

© The Author(s), under exclusive license to Springer Nature Switzerland AG 2023
F. Coccolini, F. Catena (eds.), *Textbook of Emergency General Surgery*,
https://doi.org/10.1007/978-3-031-22599-4_22

ing response with delayed regulatory loops of hypovolemic shock. Regulatory mechanisms involved are cardiac output and uterine blood flow with corresponding increase in cardiac output in the second trimester and uterine blood flow up to the end of pregnancy. Compensatory mechanisms involved in maternal hemorrhage are reduced uterine blood flow resulting in fetal distress before any maternal clinical manifestation of tachycardia and hypotension. Early maternal warning criteria represent a useful task for adequate and proper decision-making process: systolic blood pressure (<90 and >160 mmHg), diastolic blood pressure (>100 mmHg), heart rate (<50 and >100 beats/min), respiratory rate (<10 and >30/min), oxygen saturation on room air (<95%), oliguria (<35 mL/h for more than 2 h), psychological disturbances: agitation, confusion, unresponsiveness. Patients in preeclampsia report non-remitting headache and shortness of breath [3–5].

In a clinical examination of a pregnant woman with a focus on the cardiovascular system, normal conditions may include: a bounding or collapsing pulse, an ejection systolic murmur loud and audible all over the precordium, present the first heart sound loud and a third heart sound in common with ectopic beats and peripheral edema [2–7]. Due to adaptive cardiac mechanisms as normal ECG interpretation in late pregnancy we find atrial and ventricular ectopics, Q wave (small) and inverted T wave in lead III, ST-segment depression and T-wave inversion in the inferior and lateral leads, and left-axis shift of QRS [8].

Respiratory alkalosis (30 mmHg) in pregnancy corresponds to an increase in tidal volume (500–700 mL) due to increased oxygen consumption and increased resting ventilation (40%, physiological hyperventilation) thus increasing respiratory capacity mediated with increased progesterone level [6–10]. Decreased pulmonary vascular resistance (PVR) and no increase in pulmonary capillary wedge pressure (PCWP) combined to reduced capillary pressure gradient (colloid osmotic pressure is reduced by 10–15%) is making pregnant women in risk for pulmonary oedema; in clinical situations with increased cardiac preload (hypervolemia) and/or maternal hypertensive disease with increased pulmonary capillary permeability (preeclampsia) prompt that clinical and instrumental evaluation is urgently needed [8, 10–12].

Metabolic compensation via increased bicarbonate levels (19–20 MEq/L) and increased metabolic rate is enhanced for 20% with slight increase in basal body temperature. Due to physiological changes in pregnancy and compensatory mechanisms, there is a poor correlation in clinical signs significant for hypovolemia: mild tachycardia, tachypnea, narrowed pulse pressure, agitation, and normal blood pressure are warning signs for hypovolemic shock. Prompt assessment of fetal well-being including cardiotocography on gestation time is mandatory for evaluation of fetal distress [4, 10, 13].

22.2 Anatomic Changes in Pregnancy

Due to anatomic and physiologic changes of pregnancy, there is the urgent need for proper assessment, management, and prevention of trauma and critically ill circumstances [6, 7, 9].

Anatomic changes include elevated diaphragm, delayed gastric emptying, and progressive uterine growth. Uterus enlargement displaces maternal organs upwards, and in the third trimester of pregnancy, the majority of the gastrointestinal tract may be found above the inferior costal margins and subsequent elevation of the diaphragm is present as much as 4 cm.

Displacement of intra-abdominal portion of esophagus into the thorax in addition to progesterone relaxing effect causes relaxation of lower esophageal sphincter (LOS) manifesting as gastro-esophageal reflux disease of pregnancy.

Uterus enlargement compresses the vena cava and decreases venous return, resulting in a 30% drop in cardiac output ("supine hypotensive syndrome") and direct compression to ureters that in common to reduced ureteral tone and peristalsis lead to bilateral ureteral dilatation and hydronephrosis with higher incidence in the left side. As a consequence higher incidence of urinary tract infection and nephrolithiasis is present.

An increase in threshold to pain at full term and in labor corresponds to increased levels of plasma endorphins and progesterone [11–13].

Thyroid gland enlargement is a consequence of both follicular hyperplasia and increased vascularity.

To compensate for the change in center of gravity, musculoskeletal adaptive mechanisms develop, among most typical: exaggeration of lumbar lordosis with anterior flexion of neck and downward movement of shoulders. Due to hormonal (relaxin, progesterone) and mechanical effects of pregnancy, joint laxity is increased to prepare for childbirth.

Hemodynamic measurement	Term pregnancy (36–38 weeks of gestation)	Change to non-pregnant women
Heart rate	83 ± 10	↑ (10–20 beats/min)
Cardiac output (CO) (l/min)	6.2 ± 1	↑ (50%) (uterus 17%, breast 2% CO)
Systemic vascular resistance (dyne s/cm^5)	1210 ± 266	↓ (20%)
Colloid oncotic pressure (mmHg)	18 ± 1.5	↓
Pulmonary capillary wedge pressure (mmHg)	3.6 ± 2.5	No change
Central venous pressure (CVP, mmHg)	3.6 ± 2.5	No change

22.3 Physiological Changes in Pregnancy

Adaptations in pregnancy are targeted to enable sufficient oxygen and nutrient supply to growing fetus and mother. Different adaptations correspond to pregnancy timing, and for clinical implication, careful evaluation is needed; laboratory values are not in the same range to non-pregnant woman.

22.3.1 Body Fluid Homeostasis

AT the term, overall increase of body fluid volume is estimated to be 6.5–8 L, divided to fetus, placenta, and amniotic fluid for about 3.5 L and increase in maternal blood volume for 3.5 L with the rest distributed to extracellular fluid volume, adipose tissue, and breast. Increased water intake and retention are present due to lowered osmotic threshold, thus leading to sodium and potassium retention but the concentration of potassium is low (3–4 mEq/L, mmol/L) and 0.2 mEq/L (mmol/L).

22.3.2 Cardiovascular System

Adaptive cardiovascular changes in pregnancy are cardiac output (CO), heart rate, blood pressure, vascular compliance, capacitance, vascular resistance, and ventricular dimensions. [2, 12, 13]

Cardiac output is affected with maternal positioning, i.e., increased output is present in lateral recumbent and knee-chest positions. In supine position, the gravid uterus compresses inferior vena cava with possible complete venous return obstruction from lower extremities with consequent nausea, diaphoresis, headedness, and syncope; placement in the left lateral position interrupts these clinical signs [12–14].

Due to the relaxation effect of progesterone to smooth muscle, vasodilatation occurs mediated with a fall in systemic vascular resistance with lowering systemic blood pressure regardless of increased heart rate. Eccentric left ventricular hypertrophy and dilatation occur due to increased left ventricular-end diastolic volume and are pregnancy-related adaptations to enhance pumping capacity needed to increase left end-diastolic volumes [11].

22.3.3 Respiratory System

Pregnancy affects static lung volumes, gas exchange, and ventilation. Progesterone mediates upper respiratory tract edema, hyperemia, congestion persist to the term. Occasional nosebleeds are estrogen related apart to rhinitis-like symptoms. Due to the progressive growth of the uterus, the circumference of the abdomen and the diameter and circumference of the thorax increase, widening the costal angles and consequently elevates the resting position of the diaphragm up to 4–5 cm. The costal angles widen by 50%, from 68° to 103° corresponding to overall 5–7 cm increase of circumference of the lower thoracic wall. Functional adaptations to pregnancy due to structural one change static lung volumes: functional residual capacity (FRC) decreases 300–500 mL (17–20%), due to elevated diaphragm; FRC, divided to expiratory reserve volume is decreased for 100–300 mL (15–20%) and residual volume 200–300 mL (20–25%). The decrease of FRC is balanced with increase in the inspiratory capacity volume up to 100–300 mL (5–10%). Spirometry reveals normal bronchial flow [10–14]. Twenty percent increase in oxygen consumption in pregnancy covers progressively increasing metabolic demands of both, the mother and growing fetus with particular increase during labor up to 60% and is centrally regulated via increasing progesterone levels stimulating increased respiratory drive with the related increase of minute ventilation up to 30–50%, predominantly regulated via increase in tidal volume (minute ventilation = tidal volume × respiratory rate). Due to increased demands, 50–70% increase in alveolar ventilation is reached via increased minute volume combined with physiological decrease of FRC; the drive is with increasing alveolar gradient obtained with increased alveolar oxygen partial pressure (P_{AO2}) and discrete reduction of arterial partial carbon dioxide partial pressure (Pa_{CO2}), thus resulting in mild increase in blood pH [2, 10, 15]. Carbon dioxide gradient facilitates child to mother transport and with additional compensatory mechanism that involves increased renal bicarbonate excretion, compensation of mild respiratory alkalosis is balanced.

Sleep disorders in pregnancy are associated with gestational age and are progressively increasing to the term with typical sleep efficiency and continuity decrease, daytime somnolence, and night-time awakening; if snoring, excessive daytime sleepiness and self-reported or witnessed apneic attacks are present, pregnancy-related hypoventilation and obstructive sleep apnea need to be excluded due to increased risk of intrauterine growth restriction and high correlation to gestational hypertension [16, 17].

Blood gas measurement	Adult non-pregnant	Pregnant, 3rd trimester
pH	7.38–7.44	7.39–7.45
Oxygen arterial partial pressure (mmHg [kPa])	80–100	92–107
Carbon dioxide arterial partial pressure (mmHg [kPa])	35–45	25–33
Bicarbonate (mmol/L or mEq/L)	21–20	16–22

Values of arterial blood gas in pregnancy

22.3.4 Nutritional, Gastrointestinal, and Hepatobiliary Adaptations

Due to modifications of hepatobiliary and gastrointestinal systems in pregnant woman, different clinical signs may appear: (1) nausea and vomiting are the result of rising human chorionic gonadotropin levels causing estrogen production with the worse clinical manifestation in hyperemesis gravidarum, associated with vomiting, profound dehydration, electrolyte disbalance, weight loss, and the need of hospitalization; (2) gastroesophageal reflux (GERD) is mediated by lower esophageal sphincter (LES) tone reduction, increased intra-abdominal pressure and progesterone mediated smooth muscle relaxation; decrease in gastrointestinal motility tone and delayed discharge of gall bladder change bowel habits and increase the risk of gallstones, biliary colic, and cholecystitis; (3) synthetic capacity and activity of the liver are increased with increased production of total albumin (15%), fibrinogen, transferrin, ceruloplasmin, and the binding proteins, for sex steroids, including corticosteroids, and thyroid hormones [2, 11, 18]. Elevated plasma AF levels are due to release from the placenta, while the values of other liver enzymes are in the normal range. Mild subclinical cholestasis is triggered via circulating estrogen that increase acid production and secretion;

(4) estrogen-related spider angiomata, palmar erythema, lowered serum albumin, and total protein concentrations due to dilution effect might be a normal clinical presentation and not related to liver disease; (5) due to increased appetite, the pregnant woman consumes an additional 300 kcal/day average and many women complain to increased salivation with average 1–2 L of saliva (ptyalism) loss per day causing inability for swallowing normal amounts of saliva rather than overproduction.

Significant metabolic adaptation to pregnancy is present in lipid profile with increasing tendency to the term: high-density lipoprotein-cholesterol levels increase by 20%, low density lipoprotein level is increased and triglyceride level is increased up to 250% to non-pregnant women [2, 18, 19]. Metabolic adjustment of mineral and vitamin levels ensures the growth of a healthy fetus and the maintenance of pregnancy: lowering retinol (vitamin A), α-tocopherol (vitamin E) levels parallel the increase in cholesterol, 1,25-dihydroxyvitamin D increase in pregnancy, and 25-hydroxyvitamin D remains unchanged. Besides, circulating levels of trace elements depend on serum albumin level; ceruloplasmin increase due to accelerated liver synthesis and lower zinc concentration is due to lowered serum albumin concentration.

22.3.5 Genitourinary System

Hormonal related increased interstitial volume, urinary dead space, and increased renal vasculature conditional changes are the cause of the increase in kidney volume and weight. Dilatation of renal calyx, pelvis and bilateral ureter dilatation up to 2 cm in the term are typical diagnostic entities which could be misdiagnosed with ureteral obstruction. Elevation of the bladder and trigonal dilatation combined with increased vascular tortuosity are typical findings in the third trimester of pregnancy and are joined with increased incidence of microhematuria, urgency, and increased urinary frequency and stress incontinence of decreased bladder capacity. Pregnancy-related hypervolemia corresponds to 50% increase of renal plasma flow, 40–50% increase of glomerular filtration rate (GFR), and resulted relative decrease in plasma creatinine, urea, uric acid, and blood urea nitrogen concentration. Creatinine clearance is increased to 150–200 mL/min (non-pregnant 120 mL/min). Due to elevated GFR (mL/min), it consequently increases urinary excretion of glucose, proteins, amino acids which triggers the phenomenon of glycosuria, also the consequence of modified tubular resorptive capability. Up to 2.0 g of amino acid excretion, 300 mg proteinuria, and 30 mg albuminuria, excretion of 8.75–15.5 mmol/day of calcium are due to physiological adaptation to regulatory mechanisms in pregnancy [18–20].

22.3.6 Hematology and Coagulation

The increase in maternal blood volume in total is 1500–1600 mL, (of which plasma volume is 1200 mL, 300–400 mL red blood cell volume) maintain physiologically requirements of developing maternal-fetal unit and is even greater in multiparous gestation; insufficient increase in plasma volume is related to intrauterine growth retardation and preeclampsia. Regulative response to pregnancy is complex and involves hormonal mediators such as erythropoietin, human placental lactogen, estrogen, and progesterone [6, 9, 11, 18, 20, 21]. Rapid increase in maternal plasma volume in early pregnancy and delayed rise in red blood cells volume cause a drop in the hematocrit for about 10% and are named "physiological anemia of pregnancy." The increase in circulating numbers of segmental neutrophils and granulocytes representing contribute to increase in white blood count; therefore, the interpretation of the infection, especially during childbirth, is extremely demanding. In a dramatic decrease in platelet count it is necessary to exclude preeclampsia, placental abruption, and/or HELPP syndrome. The risk of thromboembolic events is increased to five-fold and is correlated to Virchow's triad: vessel wall injury, increased venous stasis, and hypercoagulability. The mechanisms involved are enlarging uterus compression to inferior vena cava and pelvic veins, pregnancy-related hypercoagulability: disbalance of procoagulant, anticoagulant, and fibrinolytic and unchanged levels of factors I (plasma fibrinogen), VII, VIII, X related to markedly increased, factors II, V, and unchanged factor IX. Pregnancy-related decreased fibrinolytic activity through an increase in plasminogen activator inhibitor 1 and 2 has procoagulable effect in addition to decreased plasma level of total protein S and no change in plasma level of protein C and antithrombin III [2, 22–24].

22.3.7 Adrenal Glands

Biochemical and metabolic changes during pregnancy maintain maternal, early embryogenic, and later fetal growth and development and are important regulatory mechanism responsible for energy turnover and nutrient transportation. Also importantly, they can have different impact to maternal and fetal outcome [2, 9, 11, 25, 26]. Adapted physiology in pregnant women is related to increased circulating cortisol levels (2 to 3-fold higher at term than to non-pregnant women), estrogen-induced increased corticosteroid binding globulin (CBG), increased cortisol half-life secondary to decrease in hepatic clearance, and placental production of cortisol-releasing hormone (CRH); adaptations are related to adrenal hypertrophy and enhanced response to synthetic ACTH administration. Adrenal disorders in pregnancy are associated with severe complications, if undiagnosed and poorly managed favor maternal and fetal morbidity and mortality. An overall increase in total serum cortisol concentration, free cortisol, aldosterone, deoxycorticosterone, corticosteroid-binding globulin (2× non-pregnant), and adrenocorticotropic hormone with increasing tendency up to the pregnancy term and diurnal pattern of cortisol is maintained. No change of catecholamines, vanillylmandelic acid, and metanephrines in urinary excretion is present. Selected diagnostic tool represents blood samples for serum electrolytes, glucose, adrenocorticotropic hormone (ACTH), and cortisol.

Assisted reproduction and advances in medical diagnostics and treatment in cases with reduced fertility significantly increased the probability of conception and pregnancy in women with preexisting adrenal disease.

22.3.8 Pancreas

Fasting hypoglycemia, postprandial hyperglycemia, and hyperinsulinemia are typically present as a result of estrogen and progesterone islet cell stimulation and enlargement, beta-cells hyperplasia, insulin secretion, and increased peripheral tissue sensitivity to insulin. These anabolic circumstances enhance increased glucose utilization, decreased gluconeogenesis, and increased glycogen storage. In the third trimester peripheral tissue insulin resistance develops due to rising levels of progesterone, cortisol, human placental lactogen, and glucagon in common to decreased insulin receptor binding. Higher postprandial glucose plasma levels and insulin resistance enhance glucose transport to the growing fetus and under-regulated results in gestational diabetes.

22.3.9 Pituitary Gland

Estrogen-mediated stimulation causes proliferation of prolactin-producing cells. Under proliferation stimulus, gland enlargement renders it more susceptible to blood supply with increasing risk for infarction. 10 times increase of prolactin in the term to non-pregnant circumstances is also prolonged in lactating women and influenced with the frequency of lactating. Also, oxytocin levels increase up to 75 ng/L at the term, representing 7.5 times magnification.

22.3.10 Thyroid Gland

Increased thyroid gland vascularity is triggering follicular hyperplasia. Thyroid -binding globulin enhanced production causes an increase in total thyroxine and total triiodothyronine concentration with a peak level in the second trimester of pregnancy. Free thyroxine concentration remains at the baseline level in the first trimester and presents 25% decrease in mean concentration in the second trimester of pregnancy. Thyrotropic effect of human chorionic gonadotropin in the first trimester triggers transient decrease in thyroid stimulating hormone and increase in free thyroxine plasma level [2, 26].

22.3.11 Immunology

Maternal and fetal adaptive mechanisms are responsible for increased women susceptibility for viral infections. The shift of T-helper type-1 mediated cellular immunity to type-2 mediated humoral immunity occurs due to altered fetal major histocompatibility complex class-1 expression and maternal uterine natural killer cells combined with a shifting effect of T-helper cells cytokine profile from type 1 to 2 [22, 25, 27].

22.4 Surgical Emergency in Pregnant Women

Surgical emergency represents a spectrum of medical conditions that relay immediate surgical intervention due to traumatic and non-traumatic pathology and is managed to acute threat to life of mother and child. Non-obstetrical surgical procedures performed each year, impacting up to 2% of all pregnancies. When immediately evaluating the clinical condition of the mother and child, it is necessary to select an appropriate diagnostic method for assessing the condition with the risks and benefits of diagnostic methodology and therapy on the mother and the fetus as taking into account the physiological adjustments in pregnancy, the age of the fetus, pregnancy-related illnesses and diseases, and any surgical procedures performed by the mother prior to pregnancy. Delayed diagnostic procedures and evaluation of surgical emergency care in pregnant women have significant impact to maternal and fetal morbidity and mortality [28–31].

Simple division of acute surgical conditions in pregnant women covers:
1. Non-gynecological and non-obstetric
2. Gynecological and non-obstetric
3. Obstetric

The incidence is 1/635 during pregnancy. The clinical examination of the pregnant woman should take into account the expanding uterus, which displaces other intra-abdominal organs and thus means the presentation of otherwise typical clinical signs at an atypical site and also, the high prevalence of nausea, vomiting, and abdominal pain routinely encountered in the normal obstetric patient. The most common non-obstetrical emergencies requiring surgery during pregnancy are acute appendicitis and cholecystitis.

Diagnostic imaging protocol during pregnancy has to point out the risks of radiation including fetal death, growth retardation, microcephaly, malformations, mental retardation, and childhood cancers.

The fetal dose of concern for teratogenesis is probably in the range of 10–20 rads and exposure of <5 rads has not been associated with an increase in fetal anomalies or pregnancy loss. Proper decision for the appropriate workup for any pregnant patient has to respect the basic principle to offer optimal care for pregnant women and growing child taking into account the duration of pregnancy, clinical circumstances, and possible specifics of each pregnancy.

Low dose abdominal CT of 0.3 rads scan can only be performed to evaluate abdominal pathology [32–37].

Ultrasound poses no known risk to the growing fetus and is used in identifying appendicitis, cholecystitis, and free fluid after abdominal trauma, also as a Fast US modality in trauma patient

MRI emerging has an important role in acute abdomen and precisely in combined maternal and child pathology. It is a mandatory diagnostic tool in urgent surgical interventions. In unclear clinical circumstances it is an important diagnostic tool for cases of acute appendicitis, ovarian torsion, uterine rupture, and small bowel obstruction (SBO), complications of inflammatory bowel disease (IBD), biliary disease, degenerating fibroids, adnexal masses, urinary tract obstruction or infection or both, and venous thromboembolic disease with the possibility of pregnancy reacutisation. Diffusion-weighted imaging DWI is a functional sequence performed during an MRI exam, and in the absence of gadolinium contrast, can increase the visibility of inflammation, abscesses, and tumors, acute pelvic pain, adnexal masses, cancer diagnosis and staging, and morbidly adherent placenta [31, 32, 37].

Radiation exposure during endoscopic retrograde cholangiopancreatography (ERCP) can be reduced to a level significantly below 5 rads and minimizing exposure is obtained with using lead shielding (placed underneath the pregnant patient), maximizing distance between the patient and the X-ray source, and decreasing fluoroscopy times. ERCP should continue to be the procedure of choice for bile duct decompression in pregnancy to prevent potentially life-threatening complications to both mother and fetus. NR-ERCP (non-radiation) with empiric biliary aspiration and CBD (common biliary duct) stenting might be used and after delivery, a repeat ERCP is performed to remove the stent and ensure CBD clearance. Stent placement without fluoroscopy might lead to the stent misplacement either in the gallbladder or before the stone, and postprocedural US is mandatory to confirm the position of the stent. Magnetic resonance cholangiopancreatography (MRCP), choledochoscopy, and endoscopic ultrasound have all been used to confirm clearance of the biliary system [37–39].

Laparoscopy is an important diagnostic and therapeutic tool, well tolerated by both mother and fetus and has minimal adverse effects in all trimesters. In the laparoscopic approach, we must take into account the fundamental features, i.e., safe trocar insertion depending on the body habitus and degree of pregnancy. Open trocar placement via Hasson technique or insertion of the Veress needle into an alternate site, Palmer's point (left upper quadrant, 3 cm below the costal margin in the medioclavicular line) is recommended to avoid injury to the uterus. In the third trimester, after 26 gestational week only open technic trocar placement is recommended in the vertical or over the point of maximal tenderness. Any manipulation of the uterus is advised against and immediate preoperative and postoperative fetal monitoring should be regular clinical practice [40–42].

22.5 Acute Abdomen in Pregnancy

Acute abdominal pain in pregnancy can occur due to obstetric factors and non-obstetric factors. The diagnostic approach of acute abdomen during pregnancy should be targeted to the gestation, concomitant diseases, and pregnancy risk factors and taking into account physiological adaptations in pregnancy. Any delay in diagnostic and therapeutic modalities can lead to adverse outcomes for both the mother and fetus [29, 40, 41].

22.6 Etiology and Incidence

Pregnancy-related (obstetric)	Non-pregnancy-related causes (non-obstetric)	Exacerbated by pregnancy	Extra-abdominal etiology
Early pregnancy	Appendicitis 1/1000	GERD	Cardiac pain
Miscarriage	Cholecystitis 1/2000	Gallbladder disease	NSAP
Ectopic pregnancy 19.7/1000	Biliary colic	Acute cystitis	Pleuritic pain
Molar pregnancy	Acute pancreatitis 3/10000	Acute pyelonephritis	Psychological drug abuse/withdrawal
Ovarian cyst (torsion, rupture) 5/10000	Peptic ulcer rare/BS	Musculoskeletal pain	Herpes zoster infection
Degeneration of uterine fibroids rare	Urolithiasis		
Round ligament pain	Intestinal obstruction 1/500		
Ruptured uterus 1/8000–15,000			
Ruptured uterus with a risk 1/1633 deliveries			
Late pregnancy	IBD		
Placental abruption	Rupture aneurysm		
AFLP	Trauma		
Abdominal pregnancy	**Medical**		
HELLP syndrome	Gastroenteritis		
Rupture uterus	Porphyria		
Fibroid degeneration	Sickle cell crisis		
Fallopian tube torsion	Deep vein thrombosis		
Uterine torsion			
Rupture of the rectus muscle			
Polyhydramnios			
Symphysiolysis			

AFLP acute fatty liver of pregnancy, *GERD* gastroesophageal reflux disease, *HELLP* hemolysis, elevated liver enzymes, and low platelet count, *IBD* inflammatory bowel disease, *NSAP* nonspecific abdominal pain

---

Dos and Don'ts
- Pain, tenderness, and muscular rigidity are clinical signs of acute abdominal pathology which require targeted multidisciplinary diagnostic evaluation and treatment in pregnant women.
- Surgical and non-surgical emergencies in pregnant women are related to concomitant diseases and nonspecific pathology and trauma—careful clinical examination, medical history, and acute care surgery indications should be evaluated.
- Knowledge of adaptation mechanisms in pregnancy enables correct interpretation of clinical investigation methods and techniques, laboratory results, and appropriate therapeutic action.
- Knowledge of physiological adaptation mechanisms is essential for the selection of appropriate investigative techniques in the mother and fetus, which provide a reliable answer to the clinical question and the fetus and the pregnant woman exposed to the smallest possible side effects of investigative methods and medications.

Take-Home Messages
- Physiological adaptations in pregnancy are the basis for the identification of acute surgical and non-surgical emergency conditions in pregnant women.
- Multidisciplinary treatment of acute conditions in pregnancy is warranted to optimize outcome for both the mother and her fetus. The sequence of diagnostic and therapeutic procedures requires knowledge of the basic adjustment mechanisms in pregnancy, recognition of clinical signs, and interpretation of the results of investigative techniques.
- Non-obstetric cause of acute abdomen during pregnancy occurs in 1/500–635 pregnancies. Predisposing factors might be related to general conditions (cholecystolithiasis, acute appendicitis), related to trauma, concomitant diseases deterioration, and violence related.
- Administration of vasopressors in pregnant women is indicated only in case of for intractable resistant to fluid resuscitation due to adverse effect to placental perfusion. After mid-pregnancy, the gravid uterus compresses inferior vena cava and manual displacement of left lateral tilt is mandatory to increase cardiac output and venous return.
- The assessment, stabilization, and care of the trauma injured pregnant women are the first priority; then, if the fetus is viable (≥23 weeks), fetal heart rate auscultation and fetal monitoring should be initiated (electronic fetal monitoring for at least 4 h) and obstetrical consultation and care initiated.
- Interpretation of adaptive physiological mechanisms in pregnancy and multidisciplinary management of traumatic and non-traumatic pregnancy emergency clinical situations should be the priority of care to obtain high standards or fetal and maternal care and improve short and long-term treatment results.
- Selection of investigative techniques must be directed; with minimal exposure to the fetus, it must provide a reliable and rapid diagnosis. Interpretation of results requires in-depth knowledge of adaptation mechanisms and pregnancy-related specifics.

Multiple Choice Questions

1. In daily clinical practice routine use of physiologically based tools
   A. Allows good risk prediction when using the one with the highest predictive value
   B. Based on a good clinical examination in practice, a rapid risk assessment can be performed
   C. **The use of prognostic indicators significantly reduces the risk of complications in the pregnant women and fetus, as on the basis of indicators we place the pregnant woman in the necessary level of intensive care; MOEWS, SOS, and OCI assessment are mandatory allocating pregnant women for the level of care**
   D. The incidence of critically ill pregnant women is about 1.37%, routine use of the calculation of risk factors for adverse disease in the mother and premature birth in the fetus does not significantly change the results of treatment.

2. Pregnant women creates the perfect surrounding of protection, development, and nourishment of the growing fetus. Bleeding protects the growing fetus against blood loss with the next mechanisms:
   A. Increased uterine flow
   B. Reduced urine output resulting in fetal distress before any maternal clinical

manifestation of tachycardia and hypotension

C. Maternal prognostic factors do not reflect the degree of risk to the fetus

D. **Physiological response to bleeding (urine excretion, blood pressure, respiration), including changes in the mental state of the pregnant woman are warning signs on the basis of which it is necessary to decide on rapid and appropriate action, i.e., intensive monitoring of the pregnant woman and fetus**

3. At the check-up in the outpatient clinic, the pregnant woman is examined at 32 weeks of pregnancy. We find shortness of breath, pretibial edema, symphysis pain, and the pregnant woman complains of increased thirst, smoked more, and drank salty fluids. She urinated less frequently than in previous days. What would be the explanation:

A. Decreased pulmonary vascular resistance (PVR) and increase in pulmonary capillary wedge pressure increase capillary pressure gradient and thus resulting in water retention

B. With increased cardiac preload (hypervolemia) and/or maternal hypertensive disease with increased pulmonary capillary permeability

C. **Decreased pulmonary vascular resistance (PVR) and no increase in pulmonary capillary wedge pressure (PCWP) combined to reduced capillary pressure gradient (colloid osmotic pressure is reduced by 10–15%) is making pregnant women in risk for pulmonary edema**

D. Increased pulmonary vascular resistance (PVR) and increase in pulmonary capillary wedge pressure (PCWP) combined to increased capillary pressure gradient is making pregnant women in risk for pulmonary oedema

4. Fetal distress is regulated via maternal metabolic compensation. 20% increase in metabolic rate there is a poor correlation to clinical signs

A. Related to hypovolemia

B. Normal blood pressure is a sufficient diagnostic tool to assess the clinical condition, as accelerated metabolism does not significantly contribute to changes in blood pressure of pregnant women

C. Tachycardia, normal pulse, and tachypnea are favorable indicators that do not indicate a risk to the fetus and pregnant women, even with moderate blood loss

D. **Fetal distress evaluation in relative stable maternal clinical situation should not be postponed due to fetal endangerment with compensatory mechanisms present**

5. Physiological changes in pregnancy, such as tachycardia, swelling of the legs, and dyspnea provide a wide overlap between the clinical symptoms of venous thromboembolism (VTE) and symptoms caused. Elevated risk of VTE with potentially fatal pulmonary embolism during pregnancy should reduce the threshold to test for pulmonary embolism during pregnancy. In clinical scenario of worsening chest pain, dyspnea with or without hemoptysis or tachycardia

A. The d-dimer level below the prespecified threshold and compression ultrasonography of both legs are safe diagnostic tool to establish diagnosis

B. **Low dose CT pulmonary angiography or ventilation-perfusion scanning without compromising safety should be performed depending on the trimester presentation**

C. Assessment of clinical probability with the use of the revised Geneva score, high-sensitivity d-dimer testing, compression ultrasonography of both legs

irrespective of symptoms represent a safe diagnostic tool irrespective to duration of pregnancy
D. Applying a d-dimer threshold on the basis of pretest probability of pulmonary embolism is a useful diagnostic tool in first trimester

6. Significant systemic immunological adaptation during pregnancy indicate highly dynamic co-operative interactions between the maternal and fetal immune system. Sepsis per se accounts for about 12.5% of all deaths in women during or within 42 days of the end of pregnancy and major concurrent physiological (e.g., circulatory changes, increased abdominal pressure) and endocrinological changes clearly modulate these risks. According to the complexity and adaptive immunological mechanisms, teasing out how specific endocrinological, physiological, and immunological factors increase the risk of infection require careful considerations. According to:
A. **Increased maternal severity is presented in invasive group *Haemophilus influenzae* infection, invasive pneumococcal disease, primary *Herpes simplex* virus infection, *Varicella Zoster* virus infection**
B. Severe adverse outcomes are related to tuberculosis and malaria
C. No correlation to toxoplasmosis, mumps, measles, rubella, and influenza was established to fetal outcomes
D. Failure to induce systemic changes related to adaptive mechanisms is not related to adverse pregnancy outcomes in healthy women; this may be more likely in women with underlying autoimmune diseases.

7. The 32-year-old pregnant woman was referred to an emergency surgery clinic for vomiting, abdominal pain, and developing shock. Relatives said she vomited a lot, took higher doses of medication than usual, and occasionally had diarrhea. Ultrasound of the abdomen showed mild bleeding in the retroperitoneum and severe electrolyte imbalance, and elevated inflammatory markers.
A. **Hemorrhage, sepsis, and adrenal vein thrombosis are highly suspicious to adrenal disease in women previously treated with steroids. Prompt intravenous saline solution should be administrated and hydrocortisone administration should be administrated in continuous infusion 200–300 mg/24 h to reduce the incidence of poor fetal and maternal outcome**
B. In women previously treated with steroids, no dose adjustment is needed in case of pregnancy
C. Sudden withdrawal of low dose steroids for systemic treatment during pregnancy is not related to adrenal crisis due to physiological response to pregnancy
D. Prompt laparoscopy is mandatory due to circulatory instability and sepsis in common to abdominal pain

8. High dose radiation exposure of pregnant patient is generally avoided but can in some cases be unintentional or unavoidable. What is your recommended algorithm for the treatment of 32 weeks of pregnant women with ultrasound-proven stones in the extremities, recurrent biliary colic and pathological liver tests, with elevated levels of amylase and lipase. Biliary colic occurs with minimal fluid intake.
A. **MRCP followed with low dose ERCP**
B. US proven choledocholithiasis, initiation of labor and ERCP as soon as possible after delivery
C. Complete parenteral nutrition and symptomatic treatment until delivery
D. Percutaneous biliary drainage

9. 28 weeks pregnant women is admitted with right upper quadrant abdominal

pain, vomiting, fever and dysuria. She says she had a cholecystectomy 2 years ago. No one else in the family got sick. Ultrasound of the abdomen shows an air-fluid collection measuring 4 × 5 × 3 cm at the height of the hepatic flexure, laboratory findings present increase in WBC, CRP, slight anemia. We opt for laparoscopy. We enter with the needle technique in umbilical region.

A. **Open trocar placement via Hasson technique or insertion of the Veress needle into an alternate site, Palmer's point (left upper quadrant, 3 cm below the costal margin in the midclavicular line) is recommended.**
B. Injury of the uterus is highly suspicious due to pregnancy duration but avoidable when trocar placement is careful
C. No laparoscopy is indicated according to pregnancy duration
D. Manipulation of the uterus might be helpful for trocar placement

10. A 42-year-old pregnant woman with a 38-week pregnancy desired epidural analgesia. Examination of blood results reveals gestational thrombocytopenia, preeclampsia, and non-functional platelets, pathologic liver tests and overt coagulopathy. What do we advise and what could be the cause?

A. Vaginal delivery and hemostasis treatment
B. **If the decision is made to place an epidural catheter, soft-tipped catheters should be used to minimize trauma to epidural vessels, and the epidural catheter should be placed in the midline. The lowest concentration of local anesthetics should be used, in order to preserve motor function. The patient should be examined every 1–2 h to assess the extent of the motor block, and these examinations should continue until after the anesthetic has worn off and the catheter has been removed.**
C. Epidural hematoma is a rare case of epidural catheter placement in pregnant women. Careful observation is needed in case of motor block
D. Acute fatty liver in pregnancy is related to coagulopathy and represents relative contraindication for epidural catheter placement

References

1. Paternina-Caicedo A, Miranda J, Bourjeily G, Levinson A, Dueñas C, Bello-Muñoz C, Rojas-Suarez JA. Performance of the Obstetric Early Warning Score in critically ill patients for the prediction of maternal death. Am J Obstet Gynecol. 2017;216(1):58.e1–8. https://doi.org/10.1016/j.ajog.2016.09.103. Epub 2016 Oct 15. PMID: 27751799.
2. Moore LE, Pereira N. Physiological changes of pregnancy. In: van de Velde M, Scholefield H, Lauren A. Plante Publisher: Cambridge University Press. https://doi.org/10.1017/CBO9781139088084.011.
3. Taranikanti M. Physiological changes in cardiovascular system during normal pregnancy: a review. Indian J Cardiovasc Dis Women. 2018;3(2/3):62–7. https://doi.org/10.1055/s-0038-1676666.
4. Bhatia P, Chhabra S. Physiological and anatomical changes of pregnancy: implications for anaesthesia. Indian J Anaesth. 2018;62(9):651–7. https://doi.org/10.4103/ija.IJA_458_18.
5. Fisgus J, Tyagaraj K, Levesque V. Trauma in pregnancy. In: Smith C, editor. Trauma anesthesia. Cambridge: Cambridge University Press; 2015. p. 623–39. https://doi.org/10.1017/CBO9781139814713.042.
6. Soma-Pillay P, Nelson-Piercy C, Tolppanen H, Mebazaa A. Physiological changes in pregnancy. Cardiovasc J Afr. 2016;27(2):89–94. https://doi.org/10.5830/CVJA-2016-021.
7. Tiwari S. Anatomical adaptation to puberty, pregnancy and menopause. In: Mukhopadhaya N, Pundir J, Arora M, editors. Part 1 MRCOG revision notes and sample SBAs. Cambridge: Cambridge University Press; 2020. p. 23–7. https://doi.org/10.1017/9781108644396.005.
8. Ananthakrishnan R, Sharma S, Joshi S, Karunakaran S, Mohanty S. ECG changes in pregnancy—an observational study. J Mar Med Soc. 2020;22:187–92.
9. Jeelani K. Anatomy of the pelvis in obstetrics. In: Mukhopadhaya N, Pundir J, Arora M, editors. Part 1 MRCOG revision notes and sample SBAs. Cambridge:

Cambridge University Press; 2020. p. 18–22. https://doi.org/10.1017/9781108644396.004.
10. LoMauro A, Aliverti A, Frykholm P, Alberico D, Persico N, Boschetti G, et al. The adaptation of lung, chest wall and respiratory muscles during pregnancy: preparing for birth. J Appl Physiol. 2019;127(6):1640–50. https://doi.org/10.1152/japplphysiol.00035.
11. Tkachenko O, Shchekochikhin D, Schrier RW. Hormones and hemodynamics in pregnancy. Int J Endocrinol Metab. 2014;12(2):e14098. https://doi.org/10.5812/ijem.14098. PMID: 24803942; PMCID: PMC4005978.
12. Hayes N, Drew T. Cardiopulmonary physiological alterations in pregnancy. In: Lapinsky S, Plante L, editors. Respiratory disease in pregnancy. Cambridge: Cambridge University Press; 2020. p. 25–33. https://doi.org/10.1017/9781108163705.004.
13. Adank MC, Broere-Brown ZA, Gonçalves R, et al. Maternal cardiovascular adaptation to twin pregnancy: a population-based prospective cohort study. BMC Pregnancy Childbirth. 2020;20:327. https://doi.org/10.1186/s12884-020-02994-w.
14. Witvrouwen I, Mannaerts D, Van Berendoncks AM, Jacquemyn Y, Van Craenenbroeck EM. The effect of exercise training during pregnancy to improve maternal vascular health: focus on gestational hypertensive disorders. Front Physiol. 2020;11:450. https://doi.org/10.3389/fphys.2020.00450.
15. Kaushik S. Biochemistry in surgical conditions. In: Mukhopadhaya N, Pundir J, Arora M, editors. Part 1 MRCOG revision notes and sample SBAs. Cambridge: Cambridge University Press; 2020. p. 192–4. https://doi.org/10.1017/9781108644396.031.
16. Gupta R, Rawat VS. Sleep and sleep disorders in pregnancy. Neurology and pregnancy: neuro-obstetric disorders, pp 169–186. https://doi.org/10.1016/b978-0-444-64240-0.
17. Silvestri R, Aricò I. Sleep disorders in pregnancy. Sleep Sci. 2019;12(3):232–9. https://doi.org/10.5935/1984-0063.20190098.
18. Zeng Z, Liu F, Li S. Metabolic adaptations in pregnancy: a review. Ann Nutr Metab. 2017;70:59–65. https://doi.org/10.1159/000459633.
19. Napso T, Yong HEJ, Lopez-Tello J, Sferruzzi-Perri AN. The role of placental hormones in mediating maternal adaptations to support pregnancy and lactation. Front Physiol. 2018;9:1091. https://doi.org/10.3389/fphys.2018.01091.
20. McCarthy F, Kenny L. Adaptations of maternal cardiovascular and renal physiology to pregnancy. In: Heazell A, Norwitz E, Kenny L, Baker P, editors. Hypertension in pregnancy (Cambridge clinical guides). Cambridge: Cambridge University Press; 2010. p. 1–18. https://doi.org/10.1017/CBO9780511902529.003.
21. Pavord S, Hunt B, editors. The obstetric hematology manual. 2nd ed. Cambridge: Cambridge University Press; 2018. https://doi.org/10.1017/9781316410837.
22. Millar C, Laffan M. Hemostatic changes in normal pregnancy. In: Cohen H, O'Brien P, editors. Disorders of thrombosis and hemostasis in pregnancy. London: Springer; 2012. https://doi.org/10.1007/978-1-4471-4411-3_1.
23. Koita-Kazi I, Serhal P. Thrombotic and hemostatic aspects of assisted conception. In: Cohen H, O'Brien P, editors. Disorders of thrombosis and hemostasis in pregnancy. London: Springer; 2012. https://doi.org/10.1007/978-1-4471-4411-3_16.
24. Aslih N, Walfisch A. Clinical approach to pregnancy-related bleeding. In: Sheiner E, editor. Bleeding during pregnancy. New York: Springer; 2011. https://doi.org/10.1007/978-1-4419-9810-1_1.
25. Parrettini S, Caroli A, Torlone E. Nutrition and metabolic adaptations in physiological and complicated pregnancy: focus on obesity and gestational diabetes. Front Endocrinol. 2020;11:611929. https://doi.org/10.3389/fendo.2020.611929.
26. Calina D, Docea A, Golokhvast K, Sifakis S, Tsatsakis A, Makrigiannakis A. Management of endocrinopathies in pregnancy: a review of current evidence. Int J Environ Res Public Health. 2019;16(5):781. https://doi.org/10.3390/ijerph16050781.
27. Abu-Raya B, Michalski C, Sadarangani M, Lavoie PM. Maternal immunological adaptation during normal pregnancy. Front Immunol. 2020;11:575197. Published 2020 Oct 7. https://doi.org/10.3389/fimmu.2020.575197.
28. Balakrishnan S. Non-obstetric imaging in pregnant women. In: Nezhat C, Kavic M, Lanzafame R, Lindsay M, Polk T, editors. Non-obstetric surgery during pregnancy. Cham: Springer; 2019. https://doi.org/10.1007/978-3-319-90752-9_3.
29. Zachariah SK, Fenn M, Jacob K, Arthungal SA, Zachariah SA. Management of acute abdomen in pregnancy: current perspectives. Int J Womens Health. 2019;11:119–34. Published 2019 Feb 8. https://doi.org/10.2147/IJWH.S151501.
30. Mukherjee R, Samanta S. Surgical emergencies in pregnancy in the era of modern diagnostics and treatment. Taiwan J Obstet Gynecol. 2019;58(2):177–82. https://doi.org/10.1016/j.tjog.2019.01.001. PMID: 30910134.
31. Kotecha HM, McIntosh LJ, Lo HS, Chen BY, Dupuis CS. What to expect when they are expecting: magnetic resonance imaging of the acute abdomen and pelvis in pregnancy. Curr Probl Diagn Radiol. 2017;46(6):423–31. https://doi.org/10.1067/j.cpradiol.2016.12.007. Epub 2016 Dec 15. PMID: 28162865.
32. Horowitz JM, Hotalen IM, Miller ES, Barber EL, Shahabi S, Miller FH. How can pelvic MRI with diffusion-weighted imaging help my pregnant patient? Am J Perinatol. 2020;37(6):577–88. https://doi.org/10.1055/s-0039-1685492. Epub 2019 Apr 12. PMID: 30978746.
33. McGory ML, Zingmond DS, Tillou A, Hiatt JR, Ko CY, Cryer HM. Negative appendectomy in pregnant women is associated with a substantial risk of fetal loss. J Am Coll Surg. 2007;205(4):534–40.
34. Babaknia A, Parsa H, Woodruff JD. Appendicitis during pregnancy. Obstet Gynecol. 1977;50(1):40–4.

35. Mantoglu B, Gonullu E, Akdeniz Y, et al. Which appendicitis scoring system is most suitable for pregnant patients? A comparison of nine different systems. World J Emerg Surg. 2020;15:34. https://doi.org/10.1186/s13017-020-00310-7.
36. Sartelli M, Baiocchi GL, Di Saverio S, Ferrara F, Labricciosa FM, Ansaloni L, et al. Prospective Observational Study on acute Appendicitis Worldwide (POSAW). World J Emerg Surg. 2018;13:19.
37. Guidelines for diagnostic imaging during pregnancy and lactation. Obstet Gynecol. 2017;130:e210–2.
38. Tolcher MC, Clark SL. Diagnostic imaging and outcomes for nonobstetric surgery during pregnancy. Clin Obstet Gynecol. 2020;63(2):364–9. https://doi.org/10.1097/GRF.0000000000000525. PMID: 32167948.
39. Kwan ML, Miglioretti DL, Marlow EC, et al. Trends in medical imaging during pregnancy in the United States and Ontario, Canada, 1996 to 2016. JAMA Netw Open. 2019;2(7):e197249. https://doi.org/10.1001/jamanetworkopen.2019.7249.
40. Ball E, Waters N, Cooper N, et al. Evidence-based guideline on laparoscopy in pregnancy: commissioned by the British Society for Gynaecological Endoscopy (BSGE) endorsed by the Royal College of Obstetricians & Gynaecologists (RCOG) [published correction appears in Facts Views Vis Obgyn. 2020 Jan 24;11(3):261]. Facts Views Vis Obgyn. 2019;11(1):5–25.
41. Newman L, Rosen M. Operative laparoscopy. In: Keder L, Olsen M, editors. Gynecologic care. Cambridge: Cambridge University Press; 2018. p. 58–66. https://doi.org/10.1017/9781108178594.008.
42. Augustin G. Isolated fallopian tube torsion. In: Acute abdomen during pregnancy. Cham: Springer; 2018. https://doi.org/10.1007/978-3-319-72995-4_13.

Geriatrics: Traumatic and Non-traumatic Surgical Emergencies

23

Kartik Prabhakaran and Rifat Latifi

23.1 Introduction

Learning Goals

- Frailty and the changes in physiology that accompany aging significantly impact the outcomes in traumatic and non-traumatic surgical emergencies in geriatric patients
- The management of trauma-related emergencies such as traumatic brain injury and thoracoabdominal injuries in geriatric patients mandates an aggressive approach that accounts for existing comorbidities, impaired physiologic reserve, and a focus on the quality of life.
- The perioperative management and operative approach to non-traumatic surgical emergencies such as hollow viscus perforation, cholecystitis, and acute mesenteric ischemia in geriatric patients are predicated on prompt diagnosis, early source control of sepsis, and anticipation of physiologic sequelae related to aging.

K. Prabhakaran · R. Latifi (✉)
Department of Surgery, Westchester Medical Center, New York Medical College, School of Medicine, Valhalla, NY, USA
e-mail: kartik.prabhakaran@wmchealth.org; rifat.latifi@wmchealth.org

This chapter will focus on both traumatic and non-traumatic surgical emergencies in geriatric patients. As geriatric patients experience a similarly broad spectrum of surgical emergencies, specific examples are highlighted in this chapter, which focuses on the frequently encountered surgical pathologies in this age group. Given the impact of frailty upon outcomes in both trauma and emergency general surgery in the elderly, a discussion of frailty precedes individual disease entities.

With a sustained increase in the proportion of the elderly (≥65 years of age) population worldwide, it has become increasingly important to understand the physiologic consequences of aging as it relates to surgical outcomes [1]. The normal aging process involves both pathologic and natural decline in organ function, which decreases the physiologic reserve in response to stressors [2]. The functional decline in organ function originates on a cellular basis in the form of homeostatic breakdown and dysregulation of regulatory pathways and molecular structures [3]. This age-related decline in organ function is associated with an increase in morbidity and mortality in geriatric surgical patients across the spectrum of human physiology. For example, the progressive loss of cardiac myocytes and decrease in arterial compliance leads to increased afterload, both systolic and diastolic dysfunction, and an overall decrease of the cardiopulmonary function and reserve of geriatric patients [4, 5]. Furthermore, senescence of the renal tubules and volume loss of the renal cortex is exacerbated by age-related comorbidities such as hypertension and diabetes, which combine to diminish normal renal physiology and place the geriatric surgical patient at increased risk for acute kidney injury and renal failure [6]. Moreover, progressive atrophy of the absorptive and secretory mechanisms of the gastrointestinal tract are compounded by decreased appetite and oral intake and create significant nutritional imbalances in the elderly, placing the geriatric patient at risk for poor wound healing and impaired response to stress [7]. Finally, yet important among these examples is the progressive cognitive decline that occurs as a consequence of neurodegeneration among the elderly. In addition to the frequent onset of dementia and neurodegenerative diseases in the aging population, normal neurophysiology is replaced with cortical atrophy and impaired cerebral blood flow in the aging brain. These changes translate into higher risks for delirium and cognitive impairment resulting from anesthesia and analgesia in the geriatric surgical patient [8].

Though the physiology of aging is well described and understood, its impact on patient and surgical outcomes is less clear given the phenotypic variance of this altered physiology. Moreover, even within the geriatric population, there is significant heterogeneity among surgical outcomes due to variation in functional independence, comorbid conditions, and overall reserve within the population [9]. This heterogeneity has created the need for other measures of vulnerability related to health-related outcomes in the elderly and has resulted in the development and use of frailty. Frailty incorporates both intrinsic and extrinsic biopsychosocial factors and is distinct from chronological age since not all frail patients may be elderly, and not all elderly patients may be frail [10, 11]. It is important to understand that frailty is an acquired syndrome that is independent of age, accumulates over the course of a lifetime, and is based upon factors that are both intrinsic (e.g., comorbidities and disability) and extrinsic (e.g., socioeconomic status and psychological well-being) to the patient. Unfortunately, there is no generally agreed upon definition of frailty. Frequently described components of frailty include weakness, appetite and muscle mass, mobility, cognitive function, psychological well-being, independence, organ system functionality, and comorbidity—all of which affect the vulnerability and risk of adverse events such as surgical complications, disability, and mortality [12]. Given that there is no consensus definition of frailty, its measurement is challenging given the innumerable available tools and indices.

One of the first instruments for measuring frailty was introduced in 2001 by Fried et al, where the authors focused on an overall "wasting" syndrome whereby deterioration in strength, fitness, balance, and ambulation translated into a cycle of low energy and impaired physiologic reserve [10]. Another important historical concept in frailty measurement was promulgated by Rockwood and Mitnitski who were contributors to the Canadian Study of Health and Aging and devised a frailty index including 70 items across several domains spanning comorbid conditions, activities of daily living, and examination of physical and neurologic function [13]. However, the computation of 70 items can be challenging and time-consuming for clinicians and therefore has given rise to modified adaptations in the form of a modified frailty index that uses 11 factors [14]. Items included in this instrument are diabetes mellitus, congestive heart failure, hypertension requiring medication, transient ischemic attack or resolved cerebrovascular accident, dependent functional status, myocardial infarction, peripheral vascular disease or rest pain, cerebrovascular accident with residual neurological deficit, chronic obstructive pulmonary disease (COPD) or pneumonia, impaired sensorium and either prior percutaneous coronary intervention, prior cardiac surgery or angina.

Whereas frailty indices are of significant academic interest, the clinical application of frailty to the practice of surgery is of the utmost importance. Surgical decision-making for the geriatric patient takes into account the necessity of surgery, preoperative optimization (if feasible), the timing of surgery, intraoperative decision-making and resuscitation, and the optimization of post-operative outcomes. To this end, traumatic and non-traumatic surgical emergencies create a unique challenge in that pre-operative optimization and risk-factor modification are often not feasible. Nonetheless, the calculation of frailty in these patient populations remains essential in understanding risk/benefit ratios, proper utilization of resources, perioperative management, and shared decision-making with patients and their families. To this end, both a trauma-specific frailty index (TSFI) and an emergency general surgery frailty index have been validated in prospective studies to accurately predict outcomes in elderly patients with both traumatic and non-traumatic emergencies [15, 16]. Both of these tools were also shown to outperform other frailty indices in the setting of both trauma and emergency general surgery.

Irrespective of the instruments or tools selected for use, the important concepts are as follows:

1. Aging results in physiologic decline on both a cellular and organ system basis;
2. The physiologic changes associated with aging affect morbidity and mortality in geriatric surgical patients;
3. Frailty is an entity distinct from age, and impacts outcomes in trauma and emergency surgery; and
4. The consideration of frailty is important in optimizing surgical approaches, outcomes, and resource utilization for geriatric patients with traumatic and non-traumatic surgical emergencies.

Both age and frailty, both taken together and independently, are significant in their effects upon diagnosis, disease course, and treatment strategies for geriatric patients with traumatic and non-traumatic surgical emergencies (Fig. 23.1). Given the predilection of elderly patients to blunt trauma in the form of falls and motor vehicle accidents, the traumatic emergencies discussed herein will focus on traumatic brain injury, thoracic injuries, and abdominal solid organ injury with special emphasis on the interplay between pre-hospital comorbidities and aging physiology upon prompt evaluation, sound surgical decision-making, and periprocedural monitoring. The emergency general surgical pathology is similarly broad, if not broader, in the geriatric patient population [17]. However, given age-related epidemiological variations in certain disease states, this chapter will focus on specific examples of non-traumatic surgical emergencies such as hollow viscus perforation, acute cholecystitis, and mesenteric ischemia.

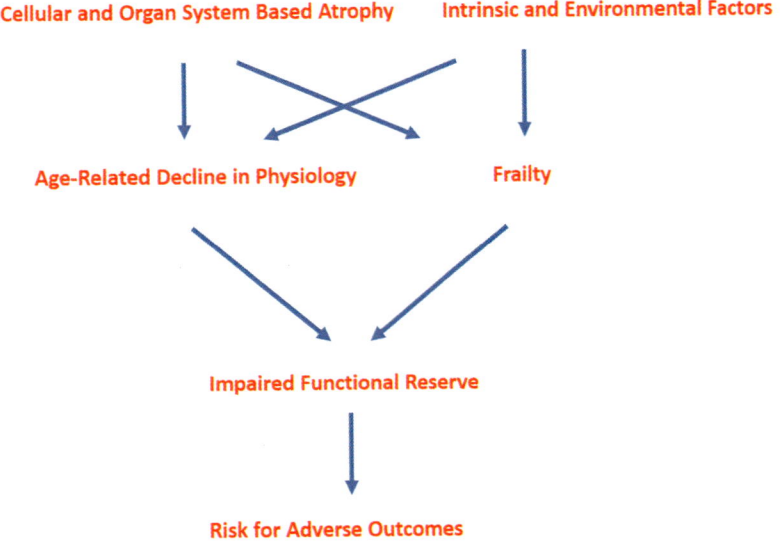

Fig. 23.1 Flowchart of interplay between aging and frailty

23.2 Traumatic Surgical Emergencies

23.2.1 Traumatic Brain Injury

The proportion of elderly individuals in the world's population continues to increase, and subsequently, trauma among the elderly is increasing [18]. The predominant mechanisms of injury in this population tend to be blunt as opposed to penetrating and are largely due to falls and motor vehicle accidents. Given the increased incidence of pre-hospital comorbid conditions, frailty, and concomitant use of medications, the geriatric trauma patient is at higher risk for in-hospital complications, debility, and mortality [19].

Traumatic brain injury (TBI) is one of the leading causes of morbidity and mortality among trauma patients at large. In elderly patients with TBI, however, both, the incidence and rate of hospitalization are higher and have worse outcomes when compared to the younger patient population [20]. The evaluation, management, resource utilization, and surgical decision-making for geriatric patients with traumatic brain injury must take into account the special considerations required of this population related to comorbidities, pre-hospital medications including anticoagulants, underlying neuropsychiatric pathology, increased susceptibility to poor functional outcomes, and end-of-life decision-making.

23.2.1.1 Diagnosis

The Glasgow Coma Scale (GCS) score remains the gold standard for standardized evaluation, classification, and prognostication of patients with TBI. The GCS measures brain function through the assessment of verbal, motor, and eye-opening responses to external stimuli and is used to classify the severity of TBI into mild (13–15), moderate (9–12), and severe (3–8) [21]. However, the application of the GCS score to the geriatric population is fraught with challenges. The prevalence of neurodegenerative disorders such as dementia, neuromuscular disease, and the use of prescription psychotropic medications may affect the clinical assessment of geriatric patients with TBI and confound the calculation of GCS scores. Recent studies have demonstrated that the presenting GCS score among elderly patients with TBI was significantly higher when compared to younger patients at each level of anatomic severity, despite a higher associated mortality rate (see if this makes sense, was not sure what you saying) [22]. These reports of age as a confounding variable in the assessment of geriatric brain injury patients have led to further studies advocating for the revision of the GCS scoring system to adjust for age, as age-adjusted scoring systems may out-perform and more accurately assess the elderly patient with traumatic brain injury [23].

The increased risk of mortality and poor outcomes in geriatric patients with traumatic brain injury has been established by both individual studies and meta-analyses [24, 25]. The widespread use of prescription anticoagulants in the elderly has compounded the effects of age in increasing risk among geriatric traumatic brain injury patients. Particularly with the increasing use of newer medications such as direct oral anticoagulants (DOAC), there are variations in the reported literature as to the relative risks of vitamin K antagonists (e.g. warfarin) versus DOACs with respect to morbidity and mortality in this population. Earlier studies demonstrated an increased risk of unfavorable outcomes in older adults with a mild traumatic brain injury that were prescribed pre-hospital warfarin or antiplatelet agents [26]. However, more recent studies have reported lower rates of mortality and intracranial hemorrhage progression with DOACs when compared to warfarin [27, 28]. With the increasing availability of viscoelastic testing to evaluate coagulopathy, as well as the availability/development of specific antidotes to anticoagulants, protocolized evaluation and treatment of the anticoagulated geriatric TBI patient is becoming increasingly important. Regardless of the relative risks of one anticoagulant versus another, the overriding theme is that patients with pre-hospital anticoagulant use are increasing in number and fare worse than their non-anticoagulated counterparts in the setting of traumatic brain injury [29].

23.2.1.2 Treatment

The procedural and surgical interventions for traumatic brain injury, irrespective of age, are aimed primarily at monitoring and relieving intracranial pressure, in order to prevent secondary brain insult. The recommendations and guidelines set forth by the Brain Trauma Foundation advocate for the placement and use of intracranial pressure (ICP) monitor in patients with survivable, severe traumatic brain injury (GCS $\leq$ 8) [30]. Whereas these guidelines have increased the overall frequency of ICP monitor use, the impact of these guidelines on patient outcomes, particularly in the elderly, is less clear. One recent study examining a United States national trauma database demonstrated an age-related disparity in the use of ICP monitors by showing that the frequency of ICP monitor use is progressively lower in older patients stratified by increasing age [31]. It is not clear, however, as to whether such disparities are due to inherent bias, or determinations of survivability and goals of care. More importantly, it is less clear as to whether there is a survival advantage of using ICP monitors in geriatric patient with severe traumatic brain injury. Although a single-institution observational study demonstrated improvement in mortality and six-month outcomes in older patients who were treated with ICP monitors [32], a larger retrospective study found that intracranial pressure monitoring was not associated with improved survival in patients above 55 years of age [33]. Similarly, questions arise as to the appropriateness and potential benefit of craniotomy and emergent surgical evacuation in this same population. Not surprisingly, studies have found that advanced age is an independent predictor for poor outcomes in patients undergoing emergent surgery for acute subdural hemorrhage [34], and that mortality significantly increases by decile of age group in elderly patients with similar presenting GCS scores that require the surgical evacuation of intracranial hemorrhage [35].

Overall, the increase in older active adults in the general population combined with both inherent and extrinsic risk factors such as anticoagulant use make traumatic brain injury a challenging problem for the healthcare system. In addition to understanding the effects of age upon outcomes, prompt, appropriate determination of survivability and impact upon the quality of life is essential in partnering with patient families to use shared decision-making so that patient autonomy, quality of life, and survival can be maximized.

> **Dos and Don'ts (Table 23.1)**
> - Do promptly reverse therapeutic anticoagulation in the setting of traumatic brain injury.
> - Do consider the patient's advance directives and the family's wishes when formulating the plan of management.
> - Don't omit the use of intracranial pressure monitoring on the basis of age alone.
> - Don't advocate for craniotomy and surgical evacuation of intracranial hemorrhage without considering the impact on quality of life.

23.2.2 Thoracic Injuries

23.2.2.1 Diagnosis

Progressive loss of muscle mass and osteoporosis place the geriatric trauma patient at significant risk for thoracic injuries including rib fractures, pneumothoraces, and hemothoraces. In addition, the physiological changes of aging place the geriatric patient with thoracic injuries at significant risk of post-injury complications such as respiratory compromise, pneumonia, empyema, and iatrogenic complications associated with analgesia. Even with low-energy traumatic mechanisms, the impact of rib fractures can be underestimated in the geriatric population. The exaggerated effects of rib fractures upon aging pulmonary physiology and the decreased functional reserve associated with both age and frailty often require the geriatric patient with rib fractures to be hospitalized for cardiopulmonary monitoring and effective analgesia. Previous studies have demonstrated that elderly patients with rib fractures have a significantly increased risk of both morbidity and

Table 23.1 Key principles of evaluation and management in geriatric traumatic emergencies

	Traumatic brain injury	Thoracic trauma	Intra-abdominal hemorrhage
Assessment	1. Recognize confounding variables such as dementia and neurologic disease that can alter the accuracy of assessment 2. A high threshold of concern is required for pre-hospital anticoagulant use	1. Even with low-energy mechanisms, thoracic trauma can occur frequently in the elderly 2. Impaired pulmonary reserve places the elderly patient at increased risk for poor outcomes	1. The diagnosis of shock is challenging in the elderly due to age-related changes in cardiovascular physiology 2. The physical exam can be unreliable in geriatric patients with intra-abdominal bleeding from solid organ injury
Management	1. Age alone should not preclude the use of intracranial pressure monitoring 2. Consider the patient's advance directives in decision-making 3. Craniotomy in the elderly is associated with a high rate of mortality and poor outcomes	1. A thoughtful multimodal approach is recommended for analgesia to minimize complications 2. Early procedural intervention for surgical rib stabilization or retained hemothorax reduces morbidity and improves outcomes	1. Advanced age should not preclude surgical control of traumatic intra-abdominal hemorrhage 2. Failure of non-operative management, using adjunctive techniques, may occur more frequently in the elderly and is associated with higher morbidity and mortality

mortality when compared to their younger counterparts, and that age is an independent predictor of poor outcomes such as pneumonia, intensive care unit admission, the requirement for mechanical ventilation and death in this population [36, 37]. Although the key elements of treatment after rib fractures are centered on appropriate pain management and respiratory support, geriatric patients with thoracic trauma and rib fractures often require monitoring in the intensive care unit setting which can lead to delirium. In fact, a recent study demonstrated that elderly patients admitted with rib fractures were at significantly higher risk for delirium independent of the mode of analgesia provided and that delirium in this population was associated with a higher rate of complications, a longer hospital stay, and a higher risk for adverse discharge disposition [38]. The triage of geriatric patients with rib fractures and ensuing resource utilization is often dependent on institutional protocols. However, specific parameters such as forced vital capacity (FVC), number of rib fractures, and frailty scores have been used as criteria for intensive care unit admission and non-invasive respiratory support among this population.

23.2.2.2 Treatment

The use of opioid analgesia in the geriatric population for the treatment of pain associated with rib fractures is fraught with concerns about lack of efficacy, and unwanted side effects. A prospective randomized trial of epidural analgesia versus intravenous opioids for patients with multiple rib fractures demonstrated a significant reduction in both ventilator days and pneumonia in those treated with epidural analgesia, despite this group being more severely injured [39]. Other retrospective studies also provide evidence in support of epidural analgesia for the treatment of multiple rib fractures, with a demonstrated reduction in mortality and pulmonary complications, particularly in the geriatric population [40]. However, the data is mixed with respect to the relative merits of epidural analgesia as other studies have shown deleterious consequences of epidural analgesia with respect to respiratory complications and length of stay [41]. Moreover, the use of epidural analgesia is fraught with concomitant considerations such as the choice of chemical DVT prophylaxis, potential for hypotension, contraindications in patients with thoracic spine fractures, and limitations on mobility.

With newer modalities of analgesia available such as ketamine and selective regional catheter-based techniques, which have shown benefit in both young and old, ultimately thoughtful consideration is required in choosing a multimodal analgesic regimen. The impact of pain and opioid medications on delirium, respiratory suppression, and gastrointestinal tract dysfunction is not only important but also exacerbated in geriatric patient with altered baseline physiology. As such, a multimodal interdisciplinary approach to analgesia with careful monitoring of pulmonary reserve and avoidance of iatrogenic medication-induced side effects is preferred and recommended.

Historically the majority of rib fractures have been managed non-operatively, but in the last few decades, an increase in surgical stabilization of rib fractures (SSRF) for patients with severe chest wall injury and flail chest injuries has occurred. Despite this, some studies have demonstrated no clear benefit in outcomes, but rather increased length of stay and cost [42]. However, other retrospective studies demonstrate a mortality benefit to SSRF specifically in the geriatric population, with added benefits of reduced incidence of pneumonia and shorter intensive care unit length of stay [43]. We believe that the management of rib fractures in the elderly should be an individual decision for each patient and that one size does not fit all. Interventions (operative and non-operative) have the most efficacy when considering patient selection. Individualized approaches to geriatric patient lead to better outcomes when considering frailty, injury severity, comorbidities, the interplay between different organ systems, and overall goals of care.

Pneumothorax and hemothorax have been found to be independent predictors of overall complications and mortality among elderly patients with blunt thoracic trauma [44]. Historically, pneumothoraces and hemothoraces arising from trauma have been treated with tube thoracostomy using large-bore chest tubes. More recently, the paradigm has shifted towards the use of smaller, 14 French pigtail catheters where studies have shown equivalent tube durations, equivalent rates of complications, and rates of failures [45]. This approach is especially attractive in the geriatric population with respect to anatomical considerations in the aging chest wall and procedural discomfort and pain. For those patients who do develop retained hemothoraces, recent literature has supported early evacuation in the form of video-assisted thoracoscopic surgery (VATS) in order to reduce the risks of empyema, pneumonia, ventilator days, and length of stay [46]. Single-center studies have supported the safety of this approach in the elderly population by demonstrating excellent results with no age-associated complications even in patients above the age of 80 [47]. In fact, others have demonstrated that direct VATS without preceding tube thoracostomy was associated with lower rates of infection and shorter durations of hospitalization in the geriatric trauma population [48]. The overriding principles in considering the choice and timing of procedural interventions for pneumothoraces and hemothoraces in the elderly population must rely on the understanding that geriatric patients with chest wall trauma have impaired pulmonary and immunologic reserve. Increased susceptibility to pain and infection, and impaired ability to wean from mechanical ventilation place the geriatric trauma patient at particular risk for poor outcomes. As such, it becomes essential to consider this subset of patients in the context of frailty and aging physiology, in order to provide the correct choice and timing of procedural intervention.

Dos and Don'ts (Table 23.1)
- Do formulate a patient-centered approach towards analgesia for the elderly patient with rib fractures.
- Do consider surgical stabilization of rib fractures as an option for geriatric patients despite advanced age.
- Don't forget the unwanted side effects of delirium and respiratory depression when choosing an analgesic regimen for the geriatric patient.
- Don't delay the early evacuation of retained hemothorax in geriatric patients with chest wall trauma.

23.2.3 Intra-abdominal Hemorrhage and Solid Organ Injury

23.2.3.1 Diagnosis

Though geriatric trauma patient is often associated with low-energy mechanisms such as falls, many of them continue to be independent and are involved in motor vehicle collisions. Moreover, the decrease in muscle mass predisposes the geriatric trauma patient to life-threatening injuries, including intra-abdominal hemorrhage even with low energy mechanisms. Taken together with a decline in functional reserve, the evaluation, and management of geriatric trauma patients with hemorrhagic shock from intra-abdominal injuries is challenging. Although there is a minimal functional decline of the adrenal glands with aging, the physiologic changes of the aging cardiovascular system create challenges for both the provider's diagnostic ability and the geriatric patient's ability to respond to shock associated with severe trauma. The widespread use of antihypertensive and chronotropic medications in the elderly population combined with the physiologic changes of the cardiovascular system associated with aging alter the hemodynamics both at baseline, and during a state of shock, of the geriatric trauma patient. To this end, studies have shown that traditional vital signs thresholds do not accurately correlate with shock and predict mortality in geriatric trauma patients when compared to their younger population [49, 50]. These studies demonstrated that hypotension should be re-defined in the elderly population with higher systolic blood pressures used as thresholds. The progressive loss of cardiac myocytes, higher peripheral vascular resistance, and lower maximum heart rate combine to limit the cardiovascular system of the geriatric trauma patient to both exhibit and compensate for hemorrhagic shock. As such, the diagnosis of shock in this patient population is challenging and warrants a high index of suspicion. Adjuncts to evaluate shock such as mentation, laboratory values for end-points of resuscitation, and liberal use of invasive and non-invasive hemodynamic monitoring are warranted in this population.

23.2.3.2 Treatment

Historically, the surgical management of blunt solid organ injury (i.e., liver and spleen) has seen a paradigm shift from operative to non-operative management beginning in the 1990s. Although operative management and hemorrhage control remain the standard for all hemodynamically unstable patients with blunt solid organ injury, hemodynamically normal patients are now managed routinely with observation, serial clinical and laboratory testing, and at times less invasive means such as angioembolization. In fact, studies have demonstrated superior outcomes for hemodynamically stable patients with blunt hepatic injury managed non-operatively [51]. Non-operative management of blunt splenic injury overall, but particularly in the hemodynamically normal patient or those with low-grade injuries has become a standard of care [52]. However, as with all management approaches, patient selection is paramount. Identifying the patients who are at high risk for failure of non-operative management is important in minimizing morbidity and mortality. Patients with high-grade blunt solid organ injuries, those with radiographic evidence of contrast extravasation suggesting active hemorrhage, and patients requiring active transfusion of blood products all represent situations where providers lean preferentially towards operative management. Similarly, underlying comorbid conditions that alter immunology, physiology, or functional reserve must be considered as indicators of possible failure of a non-operative approach. However, initial studies reported that over 90% of patients older than the age of 55 failed a conservative approach of non-operative management [53], and subsequent studies reported a failure rate of one out of every three geriatric patients [54].

The prevailing concern in the geriatric trauma patient is their ability of physiologic reserve to cope with intra-abdominal hemorrhage. However, age alone is not an independent predictor of poor outcomes for non-operative management of splenic injuries in the geriatric population [55]. It should be noted however that such studies, in addition to a multi-institutional trial of the Eastern Association for the Surgery of Trauma also demonstrated that when failure of non-operative management did occur, it was associated with increased mortality in the geriatric patient population [56].

Ultimately, the factors most predictive of success in conservative or non-operative management of blunt solid organ injury are related to the injury and presenting signs and symptoms, as opposed to the patient. The patient's hemodynamics, grade of the injury, need for transfusion, and presence/absence of contrast blush on imaging studies form the foundations of decision-making for operative versus non-operative management. Angioembolization has been shown to be effective at achieving hemorrhage control while minimizing the morbidity associated with laparotomy, however, such decisions must be guided by the patient's physiology. Particularly in geriatric patients, providers must consider that the physiology of aging places these patients at risk for under-triage because of vital signs that may mistakenly appear normal. In addition, these same physiologic changes place the geriatric patient at significant risk for morbidity and mortality because of the impaired cardiovascular and physiologic reserve with respect to the ability to respond to hemorrhage, hypotension, and shock.

> **Dos and Don'ts (Table 23.1)**
> - Do take into consideration pre-existing comorbidities and medications when triaging the elderly patient with blunt solid organ injury.
> - Do consider the risk of advanced age as a predictor of failure of non-operative management.
> - Don't avoid surgery on the basis of age alone.
> - Don't forget the use of angioembolization as an adjunct in treating blunt solid organ injury in the elderly.

23.3 Non-traumatic Surgical Emergencies

23.3.1 Intra-abdominal Sepsis from Perforated Viscus (Diverticular and Peptic Ulcer Disease)

23.3.1.1 Diagnosis

The most frequent pathologies encountered by general surgeons are composed of biliary, appendiceal, diverticular, and peptic-ulcer-related sepsis owing to obstruction, inflammation, and/or perforation. Elderly patients are a rapidly growing demographic among the general population requiring emergency general surgery for such pathology. Overall, elderly patients are known to be complex and high-risk for surgical decision-making in general with such concerns exacerbated in the setting of surgical emergencies. Whereas single-center studies have demonstrated that favorable outcomes can be achieved in geriatric patients, systems-based research has shown that advanced age is associated with significantly higher risks of complications and mortality [57, 58]. In addition to age, increased levels of frailty have also been shown to independently correlate with worse outcomes in geriatric patients undergoing emergency general surgery procedures [16]. Proper perioperative management of geriatric emergency general surgery patients is contingent upon vigilance, early recognition of complications, and minimization of iatrogenic insults. The concept of failure to rescue (FTR) was defined in the early 1990s as the rate of mortality among patients with a complication [59]. The merits of this metric lie in its cumulative approach to examining the effects of both morbidity and mortality among a population of surgical patients. In geriatric emergency general surgery patients, frailty has been shown to independently correlate with a higher incidence of FTR [60]. By recognizing the risks of FTR, prospectively assessing and calculating frailty, and understanding the impact of physiologic aging upon outcomes, a timely patient-centered approach to the geriatric emergency general surgery patient can improve outcomes and resource utilization.

23.3.1.2 Treatment

Life-threatening intra-abdominal sepsis commonly occurs as a result of perforated viscus, with diverticulitis and peptic ulcer disease as common etiologies. Similar to trauma, the recognition of perforated viscus in the elderly patient may be challenging, given the attenuated physiologic compensatory capabilities of the cardiovascular and immune systems resulting in the absence of traditional symptoms of tachycardia or fever. Earlier retrospective and post-mortem studies of elderly patients identified elderly obese females at particular risk for unrecognized intra-abdominal perforation as abdominal pain, tachycardia, and fever were encountered less frequently and with less specificity in this vulnerable population [61, 62]. Complications of diverticular disease requiring emergent surgery usually are due to either bleeding or perforation. In the setting of complicated diverticulitis associated with perforation, the geriatric patient's susceptibility to sepsis must be taken into account when determining the timing and the choice of procedure. Providers may be tempted to avoid laparotomy, or surgery altogether, in geriatric patients with complicated diverticulitis for fear of associated morbidity. However, the opposite may in fact be true: avoidance or delay in definitive treatment results in morbidity and mortality. Studies have shown that each 24-h period of delay for surgical intervention in patients with perforated diverticulitis, resulted in a significant increase in mortality for patients above the age of 65. Although providers may be more intuitively inclined to pursue minimally invasive surgical approaches in the elderly, the data indicate that percutaneous drainage of diverticular abscesses is associated with a greater risk for permanent stoma and mortality in the geriatric population [63]. Therefore, reluctance either to perform surgery or to perform maximally invasive and definitive surgery in the elderly has a significant associated cost that must be considered.

Despite the widespread use of acid-reducing medications and screening endoscopy, peptic ulcer disease continues to be a mainstay of pathology in the emergency general surgery patient population and is frequently encountered in the geriatric population. The importance of urgency in approaching perforated peptic ulcer disease is well supported by studies demonstrating a linear relationship between delays in operative intervention and increasing mortality [64]. Geriatric patients with perforated peptic ulcer disease often present with fewer signs of peritonitis and have an attenuated inflammatory response. Not surprisingly, advanced age has been shown to be an independent risk factor for post-operative mortality in patients with perforated peptic ulcer disease. The combined burden of age and comorbidities creates a significant risk for post-operative complications and morbidity. However, it should be noted that barring patient and family-driven decisions regarding advance directives, age alone is not a prohibitive factor in providing emergency surgery for such patients. Recent single-institution studies have demonstrated that a significant proportion of octogenarian and nonagenarian patients are alive more than 3 years out from emergency laparotomy including operation for perforated peptic ulcers [65, 66]. Much of the challenge in managing this patient population lies not only in the timeliness of surgical intervention, but also in peri-operative management of comorbidities, early recognition of complications, and optimization of modifiable risk factors such as nutrition. In fact, a national database study revealed that malnourished geriatric patients undergoing major abdominal surgery for intra-abdominal sepsis experienced lower rates of complications and mortality when they received surgical nutritional access at the time of index surgery [67]. Therefore, prompt diagnosis, timely surgical intervention, and a proactive approach to managing comorbidities and modifiable risk factors can lead to favorable outcomes in geriatric patients with intra-abdominal sepsis.

Table 23.2 Key principles of evaluation and management in geriatric non-traumatic surgical emergencies

	Perforated viscus	Acute cholecystitis	Acute mesenteric ischemia
Assessment	1. The diagnosis of peritonitis can be challenging in the elderly 2. Delays in intervention and failure to rescue increase morbidity and mortality	1. The prevalence of gallstone disease increases with age and delayed presentation is common in the elderly 2. The clinical signs and symptoms of acute cholecystitis may be unreliable in the elderly to establish the diagnosis	1. Despite the widespread use of anticoagulants, progressive vascular compromise places the elderly patient at elevated risk 2. Unreliable physical examinations, delays in seeking medical attention, and reluctance to perform major abdominal surgery places create elevated risks of morbidity and mortality for the geriatric patient
Management	1. Age alone should not encourage the use of minimally invasive techniques or non-operative management which are associated with a higher risk of morbidity and mortality in the elderly 2. Careful perioperative management of comorbidities, prompt recognition of complications, and early emphasis on nutrition can improve outcomes	1. Non-operative management with percutaneous cholecystostomy can be effective as a temporizing measure but can delay definitive treatment and increases morbidity 2. Laparoscopic cholecystectomy is the gold standard of surgical approaches, but conversion to open or even partial cholecystectomy for the sake of safety should not be considered a failure	1. Prompt anticoagulation, restoration of blood flow, and resection of non-viable intestines form the cornerstones of therapy 2. The risk of morbidity due to frailty and malnutrition should give rise to favoring ostomy creation over the restoration of intestinal continuity after resection in a geriatric patient who is critically ill

Dos and Don'ts (Table 23.2)

- Do perform early definitive surgery for intra-abdominal sepsis in the geriatric patient.
- Do consider the importance of perioperative management, and in particular nutritional needs and access in the geriatric patient with intra-abdominal sepsis.
- Don't delay source control and laparotomy in the geriatric patient, as delays in diagnosis and treatment confer a higher risk for morbidity and mortality.
- Don't regard age as a prohibitive risk factor for surgical control of intra-abdominal sepsis.

23.3.2 Acute Cholecystitis

23.3.2.1 Diagnosis

The prevalence of gallstones and consequently associated complications (cholecystitis, choledocholithiasis, and biliary pancreatitis) is known to increase with age, with acute cholecystitis being the most common complication requiring intervention in the geriatric population [68]. The only definitive treatment for acute cholecystitis is cholecystectomy, and both laparoscopic and open cholecystectomy have been shown to be safe surgical approaches for treatment. Moreover, cholecystectomy during index hospitalization has been shown to result in lower rates of re-admission and shorter overall hospital length of stay, with no difference in morbidity [69]. However, elderly patients with acute cholecystitis post a particular challenge as there is a tendency towards non-operative management or delay in performing surgery given the fear of poor outcomes and complications. Similar to other etiologies of sepsis, the diagnosis of acute cholecystitis can be challenging in the geriatric patient because of delays in presentation, attenuated inflammatory response, confounding causes or presenting symptoms, and unreliable abdominal examination. The hallmark of diagnosis in the modern era is ultrasound which is sensitive not only for the detection of gallstones but also for measuring the size of biliary structures and by measuring the thickness of the gallbladder wall as a surrogate for inflammation. However, studies have also shown that ultrasound can have suboptimal negative predictive value for detecting acute cholecystitis, making adjunctive clinical signs (abdominal tenderness, fever, leukocytosis, neutrophil count) and symptoms (pain, anorexia) all the more important for prompt and accurate diagnosis. Unfortunately, such clinical signs and symptoms can often be absent or unreliable in the geriatric population [70].

23.3.2.2 Treatment

Given the increased prevalence of comorbid conditions and frailty among the geriatric patient population which translates into a higher risk for perioperative morbidity and poor outcomes, prompt diagnosis is essential for the timely initiation of antibiotics and definitive treatment. The temptation to delay or defer definitive surgery is complicated by the intermediate, but non-definitive, option of percutaneous drainage of the gallbladder (percutaneous cholecystostomy). Whereas the Tokyo Guidelines recommend percutaneous cholecystostomy as the initial treatment of acute cholecystitis in critically ill patients to be followed by delayed cholecystectomy, common practice has become to use patient comorbidity and perioperative risk as indications for percutaneous cholecystostomy [71]. In turn, this approach has gained popularity in the management of the geriatric patient population with acute cholecystitis given the concerns for perioperative morbidity and mortality. Although percutaneous cholecystostomy can be effective in helping to achieve source control of sepsis in the initial phase of disease, more recent studies have shown that this approach is actually associated with lower rates of definitive surgery, higher overall mortality, and higher rates of hospital readmission [72].

Historically, performing surgery on the elderly has evolved from being the exception to being the rule, as both lifespans of individuals and the capabilities of healthcare have expanded and improved. To this end, a recent meta-analysis concluded that early cholecystectomy is safe and feasible in elderly patients with acute cholecystitis [73]. As laparoscopic cholecystectomy has become the standard of care as the initial surgical approach to cholecystitis for the overall patient population, it should be noted that a long history of cholelithiasis, delay in presentation to acute care settings, and attenuated inflammatory response may result in a higher rate of conversion from laparoscopic to open cholecystectomy in the geriatric population [74]. Moreover, in situations where the gallbladder is gangrenous or there is difficulty in recognizing anatomy due to extensive inflammation, it is important for emergency general surgeons to consider alternative strategies such as subtotal cholecystectomy as safe and feasible [75]. However, given the emphasis on patient safety, conversion from laparoscopy to open surgery or subtotal cholecystectomy should not be considered a failure. Whether laparoscopic or open, complete or subtotal, definitive source control during the index hospitalization is important in minimizing long-term morbidity, disease recurrence, impaired quality of life, and repeat hospitalizations.

Based on many of these studies, the World Society of Emergency Surgery (WSES) and the Italian Surgical Society for Elderly (SICG) recommend that laparoscopic cholecystectomy should be considered as the first line of treatment for all, irrespective of age, and that surgical risk should be calculated and considered based on the underlying disease, and not on age alone [76]. For patients of any age, prompt diagnosis, consideration of perioperative risk, open communication with patients and their families, early definitive treatment, safe technique, and excellent perioperative management are the guiding principles in the surgical management of acute cholecystitis as a surgical emergency.

> **Dos and Don'ts (Table 23.2)**
>
> - Do consider laparoscopic cholecystectomy as the first line of treatment for acute cholecystitis, irrespective of age.
> - Do remember that conversion to open cholecystectomy and subtotal cholecystectomy should be considered safe operative choices in geriatric patients with cholecystitis and difficult anatomy.
> - Don't allow age alone to serve as a prohibitive risk factor against surgery.
> - Don't pursue non-definitive treatment approaches such as percutaneous cholecystostomy based on advanced age.

23.3.3 Acute Mesenteric Ischemia

23.3.3.1 Diagnosis

Acute mesenteric ischemia encompasses a broad range of etiologies and pathology that result in impaired blood flow and oxygen delivery to the intestines (small and large), which can lead to life-threatening bowel ischemia, necrosis, and sepsis. Although the overall incidence in the general population is low, it is more frequently encountered in the critically ill population and in the elderly given the increased prevalence of risk factors in these populations. The four major subtypes of acute mesenteric ischemia are superior mesenteric artery (SMA) embolism, SMA thrombosis, superior mesenteric vein (SMV) thrombosis, and non-occlusive mesenteric ischemia (NOMI). Whereas SMV thrombosis is typically caused by intrinsic disease such as hypercoagulable states, the other three (SMA embolism, SMA thrombosis, and NOMI) are typically caused by modifiable risk factors such as arrhythmias and valvular heart disease, atherosclerosis, and chronic states of impaired blood flow. Despite the increasing and widespread use of prescription anticoagulants, the elderly population is burdened with a high incidence of these risk factors given the age-related structural and pathophysiologic changes in the cardiovascular system. Of these three, SMA embolus is the most frequently encountered etiology, and most patients with SMA embolus have a cardiac source such as atrial fibrillation, cardiomyopathy, or vascular disease which are more prevalent in the geriatric population [77]. Such patients are at particular risk given that SMA occlusion results in irreversible damage to the intestinal mucosa in as little as 6 h [78]. In comparison, SMA thrombosis occurs in patients with chronic systemic atherosclerosis which not only occurs as a natural sequela of aging but can also be exacerbated by modifiable risk factors such as tobacco use and diabetes. In these patients, deposition and rupture of plaque at the origin of the SMA can lead to critical flow-limiting stenosis, causing acute bowel ischemia. NOMI, on the other hand, typically develops as a result of impaired circulation that is frequently encountered in patients that are hospitalized and hypotensive, severely volume depleted, or on dialysis for end-stage renal failure. As the elderly patient is more susceptible to changes in intravascular volume, NOMI is frequently encountered in the geriatric patient hospitalized for general medical conditions such as heart failure and sepsis, as opposed to de novo presentation in the emergency department.

The diagnosis of acute mesenteric ischemia is challenging in the population at large irrespective of age. Although the acute phase can often be preceded by a more chronic compromise of intestinal blood flow, the critical flow-limiting insult often occurs suddenly and without warning and with time-sensitive ischemic insult. Delays in patient presentation and surgical consultation are common because of reluctance to seek medical care, the vagueness of symptoms, and unnecessary laboratory and radiographic testing. Such delays unfortunately are associated with significant morbidity and mortality. Common signs of acute mesenteric ischemia such as "pain out of proportion", are often difficult to elicit in the elderly patient, particularly if an accurate history is not available. Other signs and symptoms such as gastrointestinal bleeding, anorexia, and malaise can often be attributed to other causes that lead to a delay in diagnosis. As with other general surgical emergencies, the attenuated inflammatory response in the geriatric population may not lead to fever or leukocytosis. Unfortunately, laboratory parameters such as serum lactate can often be normal in the setting of concomitant mesenteric venous occlusion, and even when elevated represent a late finding [79]. Although the gold standards for diagnosis of angiography and multidetector-row computed tomography (CT) are highly accurate, the geriatric patient population often does not undergo such testing due to renal dysfunction. Moreover, even when such tests are feasible, the time spent obtaining them can cause significant delays in providing prompt surgical consultation and intervention.

23.3.3.2 Treatment

Once the diagnosis of acute mesenteric ischemia is made either on the basis of history, clinical exam, laboratory and radiographic testing—or some combination of these, time is of the essence in providing intervention to reduce the extent of intestinal ischemia. The hallmarks of treatment are the restoration of blood flow (through embolectomy or thrombectomy, or mesenteric artery bypass), prompt anticoagulation, and emergent laparotomy to assess bowel viability and resect the non-viable intestine. Resection of the non-viable intestine to healthy margins, restoration of blood flow, and subsequent reassessment of bowel viability with re-laparotomy form the cornerstones of surgical therapy. Restoration of bowel continuity is dependent on the individual patient's clinical status, though the elevated risks for the anastomotic leak in malnourished, septic, immune-compromised elderly patients often lead to a preference for ostomy creation. Studies examining factors influencing outcome and prognosis in patients with acute mesenteric ischemia routinely find that elderly patients have overall worse outcomes [80, 81]. Moreover, the length of intestinal necrosis and renal failure have also been shown to be predictors for mortality and poor overall outcomes[83]. Given that elderly patients are less tolerant of complications such as renal failure, short bowel syndrome, dehydration from high-output stomas, and sepsis, acute mesenteric ischemia has significant risks of mortality in the geriatric population. In addition to prioritizing early diagnosis and surgical intervention, palliative considerations must be taken into account in elderly patient with acute mesenteric ischemia. Near-total bowel necrosis, multisystem organ failure, ventilator dependence, and other fulminant conditions should prompt the emergency general surgeon and/or intensivist to engage the patient and patient families as soon as possible, in patient-centered honest discussions about goals of care and quality of life.

Dos and Don'ts (Table 23.2)

- Do be prompt in achieving a diagnosis and performing laparotomy, given that mesenteric ischemia is time-sensitive with respect to reducing morbidity and mortality.
- Do involve patients and their families, and consider advance directives and quality of life when treating patients with near-total bowel necrosis and multisystem organ failure.
- Don't forget that restoration of blood flow with prompt anticoagulation and restoration of vascular flow is essential when treating mesenteric ischemia.
- Don't hesitate to create an ostomy in elderly patients requiring bowel resection for intestinal ischemia, given that the risks for anastomotic dehiscence are higher in elderly, malnourished patients.

Take-Home Messages

- The consideration of frailty is important in optimizing surgical approaches, outcomes, and resource utilization for geriatric patients with traumatic and non-traumatic surgical emergencies (Fig. 23.1).
- Traumatic brain injury portends a significant risk of mortality in the elderly, and this can be mitigated through evidence-based treatment approaches, and open patient-centered consideration of goals of care and quality of life (Table 23.1).

- Blunt thoracic trauma and intra-abdominal hemorrhage from solid organ injury are associated with higher risks of poor outcomes in geriatric trauma patients, and treatment approaches must take into account the impact of age upon potential success or failure (Table 23.1).
- The diagnosis of non-traumatic surgical emergencies in the geriatric population is fraught with challenges due to delays in presentation, attenuated inflammatory responses, and limitations in clinical signs and symptoms.
- Emergency general surgery pathology such as perforated viscus, acute cholecystitis, and acute mesenteric ischemia is associated with higher risks of poor outcomes in the geriatric population, and patient-centered approaches to surgical management and palliative considerations can improve both outcomes and quality of life.

Multiple Choice Questions

1. Which of the following statements is accurate regarding the association of age and frailty?
   A. Frailty increases with age
   B. There is a consensus definition of frailty that can be easily tabulated
   C. **Frailty is an acquired syndrome that is multifactorial and impacts outcomes in both trauma and emergency surgery**
   D. The effects of age upon outcomes in trauma and emergency general surgery consistently portend poor outcomes
2. Which of the following is true regarding age-related changes in organ function?
   A. Increasing rates of obesity in the aging population lead to enhanced nutritional reserve
   B. The progressive loss of lean muscle mass results in a higher glomerular filtration rate
   C. Neurodegenerative atrophy results in reduced risks for delirium
   D. **Atherosclerosis and loss of cardiac myocytes result in impaired cardiac systolic function**
3. What is the impact of age upon the Glasgow Coma Scale (GCS) score in the elderly?
   A. **Elderly patients often present with higher GCS scores than their younger counterparts, even with similar radiographic severity of traumatic brain injury (TBI)?**
   B. Increasing age is associated with worse GCS scores at the time of presentation after TBI
   C. GCS score, but not age, impacts outcomes after TBI
   D. The GCS score used as threshold for intracranial pressure (ICP) monitor placement should be lower in the geriatric patient
4. The most effective approach to analgesia for rib fractures in the elderly has been shown to be:
   A. Enteral opioid analgesia
   B. **A multimodal patient-specific regimen consisting of both regional and systemic delivery**
   C. Epidural analgesia
   D. Non-opioid medications such as non-steroidal anti-inflammatory medications and ketamine
5. Which of the following is true regarding severe blunt thoracic trauma in the geriatric population?
   A. Surgical stabilization of rib fractures is contraindicated in the elderly
   B. Hemothoraces in the elderly should be managed with tube thoracostomy alone, as the risk of video-assisted thoracoscopy (VATS) is too high
   C. **Small bore pigtail catheters can be effective for the treatment of both pneumothorax and hemothorax**
   D. Age has no effect on weaning from mechanical ventilation

6. Management of intra-abdominal hemorrhage from blunt solid organ injury in the geriatric patient population should take into account which of the following special considerations?
   A. The frequency of hypertension among elderly patients allows for improved physiologic reserve in the response to hemorrhagic shock.
   B. Systolic blood pressure and heart rate are accurate parameters for the diagnosis of severe blood loss.
   C. Transfusion of blood products should be limited in the geriatric population.
   D. **Traditional dogma of non-operative management of blunt solid organ injury carries a higher risk of failure in elderly patients.**
7. Which of the following statements is true regarding perforated viscus and intra-abdominal sepsis in the elderly?
   A. The fragility of elderly patients allows for earlier diagnosis.
   B. **Percutaneous drainage of diverticular abscess as the initial approach has been shown to have a higher failure rate in the geriatric population with a greater risk for permanent stoma and mortality.**
   C. The risks outweigh the benefits of early surgical feeding access placement in geriatric patients.
   D. Extremes of age, namely octogenarians and older, represent a prohibitive risk for surgery as the majority of these patients diet within 1 year of surgical intervention.
8. The role of laparoscopy in the management of cholecystitis in elderly patients can most accurately be described as:
   A. Laparoscopy cholecystectomy is not safe in the geriatric population.
   B. Laparoscopy leads to higher rates of subtotal cholecystectomy in the setting of acute cholecystitis.
   C. Laparoscopic cholecystectomy should be deferred until the resolution of symptoms and has more favorable outcomes when performed electively after discharge.
   D. **The rate of conversion from laparoscopic to open cholecystectomy can often be higher in the geriatric population.**
9. Which of the following is true regarding acute mesenteric ischemia (AMI) in the geriatric population?
   A. The attenuated inflammatory response leads to elderly patients with AMI presenting in the early phase of the disease to the emergency room
   B. Renal failure, but not length of bowel necrosis, predicts outcomes in patients with AMI.
   C. **Near-total intestinal necrosis should prompt serious consideration regarding the goals of care and quality of life in geriatric patients.**
   D. The perioperative risks associated with surgical intervention warrant radiographic evidence of AMI prior to offering surgery.
10. Which of the following is accurate in distinguishing between the etiologies of AMI?
    A. AMI due to thrombosis of the superior mesenteric artery (SMA) typically occurs in elderly patients with valvular heart disease.
    B. **Non-occlusive mesenteric ischemia (NOMI) commonly occurs in critically ill patients who are hypotensive or on dialysis for end-stage renal disease.**
    C. Prompt laparotomy and bowel resection are more important than revascularization in the geriatric population.
    D. Arrhythmias such as atrial fibrillation lead to SMA thrombosis more often than SMA embolus.

References

1. United States Census Bureau. https://www.census.gov/.
2. Fried LP, Ferrucci L, Darer J, Williamson JD, Anderson G. Untangling the concepts of disability, frailty, and comorbidity: implications for improved targeting and care. J Gerontol A Biol Sci Med Sci. 2004;59(3):255–63. https://doi.org/10.1093/gerona/59.3.m255.
3. Holliday R. Understanding ageing, vol. 30. New York: Cambridge University Press; 1995.
4. Olivetti G, Melissari M, Capasso JM, Anversa P. Cardiomyopathy of the aging human heart. Myocyte loss and reactive cellular hypertrophy. Circ Res. 1991;68(6):1560–8. https://doi.org/10.1161/01.res.68.6.1560.
5. Knudson RJ, Lebowitz MD, Holberg CJ, Burrows B. Changes in the normal maximal expiratory flow-volume curve with growth and aging. Am Rev Respir Dis. 1983;127(6):725–34.
6. Brenner BM, Meyer TW, Hostetter TH. Dietary protein intake and the progressive nature of kidney disease: the role of hemodynamically mediated glomerular injury in the pathogenesis of progressive glomerular sclerosis in aging, renal ablation, and intrinsic renal disease. N Engl J Med. 1982;307(11):652–9. https://doi.org/10.1056/NEJM198209093071104.
7. Clegg A, Young J, Iliffe S, Rikkert MO, Rockwood K. Frailty in elderly people. Lancet. 2013;381(9868):752–62. https://doi.org/10.1016/S0140-6736(12)62167-9.
8. Dastur DK. Cerebral blood flow and metabolism in normal human aging, pathological aging, and senile dementia. J Cereb Blood Flow Metab. 1985;5(1):1–9. https://doi.org/10.1038/jcbfm.1985.1.
9. Oresanya LB, Lyons WL, Finlayson E. Preoperative assessment of the older patient: a narrative review. JAMA. 2014;311(20):2110–20. https://doi.org/10.1001/jama.2014.4573.
10. Fried LP, Tangen CM, Walston J, et al. Frailty in older adults: evidence for a phenotype. J Gerontol A Biol Sci Med Sci. 2001;56(3):M146–56.
11. Theou O, Rockwood K. Should frailty status always be considered when treating the elderly patient? Aging Health. 2012;8(3):261–71.
12. de Vries NM, Staal JB, van Ravensberg CD, Hobbelen JSM, Olde Rikkert MGM, Nijhuis-van der Sanden MWG. Outcome instruments to measure frailty: a systematic review. Ageing Res Rev. 2011;10(1):104–14. https://doi.org/10.1016/j.arr.2010.09.001.
13. Rockwood K, Song X, MacKnight C, et al. A global clinical measure of fitness and frailty in elderly people. CMAJ. 2005;173(5):489–95. https://doi.org/10.1503/cmaj.050051.
14. Farhat JS, Velanovich V, Falvo AJ, et al. Are the frail destined to fail? Frailty index as predictor of surgical morbidity and mortality in the elderly. J Trauma Acute Care Surg. 2012;72(6):1526–30; discussion 1530–1531. https://doi.org/10.1097/TA.0b013e3182542fab.
15. Joseph B, Pandit V, Zangbar B, et al. Validating trauma-specific frailty index for geriatric trauma patients: a prospective analysis. J Am Coll Surg. 2014;219(1):10–7.
16. Orouji Jokar T, Ibraheem K, Rhee P, et al. Emergency general surgery specific frailty index: a validation study. J Trauma Acute Care Surg. 2016;81(2):254–60.
17. Latifi R, editor. Surgical decision making in geriatrics. Springer Nature; 2020.
18. Bonne S, Schuerer DJE. Trauma in the older adult epidemiology and evolving geriatric trauma principles. Clin Geriatr Med. 2013;29(1):137–50. https://doi.org/10.1016/j.cger.2012.10.008.
19. Jacobs DG. Special considerations in geriatric injury. Curr Opin Crit Care. 2003;9(6):535–9. https://doi.org/10.1097/00075198-200312000-00012.
20. Czorlich P, Mader MM-D, Emami P, Westphal M, Lefering R, Hoffmann M. Operative versus non-operative treatment of traumatic brain injuries in patients 80 years of age or older. Neurosurg Rev. 2020;43(5):1305–14. https://doi.org/10.1007/s10143-019-01159-4.
21. Teasdale G, Jennett B. Assessment of coma and impaired consciousness. A practical scale. Lancet. 1974;2:81–4. https://doi.org/10.1016/s0140-6736(74)91639-0.
22. Kehoe A, Rennie S, Smith JE. Glasgow Coma Scale is unreliable for the prediction of severe head injury in elderly trauma patients. Emerg Med J. 2015;32:613–5. https://doi.org/10.1136/emermed-2013-203488.
23. Salottolo K, Panchal R, Madayag RM, et al. Incorporating age improves the Glasgow Coma Scale score for predicting mortality from traumatic brain injury. Trauma Surg Acute Care Open. 2021;6(1):e000641.
24. McIntyre A, Mehta S, Aubut J, Dijkers M, Teasell RW. Mortality among older adults after a traumatic brain injury: a meta-analysis. Brain Inj. 2013;27:31–40.
25. Mosenthal AC, Lavery RF, Addis M, Kaul S, Ross S, Marburger R, Deitch EA, Livingston DH. Isolated traumatic brain injury: age is an independent predictor of mortality and early outcome. J Trauma. 2002;52:907–11.
26. Nishijima DK, Shahlaie K, Sarkar K, Rudisill N, Holmes JF. Risk of unfavorable long-term outcome in older adults with traumatic intracranial hemorrhage and anticoagulant or antiplatelet use. Am J Emerg Med. 2013;31:1244–7.
27. Scotti P, Seguin C, Lo BWY et al. Antithrombotic agents and traumatic brain injury in the elderly population: hemorrhage patterns and outcomes. J Neurosurg. 2019;1–10.
28. Feeney JM, Santone E, DiFiori M, et al. Compared to warfarin, direct anticoagulants are associated with lower mortality in patients with blunt traumatic intracranial hemorrhage: a TQIP study. J Trauma Acute Care Surg. 2016;81(5):843–8.

29. Eibinger N, Halvachizadeh S, Hallmann B, et al. Is the regular intake of anticoagulative agents an independent risk factor for the severity of traumatic brain injuries in geriatric patients? A retrospective analysis of 10,559 patients from the TraumaRegister DGU. Brain Sci. 2020;10(11):842.
30. Bratton SL, Chestnut RM, Ghajar J, McConnell Hammond FF, Harris OA, Hartl R, Manley GT, Nemecek A, Newell DW, Rosenthal G, et al.; Brain Trauma Foundation and American Association of Neurological Surgeons. Guidelines for the management of severe traumatic brain injury. J Neurotrauma. 2007;24:S1–S106.
31. Schupper AJ, Berndtson AE, Smith A, et al. Respect your elders: effects of ageing on intracranial pressure monitor use in traumatic brain injury. Trauma Surg Acute Care Open. 2019;4(1):e000306.
32. You W, Feng J, Tang Q, et al. Intraventricular intracranial pressure monitoring improves the outcome of older adults with severe traumatic brain injury: an observational, prospective study. BMC Anesthesiol. 2016;16(1):35.
33. Liveris A, Parsikia A, Melvin J, et al. Is there an age cutoff for intracranial pressure monitoring?: a propensity score matched analysis of the national trauma data bank. Am Surg. 2022;88(6):1163–71. https://doi.org/10.1177/0003134821991985. Online ahead of print.
34. Lukasiewicz A, Grant RA, Basques BA, et al. Patient factors associated with 30-day morbidity, mortality, and length of stay after surgery for subdural hematoma: a study of the American College of Surgeons National Surgical Quality Improvement Program. J Neurosurg. 2016;124(3):760–6.
35. Kerezouids P, Goyal A, Puffer RC. Morbidity and mortality in elderly patients undergoing evacuation of acute traumatic subdural hematoma. Neurosurg Focus. 2020;49(4):E22.
36. Bulger EM, Arneson MA, Mock CN, et al. Rib fractures in the elderly. J Trauma. 2000;48(6):1040–6.
37. Battle CE, Hutchings H, Evans PA. Risk factors that predict mortality in patients with blunt chest wall trauma: a systematic review and meta-analysis. Injury. 2012;43(1):8–17.
38. Janssen TL, Hosseinzoi E, Vos DI, et al. The importance of increased awareness for delirium in elderly patients with rib fractures after blunt chest wall trauma: a retrospective cohort study on risk factors and outcomes. BMC Emerg Med. 2018;19:34.
39. Bulger E, Edwards T, Klotz P, et al. Epidural analgesia improves outcome after multiple rib fractures. Surgery. 2004;136(2):426–30.
40. Flagel BT, Luchette FA, Reed RL, Esposito TJ, Davis KA, Santaniello JM, Gamelli RL. Half-a-dozen ribs: the breakpoint for mortality. Surgery. 2005;138:717–23; discussion 723–5.
41. McKendy KM, Lee LF, Boulva K, et al. Epidural analgesia for traumatic rib fractures is associated with worse outcomes: a matched analysis. J Surg Res. 2017;214:117–23. https://doi.org/10.1016/j.jss.2017.02.057.
42. Griffard J, Daley B, Campbell M, et al. Plate of ribs: a single institution's matched comparison of patients managed operative and non-operatively for rib fractures. Trauma Surg Acute Care Open. 2020;5(1):e000519.
43. Zhu RC, de Roulet A, Ogami T, et al. Rib fixation in geriatric trauma: mortality benefits for the most vulnerable patients. J Trauma Acute Care Surg. 2020;89(1):103–10. https://doi.org/10.1097/TA.0000000000002666.
44. Sikander N, Ahmad T, Shaikh KA, et al. Analysis of injury patterns and outcomes of blunt thoracic trauma in elderly patients. Cureus. 2020;12(8):e9974. https://doi.org/10.7759/cureus.9974.
45. Kulvatunyou N, Joseph B, Friese RS, et al. 14 French pigtail catheters placed by surgeons to drain blood on trauma patients: is 14-Fr too small? J Trauma Acute Care Surg. 2012;73(6):1423–7.
46. Lin HL, Huang WY, Yang C, et al. How early should VATS be performed for retained haemothorax in blunt chest trauma? Injury. 2014;45(9):1359–64. https://doi.org/10.1016/j.injury.2014.05.036. Epub 2014 Jun 5.
47. Schweigert M, Beron M, Dubecz A, et al. Video-assisted thoracoscopic surgery for posttraumatic hemothorax in the very elderly. Thorac Cardiovasc Surg. 2012;60(7):474–9. https://doi.org/10.1055/s-0031-1298069. Epub 2012 Jan 20.
48. Huang WY, Lu IY, Yang C, et al. Efficiency analysis of direct video-assisted thoracoscopic surgery in elderly patients with blunt traumatic hemothorax without an initial thoracostomy. Biomed Res Int. 2016;2016:3741426. https://doi.org/10.1155/2016/3741426. Epub 2016 Apr 14.
49. Heffernan DS, Thakkar RK, Monaghan SF, et al. Normal presenting vital signs are unreliable in geriatric blunt trauma victims. J Trauma. 2010;69(4):813–20.
50. Zarzaur BL, Croce MA, Magnotti LJ, et al. Identifying life-threatening shock in the older injured patient: an analysis of the National Trauma Data Bank. J Trauma. 2010;68(5):1134–8.
51. Malhotra AK, Fabian TC, Croce MA, et al. Blunt hepatic injury: a paradigm shift from operative to nonoperative management in the 1990s. Ann Surg. 2000;231(6):804–13.
52. Brillantino A, Iacobellis F, Robustelli U, et al. Non operative management of blunt splenic trauma: a prospective evaluation of a standardized treatment protocol. Eur J Trauma Emerg Surg. 2016;42(5):593–8.
53. Godley CD, Warren RL, Sheridan RL, McCabe CJ. Nonoperative management of blunt splenic injury in adults: age over 55 years as a powerful indicator for failure. J Am Coll Surg. 1996;183:133–9.
54. Albrecht RM, Schermer CR, Morris A. Nonoperative management of blunt splenic injuries: factors influencing success in age >55 years. Am Surg. 2002;68:227–30.
55. Massarweh NN, Legner VJ, Symons RG, et al. Impact of advancing age on abdominal surgical outcomes. Arch Surg. 2009;144:1108–14.
56. Peitzman AB, Heil B, Rivera L, et al. Blunt splenic injury in adults: multi-institutional study of the

Eastern Association for the Surgery of Trauma. J Trauma. 2000;49:177–89.
57. Al-Refaie WB, Parsons HM, Habermann EB, et al. Operative outcomes beyond 30-day mortality. Ann Surg. 2011;253:947–52.
58. Silber JH, Williams SV, Krakauer H, Schwartz JS. Hospital and patient characteristics associated with death after surgery: a study of adverse occurrence and failure to rescue. Med Care. 1992;30(7):615–27.
59. Khan M, Jehan F, Zeeshan M, et al. Failure to rescue after emergency general surgery in geriatric patients: does frailty matter? J Surg Res. 2019;233:397–402. https://doi.org/10.1016/j.jss.2018.08.033. Epub 2018 Sep 17.
60. Fulton JD, Peebles SE, Smith GD, et al. Unrecognized viscus perforation in the elderly. Age Ageing. 1989;18(6):403–6.
61. Wroblewski M, Mikulowski P, et al. Peritonitis in geriatric inpatients. Age Ageing. 1991;20(2):90–4. https://doi.org/10.1093/ageing/20.2.90.
62. Elagili F, Stocchi L, Ozuner G, et al. Predictors of postoperative outcomes for patients with diverticular abscess initially treated with percutaneous drainage. Am J Surg. 2015;209(4):703–8. https://doi.org/10.1016/j.amjsurg.2014.05.018. Epub 2014 Jul 23.
63. Buck DL, Vester-Andersen M, Moller MH, et al. Surgical delay is a critical determinant of survival in perforated peptic ulcer. Br J Surg. 2013;100(8):1045–9. https://doi.org/10.1002/bjs.9175.
64. Lavanchy JL, Holzgang MM, Haltmeier T, et al. Outcomes of emergency abdominal surgery in octogenarians: a single-center analysis. Am J Surg. 2019;218(2):248–54. https://doi.org/10.1016/j.amjsurg.2018.11.023. Epub 2018 Nov 27.
65. Narueponjikarul N, Hwabejire J, Kongwibulwut M, et al. No news is good news? Three-year postdischarge mortality of octogenarian and nonagenarian patients following emergency general surgery. J Trauma Acute Care Surg. 2020;89(1):230–7. https://doi.org/10.1097/TA.0000000000002696.
66. Gogna S, Samson D, Choi J, et al. The role of nutritional access in malnourished elderly undergoing major surgery for acute abdomen: a propensity score-matched analysis. Am Surg. 2021;87(8):1252–8. https://doi.org/10.1177/0003134820973719.
67. Krasman ML, Gracie WA, Strasius SR. Biliary tract disease in the aged. Clin Geriatr Med. 1991;7:347–70.
68. Riall TS, Zhang D, Townsend CM, et al. Failure to perform cholecystectomy for acute cholecystitis in elderly patients is associated with increased morbidity, mortality, and cost. J Am Coll Surg. 2010;210(5):668–79.
69. Parker LJ, Vukov LF, Wollan PC, et al. Emergency department evaluation of geriatric patients with acute cholecystitis. Acad Emerg Med. 1997;4(1):51–5.
70. Chang YR, Ahn YJ, Jang JY, et al. Percutaneous cholecystostomy for acute cholecystitis in patients with high comorbidity and re-evaluation of treatment efficacy. Surgery. 2014;155:615–22.
71. Dimou FM, Adhikari D, Mehta H, et al. Outcomes in older patients with grade III cholecystitis and cholecystostomy tube placement: a propensity score analysis. J Am Coll Surg. 2017;224(4):502–511.e1.
72. Loozen CS, van Ramshorst B, van Santvoort HC, et al. Early cholecystectomy for acute cholecystitis in the elderly population: a systematic review and meta-analysis. Dig Surg. 2017;34(5):371–9.
73. Mayol J, Martinez-Sarmiento J, Tamayo FJ, et al. Complications of laparoscopic cholecystectomy in the ageing patient. Age Ageing. 1997;26:77–81.
74. Elshaer M, Gravante G, Thomas K, et al. Subtotal cholecystectomy for "difficult gallbladders": systematic review and meta-analysis. JAMA Surg. 2015;150:159–68.
75. Pisano M, Ceresoli M, Cimbanassi S, et al. 2017 WSES and SICG guidelines on acute calcolous cholecystitis in elderly population. World J Emerg Surg. 2019;14:10.
76. Martinez JP, Hogan GJ. Mesenteric ischemia. Emerg Med Clin North Am. 2004;22:909–28. https://doi.org/10.1016/j.emc.2004.05.002.
77. Klar E, Rahmanian PB, Bücker A, Hauenstein K, Jauch KW, Luther B. Acute mesenteric ischemia: a vascular emergency. Dtsch Arztebl Int. 2012;109(14):249–56.
78. Demir ED, Ceyhan GO, Friess H. Beyond lactate: is there a role for serum lactate measurement in diagnosing acute mesenteric ischemia? Dig Surg. 2012;29:226–35.
79. Kougias P, Lau D, El Sayed HF, et al. Determinants of mortality and treatment outcome following surgical interventions for acute mesenteric ischemia. J Vasc Surg. 2007;46(3):467–74.
80. Wu W, Liu J, Zhou Z, et al. Preoperative risk factors for short-term postoperative mortality of acute mesenteric ischemia after laparotomy: a systematic review and meta-analysis. Emerg Med Int. 2020;2020:1382475.
81. Akyildiz HY, Sozuer E, Uzer H, et al. The length of necrosis and renal insufficiency predict the outcome of acute mesenteric ischemia. Asian J Surg. 2015;38(1):28–32.

Further Reading

Joseph B, Pandit V, Zangbar B, et al. Validating trauma-specific frailty index for geriatric trauma patients: a prospective analysis. J Am Coll Surg. 2014;219(1):10–7.

Latifi R, editor. Surgical decision making in geriatrics. Springer Nature; 2020.

Massarweh NN, Legner VJ, Symons RG, et al. Impact of advancing age on abdominal surgical outcomes. Arch Surg. 2009;144:1108–14.

Narueponjikarul N, Hwabejire J, Kongwibulwut M, et al. No news is good news? Three-year postdischarge mortality of octogenarian and nonagenarian patients following emergency general surgery. J Trauma Acute Care Surg. 2020;89(1):230–7. https://doi.org/10.1097/TA.0000000000002696.

Pediatrics

24

Matthew P. Landman and Denis Bensard

24.1 Introduction

Learning Goals
- Pediatric surgical emergencies can present differently than adults.
- Surgeons should be able to identify signs/symptoms of child abuse.
- Non-operative management is the standard for pediatric solid organ injuries.

24.1.1 Epidemiology

The early twentieth century brought with it surgeons who steadily began focusing solely on the practice of surgery in children [1]. These surgeons increasingly recognized the unique anatomical and physiological differences that distinguish adults from pediatric patients and implemented surgical solutions with those differences in mind. Their work in establishing pediatric surgery as an independent specialty allowed for impressive improvements in pediatric conditions with previous dire outcomes.

Globally, the absolute number of children has steadily increased over the past several decades. However, in many countries, the percentage of the population made up by children under 18 years has decreased steadily [2]. While children may continually make up smaller percentages of the overall global population, their surgical needs are no less significant and, in many cases, remain unique from adult diagnoses. While there is overlap in diagnosis and treatments, it is imperative for surgeons to understand the specific burden of surgical disease in children and adolescents and to know how treatment in some cases may be different than that of adults. The breadth of pediatric diagnoses is vast and includes both acquired conditions secondary to infection, ingestion, trauma, and congenital anomalies, many of which appear at or shortly after birth.

24.1.2 Pediatric Emergency General Surgery

The breadth of pediatric emergent and urgent surgical illnesses is myriad. These surgical needs vary by age. In a 2013 study reviewing the 2009 Kids' Inpatient Database (including data from 44 of 50 US states and not including patients admitted under observation status), Somme and colleagues noted slightly more than 200,000

M. P. Landman (✉)
Indiana University School of Medicine,
Indianapolis, IN, USA
e-mail: landman@iu.edu

D. Bensard
Denver Health, University of Colorado School of Medicine, Aurora, CO, USA
e-mail: Denis.bensard@dhha.org

Table 24.1 Commonly performed pediatric surgery operations. (Adopted from Sømme S, Bronsert M, Morrato E, Ziegler M. Frequency and variety of inpatient pediatric surgical procedures in the United States. *Pediatrics*. 2013;132(6):e1466-72)

Appendectomy
Central Venous Access
Pyloromyotomy
Burn Debridement or grafting
Cholecystectomy
PDA Ligation
Bladder/ureteral reconstruction
Anti-reflux procedures
Pediatric inguinal hernia repair
Gastrostomy/jejunostomy
Intestinal resection (congenital lesions like Meckel's diverticulum, duplication cyst, meconium ileus/cyst)
Oophorectomy/salpingectomy
Decortication pleurodesis
Diagnostic laparoscopy or laparotomy
Intestinal resection/ostomy (IBD)
Pyeloplasty/UPJ reconstruction
Closure/revision/creation ostomy
Gastroschisis/omphalocele
Repair chest wall deformity
Major excision soft tissue tumor

inpatient pediatric cases. Of these cases, the top 20 procedures accounted for more than 90% of the cases (Table 24.1). Up to 40% of all inpatient pediatric cases were performed at adult general hospitals [3]. In 2006, Rabbitts et al. identified 2.3 million ambulatory anesthesia episodes (38 per 1000 children) in the United States for children less than 15 years of age, a slight increase from a previous evaluation in 1996 which noted 26 per 1000 children in the National Survey of Ambulatory Surgery [4]. The increase in ambulatory surgery, the authors note, may have resulted from shifting cases previously performed in an inpatient setting. Recognizing that children receive surgical care in a variety of environments, within many documented cases with variable outcomes, the American College of Surgeons, developed a systematic verification program based on standards established by multidisciplinary groups including pediatric surgeons, anesthesiologists, and others important in the process of children's surgical care [5]. The stated goal of this program is "to ensure pediatric surgical patients have access to high-quality care, the program verifies that resources required to achieve optimal patient outcomes for children receiving surgical care at health care facilities are met" [5].

Between 2007 and 2014, according to the National Hospital Ambulatory Medical Care Survey, there were an estimated 21.1 million unique emergency department observations for nontraumatic abdominal pain in children [6]. The general indications for admission to a hospital for pediatric patients are gastrointestinal, orthopedic, or urological diagnoses [7]. Somme and colleagues, in their 2013 report on inpatient pediatric surgical procedures, noted the following top 10 procedures in the pediatric population performed at general hospitals: Appendectomy, central venous access, cholecystectomy, burn debridement/grafting, pyloromyotomy, oophorectomy/salpingectomy, PDA ligation, pediatric inguinal hernia repair, intestinal resection (congenital lesions such as Meckel's diverticulum, enteric duplication cyst, meconium cyst/ileus) and diagnostic laparoscopy/laparotomy [3]. In this report, appendectomy was performed at a rate five times higher than the next most common procedure, central venous catheter placement, at a rate of 239 cases per 10,000 surgical admissions. This chapter will focus on pediatric surgical diagnoses most likely to be evaluated by the adult emergency general surgeon.

Pediatric appendicitis is one of the most common urgent pediatric general surgery operations performed in the United States. There are approximately 60,000 to 80,000 appendectomies performed annually with nearly half of these cases occurring in children 17 years of age and younger (www.hcup.ahrq.gov, accessed on April 13, 2021). The peak incidence of appendicitis occurs in the 10–19 years age range. Males are slightly more frequently afflicted. Other differences in incidence occur and are potentially related to socioeconomic status, race, and ethnicity [8].

Bowel obstruction presents another unique pediatric surgical diagnosis important for the adult general surgeon. Congenital, acquired, inflammatory and traumatic etiologies must be considered, and their prevalence is dependent on many factors including patient age. The rate of adhesive bowel obstruction after pediatric abdominal surgery has been estimated at 1–5% with estimates closer to 1% if previous appendectomy patients are excluded [9]. Surgical intervention is required in these patients in 35–45% of non-appendicitis-related bowel obstruction cases.

Malrotation, while possible at all ages, is much more prevalent in patients less than 1 year of age. Additionally, intussusception occurred in children younger than 6 years, classically between the ages of 6 months and 2 years of age.

24.1.2.1 Pediatric Trauma

Injury is the leading cause of death in the United States for persons aged 1–19 years old. The leading mechanism is motor vehicle crashes in patients 5–19 years while drowning is slightly higher in patients 1–4 years [10]. Annually, 9.2 million children present to US emergency departments for treatment related to injuries. These visits result in 225,000 annual hospital admissions and are a leading cause of morbidity, resource utilization, and blunted quality of life. A 2012 analysis of the National Trauma Database revealed an overall pediatric trauma mortality of 2.1%. Worldwide, as many as 1 million children die annually of injuries and as many as 10 to 30 million children suffer nonfatal injuries [10]. An estimated 17.4 million children do not have access to a pediatric trauma center within 60 min [11]. In the United States, nearly 30% of children lack prompt access to pediatric trauma care and nearly 90% of pediatric trauma patients do not receive care at a pediatric trauma hospital [12]. As with adult trauma centers, the American College of Surgeons, as well as some states, maintains guidelines for pediatric trauma level verification. As of 2021 the number of ACS designated level I/II pediatric centers is 137, more than three times the 43 in 2010 (American College of Surgeons Committee on Trauma and Trauma Quality Improvement Project Spring 2021 report). The importance of trauma-designated trauma centers for children is notable. Myers et al. found that injured children treated at a Level I pediatric trauma center were more likely to survive when compared to a Level I trauma center [13, 14]. However, as a majority of the initial evaluation and management of pediatric patients is provided outside of pediatric level I and II centers, it is imperative that adult providers understand the nuances in the treatment of pediatric trauma patients. In a 2021 analysis of pediatric trauma mortality, Pender and colleagues found a strong inverse relation between pediatric access to trauma centers and trauma-related mortality [15].

Traumatic brain injury (TBI) is a leading type of childhood injury according to the Center for Disease Control. In the United States alone children aged 0–14 years make almost half a million emergency department visits for TBI annually [16]. TBI resulting from unintentional trauma constitute the primary cause of death among children and young adults. Fortunately, most brain injuries are mild but even this level of injury is associated potentially associated with ongoing problems [17, 18]. TBI is a significant financial burden on the US economy with charges for TBI-related hospital visits being more than one billion dollars per year in the United States [19].

24.1.3 Etiology

24.1.3.1 Pediatric Emergency General Surgery

Appendicitis

Right lower quadrant pain from appendicitis is one of the most common surgical consultations in pediatric surgery. As with adults, pediatric appendicitis is related to obstruction of the blind-ending lumen of the appendix with a fecalith, lymphoid hyperplasia, parasite, or rarely, a tumor. However, obstructive etiologies are generally found in approximately 40%, and therefore environmental and genetic causes have been postulated. A positive family history of appendicitis has been shown to increase the relative risk of acute appendicitis threefold [20].

Bowel Obstruction

The underlying etiology of bowel obstruction is generally adhesions in patients with previous intra-abdominal surgery. Neonatal bowel obstructions can be from an underlying intrinsic intestinal anomaly or from external compression. Intrinsic lesions include intestinal atresia/stenosis, malrotation, duplication cyst, meconium ileus, meconium plug syndrome, small left colon syndrome, and Hirschsprung's disease [21]. In one pediatric series of patients presenting with bowel obstruction without a history of laparotomy, malrotation, intussusception, internal hernia, Meckel's diverticulum, idiopathic volvulus, inflammation, foreign body, and hamartoma, were the underlying etiologies [22]. Other important possible etiologies to consider for pediatric bowel obstruction include incarcerated inguinal hernia, malignancy, and inflammatory bowel disease.

Intestinal malrotation with volvulus is a vital consideration in pediatric patients presenting with bowel obstruction, especially those with no previous abdominal surgery. Autopsy series suggest the incidence of intestinal rotational anomalies is around 0.5% in the general population [23]. Presentation is most commonly, but not exclusively, in children less than a year of age.

Intussusception commonly occurs in pediatric patients between 3 months and 2 years and is the result of a proximal bowel segment invaginating into a distal bowel segment [24]. The worldwide incidence is estimated to be 0.74 per 1000 children. Geographical differences are present. While many pediatric cases are idiopathic; however, pathological lead points can be the source. The most common pathological lead points include Meckel's diverticulum and lymphoma with more rare etiologies being duplication cysts, polyps, or other masses.

Meckel's Diverticulum

Meckel's diverticulum is an embryological remnant of the omphalomesenteric duct and is the most common congenital anomaly of the gastrointestinal tract. It is estimated that 2% of the population has this anomaly. Meckel's diverticula can result in symptoms due to obstruction of the neck of the true diverticulum resulting in Meckel's diverticulitis, intussusception with the Meckel's diverticulum serving as a pathologic lead point, intestinal obstruction related to an associated congenital band, bleeding secondary to mucosal ulceration from heterotopic gastric tissue (present in 50–60% of cases), or less commonly intestinal perforation [25].

Inguinal Hernia

Nearly all pediatric inguinal hernias are indirect, related to a congenital patent processus vaginalis in males or canal of Nuck in females. The incidence of inguinal hernias in infants is correlated to the gestational age at birth. Anywhere from 0.8 to 5% of terms infants have an inguinal hernia whereas as many as 30% of low birthweight and premature infants may be affected [26]. The incarceration rate also differs by gestation age with a crude rate of 11% in preterm children and 7% for all children [27]. Adolescent patients presenting with inguinal hernia generally have an indirect inguinal defect [28].

24.1.3.2 Pediatric Trauma

The mechanisms of injury in pediatric trauma are largely related to the patient's age. According to the Centers for Disease Control, patients who are in their adolescence are generally more likely to be injured and/or die in motor vehicle crashes. Patients under 10 years of age tend to suffer from pedestrian-struck mechanisms and toddlers are most afflicted by falls. Falls are common in the younger patient population due to a higher center of gravity and more immature motor and cognitive skills. While penetrating mechanisms are relatively rare in pediatric patients, as patients approach adolescence, gunshot wounds and other penetrating mechanisms become more common. In an analysis of the National Inpatient Sample database, Oliver et al. noted that all pediatric trauma motor vehicle crashes remain the most important cause of pediatric trauma [29]. However, they note that in patients aged 15–19 years of age assaults, including knife and gunshot wounds were the second most common mechanism of severe injury. Overall, orthopedic injuries, in their series, were the most common injury requiring hospitalization.

24.2 Diagnosis

24.2.1 Clinical Presentation

24.2.1.1 Pediatric Emergency General Surgery

Appendicitis

The classically described presentation for patients with appendicitis is vague periumbilical pain which migrates to McBurney's point in the right lower quadrant. This is generally associated with symptoms such as fever, nausea, vomiting, and anorexia. However, it is important to note that the classic signs of appendicitis may only be present in roughly half of patients [8]. Patients may present on a spectrum from relatively minimal pain with normal vital signs to generalized peritonitis with markers of systemic inflammatory response syndrome (SIRS). Physical exam findings described in patients with appendicitis, in addition to right lower quadrant pain, include Rovsing's sign (right-sided abdominal pain from left lower quadrant palpation), obturator sign (pain with flexion and interval rotation of the right hip), psoas sign (pain with left side down right hip extension), Dunphy's sign (pain with coughing), and a positive Markle test (pain with heel drop) [8]. This is especially true in very young patients. Up to 80% of patients less than 3 years of age will present with perforated appendicitis.

Bowel Obstruction

The presenting symptoms of obstruction can be variable depending on a patient's age at presentation. Four key features of intestinal obstruction in the newborn include (1) maternal polyhydramnios, (2) bilious vomiting, (3) no meconium passage, and (4) abdominal distension [30].

The classic symptoms of obstruction include abdominal pain, bilious vomiting, abdominal distension, and obstipation. These may be relatively acute in onset or insidious in onset. Markers of volume depletion including lethargy, low urine output, tachycardia, hypotension, sunken fontanelle (in infants), and delayed capillary refill may be present. Abdominal examination may reveal point tenderness or more generalized discomfort and possibly peritonitis. Bilious vomiting is the classic presentation of intestinal malrotation with volvulus. This is especially true in the neonatal period, the most common time for the presentation of volvulus (90% of cases presenting at age 1 or younger). Older patients with intestinal volvulus commonly present with vomiting and abdominal pain and may have a history of chronic abdominal pain, dyspepsia, or early satiety [31]. Intussusception often presents with intermittent bouts of abdominal pain or fussiness and/or vomiting. Parents commonly describe patients bringing their knees to their chest during these episodes. Currant jelly stools may ensue. Abdominal examination may reveal tenderness or a mass.

Meckel's Diverticulum

Pediatric Meckel's diverticulum can present in a variety of manners. Patients with Meckel's diverticulitis may mimic patients with acute appendicitis with right lower quadrant pain, fevers, nausea, vomiting, and anorexia. Mucosal ulceration secondary to heterotopic gastric tissue may present as bright red blood per rectum, classically without abdominal pain.

Inguinal Hernia

Pediatric inguinal hernias are generally noted on clinical examination or present electively with an intermittent inguinal bulge. This bulge is generally reproducible with any Valsalva maneuver [26]. Infants and young children may not be able to participate in this examination and therefore reproduction in the examination room may not be possible making definitive diagnosis difficult. Occasionally, families have documented the finding via a picture on their smart phone. The surgeon should be astute to the differences between inguinal hernia and communicating hydrocele as this can be difficult to ascertain via history alone. Symptoms suggesting communicating hydrocele may include variable swelling depending on the time of day (generally less scrotal swelling in the morning or after a long nap) and little or no inguinal canal swelling at the location of the external inguinal ring. Incarcerated inguinal hernias present with an inguinal bulge that is generally hard and may have overlying skin changes. Patients are usually fussy and may have evidence of bowel obstruction including abdominal distension, tachycardia, and bilious vomiting. Stylianos and colleagues found that up to 35% of their patients who presented with an incarcerated hernia were known to have an asymptomatic inguinal hernia and 83% were awaiting repair [32].

24.2.1.2 Pediatric Trauma

The initial evaluation of the pediatric trauma patient proceeds identically to the adult trauma patients. Pediatric trauma patients should be evaluated by the orderly assessment dictated by the advanced trauma life support algorithms. Early intervention should focus on the diagnosis and treatment of airway, breathing, and circulation issues that may present including the management of hemorrhage. As with any trauma resuscitation, airway evaluation and management are critical periods in pediatric patients and present differently than in adults due to several anatomic differences. These anatomic differences include, particularly in infants and younger children, a prominent occiput that predisposes to the forward tilt of the patient in the supine position. This is especially true in the unconscious patient produced. Additionally, is short neck, potentially increased upper airway lymphoid tissue, and a floppy epiglottis may predispose to airway complications. Given a decreased residual capacity and functional residual capacity, pediatric patients may be at higher risk for oxygen desaturations. This makes providing supplemental oxygen important, particularly in a patient who may require additional airway interventions. Unconsciousness, combativeness, declining GCS, or shock is the most common indication for a definitive airway in an injured child and identifies a seriously injured subset of children with an increased risk of death [33]. In pediatric patients who require intubation, a video laryngoscope may be utilized to assist in the intubation. However, no definitive data on its superiority to direct laryngoscopy has been identified [34]. Rapid sequence intubation is utilized frequently in emergency airway situations. The purpose of this technique is to prevent aspiration events while obtaining rapid access airway access. Children exhibit an exaggerated vagal response to hypoxia, succinylcholine, laryngoscopy, and intubation [35]. Practitioners should be familiar with the medications used to facilitate rapid sequence intubation including medications for sedation, no muscular blockade, and also to blunt the physiological effects from excessive vagal stimulation, common in pediatric patients. An important consideration in pediatric patients undergoing intubation is the correct selection of the endotracheal tube. Importantly, unlike adults, the area of greatest narrowing of the airway in the pediatric population is the subglottic region. The selection of an endotracheal tube that is too large could result in the future development of subglottic stenosis.

Breathing is assessed similarly in adults and pediatric patients. Pediatric patients may present with respiratory distress with stridor, subcostal retractions, grunting, and or paradoxical motion of the diaphragm. Patients may, due to underdeveloped chest wall musculature and a primary diaphragmatic mechanism of breathing, tire easily. Signs of respiratory distress should prompt practitioners to consider additional airway measures in possibly the assistance of breathing. Intimated pediatric patients should be given a title volume of 6–8 mL/kg in order to reduce the risk of barotrauma. $FiO_2\%$ should be administered to maintain oxygen saturations but titrated to the lowest level possible in order to prevent hyperoxia injury. Pediatric patients with head injury are at risk for secondary traumatic brain injury due to hypotension and hypoxia. In a study of children with severe TBI (GCS <8) in level I PTC investigators found that children with the admission of $PaCO_2$ between 36 and 45 mmHg had greater discharge survival compared to those with both admission hypocarbia ($PaCO_2 \leq 35$ mmHg) and hypercarbia ($PaCO_2 \geq 46$ mmHg) [36]. In pediatric intubated patients with inadequate ventilation or hypoxia, practitioners should consider underlying etiologies including pneumothorax, hemothorax, inadequate gastric decompression, aspiration, or significant pulmonary contusion.

Classically, pediatric trauma patients can compensate for significant hemorrhage up to approximately 40% reduction in circulating blood volume before seeing changes in normal blood pressure. This compensation is a result of both increased heart rate as well as significant peripheral vasoconstriction. It is important to note that the total blood volume is approximately 80–90 mL/kg. Therefore, to reach significant levels of hemorrhage, only a small amount of absolute blood loss can be tolerated. Signs of significant hemorrhage with loss of circulating blood volume in pediatric patients include tachycardia, delayed capillary refill (less than two seconds), pallor, decreased level of consciousness, and hypotension. The Hartford consensus conference concluded that the leading cause of preventable death is bleeding and simple interventions that "Stop the bleed" can be lifesaving [37]. While no pediatric-specific data on the use of tourniquets is available in the literature, their use is generally recommended in patients with extinguishing hemorrhage from extremity wounds. The combat application tourniquet used successfully in adult patients can also be successfully utilized in pediatric patients [38]. Pediatric patients presenting with signs and symptoms of shock should be assumed to have hemorrhage until proven otherwise. Importantly, however, other types of shock may be present including cardiogenic and distributive. Notoriously, pediatric patients have difficult IV access which may be exacerbated by significant hemorrhage, hypothermia, and/or hypotension. Interosseous access should be obtained in pediatric patients in whom rapid intravenous access is unattainable. Surgeons and emergency personnel should be familiar with insertion locations and techniques importantly to prevent possible complications which can include extravasation and epiphyseal plate necrosis [39].

The possibility of physical child abuse should be forefront in the surgeon's mind when evaluating pediatric patients, particularly in the youngest age groups. Annually, three million cases of child abuse and neglect are reported to child welfare systems in the United States. One-third are substantiated (around 12 per 1000 children) [40]. An organized system of evaluation and management for potential abuse is essential to ensure equitable and complete work up for all patients. It is important to note that in many US states physicians and other healthcare providers are legally required to report concerns for abuse to the appropriate authorities. Child abuse represents 3–4% of all cases seen in pediatric trauma centers which accounts for a disproportionate share of mortality in the very young. In one recent report from two level 1 pediatric trauma centers, physical child abuse caused more than 50% of all infant trauma deaths [41]. The surgeon should be acutely astute in their history and physical examination of these patients. Suspicion may be raised if the history and extent of injury do not match. Additionally, delay in seeking medical attention may also raise a suspicion of abuse. Practitioners should understand the developmental milestones of each pediatric age group in order to understand whether the reported mechanism is possible given the developmental ability. For instance, often a fall from a crib or a couch is reported. Tarantino et al. showed that few children falling from heights of less than four feet suffer serious or life-threatening injuries, so if life-threatening injuries present with that history, the likely cause is abuse [42]. A history of repeated trauma treated at different emergency departments may be noted. Fractures from different time periods particularly under the age of 3 years should alert the clinician to the possibility of abuse.

Physical examination should look for multi-colored bruises and unique bruising patterns. Pierce et al. found that bruising was common in both groups of patients with accidental and non-accidental injuries [43]. However, bruises of the torso, ear, or neck in a child 4 years or younger and bruises in any region for an infant less than four months are predictive of abusive injury. Injuries with a distinct pattern such as demarcated burns, cigarette burns, rope marks, or bites should also be documented. Long bone fractures in children younger than three years old, multiple subdural hematomas, especially without a new skull fracture, and retinal hemorrhages are all highly predictive of abuse. Abusive head trauma is more severe and results in higher mortality than accidental injuries. The acute abdomen in a very young patient following minor trauma or of unknown etiology should raise the suspicion of injury due to trauma.

24.2.2 Tests

24.2.2.1 Pediatric Emergency General Surgery

Appendicitis
The diagnosis of appendicitis in children is generally considered to be clinical. However, additional testing can be obtained to further evaluate these patients. The white blood cell count and absolute neutrophil count in pediatric patients are generally obtained in the course of the workup for right lower quadrant pain. Importantly, the white blood cell count may be normal in up to 20% of pediatric patients presenting with abdominal pain. The sensitivity and specificity of the white blood cell count range from 70 to 80% and 60 to 68%, respectively [44]. The sensitivity and specificity of the absolute neutrophil count are similarly variable and can range from 59 to 97% and 51 to 90%, respectively. C-reactive protein generally has a limited role in the diagnosis of acute appendicitis and may be more helpful in assisting practitioners in determining complicated appendicitis if markedly high. There are a growing number of different scoring tools which incorporate both clinical and laboratory data to obtain a risk score for appendicitis. The two most commonly described scores are the Alvarado score and the pediatric appendicitis score (PAS) (Table 24.2). The Alvarado score, introduced in 1986, has six clinical items and two laboratory measurements and with scores ranging from 0 to 10 with 10 being the highest likelihood for appendicitis [45]. A score greater than 7 is generally diagnostic of appendicitis. The Pediatric Appendicitis Score (PAS) includes 10 clinic and laboratory factors with significant overlap with the Alvarado score. A PAS score greater than 6 is generally considered diagnostic of appendicitis.

Imaging in appendicitis should generally augment the physical exam and laboratory assessments of the provider and is informed by the level

Table 24.2 Components of the Pediatric Appendicitis Score (PAS) and Alvarado Score for Acute Appendicitis. (Adopted from Rentea RM, Peter SDS, Snyder CL. Pediatric appendicitis: state of the art review. *Pediatr Surg Int.* 2017;33(3):269-83)

Pediatric Appendicitis Score
Right lower quadrant tenderness to cough, percussion, or hopping
Anorexia
Fever (greater than or equal to 38.0 °C or 100.4 °F)
Nausea or vomiting
Tenderness over the right iliac fossa
Leukocytosis >10,000
Neutrophilia (ANC >7500)
Migration of pain to the right lower quadrant
Alvarado Score for Acute Appendicitis
Right lower quadrant tenderness
Elevated temperature (37.3 °C or 99.1 °F)
Rebound tenderness
Migration of pain to the right lower quadrant
Anorexia
Nausea or vomiting
Leukocytosis >10,000
Leukocyte left shift (>75% neutrophils)

of clinical risk [46]. In pediatric patients who have a high pretest probability of appendicitis, practitioners can consider the diagnosis of appendicitis without additional workup with a recommendation for treatment at that point. If additional workup for appendicitis is required, imaging can be obtained. The first line imaging modality utilized for diagnosis of appendicitis should be ultrasound given the concern for long-term deleterious effects of ionizing radiation. The normal pediatric appendix is generally considered less than 6 mm in diameter. However, this should not be considered absolute as a significant number of children will have diameters greater than that number [47]. This is particularly noted in patients with cystic fibrosis. Additional markers of appendicitis on ultrasound include increased mural thickness, non-compressibility of the appendix, thickening and hyperechogenicity of peri-appendiceal mesenteric fat, and a pathologic volume of free abdominal pelvic fluid. Nah et al., in a retrospective study of 810 pediatric patients with ultrasound scans for right lower quadrant pain, the overall rate of appendicitis in those with a non-visualized appendix on ultrasound and no evidence for inflammatory changes was less than

2% [48]. In a separate study by Williamson and colleagues of 3245 ultrasounds done in a pediatric emergency Department, 54% had non-visualization of the appendix on US [49]. Of these patients, 11.9% had acute appendicitis upon further workup. On multivariate analysis, they noted that patients who had a leukocytosis greater than 10,000/uL, an ANC value greater than 9.5, and who were male sex, had a higher likelihood of acute appendicitis.

If cross-sectional imaging is needed, most institutions will then obtain an abdominal and pelvic CT scan with IV contrast. MRI protocols are available, and their utilization is becoming more widespread. However, cost and MRI availability have hindered their widespread application [50]. For better or worse, CT scanners are nearly ubiquitous in emergency departments. Saito et al. found that CT scans were more likely to be used in the evaluation for pediatric appendicitis in community hospitals compared to children's hospitals and ultrasound was much less likely used in community hospitals [51]. These sensitivities for appendicitis were lower when they were performed at community hospitals. Doria and collaborators, in a large meta-analysis of studies evaluating the diagnostic performance of CT scans for diagnosing appendicitis in children, noted a pooled sensitivity and specificity of 88% and 94%, respectively [52]. In a retrospective review of 283 patients with a mean age of 11.3 years, Stephen et al. noted a sensitivity of preoperative CT scan with colon contrast to be 94.6% with a positive predictive value of 95.6% [53]. They concluded that a negative CT scan did not exclude the diagnosis of appendicitis. CT imaging should be reserved only for patients with unclear history and/or physical examination details.

Bowel Obstruction

Plain abdominal radiographs are the mainstay for diagnosis in pediatric patients presenting with signs and symptoms of bowel obstruction. Three-view abdominal films, supine, upright, and decubitus films can help to identify the common findings of obstruction which include air-fluid levels and little to no distal colonic gas. Pneumoperitoneum in this setting is generally an indication for operative exploration. Patients may also present with little to no gas in the intestine on imaging. In a retrospective series of patients presenting with adhesive bowel obstruction, Johnson et al. found that nearly 40% presented with a paucity of bowel gas on abdominal X-ray [54]. Half of the patients who failed nonoperative management had this radiographic finding at the time of operation, and 71% of patients had a closed loop or high-grade bowel obstruction. These authors cautioned physicians to consider these clinically important diagnoses when paucity is noted. In many patients, plain films are the only radiographic studies obtained with axial imaging used much less frequently than in adults. Abdominal CT scans in the presence of obstruction will generally recapitulate the findings of plain films. Exceptions include (1) A swirl sign that suggests volvulus or (2) a point of transition between dilated and decompressed small bowel. Factors associated with intestinal ischemia include increased bowel wall thickening, swirl signs, and/or diminished wall contrast enhancement [55]. Subtle pneumoperitoneum is generally more readily apparent on CT versus plain films. In patients with significant vomiting, hyperchloremia, hypokalemic metabolic alkalosis may be noted. However, lactic acidosis may also be present if significant intestinal ischemia and/or necrosis is present.

In patients with concerns for intussusception, the US is the diagnostic test of choice [56]. The US can diagnose with high accuracy and rapidity. The classic finding in the US is the presence of a mass with a target, doughnut, or bull's eye with multiple surrounding rings in a transverse view. The longitudinal view may show a pseudokidney, sandwich, or a hayfork sign. CT, while not utilized primarily for the diagnosis of intussusception, is 100% sensitive for its diagnosis.

The workup for intestinal malrotation with volvulus resulting in bilious vomiting generally begins with abdominal plain films. These films, however, may be nonspecific. In some cases, a paucity of bowel gas is noted and in others, a double bubble pattern may be noted. Importantly, patients may also have a normal bowel gas pattern [23]. In cases with low clinical suspicion, some pediatric centers begin with a screening US. Doppler US of the intestine in patients with intestinal malrotation, with or without volvulus, may demonstrate reversal of the normal superior mesenteric vein and artery position as well as a "whirl or whirlpool sign" with dynamic evaluation along the length of these vessels. Generally, however, the US has not reached a level of sensitivity and specificity sufficient to make this the only test for malrotation and equivocal studies should prompt additional workup [57]. The gold standard for the diagnosis of intestinal malrotation remains upper gastrointestinal contrast radiography (UGI). This study is performed to identify the location of the duodenojejunal junction which should be to the left of the midline vertebral body, inferior to the level of the pylorus, and posterior when evaluated on lateral images. Any deviation from this standard arrangement qualifies as intestinal malrotation. In patients with volvulus, contrast may not exit the duodenum and may demonstrate a birds beak sign, corkscrew sign (spiral appearance of the distal duodenum and proximal jejunum), and/or malrotated bowel configuration (small bowel loops contained in the right hemiabdomen with the colon in the left hemiabdomen) [58]. Cecal position may also be evaluated by contrast enema. However, given the wide variability of normal cecal position and fixation, abnormal cecal position alone is not diagnostic for malrotation [23]. Ultimately, clinical judgment should prevail in patients and urgent laparotomy should be carried out in patients with a history concerning malrotation with volvulus and equivocal imaging findings.

Meckel's Diverticulum

Meckel's diverticulum can present in many different manners. Patients presenting with obstruction should be evaluated with plain abdominal X-rays. Uncomplicated and asymptomatic Meckel's may be indistinguishable from the surrounding bowel on axial imaging. Meckel's diverticulitis may account for up to a third of complications related to Meckel's. In many cases, an initial US may demonstrate the thickened wall of a loop of the bowel, sonographically known as the "gut signature" sign [59]. A ^{99m}Tc-pertechnetate scan ("Meckel's scan") evaluating for heterotopic gastric mucosa can be performed in pediatric patients with hematochezia. However, given the low sensitivity, in appropriately aged patients with no other obvious source for gastrointestinal bleeding and a negative Meckel's scan, diagnostic laparoscopy should be considered.

Inguinal Hernia

Inguinal hernia is generally considered a clinical diagnosis. Ultrasound evaluation of the inguinal canal may be able to identify a hernia sac with bowel or other contents (ovary is common in females); however, this study is generally duplicative in the setting of a positive clinical examination. Ultrasound is highly sensitive to detecting a patent processus vaginalis with 98% sensitivity and 88% specificity in one recent meta-analysis [60].

24.2.2.2 Pediatric Trauma

A key component of the evaluation of trauma patients is the measure of vital signs. Practitioners should be facile with the differences in vital signs for each age group. In general, normal heart rate decreases as patients get older and blood pressure increases. As patients approach adolescence, vital signs mirror those of adult patients. The normal respiratory rate generally will decrease as patients age. Measurement of blood pressure using non-invasive cuffs in pediatrics is the standard in the trauma Bay. It is important to ensure the appropriate size blood pressure cuff to facilitate an accurate measurement, this is most important in the youngest patients [61]. Several adjuncts to the physical exam and measurement of vital signs can be obtained in pediatric trauma patients to further assist providers in their evaluation of these patients. In adult patients, the Shock Index (Heart Rate/Systolic Blood Pressure) is a simple calculation that can quantify shock and provide surgeons the opportunity to triage patients based on the risk of death [62]. Due to the changes in normal vital signs over the range of pediatric ages, an unadjusted shock index is ineffectual in providing a similar predicted value. Acker and colleagues described the Shock Index Pediatric Age-Adjusted (SIPA) to correct for these differences in patient age. Their seminal work demonstrated that SIPA is able to identify injured children with high injury severity, blood transfusion requirements within the first 24 h, high-grade solid organ injury requiring blood transfusion, and increased in-hospital mortality [63].

The routine use of screening laboratory tests, classically the complete blood count, comprehensive metabolic panel, lipase, coagulation studies, and urinalysis is not warranted in many patients and should be driven by physical exam findings, mechanism of injury, and the likelihood of intervention. No single lab test or panel of tests have been embraced as having high sensitivity and specificity in pediatric trauma patients to aid in their management.

The use of the Focused assessment with sonography from trauma (FAST) examination has been widely utilized in adult trauma evaluations. Its role in pediatric patients is not well established. In a randomized trial of FAST versus routine trauma care, Holmes and colleagues noted that routine FAST examination did not improve care in hemodynamically stable children and adolescents with blunt torso trauma [64]. Calder et al., in a multi-institutional study of 2188 children at 14 pediatric trauma centers, noted that FAST had a low sensitivity for the identification of intra-abdominal injuries and rarely changed the management of pediatric blunt abdominal trauma patients [65].

The Glasgow Come Scale is classically utilized in pediatric patients to determine their level of disability. This includes children in the preverbal stage of development. In preverbal pediatric patients, a modified pediatric Glasgow coma scale score may be applied which includes age-appropriate modifications in the verbal and motor response classifications. Both the pediatric GCS score in preverbal patients and the standard GCS score in older children have been found to be accurate in the identification of clinically significant pediatric traumatic brain injury [66].

Imaging in pediatric patients should be performed selectively and based on physical exam findings. ATLS protocols dictate the performance of a chest X-ray to rule out significant thoracic trauma. In patients with a blunt mechanism and a normal chest X-ray, chest CT does not provide additional benefit [67]. Likewise, the routine performance of abdominal CT scans is unhelpful in the setting of a normal clinical examination without vital sign abnormalities. Clinical prediction rules and treatment pathways may help decrease unnecessary imaging [68]. In patients in whom imaging is required, radiology departments should follow the principles of "as low as reasonably achievable" (ALARA) [69]. The Pediatric Emergency Care Applied Research Network (PECARN) developed a prediction rule based on 7 clinical variables which, when absent, identify low-risk pediatric patients for blunt abdominal trauma [70]. These variables include evidence of abdominal wall trauma or seat belt sign, GCS score of less than 14, abdominal tenderness, evidence of thoracic wall trauma, complaints of abdominal pain, decreased breath sounds, and vomiting (Table 24.3).

Robust clinical decision tools exist around the use of imaging in pediatric blunt head trauma. PECARN developed a prediction rule for the identification of children at very low risk of clinically important traumatic brain injury. Likewise, the Canadian Assessment of Topography for Childhood Head (CATCH) Injury rule and the Children's Head Injury Algorithm for the Prediction of Important Clinical Events

Table 24.3 Factors associated with an increased likelihood of blunt torso trauma and need for intervention. (Adapted from Holmes JF, Lillis K, Monroe D, Borgialli D, Kerrey BT, Mahajan P, et al. Identifying children at very low risk of clinically important blunt abdominal injuries. *Ann Emerg Med.* 2013;62(2):107-16.e2)

Evidence for abdominal wall trauma/seatbelt sign
GCS < 14 with blunt abdominal trauma
Abdominal tenderness
Thoracic wall trauma
Complaints of abdominal pain
Decreased breath sounds
Vomiting

(CHALICE) were created to assist in decision-making for these patients. In a large prospective study of pediatric patients with a head injury, Babl et al. found all three rules to have high sensitivity [71]. Per PECARN, children greater than or equal to 2 years with a GCS of 15 and without severe mechanisms of injury, loss of consciousness, clinical evidence for a basilar skull fracture, or vomiting can be observed without imaging as their risk of clinically significant TBI is low [72].

Patients with a concern for physical abuse should undergo a systematic evaluation for new and old fractures as well as documentation of any external signs of abuse such as bruising. This is accomplished through a physical examination, a comprehensive skeletal survey, fundoscopic retinal evaluation, and head CT. Additional imaging may be indicated pending clinical suspicion.

24.3 Treatment

24.3.1 Medical Treatment

24.3.1.1 Pediatric Emergency General Surgery

Appendicitis
Patients diagnosed with appendicitis should be started on antibiotics and fluid resuscitation without delay. Classically, appendicitis has been treated with appendectomy via the open approach and a right lower quadrant McBurney's incision. However, the technique has dramatically shifted to the laparoscopic approach in the modern era. More recently, the nonoperative management of uncomplicated appendicitis has emerged after successful application in adults [8]. In a recent systematic review and meta-analysis, Maita et al. abstracted the results of 21 articles selected from their literature search, with only one randomized controlled trial of antibiotics vs. surgery in pediatric uncomplicated appendicitis patients [73]. In this review, 92% of patients had resolution of their symptoms with antibiotic treatment. The meta-analysis found that an additional 16% (95% CI 10–22%) underwent appendectomy after that initial hospitalization. Hospital length of stay was similar between groups. In a large, multi-institutional patient-parent choice study of more than 1000 uncomplicated pediatric appendicitis, Minneci et al. found a 67.1% success rate of nonoperative management at one year and a statistically significant fewer number of disability dates after treatment in comparison to patients managed with surgery [74]. An important consideration in patients treated for appendicitis nonoperatively is that patients may potentially have higher rates of emergency department visits and parents may request interval appendectomies remote from the acute event. Predictors of failure of medical management are several including Alvarado score of 7 or higher, the presence of an appendicolith on imaging, and older patients [75].

The nonoperative management of patients with perforated appendicitis can be more complicated and nuanced. Patients are started, as with uncomplicated appendicitis, on antibiotics and fluid resuscitation. Single-agent antibiotic regimens have been shown to be as effective as the classic triple antibiotic therapy of ampicillin, gentamicin, and metronidazole/clindamycin [76]. The surgeon's choice to pursue a nonoperative strategy in patients with perforated appendicitis may rest of several characteristics, most notably those factors for which treatment failure is high. In general, appendicitis lasting more than a week should be considered for nonoperative management. Patients with generalized peritonitis, SIRS, or septic shock, should be aggressively treated with antibiotics and fluid resuscitation followed by prompt surgical source control. Studies vary on whether the presence of an appendicolith increases the risk of treatment failure. Elevated WBC count, significant bandemia (>15%), extensive inflammation/findings outside the right lower quadrant, free peritoneal fluid, and the presence of bowel obstruction, may lead the surgeon to pursue early surgical intervention.

Bowel Obstruction
Patients without a history of abdominal operation should be strongly considered for surgical intervention as should those with concern for intestinal malrotation with volvulus. Pediatric

patients with a history of abdominal operation, as with adults, are a risk for intestinal obstruction related to adhesions. Adhesive bowel obstructions, in that population, occur in less than 10% of cases [77]. Peritonitis, signs of intestinal ischemia, evidence of a closed-loop obstruction or high-grade obstruction, should prompt urgent operative intervention. As with adults, these patients can be treated with nonoperative management initially with NPO, NG tube decompression, and IV fluid resuscitation. Hyak et al., in a retrospective cohort of pediatric patients with adhesive bowel obstructions, found a 54% success rate of patients managed nonoperatively (12% required urgent operation at presentation) [77]. When urgent interventions were excluded, bowel resection was more common when the operation was delayed more than 48 h. Due to this concern for the delay in operative intervention, additional imaging tests to assist surgeons in early decision-making after presentation with adhesive bowel obstruction have been sought. Enteral water-soluble contrast has been described in the adult population as both diagnostic and therapeutic for adhesive bowel obstructions. More recently, pediatric series are emerging with promising results. Linden et al. evaluated outcomes after the implementation of a water-soluble contrast protocol at their free-standing children's hospital and found a drop in patients requiring surgery from 45 to 17% [78]. They noted that contrast presence in the cecum at 24 h had a 100% sensitivity and 90% specificity in predicting successful nonoperative management.

Ileocolic intussusception, in the absence of peritonitis, should be treated with hydrostatic or pneumatic enema under image guidance. Delayed repeat enemas for ileocolic intussusception have been shown to increase the success of nonoperative reduction, decrease bowel resections and reduce the mean hospital length of stay in pediatric patients [79]. Risk factors for the recurrence of intussusception include older age, presence of a pathological lead point, duration of symptoms greater than 48 h, presence of rectal bleeding, and the presence of a left-sided abdominal mass (vs. right) on presentation [80].

Meckel's Diverticulum

There is no role for medical management of a symptomatic Meckel's diverticulum unless an ileocolic intussusception has been diagnosed. In this case, enema reduction should be attempted in patients without peritonitis.

Inguinal Hernia

Due to the incarceration risk, pediatric patients with an inguinal hernia should undergo surgical repair.

Pediatric Trauma

The early management of pediatric trauma is centered around the identification of injuries and management to prevent sequala of shock as well as prevent secondary injury, especially secondary traumatic brain injury. Pediatric patients with signs or symptoms of hemodynamic instability should be treated initially with a 20 mL/kg bolus of 0.9% Normal Saline or lactated Ringer's solution. A Cochrane review found no evidence that resuscitation with colloids reduces the risk of death in patients with trauma [81]. Furthermore, hydroxyethyl starch may increase mortality [82]. In addition crystalloid bolus can be given yes ongoing evidence for hemodynamic instability and or bleeding is demonstrated; however, hemostatic damage control resuscitation principles dictate that blood, and its components should be delivered thereafter. In adults, the Assessment of Blood Consumption (ABC) score consists of four variables (heart rate greater than 120 bpm, systolic blood pressure less than 90 mmHg, positive FAST, and a penetrating torso injury each assigned one point). In adults, a score greater than two triggers massive transfusion protocol use and correctly classifieds most bleeding adult patients in need of MTP [83]. This score is not utilized in kids. Acker et al. created a modification of this score for children, the modified ABC score using the SIPA [84]. They found that a score greater than two poorly predicted the need for massive transfusion but a score greater than one improved the sensitivity of the need for MTP from 29 to 65%. Current evidence in adults suggests that component therapy in a one-to-one to 1:1:1 ratio should be utilized in patients with ongoing hemorrhage. However, it's important to note that while adult balance transfusion protocols are well established, the results from pediatric studies are less convincing currently. pediatrics [85].

The management of pediatric traumatic brain injury, as with adult traumatic brain injury, is centered around the prevention of secondary injury. For moderate to severe traumatic brain injury, the Brain Trauma Foundation guidelines recommend several components to care [86]. Importantly, most of these recommendations are based on moderate-to-low-quality data. These recommendations include:

- Use of ICP monitoring.
- Excluding the possibility of elevated ICP based on a normal initial (0–6 h after injury) CT examination of the brain is not suggested in comatose pediatric patients.
- Routinely obtaining a repeat CT scan greater than 24 h after the admission and initial follow-up is not suggested for decisions about neurosurgical intervention, unless there is either evidence of neurologic deterioration or increasing ICP.
- Treatment of ICP targeting a threshold of less than 20 mmHg is suggested.
- Treatment to maintain a CPP at a minimum of 40 mmHg is suggested.
- Bolus HTS (3%) is recommended in patients with intracranial hypertension. Recommended effective doses for acute use range between 2 and 5 mL/kg over 10–20 min.
- With the use of multiple ICP-related therapies, as well as appropriate use of analgesia and sedation in routine ICU care, avoiding bolus administration of midazolam and/or fentanyl during ICP crises is suggested due to risks of cerebral hypoperfusion.
- CSF drainage through an EVD is suggested to manage increased ICP.
- Prophylactic treatment is suggested to reduce the occurrence of early (within 7 days) post-traumatic seizures.
- Prophylactic severe hyperventilation to a Paco$_2$ less than 30 mmHg in the initial 48 h after injury is not suggested.
- Prophylactic moderate (32–33 °C) hypothermia is not recommended over normothermia to improve overall outcomes.
- High-dose barbiturate therapy is suggested in hemodynamically stable patients with refractory intracranial hypertension despite maximal medical and surgical management.
- Decompressive craniectomy (DC) is suggested to treat neurologic deterioration, herniation, or intracranial hypertension refractory to MM.
- Initiation of early enteral nutritional support (within 72 h from injury) is suggested to decrease mortality and improve outcomes.
- The use of corticosteroids is not suggested to improve outcome or reduce ICP.

Management of spinal cord injuries also centers on the prevention of secondary injury. Spine immobilization should be instituted immediately and preferably in the prehospital setting. Many pediatric spine fractures can be managed nonoperatively, but cord decompression and spine stabilization may be required.

Lung contusions account for nearly half of the thoracic injuries in pediatric patients. Many of these injuries can be treated with supportive therapy alone (oxygen, pain control, and chest physiotherapy). In the rare, severe contusion, ventilation-perfusion mismatch may occur with resultant hypoxia and hypercarbia. These injuries may require more intensive airway management. Judicious fluid management is also vital to prevent exacerbation of V-Q mismatch from pulmonary edema. Rib fractures, rare in children due to their compliant chest wall, are treated as in the adult population. Notably, in patients less than 2 years of age, rib fractures (especially posterior rib fractures) should raise suspicion for nonaccidental trauma. Small pneumothoraces in children can be safely observed. Chest tube placement is indicted for larger, usually symptomatic pneumothoraces or in cases where a hemopneumothorax raises concern for potential retained hemothorax with lung entrapment. In a retrospective cohort of blunt pediatric trauma patients, Osuchukwu et al. evaluated patients with asymptomatic non-occult (defined as visible on chest X-ray) pneumothoraces secondary to blunt trauma [87]. The pneumothorax sizes in their study were classified as apical (level of lung edge still above the clavicle), small (less than 10% of hemithorax per radiology report or lung edge extending just below the clavicle), and moderate (10–20% of hemithorax per radiology or lung edge located lateral to the scapula edge, with no signs of deviation of mediastinum). Sixty-three percent were observed. They concluded that patients with small to moderately sized pneumothoraces could be safely observed with decreased length of stay, decreased number of chest X-rays, and decreased overall cost. A hemothorax visible on a chest X-ray should be treated with tube thoracostomy. In a large retrospective study of adult and pediatric patients in a single Level 1 trauma center, Scott et al. evaluated risk factors for retained hemothorax [88]. Their multivariable model found that patients intubated on the day of admission and with bilateral injuries had the highest risk for retained hemothorax. They recommend the early intervention to prevent complications of RH. Tube thoracostomy size will require modification based on a patient's age and size. As with adult trauma patients, decreasing chest tube sizes have been found to successfully treat both hemo- and pneumothoraces.

Blunt abdominal injuries are common in pediatric trauma patients. This is generally related to relatively decreased abdominal musculature and lack of protection of the abdominal organs, particularly liver and spleen, by the rib cage. Abdominal injuries can be split into categories of a solid organ (liver, spleen, and kidney) vs. hollow viscus (intestine, pancreas, biliary tract, bladder, and renal collecting system). Within that framework, surgeons should evaluate patients for immediate surgical need, namely bleeding with hemodynamic instability refractory to resuscitation and/or perforation with or without peritonitis. In hemodynamically stable patients, the mainstay of treatment for pediatric solid organ injuries is nonoperative management. Blunt liver injuries are common, and the majority can be observed. The American Pediatric Surgical Association Outcomes and Evidence-Based Practice Committee performed a meta-analysis of non-operative management of solid organ injuries to reconsider the classic nonoperative treatment algorithms based solely on injury grade [89]. Based on this evaluation of the literature, they concluded that the length of hospitalization should be based on clinical findings and not based solely on injury grade. That prophylactic embolization of solid organ injuries in stable patients with known arterial extravasation was not indicated and should be reserved for patients with evidence of ongoing bleeding. Additionally, they noted that routine follow-up imaging for asymptomatic, uncomplicated, low-grade injured children with abdominal blunt trauma was not warranted [89]. Based on this systematic review, new, truncated solid organ injury management guidelines were adopted by the APSA Board of Governors (Table 24.4). Blunt injuries to the kidney, likewise, are generally managed without surgical intervention. Injuries to the collecting system may be identified on four-phase CT imaging or present later with signs/symptoms of urinoma [90]. Percutaneous and/or endoscopic intervention may be required. Extraperitoneal bladder injuries are managed similarly to adult trauma patients with urethral drainage alone. Blunt pancreatic injuries can be difficult to diagnose and may only present 24–48 h after the ini-

Table 24.4 American Pediatric Surgical Association 2019 guidelines for the management of blunt liver and spleen injuries. (Adapted from https://apsapedsurg.org/wp-content/uploads/2020/10/APSA_Solid-Organ-Injury-Guidelines-2019-2.pdf)

- Admission location (ICU vs. Ward) based on abnormal vital signs after resuscitation
- Bedrest, repeat blood counts and NPO should be used until vital signs normalize
- Transfusion for unstable vital signs after a 20 mL/kg isotonic saline bolus, low hemoglobin, or evidence of ongoing bleeding
- Intervention (angioembolization or operative exploration) is reserved for signs of ongoing bleeding despite resuscitation
- A massive transfusion protocol should be considered for uncontrolled solid organ injury bleeding
- Discharge should be based on clinical factors not only injury grade
- Activity restriction to grade plus 2 weeks is safe
- No need for additional imaging after discharge unless a patient remains symptomatic

tial injury. Low-grade injuries, as defined by the American Association for the Surgery of Trauma, are managed nonoperatively exclusively [91]. Grade 3 injuries with ductal transection, have been managed both with intervention and observation. High-grade injuries may be quite complex and require staged intervention.

24.3.2 Surgical Treatment

24.3.2.1 Pediatric Emergency General Surgery

Appendicitis

Laparoscopic appendectomy is the mainstay for the treatment of pediatric simple and complicated appendicitis [92]. This can be accomplished via the classical 3 port technique, a single port technique, or variations on those themes. The timing of surgery is dependent on the patient physiology at the time of presentation. Patients with peritonitis and/or SIRS should have prompt administration of IV fluids and antibiotics followed by urgent appendectomy. In patients without those physiologic triggers for surgery, it is generally accepted that surgery within 12–24 h is acceptable. In a systematic review of time to appendectomy, Cameron and colleagues note that appendectomy within 24 h of admission was not found to be associated with increased adverse events or resource utilization [93]. The placement of an abdominal drain at the time of surgery for complicated appendicitis is not recommended. Fujishiro et al., in a Japanese national cohort study, found that the placement of drains at the time of appendectomy showed an increase in wound dehiscence and postoperative length of stay when drains were utilized [94]. Additionally, they found no difference in the incidence of postoperative complications including organ space infections. There is no prospective evidence that extensive peritoneal lavage (compared to suction only) at the time of surgery improves postoperative outcomes [95, 96]. Postoperative antibiotics are not indicated in patients with uncomplicated appendicitis. The adult literature has clear evidence that extended-duration antibiotics for complicated appendicitis do not reduce the risk of intra-abdominal infection or skin infections [97]. The pediatric-specific data is less clear but in the setting of normalization of vital signs and improved abdominal examination, extended antibiotics may not be required. A recent NSQIP-Pediatric analysis suggested that discharge with home antibiotics may not provide significant benefit [98].

Bowel Obstruction

In patients with peritonitis or other signs of intestinal ischemia, urgent operative intervention is warranted. Patients with no history of abdominal surgery, and therefore not at risk for intraabdominal adhesions, should be considered for early surgical intervention unless intussusception has been diagnosed which can be managed with hydrostatic or pneumatic enema. In younger patients, a transverse abdominal incision will provide as much exposure as a vertical incision. Older (and taller) patients may benefit from a vertical midline incision to facilitate abdominal exploration. In select patients, laparoscopy can be performed. Miyake et al., in a systematic review and meta-analysis including three observation studies, found that postoperative complications were fewer with laparoscopy [9]. The authors did note a low quality of evidence and a lack of well-controlled studies in this area.

Meckel's Diverticulum

Laparoscopy or laparotomy can be utilized for the identification of Meckel's diverticulum [99]. With laparoscopy, the diverticulum can be managed entirely intracorporeally or via a mini-umbilical laparotomy incision. The management of the diverticulum itself includes diverticulectomy, wedge resection or segmental resection, and the selected technique is dictated by the anatomy of the diverticulum. Longer diverticula can be managed with diverticulectomy alone. Shorter diverticula can be managed with wedge resection. Segmental intestinal resection at the Meckel's should be reserved for complicated Meckel's with perforation at the base or those with bleeding. Heterotopic gastric mucosa may be present in the base of shorter diverticula (height-to-diameter less than 1.6) and therefore wedge or segmental intestinal resection is indicated [100].

Inguinal Hernia

Once diagnosed, pediatric inguinal hernias should be repaired. Incarcerated inguinal hernias refractory to reduction efforts require emergent operative intervention to prevent intestinal ischemia and, in younger male patients, testicular ischemia and atrophy. The timing of repair in patients with a reducible inguinal hernia is more nuanced. A common scenario is a premature infant convalescing in the NICU in whom an inguinal hernia is diagnosed. Data is split as to whether these need to be repaired early after the diagnosis or if they can wait until a patient is closer to discharge. A recent meta-analysis of repair prior to NICU discharge versus after NICU discharge in premature infants found that repair before discharge was associated with increased odds of recurrence but not of incarceration or surgical complications [101]. Universally, pediatric inguinal hernia repair is carried out with high ligation of the indirect inguinal hernia sac only. Most commonly this is done through an open inguinal incision. More recently, several different laparoscopic techniques have also been popularized [26]. High ligation of the hernia sac only (without mesh) is also acceptable for adolescent patients presenting with indirect inguinal hernias [28].

Pediatric Trauma

There is great overlap in the surgical management of pediatric trauma injuries of the abdomen and chest with adult surgical techniques. As previously noted, the nonoperative management of blunt solid organ injuries is the mainstay of treatment. Hemodynamically stable pediatric patients with contrast extravasation present on abdominal CT do not require prophylactic embolization. Clinical symptoms and/or hemodynamics should dictate the use of angioembolization or surgical intervention [89]. Clinical characteristics such as positive FAST, early transfusion, injury grade, pediatric-adjusted shock index, and markers of trauma-induced coagulopathy may also be associated with failure of non-operative management [102].

24.3.3 Prognosis

Generally, the prognosis for all pediatric general surgery and trauma conditions is excellent. Tzong et al., in an analysis of the Kids' Inpatient Database of surgical procedures performed in 2003, 2006, and 2009 noted a mortality of 0.8% of all surgical admissions [7]. Trauma remains the leading cause of death in pediatric patients greater than 1 year of age. Myers and colleagues examined the 2006 Healthcare Cost and Utilization Project Kids Inpatient Database to evaluate trauma mortality [13]. The overall mortality in their series was 0.9% of all admissions. Pediatric trauma populations with high morbidity and mortality remain those with traumatic brain injury and non-accidental trauma.

> **Do and Dont's**
> - Do maintain a high suspicion level in the pediatric population.
> - Do involve specialists whenever possible in the management of pediatrics, especially of the youngest ones.
> - Don't perform prosthetic hernia repair in pediatrics.
> - Don't consider children as small adults in trauma management.

> **Take-Home Messages**
> - Appendicitis is common in children, the US is the diagnostic test of choice, and surgical rather than medical management is recommended.
> - Bowel obstruction is most often due to adhesive obstruction, CT scan may prompt early diagnosis and intervention, and in cases of confirmed obstruction surgery is recommended. In the "virgin" abdomen, once the incarcerated hernia is excluded malrotation with volvulus must be excluded.
> - Meckel's diverticulum presents as painless rectal bleeding or mimics appendici-

tis. Surgery is recommended. Resection of an incidental Meckel's diverticulum is controversial but most pediatric surgeons would proceed with resection.
- Indirect inguinal hernia is the most common type of inguinal hernia in children. Surgery is recommended with simple high ligation of the sac. In general prosthetic repair is not recommended due to the risk of chronic pain or scarring of the vas deferens.
- The majority of children suffering blunt trauma enjoy a good outcome and operative intervention for torso trauma is required in less than 5% of injured children. Non-operative management is preferred unless the patient exhibits signs of hemorrhage, intestinal perforation, or pancreatic transection. Penetrating torso injury in children is associated with the poor outcome which may be in part to small blood volume and rapid exsanguination. Infants who present with signs of head trauma, rib fracture, bruising, and/or long bone fracture in the absence of a witnessed event (i.e., motor vehicle crash) NAT must be excluded.

Multiple Choice Questions

1. Hernia repair in pediatrics:
   A. should be always performed
   B. should not be performed at all
   C. **non-prosthetic techniques should be preferred**
   D. must be implemented with prosthesis use
2. Trauma management in pediatrics
   A. follows the same rules and procedures as the adult patients
   B. **must be tailored to the pediatrics with dedicated procedures and protocols**
   C. it is always operative
   D. it is always non-operative
3. Acute abdomen in pediatrics
   A. should be investigated always with Ct-scan
   B. **should be investigated with a step-up diagnostic approach**
   C. observation and antibiotic therapy are always to be undertaken
   D. surgical exploration is mandatory in almost all cases

References

1. Haller JA Jr. Why pediatric surgery? A personal journey through the first 50 years. Ann Surg. 2003;237(5):597–606.
2. O'Hare WP. The changing child population of the United States: analysis of data from the 2010 census. Report. Baltimore: The Annie E. Casey Foundation; 2010.
3. Sømme S, Bronsert M, Morrato E, Ziegler M. Frequency and variety of inpatient pediatric surgical procedures in the United States. Pediatrics. 2013;132(6):e1466–72.
4. Rabbitts JA, Groenewald CB, Moriarty JP, Flick R. Epidemiology of ambulatory anesthesia for children in the United States: 2006 and 1996. Anesth Analg. 2010;111(4):1011–5.
5. Wang KS, Cummings J, Stark A, Houck C, Oldham K, Grant C, et al. Optimizing resources in children's surgical care: an update on the American College of Surgeons' Verification Program. Pediatrics. 2020;145(5):e20200708.
6. Niles LM, Goyal MK, Badolato GM, Chamberlain JM, Cohen JS. US emergency department trends in imaging for pediatric nontraumatic abdominal pain. Pediatrics. 2017;140(4):e20170615.
7. Tzong KY, Han S, Roh A, Ing C. Epidemiology of pediatric surgical admissions in US children: data from the HCUP kids inpatient database. J Neurosurg Anesthesiol. 2012;24(4):391–5.
8. Rentea RM, Peter SDS, Snyder CL. Pediatric appendicitis: state of the art review. Pediatr Surg Int. 2017;33(3):269–83.
9. Miyake H, Seo S, Pierro A. Laparoscopy or laparotomy for adhesive bowel obstruction in children: a systematic review and meta-analysis. Pediatr Surg Int. 2018;34(2):177–82.
10. Avraham JB, Bhandari M, Frangos SG, Levine DA, Tunik MG, DiMaggio CJ. Epidemiology of paediatric trauma presenting to US emergency departments: 2006-2012. Inj Prev. 2019;25(2):136–43.
11. Nance ML, Carr BG, Branas CC. Access to pediatric trauma care in the United States. Arch Pediatr Adolesc Med. 2009;163(6):512–8.

12. Gaines BA, Hansen K, McKenna C, McMahon M, Meredith JW, Mooney DP, et al. Report from the Childress Summit of the Pediatric Trauma Society, April 22–24, 2013. J Trauma Acute Care Surg. 2014;77(3):504–9.
13. Myers SR, Branas CC, French B, Nance ML, Carr BG. A national analysis of pediatric trauma care utilization and outcomes in the United States. Pediatr Emerg Care. 2016;
14. Notrica DM, Weiss J, Garcia-Filion P, Kuroiwa E, Clarke D, Harte M, et al. Pediatric trauma centers: correlation of ACS-verified trauma centers with CDC statewide pediatric mortality rates. J Trauma Acute Care Surg. 2012;73(3):566–70; discussion 70–2.
15. Pender TM, David AP, Dodson BK, Calland JF. Pediatric trauma mortality: an ecological analysis evaluating correlation between injury-related mortality and geographic access to trauma care in the United States in 2010. J Public Health (Oxf). 2021;43(1):139–47.
16. Langlois JA, Rutland-Brown W, Thomas KE. The incidence of traumatic brain injury among children in the United States: differences by race. J Head Trauma Rehabil. 2005;20(3):229–38.
17. Quayle KS, Powell EC, Mahajan P, Hoyle JD Jr, Nadel FM, Badawy MK, et al. Epidemiology of blunt head trauma in children in U.S. emergency departments. N Engl J Med. 2014;371(20):1945–7.
18. Thornhill S, Teasdale GM, Murray GD, McEwen J, Roy CW, Penny KI. Disability in young people and adults one year after head injury: prospective cohort study. BMJ. 2000;320(7250):1631–5.
19. Schneier AJ, Shields BJ, Hostetler SG, Xiang H, Smith GA. Incidence of pediatric traumatic brain injury and associated hospital resource utilization in the United States. Pediatrics. 2006;118(2):483–92.
20. Ergul E. Heredity and familial tendency of acute appendicitis. Scand J Surg. 2007;96(4):290–2.
21. Hajivassiliou CA. Intestinal obstruction in neonatal/pediatric surgery. Semin Pediatr Surg. 2003;12(4):241–53.
22. Yoshimaru K, Kinoshita Y, Matsuura T, Esumi G, Wada M, Takahashi Y, et al. Bowel obstruction without history of laparotomy: clinical analysis of 70 patients. Pediatr Int. 2016;58(11):1205–10.
23. Langer JC. Intestinal rotation abnormalities and midgut volvulus. Surg Clin North Am. 2017;97(1):147–59.
24. Fiegel H, Gfroerer S, Rolle U. Systematic review shows that pathological lead points are important and frequent in intussusception and are not limited to infants. Acta Paediatr. 2016;105(11):1275–9.
25. Keese D, Rolle U, Gfroerer S, Fiegel H. Symptomatic Meckel's diverticulum in pediatric patients-case reports and systematic review of the literature. Front Pediatr. 2019;7:267.
26. Abdulhai S, Glenn IC, Ponsky TA. Inguinal hernia. Clin Perinatol. 2017;44(4):865–77.
27. Olesen CS, Mortensen LQ, Öberg S, Rosenberg J. Risk of incarceration in children with inguinal hernia: a systematic review. Hernia. 2019;23(2):245–54.
28. van Kerckhoven G, Toonen L, Draaisma WA, de Vries LS, Verheijen PM. Herniotomy in young adults as an alternative to mesh repair: a retrospective cohort study. Hernia. 2016;20(5):675–9.
29. Oliver J, Avraham J, Frangos S, Tomita S, DiMaggio C. The epidemiology of inpatient pediatric trauma in United States hospitals 2000 to 2011. J Pediatr Surg. 2018;53(4):758–64.
30. Pujahari AK. Decision making in bowel obstruction: a review. J Clin Diagn Res. 2016;10(11):PE07–12.
31. Dekonenko C, Sujka JA, Weaver K, Sharp SW, Gonzalez K, St Peter SD. The identification and treatment of intestinal malrotation in older children. Pediatr Surg Int. 2019;35(6):665–71.
32. Stylianos S, Jacir NN, Harris BH. Incarceration of inguinal hernia in infants prior to elective repair. J Pediatr Surg. 1993;28(4):582–3.
33. Edil BH, Tuggle DW, Jones S, Albrecht R, Kuhn A, Mantor PC, et al. Pediatric major resuscitation—respiratory compromise as a criterion for mandatory surgeon presence. J Pediatr Surg. 2005;40(6):926–8; discussion 8.
34. Vlatten A, Litz S, MacManus B, Launcelott S, Soder C. A comparison of the GlideScope video laryngoscope and standard direct laryngoscopy in children with immobilized cervical spine. Pediatr Emerg Care. 2012;28(12):1317–20.
35. Zelicof-Paul A, Smith-Lockridge A, Schnadower D, Tyler S, Levin S, Roskind C, et al. Controversies in rapid sequence intubation in children. Curr Opin Pediatr. 2005;17(3):355–62.
36. Ramaiah VK, Sharma D, Ma L, Prathep S, Hoffman NG, Vavilala MS. Admission oxygenation and ventilation parameters associated with discharge survival in severe pediatric traumatic brain injury. Childs Nerv Syst. 2013;29(4):629–34.
37. Hartford Consensus III focuses on empowering the public to serve as first responders. Bull Am Coll Surg 2015;100(6):52.
38. Harcke HT, Lawrence LL, Gripp EW, Kecskemethy HH, Kruse RW, Murphy SG. Adult tourniquet for use in school-age emergencies. Pediatrics. 2019;143(6)
39. Dornhofer P, Kellar JZ. Intraosseous vascular access. StatPearls. Treasure Island: StatPearls Publishing. Copyright © 2021, StatPearls Publishing LLC.; 2021.
40. Glick JC, Staley K. Inflicted traumatic brain injury: advances in evaluation and collaborative diagnosis. Pediatr Neurosurg. 2007;43(5):436–41.
41. Yu YR, DeMello AS, Greeley CS, Cox CS, Naik-Mathuria BJ, Wesson DE. Injury patterns of child abuse: experience of two level 1 pediatric trauma centers. J Pediatr Surg. 2018;53(5):1028–32.
42. Tarantino CA, Dowd MD, Murdock TC. Short vertical falls in infants. Pediatr Emerg Care. 1999;15(1):5–8.

43. Pierce MC, Kaczor K, Aldridge S, O'Flynn J, Lorenz DJ. Bruising characteristics discriminating physical child abuse from accidental trauma. Pediatrics. 2010;125(1):67–74.
44. Glass CC, Rangel SJ. Overview and diagnosis of acute appendicitis in children. Semin Pediatr Surg. 2016;25(4):198–203.
45. Alvarado A. A practical score for the early diagnosis of acute appendicitis. Ann Emerg Med. 1986;15(5):557–64.
46. Koberlein GC, Trout AT, Rigsby CK, Iyer RS, Alazraki AL, Anupindi SA, et al. ACR appropriateness criteria(®) suspected appendicitis-child. J Am Coll Radiol. 2019;16(5s):S252–s63.
47. Gongidi P, Bellah RD. Ultrasound of the pediatric appendix. Pediatr Radiol. 2017;47(9):1091–100.
48. Nah SA, Ong SS, Lim WX, Amuddhu SK, Tang PH, Low Y. Clinical relevance of the nonvisualized appendix on ultrasonography of the abdomen in children. J Pediatr. 2017;182:164–169.e1.
49. Williamson K, Sherman JM, Fishbein JS, Rocker J. Outcomes for children with a nonvisualized appendix on ultrasound. Pediatr Emerg Care. 2018;
50. Mervak BM, Wilson SB, Handly BD, Altun E, Burke LM. MRI of acute appendicitis. J Magn Reson Imaging. 2019;50(5):1367–76.
51. Saito JM, Yan Y, Evashwick TW, Warner BW, Tarr PI. Use and accuracy of diagnostic imaging by hospital type in pediatric appendicitis. Pediatrics. 2013;131(1):e37–44.
52. Doria AS, Moineddin R, Kellenberger CJ, Epelman M, Beyene J, Schuh S, et al. US or CT for diagnosis of appendicitis in children and adults? A meta-analysis. Radiology. 2006;241(1):83–94.
53. Stephen AE, Segev DL, Ryan DP, Mullins ME, Kim SH, Schnitzer JJ, et al. The diagnosis of acute appendicitis in a pediatric population: to CT or not to CT. J Pediatr Surg. 2003;38(3):367–71; discsussion -71.
54. Johnson BL, Campagna GA, Hyak JM, Vogel AM, Fallon SC, Shah SR, et al. The significance of abdominal radiographs with paucity of gas in pediatric adhesive small bowel obstruction. Am J Surg. 2020;220(1):208–13.
55. Chang YJ, Yan DC, Lai JY, Chao HC, Chen CL, Chen SY, et al. Strangulated small bowel obstruction in children. J Pediatr Surg. 2017;52(8):1313–7.
56. Plut D, Phillips GS, Johnston PR, Lee EY. Practical imaging strategies for intussusception in children. AJR Am J Roentgenol. 2020;215(6):1449–63.
57. Esposito F, Vitale V, Noviello D, Di Serafino M, Vallone G, Salvatore M, et al. Ultrasonographic diagnosis of midgut volvulus with malrotation in children. J Pediatr Gastroenterol Nutr. 2014;59(6):786–8.
58. Pickhardt PJ, Bhalla S. Intestinal malrotation in adolescents and adults: spectrum of clinical and imaging features. AJR Am J Roentgenol. 2002;179(6):1429–35.
59. Kotha VK, Khandelwal A, Saboo SS, Shanbhogue AK, Virmani V, Marginean EC, et al. Radiologist's perspective for the Meckel's diverticulum and its complications. Br J Radiol. 2014;87(1037):20130743.
60. Dreuning KMA, Ten Broeke CEM, Twisk JWR, Robben SGF, van Rijn RR, Verbeke J, et al. Diagnostic accuracy of preoperative ultrasonography in predicting contralateral inguinal hernia in children: a systematic review and meta-analysis. Eur Radiol. 2019;29(2):866–76.
61. Dionne JM, Bremner SA, Baygani SK, Batton B, Ergenekon E, Bhatt-Mehta V, et al. Method of blood pressure measurement in neonates and infants: a systematic review and analysis. J Pediatr. 2020;221:23–31.e5.
62. Cannon CM, Braxton CC, Kling-Smith M, Mahnken JD, Carlton E, Moncure M. Utility of the shock index in predicting mortality in traumatically injured patients. J Trauma. 2009;67(6):1426–30.
63. Acker SN, Ross JT, Partrick DA, Tong S, Bensard DD. Pediatric specific shock index accurately identifies severely injured children. J Pediatr Surg. 2015;50(2):331–4.
64. Holmes JF, Kelley KM, Wootton-Gorges SL, Utter GH, Abramson LP, Rose JS, et al. Effect of abdominal ultrasound on clinical care, outcomes, and resource use among children with blunt torso trauma: a randomized clinical trial. JAMA. 2017;317(22):2290–6.
65. Calder BW, Vogel AM, Zhang J, Mauldin PD, Huang EY, Savoie KB, et al. Focused assessment with sonography for trauma in children after blunt abdominal trauma: a multi-institutional analysis. J Trauma Acute Care Surg. 2017;83(2):218–24.
66. Borgialli DA, Mahajan P, Hoyle JD Jr, Powell EC, Nadel FM, Tunik MG, et al. Performance of the Pediatric Glasgow Coma Scale Score in the evaluation of children with blunt head trauma. Acad Emerg Med. 2016;23(8):878–84.
67. Golden J, Isani M, Bowling J, Zagory J, Goodhue CJ, Burke RV, et al. Limiting chest computed tomography in the evaluation of pediatric thoracic trauma. J Trauma Acute Care Surg. 2016;81(2):271–7.
68. Ohana O, Soffer S, Zimlichman E, Klang E. Overuse of CT and MRI in paediatric emergency departments. Br J Radiol. 2018;91(1085):20170434.
69. Sodhi KS, Krishna S, Saxena AK, Sinha A, Khandelwal N, Lee EY. Clinical application of 'Justification' and 'Optimization' principle of ALARA in pediatric CT imaging: "How many children can be protected from unnecessary radiation?". Eur J Radiol. 2015;84(9):1752–7.
70. Holmes JF, Lillis K, Monroe D, Borgialli D, Kerrey BT, Mahajan P, et al. Identifying children at very low risk of clinically important blunt abdominal injuries. Ann Emerg Med. 2013;62(2):107–16.e2.
71. Babl FE, Borland ML, Phillips N, Kochar A, Dalton S, McCaskill M, et al. Accuracy of PECARN, CATCH, and CHALICE head injury decision rules in children: a prospective cohort study. Lancet. 2017;389(10087):2393–402.

72. Kuppermann N, Holmes JF, Dayan PS, Hoyle JD Jr, Atabaki SM, Holubkov R, et al. Identification of children at very low risk of clinically-important brain injuries after head trauma: a prospective cohort study. Lancet. 2009;374(9696):1160–70.
73. Maita S, Andersson B, Svensson JF, Wester T. Nonoperative treatment for nonperforated appendicitis in children: a systematic review and meta-analysis. Pediatr Surg Int. 2020;36(3):261–9.
74. Minneci PC, Hade EM, Lawrence AE, Sebastião YV, Saito JM, Mak GZ, et al. Association of nonoperative management using antibiotic therapy vs laparoscopic appendectomy with treatment success and disability days in children with uncomplicated appendicitis. JAMA. 2020;324(6):581–93.
75. Fuhrer AE, Sukhotnik I, Ben-Shahar Y, Weinberg M, Koppelmann T. Predictive value of Alvarado Score and Pediatric Appendicitis Score in the success of nonoperative management for simple acute appendicitis in children. Eur J Pediatr Surg. 2021;31(1):95–101.
76. Howell EC, Dubina ED, Lee SL. Perforation risk in pediatric appendicitis: assessment and management. Pediatr Health Med Ther. 2018;9:135–45.
77. Hyak J, Campagna G, Johnson B, Stone Z, Yu Y, Rosenfeld E, et al. Management of pediatric adhesive small bowel obstruction: do timing of surgery and age matter? J Surg Res. 2019;243:384–90.
78. Linden AF, Raiji MT, Kohler JE, Carlisle EM, Pelayo JC, Feinstein K, et al. Evaluation of a water-soluble contrast protocol for nonoperative management of pediatric adhesive small bowel obstruction. J Pediatr Surg. 2019;54(1):184–8.
79. Lautz TB, Thurm CW, Rothstein DH. Delayed repeat enemas are safe and cost-effective in the management of pediatric intussusception. J Pediatr Surg. 2015;50(3):423–7.
80. Xie X, Wu Y, Wang Q, Zhao Y, Xiang B. Risk factors for recurrence of intussusception in pediatric patients: a retrospective study. J Pediatr Surg. 2018;53(11):2307–11.
81. Perel P, Roberts I, Ker K. Colloids versus crystalloids for fluid resuscitation in critically ill patients. Cochrane Database Syst Rev. 2013(2):CD000567.
82. Perel P, Roberts I. Colloids versus crystalloids for fluid resuscitation in critically ill patients. Cochrane Database Syst Rev. 2012;6:CD000567.
83. Nunez TC, Voskresensky IV, Dossett LA, Shinall R, Dutton WD, Cotton BA. Early prediction of massive transfusion in trauma: simple as ABC (assessment of blood consumption)? J Trauma. 2009;66(2):346–52.
84. Acker SN, Hall B, Hill L, Partrick DA, Bensard DD. Adult-based massive transfusion protocol activation criteria do not work in children. Eur J Pediatr Surg. 2017;27(1):32–5.
85. Hughes NT, Burd RS, Teach SJ. Damage control resuscitation: permissive hypotension and massive transfusion protocols. Pediatr Emerg Care. 2014;30(9):651–6; quiz 7–8.
86. Kochanek PM, Tasker RC, Bell MJ, Adelson PD, Carney N, Vavilala MS, et al. Management of pediatric severe traumatic brain injury: 2019 consensus and guidelines-based algorithm for first and second tier therapies. Pediatr Crit Care Med. 2019;20(3):269–79.
87. Osuchukwu O, Lopez J, Weaver KL, Waddell VA, Aguayo P, St Peter SD, et al. Asymptomatic non-occult pneumothorax in pediatric blunt chest trauma: chest tube versus observation. J Pediatr Surg. 2021;
88. Scott MF, Khodaverdian RA, Shaheen JL, Ney AL, Nygaard RM. Predictors of retained hemothorax after trauma and impact on patient outcomes. Eur J Trauma Emerg Surg. 2017;43(2):179–84.
89. Gates RL, Price M, Cameron DB, Somme S, Ricca R, Oyetunji TA, et al. Non-operative management of solid organ injuries in children: an American Pediatric Surgical Association outcomes and Evidence Based Practice Committee systematic review. J Pediatr Surg. 2019;54(8):1519–26.
90. Fernandez-Ibieta M. Renal trauma in pediatrics: a current review. Urology. 2018;113:171–8.
91. Moore EE, Cogbill TH, Malangoni MA, Jurkovich GJ, Shackford SR, Champion HR, et al. Organ injury scaling. Surg Clin North Am. 1995;75(2):293–303.
92. Low ZX, Bonney GK, So JBY, Loh DL, Ng JJ. Laparoscopic versus open appendectomy in pediatric patients with complicated appendicitis: a meta-analysis. Surg Endosc. 2019;33(12):4066–77.
93. Cameron DB, Williams R, Geng Y, Gosain A, Arnold MA, Guner YS, et al. Time to appendectomy for acute appendicitis: a systematic review. J Pediatr Surg. 2018;53(3):396–405.
94. Fujishiro J, Fujiogi M, Hirahara N, Terui K, Okamoto T, Watanabe E, et al. Abdominal drainage at appendectomy for complicated appendicitis in children: a propensity-matched comparative study. Ann Surg. 2020;
95. Nataraja RM, Panabokke G, Chang AD, Mennie N, Tanny ST, Keys C, et al. Does peritoneal lavage influence the rate of complications following pediatric laparoscopic appendicectomy in children with complicated appendicitis? A prospective randomized clinical trial. J Pediatr Surg. 2019;54(12):2524–7.
96. St Peter SD, Adibe OO, Iqbal CW, Fike FB, Sharp SW, Juang D, et al. Irrigation versus suction alone during laparoscopic appendectomy for perforated appendicitis: a prospective randomized trial. Ann Surg. 2012;256(4):581–5.
97. Ramson DM, Gao H, Penny-Dimri JC, Liu Z, Khong JN, Caruana CB, et al. Duration of post-operative antibiotic treatment in acute complicated appendicitis: systematic review and meta-analysis. ANZ J Surg. 2021;
98. Anderson KT, Bartz-Kurycki MA, Kawaguchi AL, Austin MT, Holzmann-Pazgal G, Kao LS, et al. Home antibiotics at discharge for pediatric compli-

cated appendicitis: friend or foe? J Am Coll Surg. 2018;227(2):247–54.
99. Chen Q, Gao Z, Zhang L, Zhang Y, Pan T, Cai D, et al. Multifaceted behavior of Meckel's diverticulum in children. J Pediatr Surg. 2018;53(4):676–81.
100. Mukai M, Takamatsu H, Noguchi H, Fukushige T, Tahara H, Kaji T. Does the external appearance of a Meckel's diverticulum assist in choice of the laparoscopic procedure? Pediatr Surg Int. 2002;18(4):231–3.
101. Masoudian P, Sullivan KJ, Mohamed H, Nasr A. Optimal timing for inguinal hernia repair in premature infants: a systematic review and meta-analysis. J Pediatr Surg. 2019;54(8):1539–45.
102. Shahi N, Shahi AK, Phillips R, Shirek G, Bensard D, Moulton SL. Decision-making in pediatric blunt solid organ injury: a deep learning approach to predict massive transfusion, need for operative management, and mortality risk. J Pediatr Surg. 2021;56(2):379–84.

Cirrhotic Patients

25

Greg Padmore and Chad G. Ball

25.1 Introduction

> **Learning Goals**
> - Understanding the complex pathophysiology of cirrhosis and how it affects the perioperative setting.
> - Preoperative assessment and management of patients with cirrhosis.
> - Intraoperative considerations and postoperative management of patient complications.

The remarkable multidisciplinary care of patients with chronic liver disease has resulted in improved survival. Additionally, improved perioperative care and operative techniques have also increased patients' eligibility for both non-hepatic and hepatic-directed surgery.

25.1.1 Epidemiology

Approximately one in every ten patients with chronic liver disease will require surgery in the final 2 years of life [1]. This relatively dated estimation does not account for the expanded surgical eligibility of cirrhotic patients due to advances in both perioperative care and operative techniques for non-hepatic and hepatic targeted operations. In the broader context of emergency general surgery, non-hepatic surgery is far more common and will present within the everyday scope of practice.

Liver failure and sepsis are major threats to incurring post-operative morbidity and mortality in patients with chronic liver disease. de Goede et al. showed in a systematic review that the overall peri-operative morbidity and mortality were 30.1% and 11.6%, respectively, and that the coexistence of portal hypertension was found to be associated with a twofold increase in mortality [2]. Teh et al., in another study of 772 cirrhotic patients, showed that the severity of hepatic dys-

---

G. Padmore
Hepatobiliary and Pancreatic Surgery, University of Calgary, Calgary, AB, Canada

C. G. Ball (✉)
Hepatobiliary and Pancreatic Surgery, Trauma and Acute Care Surgery, University of Calgary, Foothills Medical Center, Calgary, AB, Canada

function and emergency surgery were both major risk factors for postoperative mortality [3]. A Nationwide Inpatient Sample analysis of over 22,000 patients with cirrhosis also showed an increase in adjusted mortality rates in a stepwise manner with the severity of hepatic dysfunction [4]. Interestingly, this was even observed for elective procedures, and in the absence of portal hypertension.

25.1.2 Etiology

There are numerous underlying etiologies for cirrhosis which vary dramatically around the world. Mortality, in particular, is often related to the socio-demographic index of a given region [5]. Causes can further be divided into viral (hepatitis B, C, and D), fatty liver disease (alcohol or non-alcohol), autoimmune (autoimmune hepatitis, primary biliary cirrhosis, primary sclerosing cholangitis, IgG4 cholangiopathy), chronic biliary disease (recurrent bacterial cholangitis and bile duct stenosis), storage disorders (hemochromatosis, Wilson's disease, and alpha 1 antitrypsin deficiency), cardiovascular (Budd–Chiari syndrome and right heart failure), as well as less common etiologies such as various medications and porphyria.

25.1.3 Classification

The Child and Model of End-Stage Liver Disease (MELD) scoring systems represent the most helpful tools in patients with cirrhosis. In 1964, the Child-Turcotte classification system was introduced to predict mortality after portosystemic shunt surgery [6]. A modification was made to the score in 1972 by Pugh et al., where the prothrombin time (or INR) replaced the nutritional status criterion [7]. The Child-Pugh classification is based on three objective laboratories (albumin level, bilirubin level, and prothrombin time) and two subjective clinical (severity of ascites and encephalopathy) criteria which stratifies patients into class A, B, or C; with C representing the most advanced cases. This classification system is utilized in a number of surgical and medical scenarios. The predicted mortality rates range from 10%, 30%, and 80% for Child-Pugh A, B, and C, respectively [8, 9]. The limitation of this classification system, however, is the inter-observer variability of relatively subjective criteria, and therefore the stratification of a wide range of laboratory values into only three risk groups.

The MELD score, published in 2000, offers a more accurate scoring system to predict mortality after the insertion of transjugular intra-hepatic portosystemic shunts (TIPS). It is based on bilirubin, creatinine, and INR values [10]. In this sentinel publication, a MELD score of less than 8 was predictive of good post-TIPS survival, whereas a score greater than 18 translated into significantly greater mortality. The MELD score has since been validated in a number series for different operations, with slightly variable reported cutoff values for poor outcomes. In a review of the literature, Hanje and colleagues concluded that elective abdominal surgery could be recommended for MELD scores less than 10, but strongly discouraged for MELD scores greater than 15 [11]. The MELD system's current dominant use, however, has been prioritizing patients awaiting liver transplantation [12]. The addition of sodium to the MELD score (MELD-Na) has also been shown to be a helpful step forward in improving wait list outcomes for liver transplant patients [13]. For those on the Eurotransplant wait list, for example, the MELD-Na score has been validated to offer improved 90-day mortality predictions [14].

The MELD risk stratification is often preferred for risk stratification over the Child-Pugh scoring due to its more objective and detailed risk stratification with a continuum of possible scores. The limitations however are similar to the Child-Pugh score, in that the MELD is not specific to patients with surgical emergencies.

25.1.4 Pathophysiology

Cirrhosis is the end result of chronic hepatocyte injury (i.e., secondary to inflammation and fibrosis). Ultimately, the hepatic architecture becomes distorted, leading to increased resistance to portal venous flow secondary to the progressive fibrotic replacement of hepatocytes. The clinical manifestations of cirrhosis are therefore largely determined by portal hypertension and the loss of the liver's metabolic functions.

Varices and ascites are the most important clinical manifestations of portal hypertension. The increased pressure gradient from the post-hepatic venous system opens collateral portosystemic shunts in the esophagogastric and anorectal regions, umbilical veins, and retroperitoneum. As this progress, the visceral congestion increases, ascites accumulates, varices enlarge, and portal venous flow decelerates, or even reverses. The diminished delivery of hepatotrophic factors further impairs hepatic function via ongoing hepatocyte loss.

In our surgical patient cohort, this hepatic dysfunction translates into an increased risk of infection, hemorrhage, thrombosis, and a prolonged half-life of numerous drugs such as opioids and benzodiazepines. Additionally, there is a known associated imbalance of neuroendocrine mediators (e.g., vasopressin, renin-angiotensin-aldosterone system, and nitric oxide) which also potentiates sodium and fluid retention, resulting in a background hyperdynamic circulation with splanchnic venous congestion and systemic vasodilation [15].

These factors are of particular importance in emergency surgery, as the stress response to the underlying condition, anesthesia, and surgical trauma increases the risk of hepatic decompensation and associated multi-system failure. Alterations to hepatic perfusion with shock and fluid shifts further compromise hepatocellular synthetic and excretory functions. Additionally, endotoxemia from gram-negative sepsis potentiates platelet aggregation and creates a state of low-grade disseminated intravascular coagulation [16].

25.1.4.1 Renal System

The activation of the renin-angiotensin-aldosterone system, leads to the hypersecretion of vasopressin, which acts as a compensatory mechanism to preserve arterial pressure and replenish effective circulating volume when blood is pooled in the splanchnic territory. As cirrhosis progresses, the avidity of water and sodium increases, and dilutional hyponatremia results from water retention. Hepatorenal syndrome (HRS) can be the resulting outcome in advanced cases when these abnormalities are exacerbated. HRS is characterized by a rapid decline in renal function with low urinary excretion of sodium due to severe renal vasoconstriction and diminished or absent cortical perfusion. This syndrome has the potential to be reversible but carries an extremely poor prognosis [17].

25.1.4.2 Cardiovascular System

There is an increase in the cardiac output in cirrhotic patients due to the bypass of bacterial endotoxins from the splanchnic into the systemic circulation and therefore increased production of nitric oxide leading to vasodilation. In addition to this vasodilator-mediated hyperdynamic circulatory state, decreased myocardial contractility, accentuated in cases of chronic alcohol use, has been described. These events compromise mean arterial pressure and also impair the cardiac adaptive response to the resuscitative intravenous fluid expansion.

25.1.4.3 Respiratory System

Due to the presence of ascites and pleural effusions, cirrhotic patients are at increased risk of hypoxia secondary to restrictive lung disease. Diffusion abnormalities due to pulmonary arterial and venous vasodilation and shunting, and pulmonary hypertension are also problematic. Patients with large-volume ascites are further predisposed to bronchopulmonary aspiration.

25.1.4.4 Central Nervous System

Varying degrees of cognitive impairment, ranging from minimal changes to deep coma, can occur. This hepatic encephalopathy is a potentially reversible neurological condition associated with hepatic failure and portal hypertension. The driving force for this scenario is cerebral edema followed by an increased passage of ammonia through the blood-brain barrier [18]. Ammonia is produced via glutamine metabolism by enterocytes, and urea breakdown by gut flora. When there is impaired hepatocellular function and portosystemic shunting, ammonia is less likely to be converted to urea and therefore accumulates within the bloodstream. It will eventually cross the blood-brain barrier which contributes to cerebral edema and other pathological processes [19].

25.1.4.5 Coagulation System

Advanced cirrhosis leads to impairment of primary hemostasis mechanisms due to thrombocytopenia and platelet dysfunction. It is also associated with a compensatory increase in von Willebrand factor levels. Concurrent abnormalities in the platelets are the result of multiple factors. These include splenic sequestration, bone marrow suppression (secondary to alcohol, folic acid deficiency, or viral hepatitis C), decreased hepatic production of thrombopoietin, infection, and renal failure.

Upon activation, platelets trigger secondary hemostasis, generating thrombin to convert fibrinogen to fibrin. With the exception of the von Willebrand factor, all plasma clotting factors, anticoagulants, and fibrinolytic proteins are synthesized by the liver and susceptible to advancing hepatic disease. Additionally, a decrease in bile salt excretion will impair the absorption of fat-soluble vitamins and the synthesis of vitamin K-dependent clotting factors (factors II, VII, IX, and X). The liver is also responsible for clearing activated clotting factors, anticoagulants, and fibrinolytic proteins. Therefore, with such widespread effects on coagulation and anticoagulation, this will translate into an unpredictable increased risk of both bleeding and thrombosis.

25.2 Diagnosis

25.2.1 Clinical Presentation

Patients with cirrhosis often present entirely asymptomatic from a chronic liver disease point of view. Went evident, however, symptoms can include fatigue, loss of appetite, pruritus, progressive abdominal distension, hematemesis, hematochezia, decreased libido (in men), absent or irregular menses, and an alternated mental state. Physical findings may include icterus, parotid gland swelling in chronic alcohol abusers, caput medusae, ascites (evidenced by a fluid thrill and shifting dullness depending on the amount of ascites), asterixis, striae, thinning of the skin, gynecomastia (in men), and hepatomegaly.

25.2.2 Tests

Quantifying the degree of coagulopathy and thrombocytopenia within the preoperative interval can be challenging. More specifically, conventional coagulation tests, which focus on measuring defects in specific hemostatic pathways, are notoriously misleading in regards to a patient's overall clotting ability in the context of cirrhosis. Additionally, these tests are poor predictors of the risk of hemorrhage versus thrombosis [20]. Thromboelastography evaluates the viscoelastic properties of blood and therefore provides a comprehensive evaluation of the clotting process. This modality has been recommended in the global assessment of clot formation, strength, and dissolution. In a prospective study, thromboelastography differentiated cirrhotic patients from healthy volunteers (AUC = 0.921, $p < 0.001$), while conventional coagulation tests did not [21]. There is growing literature that supports the use of thromboelastography in liver transplantation, but more studies are needed for many other diagnostic tests [22–24]. Other coagulation studies such as sonorheometry, international normalized ratio calibrated for cirrhosis, and coagulation-like thrombin generation time have also been recommended, but still lack definitive prospective validation for cirrhotic patients [20].

Hypokalemia, hypocalcemia, hypomagnesemia, and dilutional hyponatremia should be predicted, monitored, and corrected. Additionally, we should always maintain a high index of suspicion for malnutrition and micronutrient deficiencies (folate, vitamins A, D, E, K, and complex B). Importantly, particularly in alcoholic liver disease, early supplementation of these nutrients is recommended. Hypoglycemia, from impaired gluconeogenesis, should also be expected and promptly corrected. Blood lactate level, a specific marker of tissue ischemia, can be significantly elevated in the context of chronic liver disease due to impaired hepatic clearance. Despite this, monitoring the trend of serial serum lactate measurement in response to resuscitation may be a useful adjunct in hemodynamic assessment. Mild increases in aminotransferases (AST and ALT) are commonly noted in chronic liver disease, reflecting active hepatic injury. Notably, however, marked elevation (greater than 1000 IU/L), suggests acute viral, alcoholic, or ischemic hepatitis. In asymptomatic patients with three or more fold increases n ALT/AST levels or any elevation in bilirubin, the incidence of undiagnosed cirrhosis ranges from 6 to 34%.

Imaging features of early cirrhosis can include hepatomegaly, widening of the porta hepatis, umbilical fissure, and pericholecystic space. The progression of cirrhosis leads to the hepatomegaly evolving into a typical nodular shrunken liver with atrophy of segment 4 and the right lobe, as well as hypertrophy of segments 2 and 3 and the caudate lobe. Bedside ultrasonography can demonstrate bright and coarse nodular texture with surface nodularity (most commonly noticed on the undersurface of the liver) [25]. Dysplastic and regenerative nodules are difficult to appreciate on CT due to their small size and isointensity. However, the identification of hyper-enhancing nodules on the arterial phase should raise suspicion for an incidental hepatocellular carcinoma [26].

The vascular manifestations of cirrhosis include signs of hepatic perfusion abnormalities and portal hypertension. Progressive hepatic fibrosis increases resistance to both arterial and venous inflow. Pathways exist for decompression of the portal venous system through portosystemic collaterals, however, there is no equivalent alternative for hepatic arterial inflow. This results in intra-hepatic vascular communications developing in the hepatic sinusoids, vasa vasorum of portal vein, and peribiliary capillaries to shunt arterial blood into the portal venous system [27]. On cross-sectional imaging, these changes present as heterogeneous delayed enhancement of hepatic parenchyma, sometimes mixed with geographic areas of arterialization. Additionally, evidence of overt portal hypertension can also be found on imaging (esophageal, gastric, and umbilical varices, prominent left gastric veins and tributaries, splenomegaly, and ascites).

25.2.3 Differential Diagnosis

The differential diagnosis for cirrhosis is wide. The search for an underlying etiology should always begin with a nuanced history and physical examination. As mentioned previously, these causes range from viral, fatty liver disease, autoimmune, chronic biliary disease, storage disorders, and cardiovascular diseases, as well as less frequent diagnoses such as atypical medications and porphyria.

25.3 Treatment

25.3.1 Medical Treatment

Potential hypovolemia is a significant preoperative concern. Fluid resuscitation should be goal-directed. Blood products (Table 25.1) should be guided where possible by hemodynamic monitoring [28]. The presence of low urine output should be interpreted with caution. Oliguria from hormonal and inflammatory changes associated with cirrhosis and the underlying emergency might mislead the clinician to volume overload the patient. Excessive crystalloid and blood product infusion, in turn, can precipitate respiratory failure and variceal hemorrhage. Being aware of the underlying cause of cirrhosis allows the implementation of specific treatments. For example, thiamine replacement with glucose infusion is indicated to prevent the progression of Wernicke encephalopathy. The risk of symptoms from alcohol withdrawal also should involve supportive measures as well as multivitamins. Those patients on chronic steroids for autoimmune hepatitis should receive a stress-dose adjustment in the perioperative period. Finally, delays in restarting anti-viral therapy for hepatitis should be avoided.

Table 25.1 Management of perioperative coagulopathy in chronic liver disease

Treatment	Comment	Dosing principles
Vitamin K	IV vitamin K can be given for patients who are severely malnourished or have malabsorption, secondary to biliary obstruction, bile salt deficiency, or the use of broad-spectrum antibiotics	The recommended dose is 10 mg IV daily for 3 days prior to surgery
Fresh frozen plasma (FFP)	The correction of INR with FFP has not been shown to decrease the risk of bleeding in cirrhotics. It is not recommended to empirically transfuse FFP for elevated INR or prothrombin time. Excessive use of FFP can lead to significant complications such as volume expansion, infection, and transfusion-associated lung injury (TRALI)	If the patient is clinically bleeding, it is recommended to transfuse FFP, at a dose of 10–15 mL/kg
Platelets	Platelet transfusion should be considered in active bleeding if platelet levels are below 50,000	The recommended dose is 1 unit per 10 kg body weight
Cryoprecipitate	Hypofibrinogenemia (<100 mg/dL) should be corrected with cryoprecipitate	The recommended dose is one bag (10 units) per 10 kg of body weight
Tranexemic acid	Tranexemic acid, an anti-fibrinolytic agent, should be used in patients with hyperfibrinolysis diagnosed by thromboelastography or patients with intractable bleeding	A loading dose of 10 mg/kg is given, repeated three times for 2–8 days
DDAVP	DDAVP is an analog of vasopressin. It releases vWF and factor VIII. Despite the high levels of vWF in cirrhosis, DDAVP has been shown to decrease bleeding time in those patients	The recommended dose is 300 μg IV
rfVIIa	rfVIIa has a high cost, transient effect, and thrombotic complications. It has been shown to reduce bleeding in the placement of intracranial pressure monitoring devices but not in any other surgical procedure. Its clinical indications are limited	If used, the dose is 40 μg/kg

25.3.2 Surgical Treatment

Careful planning of the surgical access site(s), whether open or laparoscopic is essential. Fixed retractor placement also demands contemplation. It is essential to avoid engorged abdominal wall veins and to optimize surgical exposure in anticipation of the most critical operative steps. Despite the lack of definitive evidence, the authors believe that bipolar and ultrasonic energy devices, mechanical vascular staplers, and topical hemostatics are useful adjuncts in attempting to decrease both operating time and blood loss [29]. Postoperative coagulopathy can easily facilitate bleeding from initial minor sources, so extra attention to hemostasis is required.

The use of intra-abdominal drains to help control postoperative ascites and prevent surgical wound complications is a controversial topic. Even though a more restrictive policy for the placement of surgical abdominal drains has gained growing support in the literature, its associated safety in the context of cirrhosis remains poorly explored [30]. A rationale for improved control of postoperative ascites and potential associated wound complications is compelling, but the risk of infectious contamination of ascites and increased postoperative fluid shifts must also be considered. Notably, a small clinical trial in the early 2000s showed increased morbidity due to wound complications in cirrhotic patients randomized to prophylactic drainage after liver resection [31]. It is the opinion of the authors of this chapter that routine use of surgical drains should be avoided in cirrhotic patients, and if indicated, early removal should be aggressively pursued.

As a general rule, the most expeditious and least invasive operation should be utilized, which includes a laparoscopic approach were feasible and safe. Historically, the safety of laparoscopy in cirrhotic patients has been challenged due to the theoretical risks of hemorrhage from abdominal wall varices during port placement, detrimental effects of pneumoperitoneum on hepatic perfusion, and technical limitations to approaching intraoperative hemorrhage. Over the years, however, these concerns have been vastly mitigated, with multiple reports now attesting to the safety of laparoscopy, as well as suggesting some useful technical tips (Table 25.2).

Laparoscopic cholecystectomy in cirrhotic patients has been shown to be superior to open approaches in regards to operative blood loss, surgical time, post-operative pain, morbidity, and hospital length of stay [32, 33]. Technical difficulties must be expected in retracting the liver and identifying anatomic landmarks due to hepatic distortion. Identification of regional anatomy markers is essential (sulcus of Rouviere, umbilical fissure, hepatic artery, duodenum, common bile duct).

The expectation of increased intraoperative bleeding in cirrhotic patients is a tenant that must always be considered. In the conduct of laparoscopic surgery, the use of additional ports and meticulous operative techniques, both assist in preventing iatrogenic injuries. Venous hemorrhage can be temporized by brief increases in pneumoperitoneum pressure and compression with sponges. For gallbladder bed bleeding, if electrocautery use is considered, a high setting (100 ECU units on spray) and precise contact to the site of bleeding are recommended. In scenarios where this technique does not arrest ongoing bleeding, placement of a clip immediately beside the site of hemorrhage (i.e., into the liver in a perpendicular manner) can be helpful as an ignition tool for cauterization.

The use of laparoscopy has also been recommended for cirrhotic patients with acute appendicitis. This was demonstrated by Tsugawa and colleagues, who compared open (25 patients) to laparoscopic appendectomy (15 patients) in a retrospective series. Laparoscopy was compared favorably with open surgery with respect to blood loss, ascites formation, wound complications, hospital length of stay, postoperative pain, and liver function [34].

Patients with chronic liver disease are predisposed to ventral hernias due to ascites. Umbilical hernias occur in up to 20% of all patients with cirrhosis [35]. The indications for surgery are debatable in non-complicated cases due to the high risk of postoperative morbidity and a 60% risk of recurrence in patients with persistent ascites [36]. The conservative approach, however, imposes a risk of hernia strangulation and rupture of overlying skin, with even poorer surgical outcomes. In the scenario of an emergency, however, timely surgical treatment and clinical management of ascites are mandatory. There are concerns about the increased risk of surgical site infection, ascites leakage, and mesh displacement, which mandate judicious planning of the

Table 25.2 Laparoscopic strategies in advanced liver disease

Port placement	As a general rule, an open Hasson technique is recommended for entry into the peritoneal cavity [32]. To avoid abdominal wall varices from the umbilical vein and falciform ligament, several authors have recommended port placement to the right of the midline, especially the subxiphoid port in laparoscopic cholecystectomy [33, 34]
Pneumoperitoneum	Blunting of the hepatic arterial buffer response is a theoretical risk. There is no report in the literature of liver failure related to pneumoperitoneum in a cirrhotic patient [35, 36]. Some authors reduce their intra-abdominal pressure in cirrhotic patients [37]
Bleeding risk	There are few reports of bleeding during laparoscopic procedures in cirrhotic patients. Cobb et al. describes an 8% transfusion rate, with only one patient requiring transfusion for bleeding [38]. In a retrospective study of 68 patients undergoing laparoscopic cholecystectomy, only one patient received blood transfusion [36]. Laparoscopic hemostatic devices such as ultrasound knife, Ligasure, and harmonic scalpel can significantly improve hemostasis and are recommended by many authors [33, 37]
Conversion	The published conversion rate for laparoscopic cholecystectomy is between 4 and 6%, which is similar to the non-cirrhotic patient population [33, 36–38]
Immune function	Li et al. report a reduced risk of bacterial seeding with laparoscopy, with a subsequent decreased risk in spontaneous bacterial peritonitis [37]

repair technique by the acute care surgeon. To minimize the risk of these complications, when a repair with mesh is indicated, pre-peritoneal placement has been favored over an onlay technique. A laparoscopic approach has also been proven safe in multiple surgical series [36–38].

25.3.3 Prognosis

Any resuscitative and therapeutic efforts which were initiated preoperatively (i.e., careful volume resuscitation, correction of electrolyte abnormalities, coagulopathy reversal), must continue in the postoperative period. A high degree of vigilance for evidence of postoperative hepatic decompensation is also critical. Liver failure can result from either the inflammatory response to surgery and/or the underlying emergency condition. The possibility of additional precipitating factors (e.g., constipation, fluid and electrolyte abnormalities, gastrointestinal hemorrhage, and spontaneous bacterial peritonitis) should also be considered.

25.3.3.1 Ascites

The presence of large-volume ascites after abdominal surgery increases the risk of abdominal wall dehiscence and herniation. It also contributes to atelectasis, aspiration, and pneumonia. Associated fluid shifts may precipitate electrolyte imbalances, hypovolemia, and acute kidney injury. Management is based on sodium restriction and judicious use of diuretics, with close monitoring of electrolytes and renal function. The use of therapeutic paracentesis should be reserved for refractory cases and limited to symptomatic relief. A high index of suspicion for spontaneous bacterial peritonitis is also critical.

25.3.3.2 Hepatic Encephalopathy

Investigating additional possible causes of global neurologic decline such as hypoxia, hypercapnia, hypoglycemia, uremia, medications, delirium tremens, seizures, and intracranial hemorrhage should be considered. Although the correlation with actual disease severity is poor, the presence of elevated blood ammonia levels, which are found in over 90% of cases, corroborates a clinical diagnosis. Furthermore, monitoring blood ammonia levels has been shown to be inferior to a comprehensive clinical assessment, and is therefore not recommended in asymptomatic patients [39]. When chemical restraint is required, haloperidol should replace the use of benzodiazepines.

The current literature does not support the use of the classic protein-restricted diet because most patients do not tolerate high-food/calorie intake [40]. Malnutrition is a much more significant concern, and the use of branched amino acid supplementation may also be beneficial [41]. Cathartics and oral antibiotics are other adjuncts are recommended in an attempt to decrease the intestinal production of ammonia due to bacterial overgrowth.

Lactulose is a non-absorbable sugar that creates osmotic diarrhea and has been traditionally used to treat hepatic encephalopathy. It works by acidifying the colon and promoting the conversion of ammonia to ammonium, which is not reabsorbed [42]. The dosing of lactulose should be titrated to two to three bowel movements per day. The known side effects include electrolyte imbalances, nausea, and bloating.

A semisynthetic drug derivative of rifampin, known as rifaximin, was originally employed as a second-line treatment for hepatic encephalopathy. This agent was the subject of a 2012 meta-analysis of 12 randomized controlled trials which stated that rifaximin had similar effectiveness to lactulose, with fewer side effects [43]. Another meta-analysis also supports its use but highlights its high associated cost when compared to lactulose [44].

25.3.3.3 Hepatorenal Syndrome

Ensuring euvolemia and electrolyte homeostasis via strict clinical and laboratory monitoring is essential. Evidence of acute kidney injury in the absence of hemodynamic instability, use of nephrotoxic drugs, or parenchymal renal disease suggests a diagnosis of hepatorenal syndrome. Additional criteria to confirm this diagnosis include no improvement in renal function after volume expansion with albumin and diuretic withdrawal. The treatment of hepatorenal syndrome requires the use of splanchnic vasoconstrictors (terlipressin, noradrenaline, or midodrine) and albumin infusion. Improvement in renal function has been demonstrated with medical treatment, but a mortality benefit is only ultimately achieved with liver transplantation [28]. TIPS placement and renal and hepatic replacement therapies can also be utilized as potential bridging strategies.

25.3.3.4 Variceal Hemorrhage

Hemorrhage from esophageal varices can be precipitated by increased portal pressures from perioperative volume overload. Postoperative hepatic dysfunction, in addition to portal vein thrombosis, is additional factors that may contribute to variceal bleeding. Variceal hemorrhage is life-threatening, and often requires management in the intensive care unit [45].

Rapid resuscitative efforts are critical to ensure the preservation of the respiratory and circulatory systems. Restrictive transfusion strategies, aiming for a target hemoglobin of 7-9 g/dL have been associated with decreased re-bleeding and mortality rates [46]. Given the associated increased risks of bacterial infections, as well as decreased risk of re-bleeding and mortality, antibiotic prophylaxis with ceftriaxone is indicated for up to 7 days [47]. Infusion with vasoactive agents (somatostatin, octreotide, and terlipressin) for 2–5 days has also been associated with lower mortality and transfusion requirements [48].

Identification of the specific source of bleeding is essential. Upper endoscopy should occur within 12 h of presentation [45]. Various endoscopic options for hemorrhage control include elastic band ligation as the first-line maneuver for esophageal varices. Sclerotherapy is also an alternative for difficult cases [49]. It must be noted however that elastic band ligation has been shown to be more effective than sclerotherapy in terms of the number of required sessions, as well as re-bleeding and mortality rates [46, 50]. Non-specific beta-blockers, such as nadolol or propranolol, are also indicated after the vasoactive infusion is discontinued.

The use of balloon tamponade should be reserved for temporary control of ongoing variceal bleeding while awaiting definitive therapy. In high-risk patients, TIPS should be considered preemptively, or in refractory or recurrent hemorrhage cases. These approaches have been shown to be associated with improved mortality [51].

25.3.3.5 Venous Thromboembolism Prophylaxis

Cirrhosis is associated with an increased risk of both venous thromboembolism and hemorrhage as a result of multimodal impacts on the coagulation system. As previously mentioned, conventional coagulation tests do not reflect many of these risks. Furthermore, an increased INR is rarely evidence of protection from thromboembolic events. Detailed guidelines remain unavailable, however, thromboprophylaxis is highly recommended in most patients, and certainly in all high-risk scenarios.

> **Dos and Don'ts**
> - Do not over-resuscitate your patient.
> - Do review all preoperative laboratory investigations and imaging for features of portal hypertension.
> - Do plan carefully your surgical access route to avoid torrential hemorrhage from engorged abdominal wall veins.

> **Take-Home Messages**
> - In acute care surgery, we are more likely to encounter cirrhotic patients in need of emergency, non-hepatic procedures.
> - Cirrhosis affects a variety of organ systems and it is prudent to have a good understanding of the physiological changes within each of these systems, as it will correlate with optimal perioperative management.
> - Classify the patient using the Child-Pugh and MELD scoring systems. This will assist with prognostication.
> - Be prepared for a possibly challenging post-operative course. Successful outcomes can be achieved with a strong collaborative multi-disciplinary approach.

Questions

1. What estimate is quoted in regards to the chances of a patient with cirrhosis requiring surgery?
   A. 5 in 10 patients in the final 2 years of life
   B. 1 in 10 patients in the final 2 years of life
   C. 8 in 10 patients in the final 2 years of life
   D. 4 in 10 patients in the final 2 years of life
2. Which parameters are included in the MELD score?
   A. Urea, platelet, bilirubin
   B. Bilirubin, creatine, sodium
   C. Bilirubin, creatine, INR
   D. Sodium, platelet, creatine
3. Liver changes in cirrhosis can result in:
   A. Atrophy of the left lobe
   B. Hypertrophy of segments II and III
   C. Atrophy of segment I
   D. No changes to the liver
4. What is the rate of conversion to an open approach during a laparoscopic cholecystectomy in a patient with cirrhosis?
   A. 4–6%
   B. 10–15%
   C. 20–25%
   D. 30–35%
5. When ventral hernia repair is necessary in a cirrhotic patient, which mesh location is favored?
   A. On-lay
   B. Pre peritoneal
   C. Inlay
   D. No mesh should be used
6. Lactulose dosing should be titrated to:
   A. 2–3 bowel movements a day
   B. 9–10 bowel movements a day
   C. 4–5 bowel movements a day
   D. 6–8 bowel movements a day
7. Transfusion targets for hemoglobin are:
   A. 10–12 g/dL
   B. 9–10 g/dL
   C. >12 g/dL
   D. 7–9 g/dL
8. For upper GI bleeding due to varices, what is the recommended first line endoscopic intervention?
   A. Elastic band ligation
   B. Sclerotherapy
   C. Clips
   D. Argon beam coagulation
9. Hepatorenal syndrome is characterized by:
   A. Rapid decline in renal function and low urinary excretion of potassium
   B. Rapid decline in renal function and low urinary excretion of sodium
   C. Rapid decline in renal function and low urinary excretion of magnesium
   D. Easy recovery of renal function
10. Post-operative ventral hernia recurrence rate after emergency repair in cirrhotic patients can be as high as?
    A. 60%
    B. 20%
    C. 10%
    D. 5%

Answers
1. B
2. C
3. B
4. A
5. B
6. A
7. D
8. A
9. B
10. A

References

1. Jackson FC, Christophersen EB, Peternel WW, Kirimli B. Preoperative management of patients with liver disease. Surg Clin North Am. 1968;48(4):907–30.
2. de Goede B, Klitsie PJ, Lange JF, Metselaar HJ, Kazemier G. Morbidity and mortality related to non-hepatic surgery in patients with liver cirrhosis; A systematic review. Best Pract Res Clin Gastroenterol. 2012;26(1):47–59.
3. Teh SH, Nagorney DM, Stevens SR, Offord KP, Therneau TM, Plevak DJ, et al. Risk factors for mortality after surgery in patients with cirrhosis. Gastroenterology. 2007;132(4):1261–9.
4. Csikesz NG, Nguyen LN, Tseng JF, Shah SA. Nationwide volume and mortality after elective surgery in cirrhotic patients. J Am Coll Surg. 2009;208(1):96–103.
5. Sepanlou SG, Safiri S, Bisignano C, Ikuta KS, Merat S, Saberifiroozi M, et al. The global, regional, and national burden of cirrhosis by cause in 195 countries and territories, 1990–2017: a systematic analysis for the Global Burden of Disease Study 2017. Lancet Gastroenterol Hepatol. 2020;5(3):245–66.
6. Child CG, Turcotte JG. Surgery and portal hypertension. The liver and portal hypertension 1964;50–64.
7. Pugh RNH, Murray-Lyon IM, Dawson JL, Pietroni MC, Williams R. Transection of the oesophagus for bleeding oesophageal varices. Br J Surg. 1973;60(8):646–9.
8. Garrison RN, Cryer HM, Howard DA, Polk HC. Clarification of risk factors for abdominal operations in patients with hepatic cirrhosis. Ann Surg. 1984 Jun;199(6):648–55.
9. Mansour A, Watson W, Shayani V, Pickleman J. Abdominal operations in patients with cirrhosis: still a major surgical challenge. Surgery. 1997;122(4):730–5; discussion 735–736.
10. Malinchoc M, Kamath PS, Gordon FD, Peine CJ, Rank J, ter Borg PC. A model to predict poor survival in patients undergoing transjugular intrahepatic portosystemic shunts. Hepatology. 2000;31(4):864–71.
11. Hanje AJ, Patel T. Preoperative evaluation of patients with liver disease. Nat Clin Pract Gastroenterol Hepatol. 2007;4(5):266–76.
12. Wiesner RH, McDiarmid SV, Kamath PS, Edwards EB, Malinchoc M, Kremers WK, et al. MELD and PELD: application of survival models to liver allocation. Liver Transpl. 2001;7(7):567–80.
13. Nagai S, Chau LC, Schilke RE, Safwan M, Rizzari M, Collins K, et al. Effects of allocating livers for transplantation based on model for end-stage liver disease-sodium scores on patient outcomes. Gastroenterology. 2018;155(5):1451–1462.e3.
14. Goudsmit BFJ, Putter H, Tushuizen ME, de Boer J, Vogelaar S, Alwayn IPJ, et al. Validation of the Model for End-stage Liver Disease sodium (MELD-Na) score in the eurotransplant region. Am J Transplant [Internet]. [cited 2020 Dec 20];n/a(n/a). http://onlinelibrary.wiley.com/doi/abs/10.1111/ajt.16142.
15. Moore CM, Van Thiel DH. Cirrhotic ascites review: pathophysiology, diagnosis and management. World J Hepatol. 2013;5(5):251–63.
16. Blasi A. Coagulopathy in liver disease: lack of an assessment tool. World J Gastroenterol WJG. 2015;21(35):10062–71.
17. Arroyo V, Terra C, Ginès P. Advances in the pathogenesis and treatment of type-1 and type-2 hepatorenal syndrome. J Hepatol. 2007;46(5):935–46.
18. Patidar KR, Bajaj JS. Covert and overt hepatic encephalopathy: diagnosis and management. Clin Gastroenterol Hepatol. 2015;13(12):2048–61.
19. Dhiman RK. Gut microbiota and hepatic encephalopathy. Metab Brain Dis. 2013;28(2):321–6.
20. Amarapurkar PD, Amarapurkar DN. Management of coagulopathy in patients with decompensated liver cirrhosis. Int J Hepatol. 2011;2011:695470. https://www.ncbi.nlm.nih.gov/pmc/articles/PMC3227517/.
21. Branco BC, Inaba K, Ives C, Okoye O, Shulman I, David J-S, et al. Thromboelastogram evaluation of the impact of hypercoagulability in trauma patients. Shock. 2014;41(3):200–7.
22. Coakley M, Reddy K, Mackie I, Mallett S. Transfusion triggers in orthotopic liver transplantation: a comparison of the thromboelastometry Analyzer, the thromboelastogram, and conventional coagulation tests. J Cardiothorac Vasc Anesth. 2006;20(4):548–53.
23. Feltracco P, Barbieri S, Cillo U, Zanus G, Senzolo M, Ori C. Perioperative thrombotic complications in liver transplantation. World J Gastroenterol WJG. 2015;21(26):8004–13.
24. Pietri LD, Bianchini M, Montalti R, Maria ND, Maira TD, Begliomini B, et al. Thrombelastography-guided blood product use before invasive procedures in cirrhosis with severe coagulopathy: a randomized, controlled trial. Hepatology. 2016;63(2):566–73.
25. Yeom SK, Lee CH, Cha SH, Park CM. Prediction of liver cirrhosis, using diagnostic imaging tools. World J Hepatol. 2015;7(17):2069–79.
26. Sangster GP, Previgliano CH, Nader M, Chwoschtschinsky E, Heldmann MG. MDCT imaging findings of liver cirrhosis: spectrum of hepatic and extrahepatic abdominal complications. HPB Surg [Internet]. 2013 [cited 2020 Dec 28];2013. https://www.ncbi.nlm.nih.gov/pmc/articles/PMC3748773/.
27. Wachsberg RH, Bahramipour P, Sofocleous CT, Barone A. Hepatofugal flow in the portal venous system: pathophysiology, imaging findings, and diagnostic pitfalls. Radiographics. 2002;22(1):123–40.
28. Davenport A, Ahmad J, Al-Khafaji A, Kellum JA, Genyk YS, Nadim MK. Medical management of hepatorenal syndrome. Nephrol Dial Transplant. 2012;27(1):34–41.
29. Moggia E, Rouse B, Simillis C, Li T, Vaughan J, Davidson BR, et al. Methods to decrease blood loss during liver resection: a network meta-analysis. Cochrane Database Syst Rev [Internet]. 2016 [cited

2020 Dec 29];2016(10). https://www.ncbi.nlm.nih.gov/pmc/articles/PMC6472530/.
30. Wong-Lun-Hing EM, van Woerden V, Lodewick TM, Bemelmans MHA, Olde Damink SWM, Dejong CHC, et al. Abandoning prophylactic abdominal drainage after hepatic surgery: 10 years of no-drain policy in an enhanced recovery after surgery environment. Dig Surg. 2017;34(5):411–20.
31. Liu C-L, Fan S-T, Lo C-M, Wong Y, Ng IO-L, Lam C-M, et al. Abdominal drainage after hepatic resection is contraindicated in patients with chronic liver diseases. Ann Surg. 2004;239(2):194–201.
32. El-Awadi S, El-Nakeeb A, Youssef T, Fikry A, Abd El-Hamed TM, Ghazy H, et al. Laparoscopic versus open cholecystectomy in cirrhotic patients: a prospective randomized study. Int J Surg. 2009;7(1):66–9.
33. Puggioni A, Wong LL. A metaanalysis of laparoscopic cholecystectomy in patients with cirrhosis. J Am Coll Surg. 2003;197(6):921–6.
34. Tsugawa K, Koyanagi N, Hashizume M, Tomikawa M, Ayukawa K, Akahoshi K, et al. A comparison of an open and laparoscopic appendectomy for patients with liver cirrhosis. Surg Laparosc Endosc Percutan Tech. 2001;11(3):189–94.
35. Belghiti J, Durand F. Abdominal wall hernias in the setting of cirrhosis. Semin Liver Dis. 1997;17(3):219–26.
36. Belli G, D'Agostino A, Fantini C, Cioffi L, Belli A, Russolillo N, et al. Laparoscopic incisional and umbilical hernia repair in cirrhotic patients. Surg Laparosc Endosc Percutan Tech. 2006;16(5):330–3.
37. Yu BC, Chung M, Lee G. The repair of umbilical hernia in cirrhotic patients: 18 consecutive case series in a single institute. Ann Surg Treat Res. 2015;89(2):87–91.
38. Cobb WS, Heniford BT, Burns JM, Carbonell AM, Matthews BD, Kercher KW. Cirrhosis is not a contraindication to laparoscopic surgery. Surg Endosc. 2005;19(3):418–23.
39. James J, Liou IW. Comprehensive care of patients with chronic liver disease. Med Clin North Am. 2015;99(5):913–33.
40. Cabral CM, Burns DL. Low-protein diets for hepatic encephalopathy debunked: let them eat steak. Nutr Clin Pract. 2011;26(2):155–9.
41. Gluud LL, Dam G, Les I, Córdoba J, Marchesini G, Borre M, et al. Branched-chain amino acids for people with hepatic encephalopathy. Cochrane Database Syst Rev. 2015;(2):CD001939.
42. Patil DH, Westaby D, Mahida YR, Palmer KR, Rees R, Clark ML, et al. Comparative modes of action of lactitol and lactulose in the treatment of hepatic encephalopathy. Gut. 1987;28(3):255–9.
43. Eltawil KM, Laryea M, Peltekian K, Molinari M. Rifaximin vs conventional oral therapy for hepatic encephalopathy: a meta-analysis. World J Gastroenterol WJG. 2012;18(8):767–77.
44. Kimer N, Krag A, Møller S, Bendtsen F, Gluud LL. Systematic review with meta-analysis: the effects of rifaximin in hepatic encephalopathy. Aliment Pharmacol Ther. 2014;40(2):123–32.
45. Garcia-Tsao G, Abraldes JG, Berzigotti A, Bosch J. Portal hypertensive bleeding in cirrhosis: risk stratification, diagnosis, and management: 2016 practice guidance by the American Association for the study of liver diseases. Hepatology. 2017;65(1):310–35.
46. Villanueva C, Colomo A, Bosch A, Concepción M, Hernandez-Gea V, Aracil C, et al. Transfusion strategies for acute upper gastrointestinal bleeding. N Engl J Med. 2013;368(1):11–21.
47. Chavez-Tapia NC, Barrientos-Gutierrez T, Tellez-Avila F, Soares-Weiser K, Mendez-Sanchez N, Gluud C, et al. Meta-analysis: antibiotic prophylaxis for cirrhotic patients with upper gastrointestinal bleeding—an updated Cochrane review. Aliment Pharmacol Ther. 2011;34(5):509–18.
48. Wells M, Chande N, Adams P, Beaton M, Levstik M, Boyce E, et al. Meta-analysis: vasoactive medications for the management of acute variceal bleeds. Aliment Pharmacol Ther. 2012;35(11):1267–78.
49. Bari K, Garcia-Tsao G. Treatment of portal hypertension. World J Gastroenterol. 2012;18(11):1166–75.
50. Avgerinos A, Armonis A, Stefanidis G, Mathou N, Vlachogiannakos J, Kougioumtzian A, et al. Sustained rise of portal pressure after sclerotherapy, but not band ligation, in acute variceal bleeding in cirrhosis. Hepatology. 2004;39(6):1623–30.
51. Garcia-Pagán JC, Di Pascoli M, Caca K, Laleman W, Bureau C, Appenrodt B, et al. Use of early-TIPS for high-risk variceal bleeding: results of a post-RCT surveillance study. J Hepatol. 2013;58(1):45–50.

Further Reading

Amarapurkar PD, Amarapurkar DN. Management of coagulopathy in patients with decompensated liver cirrhosis. Int J Hepatol. 2011;2011:695470. https://www.ncbi.nlm.nih.gov/pmc/articles/PMC3227517/

de Goede B, Klitsie PJ, Lange JF, Metselaar HJ, Kazemier G. Morbidity and mortality related to non-hepatic surgery in patients with liver cirrhosis; A systematic review. Best Pract Res Clin Gastroenterol. 2012;26(1):47–59.

James J, Liou IW. Comprehensive care of patients with chronic liver disease. Med Clin North Am. 2015;99(5):913–33.

Management of Animal Bites: A Global Perspective

26

Saleh Abdel-Kader, Ihab M. Abbas, and Fikri M. Abu-Zidan

26.1 Introduction

The relationship between humans, animals, and environment has been delicate and balanced since human existence. Man depended on agricultural activities and domestic animals for living and transportation. This balance has been affected by industrialization. A "one globe, one health approach" is essential to address major threats to humans like the current SARS-CoV-2 (COVID-19) pandemic [1, 2]. Animal bites on humans is a major neglected global health problem with 10 million dog bites and 5 million snake bites every year [3]. These bites can cause major tissue damage, severe bacterial and viral infections, and long-term psychological effects. Rabies from dog bites cause tens of thousands of annual deaths globally mainly in Africa and Asia. 40% of rabies patients are children. About 1% of emergency room visits in the USA are related to animal bites [4]. Rabies costs the world 8.6 billion US dollars annually [5]. The world health organization has stressed the need to address this global burden. The type of animal bite varies globally depending on the existence of the animals and their interaction with humans. Dog and cat bites are most common in the USA and Europe [6], snake bites in southeast Asia [3], crocodile and camel bites in Africa where 80% of camels live [7, 8]. It is extremely difficult to cover all aspects of animal bites in a single book chapter. It took the senior author (FAZ) more than 20 years to understand the biomechanism and effects of camel bites. We aimed in this concise book chapter to lay out the principles of managing the bites of dogs, cats, snakes, crocodiles, and camels to humans taking into consideration the geographical variation and our own experience in camel and snake bites.

> **Learning Objectives**
> - To highlight that animal bites are a neglected global health problem that should be addressed.
> - To lay the general principles of managing animal bites taking into consideration the geographical variation and local experience.
> - To highlight the importance of the prevention of animal bites and their viral and bacterial infections.

S. Abdel-Kader
Department of Surgery, Ain Shams University, Cairo, Egypt

I. M. Abbas
Department of Surgery, Tawam Hospital, Al-Ain, United Arab Emirates
e-mail: ihabbas@seha.ae

F. M. Abu-Zidan (✉)
The Research Office, College of Medicine and Health Sciences, United Arab Emirates University, Al-Ain, United Arab Emirates
e-mail: fabuzidan@uaeu.ac.ae

26.1.1 Epidemiology

The incidence and type of animal bites are affected by geography, community development, and culture. Approximately half of the population in high-income countries are bitten by an animal at least once during their life. Animal bites are underreported in some countries despite being a common injury [6]. The incidence of animal bites ranges between 50 and 200 per 100,000 population per year [9, 10]. Males are more commonly affected by dog bites compared with females (a ratio of 2:1) who are more commonly affected by cat bites compared with males (a ratio of 2:1) [11, 12].

Giant dogs cause more severe bite injuries. Specific aggressive breeds like the Pit Bull and the German Shepherd may cause fatal injuries. The victims are usually small children and elderly persons because they cannot properly defend themselves [13, 14]. These injuries have no socioeconomic barriers [14]. Extensive injuries may occur when the victim is attacked by more than one animal at the same time [13].

The time of injury depends on the behavior and activity of the animal. For example, cobra and viper snakes bite on the daytime, rats bite at night, and Nile crocodiles bite during the hot season [15]. Camel bites are more common during cold weather. This is the rutting season in which sexually active male camels are more aggressive and difficult to handle. They can be recognized by the "Dulla," which is a long pink diverticulum of the soft palate protruding from the mouth and covered by froth. These camels should be handled carefully during that period [16, 17].

The Nile crocodile is the biggest man-killer in Africa. It is common in the water resources of humans [15, 18]. The majority of crocodile attacks occur in the water or near the water edge because humans are slower than crocodiles in water [15, 18–20]. Its death rate is more than the motor vehicle collision death rates of some developed countries [7]. Their bites have a mortality of around 65% [18]. Camels cause around 80% of animal-related injuries in our city [20] of which 25% are caused by bites [21] having a mortality of 3% [16]. Snake bites are life-threatening injuries. They usually affect poor farmers and fishers who sleep on the floor when exhausted from work. That is why snake bites usually affect young males [22]. Viper snakes are the most dangerous snakes in Europe, and the Middle East [22, 23].

26.1.2 Animal Behavior and Biomechanism of Injury

Male dogs, which are more aggressive than females, cause 75% of dog bites. When the dog or cat is disturbed while eating or frightened, they tend to bite its owner. This is more common if the disturbing individuals are children because dogs consider them as a competitor [24]. Dogs become more aggressive when they get sick which is often unnoticed by their caregivers. A regular veterinary checkup is recommended even if the dog is apparently healthy. A veterinary behaviorist should be consulted if the dog has a history of aggressiveness or nervousness so as to avoid future bites [25].

The localized force of the animal bite on the body of the victim causes a crushing injury with tissue devitalization [6]. Such injuries vary in severity including superficial abrasions, tears, crush wounds, degloving injuries, tissue loss (Fig. 26.1), avulsion injuries of the skull, and bone fractures [26]. Dog bites are commonly complicated by cellulitis and fractures and often require invasive surgical procedures. Punctate wounds with deep inoculation of feline saliva are usually noticed with cat bites. Frequently, an inaccurate estimation of the depth of the injury occurs, and it is attributed to the sliding movement of the deep anatomical layers of the injured soft tissue over each other during the bite and then immediately returning back to its normal position [6]. Serious and fatal injuries from large dog bites may cause extensive tissue damage or exsanguinating bleeding [11]. Less common fatalities are caused by asphyxia, sepsis, or craniocerebral trauma [27].

Snake bites have special considerations [22]. The injected venom circulates through the lymphatic system of the body of the victim.

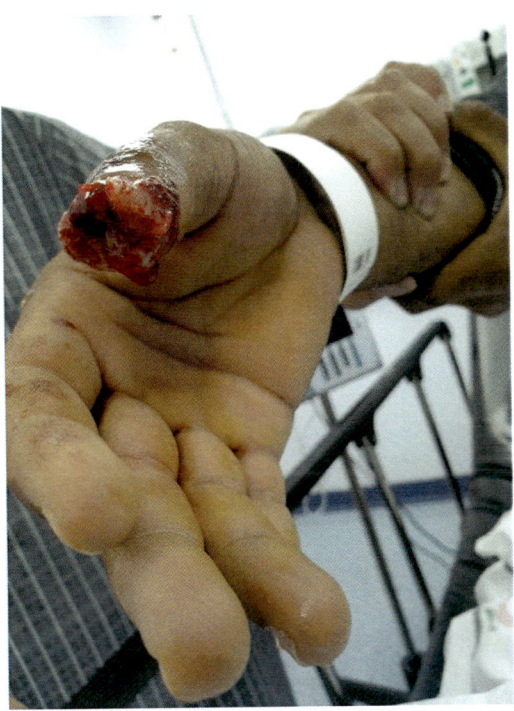

Fig. 26.1 A 32-year-old man was bitten by his own dog and sustained a partial loss of the distal tip and pulp soft tissue of the right thumb (Courtesy of Dr. Mauro D'Arcangelo, Consultant Plastic Surgeon, Tawam Hospital, Al-Ain, United Arab Emirates)

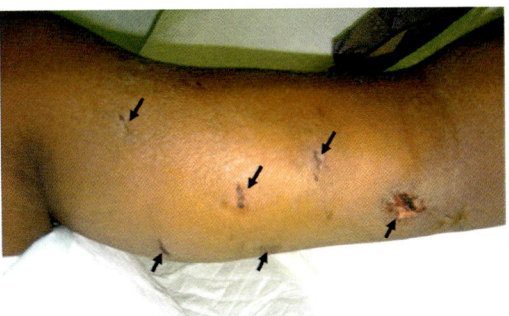

Fig. 26.2 Camel bites are caused by its long 4 canine teeth. It has a classical 4 dot sign (punctures, black arrows). The camel attacks the thin regions of the body like the forearm and neck. Having more than 4 punctures is evidence of repeated bites and indicates the aggressiveness of the camel (Courtesy of Professor Fikri Abu-Zidan, Consultant Acute Care Surgeon, Al-Ain Hospital, Al-Ain, United Arab Emirates)

Accordingly, first-aid immobilization with pressure bandages of the injured limb can reduce the systemic dissemination of the venom [22, 23]. Edema of extremity tissues may cause a limb-threatening compartment syndrome which should be urgently addressed [22, 23, 28].

Crocodile and camel bites have complex mechanism, which includes penetrating, crushing, and blunt injuries [16, 18]. The high force of a crocodile bite can transect an adult human body into two [18]. The crocodile may suddenly grab its victim from the edge of a river using its strong sharp teeth, shakes the victim by swiftly rolling his/her body over (death roll), and then take the victim underwater as a source of food [18, 29]. The head of the victim can be completely decapitated by this movement. The camel may lift its victim by its canine teeth, crushing the body by the side movements of the jaw, and finally throwing the victim through the air to strongly land on the ground. Each camel canine tooth is around 4 cm long. The two opposing teeth work together as a knife (Fig. 26.2). Although they leave trivial marks on the skin, they may cause serious life-threatening injuries to the major superficial vessels. Camels may then use their hooves to step on the victims with their heavy bodies [16, 17].

Viper snakes venom has proteolytic, neurotoxic, coagulopathic, and hemorrhagic effects which cause pain, swelling, blistering, bleeding, and tissue necrosis [22, 23]. In contrast, the Cobra venom contains presynaptic toxins which damage the nerve endings and postsynaptic neurotoxins which block the acetylcholine receptors of the neuromuscular junction to paralyze the victim [23, 30].

26.1.3 Anatomical Regions of Injury

Bites located on the hands, arms, and legs comprise 70–80% of animal bites. The head and neck are involved in 10–30%, and in 90% of children under the age of 5 years [31]. This occurs because of the relatively big size of the head in children, their risk-taking behavior, unawareness of how to deal with animals, short stature of children, and their tendency for crawling and playing on the floor. Children older than 9 years are usually bitten at their extremities because of their height, increased maturity, and ability to protect themselves [14]. The human infant skull is small, and a large dog can take it between its jaws. If the dog shakes it forcefully, then it can tear off. The outcome is then usually fatal because of bleeding, brain injury, decapitation, or air embolism [32]. The most frequent bite site of snakes is the lower extremity. Nevertheless, head and trunk bites may occur for floor sleepers [22].

26.1.4 Infection of Bite Wounds

The occurrence of wound infection depends on the nature and location of the wound, the patient's immunity, and the type of attacking animal. Cat bites with deep punctures have a high infection rate (Fig. 26.3). Wound infection increases in contaminated edematous poorly perfused wounds with destructive nature especially in the face, hands, feet, joints, bones, and genitalia [33]. Neonates and infants are at higher risk of wound infection compared with other ages. Immunosuppressed patients have a higher risk of infection, including those having AIDS, liver disease/alcoholism, malignancy, neutropenia, diabetes, and those on corticosteroids or immunosuppressant therapy [34]. Nevertheless, severe bite wound infection may occur without any predisposing factors.

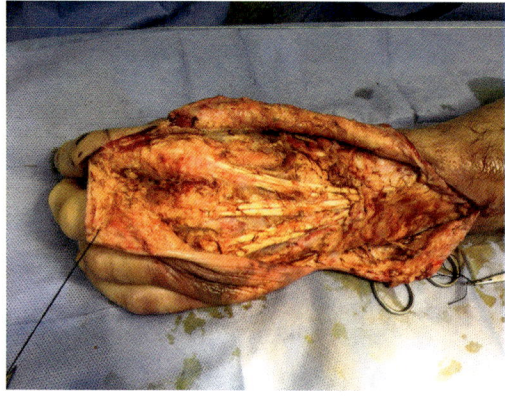

Fig. 26.3 The left hand of a 67-year-old man who was bitten by his own cat. The bite caused severe necrotizing fasciitis of the left upper limb that required repeated debridement to save the limb (Courtesy of Dr. Mauro D'Arcangelo, Consultant Plastic Surgeon, Tawam Hospital, Al-Ain, United Arab Emirates)

26.1.5 Bacteriology

The most common causative pathogens of wound infection are mixed aerobic and anaerobic bacteria originating from the oral flora of the biting animal [35]. Two to five different pathogens usually grow in cat or dog bite wounds [36]. The type and severity of wound infection determine the number of pathogens. The median number of bacteria is 7.5 in abscesses, 5 in purulent wound secretions, and 2 in non-purulent wounds [33]. The commonly isolated pathogens in animal bites include *Staphylococcus*, *Streptococcus*, *Capnocytophaga canimorsus*, anaerobes, *Pasteurella*, *Bacteroides*, and *Porphyromonas* [6]. Necrotizing fasciitis wounds following snake bites usually grow Enterococci and *Morganella morganii* [23, 30]. Normal camel saliva can grow different bacterial species including, *Staphylococcus*, *Streptococcus*, *Escherichia coli*, *Klebsiella pneumoniae*, *Bacillus* spp., and *Pseudomonas aeruginosa* [37].

26.2 Diagnosis

26.2.1 History and Physical Examination

A detailed history should collect information on the injury pattern and circumstances, mechanism of injury, the attacking animal, tetanus vaccination, and risk of rabies [38]. The most important factor in diagnosing a snake bite is to identify the snake type which helps to define the proper antivenom for treatment [22, 23, 28, 30, 39].

Signs suggesting wound infection include wound tenderness, swelling, redness, and purulent discharge. Fever and malaise may occur in severe infection [26]. Symptoms of wound infection usually occur within 12–24 h with *Pasteurella multocida* infection and in around 5–8 days with other infections [40]. The bitten patient may present with cellulitis, abscess formation, lymphadenopathy, or pyogenic arthritis [22]. Severe infections may include endocarditis, meningitis, osteomyelitis, endophthalmitis, and distant organ abscesses involving the brain, lung, or liver [9]. Local infection in a bite wound of immune-compromised patients is likely to progress to systemic sepsis. This particularly occurs in *Capnocytophaga canimorsus* infection. The infection may cause tissue gangrene which may progress to multiorgan failure including renal failure, adult respiratory distress syndrome, disseminated intravascular coagulation, and possibly death [41].

Severe cases of snake bites may present with generalized symptoms including headache, dizziness, irritability, confusion, sweating, nausea, vomiting, cyanosis, difficulty in breathing or swallowing, hypotension, muscle cramps, paralysis, and disseminated intravascular coagulation [22, 23, 28, 30, 39].

26.2.2 Radiological Workups

Plain X-ray and computed tomography are indicated if there was a suspected bone fracture. Ultrasonography is useful to assess soft tissue injury, abscesses and adjacent arteries. Magnetic resonance imaging (MRI) is indicated for a patient with suspected spinal cord or brain injuries, and extensive injuries of the extremities near the joints [6].

26.2.3 Laboratory Investigations

If a patient is suspected to have wound infection, swab/culture and sensitivity, blood cell count, C-reactive protein, and coagulation profile should be requested. A detailed history should be provided to the laboratory because special culture techniques including anaerobic culture or long incubation time may be required. Swabs for the bacterial culture of the saliva and stool culture of the offending animal may be required [42]. Cerebrospinal fluid (CSF) analysis should be performed in cases of suspected meningitis [6].

26.3 Treatment

26.3.1 General Management

General principles of management should be the same as managing multiple trauma patients which usually follows the Advanced Trauma Life Support Guidelines in most of the countries. Nevertheless, stopping the bleeding may become the first priority in cases of severe bleeding involving major vessels away from the airway (like the femoral artery). Life-threatening injuries should be addressed before performing the secondary survey and before a proper assessment of the bite wound is performed. First aid for managing snake bites should include recognizing the type of biting snake, immobilization of the affected limb, and rapid prehospital transportation to an appropriate treating center. Wound assessment may be done under general anesthesia if needed and should include the extent of tissue injury and spread of infection [35].

Rabies spreads by contact with the saliva of an infected animal, usually through a bite. The disease is universally fatal. Dogs are the primary cause of rabies transmission. Deep lacerated devitalized tissues which are caused by animal bites when contaminated by the soil have the risk of developing tetanus [43].

Proper management guidelines for snake bites cannot be properly applied because of a lack of antivenoms that cover important venomous snakes [22]. Treating a patient with an antivenom may decrease the neurotoxic and hemorrhagic effect of the venom but it does not affect the bacterial growth and does not affect the risk of necrotizing fasciitis or compartment syndrome [30].

26.3.2 Local Wound Management

The main objective of wound management is to prevent wound infection. All animal bites are potentially infectious and should be thoroughly irrigated with sterile normal saline or alternatively tap water as first aid. High-pressure irrigation is not recommended so as not to spread the infection into deeper structures. Slight wound bleeding helps to reduce contamination and remove foreign bodies [38]. Debridement of devitalized tissues of the wound is essential.

Antimicrobial therapy is important in high-risk wounds. These include animal bites in the elderly, full-thickness wounds, and those that require debridement. Wounds with localized infection and puncture wounds should be given antibiotics and reviewed within 2 days. Bacterial infection is common following snake bites which needs antibiotics treatment [22, 28, 39].

Although there is evidence supporting the primary closure of bite wounds [44], we advocate the "pay off approach" of keeping the wound open for healing by secondary intention because of the risk of life-threatening infections. This weighs the cosmetic gain. A recent Cochrane database systematic review showed that the evidence for primary wound closure for animal wounds is not strong. This review identified three trials which included 878 participants that compared no closure with primary closure and another trial of 120 participants which compared early with delayed closure. All four studies were for dog bites [45]. The study recommended performing better future-designed clinical trials with larger numbers.

Simple lacerations can be managed in the Emergency Department under local anesthesia while complex lacerations, especially for children, may need surgery under general anesthesia. Bite wounds older than 24 h and infected wounds should be kept open to heal by secondary intention [6]. Repeated surgery and debridement can be essential, especially in cases of necrotizing fasciitis (Fig. 26.4).

Children may have more severe injuries requiring reconstructive surgery. This may

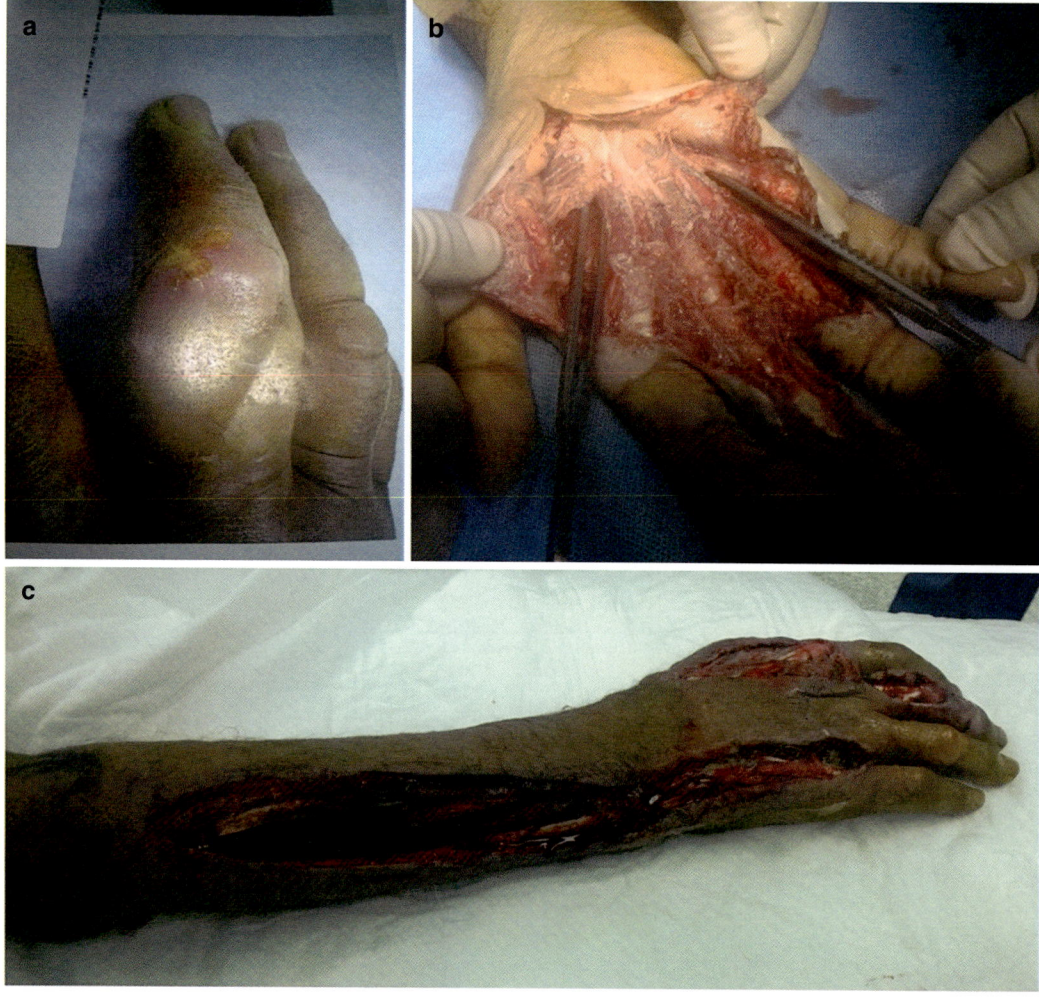

Fig. 26.4 49-year-old farmer had a snake bite in his right middle finger (**a**) when he was sleeping. The patient developed necrotizing fasciitis and needed repeated debridement of his right hand (**b**) and forearm (**c**) to save his limb (Courtesy of Dr. Ihab Marwan, Consultant Orthopedic Surgeon, Tawam Hospital, Al-Ain, United Arab Emirates)

include repeated wound debridement and repair under general anesthesia and skin grafts or flaps [24]. Injuries involving the head and neck, require a multidisciplinary team including a plastic reconstructive surgeon to have the best possible functional and cosmetic outcome that can reduce the long-term physical and psychological effects [46].

> **Treatment Do and Don't**
>
> - Take a proper medical history of the animal bite injury including the details of the incident and animal behavior.
> - Address tetanus and rabies risk, antibiotic administration, and the need for antivenom.
> - Take care of the wounds by irrigation and proper debridement; aim at delayed primary using VAC dressing if available.
> - Review the wound and re-debride as needed taking into consideration the risk of necrotizing fasciitis and compartment syndrome.
> - Once the wound becomes clear consider delayed closure/skin graft and fracture management.

26.4 Psychological Impact

The animal bite experience of being attacked by an aggressive animal may not be forgotten. Furthermore, major facial scars may have long-term psychological effects. This may lead to emotional distress, anxiety, fear, and post-traumatic stress disorder. This may also have a long-term economic impact on work and personal relationships [47]. Parents of injured children observe a change in the behavior of their children including fear of animals, separation anxiety, and changing the favored toys to play with. Parents may also develop a feeling of anxiety, fear, guilt, and responsibility for what happened to their children [48].

26.5 Injury Prevention

The Haddon matrix is a very useful tool for injury prevention. It includes preventing the animal bite before it occurs, reducing its impact if it occurs, and treating it properly after it occurs. Animals are the vector, humans are the host, and both share the same environment [29]. The environment should be modified to accommodate both humans and animals, so they do not compete. Muzzles can be used to cover the animal's mouth to prevent bite injuries [16].

Local inhabitants of Australia and Africa recognized that poking the eye of the attacking crocodile or camel during the bite would force the animal to leave the victim, which reduces the severity of injury [16, 17, 20, 29].

Very young children are immature and have a short memory for injury prevention and educational activities against animal bites. Accordingly, parents or caregivers should be targeted in such activities [24]. Detailed data collection and studies of animal bites including the cause, biomechanism of injury, time of injury, type of the animal and its sex, the change of behavior of the animal, and how to prevent them are helpful to build up injury prevention programs aiming to reduce the impact of animal bites [38]. The local communities, who are aware of their own circumstances and beliefs, are more capable of achieving this target by developing accepted injury prevention educational programs [19].

> **Take Home Messages**
>
> - Animal bites are a neglected global health problem that should be addressed properly.
> - The severity of animal bite injuries varies globally depending on the animal, its behavior, biomechanism of injury, and risk of viral and bacterial infection.
> - Injury prevention is an important component of addressing this global problem. The "one globe one health approach" should be adopted. Acute care surgeons should be part of this approach.

Multiple Choice Questions

1. **The most common injured region in snake bites is**
   A. The head and neck
   B. The upper limb
   C. The trunk
   D. The lower limbs
2. **First aid local wound management of animal bites include all of the following except**
   A. Irrigation with sterile normal saline
   B. Irrigation with tap water
   C. High-pressure irrigation
   D. Allow slight bleeding from the wound
3. **The head and neck are commonly involved in animal bites of**
   A. Adolescents
   B. Toddlers
   C. Adults
   D. Geriatrics
4. **The most probable bacteria that can cause generalized sepsis after animal bites in immune-compromised patients is**
   A. Staphylococcus
   B. Capnocytophaga canimorsus
   C. Streptococcus
   D. Bacteroides
5. **The highest human mortality following animal bites occurs after:**
   A. Camel bites
   B. Snake bites
   C. Dog bites
   D. Crocodile bites
6. **The median number of bacteria species is in purulent animal bite wounds is**
   A. 3
   B. 4
   C. 5
   D. 6
7. **Which of these animals has a different behavior for biting humans**
   A. Camels
   B. Snakes
   C. Dogs
   D. Crocodiles
8. **How many cells does the Haddon matrix have**
   A. 4
   B. 9
   C. 12
   D. 16
9. **The most common animal bites to humans are**
   A. Camel bites
   B. Snake bites
   C. Dog bites
   D. Crocodile bites
10. **Which of these animals tend to bite humans in winter**
    A. Camels
    B. Snakes
    C. Dogs
    D. Crocodiles

Answers
1. D
2. C
3. B
4. B
5. D
6. C
7. D
8. B
9. C
10. A

Conflict of Interest None declared by all authors.

References

1. Babo Martins S, Bolon I, Chappuis F, Ray N, Alcoba G, Ochoa C, et al. Snakebite and its impact in rural communities: the need for a One Health approach. PLoS Negl Trop Dis. 2019;13(9):e0007608. https://doi.org/10.1371/journal.pntd.0007608.
2. Khan G, Sheek-Hussein M, Al Suwaidi AR, Idris K, Abu-Zidan FM. Novel coronavirus pandemic: a global health threat. Turk J Emerg Med. 2020;20(2):55–62.

3. World Health Organization. Animal bites. 5 February 2018. https://www.who.int/news-room/fact-sheets/detail/animal-bites. Accessed 2021 May 4.
4. Ellis R, Ellis C. Dog and cat bites. Am Fam Physician. 2014;90:239–43.
5. World Health Organization. Animal bites. 17 May 2021. https://www.who.int/news-room/fact-sheets/detail/rabies. Accessed 2021 May 29.
6. Rothe K, Tsokos M, Handrick W. Animal and human bite wounds. Dtsch Arztebl Int. 2015;112(25):433–43.
7. Abu-Zidan FM. Crossroad between camel bites and crocodile bites. Afr Health Sci. 2015;15:i–iv.
8. Faye B. The Camel today: assets and potentials. Anthropozoologica. 2014;49:15–24. https://doi.org/10.5252/az2014n2a01. Accessed 28 May 2021.
9. Norton C. Animal and human bites. Emerg Nurse. 2008;16(6):26–9.
10. Ostanello F, Gherardi A, Caprioli A, La Placa L, Passini A, Prosperi S. Incidence of injuries caused by dogs and cats treated in emergency departments in a major Italian city. Emerg Med J. 2005;22(4):260–2.
11. Holzer KJ, Vaughn MG, Murugan V. Dog bite injuries in the USA: prevalence, correlates and recent trends. Inj Prev. 2019;25(3):187–90.
12. Schalamon J, Ainoedhofer H, Singer G, Petnehazy T, Mayr J, Kiss K, et al. Analysis of dog bites in children who are younger than 17 years. Pediatrics. 2006;117(3):e374–9.
13. Heinze S, Feddersen-Petersen DU, Tsokos M, Buschmann C, Püschel K. Fatal dog attacks on children. Rechtsmedizin. 2014;24:37–41.
14. Dhillon J, Hoopes J, Epp T. Scoping decades of dog evidence: a scoping review of dog bite-related sequelae. Can J Public Health. 2019;110(3):364–75.
15. Lamarque F, Anderson J, Fergusson R, Lagrange M, Osei-Owusu Y, Bakker L. Human-wildlife conflict in Africa: Causes, consequences and management strategies. FAO Forestry Paper 157. Rome: Food and Agriculture Organization of the United Nations; 2009. http://www.fao.org/docrep/012/i1048e/i1048e00.pdf. Accessed on 16 Feb 2015.
16. Abu-Zidan FM, Eid HO, Hefny AF, Bashir MO, Branicki F. Camel bite injuries in United Arab Emirates: a 6 year prospective study. Injury. 2012;43:1617–20.
17. Abu-Zidan FM, Abdel-Kader S, El Husseini R. Common carotid artery injury caused by a camel bite: case report and systematic review of the literature. Ulus Travma Acil Cerrahi Derg. 2014;20:59–62.
18. Caldicott DG, Croser D, Manolis C, Webb G, Britton A. Crocodile attack in Australia: an analysis of its incidence and review of the pathology and management of crocodilian attacks in general. Wilderness Environ Med. 2005;16:143–59.
19. Scott R, Scott H. Crocodile bites and traditional beliefs in Korogwe District, Tanzania. BMJ. 1994;309:1691–2.
20. Eid HO, Hefny AF, Abu-Zidan FM. Epidemiology of animal-related injuries in a high-income developing country. Ulus Travma Acil Cerrahi Derg. 2015;21(2):134–8.
21. Abu-Zidan FM, Hefny AF, Eid HO, Bashir MO, Branicki FJ. Camel-related injuries: prospective study of 212 patients. World J Surg. 2012;36:2384–9.
22. Alirol E, Tsai SK, Bawaskar HS, Kuch U, Chappuis F. Snake bite in South Asia: a review. PLoS Negl Trop Dis. 2010;4(1):e603.
23. Tsai YH, Hsu WH, Huang KC, Yu PA, Chen CL, Kuo LT. Necrotizing fasciitis following venomous snakebites in a tertiary hospital of southwest Taiwan. Int J Infect Dis. 2017;63:30–6. https://doi.org/10.1016/j.ijid.2017.08.005.
24. Cook JA, Sasor SE, Soleimani T, Chu MW, Tholpady SS. An epidemiological analysis of pediatric dog bite injuries over a decade. J Surg Res. 2020;246:231–5.
25. Newman J, Christley RM, Westgarth C. Risk factors for dog bites-an epidemiological perspective. In: Mills DS, Westgarth C, editors. Dog bites: a multidisciplinary perspective. Sheffield, UK: 5m Publishing; 2017. p. 133–58.
26. Pfortmueller CA, Efeoglou A, Furrer H, Exadaktylos AK. Dog bite injuries: primary and secondary emergency department presentations—a retrospective cohort study. Scientific World Journal. 2013:393176.
27. Lone KS, Bilquees S, Salimkhan M, Haq IU. Analysis of dog bites in Kashmir: an unprovoked threat to population. Natl J Commun Med. 2014;5(1):66–8.
28. Hifumi T, Sakai A, Kondo Y, Yamamoto A, Morine N, Ato M, et al. Venomous snake bites: clinical diagnosis and treatment. J Intensive Care. 2015;3(1):16.
29. Gruen RL. Crocodile attacks in Australia: challenges for injury prevention and trauma care. World J Surg. 2009;33:1554–61.
30. Stewart CJ. Snake bite in Australia: first aid and envenomation management. Accid Emerg Nurs. 2003;11(2):106–11. https://doi.org/10.1016/s0965-2302(02)00189-3.
31. Freeman AJ, Senn DR, Arendt DM. Seven hundred seventy eight bite marks: analysis by anatomic location, victim and biter demographics, type of crime and legal disposition. J Forensic Sci. 2005;50(6):1436–43.
32. Tsokos M, Byard RW, Püschel K. Extensive and mutilating craniofacial trauma involving defleshing and decapitation: unusual features of fatal dog attacks in the young. Am J Forensic Med Pathol. 2007;28(2):131–6.
33. Talan DA, Citron DM, Abrahamian FM, Moran GJ, Goldstein EJ. Bacteriologic analysis of infected dog and cat bites. Emergency medicine animal bite infection study group. N Engl J Med. 1999;340(2):85–92.
34. Jaindl M, Grünauer J, Platzer P, Endler G, Thallinger C, Leitgeb J, et al. The management of bite wounds in children – a retrospective analysis at a level I trauma centre. Injury. 2012;43(12):2117–21.
35. Greene SE, Fritz SA. Infectious complications of bite injuries. Clin North Am. 2021;35(1):219–36.
36. Abrahamian FM, Goldstein EJC. Microbiology of animal bite wound infections. Clin Microbiol Rev. 2011;24(2):231–46.

37. Badejo OA, Komolafe OO, Obinwogwu DL. Bacteriology and clinical course of camel-bite wound infections. Eur J Clin Microbiol Infect Dis. 1999;18:918–9.
38. Jakeman M, Oxley JA, Owczarczak-Garstecka SC, Westgarth C. Pet dog bites in children: management and prevention. BMJ Paediatrics Open. 2020;4:e000726. https://doi.org/10.1136/bmjpo-2020-000726.
39. Türkmen A, Temel M. Algorithmic approach to the prevention of unnecessary fasciotomy in extremity snake bite. Injury. 2016;47(12):2822–7. https://doi.org/10.1016/j.injury.2016.10.023.
40. Myers JP. Bite wound infections. Curr Infect Dis Rep. 2003;5:416–25.
41. Stiegler D, Gilbert JD, Warner MS, Byard RW. Fatal dog bite in the absence of significant trauma. Capnocytophaga canimorsus infection and unexpected death. Am J Forensic Med Pathol. 2010;31(2):198–9.
42. Medeiros I, Saconato H. Antibiotic prophylaxis for mammalian bites. Cochrane Database Syst Rev. 2001;(2):CD001738.
43. Radjou A, Hanifah M, Govindaraj V. Tetanus following dog bite. Indian J Community Med. 2012;37(3):200–1.
44. Chen E, Hornig S, Shepherd SM, Hollander JE. Primary closure of mammalian bites. Acad Emerg Med. 2000;7(2):157–61.
45. Bhaumik S, Kirubakaran R, Chaudhuri S. Primary closure versus delayed or no closure for traumatic wounds due to mammalian bite. Cochrane Database Syst Rev. 2019;12:CD011822.
46. Gurunluoglu R, Glasgow M, Arton J, Bronsert MN. Retrospective analysis of facial dog bite injuries at a level I trauma center in the Denver metro area. J Trauma Acute Care Surg. 2014;76(5):1294–300.
47. Dixon CA, Mahabee-Gittens EM, Hart KW, Lindsell CJ. Dog bite prevention: an assessment of child knowledge. J Pediatr. 2012;160(2):337–41.
48. Boat BW, Dixon CA, Pearl E, Thieken L, Bucher SE. Pediatric dog bite victims: a need for a continuum of care. Clin Pediatr. 2012;51(5):473–7.

Selected References

Abu-Zidan FM. Crossroad between camel bites and crocodile bites. Afr Health Sci. 2015;15:i–iv.

Abu-Zidan FM, Eid HO, Hefny AF, Bashir MO, Branicki F. Camel bite injuries in United Arab Emirates: a 6 year prospective study. Injury. 2012;43:1617–20.

Babo Martins S, Bolon I, Chappuis F, Ray N, Alcoba G, Ochoa C, et al. Snakebite and its impact in rural communities: the need for a One Health approach. PLoS Negl Trop Dis. 2019;13(9):e0007608. https://doi.org/10.1371/journal.pntd.0007608.

Ellis R, Ellis C. Dog and cat bites. Am Fam Physician. 2014;90:239–43.

Rothe K, Tsokos M, Handrick W. Animal and human bite wounds. Dtsch Arztebl Int. 2015;112(25):433–43.

Burns, Inhalation, and Lightning Injury

27

Mariëlle Vehmeijer-Heeman and Edward Tan

27.1 Introduction

Learning Goals
- To take care of the initial assessment of major burn patients according to a modified ATLS principle, the cABCDEffp method.
- Recognize signs of an inhalation injury and rapid airway compromise.
- Assessment and classification of burn wounds.
- Understand the pathophysiology of the burn injury.
- Recognize the patterns of child abuse.
- Knowledge about the different types of lightning injuries.

M. Vehmeijer-Heeman
Department of Plastic Surgery, Radboud University Medical Center, Nijmegen, The Netherlands
e-mail: Marielle.vehmeijer-heeman@radboudumc.nl

E. Tan (✉)
Department of Traumasurgery, Radboud University Medical Center, Nijmegen, The Netherlands
e-mail: Edward.tan@radboudumc.nl

27.1.1 Epidemiology

An estimated 180,000 fatal burns occur annually, mostly in low-income countries. According to the World Health Organization's fact sheet, over 400,000 burn injuries occurred in the United States, with approximately 10% (40,000) requiring hospitalization [1, 2]. In the United States, 10–20% of burn center patients have sustained inhalation injuries. An inhalation injury both in adults and children leads to an increase in morbidity and mortality [3]. Burns in children often (80%) occur in and around the house in a moment of inattention. Scalds (tea, soup, bath water) are the cause of burns in 75% of cases in 0- to 4-year-old (Fig. 27.1).

27.1.2 Etiology

Burns are usually caused by heat commonly by scalds, flames, or contact with a hot object. Burns may also be inflicted by chemicals, electricity, radiation, or cold causing frostbite. In children, these different types of burns vary according to the different age groups. About 70% of pediatric burns under 4 years old are caused by scalds. A child's motor skills are often underestimated by parents. Although exact numbers are not known, it appears that in the United States, injuries to 10% of children admitted to a burn center are caused by child abuse [4].

© The Author(s), under exclusive license to Springer Nature Switzerland AG 2023
F. Coccolini, F. Catena (eds.), *Textbook of Emergency General Surgery*,
https://doi.org/10.1007/978-3-031-22599-4_27

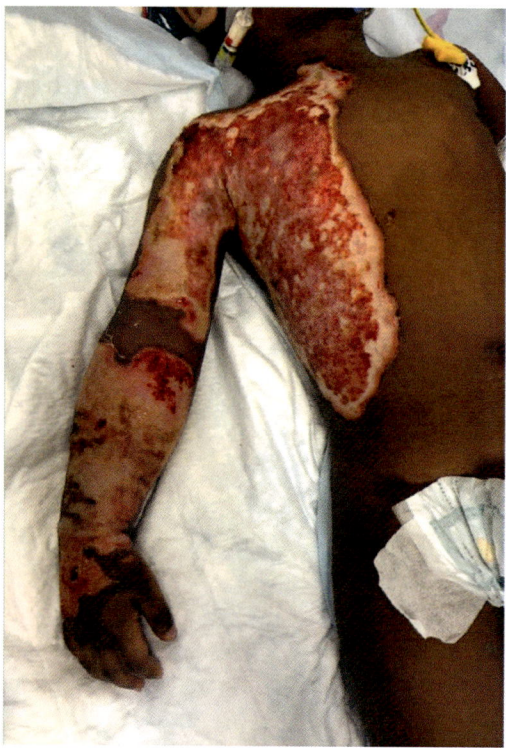

Fig. 27.1 Scalds in a 2-year-old boy

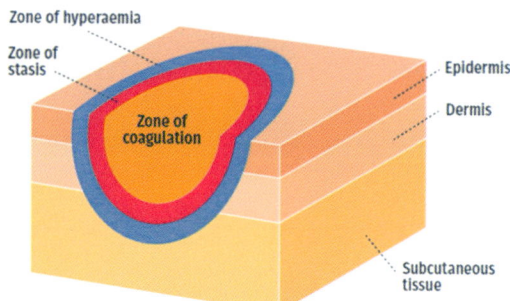

Fig. 27.2 Jackson's model was described in 1947. Illustration by Stephan van Raay

27.1.3 Classification

Burns are classified according to depth and TBSA (Total Burn Surface Area). The depth of the burn is determined by the temperature, the duration of impact, the nature of the agent, and the presence of pressure.

For indicating the depth of the burn injury, the classification of first-, second-, and third-degree has still been used. The terms of superficial, superficial partial, deep partial, and full-thickness describe the depth of the injury much better. These more comprehensive terms explain the wound healing and the implications on the method of treatment.

27.1.4 Pathophysiology

Jackson's model (Fig. 27.2) schematically describes the acute burn with its dynamic character. In Jackson's model, the burn is represented by three concentric areas. Central to these is *the zone of necrosis* (coagulation). This is irreversible tissue damage caused by the most intensive contact with the heat source. Around it, *the zone of stasis* develops and is caused by inflammatory mediators and microvascular closure (coagulation of the small capillaries). This is a progressive lesion within a period of 24–48 h. The treatment of burns aims to optimize this ring of stasis so that no secondary deepening of the burn occurs. Prevent vasoconstriction due to extreme cooling, prevent edema due to overfilling, prevent hypotension, and prevent infections. The outer ring is *the zone of hyperemia*. This is vital tissue and not a burn. The inflammatory mediators released in this area cause maximum dilation of the capillary blood vessels. In burns of more than 20% TBSA, the zone of hyperemia may involve the whole body.

An acute burn is dynamic. Burns evolve greatly over the first 72 h. Desiccation of the wound bed, hypothermia as well as infection may contribute to or lead to wound conversion. Wound management should limit dehydration of the wound and keep the wound colonization low.

27.2 Diagnosis

27.2.1 Clinical Presentation

First aid at the accident site consists of self-protection of the rescuer(s), stop the burning process, and bringing the victim to safety. Remove the source, by extinguishing the flames using a fire blanket, switching off the power in the event of an electrical injury and in scalds remove soaked clothes and also the nappy (acts as a reservoir of heat). In case of a chemical burn, all soaked clothing must be removed immediately with due regard for your own safety. If the patient is not breathing, resuscitation is started immediately. If the patient is breathing spontaneously, it is recommended to cool the burn (not the whole patient) with lukewarm running tap water for 10 min [5]. If cooling has not yet occurred, hydrogel-impregnated cooling blankets, which are available in the ambulance, can be used. If the burn has already been sufficiently cooled, the cooling blankets are not recommended because of the risk of hypothermia. Leave adherent clothes in place. After cooling, the burn can be covered with cling film, clean bandages, sheets, or tea towels. The idea behind cooling the burn is to limit the depth of the burn and the edema and to reduce pain (by inactivating the inflammatory mediators that influence the perfusion of the burn). It is still useful to start cooling up to three hours after the burn occurred. Be aware of hypothermia in children, especially if a large percentage of the body surface is burnt. Ice should not be used because, in addition to hypothermia, it causes vasoconstriction and therefore secondary deepening of the burn. In case of chemical (acid and alkali) burns irrigate with water for 30 min. In alkali burns irrigate for 1 h.

27.2.1.1 In Hospital at the Emergency Department

Management consist of the cABCDEffp protocol [6–10] starting with the Primary Survey

c: Catastrophic Bleeding
Stop the bleeding. This can be done by direct pressure, or if available and applicable to the bleeding body part by applying a tourniquet.

A: Airway and c-spine
Diagnosis of inhalation injury can be suspected on history and clinical criteria. Clinical signs consist of stridor, hoarseness and swallowing problems, shortness of breath, difficulty breathing, weak voice, and a deep hoarse cough. Obstruction due to the development of edema can develop very rapidly. Rapid intubation (with stabilization of the cervical spine) can prevent life-threatening problems. By inspection of the oral cavity and throat, the presence of soot particles or redness due to inhalation of hot air and smoke can be determined. This may indicate an inhalation injury with a risk of worsening of airway permeability over time.

The diagnosis is established by inspection of the oral cavity and by laryngoscopy or bronchoscopy. Inhalation injury of the upper respiratory tract does not indicate the presence of damage to the lower respiratory tract. Inhalation injury is found in 10% of facial burns. Airway obstruction can also be caused by circular semicircular full-thickness burns of the neck. An escharotomy is indicated.

B. Breathing
Any patient with severe burns should be oxygenated from the start using a non-rebreathing mask (flow rate greater than 10 L/min).

Expose the thorax and assess whether there are symmetrical supine chest movements with a normal respiratory rate. In case of full-thickness ventral or semi-circumferential burns of the chest, an escharotomy needs to be performed. In children breathing by diaphragmatic movement is more important than in adults, so even semicircular burns to the chest and upper abdomen that causes ventilation restriction need an escharotomy.

Damage to the lower respiratory tract can be caused by inhaling smoke constituents. Smoke particles cause a *chemical tracheobronchitis: classic smoke inhalation*. This may cause bronchospasm or pulmonary edema (asthmatics are at increased risk of this) and may lead to respiratory failure.

Thermal injury of the lower airways may rarely occur from direct fire contact and from inhalation of steam.

The diagnosis of lower respiratory tract inhalation injury is confirmed by bronchoscopy, endobronchial redness, swelling, and the presence of soot. A bronchial lavage should be performed to remove as much harmful substances and the resulting secretions from the airways as possible.

In the case of carbon monoxide intoxication, the pulse oximeter is not reliable, as it may wrongly give normal values. Special pulse oximeters already exist that can measure SPO_2 as well as SPCO (carbon monoxide) and SPMET (methemoglobin). Cyanide intoxication is suspected especially from burning plastic in a closed space.

C. Circulation

In severe burns, two peripheral intravenous catheters are inserted, preferably located outside the burnt area. If a peripheral intravenous catheter is technically not possible, intraosseous access is a good alternative for resuscitation. A central line becomes soon contaminated and is therefore not the first choice. Blood samples and if possible blood gases are taken after iv access. If a disturbed circulation/shock is detected, a fluid bolus of crystalloids (Ringer's lactate or NaCl 0.9%) is started, max. 20 mL/kg for children. The calculation of the required quantity follows at f fluids.

D. Disability

Check the neurological status and level of consciousness (AVPU) of the patient. Carbon monoxide (CO) or cyanide intoxication (CN) (or inhalation of other toxic gases) can cause confusion, dizziness, headache, agitation, and insults. Patients may be confused, drowsy, and agitated based on hypoxia. In young children, always consider hypoglycemia as a cause of disturbance of consciousness.

E. Exposure

Determination of the total body surface area burned (TBSA) and depth of the burns. This involves completely stripping the patient of clothing, footwear, rings, watches, etc. If remnants of clothing, often synthetic material, sticks to the body, they should be left in place, as often there is deeper burned skin underneath. TBSA can be determined globally using the rule of nine or the hand rule. First-degree (Superficial) burns do not count in the TBSA calculation. Therefore, the TBSA is often overestimated.

The Wallace rule of nines (Fig. 27.3) can be used to asses TBSA.

27.2.1.2 The Rule of 9

For extensive burns, the rule of 9 can be used. The rule of 9 according to Wallace is mainly used for adults and for children older than 10 years. It divides the body into compartments of 9% or multiples thereof. The head and neck area is 9% TBSA, a full arm is 9%. The front of the torso is 18%, the back of the torso is 18% and one leg is 18%. The perineum and genital area are 1% of the body surface. Smaller children have different body proportions: a baby's head is 18% and a leg is 14%. Every year of life, 1% is subtracted from the head and 0.5% is added to each leg. Around the age of ten, the body proportions of children are the same as those of adults.

27.2.1.3 The Hand Rule

One side of the patient's hand with fingers joined and stretched is equivalent to 1% of the body surface area (not the palm of the hand).

27.2.1.4 Lund and Browder

The Lund and Browder chart takes into account the age of the patient and is more accurate, especially in children.

27.2.1.5 Depth of the Burn

Check on the presence of blisters, the wound aspect, flexibility, capillary refill, and painfulness of the wound (the so-called prick test is obsolete) (Table 27.1). In 60–75% of the cases, clinical evaluation of the burn depth has been accurate [11]. A wide range of different techniques is used, for example, laser Doppler imaging, and thermography to assess the depth of the burn. A burn can be heterogeneous. The burn is not equally deep everywhere, and shallower and deeper areas alternate. In particular, hot water burns are often mixed burns.

Fig. 27.3 The Wallace rule of nines. Illustration by Stephan van Raay

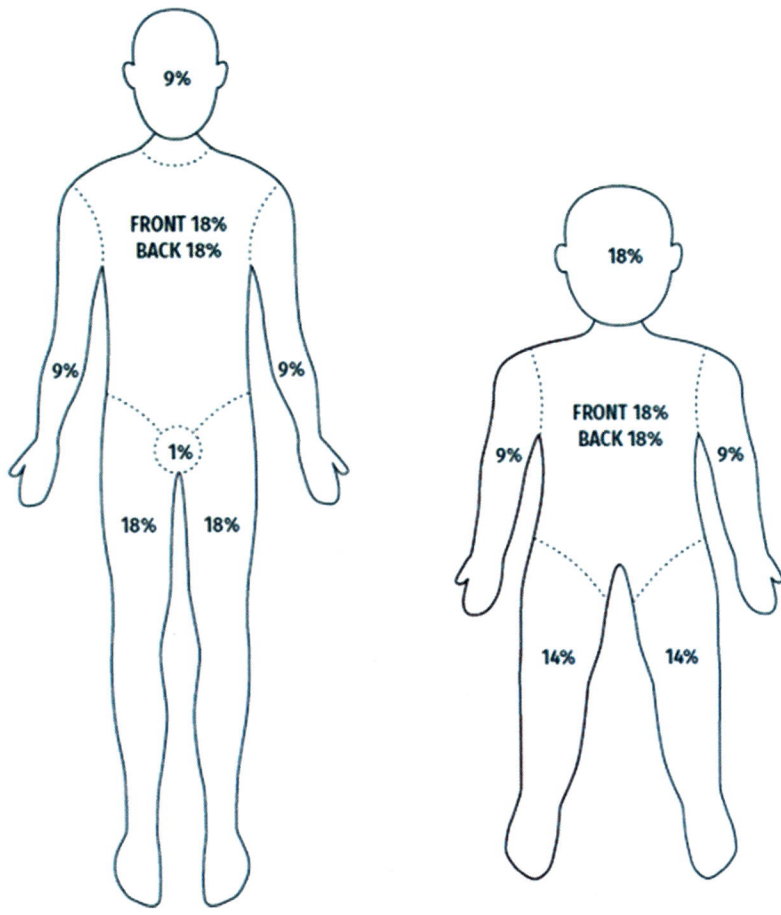

Table 27.1 Assessment of burn depth

Depth	Appearance	Areas of destruction	Blanching
Superficial burn	Dry, Red No Blisters	Epidermis, (no burnwound, erythema)	Present Pronounced
Superficial partial thickness burn	Red or bright pink Blisters Moist Soft and elastic	Epidermis and portions of the papillary dermis	Present Pronounced
Deep partial thickness burn	Mottled red or white, patchy Ruptured blisters Dry looking wound	Epidermis, papillary dermis, and significant portions of the reticular dermis (hair follicles, sweat glands, are affected)	Diminished
Full thickness burn	White, tan, or brown-black waxy Dry, leathery texture Wound rigid, non-elastic	Entire epidermis and all layers of the dermis	Absent
Classic conductive electrical burn	Variable, dependent on voltage and duration of contact Entry wound charred and depressed Exit wound dry with depressed edges, explosive appearance	Variable surface area from small to very large. Deep soft tissue damage to fat, muscle, and bone (not always apparent immediately) Blood vessels thrombosed Nerves may be damaged along the path of electricity	Absent

27.2.1.6 Fluids

Resuscitation

Patients with severe burns require substantial amounts of fluid to prevent underfilling and maintain perfusion of all organs. In children, resuscitation is initiated with more than 10% deep burns, and in adults with more than 15% deep burns. In order to calculate the patient's fluid requirements, it is necessary to properly estimate the depth of the burns.

A commonly used formula is the modified Parkland formula: 4 mL × kg × % TBSA per 24 h, with the first half given in the first 8 h after the time of burn (not the time of admission) and the second half spread over the next 16 h.

The plasma loss is greatest in the first eight hours after the burn. This is the reason why half of the calculated amount of fluid, is given in the first 8 h after the accident and the rest in the following sixteen hours. Due to the increased permeability of the capillary wall, fluid exits the blood vessels. The capillary leak is even permeable to molecular proteins such as albumin. For this reason, as well as others, Ringer's lactate is given in the first period and colloidal fluids and albumin are not given.

For children up to 30 kg, a so-called maintenance fluid should be given in addition to the above volume. Because children are especially susceptible to hyponatremia, this maintenance fluid should contain sufficient sodium. The maintenance fluid or children up to 30 kg is calculated as follows:

$$100\,\text{mL per kg for the first}\,10\,\text{kg}$$
$$+50\,\text{mL per kg for the second}\,10\,\text{kg}$$
$$(\text{i.e., from}\,10\,\text{to}\,20\,\text{kg}) + 20\,\text{mL per kg for each}$$
$$\text{kg above}\,20\,\text{kg}\,(\text{up to a maximum of}\,30\,\text{kg})$$

The total amount of maintenance liquid is given over 24 h. Very young children often also require glucose administration.

Starting a resuscitation regimen includes placing a bladder catheter.

It is more important to properly monitor and adjust the fluid policy than an initial calculation. Fluid management should be guided not only by diuresis but particularly by the clinical picture, heart rate, and blood pressure. Laboratory sodium, potassium, chloride, and renal function and glucose should be measured and advanced monitoring through PiCCO (advanced hemodynamic monitor) should be considered. One of the parameters to monitor the effect of fluid resuscitation is to check urine output. The Emergency Management of Severe Burns (EMSB) course recommends a desirable urine output of 1 mL/kg/h for children up to 30 kg (in adults, we assume an output of at least 0.5 mL/kg/h or 30–50 mL/h) [12]. To prevent a so-called hyperchloremic acidosis, Ringer's lactate and not NaCl 0.9% is recommended. Because of all the complications due to over resuscitation, called fluid creep, there are new insights regarding this fluid policy. A recent article shows that 3 ml/kg/TBSA% (24 hours) can be sufficient in children [13–15].

27.2.1.7 Myoglobinurea

The diagnosis of myoglobinurea is made clinically because the urine is dark red in color. Myoglobinurea is caused by massive muscle destruction. A high level of breakdown products such as hemoglobin and myoglobin may end up in the urine. In the blood, the creatine phosphokinase and potassium are elevated. Muscle destruction occurs in electrical burns, circular deep burns with ischemia, crush injuries, and compartment syndrome with muscle necrosis. To prevent these products from precipitating in the renal tubules causing renal failure, forced diuresis (increasing the flow in the tubules) is indicated. Alkalizing the urine also might prevent renal impairment.

27.2.1.8 Fahrenheit

Burn patients may have severely impaired body thermoregulation. If a large percentage of body surface area is affected, it is essential to prevent hypothermia which in combination with hypovolemia may lead to fatal acidosis and coagulation disorders.

Warm IV fluids, warm blankets, and increased ambient temperature in the examination room are desirable. One should recover the patient with warm blankets after the examination

27.2.1.9 Pain
Pain medication is given as soon as possible [16]. Cooling and covering the burns provides significant pain relief.

27.2.1.10 First Option Without Intravenous Access
Fentanyl intranasal 1–2 microgram/kg (max 100 mcg)

S-ketamine intranasal 0.5–1 mg/kg

27.2.1.11 First Option with Venous or Intraosseous Access
Fentanyl 1–2 microgram/kg intravenous, titrate

Morphine 10–30 microgram/kg/h intravenously

Paracetamol 20 mg/kg intravenously, then 4 dd 15 mg/kg intravenously

27.2.1.12 Radiology
After the initial examination, in accordance with the usual trauma screening, X-ray examination takes place in the form of photographs of the chest, cervical spine, and pelvis.

27.2.1.13 Secondary Survey
The head-to-toe examination begins with the history in which AMPLE history is obtained.

- A. Allergies
- M. Medications
- P. Past medical history, illnesses, and pregnancies
- L. Last meal
- E. Events/Environment and exposure related to the injury. The circumstances under which the injury occurred, the type of burn: flame, hot liquid, chemical, etc., the duration of exposure, and first aid measures already taken.

This is followed by the secondary survey, consisting of an examination from head to toe. For example, also check the tympanic membranes in case of an explosion. Check the tetanus vaccination status. If necessary, additional X-ray examination or toxicology tests are performed. Prophylactic antibiotics are not indicated.

27.2.1.14 Non-accidental Burns
Non-accidental injuries should be considered in burns, especially in children. The incidence of non-accidental burns varies widely. Besides the intentional inflicted injuries, burns can also occur due to neglect, unsafe home situations, or in a moment of inattention. Suspicion of child abuse exists if the type of burn does not match the history, there is a delay in the presentation of the child; adequate measures have not been taken; old injuries are visible (broken bones, bruises, and old burns); there is an inconsistent narrative.

Child abuse burns often have a sharp demarcation (boundary) and the location of the burn is suspect (palm, inside of fingers, sole of foot, buttocks, and between the legs).

The burn is of equal depth everywhere as opposed to a hot water burn from an accident which produces many splashes and burns of varying depths. Deliberate immersion of a child's hands or feet in hot water has a typical glove or sock distribution. The child being pressed with his buttocks on the bottom (relatively cold) of a bath of hot water has recesses of deep burns on the buttocks (the so-called "donut-sign," Fig. 27.4). A deep non-heterogeneous contact burn (equally deep everywhere) with an imprint pattern (iron, lighter, and hair straightener) is also very characteristic of child abuse.

27.2.1.15 Toxic Gases

Carbon Monoxide (CO)
Carbon monoxide (CO) is a colorless and odorless gas. CO is produced by incomplete combustion (oxidation) of carbon. After inhalation, CO

Fig. 27.4 Sock en donut sign in child abuse. Illustration by Stephan van Raay

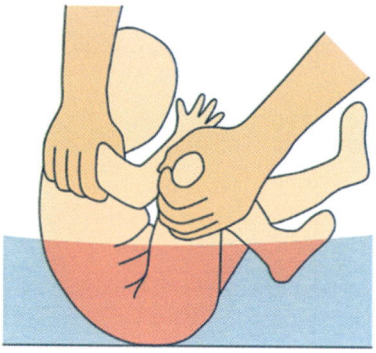
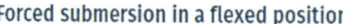
Forced submersion in a flexed position

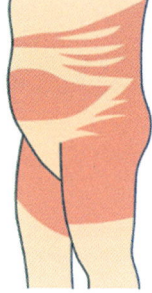
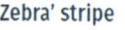
'Zebra' stripe

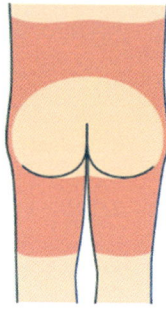
'Doughnut hole' sparing

binds to hemoglobin in the blood and forms carboxyhemoglobin (COHb). The affinity of CO to Hb is 200–250 times greater than that of oxygen (O_2). CO displaces oxygen from hemoglobin. CO also easily penetrates the cell causing disruption of cellular functions. COHb concentrations of 30–40% cause clinical symptoms, such as decline in judgment and vision, drowsiness, dizziness, headache, nausea, palpitations, and collapse. COHb concentrations above 50% lead to coma and increased risk of death. The use of transcutaneous oxygen saturation measurement as a measure of oxygenation is unreliable. Also, arterial blood gases analysis gives a biased picture. The treatment of carbon monoxide intoxication is to administer high concentrations of oxygen as early as possible. This is because the half-life for COHb in outdoor air is about 250 min and in 100% oxygen 40–60 min. If the victim is unconscious, not breathing adequately or the airway is obstructed, intubation should be considered so that 100% oxygen can be administered.

Cyanide

A second serious and often unnoticed or measurable intoxication involves cyanide poisoning. Cyanide compounds are primarily released during the combustion of plastics and are also rapidly absorbed through the lungs. Cyanide, also called hydrocyanic acid gas (HCN), is released during the combustion of nitrogen-containing polymers, for example, polyamide (nylon) and polyurethane. Cyanide is highly toxic. It prevents the cells from utilizing the available oxygen, causing tissue anoxia (absolute oxygen deficiency). High concentrations of cyanide (>2.5 mg/L) leads to coma and death within an hour. Diagnosis at the accident site is difficult. Inhalation of cyanide causes rapid onset of drowsiness, nausea, headache, muscle weakness, coma, and eventually death. In the early stages, chemical stimulation of the respiratory center increases respiratory minute volume. This can enhance the rate of poisoning as more cyanide is inhaled. Sometimes the smell of bitter almonds (cyanide smells like almonds) can be smelled in the victim's exhaled air. An ECG shows ST elevations, indicative of cardiac ischemia. Ampoules of 2.5 g of hydroxocobalamin (vitamin B12) can be administered intravenously (70 mg/kg (max 5 g)) in 15 min. This binds to cyanide (cyanocobalamine), which is excreted renally. As the second step in a persistent coma and/or severe lactate acidosis, sodium thiosulfate (400 mg/kg in max 100 mg/min iv) should be administered. This produces thiocyanate which is then excreted via the urine.

Electrical Injury

Electricity-related burns can be divided into high-voltage (>1000 volts), low-voltage (<1000 volts), and lightning injuries. An electricity injury is defined as an injury caused by the passage of electricity or by lightning. A distinction has to be made between high-voltage and low-voltage electrical injuries.

Low-Voltage Injury

A low-voltage injury involves a voltage of less than 1000 volts. This may lead to deep skin burns. Cardiac arrhythmias may occur in low-voltage injuries.

High-Voltage Injury

A high-voltage injury is a voltage in excess of 1000 volts, but can also be between 10,000 and 30,000 volts. In high-voltage electrical injuries, the visible third-degree burns are relatively limited in size, while the extensive necrosis of the muscle groups, vessels, and bones is underneath the skin as a result of current passage through the body.

Watch for neurological, respiratory, and cardiac (arrhythmia and cardiac arrest) problems. It is important to take an ECG. Locate both the site of entry and the site of exit. This is because it gives an indication where there may be severe necrosis (subcutaneous). It is also an indication of a greater fluid requirement than the calculation based on the % TSBA. Fasciotomy is indicated if a compartment syndrome develops or is expected to develop.

Lightning Injury

It is estimated that worldwide approximately 24,000 fatalities and even ten times more injuries occur annually due to lightning [17]. Men are at greater risk of suffering lightning injuries with a male: female ratio of 5:1 [18]. The incidence of lightning strikes worldwide is estimated to be 0.09–0.12/100,000 people. Mortality is estimated to be 0.2–1.7 deaths per million people per year worldwide. Approximately 10–30% of the patients struck by lightning die and 76% present some permanent sequela [19].

Lightning is a sudden high-voltage discharge of electricity that occurs within a cloud, between clouds, or between a cloud and the ground. Globally, there are about 40–50 flashes of lightning every second, or nearly 1.4 billion flashes per year. The electric current involved in lightning strikes is direct current (DC) and in the order of 30,000–50,000 A, far greater than that produced by AC electricity. The duration of exposure is generally very short approximately 10–100 ms. This current causes the release of a tremendous amount of heat, raising temperatures to approximately 30,000 K. This brief temperature effect causes a "thermoacoustic blast wave," or thunder. The overpressure generated by thunder at the source may approach 100 atm [20]. Approximately 20% of those electric discharge result in ground strikes.

Types of lightning strikes and its injuries can be classified as;

- Direct strike: lightning strikes the victim and the current passes through the body (Fig. 27.5a); the highest mortality.
- Contact injury: lightning strikes into an object that is touched by the victim (Fig. 27.5b).
- Side splash: lightning strikes a near object (e.g., a three) and flashes over to the victim (Fig. 27.5c).
- Ground strike: lightning strikes into the ground near the victim. Lightning energy decreases from the strike point. A potential difference can be generated between a part of the body closer to the strike and that further away, setting up current through the body (Fig. 27.5d1) Step voltage or ground current traveling through the ground (Fig. 27.5d2), and ground arcing across the mouth of a cave (Fig. 27.5d3).
- Upward streamer: electrical stream heads upward into the sky but does not reach sky lightning and thus does not complete a connection. Nevertheless, it may carry current causing electrical injury (Fig. 27.5e).
- Blunt injury: due to the explosive force that occurs as the surrounding air is superheated and rapidly cooled.

Lightning has four main physical components which can cause injury; light, heat, electricity, and barotrauma [22]. Which further injuries will occur are determined by: voltage, current (amperage), type of current (alternating or direct), the path of current flow across the body, duration of contact, and individual vulnerability? Therefore, injuries vary from a headache, to burns to cardiac arrest.

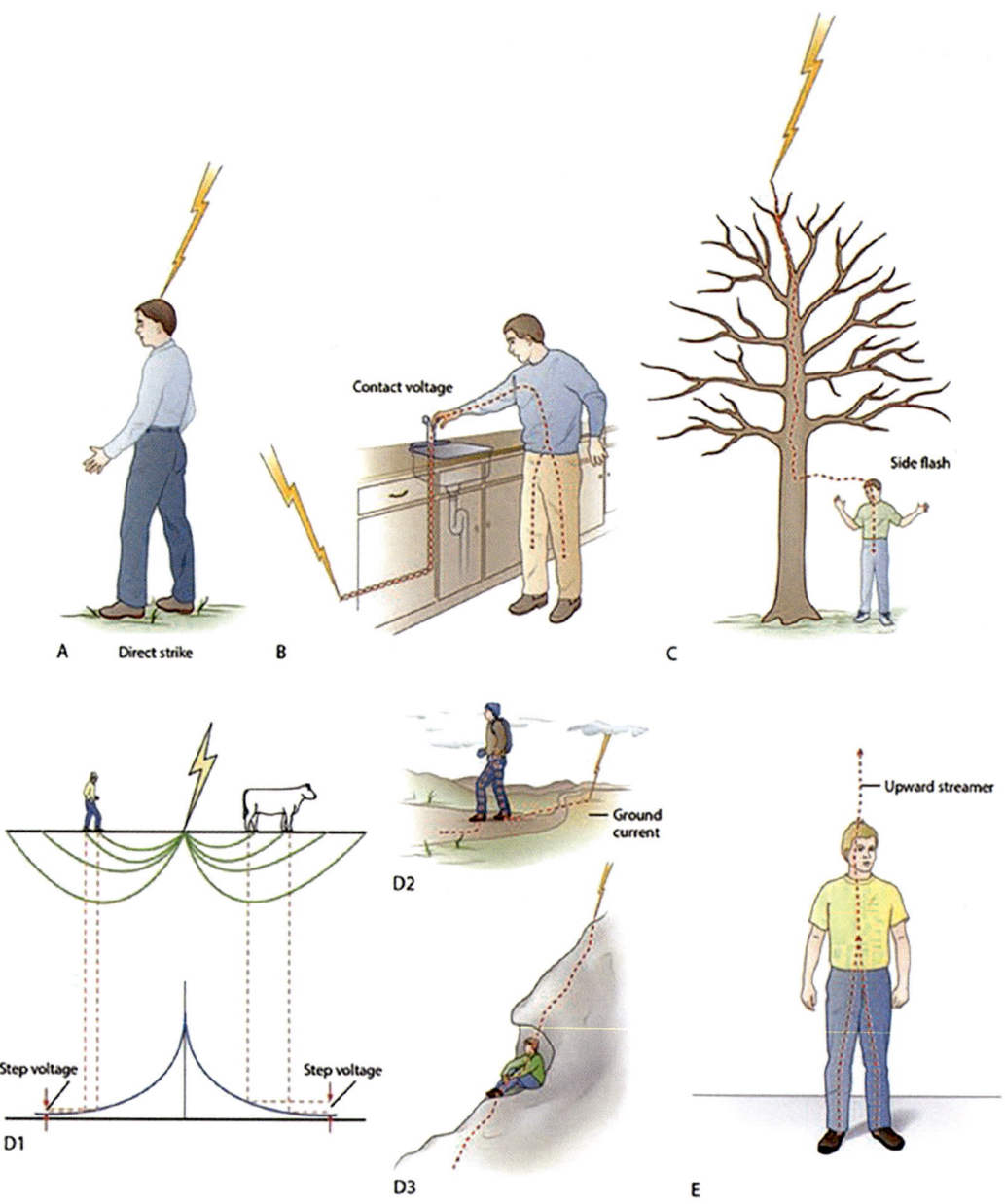

Fig. 27.5 Mechanisms of lightning injury. (**a**) Direct. (**b**) Contact. (**c**) Sidesplash/flash. (**d1**) As lightning energy spreads out from the strike point, the energy decreases. A potential difference can be generated between a part of the body is closer to the strike and that further away, setting up a current through the body. (**d2**) Step voltage or ground current traveling through the ground. (**d3**) Ground arcing across the mouth of a cave. (**e**) Upward streamer . (Cooper et al. 2017 with permission of Elsevier) [21]

Specific Burns Related to Lightning Injury
- Lichtenberg figures—transient ferning or feathering patterns pathognomonic of a lightning strike (onset <1 h, duration <24 h).
- Linear–"flashover" (sweat turns to steam).
- Punctate burns–multiple circular burns due to current leaving the body, for example, tip-toe sign.
- Full-thickness contact burns—due to fire or heated object in contact with skin (NB. Deep thermal burns are rare, unlike HV electrical injuries).

Management
The clinical features of the lightning victim are very variable and involve complaints of the cardiovascular tract (cardiac dysfunction, dysrhythmias, asystole, ventricle fibrillation), neurological complaints (headache, paresthesia, loss of consciousness, intracranial hemorrhages, spinal cord injury, movement disorders), burns and ENT symptoms (deafness, tympanic membrane rupture, cataract) [23].

Initial assessment consists of a full trauma screening of all lightning patients according to ATLS principles [10]. Consider traumatic injuries, brain, and heart damage. Therefore, ECG including cardiac markers are advised. The main treatment goal is to supply supportive care and monitoring.

Note
If multiple lightning victims are present, initial triage and treatment should follow a "reverse triage" system; a patient may appear dead (fixed dilated pupils with respiratory arrest) but may develop ROSC and may make a full recovery. All patients with high-risk features such as loss of consciousness of neurological symptoms, or major trauma should be presented to the ER [10, 24]. Lightning injuries can be prevented following lightning safety guidelines (e.g., avoid being outside in open spaces during thunderstorms).

27.3 "Acute" Surgical Treatment

27.3.1 Escharotomy

An escharotomy is part of a decompression process [25]. An escharotomy is a surgical incision through the eschar to relieve pressure caused by a rigid eschar. An escharotomy can be indicated for the extremities, the neck, chest, and abdomen (Figs. 27.6 and 27.7). In combination with edema in the surrounding tissues, the rigid eschar acts like a tourniquet leading to impaired perfusion of the extremities. In limbs, this occurs gradually and does not become manifest until hours after a burn. Escharotomies are almost always performed under general anesthesia in the operating room. The incision by diathermy is extended a few centimeters into healthy tissue, the unaffected skin, or the superficially burned skin. In terms of depth, the incision extends into the underlying unburned subcutaneous fat and the muscle fascia remains intact. After the incision, the eschar will expand open and the subcutaneous fat will be seen. To detect restricting areas of dermal remnants run a finger along the incision. Although minor bleeding will occur, secure hemostasis. Escharotomies are not closed, but covered with burn dressings until they will be included in the excision of the burn wound.

The incisions of the trunk are performed on the lateral sides. To ensure free breathing movements, transverse incisions are also made on the trunk, at the border of chest and abdomen and under the neck.

The location of the escharotomy incisions of the neck is along the border of the sternocleidomastoid muscle up to the ear.

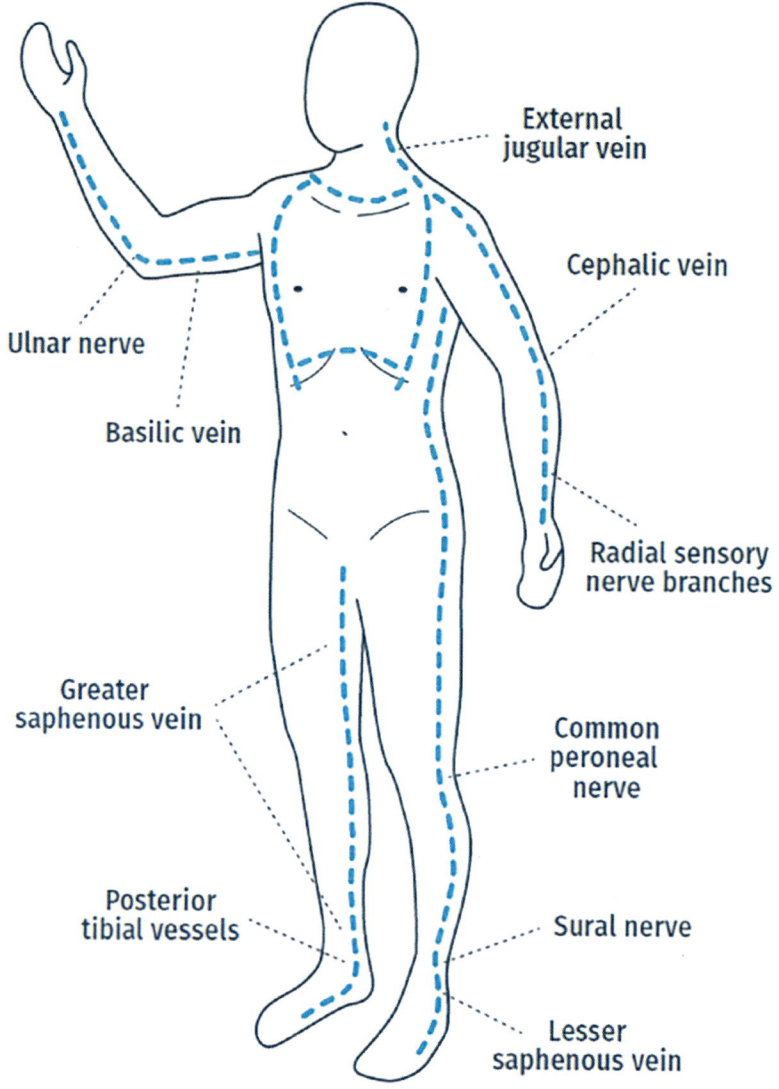

Fig. 27.6 Escharotomy incisions, avoid damage to subcutaneous veins or nerves. Illustration by Stephan van Raay

The arm is positioned in the anatomical position. A longitudinal incision is made on the lateral and on medial side of the upper extremity until the base of the fifth finger and the thumb. On the medial side, the incision runs ventral to the medial epicondyle to avoid damaging the ulnar nerve. Extremities are elevated after an escharotomy. In the lower extremity, the incisions are made midlaterally and, with care taken of the head of the fibula to avoid damaging the peroneal communal nerve. The incision follows the anterior of the malleolus until the base of the first en fifth toe. At all locations, damage to subcutaneous veins should be avoided as much as possible (e.g., the vena saphena magna on the medial side).

On the middle hand, the incisions run on ulnar and radial sides. For the fingers, a longitudinal incision is sufficient. For the little finger, the incision is best placed on the radial side.

27.3.2 Fasciotomy

A release of the fascial compartments is not often necessary in burns. Fasciotomies are required in case of high-voltage electrical burns, or very deep thermal burns. In the presence of overlying thermal burns, escharotomy incisions can be done such that subsequent fasciotomies, if needed, can be done through the same incision.

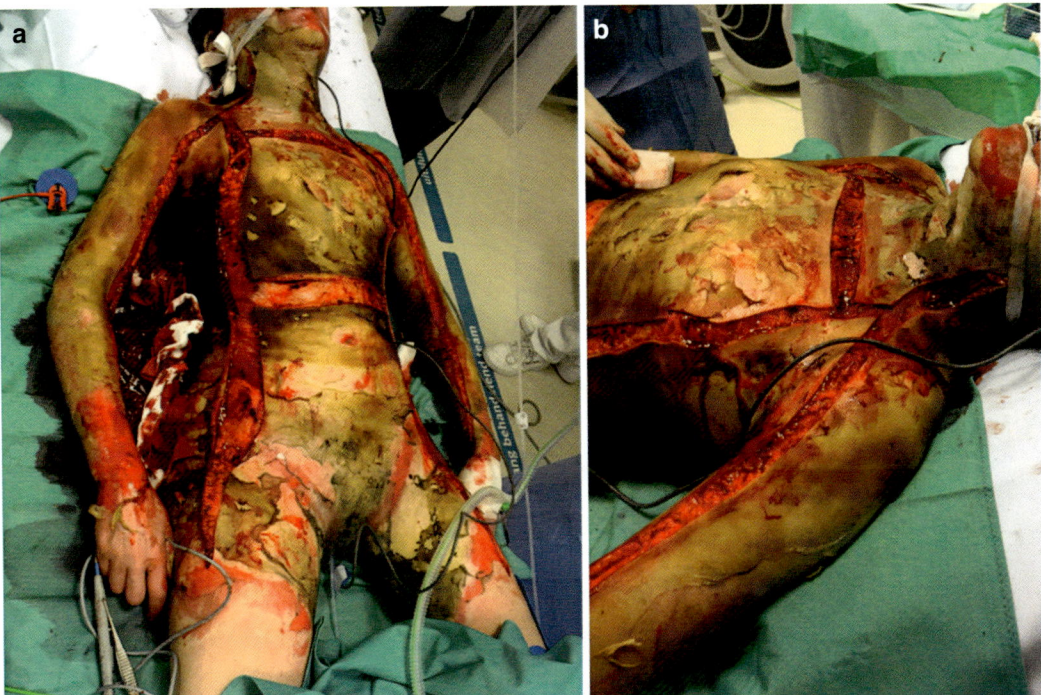

Fig. 27.7 (**a**, **b**) Escharotomy incisions after flame burn

27.3.3 Surgical Treatment

27.3.3.1 Excision of the Burn Eschar

In patients with large TBSA deep burns, morbidity and mortality are significantly reduced if the burn eschar is excised early [26, 27]. Primary surgery or early excision has become established as the gold standard burn care [28, 29]. Although the exact timing is still under debate, the burn excision of large deep burns occurs preferably in the first 24 h after the accident. Early excision of the burn scar and prompt wound coverage is important for a functioning immune system. At primary surgery, a still intact burn crust exists that is barely colonized with microorganisms. Within 48 h burns become colonized by Gram-positive organisms and after a week with Gram-negative organisms [30]. Early excision helps reduce the incidence of infection and sepsis.

Tangential excision is the method of sequentially shaving the eschar from the wound surface until a viable vascular bed is achieved. Small hand dermatomes (a Weck knife) and large hand dermatomes (a Humbyknife) may be used. The eschar can be excised with electric or compressed air-powered dermatomes (the thickness of the excision can be adjusted on the device). Hydrosurgery enables a surgeon to precisely select, excise, and evacuate nonviable tissue. A precise excision with selective preservation of the dermis is possible. It gives less blood loss and less contour loss. Hemostasis is achieved by the immediate topical application of gauze with a solution containing adrenalin mixed in 0.9% saline.

27.3.3.2 Skin Graft

The excised wound is usually closed with a split-thickness skin graft (autologous skin). The STSG is removed with a (electrical) dermatome. There are various donor sites. In adults, the thigh is the preferred site whereas in children, the scalp. Infiltration of a tumescent solution into the subgaleal plane makes harvesting of the scalp more feasable. The scalp as a donor site is less painful and not visible after the regrowth of hair [31].

The donor site can be treated with different temporary wound coverage materials. As the donor sites are healed they can be reharvested. Complications (infection and delayed wound healing) in donor site healing are the result of incorrect wound treatment methods or removing the donor skin too deeply.

The mesh technique is the most commonly used method for obtaining surface enlargement in an STSG. The desired enlargement of 1:1.5-1:2-1:3 mesh is created. The choice depends on the number of available donor sites and TBSA. Smaller mesh ratios give a better aesthetic result. Therefore, a full sheet STSG is used for the face.

The graft is fixed to the wound surface with staples, glue, or a suture (tie-over) or with vacuum-assisted closure (VAC) to prevent the graft from slipping. The STSG takes about five days to attach, which is why a splint is used for transplants over joints (24 h a day for 5 days).

In very extensive burns, there is sometimes not enough skin to transplant. Wider meshing to cover larger surface areas will result in dried-out or desiccated interstices. To avoid this an allograft may be applied as a biological dressing. A second method when there is a shortage of donor skin is the Meek-Wall technique [32]. Here the skin is cut into small 3 × 3 mm blocks and applied to the wound using a nylon gauze folded in two directions. With the use of the Meek-Wall technique, a higher expansion is possible and appropriate for a large percentage of TBSA and poor wound bed areas.

27.3.3.3 Full-Thickness Grafts

The transplantation of split-thickness skin grafts often results in hypertrophic scarring, due to a lack of dermal components. Hyperthrophic scarring over a joint may result in contractures. Full-thickness skin grafts (FTSG) offer a solution, but are only suitable for very small areas, as the donor site does not heal and has to be closed primarily. Deep burns to the hands, fingers, and eyelids could be treated with a full-thickness graft. The donor site is behind the ear, the inside of the upper arm, the groin, or at the base of the neck.

27.3.3.4 Dermal Substitutes

Dermal components deliver mechanical stability and structural integrity to the regenerating epidermal tissues. Therefore, both a STSG and a dermal component are required in the acute as well as delayed treatment of full-thickness and deep dermal burns. The use of dermal substitutes may give better (than just an STSG) functional and cosmetic results [33]. High costs and a learning curve are known drawbacks.

> **Dos and Don'ts**
> - Do not postpone intubation when the diagnosis of inhalation injury is suspected on history and clinical criteria.
> - Prevent prolonged cooling.
> - Be aware of over-fluid resuscitation, formulas are only a guide.
> - In extensive deep burns excision and grafting has to be performed early.
> - Do not use systemic antibiotics prophylactically.
> - Elevate burned limbs.
> - Perform an escharotomy in circular full-thickness burns of the extremities.

> **Take-Home Messages**
> - Be aware of the combined burn / trauma patient.
> - Take care of the burn patient according to the cABCEffp-method.
> - Inhalation injury is potentially fatal.
> - Unconsciousness in an enclosed area is very suspect for CO intoxication but is also considered a head trauma after a fall and hypoglycemia in children.
> - Standard pulse oximetry may be normal with significant carbon monoxide toxicity and therefore unreliable.
> - Be aware of hemorrhagic shock within the first hour, a burn shock does not occur within the first hour.
> - Fluid resuscitation must be based on frequent reassessment.

- Suspect nerve and deep muscle injury after a high voltage electrical injury.
- Suspect myoglobinuria after a fall from a high-tension cable and dark red-colored urine.
- Treat lightning injuries according to standard ATLS guidelines, with a specific focus on possible sequelae of lightning injuries.
- In a flash injury, no current passes through the patient's body.

Questions

1. At what moment do you calculate the patient's fluid requirements?
   A. Pre-hospital
   B. During the C of circulation,
   C. After the second IV access
   D. **After performing the ABCDE assessment**
2. In which case would you not intubate immediately?
   A. **Singed nasal hairs caused by a flashburn (from the BBQ)**
   B. Hoarseness
   C. Fire in an enclosed space
   D. Uconsciousness
3. Which of the following characteristics belong to deep dermal burns
   A. Intact blisters
   B. No capillary refill
   C. Leathery
   D. **Can lead to significant scarring**
4. In case resuscitation is needed, which infusion therapy is used in burn patients?
   A. **Ringer's lactate**
   B. Colloidal fluids
   C. Albumin
   D. Artificial colloid
5. Myoglobinurea (dark red urine) is not caused by
   A. Electrical burns
   B. Circular deep burns
   C. Compartment syndrome
   D. **A bladder injury**
6. A child of 8 years old got sunburned leading to redness of his total back, what is the TBSA?
   A. 9%
   B. 18%
   C. **0%**
   D. 14%
7. Which of the following is the most likely cause of immediate death resulting from a lightning strike?
   A. Severe burn injury
   B. **Cardiac arrest**
   C. Brain damage
   D. Respiratory arrest
8. Lichtenberg figures are seen in?
   A. heat stroke
   B. **Lightning**
   C. Radiation injury
   D. Electrocution
9. Which of the following is another way lightning can injure a person?
   A. **Being near an item that has been struck by lightning**
   B. Standing on a charred spot on the ground where lightning has struck
   C. Helping carry a lightning victim to safety
   D. Touching someone who has been struck by lightning
10. What is advised not to do for preventing lightning injuries when indoors?
    A. Avoid contact with any hard-wired device.
    B. Unplug electrical equipment before the storm.
    C. **Take a shower.**
    D. Use a cell phone.

References

1. WHO fact sheet. World Health Organization https://www.who.int/en/news-room/fact-sheets/detail/burns
2. Mock C, Peck M, Krug E, Haberal M. Confronting the global burden of burns: a WHO plan and a challenge. Burns. 2009;35(5):615–7.
3. Palmieri T, Warner P, Mlcak R, Sheridan R, Kagan R, et al. Inhalation injury in children: a 10 year experience at Shriners Hospitals for Children. J Burn Care Res. 2009;30(1):206–8.
4. Burn Injuries in child abuse. U.S. Department of Justice. Office of Justice Programs. Office of Juvenile Justice and Delinquency Prevention. https://www.ojp.gov/pdffiles/91190-6.pdf
5. Cuttle L, Kempf M, Liu P, Kravchuk O, Kimble R. The optimal duration and delay of first aid treatment for deep partial thickness burn injuries. Burns. 2010;36(5):673–9.
6. Santaniello JM, Luchette FA, Esposito TJ, Gunawan H, Reed RL, Davis KA, Gamelli RL. Ten year experience of burn, trauma, and combined burn/trauma injuries comparing outcomes. J Trauma. 2004;57(4):696.
7. Advanced Trauma Life Support® (ATLS®). ATLS for doctors student course manual. 8th ed. Chicago: American College of Surgeons; 2010.
8. Acute Pediatric Burns Course (APBC). APBC course manual. The Netherlands: Radboud University Hospital; 2020.
9. Suma A, Owen J. Update on the management of burns in paediatrics. BJA Educ. 2020;20(3):103–10.
10. van Ruler R, Eikendal T, Kooij FO, Tan ECTH. A shocking injury: A clinical review of lightning injuries highlighting pitfalls and a treatment protocol. Injury. 2022;53(10):3070–77. https://doi.org/10.1016/j.injury.2022.08.024. Epub 2022 Aug 17. PMID: 36038387
11. Monstrey S, Hoeksema H, Verbelen J, Pirayesh A, Blondeel P. Assessment of burn depth and burn wound healing potential. 2008;34(6):761–9.
12. Emergency Management of Severe Burns(EMSB): Australian and New Zealand Burn Association. Education Committee.
13. Barrow RE, Jeschke MG, Herndon DN. Early fluid resuscitation improves outcomes in severely burned children. Resuscitation. 2000;45:91–6.
14. Rogers AD, Karpelowsky J, Millar AJW, et al. Fluid creep in major pediatric burns. Eur J Pediatr Surg. 2010;20:133–8.
15. Pruitt BA. Protection from excessive resuscitation 'Pushing The Pendulum Back'. J Trauma. 2000;49:567–8.
16. Richardson P, Mustard L. The management of pain in the burns unit. Burns. 2009;35:921–36.
17. Ritenour A, et al. Lightning injury: a review Burns. 2008;34:585–94.
18. Jensen JD, Thurman J, Vincent AL. Lightning injuries. StatPearls. Treasure Island, FL: StatPearls Publishing.
19. Pfortmueller C, et al. Injuries, sequelae and treatment of lightning-induced injuries: 10 years of experience at a Swiss trauma center. Emerg Med Int. 2012;167698
20. Whitecomb D, Martinez JA, Daberkow D. Lightning injuries. South Med J. 2002;95:1331–4.
21. Cooper MA, Hole RL. Reducing lightning injuries worldwide. Springer. p. 165–77. https://doi.org/10.1007/978-3-319-77563-0.
22. Blumenthal R. Lightning and the forensic pathologist. Acad Forensic Pathol. 2018;8(10):98–111.
23. Forster, et al. Lightning burn—review and case report. Burns. 2013;39(2):e8–12.
24. https://litfl.com/lightning-injury/
25. Sheridan RL, Chang P. Acute burn procedures. Surg Clin North Am. 2014;94(4):755–64.
26. Greenwood JE. Advantages of immediate excision of burn eschar. Anaesth Intensive Care. 2020;48(2):89–92.
27. Barret JP, Herndon DN. Effects of burn wound excision on bacterial colonization and invasion. Plast Reconstr Surg. 2003;111(2):744–50; discussion 751–2.
28. Muller M, Gahankari D, Herndon DN. Operative wound management. Total Burn Care (Third Edition), W.B. Saunders, 2007;177–195. ISBN 9781416032748, https://doi.org/10.1016/B978-1-4160-3274-8.50016-7. (https://www.sciencedirect.com/science/article/pii/B9781416032748500167).
29. Orgill DP. Excision and skin grafting of thermal burns. N Engl J Med. 2009;360:893–901.
30. Gill P, Falder S. Early management of paediatric burn injuries. Paediatr Child Health. 2017;27:406–14.
31. van Niekerk G, Adams S, Rode H. Scalp as a donor site in children: is it really the best option? 2018;44(5):1259–68.
32. Medina A, Riegel T, Nystad D, Tredget EE. Modified meek micrografting technique for wound coverage in extensive burn injuries. J Burn Care Res. 2016;37(5):305–13.
33. Shahrokhi S, Arno A, Jeschke M. The use of dermal substitutes in burn surgery: acute phase. Wound Repair Regen. 2014;22(1):14–22.

Blast: Mechanisms of Injury and Implications upon Treatment

28

Itamar Ashkenazi and Yoram Kluger

Learning Goals
- Understand the different mechanisms of trauma in patients injured by blast injury.
- Understand the possible interactions between the different mechanisms of trauma created by the blast.
- Recognize the correct approach and possible pitfalls in evaluating and treating victims injured following an explosion.

28.1 Introduction

It is said that gunpowder, which is a mixture of potassium nitrate, sulfur, and carbon, was first produced by alchemists in China in the middle of the ninth century AD [1]. Primarily used for firecrackers and as an incendiary, with time, it was learned that upon incineration, gunpowder could produce enough pressure to propel a bullet out of a gun's barrel. One thousand years after the invention of gunpowder, around 1850, dynamite and guncotton were discovered. Unlike gunpowder, both dynamite and guncotton could deliver an immense amount of energy during a short time. The inventions of trinitrotoluene (TNT), RDX, and other types of explosives quickly followed. These include non-nitrogenous based explosives, such as triacetone triperoxide (TATP), which are difficult to detect by systems tuned to nitro-based explosives and are prevalent in acts of terrorism [2].

In this chapter, we wish to describe the mechanisms of injury encountered following the blast. We also want to highlight those injuries that may be encountered and emphasize the similarities and differences compared to other mechanisms of trauma that are commonly experienced in the civilian setting, mainly blunt trauma and penetrating trauma.

28.2 Mechanisms of Injury

Apart from thermal energy released by the explosion, the main destructive effect is related to a sudden increase in pressures at the explosion site. These compress the surrounding medium resulting in an outward propagation of a positive pressure wave [3, 4]. This first wave is followed by a second negative-pressure wave caused by the medium being drawn back to the point of detonation.

The intensity of the positive pressure wave to which a casualty may be exposed depends on several factors [4]. The explosion releases a cer-

I. Ashkenazi · Y. Kluger (✉)
General Surgery Division, Rambam Medical Center, Haifa, Israel
e-mail: y_kluger@rambam.health.gov.il

tain amount of energy dependent on the type and amount of explosives detonated. Higher energies released will result in higher peaks of overpressures. In an ideal blast model, the positive pressure expands circumferentially away from the detonated explosive. The peak overpressure decreases in its intensity as the distance from the detonated explosive increases and with it the possibility for bodily harm. One individual will be exposed to overpressures nine times higher than a second individual whose distance from the explosion is twice as much. Increased duration of overpressures diminishes the peak overpressure needed to induce organ injury [5]. In the real world, blast waves may reflect off the ground and other solid surfaces creating reflected waves that further augment the overpressures created by the primary positive-pressure wave. Thus, explosions occurring within enclosed environments may lead to higher overpressures compared to explosions occurring in open fields. The type of medium is also crucial. Underwater explosions result in overpressure waves that travel faster and induce injury at greater distances when compared to air explosions.

Blast injuries may be caused by several different mechanisms [3]. These include bodily harm caused by the explosions' pressure wave as described above. However, injury can also be caused by penetrating fragments propagated by the blast. The body may be forcefully displaced against other hard objects. Finally, an injury may be caused by other effects like fire, toxic gas, or biological material. Following is a detailed description of each of these mechanisms.

28.2.1 Primary Blast Injury

Primary blast injury (PBI) occurs when a casualty is exposed to the pressure wave generated by a detonation of an explosive [6]. Organs containing air-fluid interfaces are more susceptible to barotrauma since overpressure affects water and air differently. Following an explosion, the classical injuries are blast lung injury (BLI), tympanic membrane perforation (TMP), and bowel injury. However, primary blast injury to solid organs has been suspected as well. Following is a discussion of the different PBIs, their clinical implications, and treatment.

28.2.1.1 Blast Lung Injury

BLI is characterized by severe alveolar overdistention with evident thinning and rupture of alveolar septae and enlargement of alveolar spaces [7]. Subpleural, intra-alveolar, and perivascular hemorrhages coexist. These hemorrhages form the typical perihilar patchy infiltrates in a "butterfly" distribution observed in chest radiographs of victims of explosion (Fig. 28.1) [8]. The main clinical manifestations include hypoxia and hemoptysis. Following an explosion, both lungs will be affected.

In 1978, Hadden et al. published their experience with 1532 explosion victims treated in the Royal Victoria Hospital during the civil disturbances in Northern Ireland [9]. Only two patients had BLI. In contrast with survivors, BLI was observed in 45% of the autopsies performed in those who died on site.

On February 25 and March 3 in 1996, two bombs exploded on civilian buses in Jerusalem. Overall, 24 immediate surviving victims with varying degrees of BLI were treated in two of the main hospitals in Jerusalem [10, 11]. In most of

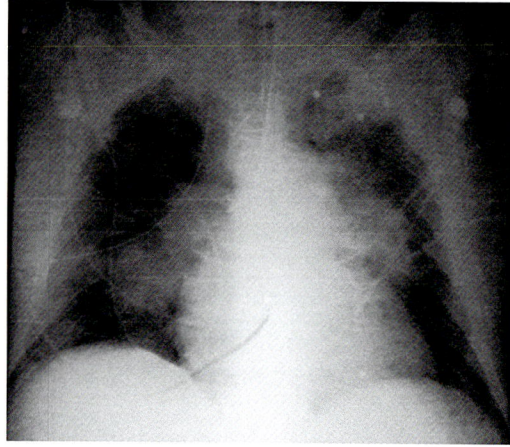

Fig. 28.1 An elderly patient injured following a bomb explosion carrying metal pellets in an enclosed environment. Legend: Notice the butterfly pattern of perihilar pulmonary infiltrates typically encountered in patients suffering from BLI

these patients, BLI was their principal, if not their only significant injury. These represent one of the largest groups of survivors with BLI we are aware of. The discrepancy between this experience to the rarity of BLI following explosions in Northern Ireland deserves an explanation.

Perpetrators of explosion attacks in Northern Ireland were aware of the added benefit of adding metallic fragments of all types to their bombs in increasing their destructive potential. Both Cooper et al. and Mellor et al. hypothesized that sufficient proximity to an explosion from an improvised device needed to initiate BLI would more likely lead to the victim's death from blast-energized penetrating and nonpenetrating missiles [5, 12]. Thus, the patient whose X-ray is presented in Fig. 28.1 is an example of the exception rather than the rule. With the increasing addition of metallic fragments to bombs, BLI has become infrequent, even in our own experience. Over the years, we have treated many patients with significant injuries following explosions containing additional metal fragments such as nails, nuts, and metal pellets. Still, most did not have any clinical evidence of BLI.

As mentioned above, the most common manifestations of clinically significant BLI are hypoxia, hemoptysis, and radiological evidence of diffuse lung opacities. Most patients with hypoxia will respond to oxygen supplementation. Oxygen provided by nasal prongs or a mask may be sufficient for the minority of patients with mild BLI. However, mechanical ventilation and positive pressure ventilation are the rule in the majority of the patients who will present with evidence of either moderate or severe acute lung injury, manifested by a PaO_2/FIO_2 ratio of 200 or less [10]. In many of these patients, oxygenation through mechanical ventilation using parameters advocated by the ARDS protocol may be sufficient [13]. However, in others, even this intervention may prove insufficient. In these other patients, significant proportions of their lungs are contused, and the remaining functional reserves are low. Appropriate oxygenation is not possible without increasing PEEP to levels that may theoretically exacerbate barotrauma. PEEP levels exceeding 10 cm H_2O were not uncommon and temporary levels as high as 20 cm H_2O in survivors were reported [10, 11, 14].

Significant increases in PEEP and PIP levels during positive pressure ventilation in patients with low lung compliance may demand alternative approaches. These include the institution of permissive hypercapnia ventilation and inhaled nitric oxide (iNO) [10, 11, 15]. Permissive hypercapnia allows for decreasing airway pressures by decreasing the tidal volumes while compensating for low arterial pH by increasing the respiratory rates [15]. iNO is a pulmonary vasodilator. It reduces the shunt by improving the blood flow in ventilated lung regions. Once systemically absorbed, iNO is quickly scavenged by hemoglobin, and systemic dilatation is avoided [16]. The authors' limited experience with iNO superimposed with positive pressure ventilation was that it provided a bridge in complicated patients, improving the shunt and oxygenation in these until respiratory function improved several days later (Fig. 28.2).

Other techniques for improving oxygenation will be briefly mentioned. Non-invasive positive pressure ventilation techniques may avoid the need for mechanical ventilation. Nevertheless, hemoptysis, which is commonly encountered in BLI patients, may preclude this option. High-flow nasal cannula oxygen therapy was unavailable when the authors experienced their BLI patients during the 1990s and the first decade of this century. High-flow nasal cannulas provide humidified warm air of up to 60 L/min [17]. In severely hypoxemic patients, in whom conventional respiratory techniques proved insufficient, high-frequency jet ventilation, ECMO, and one-lung ventilation were suggested. High-frequency jet ventilation with superimposed positive pressure ventilation was used in several patients with reported improvements manifested in the PaO_2/FIO_2 ratio. Still, due to increased mortality observed in ARDS patients treated by this mode of ventilation compared to conventional methods of ventilation, high-frequency jet ventilation in adults has been abandoned [18]. The availability of respirators with this mode of ventilation is probably limited. ECMO was only sporadically used. Twenty years ago, this oxygenation method

Fig. 28.2 Respiratory parameters in one patient with BLI ultimately treated with iNO. Legend: On admission, the tube was repositioned due to one lung intubation performed prehospital. On FIO_2 1.0, the patient remained hypoxic, even when PEEP was increased to 10 cm H_2O. Only when PEEP was increased to 15 did SO_2 increase to 87.5%. A decrease of FIO_2 to 0.7 was followed by an SO_2 decrease to 82%. FIO_2 was increased to 0.8, and PEEP was increased to 17 cm H_2O. This resulted in an SO_2 of 97%. This was the first time SO_2 measured over 90%, and this was achieved following 9 h of treatment. A decrease of FIO_2 to 0.5 led to a decrease in PaO_2 from 126 mmHg to 62 mmHg (SO_2 was not recorded). iNO was initiated at 13.5 h resulting in an SO_2 of 96.5% with FIO_2 0.5 and PEEP 17. PEEP was slowly decreased to 10 cm H_2O and FIO_2 to 45 over the next 10 h

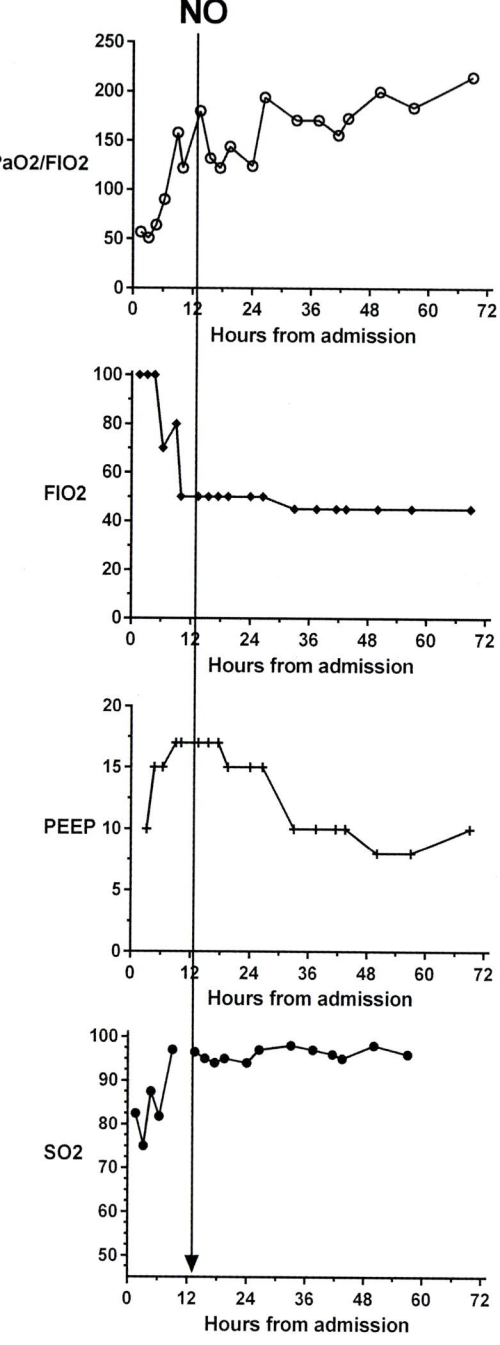

was limited due to the need to fully anticoagulate the patients, some of whom suffered from hemoptysis. Nevertheless, dry ECMOs are currently available and should be considered when all other options fail. We did not experience one-lung ventilation in patients with severe BLI. It must be remembered that BLI is bilateral disease, and both lungs are affected. Still, one lung intubation is a viable option in patients with severe one-sided bronchopleural fistulas.

Certain controversial issues concerning BLI require elaboration. These include a discussion of air emboli, tension pneumothorax, and the time needed for respiratory failure to develop following the blast.

Arterial air embolism has been cited as a common cause of mortality following BLI, especially in patients undergoing positive pressure ventilation [19]. We have not encountered clinically significant air embolisms in our patients, including those treated with positive pressure ventilation. Neither Mellor et al., who discussed 828 service members either killed or injured by an explosion in Northern Ireland [12]. Air embolism has been demonstrated experimentally and in case reports [20–22]. It may have been the cause of transient paralysis described in patients treated in seven hospitals following the Madrid 2004 terror bombings [23]. In our opinion, fear of air embolism should not prevent mechanical ventilation and positive pressure ventilation in patients with BLI who are hypoxic or need emergency surgery under general anesthesia.

Patients with severe BLI may present in an agonal state. The current teaching is to drain both hemithoraces counteracting possible tension pneumothoraces immediately. We wish to discuss specific technical aspects that should be considered when approaching victims following explosions with suspected pneumothorax. Decreased air entry to the hemithorax may be secondary to a pneumothorax, but it may also be secondary to a severely contused lung. In severe BLI, the contused lung does not collapse, even if a tension pneumothorax develops. Tracheal displacement will not happen if both lungs are severely contused. When inserting a chest tube, one should consider that the lung may be severely contused, and contused lungs are highly brittle. All precautions should be taken following the incision of the pleura. A finger should be gently inserted into the pleural cavity allowing one to evaluate the pathology. Only then should the chest tube be inserted.

Several authors have cautioned that significant BLI may develop gradually within 24 h or even after a latent period that can extend up to 48 h after the explosion [24, 25]. Brismar et al. even recommended performing chest X-rays routinely in all casualties on admission following a blast since this will often reveal pulmonary lesions that are not suspected clinically [24]. These recommendations are based on several reports published in the literature on patients diagnosed with delayed presentation of hemothorax, pneumohemothorax, and even respiratory failures following 36 and 48 h from the explosion [22, 26]. However, careful analysis of one of these accounts reveals that in two of the cases, both were symptomatic on admission [26]. Both had abnormal chest X-rays on admission. Furthermore, both had associated abdominal injuries. Weiler-Ravell et al. describe 13 male soldiers injured by an underwater explosion while swimming [22]. All but one either died within minutes or were severely wounded. The authors report one patient who initially seemed well and had remained under the supervision of his local physician. He had been up to his knees in the water at the time of the explosion. Forty-eight hours later, he began to behave strangely and was referred for a psychiatric consultation. Within a short time, signs of severe pulmonary insufficiency developed. He underwent an urgent tracheostomy, after which he was ventilated for ten days. He eventually recovered.

Counteracting the possibility of delayed diagnosis and delayed presentation of BLI may have logistical consequences. Bomb explosions aimed at civilians commonly result in mass casualty incidents. Hospitalizing all incoming patients for observation over a couple of days is not practically feasible. Neither is performing chest X-rays or taking blood gases to rule out "asymptomatic BLI", which may eventually manifest as respiratory failure hours or days later. Having analyzed the course of clinical events in hundreds of patients following explosions, we have not encountered any case of delayed presentation of significant BLI. Neither have other authors who have summarized their experience with almost one thousand patients, of which over 83 were reported to have BLI [10, 27, 28]. In our experience, most patients who developed respiratory failure in need of intubation either manifested immediately following the blast or once they were admitted to the emergency department. In one mass casualty incident, we encountered a young patient who gradually deteriorated and was eventually intubated three hours after the explosion. However, he was both dyspneic and suffering from hemoptysis on admission. Relying on this experience, we discharged patients without significant injury following a couple of hours of observation. On admission and before discharge, we evaluated the patients for their vital signs and the presence of hemoptysis. We did not rule out BLI by performing chest X-rays or taking arterial blood gases. At most, we measured SO_2 at room air.

Hemoptysis is a hallmark of BLI. In most cases, it is self-limiting, and most cases were therefore treated by observation only. Overzealous deep airway suction should be avoided since it only serves to exacerbate airway bleeding further. Frequent exchange of their filters better served mechanically ventilated patients with significant hemoptysis. Successful treatment with Factor VIIa was reported in one patient only (unpublished data). Factor VIIa has been used successfully in treating hemoptysis in other nontrauma settings, such as in diffuse alveolar hemorrhage [29]. A possible treatment alternative is inhaled tranexamic acid. We are not aware of BLI patients with hemoptysis so treated. Inhaled tranexamic acid has shown efficacy in patients bleeding from the lung secondary to cancer and bronchiectasis, with very few adverse events [30, 31]. There is a theoretical advantage for tranexamic acid over factor VIIa due to its low price and safety profile.

In summary, BLI is an uncommon injury affecting both lungs. It is manifested in hypoxic failure. Some of the severely injured patients are extremely difficult to oxygenate. However, our experience in those surviving the injury, recovery to a fully functional life is the rule.

28.2.1.2 Tympanic Membrane Perforation

The overpressures needed to develop TMP are about one-fifth of those with the same duration required to develop BLI [32]. TMP is therefore commonly diagnosed following explosions. Of 775 patients treated in 7 hospitals in Madrid following the March 2004 terrorist attack, 240 (31%) were diagnosed with TMP, of which 60% (144/240) were bilateral, and 40% (96/240) were unilateral [23]. Following an explosion, most perforations are large, and many require operative intervention. Of US service members with TMP analyzed by the United States Army Institute of Surgical Research, only 48% of TMP healed spontaneously [33].

TMP has been suggested as a marker of barotrauma caused by blast [34]. The presence of TMP could theoretically identify those who were most exposed to the blast overpressures, while the absence of TMP could rule out this exposure. Leibovici analyzed 647 survivors treated in hospitals following 11 terrorist bombing attacks [28]. Of these, 193 (29.8%) were diagnosed with primary blast injuries: 142 with TMP, 18 with BLI, 31 with combined TMP and BLI, and 2 with intestinal blast injury. Thus, in this study, the positive predictive value of TMP in identifying BLI and intestinal blast injury was only 0.18 (95% CI 0.13 to 0.24), and the negative predictive value was 0.96 (95% CI 0.94 to 0.97). Using TMP as a marker, 18 of 49 BLIs would have been missed.

28.2.1.3 Blast Intestinal Injury

Intestinal injuries due to overpressures created by the blast wave are uncommon. These injuries are more commonly encountered in survivors of underwater explosions [35]. Injuries encountered include serosal tears, intramural hemorrhages, as well as perforations [36]. Though a predilection to the small intestine near the ileocecal valve has been described, both small bowel and large bowel may be involved [35, 36].

The exact prevalence of injury secondary to overpressures is unknown since primary blast intestinal injury cannot be reliably differentiated from displacement injuries to the abdomen (the third mechanism of blast injury). Nevertheless, the clinical approach is similar in both cases.

Patients commonly present with abdominal pain. This may be apparent immediately following admission to the emergency department. However, abdominal pain may also appear hours and days following the explosion. In a series described by Paran et al., abdominal pain and peritonitis became evident on admission, 20 h after admission, and 48 hours after admission in three patients, respectively [37]. During laparotomy in the latter two patients, circular hematomas were encountered in the ileum within which perforations were found. There was minimal contamination, indicating these were recent perforations that gradually evolved rather than a delayed diagnosis. Katz et al. described two patients with an ileal perforation and colonic perforation identified 3 and 7 days following an explosion in a bus [36]. According to the authors, in both cases, the diagnosis was delayed since none of the treating physicians considered the possibility of primary bowel blast injury. Up until then, primary blast injuries to the bowel were only described in victims surviving underwater explosions.

With or without free air on imaging, evidence of peritonitis demands an exploratory laparotomy in patients developing abdominal pain following an explosion. Bowel segments with evident perforation should be resected. Bowel segments with contusions may be at risk for late perforation. Very small hematomas may be imbricated. Experimental models reveal that antimesenteric contusions with diameters of less than 15 mm may be observed, while larger contusions and those affecting the mesenteric border should be excised [38]. Whether to perform a primary anastomosis or not depends on the degree of peritoneal contamination and the patient's general condition. A second-look laparotomy may be advised whenever several contusions are spread across a large segment of the intestine that would otherwise demand a significant resection.

28.2.1.4 Primary Blast Injury of Solid Organs

Though the pathognomonic injuries of PBI involve organs with an air-fluid interface, some solid organ injuries have been attributed to this mechanism as well. We will briefly describe primary blast neurotrauma, primary blast facial injury, and primary blast extremity injury.

Improvised explosive devices were commonly employed against the coalition forces in both Iraq and Afghanistan. It soon became clear the many service members surviving these explosions without any evidence of physical impact developed a chronic neurological disorder characterized by PTSD and other PTSD-related disorders such as depression, anxiety, memory and attention disorders, sleep problems, and emotional disturbances [39]. Indeed, "Shell Shock," described in the First World War, was identified throughout the wars that broke out since then. However, the psychological sequel was attributed to contributing stressful experiences during combat coupled with other contributing factors such as lack of support [40]. Only in the last decades has it been realized that the psychological symptoms in those exposed to blast from improvised explosive devices seem to parallel chronic symptomatology observed in some of the casualties following mild traumatic brain injury secondary to impact [39, 41]. MRI studies and several postmortem findings suggest corresponding brain tissue changes secondary to the blast [42]. Significant research is underway to understand these phenomena better, evaluate their underlying pathophysiology, and improve the diagnosis and treatment of this insult.

PBI produces a unique form of mandibular fracture that affects the mandibular body and is transverse in its orientation [43]. These transverse fractures may be single or multiple. Fractures may be associated with the transection of the teeth below the gingival margin at the cementoenamel junction.

Blowout fractures of the orbit in victims of explosion without any other external injuries have also been described [44]. The coexistence of TMP suggested PBI as the primary mechanism of injury. The eye globe exposed to the pressure wave is capable of withstanding the increased pressure. However, following the blast, it may be pushed back into its socket. Compression of the orbital contents will cause a rise in the intraorbital pressures. The orbital floor and the lamina papyracea are prone to fracture. The clinical signs of this type of fracture include enophthalmos, diplopia, and restricted upward gaze movement of the eye globe.

Though the tertiary blast mechanism predominates as a cause of extremity fractures, PBI has also been implicated [45]. The proximal third of the tibia and the femur are the most commonly affected. Due to these bones' geometry and the differential movement allowed by the ankle, knee, and hip joints, specific areas in the femur and tibia are affected by bending forces created by the blast. The clinical approach to these fractures is independent of the mechanism of injury. It depends on the type of fracture and the associated vascular, neurological and soft tissue injuries.

28.2.2 Secondary Blast Injury

The most common mechanism of trauma leading to significant injuries in immediate survivors of an explosion is probably caused by penetrating fragments propagated by the blast. Henry Shrapnel was an English artillery officer that developed a unique artillery shell that contained an explosive charge with spherical lead bullets [46]. A time fuze set off the explosive at the latter part of the shell's flight. This explosion brought about the dispersion of the spherical bullets and fragments of the shell's case. It was later discovered that increasing the power of the explosive charge would break up the shell's iron casing into small fragments. Thus, adding the bullets was unnecessary.

The concepts underlying Henry Shrapnel's invention and its later modification serve as the basis to understand the underlying mechanism leading to penetrating injuries observed following exposure to the blast. It may be that the projectiles are primary fragments that originate from the case of the weapon used as the explosive. This may be the case when grenades and shells explode. Similar to the original idea proposed by Henry Shrapnel, it may be that different types of metallic objects are added to the explosive, such as nails, screws, screw nuts, and metal pellets. These have been the primary type of bombs employed in terrorist bombings to which we have responded [47]. Finally, the projectiles may be secondary fragments that result from the surroundings of where the bomb exploded. This was the case in the bombings aimed at the US in Nairobi in 1998, where many were injured from flying glass from the shattered windows [48]. It was also the case in the Tower of London bombing in 1974. Many of the injuries resulted from penetrating wooden splinters that originated from a large wooden cannon carriage next to which the explosive device was placed [5]. Just about anything at the vicinity of the bomb can turn into a penetrating projectile, as exemplified by remnants of a watch that penetrated one surviving victim's neck in Jerusalem, and bone fragments originating from other victims described in other cases in Israel and London [49–52]. The biological implications of the latter will be discussed later.

The projectiles propelled by the explosion rapidly decelerate and lose their kinetic energy. Their irregular shapes increase their friction with the surrounding medium through which they move [5]. The skin forms a protective barrier against low-energy projectiles. These characteristics limit the distance from the explosion within which the projectiles may cause serious injury. However, for those casualties within the effective perimeter of the bomb, penetrating injury is a source of much morbidity and mortality, which may mislead even those most experienced with trauma management.

Casualties commonly present with multiple skin wounds of different sizes, apparent external injuries coupled with dust tattooing, external ash, and bloodstains (Fig. 28.3). Numerous body

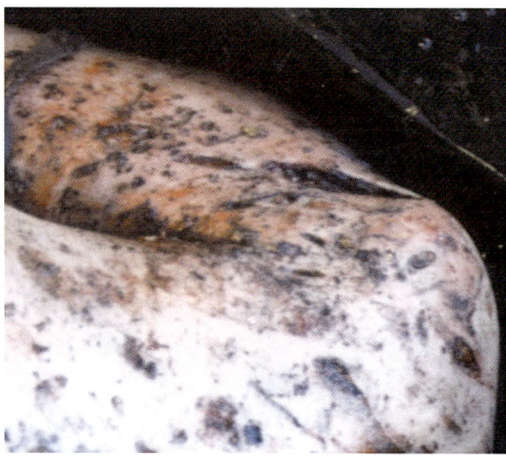

Fig. 28.3 A casualty with multiple penetrating fragment wounds, dust tattooing, and external ash

areas are affected [53]. Whether certain projectiles penetrated deeply or not is not always easy to assess [54]. This is further compounded by the multiplicity of wounds that may distract one's attention from another injury that may be life-threatening. Thus, a severe periorbital hematoma may portray a significant eye globe injury. However, it could also be the port of entry for a penetrating injury to the brain. A significant flash burn affecting the face of a young girl distracted the attention away from a large nail that penetrated the heart through an otherwise innocent-looking skin injury in the trunk [55]. A severe facial injury and upper extremity injury distracted the attention away from a deeply penetrating projectile that caused small and large bowel lacerations and a tear in the mesenteric vessels that eventually led to hemorrhagic shock. Some of these cases have been published; others have not. All the cases portray the difficulty in identifying the real severity of the injury of patients in whom most, if not all, penetrating skin wounds may be secondary to projectiles that ended up lodging superficially within the soft tissue.

For this reason, we question recommendations made by some of our colleagues as to the workup of these patients who suggest screening patients with eFAST regardless of their hemodynamic status while limiting CT scans to evaluate possible head injury [56, 57]. This policy led to nontherapeutic laparotomies due to false-positive eFAST [27, 56]. We recommend not changing current guidelines when evaluating patients with evidence of injuries to multiple body areas, even within the context of a mass casualty incident. eFAST should be conserved to evaluate hemodynamically unstable patients for possible sources of life-threatening bleeding. Total body CT is the recommended imaging modality to work up hemodynamically stable patients who suffer from injuries to multiple body areas.

Surgical removal of retained foreign bodies should consider the possible benefits against the morbidity of surgical exploration. Surgical removal is recommended if the foreign bodies are easily accessible, if they are symptomatic, composed of organic material and if their location may eventually lead to secondary damage to nearby structures. Organic foreign bodies such as cloth and wood splinters from explosions cause an inflammatory response that may become complicated by a secondary infection. Non-organic foreign bodies may pose a lower risk of infection. Still, they may lodge within joints, within the eye globe, adjacent to nerves and blood vessels, leading to symptoms on presentation or delayed symptoms by secondary damage [58–60]. Otherwise, most of the foreign bodies cause superficial wounds on the skin and underlying soft tissue. Many of these can be managed nonsurgically with antibiotics and dressing. Bowyer reported only two casualties who developed infection out of 63 casualties, with over 850 soft tissue fragment wounds treated this way [61]. Surveillance of patients like these is advised since the accurate composition of the foreign bodies is unknown, and the long-term risks of metals embedded within the body have not been defined [62].

Imaging should precede surgery. Radiography and CT scan help localize foreign bodies such as metal fragments, glass, and bones. Ultrasound may identify the precise location of glass and wood. Both imaging modalities can then be used intraoperatively in deeply penetrating foreign bodies [63].

28.2.3 Tertiary Blast Injury

Significant displacement of the whole body away from the explosion against hard surfaces carries a high risk of injury. Many head injuries and extremity fractures may be attributed to this mechanism of trauma [5]. All body areas are susceptible to blunt injury. The approach to the casualties should resemble that of other blunt trauma scenarios secondary to high impacts such as falls from height and motor vehicle accidents.

Similar to what was described above, the multiplicity of body areas injured may distract the attention away from a life-threatening injury. Careful history-taking may reveal this mechanism of injury. Take, for example, the recollection of one casualty with a pancreatic transection in whom this injury was missed during the primary evaluation:

"... suddenly there was an explosion. My hands flew up in the air, and I fell backward ...".

Though similar to other high-impact blunt trauma mechanisms, we wish to emphasize one aspect that may be different. Severe loss of soft tissue is not uncommon in these casualties with extremity injuries. These may result from the displacement of the whole body against hard objects or the displacement of large objects against the extremities. Whatever the mechanism, these injuries tend to bleed significantly, much more when compared to extremity injuries from either blunt trauma or penetrating trauma from non-explosion scenarios. Bleeding may be arrest on its own, following bandaging or placement of a tourniquet.

Significant blood loss from the extremities during the prehospital phase may be underestimated when rushing the patient to the operating room for debridement and external fracture fixation. One of the authors experienced two elderly patients who hemodynamically decompensated during surgery for their extremity injuries. One died intraoperatively with evidence of acute myocardial ischemia. The other died following several days from multiple organ failure. Non-therapeutic laparotomies due to a similar underlying cause were described following the bombings in London in 2005 [64, 65]. Several patients with significant limb injuries decompensated during their surgery leading the surgeons to perform these laparotomies to rule out intra-abdominal bleeding.

At times it is difficult to differentiate whether displacement or other blast mechanisms of trauma are the underlying cause of injury in explosion casualties. We discussed above PBI as a cause of extremity fractures and intestinal injuries. DeCeballos et al. compared patients with blast injury to other patients with lung contusions coupled with fractures of their chest wall (ribs, sternum, and/or scapula) [27]. Patients with lung damage associated with fractures of the chest wall tended to have a long course of ventilation and high ventilator-associated pneumonia rates. These examples question the need to differentiate between blast and displacement as the cause of explosion-related injuries since their treatment and outcome may be similar.

28.2.4 Quarternary Blast Injury

The quarternary blast injury mechanism encompasses various types of injuries caused by explosions unrelated to each other. These include burn injuries, inhalational injuries, and toxic poisoning, among others.

Explosions release thermal injury that usually results in flash burns but may result in a fire with significant burns and inhalational injuries. Such was the case in the bombing attack in Bali, Indonesia, in 2002. Two nearby bars were targeted. The second, larger explosion led to a fire breaking out in a number of nearby buildings [66]. As reported in Sanglah Hospital that admitted 40% of the victims, burn injuries predominated.

Explosions may also result from industrial substances. Apart from the classical blast wave and projectiles, explosions may lead to fires and the release of toxic chemicals such as chlorine and phosgene [67]. Any explosion has the potential to be associated with contaminants, whether these are chemical, biological, or radioactive. The involvement of toxic material should be taken into consideration and ruled out by responders.

Kluger et al. reported on four surviving casualties who developed a unique hyperinflammatory state following an explosion manifested as hyperpyrexia, sweating, low central venous pressure, and positive fluid balance [68]. The underlying injuries did not explain the manifestations observed. The authors hypothesized that this clinical manifestation could have resulted from unconventional materials used to manufacture the explosive.

In 2001, following a suicide bombing in a mall near the hospital where one of the authors previously worked, one of the mildly injured casualties was diagnosed with four superficially penetrating bone fragments that were eventually removed. Assuming these bones emanated from the suicide bomber, his remains were examined, and serology was found to be positive for hepatitis B. Discussions within the Israel Ministry of Health followed, and a recommendation to vaccinate victims of explosion with hepatitis B vaccine was adopted in Israel and other countries [69]. Since then, other cases of penetrating bone fragments in victims of the explosion have been described [50–52]. A review of the literature reveals that penetrating bone fragments was also reported following other trauma scenarios [70–73].

A detailed discussion of the Israel Ministry of Health's decision is beyond the scope of the manuscript. However, it is essential to emphasize that this decision was criticized for several reasons. The reliability of the conventional serology test on dead tissue has probably never been verified. The bone projectiles created by the explosion are exposed to extreme temperatures questioning whether these retain any infectious potential. Assuming there remains a potential for infection, the committee did not recommend adding hepatitis B immune globulin for postexposure prophylaxis. Finally, the Ministry of Health's expert committee avoided discussing the possibility that the bone fragments might emanate from a hepatitis C or HIV carrier. Still, the hepatitis B vaccine is safe. HIV prophylaxis should be considered after weighing the side effects of prophylaxis against the odds that the perpetrator of the bomb was indeed an HIV carrier. The average risk for HIV transmission has been estimated to be approximately 0.3% after percutaneous exposure to HIV-infected blood [69]. In a country with a 5% prevalence of HIV within its population, the overall hazard for infection will be 0.014%. The hazard–benefit ratio for post-exposure prophylaxis is minimal.

> **Do's and Don'ts**
> - Do not fear arterial air emboli. Intubate hypoxic patients if needed and apply PEEP as necessary.
> - In patients with BLI complicated by pneumothorax, who do not respond to primary treatment, consider bilateral pathologies. Be extra careful when introducing chest tubes in patients with BLI.
> - Do not use eFAST to screen for trunkal injuries in hemodynamically stable patients with evidence of significant exposure to the blast. If imaging is needed, use a CT scan.
> - Request information on the explosion scene since it may uncover important information on other possible vectors of injury.
> - Be thorough. Life-threatening injuries may be masked by other significant distracting injuries.

> **Take-Home Messages**
> - Explosions result in injuries to multiple body areas.
> - Multiple mechanisms of injury may be involved. However, elucidating the actual mechanism at the time of primary evaluation may be unclear.
> - When treating BLI, think of bilateral pathologies.
> - When evaluating an unstable patient with evidence of multiple skin fragment wounds, bleeding should be considered the cause of instability until ruled out.
> - eFAST should be used to evaluate trunkal pathologies only in hemodynamically unstable patients. Hemodynamically stable patients in need of imaging for possible trunkal pathologies should undergo CT.

Questions
1. Which of the following mechanisms of trauma best explains a pancreatic neck transection?
    A. the first mechanism
    B. the second mechanism
    C. the third mechanism
    D. the fourth mechanism

2. Which sentence best describes the epidemiology of blast lung injury and tympanic membrane perforation?
   A. all patients with blast lung injury have tympanic membrane perforation
   B. all patients with tympanic membrane perforation have blast lung injury
   C. blast lung injury may occur without tympanic membrane perforation
   D. this issue has never been evaluated
3. A 50-year-old male patient is seen in the emergency department following an explosion. The patient is asymptomatic and vital signs are normal. When can the patient be discharged?
   A. following 48 h of observation
   B. following a normal chest X-ray
   C. following a normal blood gases report
   D. after a couple of hours observation, if he remains asymptomatic and vital signs are normal
4. A 25-year-old female following an explosion has hemoptysis and is tachypneic even with a rebreathing mask. Her vital signs show heart rate—114, blood pressure 115/85, respiratory rate 40. Her blood gases show pO_2 50. How should this patient be oxygenated?
   A. continue rebreathing mask
   B. BiPAP
   C. CPAP
   D. oral tracheal intubation with positive pressure ventilation
5. A 40-year-old intubated patient is still hypoxic though FIO_2 is 1.0 and PEEP is 10 cm H_2O. What should be the next step to improve oxygenation?
   A. bilateral chest tubes
   B. increase FIO_2
   C. increase PEEP
   D. blood transfusions
6. For the patient in the previous question, what other adjunct treatment in the ICU in common use could improve the oxygenation?
   A. none
   B. inhaled nitric oxide
   C. high-frequency jet ventilation
   D. humidified air
7. A 30-year-old male was admitted following an explosion of a gas tank in his factory. On admission, he is tachycardic and tachypneic. He has hemoptysis, and SO_2 is low. There are no signs of penetrating injuries. The breath sounds are diminished in both hemithoraces. What is the most probable diagnosis?
   A. bilateral pneumothorax
   B. bilateral hemothorax
   C. bilateral chest wall edema
   D. bilateral pulmonary contusions
8. You are informed that the patient in the previous question was rescued after almost half an hour from the explosion due to a fire that developed in the factory. The factory manufactures plastic bottles. What could be a possible toxic material involved in this case?
   A. Manganese
   B. carbon dioxide
   C. phosgene
   D. O_3
9. A 30-year-old male patient is brought to the emergency department following a nail-bomb explosion. The patient is tachycardic, hypotensive and oxygen saturations are low. External evaluation reveals multiple penetrating injuries to the trunk and limbs with significant soft tissue loss. What is the **least** probable reason for hypoxia in this patient?
   A. blast lung injury
   B. bilateral massive pneumothoraces
   C. bilateral massive hemothoraces
   D. significant bleeding either within the abdomen or from the limbs

10. What should be the next diagnostic step in the patient described in the previous question?
    A. blood gases
    B. chest X-ray
    C. eFAST
    D. CT scan

Answers: 1-c; 2-c; 3-d; 4-d; 5-c; 6-b; 7-d; 8-c; 9-a; 10-c

Acknowledgment The authors wish to thank Michael Alkan and Boris Isakovitch for their advice concerning different issues discussed in this chapter.

References

1. Brown GI. Explosives. History with a bang. Gloucestershire, Great Britain: The History Press; 2010.
2. Bannister WW, Oxley JC. Potential detection problems: nonnitrogen-based explosives. In: Society of Photo-Optical Instrumentation Engineers (SPIE) Conference Series. 1 December 1992, Volume 10264. doi: https://doi.org/10.1117/12.141387.
3. Lennquist S. Chapter 7: Incidents caused by physical trauma. In Lennquist S, editor. Medical response to major incidents and disasters. A practical guide for all medical staff. Springer-Verlag Berlin Hidelberg 2012. pp 111-196. doi: https://doi.org/10.1007/978-3-642.21895-8
4. Cernak I. Chapter 45: Blast injuries and blast-induced neurotrauma: overview of pathophysiology and experimental knowledge models and findings. In: Kobeissy FH, editor. Brain neurotrauma: molecular, neuropsychological, and rehabilitation aspects. Boca Raton, FL: CRC Press/Taylor & Francis; 2015.
5. Cooper GJ, Maynard RL, Cros NL, Hill JF. Casualties from terrorist bombings. J Trauma. 1983;23(11):955–67. https://doi.org/10.1097/00005373-198311000-00001.
6. Argyros GJ. Management of primary blast injury. Toxicology. 1997;121(1):105–15. https://doi.org/10.1016/s0300-483x(97)03659-7.
7. Tsokos M, Paulsen F, Petri S, Madea B, Püschel K, Türk EE. Histologic, immunohistochemical, and ultrastructural findings in human blast lung injury. Am J Resp Crit Care Med. 2003;168(5):549–55. https://doi.org/10.1164/rccm.200304-528OC.
8. Shaham D, Sella T, Makori A, Appelbum L, Rivkind AI, Bar-Ziv J. The role of radiology in terror injuries. Isr Med Assoc J. 2002;4(7):564–7.
9. Hadden WA, Rutherford WH, Merrett JD. The injuries of terrorists bombing: a study of 1532 consecutive patients. Br J Surg. 1978;65(8):525–31. https://doi.org/10.1002/bjs.1800650802.
10. Pizov R, Oppenheim-Eden A, Matot I, Weiss YG, Eidelman LA, Rivkind AI, Sprung CL. Blast lung injury from an explosion on a civilian bus. Chest. 1999;115(1):165–72. https://doi.org/10.1378/chest.115.1.165.
11. Avidan V, Hersch M, Armon Y, Spira R, Aharoni D, Reissman P, Schecter WP. Blast lung injury: clinical manifestations, treatment, and outcome. Am J Surg. 2005;190(6):945–50. https://doi.org/10.1016/j.amjsurg.2005.08.022.
12. Mellor SG, Cooper GJ. Analysis of 828 servicemen killed or injured by explosion in Northern Ireland 1970-84; the Hostile Action Casualty System. Br J Surg. 1989;76(10):1006–10. https://doi.org/10.1002/bjs.1800761006.
13. Amato MB, Barbas CS, Medeiros DM, Magaldi RB, Schettino GP, Lorenzi-Filho G, Kairalla RA, Deheinzelin D, Munoz C, Oliveira R, Takagaki TY, Carvlaho CR. Effect of a protective-ventilation strategy on mortality in the acute respiratory distress syndrome. N Engl J Med. 1998;338(6):347–54. https://doi.org/10.1056/NEJM199802053380602.
14. Uretzky G, Cotev S. The use of continuous positive pressure airway pressure in blast injury of the chest. Crit Care Med. 1980;8(9):486–9. https://doi.org/10.1097/00003246-198009000-00002.
15. Sorkine P, Szold O, Kluger Y, Halpern P, Weinbroum A, Fleishon R, Silbiger A, Rodrick V. Permissive hypercapnia ventilation in patients with severe pulmonary blast injury. J Trauma. 1998;45(1):35–8. https://doi.org/10.1097/00005373-199807000-00006.
16. Yu B, Ichinose F, Bloch DB, Zapol WM. Inhaled nitric oxide. Br J Pharmacol. 2019;176(2):246–55. https://doi.org/10.1111/bph.14512.
17. Nishimura M. High-flow nasal cannula oxygen therapy in adults. J Intensive Care. 2015;3(1):15. https://doi.org/10.1186/s40560-015-0084-5.
18. Ferguson ND, Cook DJ, Guyatt GH, Mehta S, Hand L, Austin P, Zhou Q, Matte A, Walter SD, Lamontagne F, Ganton JT, Arabi YM, Arroliga AC, Stewart TE, Slutsky AS, Meade MO. OSCILLATE Trial Investigators, Canadian Critical Care Trials Group. High-frequency oscillation in early acute respiratory distress syndrome. N Engl J Med. 2013;36(9):795–805. https://doi.org/10.1056/NEJMoa1215554.
19. Wightman JM, Gladish SL. Explosions and blast injuries. Ann Emerg Med. 2001;37(6):664–78. https://doi.org/10.1067/mem.2001.114906.
20. Mayorga MA. The pathology of primary blast overpressure injury. Toxicology. 1997;121(1):17–28. https://doi.org/10.1016/s0300-483x(97)03652-4.
21. Freund U, Koplovic J, Durst AL. Compressed air emboli of the aorta and renal artery in blast injury. Injury. 1980;12(1):37–8. https://doi.org/10.1016/0020-1383(80)90072-8.
22. Weiler-Ravell D, Adatto R, Borman JB. Blast injury of the chest: review of the problem and its treatment. Israel J Med Sci. 1975;11(2-3):268–74.

23. Turegano-Fuentes F, Caba-Doussoux P, Jover-Navalon JM, Martin-Perz E, Fernandez-Luengas D, Diez-Valladares L, Perez-Diaz D, Yuste-Garcia P, Guadalajara Labajo H, Rios-Blanco R, Hernando-Trancho F, Garcia-Moreno Nisa F, Sanz-Sanchez M, Garcia-Fuentes C, Martinez-Virto A, Leon-Baltasar JL, Vasquez-Estevez J. Injury patterns from major urban terrorist bombings in trains: the Madrid experience. World J Surg. 2008;32(6):1168–75. https://doi.org/10.1007/s00268-008-9557-1.
24. Brismar B, Bergenwald L. The terrorist bomb explosion in Bologna, Italy, 1980: An analysis of the effects and injuries sustained. J Trauma. 1982;22(3):216–20. https://doi.org/10.1097/00005373-198203000-00007.
25. Institute of Medicine. 2014. Gulf war and health. In: Volume 9: Long-term effects of blast exposures. Washington, DC: The National Academies Press. doi: https://doi.org/10.17226/18253.
26. Hirsch M, Bazini J. Blast injury of the chest. Clin Radiol. 1969;20(4):362–70. https://doi.org/10.1016/s0009-9260(69)80087-5.
27. Gutierrez de Ceballos JP, Turégano Fuentes F, Perez Diaz D, Sanz Sanchez M, Martin Llorente C, Guerrero Sanz JE. Casualties treated at the closest hospital in the Madrid, March 11, terrorist bombings. Crit Care Med. 2005;33(1 Suppl):S107–12. https://doi.org/10.1097/01.ccm.0000151072.17826.72.
28. Leibovici D, Gofrit ON, Shapira SC. Eardrum perforation in explosion survivors: Is it a marker of pulmonary blast injury? Ann Emerg Med. 1999;34(2):168–72. https://doi.org/10.1016/s0196-0644(99)70225-8.
29. Heslet L, Nielsen JD, Nepper-Christensen S. Local pulmonary administration of factor VIIa (rFVIIa) in diffuse alveolar hemorrhage (DAH)—a review of a new treatment paradigm. Biologics. 2012;6:37–46. https://doi.org/10.2147/BTT.S25507.
30. Solomonov A, Fruchter O, Zuckerman T, Brenner B, Yigal M. Pulmonary hemorrhage: a novel mode of therapy. Resp Med. 2009;103(8):1196–200. https://doi.org/10.1016/j.rmed.2009.02.004.
31. Segrelles Calvo G, De Granada-Orive I, Lopez PD. Inhaled tranexamic acid as an alternative for hemoptysis treatment. Chest. 2016;149(2):604. https://doi.org/10.1016/j.chest.2015.10.016.
32. Mellor SG. The pathogenesis of blast injury and its management. Br J Hosp Med. 1988;39(6):536–9.
33. Ritenour AE, Weakley A, Ritenour JS, Kriete BR, Blackbourne LH, Holcomb JB, Wade CE. Tympanic membrane perforation and hearing loss for blast overpressure in Operation Enduring Freedom and Operation Iraqi Freedom wounded. J Trauma. 2008;64(2 Suppl):S174–8. https://doi.org/10.1097/TA.0b013e318160773e.
34. DePalma RG, Burris DG, Champion HR, Hodgson MJ. Blast injuries. N Engl J Med. 2005;352(13):1335–42. https://doi.org/10.1056/NEJMra042083.
35. Huller T, Bazini Y. Blast injuries of the chest and abdomen. Arch Surg. 1970;100(1):24–30. https://doi.org/10.1001/archsurg.1970.01340190026008.
36. Katz E, Ofek B, Adler J, Abramowitz HB, Krausz MM. Primary blast injury after a bomb explosion in a civilian bus. Ann Surg. 1989;209(4):484–8. https://doi.org/10.1097/00000658-198904000-00016.
37. Paran H, Neufeld D, Shwartz I, Kidron D, Susmallian S, Mayo A, Dayan K, Video I, Sivak G, Freund U. Perforation of the terminal ileum induced by blast injury: delayed diagnosis or delayed perforation? J Trauma. 1996;40(3):472–5. https://doi.org/10.1097/00005373-199603000-00029.
38. Crips NPJ, Cooper GJ. Risk of late perforation in intestinal contusions caused by explosive blasts. Br J Surg. 1997;84(9):1298–303.
39. Chen Y, Huang W, Constantini S. Concepts and strategies for clinical management of blast-induced traumatic brain injury and posttraumatic stress disorder. J Neuropsychiatr Clin Neurosci. 2013;25(2):103–10. https://doi.org/10.1176/appi.neuropsych.12030058.
40. Fontana A, Rosenheck R. Posttraumatic stress disorder among Vietnam Theater Veterans. A casual model of etiology in a community sample. J Nerv Ment Dis. 1994;182(12):677–84. https://doi.org/10.1097/00005053-199412000-00001.
41. McDonald SC, Walker WC, Cusack SI, Yoash-Gantz RE, Pickett TC, Cifu DX, VA Mid-Atlantic Mirecc Workgroup, Tupler LA. Health symptoms after war zone deployment-related mild traumatic brain injury: contributions of mental disorders and lifetime brain injuries, Brain Injury. Published online: 20 Sep 2021. doi: https://doi.org/10.1080/02699052.2021.1959058.
42. De Palma RG, Hoffman SW. Combat blast related brain injury (TBI): Decade of recognition; promise of progress. Behav Brain Res. 2018;340:102–5. https://doi.org/10.1016/j.bbr.2016.08.036.
43. Shuker ST. The effect of blast on the mandible and teeth. transverse fractures and their management. Br J Oral Maxillofac Surg. 2008;46(7):547–51. https://doi.org/10.1016/j.bjoms.2008.03.014.
44. Shamir D, Ardekian L, Peled M. Blowout fracture of the orbit as a result of blast injury: case report of a unique entity. J Oral Maxillofac Surg. 2008;66(7):1496–8. https://doi.org/10.1016/j.joms.2007.12.015.
45. Ramasamy A, Hill AM, Masouros S, Gibb I, Bull AMJ, Clasper JC. Blast-related fracture patterns: a forensic biomechanical approach. J Royal Soc Interface. 2011;8(58):689–98. https://doi.org/10.1098/rsif.2010.0476.
46. Britannica, The Editors of Encyclopaedia. [Internet]. "Shrapnel". Encyclopedia Britannica; 31 Oct 2018 [cited 2021 September 17]. https://www.britannica.com/technology/shrapnel-weaponry.
47. Kluger Y, Mayo H, Hiss J, Ashkenazi I, Bendahan J, Blumenfeld A, Michaelson M, Stein M, Simon D, Schwartz I, Alfici R. Medical consequences of terrorist bombs containing spherical metal pellets: analysis of a suicide terrorism event. Eur J Emerg Med. 2005;121(1):19–23. https://doi.org/10.1097/00063110-200502000-00006.

48. Odhiambo WA, Guthua SW, Macigo FG, Ahama MK. Maxillofacial injuries caused by terrorist bomb attack in Nairobi. Kenya. Int J Oral Maxillofac Surg. 2002;31:374–7. https://doi.org/10.1054/ijom.2001.0199.
49. Ad-El DD, Eldad A, Mintz Y, Berlatzky Y, Elami A, Rivkind AI, Almogy G, Tzur T. Suicide bombing injuries: The Jerusalem experience of exceptional tissue damage posing a new challenge for the reconstructive surgeon. Plast Reconstr Surg. 2006;118(2):383–7. https://doi.org/10.1097/01.prs.0000227736.91811.c7.
50. Leibner ED, Weil Y, Gross E, Liebergall M, Mosheiff R. A broken bone without a fracture: traumatic foreign bone implantation resulting from a mass casualty bombing. J Trauma. 2005;58(2):388–90. https://doi.org/10.1097/01.ta.0000152534.80952.2f.
51. Eshkol Z, Katz K. Injuries from biologic material of suicide bombers. Injury. 2005;36(2):271–4. https://doi.org/10.1016/j.injury.2004.06.016.
52. Wong JM, Marsh D, Abu-Sitta G, Lau S, Mann HA, Nawabi DH, Patel H. Biologic foreign body implantation in victims of the London July 7th suicide bombings. J Trauma. 2006;60(2):402–4. https://doi.org/10.1097/01.ta.0000203715.31280.65.
53. Sheffy N, Mintz Y, Rivkind AI, Shapira SC. Terror-related injuries: a comparison of gunshot wounds versus secondary-fragments-induced injuries from explosives. J Am Coll Surg. 2006;203(3):297–303. https://doi.org/10.1016/j.jamcollsurg.2006.05.010.
54. Almogy G, Belzberg H, Mintz Y, Pikarsky AK, Zamir G, Rivkind AI. Suicide bombing attacks. Update and modifications to the protocol. Ann Surg. 2004;239(3):295–300. https://doi.org/10.1097/01.sla.0000114014.63423.55.
55. Georghiou GP, Birk E, Nili M, Stein M, Vine BA, Erez E. Direct nail injury to the heart without functional or hemodynamic compromise. Circulation. 2003;107(14):e92–3. https://doi.org/10.1161/01.CIR.0000059740.00763.89.
56. Gaarder C, Jorgensen J, Magne Kolstadbraaten K, Steinar Isaksen K, Skattum J, Rimstad R, Gundem T, Holtan A, Walloe A, Pillgram-Larsen J, Aksel NP. The twin terrorist attacks in Norway on July 22, 2011: the trauma center response. J Trauma Acute Care Surg. 2012;73(1):269–75. https://doi.org/10.1097/TA.0b013e31825a787f.
57. KAMEDO report 97: The bomb attack in Oslo and the shootings at Utøya, 2011 [Internet]; 2012. [cited 2021 September 17]. https://www.socialstyrelsen.se/globalassets/sharepoint-dokument/artikelkatalog/ovrigt/2012-12-23.pdf
58. Justin GA, Baker KM, Brooks DI, Ryan DS, Weichel ED, Colyer MH. Intraocular foreign body trauma in operations Iraqi Freedom and Operation Enduring Freedom: 2002 to 2011. Ophthalmology. 2018;125(11):1675–82. https://doi.org/10.1016/j.ophtha.2018.06.006.
59. Symonds RP, Mackay C, Morley P. The late effects of granade fragments. JR Army Med Corps. 1985;131(2):68–9. https://doi.org/10.1136/jramc-131-02-03.
60. Johnston AMD, West AT, Kendrew JM, Steyn RS, Kalkat MS, Graham TR. Delayed haemoptysis from explosive device fragments. Lancet. 2013;382(9898):1152. https://doi.org/10.1016/S0140-6736(13)61651-7.
61. Bowyer GW. Management of small fragment wounds: experience from the Afghan border. J Trauma. 1996;40(3 Suppl):S170–2. https://doi.org/10.1097/00005373-199603001-00037.
62. Gaitens JM, Centeno JA, Squibb KS, Condon M, McDiarmid MA. Mobilization of metal from retain embedded fragments in a blast-injured Iraq War veteran. Mil Med. 2016;181(6):e625–9. https://doi.org/10.7205/MILMED-D-15-00432.
63. Mosheiff R, Weil Y, Khoury A, Liebergall M. The use of computerized navigation in the treatment of gunshot and shrapnel injury. Comput Aided Surg. 2004;9(1-2):39–43. https://doi.org/10.3109/10929080400006382.
64. Aylwin CJ, Konig TC, Brennan NW, Shirley PJ, Davies G, Walsh MS, Brohi K. Reduction in critical mortality in urban mass casualty incidents: analysis of triage, surge, and resource use after the London bombings on July 7, 2005. Lancet. 2006;368(9554):2219–25. https://doi.org/10.1016/S0140-6736(06)69896-6.
65. Turegano-Fuentes F, Perez-Diaz D. Medical response to the 2005 terrorist bombings in London. Lancet. 2006;368(9554):2188–9. https://doi.org/10.1016/S0140-6736(06)69871-1.
66. KAMEDO report 89: The terror attack on Bali, 2002. [Internet]; 2012. [cited 2021 September 17]. https://www.socialstyrelsen.se/globalassets/sharepoint-dokument/artikelkatalog/ovrigt/2007-123-35_200712335.pdf
67. Abbasi T, Abbasi SA. The boiling liquid expanding vapour explosion (BLEVE): mechanism, consequence assessment, management. J Hazard Mater. 2007;141(3):489–519. https://doi.org/10.1016/j.jhazmat.2006.09.056.
68. Kluger Y, Nimrod A, Biderman P, Mayo A, Sorkin P. The quinary pattern of blast injury. Am J Disaster Med. 2007;2(1):21–5.
69. Chapman LE, Sullivent EE, Grohskopf LA, Beltrami EM, Perz JF, Kretsinger K, Panlilio AL, Thompson ND, Ehrenberg RL, Gensheimer KF, Duchin JS, Kilmarx PH, Hunt RC, Centers for Disease Control and Prevention (CDC). Recommendations for postexposure interventions to prevent infection with hepatitis B virus, hepatitis C virus, or human immunodeficiency virus, and tetanus in persons wounded during bombings and other mass-casualty events—United States, 2008: recommendations of the Centers for Disease Control and Prevention (CDC). MMWR Recomm Rep. 2008;57(RR-6):1–21.
70. Ziperman HH, McGinty JB. Case report: traumatic intrathoracic tibia. J Trauma. 1964;4:400–7.

71. Lynch AF. The broken bone without a fracture: a case report. Injury. 1980;12(3):256–7. https://doi.org/10.1016/0020-1383(80)90018-2.
72. Bilinski PJ, Pawloski P, Talkowski J. Extraordinary case of shoulder trauma caused by a foreign bone. J Trauma. 1999;47(6):1148. https://doi.org/10.1097/00005373-199912000-00030.
73. Suzuki A, Nough F, Soeharno H, Jansen S. Traumatic allogenic bone implantation. Eur J Trauma Emerg Surg. 2009;35(2):190–1. https://doi.org/10.1007/s00068-008-8110-0.

Major Bleeding Management and REBOA

29

Amelia Pasley, Victoria Sharp, Jason Pasley, and Megan Brenner

29.1 Introduction

> **Learning Goals**
>
> - Discuss REBOA origins and indications for use in the trauma and non-trauma population.
> - Discuss medical management of the exsanguinating patient.
> - Describe the technique of REBOA, including deployment and removal, with associated pitfalls.

29.1.1 Epidemiology

Resuscitative Balloon Occlusion of the Aorta (REBOA) is a minimally invasive technique that can be used to temporize hemorrhage in non-compressible torso bleeding while augmenting proximal cerebral and coronary perfusion [1]. Balloon occlusion has been used for a variety of indications including hemorrhage control in the setting of ruptured aortic aneurysms [2], postpartum bleeding [3], and hypotension associated with hemorrhagic shock from all etiologies [1, 4]

29.1.1.1 History of REBOA

Temporary balloon occlusion of the aorta for aortic hemorrhage control was first described in the Korean war [5]. More recently, with advances in endovascular surgery, proximal aortic balloon occlusion became the standard of care for ruptured abdominal aortic aneurysms [6], as well as an adjunct for hemorrhage during complicated pelvic procedures and postpartum hemorrhage [7]. Other countries across the globe have published their experiences with REBOA, particularly Japan, where the resources and subspecialty training of EM physicians has provided an ideal setting for endovascular hemorrhage control [8]. Due to continued improvements in endovascular technology, REBOA use has been standardized into clinical algorithms [9], published in multiple case series [10, 11] and formal training platforms have been created [12, 13]. While REBOA has

---

A. Pasley (✉)
Michigan State University College of Osteopathic Medicine, Beaumont Farmington Hills, Farmington Hills, MI, USA
e-mail: Amelia.pasley@beaumont.org21

V. Sharp
St Joseph Mercy Hospital, Ann Arbor, MI, USA

J. Pasley
Michigan State University College of Osteopathic Medicine, McLaren Oakland Hospital, Pontiac, MI, USA
e-mail: jason.pasley@mclaren.org

M. Brenner
University of California, Riverside School of Medicine, Riverside, CA, USA
e-mail: m.brenner@ruhealth.org

been used for decades in hemorrhage control, only in the past 8 years has it become a procedure performed by acute care surgeons without formal endovascular certification.

29.1.1.2 Trauma Patients

Compressible and non-compressible torso hemorrhage have been reported to be the leading causes of preventable mortality in both civilian and military trauma casualties. As early as the mid-1980s the precursor to today's REBOA catheter, the Percluder™, was compared to Military Antishock Trousers (MAST™) in the setting of fifteen trauma cases, five ruptured abdominal aortic aneurysms, and three other unspecified sources of bleeding. The overall survival rate was 26%, including two of the trauma patients and four of the aneurysms in the setting of Percluder™ use [14]. The use of aortic balloon occlusion was abandoned due to high complication rates partially due to the large devices available at the time, and those with specific training were not immediately at the bedside. Several decades later, US military vascular surgery pioneers Dr. Todd Rasmussen and Dr. Jonathan Eliason commanded the effort to standardize and implement REBOA into clinical use for trauma [15]. The partnership between military and civilian vascular trauma surgeons lead to training and early adoption by a few trauma centers in the United States. In 2013 the first case series of REBOA use by trauma surgeons in trauma patients in the United States was published. REBOA resulted in increased blood pressure with no REBOA-related complications and no hemorrhage-related death, demonstrating that REBOA is a feasible method of hemorrhage control for both blunt and penetrating trauma [10].

29.1.1.3 Acute Care Surgery

The application of REBOA in non-trauma has been described in the literature for upper gastrointestinal hemorrhage, ruptured visceral aneurysm, hemorrhagic pancreatitis, sacral/pelvic tumor surgery, and surgical oncology cases. A natural progression of training and use of REBOA by acute care surgeons resulted in its applications for non-traumatic hemorrhage. In one series of eleven patients, most suffered from bleeding originating from ruptured visceral aneurysms or the upper GI tract. All but one patient was able to be temporized with REBOA to allow for transfer to the operating room or interventional radiology for intervention without any access complications. This demonstrated that REBOA could be performed by acute care surgeons in non-trauma patients and lead to the development of a clinical algorithm [4]. Case reports for its use in iatrogenic intra-abdominal hemorrhage have also been published, notably in the setting of visceral revascularization attempts that resulted in the dissection of the celiac artery [16]. Recently, a multi-institution experience demonstrated the use of REBOA in thirty-seven patients with acute hemorrhage from non-trauma sources. The most common indications were gastrointestinal and peripartum bleeding, however, additional sources included ruptured abdominal aortic aneurysms, ruptured splenic artery aneurysm, unknown sources of massive hemorrhage in patients in extremis, and complications of a sacral decubitus ulcer ($n =$). In the 30 cases of balloon inflation, 24 of 30 (80%) resulted in improved hemodynamics. Eleven of 30 patients (37%) died before discharge. One patient developed a distal embolism, but there were no reports of limb loss. Twelve patients (40% of all REBOAs and 63% of survivors) were discharged to home [17].

29.1.1.4 Obstetrical and Gynecologic Patients

Given the origin of hemorrhage which can be temporized by zone 3 REBOA (between the renal arteries and the aortic bifurcation), there is increasing use for this technique in peripartum hemorrhage, particularly for placental abnormalities. A case series over more than 2 years was reviewed in which pregnant women with morbidly adherent placenta undergoing elective cesarean delivery had prophylactic REBOA placement. Of the 12 patients who fell into this category, there was lower intraoperative hemorrhage and lower blood transfusion requirements compared to the control group, with all 12 surviving at 28 days, demonstrating that prophylactic use in women afflicted by morbidly adherent placenta may benefit from its use [18]. A similar study by Riazanova et al in 2021 demonstrated improved outcomes and decreased transfusion needs in the setting of REBOA for placenta accreta when used instead of open bilateral common iliac artery occlusion. In the REBOA group, there was lower blood loss, allowing for decreased transfusion needs and decreased need for hysterectomy [19]. Knowing the potential benefit of placement for placenta accreta, the question arose should REBOA catheters be placed prophylactically in these women prior to cesarean delivery? Whittington et al evaluated this possibility in 2020 with a retrospective review of patients with placenta accreta spectrum over a three-year period. They found no complications occurring in the group who had the balloon catheter inserted prophylactically but did find three of four who underwent emergent placement developed a vascular access complication that required intervention. They concluded from this data that prophylactic use of REBOA in this setting could decrease potential vascular access complications in placenta accreta patients [20]. A recent case-matched series of 17 patients described the prophylactic use of REBOA for placental disease and demonstrated reduced blood loss, decreased length of hospital stays, lower rates of ileus [21]. Thrombotic complications occurred in 11% of patients, but no limb loss or functional deficit resulted. Thrombotic complications in this population are higher than in trauma patients and are likely due to the complex and highly sophisticated coagulation cascade of pregnancy, which is not completely understood. Lower-profile devices may reduce these complications in the future.

Aortic Occlusion for Temporization of Hemorrhage from Vascular DiseaseRuptured abdominal and para-visceral aortic aneurysms have significant morbidity and mortality which has decreased over the past decades with the use of proximal aortic balloon occlusion [2]. Some case reports and systematic reviews have been completed including a recent article in 2018 European Journal of Trauma and Emergency Surgery. This study evaluated mortality and morbidity associated with REBOA in hemodynamically unstable patients due to blood loss, both traumatic and non-traumatic in etiology [22]. Fifty studies evaluated REBOA use in ruptured AAA. The mortality of ruptured AAA in these studies was 39.1%.

29.1.2 Etiology

The etiology of hemorrhage that causes shock has many sources. In the setting of trauma, examples include blunt or penetrating trauma to the thorax, abdomen, or junctional area when the injury to the extremity is too proximal to allow for tourniquet application.

Acute care surgery and vascular surgery etiologies include hemorrhagic pancreatitis, massive gastrointestinal bleeding from celiac and SMA branches, and ruptured aneurysms of the aorta and visceral arteries. Post-operative complications such as ruptured anastomoses from transplanted organs, infectious complications causing ruptured arteries, and oncologic resections have all been temporized with REBOA [4].

Obstetric and gynecologic etiologies include bleeding from placental abnormalities such as morbidly adherent placenta and placenta accrete [18–20]. REBOA can be used with or without a uterine tamponade balloon to temporize hemorrhage until embolization or surgical control of bleeding can occur.

29.1.3 Classification

Patients in extremis from non-compressible torso hemorrhage can be classified by the four stages of hemorrhagic shock.

29.1.3.1 Hemorrhagic Shock

The four stages of hemorrhagic shock as classified by the American College of Surgeons are divided into four classes which are based on heart rate, blood pressure, pulse pressure, respiratory rate, mental status, and urine output [23]. These factors combine to indicate the volume of blood loss and what resuscitative fluids will be required.

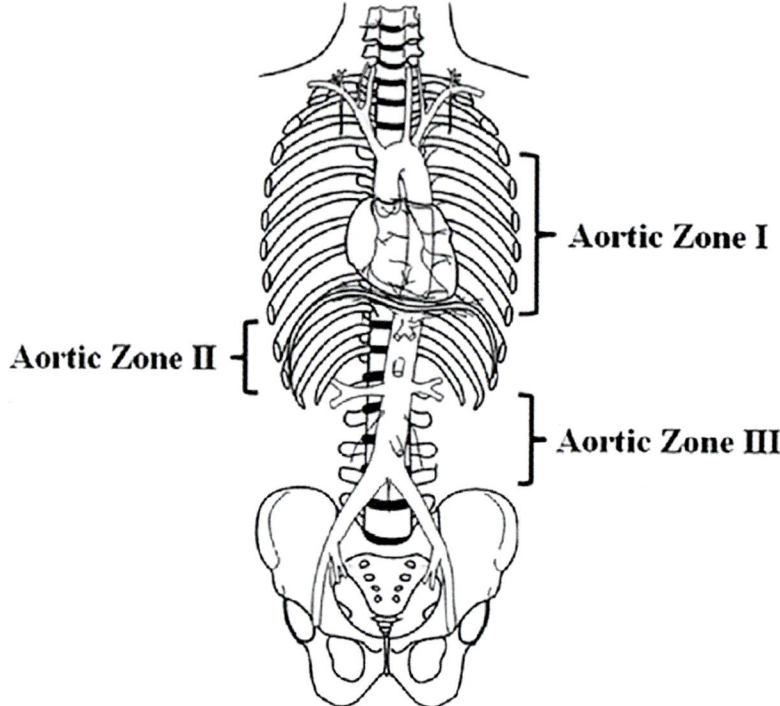

Fig. 29.1 Zone 1 is the descending thoracic aorta between the origin of the left subclavian artery to the celiac trunk. Zone 2 is the celiac trunk to the lowest renal artery and is a not used/"no-occlusion" zone. Zone 3 is the infrarenal abdominal aorta between the lowest renal artery to the aortic bifurcation. The decision on which zone to place the REBOA is determined by chest x-ray, FAST examination, and the presence of pelvic fractures in hypotensive patients. When the FAST is positive, the REBOA should be positioned in zone 1. If the FAST is negative but there is suspicion of pelvic hemorrhage, a pelvic x-ray should be obtained. If the pelvic x-ray shows concern for fractures, in a patient who is hypotensive the REBOA should be placed in zone 3 [15]

29.1.4 Pathophysiology

While the etiology of hemorrhagic shock can vary as listed above, the pathophysiology of hemorrhagic shock is the same. Its management depends on the cause and location of the bleeding. In regard to REBOA use, there are three thoracoabdominal zones that are important for the appropriate application of the aortic occlusion balloon, as described by Stannard et al [15]. These are listed here.

Abdominal zones

- Zone 1
  - From the left subclavian artery to the celiac trunk
- Zone 2
  - Celiac trunk to the lowest renal artery (this zone is not used)
- Zone 3
  - From lowest renal artery to aortic bifurcation (Fig. 29.1).

29.2 Diagnosis

29.2.1 Clinical Presentation

Hemorrhagic shock is the most common cause of preventable death after injury [24]. Shock secondary to blood loss is most likely to occur in the second phase of the trimodal distribution of death and rapid hemorrhage control is crucial to alter patient morbidity and mortality. Mortality rates during the "golden hour" of trauma intervention historically noted to be approximately 60% with a preventable death rate nearing 35% have been substantially decreased to <10% with rapid assessment and intervention in these life-threatening scenarios [24].

The patient's clinical presentation may vary from an obvious traumatic amputation with frank bleeding to concealed bleeding within the thorax, abdominal cavity, or pelvis. Mental status changes may range from anxiousness to coma. Depending on the stage of shock, tachycardia is typically present. Bradycardia may be seen before the catastrophic cardiovascular collapse.

29.2.2 Tests

While hemorrhagic shock is more of a clinical diagnosis based on examination, there are crucial laboratory and imaging supplements that can assist in diagnosing sources of hemorrhage. Complete blood count for hemoglobin and platelet levels provides information about baseline values. The lethal triad consists of hypothermia, acidosis, and coagulopathy, all of which can lead to worsening morbidity and mortality. Laboratories evaluating for coagulopathy should be ordered such as PT, INR, PTT, and Fibrinogen. Thromboelastography in the form of ROTEM or TEG has emerged that evaluates clot strength, duration, and breakdown, allowing for more specific transfusion guidance.

Imaging modalities also assist in the diagnosis and management of hemorrhagic shock, including chest x-ray, pelvis x-ray, and Focused Abdominal Sonography for Trauma (FAST) ultrasound exams, all of which can be done in the trauma bay or at the bedside. In stable patients, CT scans can also be used for further evaluation of these patients, especially in regard to areas not well-visualized by plain films and ultrasound, such as the retroperitoneum.

> **Differential Diagnosis—Based on Zone**
> Five places account for the majority of major blood loss and include the thorax, the abdomen, pelvic fractures, long bones, and external blood loss [24]. Advances in community outreach programs such as the Stop the Bleed campaign and tourniquet application have helped immensely with external blood loss sources and long bone fractures. Resuscitative Endovascular Balloon Occlusion of the Aorta (REBOA) has evolved as a less invasive method of hemorrhage control for the thorax, abdomen, pelvis, and even proximal lower extremities.
>
> Differential diagnoses for bleeding are based on what zone the hemorrhage is coming from. Picture 1 demonstrates each of the zones for REBOA and understanding the anatomy is critical for the appropriate placement of the balloon. Zone 1 is located at the distal thoracic aorta and is occluded for intra-abdominal or retroperitoneal hemorrhage [15] and in the setting of traumatic arrest [25, 26]. Zone 2 contains the renal arteries and should be avoided during balloon occlusion. Zone 3 is located at the distal abdominal aorta and can be occluded for bleeding in the pelvis or proximal lower extremities that are not controllable with a tourniquet application [26].

29.3 Treatment

29.3.1 Medical Treatment

A multi-modal approach to hemorrhage control is necessary and begins with blood component therapy, consideration of whole blood transfusion (if available) reversal of any coagulopathy, and administration of tranexamic acid.

Current blood transfusion therapy is based on the PROPPR trial, with the administration of plasma, platelets, and red blood cells in a 1:1:1 ratio because hemostasis was achieved more rapidly with fewer deaths due to exsanguination at 24 h [27].

Whole blood transfusions have been used in the military with success and this has similarly been shown in the civilian literature with improved hemostasis and trauma bay mortality [28].

The combination of TXA with blood component-based resuscitation has been shown in the military to result in the improvement of coagulopathy and a survival benefit, particularly in patients requiring massive transfusion [29].

Additional studies have shown some promise with use in civilian trauma. further randomized clinical trials can help identify the subset of trauma patients who may benefit from TXA administration [30].

29.3.2 Surgical Treatment of Hemorrhage

Surgical treatment of hemorrhage includes both initial temporization methods as well as definitive management. A joint statement from the American College of Surgeons Committee on Trauma (ACS COT) and the American College of Emergency Physicians (ACEP) was made with recommendations regarding the application of REBOA [31]. It is indicated for a variety of trauma patients with either known life-threatening hemorrhage below the diaphragm or those suspected of it, who transiently or do not respond to resuscitation, in the setting of profound refractory shock or during arrest [13]. Recommendations from the statement stress the importance of using REBOA for short periods of time, and only where definitive control of bleeding can occur (Fig. 29.2).

The catheter has a curved P-tip that protects the vessel lumen as the catheter is inserted. There is an arterial line port that allows for blood pressure monitoring, a balloon lumen that is inflated once the catheter is appropriately positioned, and two radiopaque markers on either side of the balloon that allow it to be seen more easily via radiography. A peel-away sheath is used for ease of insertion into the dilator. The ER-REBOA™ catheter has been recently replaced by the ER-REBOA PLUS™. The newer catheter is able to be exchanged over a guidewire and has a tag attached to document inflation volume and time, as well as insertion distance.

The procedure begins by obtaining common femoral artery access, either percutaneously or via cutdown onto the vessel. Cutdown may allow for more rapid access in those patients who do not have a palpable pulse. Placing a common femoral arterial line in patients who are at risk for hemorrhagic shock or with unstable physiology allows for a more rapid transition to a REBOA catheter. More importantly, the line transduces a more accurate blood pressure than a standard extremity cuff which is critical to guide resuscitation in unstable patients. This femoral arterial line can then be upsized to a 7 French sheath for REBOA insertion. It is then necessary to measure the catheter length for placement and document this to allow for monitoring of catheter migration during transport and continued care. If the goal is zone 1 insertion, the catheter should be measured from the insertion site to the level of the sternal notch and for zone 3 the catheter is measured to the xiphoid process. Insertion distances and inflation volumes vary significantly between patients, therefore external landmarks are used [32]. The balloon should be completely deflated by pulling on the syringe attached for five seconds and the stopcock closed to hold vacuum suction [13]. In earlier iterations of the catheter, it is necessary to slide the peel-away sheath over the balloon, and in newer versions, the sheath is in place over the balloon when the kit is opened. The arterial line should be flushed. The sheath should be inserted into the valve approximately 5 mm and the blue catheter advanced, removing the sheath after the balloon is felt to pass the valve [13]. Prior to the inflation of the balloon, a chest x-ray or fluoroscopy should be used to confirm the position of the radiopaque markers. In the case of traumatic cardiac arrest, CPR should not be paused for

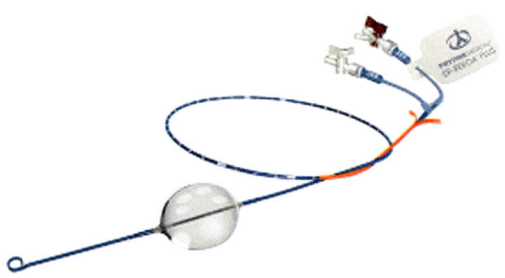

Fig. 29.2 ER-REBOA PLUS™ catheter. Photo courtesy of Prytime Medical, Borne, TX

radiographic confirmation, this can be obtained if/once the patient regains spontaneous circulation [25]. After proper positioning is ensured the balloon can be inflated, and monitoring for blood pressure changes/improvement on the arterial waveform indicates proper arterial occlusion [13]. The time that the balloon is inflated should be noted to prevent prolonged inflation. To prevent end-organ ischemia and other complications associated with prolonged balloon insufflation, it is recommended that zone 1 REBOA be inflated no longer than 30 min and zone 3 no longer than 60 min [24, 33–35]. The catheter should be secured well to prevent complications associated with shear injury or catheter migration and the patient should be immediately transported to the location where definitive hemorrhage can occur. Clear documentation should be made of the time of catheter insertion, duration of balloon inflation throughout the patient's course, and mean arterial pressure (MAP) prior to and after inflation.

It is important to remember that REBOA insertion is not a definitive hemorrhage control procedure, but a temporizing measure to allow further resuscitation and transfer of the patient to operative and/or interventional hemostasis As long as the sheath remains in place the access groin should remain in full extension with hourly neurovascular checks of the bilateral lower extremities. After hemorrhage control is obtained definitively, the catheter should be removed as early as possible to prevent thrombogenic complications and direct pressure held at the access site for no fewer than 30 min. Prior to removal, the balloon should be completely deflated by turning the three-way stopcock and slowly removing the saline while closely monitoring the blood pressure changes. Communication with anesthesia is critical prior to balloon deflation, and the resuscitation strategy should prepare for reperfusion injury both in the immediate operative period and beyond.

29.3.2.1 Timing

Translational research suggests that inflation of the balloon for up to 60 min in zone 1 and for 90 min in zone 3 is survivable, and preliminary data suggest that zone occlusion times of less than 60 min appear to be tolerated in most patients [1, 36]. The ACS statement has listed specific criteria for the duration of aortic occlusion based on extrapolation from rAAA experience, clinical and translational data, and expert opinion. Attempts to lengthen the time limits for occlusion while minimizing distal ischemia have led to the development of partial REBOA in which the balloon is deflated slightly, allowing some blood flow past the balloon occlusion for some perfusion, while maintaining target pressures above the balloon [37, 38].

Translational and clinical data is sparse for the use of partial REBOA, and its benefit has not been uniformly demonstrated [39].

29.3.2.2 Complications

Access and procedural complications are not unique to REBOA and can be usually correlated with specific steps of the procedures. Systemic complications result from the complex sequelae of ischemia and subsequent reperfusion.

Access complications can be potentially limb-threatening, depending on the location of the access site as well as the duration of aortic occlusion and/or in-dwelling sheath [40]. Ideal arterial access for the femoral sheath is in the common femoral artery (CFA) due to its diameter, as more distal cannulation in the superficial femoral artery (SFA) has a higher risk of arterial thrombosis due to the smaller caliber of the vessel. If access is placed too proximal into the external iliac artery, uncontrolled, non-compressible bleeding can ensue after sheath removal. Therefore, the preferred method for successful, accurate sheath placement into the CFA should occur with ultrasound guidance, open cutdown, or using anatomic landmarks.

Balloon malposition and rupture can occur due to improper initial positioning or migration of the device [41]. Depending on the location of the balloon and the degree of inflation, this can cause significant complications. If the balloon is placed too proximal in the proximal aortic arch or heart, this can cause excessive ventricular afterload, occlusion of aortic arch, or occlusion of cardiac vessels. If the device has cannulated one of the vessels off of the arch, inflation can lead to vessel rupture and ischemia. Distally, inflation in the ipsilateral iliac artery can result in balloon rupture. Over inflation in any position can lead to balloon or arterial rupture as well as local vascular injury. Catheter malposition can occur leading to inadvertent cannulation of branch vessels. This can be rapidly identified and corrected by imaging after insertion, and prior to inflation.

Sheath management is a key component in limiting complications for REBOA. Removal should be done as soon as possible, once hemostasis is obtained and coagulopathy improved. Smaller sheaths are noted to have fewer complications even when left in place for twenty-four hours, however expert opinion recommends removing them as soon as possible to avoid any issues with limiting flow to the extremity. Arterial thrombus has been noted on the catheter and clot through the side port of even small sheaths, therefore some authors recommend on-table femoral angiography prior to sheath removal [37]. Prior to sheath removal, negative pressure can be held through the side port in attempt to remove any possible clot. Upon sheath removal, palpation of a distal pulse in the ipsilateral leg must be noted. This should be compared to the contralateral side as well. Any discrepancy should be concerning, and further investigation should be undertaken. An angiogram or exploration and thrombectomy should be considered. A groin duplex ultrasound is recommended 24–48 h from sheath removal, to check for any evidence of pseudoaneurysm or other local site complications. Limb loss after REBOA has been reported, but amputations are attributable to the initial traumatic mechanism in these polytrauma patients [42, 43].

In multi-institutional trials in the United States, REBOA has demonstrated improved survival from the time of Emergency room evaluation to discharge when compared to the emergency resuscitative thoracotomy in the setting of trauma patients who have not had a cardiac arrest [1].

Access complications such as thrombosis and outcomes have significantly improved with the introduction of lower-profile devices [44]. Newly FDA-approved balloon catheters compatible with 4Fr introducer sheaths may improve the safety profile of REBOA in the future [44]

Systemic complications with REBOA are not a direct cause and likely expected sequelae of a combination of factors including hemorrhagic shock, aortic occlusion, and reperfusion ischemia. One AORTA study demonstrated only a 4.3% rate of AKI in the 46 patients who received REBOA [45]. With the continued adoption of REBOA, higher rates of AKI are being reported. Physiologically it is known that reduction of antegrade flow by AO at zone 1 reduces visceral perfusion, specifically renal blood flow by up to 94%, and results in AKI [46]. Animal models of hemorrhagic shock have demonstrated that the renal arteries are the most sensitive to flow reduction, never returning to baseline even after hours of reperfusion [47]. Early studies of patients undergoing aortic surgery estimate transient renal dysfunction rates of up to 35% with AO at zone 1 but only 10% at zone 3 [47, 48]. This argues for a more complex pathophysiology of AKI than simply reduction of inflow, compounded by profound hemorrhagic shock. Potential additional insults contributing to renal dysfunction in patients with REBOA include CT scanning using IV contrast, the use of IV contrast for angiography during procedures for hemostasis, and medications. Renal protection strategies used during aortic surgery include sodium bicarbonate, mannitol, crystalloid resuscitation, vasopressors, and others [49, 50], but these agents have not been studied in REBOA patients.

The rate of ARDS has also increased substantially with the increased use of REBOA [1, 45]. It is unclear whether survival bias plays a role in the incidence of this or any other complication. It is known that multiple factors contribute to pulmonary dysfunction after AO, including the release of thromboxane, leukocyte priming and activation, complement C3 and C5 activation, and TNF synthesis. The end products of these pathways may have direct and indirect effects on the lungs [51].

One of the many currently unanswered questions regarding REBOA is the safe duration of AO in trauma patients. While recommendations exist based on elective aortic surgery data, conclusive evidence to support AO duration does not exist in trauma patients. Clinical studies have demonstrated the duration of AO at zone 1 to be between 20 and 74 minutes [45], but no direct correlation with mortality has been demonstrated at any time period. A study of elective aortic abdominal aneurysm repairs demonstrated that durations of AO beyond 90 min were associated with higher mortality [52]. The second edition of the joint clinical statement lead by the American College of Surgeons Committee on Trauma recommends a maximum target occlusion time at zone 1 of 30 min, and at zone 3 of 60 min in order to reduce complications [26]. These durations of AO may be lengthened by partial or intermittent occlusion strategies; however, no clinical data exists to direct this practice.

Propensity-score matching has been used to examine complications in patients who have received REBOA. More recent studies from Japan have demonstrated that with a more refined study design, outcomes with the use of REBOA are superior to no REBOA [53, 54]. NTDB data in the United States has demonstrated that limb amputations originally linked to REBOA patients are attributed to initial injury rather than REBOA [42]. Further studies with REBOA-specific data points are required to help determine the optimal use for this procedure in trauma [55].

Pearls Do's and Don'ts

- Hold the catheter securely before, during, and after inflation to prevent migration and intimal shear injury of the vessel.
- Remove all fluid and air from the balloon prior to removal. If stuck, insert the balloon past the sheath and apply negative pressure to the balloon rather than pulling the catheter and sheath out together (which risks causing further damage to the arteriotomy).
- Remove the catheter and sheath, not necessarily at the same time, but as soon as possible to reduce complications.
- Check distal pulses via Doppler if needed to rule out distal thromboembolism

Take-Home Messages

- REBOA can be used to temporize abdominal, pelvic, and junctional bleeding from multiple etiologies
- Replacement of blood products and a balanced strategy is a key adjunct to surgical temporization and definitive management of bleeding
- Rapid transport of patients to definitive hemostasis is critical to reduce complications associated with hemorrhagic shock after aortic occlusion

Multiple Choice Questions

1. Which patient would be least likely to benefit from REBOA insertion?
   A. A 24-year-old female has delivered a baby and becomes hypotensive with persistent vaginal bleeding uncontrolled by medical management in post-partum.
   B. A 78-year-old male who presents after motor vehicle collision with a seatbelt sign, hypotension, and a positive abdominal FAST examination is a non-responder to fluids.
   C. A 30-year-old hypotensive male with an open fracture of the right femur that has non-compressible arterial bleeding noted from the wound.
   D. A 60-year-old female who feel from her horse with complaints of significant pelvic pain, an open book pelvic fracture, and tachycardia unresponsive to blood transfusion.

Answer to 1: C
REBOA can be used in all hemorrhagic shock that occurs as a result of bleeding in the chest, abdomen, pelvis, and even proximal lower extremities. In this patient with a lower extremity open fracture, a tourniquet would be a faster and more effective method of hemorrhage control.

2. For balloon placement in zone 1, where should the P-tip be measured prior to insertion at what external anatomic location?
   A. The xiphoid process.
   B. The sternal notch.
   C. The umbilicus.
   D. The pelvic brim.

Answer to 2: B

The sternal notch

3. Which step is not necessary prior to balloon inflation?
   A. Confirm balloon location with a chest x-ray or fluoroscopy, or manually in a patient in arrest.
   B. Measure the catheter length prior to insertion at the external anatomic location based on the zone.
   C. Secure the catheter.
   D. Flush the arterial line port.

Answer to 3: A

Confirmation of catheter placement can be delayed until after ROSC has occurred if the procedure was without difficulty. CPR should be continued throughout the REBOA procedure and after inflation until ROSC occurs.

4. Based on the ACS-COT recommendations, which of the below is NOT a criterion to place REBOA?
   A. The catheter should be inserted by an Acute Care Surgeon, and Interventional Radiologist, or a Vascular Surgeon trained in REBOA.
   B. REBOA should only be deployed if surgical intervention is immediately available.
   C. REBOA may be used if there is a concern for hemorrhage below the diaphragm.
   D. REBOA may be placed without prior training in REBOA insertion.

Answer to 4: D

The ACS-COT recommends that Acute Care Surgeons and Interventionalists (Interventional Radiology or Vascular Surgery) who have been trained in REBOA are eligible to insert it. They also recommend that EM physicians with additional critical care medicine training and REBOA training are also eligible. It should only be deployed if immediate surgical intervention is available and is indicated in the setting of hemorrhage below the diaphragm.

5. Which of the following is a true statement?
   A. Cutdown onto the common femoral artery is a viable alternative to the percutaneous approach.
   B. REBOA has replaced resuscitative thoracotomy in unstable trauma patients.
   C. If the catheter does not come out with initial attempts, pull harder.
   D. Zone 2 is safe for balloon inflation.

Answer to 5: A

Cutdown is a viable alternative to percutaneous common femoral artery access and may be more successful in the setting of cardiac arrest or profound shock where pulses can be difficult to palpate. REBOA has not replaced ED thoracotomy but is a non-inferior alternative for unstable patients with exsanguination from below the diaphragm. Pulling harder when feeling resistance during removal can lead to disruption of the vessel wall and irreparable damage. Zone 2 is where the renal arteries lie and balloon insufflation in this area should be avoided.

6. Which of the following is FALSE?
   A. REBOA is a definitive management for hemorrhage control.
   B. Zone 1 REBOA should be inflated no longer than 30 min.
   C. Zone 3 REBOA should be inflated no longer than 60 min.
   D. REBOA catheters should be removed as soon as clinically able.

Answer to 6: A

REBOA is NOT a definitive management for hemorrhage control. It is a temporizing measure to get the patient to a more definitive intervention like Interventional Radiology or the Operating room. The balloon should be inflated no longer than 30 min in zone 1 and 60 min in zone 2. REBOA catheters are theoretically thrombogenic and should be removed as soon as able.

7. The following is TRUE with regards to REBOA use in Gynecologic patients:
   A. There is no difference in transfusion needs with REBOA vs open bilateral iliac artery occlusion in the setting of extensive placenta accreta.
   B. Consideration of prophylactic REBOA placement for placenta accreta may decrease vascular access complications.
   C. There is no indication of its use in morbidly adherent placenta.
   D. There is no difference in hysterectomy rates when using REBOA over open bilateral iliac artery occlusion in the setting of extensive placenta accreta.

Answer to 7: B

Whittington et al in 2020 demonstrated increased vascular access-associated injury when REBOA was placed emergently over prophylactically in the setting of placenta accreta spectrum. REBOA has demonstrated decreased hysterectomy rates and transfusion rates in the setting of placenta accreta over open bilateral iliac artery occlusion and improved transfusion rates in the morbidly adherent placenta.

8. What is the recommended maximum occlusion time for zone 1?
   A. 30 min
   B. 60 min
   C. 90 min
   D. Until hypotension is resolved

Answer to 8: A

When deciding which zone to place the REBOA which of the following is false?
9. It is highly recommended to obtain a chest x-ray prior to placement
   A. If the FAST exam is a positive place in zone 3 even if the SBP does not increase after AO
   B. In a hypotensive patient who's FAST is negative obtain pelvic x-rays to rule out fractures
   C. Zone 2 is ideally a "no-occlusion" zone

Answer to 9: B

The initial FAST exam can be falsely negative. If a patient with a mechanism consistent with possible abdominal hemorrhage does not respond to AO at zone 3, deflate the balloon and inflate at zone 1.

10. REBOA has shown feasibility for hemorrhage control in which patient population(s)?
    A. Gynecologic
    B. Acute Care Surgery
    C. Trauma
    D. All of the above

Answer to 10: D

References

1. Brenner M, Inaba K, Aiolfi A, et al. Resuscitative endovascular balloon occlusion of the aorta and resuscitative thoracotomy in select patients with hemorrhagic shock: early results from the american association for the surgery of trauma's aortic occlusion in resuscitation for trauma and acute care surgery registry [published correction appears in J Am Coll Surg. 2018 Oct;227(4):484]. J Am Coll Surg. 2018;226(5):730–40. https://doi.org/10.1016/j.jamcollsurg.2018.01.044.
2. Mayer D, Pfammatter T, Rancic Z, et al. 10 years of emergency endovascular aneurysm repair for ruptured abdominal aortoiliac aneurysms: lessons learned. Ann Surg. 2009;249(3):510–5. https://doi.org/10.1097/SLA.0b013e31819a8b65.
3. Manzano-Nunez R, Escobar-Vidarte MF, Orlas CP, et al. Resuscitative endovascular balloon occlusion of the aorta deployed by acute care surgeons in patients with morbidly adherent placenta: a feasible

solution for two lives in peril. World J Emerg Surg. 2018;13:44. Published 2018 Sep 24. https://doi.org/10.1186/s13017-018-0205-2.
4. Hoehn MR, Hansraj NZ, Pasley AM, et al. Resuscitative endovascular balloon occlusion of the aorta for non-traumatic intra-abdominal hemorrhage. Eur J Trauma Emerg Surg. 2019;45(4):713–8. https://doi.org/10.1007/s00068-018-0973-0.
5. Hughes CW. Use of intra-aortic balloon catheter tamponade for controlling intra-abdominal hemorrhage in man. Surgery 1954 Jul;36(1):65-58.
6. Greenberg RK, Srivastava SD, Ouriel K, et al. An endoluminal method of hemorrhage control and repair of ruptured abdominal aortic aneurysms. J Endovasc Ther. 2000;7(1):1–7. https://doi.org/10.1177/152660280000700101.
7. Varga S. Resuscitative Endovascular Balloon Occlusion of the Aorta (REBOA). In: Scalea TM, editor. The shock trauma manual of operative techniques. Springer; 2021. p. 499–517.
8. Shoji T, Tarui T, Igarashi T, et al. Resuscitative endovascular balloon occlusion of the aorta using a low-profile device is easy and safe for emergency physicians in cases of life-threatening hemorrhage. J Emerg Med. 2018;54(4):410–8. https://doi.org/10.1016/j.jemermed.2017.12.044.
9. Tran TL, Brasel KJ, Karmy-Jones R, et al. Western trauma association critical decisions in trauma: management of pelvic fracture with hemodynamic instability-2016 updates. J Trauma Acute Care Surg. 2016;81(6):1171–4. https://doi.org/10.1097/TA.0000000000001230.
10. Brenner ML, Moore LJ, DuBose JJ, et al. A clinical series of resuscitative endovascular balloon occlusion of the aorta for hemorrhage control and resuscitation. J Trauma Acute Care Surg. 2013;75(3):506–11. https://doi.org/10.1097/TA.0b013e31829e5416.
11. Moore LJ, Martin CD, Harvin JA, Wade CE, Holcomb JB. Resuscitative endovascular balloon occlusion of the aorta for control of noncompressible truncal hemorrhage in the abdomen and pelvis. Am J Surg. 2016;212(6):1222–30. https://doi.org/10.1016/j.amjsurg.2016.09.027.
12. Villamaria CY, Eliason JL, Napolitano LM, Stansfield RB, Spencer JR, Rasmussen TE. Endovascular Skills for Trauma and Resuscitative Surgery (ESTARS) course: curriculum development, content validation, and program assessment. J Trauma Acute Care Surg. 2014;76(4):929–36. https://doi.org/10.1097/TA.0000000000000164.
13. Brenner M, Hoehn M, Pasley J, Dubose J, Stein D, Scalea T. Basic endovascular skills for trauma course: bridging the gap between endovascular techniques and the acute care surgeon. J Trauma Acute Care Surg. 2014;77(2):286–91. https://doi.org/10.1097/TA.0000000000000310.
14. Low RB, Longmore W, Rubinstein R, Flores L, Wolvek S. Preliminary report on the use of the Percluder occluding aortic balloon in human beings. Ann Emerg Med. 1986;15(12):1466–9. https://doi.org/10.1016/s0196-0644(86)80945-3.
15. Stannard A, Eliason JL, Rasmussen TE. Resuscitative endovascular balloon occlusion of the aorta (REBOA) as an adjunct for hemorrhagic shock. J Trauma. 2011;71(6):1869–72. https://doi.org/10.1097/TA.0b013e31823fe90c.
16. Goodenough CJ, Cobb TA, Holcomb JB. Use of REBOA to stabilize in-hospital iatrogenic intra-abdominal hemorrhage. Trauma Surg Acute Care Open. 2018;3(1):e000165. Published 2018 Oct 1. https://doi.org/10.1136/tsaco-2018-000165.
17. Hatchimonji JS, Chipman AM, McGreevy DT, et al. Resuscitative endovascular balloon occlusion of aaorta use in nontrauma emergency general surgery: a multi-institutional experience. J Surg Res. 2020;256:149–55. https://doi.org/10.1016/j.jss.2020.06.034.
18. Ordoñez CA, Manzano-Nunez R, Parra MW, et al. Prophylactic use of resuscitative endovascular balloon occlusion of the aorta in women with abnormal placentation: A systematic review, meta-analysis, and case series. J Trauma Acute Care Surg. 2018;84(5):809–18. https://doi.org/10.1097/TA.0000000000001821.
19. Riazanova OV, Reva VA, Fox KA, et al. Open versus endovascular REBOA control of blood loss during cesarean delivery in the placenta accreta spectrum: a single-center retrospective case control study. Eur J Obstet Gynecol Reprod Biol. 2021;258:23–8. https://doi.org/10.1016/j.ejogrb.2020.12.022.
20. Whittington JR, Pagan ME, Nevil BD, et al. Risk of vascular complications in prophylactic compared to emergent resuscitative endovascular balloon occlusion of the aorta (REBOA) in the management of placenta accreta spectrum [published online ahead of print, 2020 Aug 11]. J Matern Fetal Neonatal Med. 2020:1–4. https://doi.org/10.1080/14767058.2020.1802717.
21. Burriss S et al. TSACO 2021 in press, awaiting details will get complete reference
22. Borger van der Burg BLS, van Dongen TTCF, Morrison JJ, et al. A systematic review and meta-analysis of the use of resuscitative endovascular balloon occlusion of the aorta in the management of major exsanguination. Eur J Trauma Emerg Surg. 2018;44(4):535–50. https://doi.org/10.1007/s00068-018-0959-y.
23. Advanced trauma life support: student course manual. 10th ed. American College of Surgeons, p. 49; 2018.
24. Mattox KL, Feliciano DV, Moore EE. Trauma. New York: Appleton & Lange; 2000. p. 157.
25. Brenner M, Moore L, Dubose J, Scalea T. Resuscitative endovascular balloon occlusion of the aorta (REBOA) for use in temporizing intra-abdominal and pelvic hemorrhage: physiologic sequelae and considerations. Shock. 2020;54(5):615–22. https://doi.org/10.1097/SHK.0000000000001542.
26. Bulger EM, Perina DG, Qasim Z, et al. Clinical use of resuscitative endovascular balloon occlusion of the aorta (REBOA) in civilian trauma systems in

the USA, 2019: a joint statement from the American College of Surgeons Committee on Trauma, the American College of Emergency Physicians, the National Association of Emergency Medical Services Physicians and the National Association of Emergency Medical Technicians. Trauma Surg Acute Care Open. 2019;4(1):e000376. Published 2019 Sep 20. https://doi.org/10.1136/tsaco-2019-000376.

27. Holcomb JB, Tilley BC, Baraniuk S, et al. Transfusion of plasma, platelets, and red blood cells in a 1:1:1 vs a 1:1:2 ratio and mortality in patients with severe trauma: the PROPPR randomized clinical trial. JAMA. 2015;313(5):471–82. https://doi.org/10.1001/jama.2015.12.

28. Hazelton JP, Cannon JW, Zatorski C, et al. Cold-stored whole blood: a better method of trauma resuscitation? J Trauma Acute Care Surg. 2019;87(5):1035–41. https://doi.org/10.1097/TA.0000000000002471.

29. Morrison JJ, Dubose JJ, Rasmussen TE, Midwinter MJ. Military application of tranexamic acid in trauma emergency resuscitation (MATTERs) study. Arch Surg. 2012;147(2):113–9. https://doi.org/10.1001/archsurg.2011.287.

30. Khan M, Jehan F, Bulger EM, et al. Severely injured trauma patients with admission hyperfibrinolysis: Is there a role of tranexamic acid? Findings from the PROPPR trial. J Trauma Acute Care Surg. 2018;85(5):851–7. https://doi.org/10.1097/TA.0000000000002022.

31. Brenner M, Bulger EM, Perina DG, et al. Joint statement from the American College of Surgeons Committee on Trauma (ACS COT) and the American College of Emergency Physicians (ACEP) regarding the clinical use of Resuscitative Endovascular Balloon Occlusion of the Aorta (REBOA). Trauma Surg Acute Care Open. 2018;3(1):e000154. Published 2018 Jan 13. https://doi.org/10.1136/tsaco-2017-000154.

32. Meyer DE, Mont MT, Harvin JA, Kao LS, Wade CE, Moore LJ. Catheter distances and balloon inflation volumes for the ER-REBOA catheter: a prospective analysis. Am J Surg. 2020;219(1):140–4. https://doi.org/10.1016/j.amjsurg.2019.04.019.

33. Reva VA, Matsumura Y, Hörer T, et al. Resuscitative endovascular balloon occlusion of the aorta: what is the optimum occlusion time in an ovine model of hemorrhagic shock? Eur J Trauma Emerg Surg. 2018;44(4):511–8. https://doi.org/10.1007/s00068-016-0732-z.

34. Kauvar DS, Dubick MA, Martin MJ. Large animal models of proximal aortic balloon occlusion in traumatic hemorrhage: review and identification of knowledge gaps relevant to expanded use. J Surg Res. 2019;236:247–58. https://doi.org/10.1016/j.jss.2018.11.038.

35. Bekdache O, Paradis T, Shen YBH, et al. Resuscitative endovascular balloon occlusion of the aorta (REBOA): indications: advantages and challenges of implementation in traumatic non-compressible torso hemorrhage. Trauma Surg Acute Care Open. 2019;4(1):e000262. Published 2019 Apr 15. https://doi.org/10.1136/tsaco-2018-000262.

36. Ribeiro Junior MAF, Feng CYD, Nguyen ATM, et al. The complications associated with Resuscitative Endovascular Balloon Occlusion of the Aorta (REBOA). World J Emerg Surg. 2018;13:20. Published 2018 May 11. https://doi.org/10.1186/s13017-018-0181-6.

37. DuBose JJ. How I do it: Partial resuscitative endovascular balloon occlusion of the aorta (P-REBOA). J Trauma Acute Care Surg. 2017;83(1):197–9. https://doi.org/10.1097/TA.0000000000001462.

38. Johnson MA, Neff LP, Williams TK, DuBose JJ, EVAC Study Group. Partial resuscitative balloon occlusion of the aorta (P-REBOA): clinical technique and rationale. J Trauma Acute Care Surg. 2016;81(5 Suppl 2):S133–7. Proceedings of the 2015 Military Health System Research Symposium. https://doi.org/10.1097/TA.0000000000001146.

39. Russo RM, Neff LP, Lamb CM, et al. Partial resuscitative endovascular balloon occlusion of the aorta in swine model of hemorrhagic shock. J Am Coll Surg. 2016;223(2):359–68. https://doi.org/10.1016/j.jamcollsurg.2016.04.037.

40. Taylor JR 3rd, Harvin JA, Martin C, Holcomb JB, Moore LJ. Vascular complications from resuscitative endovascular balloon occlusion of the aorta: life over limb? J Trauma Acute Care Surg. 2017;83(1 Suppl 1):S120–3. https://doi.org/10.1097/TA.0000000000001514.

41. Davidson AJ, Russo RM, Reva VA, et al. The pitfalls of resuscitative endovascular balloon occlusion of the aorta: Risk factors and mitigation strategies [published correction appears in J Trauma Acute Care Surg. 2018 Mar;84(3):544]. J Trauma Acute Care Surg. 2018;84(1):192–202. https://doi.org/10.1097/TA.0000000000001711.

42. Levin SR, Farber A, Burke PA, et al. The majority of major amputations after resuscitative endovascular balloon occlusion of the aorta are associated with preadmission trauma [published online ahead of print, 2021 Feb 4]. J Vasc Surg. 2021:S0741-5214(21)00168-3. https://doi.org/10.1016/j.jvs.2020.12.107.

43. Wasicek PJ, Teeter WA, Yang S, et al. Life over limb: lower extremity ischemia in the setting of resuscitative endovascular balloon occlusion of the aorta (REBOA). Am Surg. 2018;84(6):971–7.

44. Power A, Parekh A, Scallan O, et al. Size matters: first-in-human study of a novel 4 French REBOA device. Trauma Surg Acute Care Open. 2021;6(1):e000617. Published 2021 Jan 8. https://doi.org/10.1136/tsaco-2020-000617.

45. DuBose JJ, Scalea TM, Brenner M, et al. The AAST prospective Aortic Occlusion for Resuscitation in Trauma and Acute Care Surgery (AORTA) registry: data on contemporary utilization and outcomes of aortic occlusion and resuscitative balloon occlusion of the aorta (REBOA). J Trauma Acute Care

46. Gelman S. The pathophysiology of aortic cross-clamping and unclamping. Anesthesiology. 1995;82(4):1026–60. https://doi.org/10.1097/00000542-199504000-00027.
47. Hoehn MR, Teeter WA, Morrison JJ, et al. Aortic branch vessel flow during resuscitative endovascular balloon occlusion of the aorta. J Trauma Acute Care Surg. 2019;86(1):79–85. https://doi.org/10.1097/TA.0000000000002075.
48. Dubois L, Durant C, Harrington DM, Forbes TL, Derose G, Harris JR. Technical factors are strongest predictors of postoperative renal dysfunction after open transperitoneal juxtarenal abdominal aortic aneurysm repair. J Vasc Surg. 2013;57(3):648–54. https://doi.org/10.1016/j.jvs.2012.09.043.
49. Yeung KK, Groeneveld M, Lu JJ, van Diemen P, Jongkind V, Wisselink W. Organ protection during aortic cross-clamping. Best Pract Res Clin Anaesthesiol. 2016;30(3):305–15. https://doi.org/10.1016/j.bpa.2016.07.005.
50. Lennon GM, Ryan PC, Fitzpatrick JM. Ischaemia-reperfusion injury in the rat kidney: effect of a single dose of sodium bicarbonate. Br J Surg. 1993;80(1):112–4. https://doi.org/10.1002/bjs.1800800137.
51. Caty MG, Guice KS, Oldham KT, Remick DG, Kunkel SI. Evidence for tumor necrosis factor-induced pulmonary microvascular injury after intestinal ischemia-reperfusion injury. Ann Surg. 1990;212(6):694–700. https://doi.org/10.1097/00000658-199012000-00007.
52. Mackenzie S, Swan JR, D'Este C, Spigelman AD. Elective open abdominal aortic aneurysm repair: a seven-year experience. Ther Clin Risk Manag. 2005;1(1):27–31. https://doi.org/10.2147/tcrm.1.1.27.53602.
53. Aoki M, Abe T, Hagiwara S, Saitoh D, Oshima K. Resuscitative endovascular balloon occlusion of the aorta may contribute to improved survival. Scand J Trauma Resusc Emerg Med. 2020;28(1):62. Published 2020 Jun 30. https://doi.org/10.1186/s13049-020-00757-2.
54. Yamamoto R, Cestero RF, Suzuki M, Funabiki T, Sasaki J. Resuscitative endovascular balloon occlusion of the aorta (REBOA) is associated with improved survival in severely injured patients: a propensity score matching analysis. Am J Surg. 2019;218(6):1162–8. https://doi.org/10.1016/j.amjsurg.2019.09.007.
55. Brenner M, Moore L, Teeter W, et al. Exclusive clinical experience with a lower profile device for resuscitative endovascular balloon occlusion of the aorta (REBOA). Am J Surg. 2019;217(6):1126–9. https://doi.org/10.1016/j.amjsurg.2018.11.029.

Further Reading

Brenner ML, Moore LJ, DuBose JJ, et al. A clinical series of resuscitative endovascular balloon occlusion of the aorta for hemorrhage control and resuscitation. J Trauma Acute Care Surg. 2013;75(3):506–11. https://doi.org/10.1097/TA.0b013e31829e5416.

Hatchimonji JS, Chipman AM, McGreevy DT, et al. Resuscitative endovascular balloon occlusion of aaorta use in nontrauma emergency general surgery: a multi-institutional experience. J Surg Res. 2020;256:149–55. https://doi.org/10.1016/j.jss.2020.06.034.

Holcomb JB, Tilley BC, Baraniuk S, et al. Transfusion of plasma, platelets, and red blood cells in a 1:1:1 vs a 1:1:2 ratio and mortality in patients with severe trauma: the PROPPR randomized clinical trial. JAMA. 2015;313(5):471–82. https://doi.org/10.1001/jama.2015.12.

Stannard A, Eliason JL, Rasmussen TE. Resuscitative endovascular balloon occlusion of the aorta (REBOA) as an adjunct for hemorrhagic shock. J Trauma. 2011;71(6):1869–72. https://doi.org/10.1097/TA.0b013e31823fe90c.

Varga S. Resuscitative Endovascular Balloon Occlusion of the Aorta (REBOA). In: Scalea TM, editor. The shock trauma manual of operative techniques. Springer; 2021. p. 499–517.

Robotics

30

Giorgio Bianchi, Aleix Martínez-Pérez, and Nicola de'Angelis

> **Learning Goals**
> - To know the history of robotics in surgery and the current trends in robotic surgery.
> - To understand the potential advantages and disadvantages of this technology.
> - To revise the current and future applications of robotics in emergency surgery

30.1 Introduction

Robotics represents the latest evolution in laparoscopic surgery and enhances the advantages of a minimally invasive surgical (MIS) approach. Its applications continue to expand as each time more hospitals are equipped with a robotic platform. To fully appreciate the current widespread applications of robotic surgery and its implementation in specific surgical fields, we need to understand the history and evolutions of robotic platforms in surgery.

30.1.1 Historical Overview of Robotics in Surgery

The word "robot" appeared for the first time in 1920 in a Czech play called *Rossum's Universal Robots* by Karel Capek and became a popular term with the novels *Runaround* and *I, Robot* by Isaac Asimov. The word robot derives from the Czech word "robota" meaning "labor" and was used to describe a fictional humanoid [1–3]. However, the first appearance of a robot mimicking human movements is dated centuries earlier, being attributed to Leonardo da Vinci in 1495 with his metal-plated warrior. This was followed by a significant creation by Gianello Torriano, who built a robotic mandolin-playing lady in 1540 [4]. In the late eighteenth century, in *The Writer* from Jaquet-Droz appeared a programmable robot with the human aspect that was capable of writing complete sentences and could replicate tasks previously performed only by humans [4]. More recently, in 1978, after the development of the first industrial robot, namely Unimate® by Unimation Inc., capable of 6

G. Bianchi
Colorectal and Digestive Surgery Unit, Beaujon University Hospital (AP-HP), Clichy, France

A. Martínez-Pérez
Colorectal and Digestive Surgery Unit, Beaujon University Hospital (AP-HP), Clichy, France

Valencian International University, Valencia, Spain

N. de'Angelis (✉)
Colorectal and Digestive Surgery Unit, Beaujon University Hospital (AP-HP), Clichy, France

University Paris Cité, Paris, France

degrees of freedom, Victor Scheinmann applied the concept of a robotic arm to replace human movements and invented the first truly flexible medical robotic arm called PUMA (Programmable Universal Manipulation Arm) [5].

The first robotic medical procedure, a brain biopsy carried out under computer-tomography (CT) guidance, was performed by Kwoh in 1985 with the help of the PUMA 560® robotic arm. By providing a more accurate and steady guidance compared to a human hand, the PUMA 560® helped to open the future field for robots in surgery [5]. As a proof of its success, the first robotic-assisted laparoscopic cholecystectomy was performed in 1987 [6]. In the late 1980s, the Imperial College of London developed an active robotic system named PROBOT® to assist in transurethral prostatectomies [3]. In 1992, another active robot called ROBODOC® (Integrated Surgical Systems, Sacramento, CA, USA) revolutionized orthopedic surgery by assisting in total hip arthroplasty [7].

Currently, there are three types of robotic systems in use: active, semi-active, and master–slave systems. Active systems work essentially autonomously (while remaining under the control of the operative surgeon) and undertake pre-programmed tasks. Semi-active systems allow for a surgeon-driven element to complement the pre-programmed element of active robot systems, whereas master-slave systems are totally dependent on the surgeon's activity.

In 1994 the Food and Drug Administration (FDA) approved, for the first time in history, the AESOP 1000® (Computer Motion, Santa Barbara, CA, USA) as the first laparoscopic table-mounted camera holder. The AESOP® was initially regulated by hand/foot controls, and then, in its later version, by voice commands. It had the advantage of a more stable view of the operative field while replacing the need for a surgical assistant. In 1996, Geis et al. documented 24 successful solo-surgeon AESOP®-assisted laparoscopic inguinal hernia repairs, cholecystectomies, and Nissen fundoplications [8].

In the meantime, Computer Motion (Santa Barbara, CA, USA) went on with the development of a robotic platform and in 1998 started to commercialize ZEUS®, a master-slave type surgical robot composed of three arms independently attached to the surgical table (i.e., one camera holder and two operative arms) and a console, where the surgeon can sit and control the robot at a distance from the surgical table. Using the ZEUS® platform, and with the help of a fiber-optic cable, Marescaux et al. in 2001 performed long-range telesurgery, a robotic cholecystectomy on a patient in Strasbourg (France) while being in New York (USA) [9].

In 1995, Intuitive Surgical, the company which developed the da Vinci® Surgical System, was founded as a project of the Stanford Research Institute financed by the Defense Advanced Research Projects Agency (DARPA) with the aim to build systems that allow surgeons to operate remotely on soldiers wounded on the battlefield. As the ZEUS®, the da Vinci system was conceived as a master-slave robotic platform; it obtained FDA approval for general laparoscopic procedures in 2000 and then become the first operative surgical robot in the United States.

The ZEUS® and da Vinci® systems were effectively unified when Computer Motion and Intuitive Surgical merged in 2003. As a result, further innovations and improvements were centered on the da Vinci® platform and its ability to improve dexterity, enhance visualization, and boost its advantages when compared to the conventional laparoscopic approach. In 2019, the company registered a growth year-over-year of almost 20% of procedures and subsequently revenues. In the scientific literature, there are over 21,000 peer-reviewed articles that, taken together, support the safety, efficacy, and benefits of the da Vinci surgical system for robotic surgery procedures [10].

In 2006 another company, TransEnterix, Inc. (NYSE American:TRXC), entered the market of robotic surgery. The main goal of TransEnterix was to digitize the interface between the surgeon and the patient and to create a platform that could reduce the costs of the laparoscopic and robotic devices in the current value-based healthcare environment [11]. TransEntrix developed Senhance®, a master-slave robot composed of a console and three independent cart-mounted robotic arms; it represented the first laparoscopic robot with a haptic force feedback. With around 1600 surgical procedures in 2019 and 16 peer-reviewed clinical papers published evaluating the system, Senhance® became the main competitor of the da Vinci® surgical system [12].

30.1.2 Current Trends in Robotic Surgery

Robotic surgery represents an evolution of laparoscopy, therefore it offers all the advantages of a minimally invasive surgical (MIS) approach. Currently, it is well demonstrated that MIS is associated with several benefits for the patients, including reduced blood loss, decreased postoperative pain, less postoperative morbidity, earlier bowel recovery, and shorter hospital stay when compared with the standard laparotomic approach [13–16]. For certain operations, such as oncological colectomies, laparoscopy showed adequate pathologic and long-term oncologic outcomes, comparable to those obtained with open surgery [13, 14]. Nevertheless, laparoscopic surgery is a challenging technique with a steep learning curve [17, 18].

In this perspective, robotic surgery was introduced to overcome the difficulties and drawbacks of conventional laparoscopy by offering a 10x magnification, a 3D stereoscopic vision, much higher precision with tremor control, motion scaling, and also an ergonomically efficient position for the surgeon. Moreover, robotic surgery appeared to have a shorter learning curve than laparoscopy for certain procedures, like right hemicolectomy [19]. Thus, there has been an increasing demand to access robotic surgery platforms from both surgeons and patients, which resulted in an exponential growth in the number of hospitals investing in robotic surgery, despite its higher costs. A recent survey focusing on the public perception of robotic surgery conducted in 2016 in the United States on approximately 800 participants (13% physicians), showed that 53% of respondents thought that hospitals offering robotic surgery were better than those that did not; 72% of the interviewed people also indicated that robotic surgery was faster, safer and less painful. Moreover, 45% preferred to be operated on by robotic surgery rather than by conventional MIS techniques. Interestingly, 50% of respondents would prefer remote robotic surgery performed by a renowned surgeon they had never met over having robotic surgery by a local, non-expert surgeon [20].

Despite its widespread, evidence that supports clinically relevant advantages of robotic surgery over conventional laparoscopy are generally lacking, whereas literature is consistent in demonstrating that the costs associated with the acquisition, maintenance, and routine use of a robotic platform are superior to those of standard laparoscopy. The only surgical field in which strong clinical data to support the advantages of robotics are available in the field of urologic surgery. In 2016 the National Health Service in the UK recommended the use of robot-assisted surgery for radical prostatectomies [21] and the treatment of early-stage kidney cancer [22]. One possible explanation was advanced by Randell et al. who suggested, in a report published in 2014, that many hospitals may have purchased the robotic platform but then encountered several difficulties in running it leading to a general underuse of the robot. This situation contributes to mask and limit a real estimation of the benefits related to the application of robotic surgery [23]. Indeed, an actual utilization below the potentialities of the platform was also confirmed by the annual report from Intuitive Surgical [24].

Because the cost/effectiveness of a robot-assisted surgery depends on the number of operations for which the robot is used [25], it is expected that hospitals that have purchased a robotic platform will seek to maximize its applications. However, the implementation of robot-assisted surgery is challenging and requires specific training not only for the operating surgeons and nursing staff but also for the whole healthcare service that will need to apply a new and specific organization [24, 25].

While operating with the robot, the surgeon is distant from the patient and the surgical field, which are managed by the assistant surgeon with the operative theatre team. Thus, this is crucial to guarantee the appropriate training and to build dedicated robotic surgical teams, in, ideally, dedicated robotic operative theaters [26]. Indeed, the implementation of robotic platforms in the operative theater may contribute to interrupt or disrupt the existing workflow leading to a rearrangement of the operative theater activity. This passes through a new way of communication. Studies focused on this topic showed the importance for the whole surgical team to have access to the same information in order to have the same shared situation awareness of what is going on in the operative theater. Interestingly, these studies demonstrated a direct relationship between communication and patient safety [27, 28]. It must be also acknowledged that a learning curve is expected for the whole team [29], and not only for the operating surgeon [30].

As a result, it is of upmost importance to establish a "robotic program" when equipping the operative theater with a robotic platform, which encompasses specific training for the surgeons and also for the whole operational theater personnel, in order to be successful and efficient in robotic surgery [31]. As highlighted in a recent review based on 30 articles, a wide range of barriers to safety and efficiency can be encountered in robotic surgery, and these are mainly not related to technical skills, as, for instance, management tasks, communication breakdowns, coordination failures, and technology management. The authors of this review suggested that an improvement in these fields may subsequently lead to improved dynamics in the operative theater associated with greater efficiency, reduced costs, and better systems-level outcomes [32].

30.2 Robotics in Emergency Surgery

30.2.1 Background

As the technology evolves, more hospitals are equipped with a robotic platform and more operations are assisted by a robot. In the field of general surgery, during the period 2010–2014 in the United States, there was a fivefold increase in oncological robotic procedures and this trend was observed in all states and regions, despite achieving similar outcomes in terms of length of hospital stay and rate of complications than conventional laparoscopy [33]. However, robotic surgery has been always associated with elective surgery performed in the daytime. This is mainly due, as mentioned before, to the complexity of this new technology that requires staff members in the operating theater who are familiar with the setup and use of the robot and who share the perception of the potential benefits provided by the use of robotics (Fig. 30.1).

An increased competition to access the robotic platform and the need to optimize its use to become cost-effective bring up the hypothesis of a possible application of robot surgery also during the night shifts or in the weekends as well as for emergency interventions [34]. In this latter setting, the robotic approach may allow to overcome some technical difficulties often encountered in emergency laparoscopy that would frequently lead to conversion to open surgery. Avoiding or reducing the need to convert and enlarging the panel of emergency interventions approached by MIS will ultimately lead to lower morbidity rates and to reduce hospital stay, making the application of robotics in emergency settings highly interesting [35] (Table 30.1).

30.2.2 Literature Reports

The first report of an emergency robotic procedure in general surgery was published by Sudan et al. in 2012. The authors reported two cases of patients who developed post-operative complications after robotic biliopancreatic diversion with duodenal switch and required re-intervention to manage the complication. Those complication were successfully treated by robotic approach, which was opted by the operating surgeons to avoid laparotomy and then loose the benefits from the MIS approach. Moreover, the authors reported that the robotic technology may facilitate the identification of the damage, and its repair [34].

Fig. 30.1 (**a**) Schema of robotic cart placement and patient's positioning. (**b**) Operative theater setting during an emergency robotic procedure for the treatment of a hiatal hernia. Robotic platform: da Vinci Xi Surgical System® (Intuitive Surgical, Sunnyvale, USA). [Courtesy of Nicola de'Angelis]

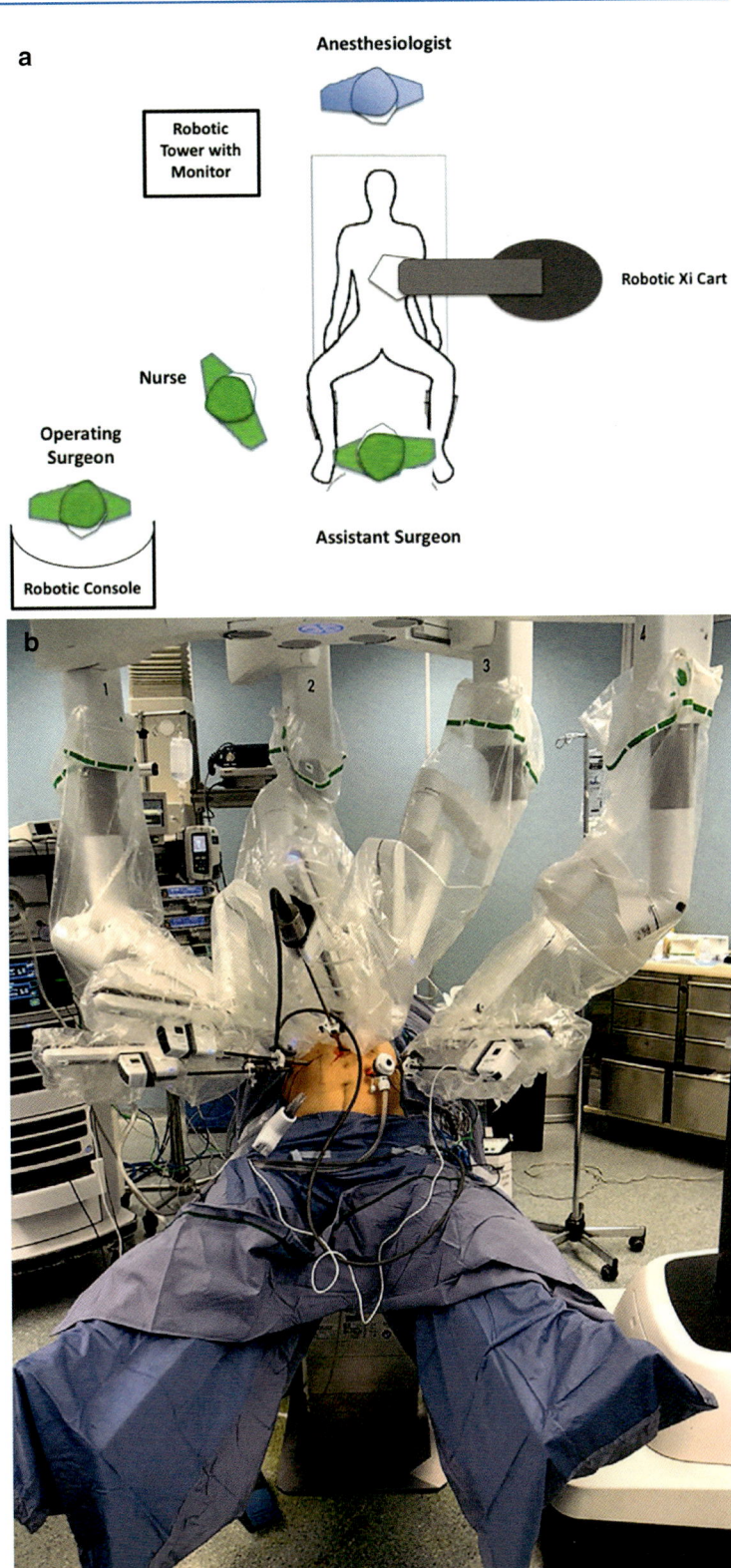

Table 30.1 Advantages and disadvantages of robotic approach in emergency surgery

Advantages	Disadvantages
• Might overcome technical difficulties that in laparoscopy could be resolved only by a conversion to open surgery	• Highly dependent on the surgeon's experience and attitude
• Enhanced visualization and ergonomics of the robot compared to laparoscopy, particularly useful for technically demanding operations involving friable, inflamed tissues	• Possible only in highly selected patients
	• Needs equipped operating theater and trained nursing staff
• Alleviate scheduling conflicts and expand the application of robot surgery	
• Reasonable option in challenging situations in stable patients	• Higher costs compared to laparoscopy

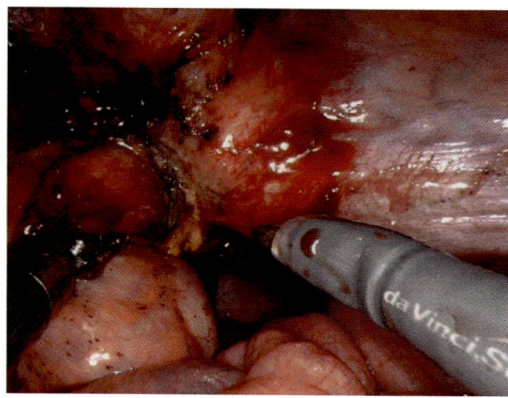

Fig. 30.2 Robotic sigmoidectomy for a vescico-sigmoid fistula using the da Vinci Xi Surgical System®. [Courtesy of Nicola de'Angelis]

In 2014, Felli et al. described for the first time an emergency robotic right colectomy performed in an 86 years-old patient presenting with right colon cancer with active bleeding. Both the surgery and postoperative period were uneventful [36].

In upper gastrointestinal surgery, three patients were treated with robotic surgery for a complicated giant hiatal hernia. In all the cases, the content of the hernia was reduced, the sac was removed, and a hiatoplasty was performed. In two cases, the surgery was completed with a Nissen fundoplication, whereas the other was completed with a Toupet one[37].

In 2018, the Metabolic and Bariatric Surgery Accreditation and Quality Improvement Program (MBSAQIP®) database showed that the robotic approach was used in 9.4% of all bariatric surgeries; concerning the emergency procedures, only 2.1% (corresponding to 44 patients) were carried out using the robot [38].

Recently, a comparative study was published reporting the outcomes of emergency robotic vs laparoscopic surgery for gastro-jejunal perforation, as complication of Roux-en-Y gastric bypass. The authors compared operative and short-term postoperative outcomes of 24 patients who underwent robotic surgery repair vs. 20 patients who underwent laparoscopic repair. The results demonstrated that the use of robotic surgery was non-inferior to laparoscopy but significantly more expensive. The only outcome that was significantly different between the two surgical approaches was the in-room-to-surgery-start time, which was significantly shorter in the robotic surgery group. Interestingly, 23 out of 24 robotic procedures were performed by the same and unique operator, suggesting a dependence on the surgeon's attitude. Moreover, improved visualization and ergonomics were described for the robotic procedures, in particular during technically challenging steps involving friable and inflamed tissue (Fig. 30.2). Overall, this study supports earlier trends and affirms that robotic surgery should not be contraindicated for emergency general surgery *a priori*; rather, its application, in selected patients and by experienced surgeons, may be associated with improved outcomes [39].

30.2.3 Advantages and Disadvantages of Robotic Emergency Surgery

Today, in a robotic surgery operative theater with trained personnel, the biggest obstacle that remains to be overcome is likely to be the dogma that the robot is used only for surgery operations. Indeed, all the staff needs to accept that the robot could be a reasonable and effective option also in emergency surgery.

As shown in 2019 in the "European consensus on the standardization of robotic total mesorectal excision for rectal cancer", the robotic platform could facilitate the process of standardization of the different surgical stages, including patient positioning, port placement, and procedural steps [40].

The potential advantages of robotic surgery in emergency settings are the following:

- Enhanced visualization and improved ergonomics compared to laparoscopy and open surgery, particularly useful for technical operations involving friable and inflamed tissues.
- Enhanced dexterity compared to conventional laparoscopy, which can facilitate some technically demanding steps reducing the risk of conversion to open surgery to complete the intervention.
- Eased standardization of the surgical steps, as performed during elective surgery, which ultimately contributes to overcome the technical difficulties more often encountered during emergency.
- Mitigation of scheduling conflicts and expansion of the application of robotic surgery in a cost/efficient manner.

On the other hand, the potential drawbacks that could preclude the application of robotic surgery in emergency setting are:

- The necessity of an equipped operative theater and trained nursing staff.
- The need of surgeons' and collaborators' intent and experience.
- The higher costs, today not counterbalanced by clear evidence of superior clinical outcomes of robotics over laparoscopy.

In general, the evidence supporting of robotic surgery in emergency settings is still low. The current literature is limited to few reports of single centers' experience. Robotic surgery is being performed in an emergency setting only in highly selected patients, hemodynamically stable, presenting with a clear diagnosis, and not requiring wide exposure during the surgery [36, 39].

30.3 Future Applications and Research Perspectives

30.3.1 Fluorescence-Based Surgery

Near-infrared fluorescence (NIRF) imaging is a promising tool that is being explored as a method to enhance visualization during surgery. Fluorescence is the property of certain molecules called fluorochromes (e.g. indocyanine green), able to emit fluorescent radiation when excited by a laser beam or exposed to near-infrared light at specific wavelengths [41]. Thus, the fluorescence can be detected using specific scopes and cameras.

Despite the lack of evidence supporting a routine use of NIRF, this technique is nowadays largely utilized in general surgery, mainly to asses esophageal, gastric, or colorectal perfusion with the objective of reducing the incidence of anastomotic leaks (Fig. 30.3). Recently, three

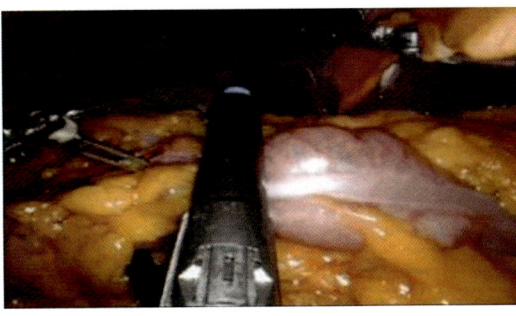 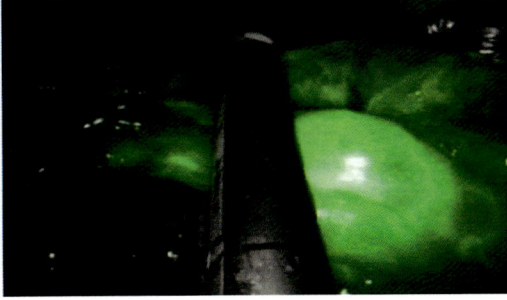

Fig. 30.3 Indocyanine Green Fluorescence Angiography is used to assess bowel perfusion during a robotic right hemicolectomy using the da Vinci Xi Surgical System®. [Courtesy of Nicola de'Angelis]

systematic reviews explored the role of NIRF imaging in the assessment of bowel perfusion in colorectal resection and recognized a great potential in the prevention of anastomotic leaks but without a definitive conclusion to support its routine use in gastrointestinal surgery [42–44]. Data from a European-based prospective registry of more than 1000 patients, showed that the NIRF technique was safe and then applied in a considerable number of cases. This technology provides the majority of the operators a high sense of confidence while performing the anastomosis [45]. NIRF imaging has also been used to perform near-infrared fluorescent cholangiography (NIFC) and has been shown to increase the visualization and identification of extrahepatic biliary structures [46]. NIFC consists of preoperative intravenous administration of indocyanine green (ICG) fluorescent dye and then intraoperative visualization of the extrahepatic bile ducts with a fluorescence imaging system. Recently, a randomized trial conducted on more than 600 patients demonstrated that NIFC was superior to white light alone in visualizing extrahepatic biliary structures before surgical dissection during laparoscopic cholecystectomy [46]. NIFC has been successfully proposed in adjunct to emergency laparoscopic cholecystectomy to help maintain a low complication rate [47].

NIRF imaging technology is already included in all robotic platforms, and its use can be easily systematic. Being a safe and feasible method, it could assist surgeons during both elective and emergency surgery.

30.3.2 Telemedicine

Telemedicine describes remote clinical services, such as diagnosis and monitoring, via electronic information and telecommunication technologies. It represents nowadays a fast-growing sector that plays an important role in medical practice and education. In surgery, it can be divided into two main components according to the increasing level of interaction: telementoring and telesurgery [48]. Telementoring is a concept within telemedicine in which an expert physician guides another physician at a different geographical location. Instructions from the mentor could be as simple as verbal guidance while the mentor is watching a real-time video of the operation or, in more evolved interfaces, could progressively involve indicating target areas on the local monitor screen (telestration) or taking over as the assistant by controlling the operative camera or an instrument via robotic arms (tele-assisted surgery) [49]. Telesurgery is defined as a remote intervention carried through the use of a surgical robot actively controlled by a distant operator. Telesurgery has only been made possible by the advent of robotic-assisted surgery. Since the first telesurgery intervention by Marescaux in 2001 with the help of the ZEUS robotic system, there have been a number of further trials of various procedures [9] and even the first telerobotic surgical service between a teaching hospital and a rural hospital, both placed in Ontario (USA). In this latter case, the delivery of telerobotic surgery aimed to aid local surgeons in providing a variety of advanced laparoscopic surgery to their community patients [50]. These applications are all very interesting and promising but still blunted by some technical difficulties, such as the delays in sending and receiving the audio-visual feed, known as the latency time, major safety drawbacks for telesurgery. Indeed, a number of studies have examined the effect of the time latency on the surgical performance and they showed an exponential reduction in the surgical performance as the latency times increase. A latency of less than 300 ms has been found to be generally acceptable by the surgeons, with a minimal effect on the surgical intervention [51].

Despite these technical limitations, surgical teams across the world have been working to increase the scope of telesurgery. The spread of telesurgery to remote and hostile environments represents a great potential for development. There are considerable advantages in being able to offer advanced surgical treatments within their communities, not only to the patients but also to the health system in general.

A systematic review published in 2017 observed an increasing interest and technological growth in telesurgery and telemedicine in MIS. However, today safety, legal and ethical issues limit its widespread use and application. With the advent of favorable legislation and favored by an extensive collaboration with telecommunications engineers, we can expect in a near future the development of safe and cost-effective services of robotic telementoring and telesurgery [49].

30.3.3 Artificial Intelligence in Surgery

In computer sciences, the term artificial intelligence (AI) refers to any human-like intelligence exhibited by a computer, robot, or other machines. AI is already part of our everyday lives (e.g. speech recognition, image recognition, or autopilot technology) and is advancing rapidly with a wide range of applications. In medicine, AI has already found its role mainly with image recognition tasks and clinical decision support in the field of radiology, pathology, cardiology, and gastroenterology [52]. The development and use of AI in surgery have been slower, mainly due to the complexity of interaction and the lack of evidence and awareness of the potential capabilities of computational approaches in surgical practice. The current tendency is to consider AI in surgery as complement of human skills in two main areas: the surgical decision-making process and the operative surgery. The accessibility to large and varied stores of 'big data' will allow to develop algorithms able to cross-talk between data stores and finally provide a solution to a specific clinical case. Future systems will predict surgical outcomes based on biochemical, radiological, and sequencing data available from the preoperative assessment [53]. Realistically, this trend towards robotic-assisted surgery supported by advanced technology will continue to increase. Bio-informatic pattern-recognition algorithms from past saved procedures will be incorporated into new programming in a rapid manner, further enhancing automated surgical procedures support. Importantly, deciding when to allow the technology to "move" on its own sensors will be essential to guarantee its usefulness and safety in medicine [54].

30.3.4 Coming-Soon Technologies

The increasing demand in robotic surgery has brought new competitors challenging the da Vinci Surgical System, such as Medtronic or CMR Surgical, who are all developing their next-generation surgical robot. This expanding market will favor the widespread application of robotic surgery and ultimately it will contribute at improving value and quality as well as lowering costs. In 2020, TransEnterix, Inc. (NYSE American:TRXC) announced that the company received the CE Mark approval for the Intelligent Surgical UnitTM (ISUTM), which enables machine vision capabilities on the Senhance® Surgical System. ISU's machine vision capabilities will be able to recognize certain objects and locations in the surgical field. This will enhance visualization and camera control compared with the currently available surgical technology, and will also provide the base for additional augmented intelligence capabilities. Eventually, the system could have an overwatch feature in which the system would use scene cognition and image analytics to provide the surgeon suggestions based on accumulated laparoscopic experience around Senhance® [12]. In the most recent yearly report by Intuitive Surgical, it was announced that consistent investments were made in informatics comprising: (a) big data capability; (b) Intuitive Cloud computing and telemedicine; (c) machine learning; and (d) training technologies [10]. Finally, Verb Surgical, a joint venture between Johnson & Johnson and Google, was founded in 2015 to develop "a digital surgery platform that combines robotics, advanced visualization, advanced instrumentation, data analytics, and connectivity." The main objective was to advance robotic surgery by making technology and information available to more patients and thus reduce overall costs of cares [55].

In this panorama, the continuous evolution of the robotic platforms and the introduction of new technologies are likely to provide the operating surgeons with advanced assistance to push further the limits of MIS.

Dos and Don'ts

(List what should and should not be done when treating patients)

- Robotic surgery, as an advanced technology for MIS, provides clinically relevant benefits that could be observed also for emergency surgery in highly selected patients.
- However, do not consider the robotic approach in emergency settings if there is not adequate training and sufficient experience of all operating surgeons and nursing staff in the operative theater.

Take-Home Messages

- Robotic surgery will continue to expand
- Robotic surgery in emergency settings could be considered in selected cases, as successful outcomes have been considered in stable patients, and with appropriately trained staff and experienced surgeons
- Robotic surgery may be a useful technology to facilitate the completion of complex intervention
- In the future, telesurgery could help improving surgical training (telementoring) and provide surgical expertise in remote locations for both elective and emergency surgery
- Artificial Intelligence could enter in operative theater during the decision-making process and, maybe, helping during the intervention

[Diagnosis: NOT APPLICABLE]

Multiple Choice Questions

1. Which was the first robotic-assisted surgical procedure performed?
   A. A brain biopsy (true)
   B. Laparoscopic cholecystectomy (false)
   C. Transurethral prostatectomy (false)
   D. Total hip arthroplasty (false)
2. Robotic platforms ZEUS® and da Vinci® surgical system are:
   A. Active (false)
   B. Semi-active (false)
   C. Master-slave (true)
   D. Autonomous (false)
3. Compared to laparoscopy, robotic platforms offer:
   A. A shorter learning curve (false)
   B. Better results in terms of long-term oncological outcomes (false)
   C. Higher precision, tremor filtration, and haptic force feedback (false)
   D. A + C (true)
4. The advantages of robotic approach over laparoscopy:
   A. Are well documented with randomized control trials (false)
   B. Are still lacking (false)
   C. Are well described only in urologic surgery (false)
   D. B + C (true)
5. Robotic approach in emergency:
   A. is contraindicated (false)
   B. is routinely used (false)
   C. There are no reports on the subject (false)
   D. It has been described for selected patients (true)
6. The major problem to approach emergency with robotic surgery is:
   A. The need of an equipped operative theater and trained nursing staff (false)

B. The elevated costs (false)
C. The requirement of surgeon's and collaborator's intent and experience (false)
D. A + B + C (true)
7. The robotic approach in emergency:
   A. could overcome some technical difficulties (true)
   B. is currently utilized by dedicated robotic teams (false)
   C. is indicated for most of general surgery emergencies (false)
   D. is indicated for the most urologic surgery emergencies (false)
8. Telemedicine:
   A. can be divided into two main components: Telestration and Tele-assisted surgery (false)
   B. is the integration of communication technologies in medicine (true)
   C. is a kind of autonomous robot (false)
   D. is already in use in all the robotic platforms (false)
9. Telesurgery:
   A. is possible without the robotic platform (false)
   B. is already possible with most of the available internet connections (false)
   C. is possible with a latency time of 0.5 s (false)
   D. is a fast-growing sector but its routine clinical use is not yet possible (true)
10. Artificial intelligence:
    A. is already routinely used in surgery (false)
    B. In surgery, it could complement human skills mainly in two areas: surgical decision-making and operative surgery (true)
    C. has already been developed in some field of medicine (false)
    D. can already perform some kind of surgical interventions (false)

References

1. Kalan S, Chauhan S, Coelho RF, et al. History of robotic surgery. J Robot Surg. 2010;4:141–7.
2. Asimov I. I, Robot. Fawcett, Greenwich, CT; 1950.
3. Runaround AI. Austonding science fiction. New York: Street & Smith Pubblication Inc.; 1942.
4. García-Diego J. Los relojes y autómatas de Juanelo Turriano. Monografías Españolas de Relojería. Tempvs Fvgit, Madrid, pp L V–LX, Wgs 6.3–6.9; 1982.
5. Kwoh YS, Hou J, Jonckheere EA, Hayati S. A robot with improved absolute positioning accuracy for CT guided stereotactic brain surgery. IEEE Trans Biomed Eng. 1988;35:153–60.
6. Samadi D. History and the future of robotic surgery. Robotic Oncology. [Online]; 2018. http://www.robot-iconcology.com/history-of-robotic-surgery/.
7. Paul HA, Bargar WL, Mittlestadt B, et al. Development of a surgical robot for cementless total hip arthroplasty. Clin Orthop Relat Res. 1992:57–66.
8. Geis WP, Kim HC, Brennan EJ Jr, et al. Robotic arm enhancement to accommodate improved efficiency and decreased resource utilization in complex minimally invasive surgical procedures. Stud Health Technol Inform. 1996;29:471–81.
9. Marescaux J, Leroy J, Gagner M, et al. Transatlantic robot-assisted telesurgery. Nature. 2001;413:379–80.
10. Intuitive. Surgical. Annual report 2019 Intuitive Surgical Inc.; 2020.
11. Schreuder HW, Verheijen RH. Robotic surgery. BJOG. 2009;116:198–213.
12. Transenterix. Annual report. Morrisville:Transenterix, Inc.; 2020.
13. Guillou PJ, Quirke P, Thorpe H, et al. Short-term endpoints of conventional versus laparoscopic-assisted surgery in patients with colorectal cancer (MRC CLASICC trial): multicentre, randomised controlled trial. Lancet. 2005;365:1718–26.
14. Jayne DG, Guillou PJ, Thorpe H, et al. Randomized trial of laparoscopic-assisted resection of colorectal carcinoma: 3-year results of the UK MRC CLASICC Trial Group. J Clin Oncol. 2007;25:3061–8.
15. Fleshman J, Sargent DJ, Green E, et al. Laparoscopic colectomy for cancer is not inferior to open surgery based on 5-year data from the COST Study Group trial. Ann Surg. 2007;246:655–62; discussion 662–654.
16. Ohtani H, Tamamori Y, Arimoto Y, et al. A meta-analysis of the short- and long-term results of randomized controlled trials that compared laparoscopy-assisted and open colectomy for colon cancer. J Cancer. 2012;3:49–57.
17. Reissman P, Cohen S, Weiss EG, Wexner SD. Laparoscopic colorectal surgery: ascending the learning curve. World J Surg. 1996;20:277–81; discussion 282.
18. Tekkis PP, Senagore AJ, Delaney CP, Fazio VW. Evaluation of the learning curve in laparoscopic

19. Bokhari MB, Patel CB, Ramos-Valadez DI, et al. Learning curve for robotic-assisted laparoscopic colorectal surgery. Surg Endosc. 2011;25:855–60.
20. Joshua A, Boys ETA, DeMeester MJ, Worrell SG, Oh DS, Hagen JA, DeMeester SR. Public perceptions on robotic surgery, hospitals with robots, and surgeons that use them. Surg Endosc. 2015;30:1310–6.
21. NHS. England Specialised Commissioning Team. Clinical commissioning policy: robotic-assisted surgical procedures for prostate cancer; 2015.
22. NHS. England Specialised Commissioning Team. Clinical Commissioning Policy: robotic assisted surgery for early kidney cancers that are unsuitable for conventional laparoscopic surgery; 2016.
23. Trehan A, Dunn TJ. The robotic surgery monopoly is a poor deal. BMJ. 2013;347:f7470.
24. Jones A, Sethia K. Robotic surgery. Ann R Coll Surg Engl. 2010;92:5–6.
25. Scales CD Jr, Jones PJ, Eisenstein EL, et al. Local cost structures and the economics of robot assisted radical prostatectomy. J Urol. 2005;174:2323–9.
26. Randell R, Honey S, Alvarado N, et al. Factors supporting and constraining the implementation of robot-assisted surgery: a realist interview study. BMJ Open. 2019;9:e028635.
27. Hull L, Arora S, Aggarwal R, et al. The impact of non-technical skills on technical performance in surgery: a systematic review. J Am Coll Surg. 2012;214:214–30.
28. Fuji L, Eileen E. Robotic surgery and the operating room team. Proceeding of the human factors and ergonomics society 49th annual meeting; 2005.
29. Smith AL, Krivak TC, Scott EM, et al. Dual-console robotic surgery compared to laparoscopic surgery with respect to surgical outcomes in a gynecologic oncology fellowship program. Gynecol Oncol. 2012;126:432–6.
30. Smith AL, Scott EM, Krivak TC, et al. Dual-console robotic surgery: a new teaching paradigm. J Robot Surg. 2012;7:113–8.
31. Zhao B, Lam J, Hollandsworth HM, et al. General surgery training in the era of robotic surgery: a qualitative analysis of perceptions from resident and attending surgeons. Surg Endosc. 2019;34:1712–21.
32. Kanji F, Catchpole K, Choi E, et al. Work-system interventions in robotic-assisted surgery: a systematic review exploring the gap between challenges and solutions. Surg Endosc. 2021;35:1976–89.
33. Stewart CL, Ituarte PHG, Melstrom KA, et al. Robotic surgery trends in general surgical oncology from the National Inpatient Sample. Surg Endosc. 2019;33:2591–601.
34. Sudan R, Desai SS. Emergency and weekend robotic surgery are feasible. J Robot Surg. 2011;6:263–6.
35. Koh FH, Tan KK, Tsang CB, Koh DC. Laparoscopic versus an open colectomy in an emergency setting: a case-controlled study. Ann Coloproctol. 2013;29:12–6.
36. Felli E, Brunetti F, Disabato M, et al. Robotic right colectomy for hemorrhagic right colon cancer: a case report and review of the literature of minimally invasive urgent colectomy. World J Emerg Surg. 2014:9.
37. Ceccarelli G, Pasculli A, Bugiantella W, et al. Minimally invasive laparoscopic and robot-assisted emergency treatment of strangulated giant hiatal hernias: report of five cases and literature review. World J Emerg Surg. 2020:15.
38. Metabolic and Bariatric Surgery Accreditation and Quality Improvement Program. https://www.facs.org/quality-programs/mbsaqip/registry-request; 2020.
39. Robinson TD, Sheehan JC, Patel PB, et al. Emergent robotic versus laparoscopic surgery for perforated gastrojejunal ulcers: a retrospective cohort study of 44 patients. Surg Endosc. 2021;
40. Miskovic D, Ahmed J, Bissett-Amess R, et al. European consensus on the standardization of robotic total mesorectal excision for rectal cancer. Colorectal Disease. 2019;21:270–6.
41. Alander JT, Kaartinen I, Laakso A, et al. A review of indocyanine green fluorescent imaging in surgery. Int J Biomed Imaging. 2012;2012:940585.
42. van den Bos J, Al-Taher M, Schols RM, et al. Near-infrared fluorescence imaging for real-time intraoperative guidance in anastomotic colorectal surgery: a systematic review of literature. J Laparoendosc Adv Surg Tech A. 2018;28:157–67.
43. Blanco-Colino R, Espin-Basany E. Intraoperative use of ICG fluorescence imaging to reduce the risk of anastomotic leakage in colorectal surgery: a systematic review and meta-analysis. Tech Coloproctol. 2018;22:15–23.
44. Shen R, Zhang Y, Wang T. Indocyanine green fluorescence angiography and the incidence of anastomotic leak after colorectal resection for colorectal cancer: a meta-analysis. Dis Colon Rectum. 2018;61:1228–34.
45. Spota A, Al-Taher M, Felli E, et al. Fluorescence-based bowel anastomosis perfusion evaluation: results from the IHU-IRCAD-EAES EURO-FIGS registry. Surg Endosc. 2021;
46. Dip F, LoMenzo E, Sarotto L, et al. Randomized trial of near-infrared incisionless fluorescent cholangiography. Ann Surg. 2019;270:992–9.
47. Di Maggio F, Hossain N, De Zanna A, et al. Near-infrared fluorescence cholangiography can be a useful adjunct during emergency cholecystectomies. Surg Innov. 2020;
48. Raison N, Khan MS, Challacombe B. Telemedicine in surgery: what are the opportunities and hurdles to realising the potential? Curr Urol Reports. 2015;16
49. Hung AJ, Chen J, Shah A, Gill IS. Telementoring and telesurgery for minimally invasive procedures. J Urol. 2018;199:355–69.

50. Anvari M, McKinley C, Stein H. Establishment of the world's first telerobotic remote surgical service: for provision of advanced laparoscopic surgery in a rural community. Ann Surg. 2005;241:460–4.
51. Xu S, Perez M, Yang K, et al. Determination of the latency effects on surgical performance and the acceptable latency levels in telesurgery using the dV-Trainer((R)) simulator. Surg Endosc. 2014;28:2569–76.
52. Mintz Y, Brodie R. Introduction to artificial intelligence in medicine. Minim Invasive Ther Allied Technol. 2019;28:73–81.
53. Mirnezami R, Ahmed A. Surgery 3.0, artificial intelligence and the next-generation surgeon. Br J Surg. 2018;105:463–5.
54. Stefano GB. Robotic surgery: fast forward to telemedicine. Med Sci Monitor. 2017;23:1856.
55. Verb Surgical. Our Story. Verb Surgical. Available online: http://www.verbsurgical.com/about/; 2018.

Further Reading

Kalan S, Chauhan S, Coelho RF, et al. History of robotic surgery. J Robot Surg. 2010;4:141–7.

Robinson TD, Sheehan JC, Patel PB, et al. Emergent robotic versus laparoscopic surgery for perforated gastrojejunal ulcers: a retrospective cohort study of 44 patients. Surg Endosc. 2021;

Raison N, Khan MS, Challacombe B. Telemedicine in surgery: what are the opportunities and hurdles to realising the potential? Curr Urol Reports. 2015;16

Dip F, LoMenzo E, Sarotto L, et al. Randomized trial of near-infrared incisionless fluorescent cholangiography. Ann Surg. 2019;270:992–9.

Mintz Y, Brodie R. Introduction to artificial intelligence in medicine. Minim Invasive Ther Allied Technol. 2019;28:73–81.

Emergency and Trauma Surgery During Epidemia and Pandemia

31

Belinda De Simone, Elie Chouillard, and Fausto Catena

Learning Goals
- Management of trauma victims and surgical patients at admission in the emergency department to limit the in-hospital spreading of a pandemic.
- Personal Protective Equipment and operating theatre set up.
- Preoperative management of surgical urgent patients during a pandemic.
- Decision-making for non-operative or operative management in the emergency setting during a pandemic.
- Operative management of a surgical patient.
- Multidisciplinary postoperative management of surgical patients and discharge policies.

31.1 Introduction

The outbreak of a global pandemic is considered a mass casualty for the high number of confirmed cases and deaths and the high transmissibility of the virus. Critically ill infected patients require intensive care unit (ICU) admission. Hospitals are overwhelmed. During the COVID-19 pandemic, at the earliest phase, surgical theatres were converted into additional ICUs and non-urgent, non-cancer surgical procedures were cancelled. Medical and paramedical staff were relocated to provide care and ventilatory support for patients with COVID-19 pneumonia.

Lack of beds in ICUs, of a dedicated path for infected patients, of protective personal equipment (PPE), of education of healthcare personnel, contributed to an increase in the number of deaths due to the virus among patients and healthcare workers.

This catastrophic scenario of the COVID-19 pandemic reflected errors in disaster evaluation and management and we experienced and learned from it.

People were recommended to keep social distancing with the closure of all non-essential businesses until to comply with lockdown orders and mandatory mask requirements to reduce the transmission rate and the severity of the pandemic's impact.

Several articles addressed the re-organization of scheduled surgical activity during the COVID-19 pandemic because it was essential to

Supplementary Information The online version contains supplementary material available at https://doi.org/10.1007/978-3-031-22599-4_31.

B. De Simone (✉) · E. Chouillard
Department of Emergency, Digestive and Metabolic Minimally Invasive Surgery, Centre Hospitalier Intercommunal de Poissy et Saint Germain en Laye, Poissy, France

F. Catena
Department of Emergency and Trauma Surgery, Bufalini Hospital, Cesena, Italy

ensure the management of patients presenting with surgical diseases and oncological complicated patients and trauma victims.

Acute care and emergency surgeons recognized immediately their crucial role in a pandemic and provided essential information for surgical practice.

31.2 Personal Protective Equipment and Healthcare Workers' Infection

The first wave of the COVID-19 pandemic showed the entity of governments and world institutions' unpreparedness in managing a mass casualty disaster such as a viral pandemic.

The key to a public health emergency response lies in the abundance of reserves, proper allocation of emergency medical supplies, and rapid distribution.

In an early pandemic, insufficient accurate scientific data on the virus responsible including its virulence factors, survival outside a host, resistant strains, incubation period, and infection pathophysiology, associated with the incapability to have a screening test for all patients admitted in the emergency departments and the lack of specialized PPE and education, are factors that contribute to a high spreading of the virus in the general population and among healthcare workers (HCWs). Moreover, stressful working environments, long working hours leading to fatigue and isolation with related psychological issues, increase the HCWs' risk of infection.

General measures to limit transmission of a virus provide promptly the careful implementation of basic hand hygiene practice, including frequent hand washing, the use of portable hand sanitizer, wearing specific PPE, and avoiding contact with face and mouth after interacting with a possibly contaminated environment and patients.

The inadequate availability and improper use of PPE was a critical harmful factor in the high COVID-19 infection rate in HCWs. Furthermore, RT-PCR testing for the identification of the virus wasn't readily available at all healthcare facilities and for all suspected patients.

For containing the in-hospital spreading of SARS-CoV-2, it was recommended to screen for COVID-19 infection at the emergency department, all surgical patients with clinical and epidemiological features suspect of COVID-19 disease, waiting for hospital admission and urgent surgery [1].

During a pandemic, appropriate PPE depends on exposure risk, according to three categories of transmission-based precautions:

1. Contact and droplet;
2. Airborne and droplet;
3. High-risk aerosol generating medical procedures.

The established minimum recommended PPE for any staff caring for a patient with confirmed/suspected/undetermined viral infection is summarized in Table 31.1 and includes wearing a fitted, NIOSH-certified N95 respirator, eye protection (either goggles or full-face shield),

Table 31.1 Minimum standard of PPE in a pandemic for any staff caring for highly symptomatic patients with confirmed/suspected viral infection and practising in high-prevalence settings who need to be close to patients' respiratory tracts (positive pressure ventilation, high-flow oxygen, coughing, heavy breathing, and spirometry), even in the absence of traditionally defined aerosol-generating procedures [2]

Recommended PPE	Why
NIOSH-certified N95 respirator	Filters at least 95% of airborne particles
Eye protection (either goggles or full-face shield)	To avoid contact of droplets with mucosa and conjunctiva
Cap	To avoid contact with contaminated surfaces or biological liquids
Gown	To avoid contact with contaminated surfaces or biological liquids
Gloves (Double gloves may be considered and the outer pair should be changed when contaminated.)	To avoid contact with contaminated surfaces or biological liquids
Powered air-purifying respirator (PAPR)	Especially in aerosol-generating procedures (such as during induction of anesthesia and intubation) when available

cap, gown, and gloves. As transmission remains possible despite N95 protection, staff participating in aerosol-generating procedures (AGP) should wear a powered air-purifying respirator (PAPR) [2].

Concerning the definition of AGP, the World Health Organization (WHO) stipulated that intubation, noninvasive positive pressure ventilation, tracheotomy, cardiopulmonary resuscitation, bronchoscopy, and sputum induction are definite AGPs because they were associated with a greater risk of infection for HCWs [3].

The transmission risk during medical procedures is related to the forced air, symptoms and disease severity of the patient, the distance of the HCW, and the duration of the exposition to the virus. Oro-tracheal intubation in the operating room (OR) was claimed as a high-risk AGP and associated with increased risk of infection for HCWs, but it is not this procedure per se that generates aerosols and facilitates transmission but the circumstances surrounding the procedure, including patient factors (e.g., severe illness, high viral loads, coughing, heavy breathing, and super emissions) as well as forced air, profound proximity to the respiratory tract, and for some procedures, prolonged exposure [4].

For care not involving high-risk aerosol-generating medical procedures use droplet and contact precautions which include a surgical mask with face shield, an Association for the Advancement of Medical Instrumentation (AAMI) level 2 gown and gloves that overlap the gown sleeve enough to prevent wrist exposure during movement.

PPE for airborne, droplet, and contact precautions consists of head covering, eye protection, N95 respirator, an AAMI level 2 (or higher) gown, and a single pair of gloves overlapping the gown sleeve enough that movement does not expose the wrists.

For high-risk AGP, in addition to the airborne, droplet, and contact precautions, a neck covering, a gown with AAMI level 2 (or higher), and two sets of gloves that overlap the gown sleeve enough to prevent wrist exposure during movement are recommended [5] (Table 31.2).

Table 31.2 The Association for the Advancement of Medical Instrumentation level of protection

AAMI level	Type of protection
I	Minimal level of fluid barrier protection
II	Low level of fluid barrier protection
III	Moderate level of fluid barrier protection
IV	Highest level of fluid and viral barrier protection

Routine care of low-risk patients (no fever or respiratory symptoms in a setting with low virus prevalence) requires only the use of a simple surgical mask to protect against droplet transmission.

31.3 Diagnosis: Emergency Surgery and Trauma Care During a Pandemic

In the first phase of a pandemic, the primary aim is to contain the admission rate of infected people to preserve resources, protective equipment, and limit the in-hospital transmission of the virus.

During the COVID-19 pandemic, governments instructed individuals to stay home except for medical and compassionate reasons, work, or education that was not possible remotely. Home isolation was recommended for individuals elder than 70 years. The lockdown policy, travel restrictions, and reduced industrial work had an impact in decreasing significantly the overall number of trauma-related admissions during the COVID-19-related period of societal restrictions and lockdown, resulting also in a decrease in minor traumas, falls, and road traffic collisions. Over time these restrictions caused high isolation and psychological stress, and barriers to non-emergent physical and mental health treatment with an increase in suicidal ideation, drug abuse, and domestic violence.

Early reports after the onset of the COVID-19 pandemic from individual trauma centers around the world [6–9] described a decrease in overall trauma volume but an increase in the amount of penetrating trauma due to a person-to-person violent mechanism of injury usually involving a sharp instrument or less commonly a firearm and self-harm injuries, mostly localized at head and neck regions.

The COVID-19 pandemic impacted also emergency surgery activity. Several studies reported a decrease in the number of emergency surgical patients admitted and an increase in more severe septic diseases to manage. This could be the result of the fear of patients to become infected with SARS-CoV-2 and consecutive delayed hospital admission and diagnosis due to overcrowded hospitals. There was also to consider a critical delay in time-to-diagnosis and time-to-intervention due to changes in in-hospital logistics and operating theatres as well as intensive care capacities [10, 11].

During a pandemic, the decision of operating or delaying an urgent surgical procedure depends on the acute care surgeon/emergency surgeon's evaluation.

If an urgent surgical procedure is needed, (life-threatening surgical disease, high-risk patients, hemodynamic compromise, or shock), the emergency surgeon should check promptly the availability of a dedicated operating room with functional and suitable human and technical resources for infected and negative patients, and involve the smallest number of healthcare staff, correctly educated and protected.

The first step in the management of a surgical patient or trauma victim during a pandemic is to confirm the infection as early as possible to decide for the isolation of the patient and put in place all the mandatory measures to limit contact and manage the patient and resources correctly.

The diagnosis of COVID-19 infection is made by:

- The COVID-19 RT-PCR swab test that provides nucleic acid detection in the nasal and throat swab sampling and confirms the infection; a positive RT-PCR test for COVID-19 has more weight than a negative test because it has high specificity but moderate sensitivity [12].
- CHEST IMAGING to assess the severity of the pneumonia; It includes chest radiograph, computed tomography (CT) scan, or lung ultrasound demonstrating bilateral opacities (lung infiltrates >50%), lobar, or lung collapse. Multiple patchy ground-glass opacities in bilateral multiple lobular with periphery distribution are typical chest CT imaging features of COVID-19 pneumonia.

During the COVID-19 pandemic, patients who are not yet being routinely tested for COVID-19, even if they are asymptomatic should be considered as possibly COVID-19 positive to limit the contamination of HCWs.

In case of unavailability of the diagnostic test to confirm the infection, a surgical patient has to be considered potentially infected and managed like a positive patient, even if he/she is asymptomatic, to limit the spreading of virus in the hospital and allocate properly resources.

During a pandemic, it is recommended to assess patients needing hospital admission with the screening test as soon as possible; if it is not possible, the suspected/uncertain patient has to be managed such an infected one with all the mandatory precautions, that include all the protective measures and a dedicated pathway for the operating room, to decrease the risk of environmental contamination and health personnel exposure. If a dedicated pathway for infected patients is not available in the hospital, it should be an option to transfer hemodynamic stable patients to the nearest designed HUB hospital for the appropriate management [1].

Concerning the COVID-19 disease, in case of RT-PCR test and chest CT scan unavailability, it was suggested to screen the patient for COVID-19 pneumonia with Chest XR or lungs ultrasound that can help to assess viral pneumonia radiological signs and severity before surgery. In this case, SARS-CoV-2 infection can only be suspected [1].

Insufficient precaution in managing a non-assessed patient for the infection could cause the contagion of nurses, surgeons, and negative patients; consequently, a single negative screening test should not be used to rule out the infection in patients with strongly suggestive symptoms but it has to be repeated.

In clinical practice, during a pandemic, it means that suspected/uncertain patients should be isolated to ensure the limiting of exposure and contagion [1].

In patients with life-threatening injuries, there is a limited time available for preoperative evaluation and these patients should be managed as suspected infected patients with all the mandatory precautions.

A dedicated triage area is essential for the care of trauma victims. There should be the ready availability of supplies, easy accessibility of PPE, and a limited number of healthcare workers and physicians in this area.

On the arrival at the emergency department (ED), all trauma victims should be considered positive for the viral infection responsible of the pandemic, and necessary precautions should be implemented. Initial assessment and management are done following Advanced Trauma Life Support protocol and taking into consideration that procedures like airway suctioning, endotracheal intubation, non-invasive ventilation, bronchoscopy, chest tube insertion, and tracheostomy are AGPs. An unstable trauma patient might require urgent airway management in the ED where preparedness and teamwork are of utmost importance. Strategies to reduce the infection risk include intubation by an experienced person, rapid sequence induction, and videolaryngoscope facilitated intubation using level three precautions.

Cardiopulmonary resuscitation should be avoided in acute major trauma (blunt or penetrating trauma) unless it was preceded by medical events such as dysrhythmia, pulmonary embolism, or myocardial infarction. Level 3 precautions should be implemented before initiating manual ventilation or chest compressions. Early tracheal intubation using a cuffed endotracheal tube to secure the airway and reduce aerosol generation is recommended. The use of an external chest compression mechanical device and bag valve mask with a high-efficiency particulate air filter reduces the risk of infection to the HCWs [13].

For urgent surgical patients, early clinical diagnosis, adequate source control to stop ongoing contamination, appropriate antimicrobial therapy, and prompt resuscitation in critically ill patients are the cornerstones in the management of intra-abdominal infections.

Under a pandemic, forced to limited access to hospital resources, it could be better to evaluate to postpone an urgent surgical procedure if it is possible. The triage of the patients is fundamental to assess the severity of the intra-abdominal disease underlying the acute abdominal pain and decide on a non-operative (NOM) or operative management (OM), following the international guidelines recommendations.

The hemodynamic stability or instability after adequate resuscitative maneuvers is the main tool to risk-stratify patients for immediate surgery or not.

Furthermore, general, or more specific, clinical scores (such, e.g., the American Society of Anesthesiologists' (ASA) score, Alvarado's score in case of acute appendicitis, Sequential Organ Failure Assessment (SOFA) Score for sepsis, etc.), the age of the patient and the presence of co-morbidities such as obesity, diabetes, chronic obstructive pulmonary disease (COPD), can assist the emergency surgeon decision-making process, associated with clinical (signs of localized or generalized peritonitis at abdominal examination) and biological parameters (inflammatory biomarkers such as C-reactive protein, procalcitonin, lactates).

The timing of acute care surgery (TACS) classification [14] is a useful tool to prioritize patients admitted to ED with a potential surgical condition. It was proposed by a group of expert acute care surgeons such as a color-coded triage system of emergency and trauma surgical cases based on simple hemodynamic and clinical data, as it is shown in Table 31.3.

In evaluating the necessity to perform an emergent/urgent surgical procedure during a pandemic, it is recommended to comply with international guidelines about immediate surgery or non-operative strategies, evaluating case by case and resources.

The TACS classification could support in triaging surgical patients for operating room (OR) access. According to the TACS classification, classes red and orange patients require surgical treatment in a very short delay and the NOM has not to be considered [1].

Table 31.3 Timing of acute care surgery (TACS) classification [14]

Timing- iTTS from diagnosis	Possible Clinical Scenarios (TACS)	Color code	Note
Immediate surgery	Bleeding emergencies	Red	Immediate life saving surgical intervention, resuscitative laparotomy
Within an hour	Incarcerated hernia, perforated viscus, diffuse peritonitis, soft tissue infection accompanied with sepsis	Orange	Surgical Intervention as soon as possible but only after resuscitation (within 1 to 2 hours). administration of antibiotics upon diagnosis- no delay
Within 6 hours	Soft tissue infection (abscess) not accompanied with sepsis	Yellow	Administration of antibiotics upon diagnosis- no delay
Within 12 hours	Appendicitis (local peritonitis), cholecystitis (optional)	Green	Administration of antibiotics upon diagnosis- no delay
Within 24 or 48 hours	Second-look laparotomy	Blue	Schedule in advance. Intervention should occur during day time

The last available data about the ongoing pandemic showed that postoperative pulmonary complications occur in half of the patients with peri-operative SARS-CoV-2 infection and they are associated with high mortality, particularly in men aged 70 years and older [15].

Consequently, if the intra-abdominal disease is uncomplicated (i.e., involving the organ and not the peritoneum), the NOM could be a valid option to be considered on a case-by-case basis to decrease the postoperative mortality rate in SARS-CoV-2 infected patients.

In the case of NOM, it is crucial to plan close clinical and radiological monitoring of the patient at 12- to 24-hrs intervals from the beginning of the intravenous antibiotic therapy until the situation is under control.

Patients who have failed NOM for a surgical condition or who present with hemodynamic instability should be considered for immediate surgery [1].

If a suspected/uncertain patient needs to undergo immediate surgery, it is recommended to manage him/her as a confirmed infected patient and isolate the patient after surgery, until the diagnosis is confirmed by the diagnostic test.

31.4 Treatment: The Management of an Infected Patient for an Emergency Surgical Procedure after Admission

31.4.1 The Transfer of the Infected Patient to the Operating Room

The transfer of the patient, wearing a surgical mask, from the ward to the OR will have to be done by the ward nurses in full PPE including a well-fitting N95 mask, goggles or face shield, splash-resistant gown, and boot covers [16].

For patients coming from ICU, a dedicated transport ventilator can be used. To avoid aerosolization, the gas flow is turned off and the endotracheal tube is clamped with forceps during the switching of the ventilator. The ICU personnel has to wear full PPE with a PAPR for the transfer.

The patient should be transported from the isolation unit to the OR along a designated route with minimal contact with others patients and HCWs [17].

The Safety and Health officers in the hospital are responsible for clearing the route from the ward or ICU to the OR, including the elevators.

All personnel who come into contact with the patient must perform hand hygiene and are required to wear all PPE including an FFP2 mask, oversized waterproof long-sleeved gown, knee-high shoe protection, cap, eye protection, and double-pair gloves. HCWs are advised against touching their eyes, nose, or mouth.

31.4.2 The Operating Room Set Up

All the surgical procedures involving an infected patient have to be performed in a negative pressure environment to reduce the dissemination of the virus beyond the OR; if it is not possible, a high frequency of air changes (25 per hour) in a standard positive pressure OR can reduce the viral load [18].

The OR doors will be closed for the duration of the surgical procedure.

Only selected equipment and drugs should be brought into the OR to reduce the number of items that need cleaning or discarding following the procedure; a runner will be stationed outside the OR if additional drugs or equipment are needed. These are placed onto a trolley that will be left in the anteroom for the OR team to retrieve. This same process in reverse is used to send out specimens such as arterial blood gas samples and frozen section specimens. The runner wears PPE when entering the anteroom.

Single-use equipment should be selected where possible.

Anesthetic monitors, laptop computers, and ultrasound machine surfaces are covered with plastic wrap to decrease the risk of contamination and to facilitate cleaning.

31.4.3 The Timing of Anesthesia

The surgical-infected patient should be reviewed, induced, and recovered within the dedicated OR. The number of staff involved in the surgery should be limited. The movement of staff in and out of the OR should also be restricted.

The surgical team will perform the surgical dressing according to the procedure for performing surgery, replacing the surgical mask with a FFP2 mask, wearing high shoes protection, and a waterproof gown. Eye protection (goggles) or facial protection (face shield) should be always worn.

If sedation is administered, supplemental oxygen may be administered via nasal prongs underneath the surgical mask. Non-invasive positive pressure ventilation and high-flow nasal cannulae such as the trans-nasal humidified rapid-insufflation ventilatory exchange should be avoided to reduce the risk of viral aerosolization [19].

Before anesthesia induction, a HEPA filter should be connected to the patient end of the breathing circuit, and another between the expiratory limb and the anesthetic machine. Equipment should be prepared to reduce the need for circuit disconnections. A definitive airway with an endotracheal tube is preferred over a supra-glottic airway device because it has a better seal. A video-laryngoscope is recommended because a PAPR hood or goggles may hamper the vision during direct laryngoscopy. A video-laryngoscope also keeps the physician far from the patient's airway during intubation [16].

Fast induction of anesthesia with adequate muscle relaxation is recommended to prevent cough. The order of administration should be muscle relaxation drugs, intravenous general anesthetic, and opioids to avoid cough. Mask pressurization ventilation should be avoided before the patient loses consciousness. During anesthesia maintenance, a small tidal volume of lung-protective ventilation strategy should be adopted to reduce ventilator-related lung injury [9].

During a pandemic, it is recommended to reduce to the minimum the number of healthcare staff present at intubation and extubation maneuvers if it is possible [1].

31.4.4 The Surgical Procedure

Since the COVID-19 outbreak, many authors suggested great care when carrying out a laparoscopic procedure in surgical SARS-CoV-2 infected patients, based on a theoretical risk of occupational exposure and infection of the operating theatre staff. To the best of our knowledge, there are no studies that have firmly confirmed the correlation between laparoscopy, the artificial pneumoperitoneum and the infection rate of the OR staff [20–24].

Several previous studies have demonstrated that electrosurgical devices can produce aerosolized bacteria and viruses with several studies demonstrating a risk of oral papillomatosis due to occupational exposure during open surgery [24–30].

At the early stage of the COVID-19 pandemic, in the lack of strong evidence, many international societies were nearly to prohibit laparoscopy, except in ultra-selected cases.

More carefully, several authors [20–22] proposed different techniques to perform a safe laparoscopy, based on the principle of limiting the leakage of gas as summarized in Table 31.4.

During a pandemic, minimally invasive techniques should include constant pressure insufflators to reduce the aerosol effect of insufflation and central aspirator systems to drain the smoke. Special attention should be paid to evacuating residual pneumoperitoneum from the container and the abdominal cavity before removing the trocars.

For some authors, during a pandemic, a laparoscopic approach should be avoided because it could be associated with longer operative time (and therefore increased risk of exposure and occupational time of OR), especially in an emergency setting [20]. For others, laparoscopic procedures create a functional barrier between the surgeon and biological fluids because the abdomen is not opened, reducing HCWs' exposure to the virus compared with open surgery [20, 21].

Considering available evidence since now, both laparoscopic and open approaches could be considered AGPs and could contribute to environmental contamination and virus exposure.

Taking into consideration patient safety and infection prevention, on a case-by-case evaluation, the emergency surgeon has to select the appropriate surgical technique for that patient with the available resources.

The availability of adapted surgical equipment, all PPE, and trained HCWs are essential to perform a safe surgical procedure.

Generally, OR exposure to the virus and the risk of environmental contamination could be minimized by employing negative-pressure ventilation (preventing cross-contamination between rooms),

Table 31.4 Tips and tricks to perform a safe surgical procedure during a pandemic [2]

Performing a safe laparoscopic approach	Performing a safe laparotomy
Check if a closed suction system is available	Avoid huge incision causing loss of biological fluids and staff contamination
Create suitable surgical incisions for the introduction of leak-free trocars such as balloon trocars if available	Think to protect the incision with a double ring wound protector, if it is available according to recommendations for SSI control
Be sure not to contribute to increasing the OR air contamination by creating a leak in the presence of smoke obstructing the intervention	The power settings of the electrocautery should be as low as possible
Aspirate the entire pneumoperitoneum before making an auxiliary incision to extract the specimen, at the end of the procedure before removing the trocars, or before converting the intervention to laparotomy	Avoid long dissecting times on the same spot by electrocautery or ultrasonic scalpels to reduce surgical smoke
Keep intraoperative pneumoperitoneum pressure and CO_2 ventilation at the lowest possible levels without compromising the surgical field exposure	Use the suction devices to remove the surgical smoke
Reduce the Trendelenburg position time as much as possible. This minimizes the effect of pneumoperitoneum on lung function and circulation, to reduce pathogen susceptibility	Special attention is warranted to avoid sharp injury or damage to protective equipment, in particular gloves and body protection
Avoid long dissecting times on the same spot by electrocautery or ultrasonic scalpels to reduce surgical smoke	Minimize the use of drainage

decreasing time and exposure during intubation, using surgical masks such as FFP2 (minimum) or FFP3, improving the energy devices/electrocautery use among other measures to minimize operative staff exposure to aerosolized particles, as well as smoke evacuation/suction systems both in laparoscopic approach and emergency laparotomy.

Contraindications to laparoscopy are not evidence-based since aerosolization is produced during both open and laparoscopic surgical procedures. However, personal protective equipment is the key for the infection prevention [1, 2].

Moreover, the laparoscopic approach has the main advantage of decreasing the length of hospital stay of a surgical patient, decreasing the risk of in-hospital infection of a negative patient, in a period of limited availability of beds.

According to these data, it is suggested to both in laparoscopic and in laparotomy, carefully balance the risk of potential viral exposure and transmission in that particular situation and the clinical benefits of a minimally invasive approach or a laparotomy for that patient [2].

Damage control surgery may have a role in hemodynamically compromised patients with minimum manipulation and short surgical duration. Patients treated with either damage control surgery or open abdomen will need to be admitted to the ICU. However, as ICUs are overwhelmed because of the pandemic, the indications for performing open abdomen surgery should be carefully evaluated on a case-by-case basis [2].

During a pandemic, the technique to perform the surgery has to be selected considering the benefits for the patient, with the aim of reducing the occupational time of the operating room, and the risk of environmental contamination.

Experts recommend being careful in the establishment and management of the artificial pneumoperitoneum, in the management of the hemostasis and of surgical incisions to prevent any loss of biological fluids and contamination of the surgical staff during a pandemic and using of all available devices to remove smoke and aerosol during the surgical procedure both in laparoscopy and open approach [1].

In the lack of PPE and general measures to prepare the operating theatre for an infected patient, and in the impossibility to perform surgery in a safe and protected environment, it is recommended do not underestimating the highest risk of contamination and infection for HCWs and dissemination of the virus in the hospital and to consider transferring hemodynamically stable surgical patients in a designed HUB hospital for the appropriate management [1].

31.4.5 After the Surgical Procedure

At the end of the surgical procedure, surgeons and all the staff who are not implicated in the transfer of the patient will leave the OR to perform the undressing procedure in the ante-OR area [14, 16].

The recommended PPE removal sequence provides:

1. to remove the first pair of gloves not touching the ones below;
2. to untie the closing laces of the gown:
3. to remove the gown taking care not to touch its external anterior part by turning it over so that the contaminated external part remains inside;
4. to remove the shoes protection;
5. to remove the second pair of gloves;
6. to perform hands hygiene with antiseptic soap;
7. to wear a pair of clean gloves;
8. to remove the eye-protective disposal proceeding from the non-contaminated part;
9. to remove the FFP2/FFP3 mask being careful to touch only the elastics and not the contaminated surface;
10. to remove the cup, proceeding from the back of the head;
11. to perform hand hygiene with antiseptic soap.

All staffs have to shower and change into a clean set of scrubs before resuming their regular duties.

Names of all participating staff members are recorded to facilitate contact tracing.

The PPE used must be disposed of inside the containers for special waste at risk of infection.

Personnel who continue to assist the patient and who will take the patient to the ward/ICU will leave the operating theatre following the access path backward taking care to change the gloves before the transport.

The operating room must be sanitized as soon as possible. For example, after confirmed COVID-19 cases management, a hydrogen peroxide vaporizer will be used to decontaminate the OR, infact it is well known that human coronaviruses such as SARS-CoV, MERS coronavirus, or endemic human coronaviruses can persist on inanimate surfaces such as metal, glass, or plastic for up to nine days; these can be efficiently inactivated by surface disinfection procedures with 62–71% ethanol, 0.5% hydrogen peroxide or 0.1% sodium hypochlorite within one minute. Other biocidal agents such as 0.05–0.2% benzalkonium chloride or 0.02% chlorhexidine digluconate are less effective [15, 18].

31.4.6 The Postoperative Management and Discharge of the Patient

During a pandemic, surgical patients with confirmed infection require a multidisciplinary approach and management, in the lack of a specific treatment because of the multisystemic syndrome showed by the infectious disease, to decrease morbidity and mortality rates related to the emergent surgical procedure and the infectious disease.

Infected patients need to be isolated from negative patients to decrease the in-hospital risk of virus transmission and environmental contamination and to be cared for by a trained and skilled workforce with adequate PPE to preserve negative surgical patients from contagion because of the high risk of coming in contact with droplets and biological fluids.

During the COVID-19 pandemic, after an emergency surgical procedure, patients with severe COVID-19 pneumonia have to be re-admitted to Covid-ICU for management, monitoring, and early detection of postoperative complications.

For stable asymptomatic or mildly symptomatic patients, it would be better to create a surgical dedicated ward to avoid any contamination of negative patients and to limit the in-hospital exposure to the virus to a dedicated and trained team [1].

Concerning COVID-19 disease, there is not a specific available treatment for COVID-19 disease. The current Centers for Disease Control (CDC) and Prevention recommended the prompt implementation of infection prevention and control measures and supportive management of complications for all infected patients [31]. Similarly, WHO stated the importance of the role of supportive care based on the severity of illness, ranging from symptomatic treatment for mild disease to evidence-based ventilatory management for ARDS and early recognition and treatment of bacterial infections and sepsis in critically ill patients [32].

As to antibiotics management, initial prompt antibiotic therapy for intra-abdominal infections in surgical negative and positive patients is typically empirical and depends on the underlying severity of infection, the pathogens presumed to be involved, and the risk factors indicative of major resistance patterns. Antimicrobial treatment should be targeted to results from cultures from the site of infections or hemocultures with de-escalation of treatment as early as possible, in accordance with international guidelines [33, 34].

Empirical anti-fungal treatment should only be considered in critically infected patients, presenting fever of unknown origin, with a new pulmonary infiltrate superimposed on a viral pneumonitis pattern, to confirm the diagnosis by invasive techniques and/or the use of fungal biomarkers [1].

COVID-19 patients showed a high risk to develop venous thromboembolism events because of severe hypercoagulability induced by the virus. Early anticoagulation may block clotting formation and reduce micro-thrombus, thereby reducing the risk of major organ damage. Prophylactic-dose low-molecular weight heparin (LMWH) should be initiated in all surgical patients with COVID-19 disease admitted to the hospital to decrease thromboembolic risk related to the infection and emergency surgery, in accord with the risk of bleeding related to the patient himself and the surgical procedure [35].

LMWH should be given at a dosage approved for high-risk patients (e.g., body mass index > 30 kg/m^2, history of Venous Thromboembolism (VTE), known thrombophilia, active cancer) or requiring ICU admission or with rapidly increasing D-dimer levels, taking into account renal function and bleeding risk. In case of contraindications for anticoagulation, physical measures should be used (e.g., medical compression stockings).

Carfora et al [36] developed an algorithm for anticoagulation management in COVID-19 patients. It provides that in Mild cases of Covid pneumonia, Padua or Caprini scores should be evaluated; if Padua score is ≥4 and/or Caprini score is ≥10, LMWH (4000 IU q24h) should be started in the absence of contraindications. In Moderate cases, LMWH (4000–6000 IU q24h) should be started, irrespective of VTE risk assessment scores, in the absence of contraindications. In Severe and Critical cases, the International Society of Thrombosis and Hemostasis-Disseminated Intravascular Coagulation (ISTH-DIC) score should be evaluated; in case of ISTH-DIC score <5, LMWH (4000–6000 IU q24h) should be started, in the absence of contraindications; if the ISTH-DIC score is ≥5, it was suggested to use full-dose LMWH (100 IU/kg q12h), in the absence of contraindications.

During a pandemic, in the case of an infectious disease that induces hypercoagulability, it is suggested to administer prophylactic anticoagulation with LMWH as soon as possible in surgical patients to reduce the thromboembolic risk related to the virus, sepsis, and emergency surgery. The dosage of the anticoagulant therapy has to be adjusted according to the risk of surgical bleeding, renal function, and weight of the patient. In high-risk conditions for bleeding, when is contraindicated to administer antithrombotic prophylaxis, it is suggested to consider intermittent pneumatic compression, in case of an immobilized patient, and to mobilize the patient as soon as possible after surgery [1].

In an unusual scenario of a limited number of beds, the discharge from the hospital of uncertain/suspected or confirmed, asymptomatic or mild symptomatic surgical patients—if clinically appropriate, after recovery from the intra-abdominal infection—may be considered as soon as possible.

After hospital discharge, all the confirmed infected asymptomatic patients should be kept in isolation limiting the risk of exposure for the other household members (e.g., single room with good ventilation, face-mask wear, reduced close contact with family members, separate meals, good hand sanitation, and no outdoor activities) for at least 2 weeks have passed since the date of their first positive diagnostic test.

The decision to remove precautions is based on two general strategies: a test-based strategy that requires negative diagnostic tests obtained after the resolution of symptoms, and a symptom-based strategy that recommends keeping patients on contact precautions until a fixed period has elapsed from symptom recovery.

During the COVID-19 pandemic, experts have recommended obtaining a negative RT-PCR nasopharyngeal swab test before discontinuing isolation and precautions earlier than 14 days after the confirmed diagnosis of COVID-19 [1].

The lockdown and isolation required to contain the COVID-19 pandemic have increased the implementation of telemedicine platforms in clinical practice. Telemedicine allowed caring for asymptomatic and stable patients virtually through non-physical encounters with the use of videoconferencing and telephone communications, ensuring the safety of patients and healthcare workers during the crisis [37]

Post-operative follow-ups using video calls, or a combination of phone calls and wound images taken by patients can limit the circulation of patients and showed to be safe and effective ways of detecting early postoperative complications [38].

Tele-rehabilitation for trauma patients which includes home-based rehabilitation programs and video-based rather than direct physical training will also decrease in-hospital stay and expedite safe home discharge [39].

Dos and Don'ts
- All surgical and trauma victims have to be considered as infected as long as they are not screened for the disease responsible for the pandemic.
- All the positive patients have to be managed with all the mandatory precautions against viral infection, which include all the protective measures, isolation, and a dedicated pathway for the operating room.
- If a dedicated pathway for infected patients is not available in the hospital and the lack of required personal protective equipment, is better to evaluate to transfer of clinically stable patients to the nearest designed HUB hospital for the appropriate management.
- In evaluating the necessity to perform an emergent/urgent surgical procedure, it is recommended to comply with international guidelines about immediate surgery or non-operative strategies, evaluating case by case and resources.
- In performing a surgical procedure, reduce the number of healthcare staff to the minimum, and be careful in the establishment and management of the artificial pneumoperitoneum (low pressure and aspiration system), in the management of the hemostasis and of surgical incisions to prevent any loss of biological fluids and contamination.
- Antibiotics should be carefully administrated for the high risk of selecting resistant bacteria, especially in patients admitted to the ICU for mechanical ventilation.
- Early empirical antibiotic treatment should be targeted to results from cultures, with de-escalation of treatment as soon as possible.
- Do not prescribe empirical anti-fungal treatments in all surgical patients but only in critically ill patients, presenting fever of unknown origin, with new pulmonary infiltrate superimposed on a viral pneumonitis pattern, to confirm the diagnosis by invasive techniques and/or the use of fungal biomarkers.
- Administer prophylactic anticoagulation with LMWH as soon as possible in surgical patients or intermittent pneumatic compression.
- Patients should be discharged as soon as possible and followed up by video and phone calls to limit access to the hospital.

Take-Home Messages
- Emergency and acute care surgeons need to ensure the management of surgical patients and trauma victims with a high standard of care during a pandemic.
- We have learned from the COVID-19 pandemic that, all trauma and surgical patients who are waiting for hospital admission have to be screened for the infectious disease responsible for the pandemic to limit the diffusion of the virus in the hospitals. The management of positive/infected patients is multidisciplinary and requires a well-defined protocol of care.
- Emergency surgeons must evaluate whether it is possible to postpone a surgical treatment until the patient is no longer considered potentially infectious or at risk of perioperative and postoperative complications. If an emergency surgical procedure, both in laparoscopy or in an open approach, is necessary, the emergency surgeon must supervise the implementation of safety measures in the operating theatre. Trained staff, adequate instruments and strict application of the recommendations are crucial to avoid the increase of the risk of contamination and the dissemination of the disease.

References

1. De Simone B, Chouillard E, Sartelli M, Biffl WL, Di Saverio S, Moore EE, Kluger Y, Abu-Zidan FM, Ansaloni L, Coccolini F, Leppäniemi A, Peitzmann AB, Pagani L, Fraga GP, Paolillo C, Picetti E, Valentino M, Pikoulis E, Baiocchi GL, Catena F. The management of surgical patients in the emergency setting during COVID-19 pandemic: the WSES position paper. World J Emerg Surg. 2021;16(1):14. https://doi.org/10.1186/s13017-021-00349-0.
2. De Simone B, Chouillard E, Di Saverio S, Pagani L, Sartelli M, Biffl WL, Coccolini F, Pieri A, Khan M, Borzellino G, Campanile FC, Ansaloni L, Catena F. Emergency surgery during the COVID-19 pandemic: what you need to know for practice. Ann R Coll Surg Engl. 2020;102(5):323–32. https://doi.org/10.1308/rcsann.2020.0097. Epub 2020 Apr 30.
3. World Health Organization. Infection prevention and control during health care when coronavirus disease (COVID-19) is suspected or confirmed. Published June 29, 2020. Accessed November 2, 2020. https://www.who.int/publications/i/item/WHO-2019-nCoV-IPC-2020.4.
4. Klompas M, Baker M, Rhee C. What is an aerosol-generating procedure? JAMA Surg. 2021;156(2):113–4. https://doi.org/10.1001/jamasurg.2020.6643.
5. Lockhart SL, Duggan LV, Wax RS, Saad S, Grocott HP. Personal protective equipment (PPE) for both anesthesiologists and other airway managers: principles and practice during the COVID-19 pandemic. Can J Anaesth. 2020;67(8):1005–15. https://doi.org/10.1007/s12630-020-01673-w. Epub 2020 Apr 23.
6. Jacob S, Mwagiru D, Thakur I, Moghadam A, Oh T, Hsu J. Impact of societal restrictions and lockdown on trauma admissions during the COVID-19 pandemic: a single-centre cross-sectional observational study. ANZ J Surg. 2020;90(11):2227–31. https://doi.org/10.1111/ans.16307. Epub 2020 Sep 29.
7. Yeates EO, Grigorian A, Barrios C, Schellenberg M, Owattanapanich N, Barmparas G, Margulies D, Juillard C, Garber K, Cryer H, Tillou A, Burruss S, Penaloza-Villalobos L, Lin A, Figueras RA, Brenner M, Firek C, Costantini T, Santorelli J, Curry T, Wintz D, Biffl WL, Schaffer KB, Duncan TK, Barbaro C, Diaz G, Johnson A, Chinn J, Naaseh A, Leung A, Grabar C, Nahmias J. Changes in traumatic mechanisms of injury in Southern California related to COVID-19: penetrating trauma as a second pandemic. J Trauma Acute Care Surg. 2021;90(4):714–21. https://doi.org/10.1097/TA.0000000000003068.
8. Olding J, Zisman S, Olding C, Fan K, et al. Surgeon. 2021;19(1):e9–e13. https://doi.org/10.1016/j.surge.2020.07.004. Epub 2020 Jul 30.
9. Chodos M, Sarani B, Sparks A, Bruns B, Gupta S, Michetti CP, Crane J, Hall E, Trankiem CT, Abouassaly C, Haut ER, Etchill E, Kovler ML, Williams M, Zeineddin A, Estroff J. Impact of COVID-19 pandemic on injury prevalence and pattern in the Washington, DC metropolitan region: a multicenter study by the American College of Surgeons Committee on Trauma, Washington, DC. Trauma Surg Acute Care Open. 2021;6(1):e000659. https://doi.org/10.1136/tsaco-2020-000659.
10. Reichert M, Sartelli M, Weigand MA, Doppstadt C, Hecker M, Reinisch-Liese A, Bender F, Askevold I, Padberg W, Coccolini F, Catena F, Hecker A. WSES COVID-19 emergency surgery survey collaboration group. Impact of the SARS-CoV-2 pandemic on emergency surgery services-a multi-national survey among WSES members. World J Emerg Surg. 2020;15(1):64. https://doi.org/10.1186/s13017-020-00341-0.
11. Kurihara H, Marrano E, Ceolin M, Chiara O, Faccincani R, Bisagni P, Fattori L, Zago M, Lombardy Emergency Surgery Group During Covid19 Outbreak. Impact of lockdown on emergency general surgery during first 2020 COVID-19 outbreak. Eur J Trauma Emerg Surg. 2021;47(3):677–82. https://doi.org/10.1007/s00068-021-01691-3. Epub 2021 May 4.
12. Watson J, Whiting PF, Brush JE. Interpreting a covid-19 test result. BMJ. 2020;369:m1808. https://doi.org/10.1136/bmj.m1808.
13. Sawhney C, Singh Y, Jain K, Sawhney R, Trikha A. Trauma care and COVID-19 pandemic. J Anaesthesiol Clin Pharmacol. 2020;36(Suppl 1):S115–20. https://doi.org/10.4103/joacp.JOACP_272_20. Epub 2020 Jul 31.
14. Kluger Y, Ben-Ishay O, Sartelli M, et al. World society of emergency surgery study group initiative on Timing of Acute Care Surgery classification (TACS). World J Emerg Surg. 2013;8:17. https://doi.org/10.1186/1749-7922-8-17.
15. COVIDSurg Collaborative. Mortality and pulmonary complications in patients undergoing surgery with perioperative SARS-CoV-2 infection: an international cohort. Lancet. 2020;396:27–38.
16. Coccolini F, Perrone G, Chiarugi M, Di Marzo F, Ansaloni L, Scandroglio I, Marini P, Zago M, De Paolis P, Forfori F, Agresta F, Puzziello A, D'Ugo D, Bignami E, Bellini V, Vitali P, Petrini F, Pifferi B, Corradi F, Tarasconi A, Pattonieri V, Bonati E, Tritapepe L, Agnoletti V, Corbella D, Sartelli M, Catena F. Surgery in COVID-19 patients: operational directives. World J Emerg Surg. 2020;15(1):25. https://doi.org/10.1186/s13017-020-00307-2.
17. Fransvea P, Sganga G, Cozza V, Di Grezia M, Fico V, Tirelli F, Pepe G, La Greca A. Set up of a dedicated COVID-19 surgical pathway and operating room for surgical emergencies. J Trauma Acute Care Surg. 2020;89(4):e97–e100. https://doi.org/10.1097/TA.0000000000002852.
18. Ti LK, Ang LS, Foong TW, Ng BSW. What we do when a COVID-19 patient needs an operation: oper-

19. Peng PWH, Ho PL, Hota SS. Outbreak of a new coronavirus: what anaesthetists should know. Br J Anaesth. 2020;124(5):497–501. https://doi.org/10.1016/j.bja.2020.02.008. Epub 2020 Feb 27.
20. Yu GY, Lou Z, Zhang W. Several suggestions of operation for colorectal cancer under the outbreak of corona virus disease 2019 in China. Zhonghua Wei Chang Wai Ke Za Zhi. 2020;23:208–11.
21. Di Saverio S, Pata F, Gallo G, Carrano F, Scorza A, Sileri P, Smart N, Spinelli A, Pellino G. Coronavirus pandemic and colorectal surgery: practical advice based on the Italian experience. Colon Dis. 2020;22(6):625–34. https://doi.org/10.1111/codi.15056.
22. Di Saverio S, Khan M, Pata F, Ietto G, De Simone B, Zani E, Carcano G. Laparoscopy at all costs? Not now during COVID-19 outbreak and not for acute care surgery and emergency colorectal surgery. J Trauma Acute Care Surg. 2020;88(6):715–8. https://doi.org/10.1097/TA.0000000000002727.
23. Coccolini F, Tartaglia D, Puglisi A, et al. SARS-CoV-2 is present in peritoneal fluid in COVID-19 patients. Ann Surg. 2020;272(3):e240–2. https://doi.org/10.1097/SLA.0000000000004030.
24. Baggish MS, et al. Presence of human immunodeficiency virus DNA in laser smoke. Lasers Surg Med. 1991;11(3):197–203. https://doi.org/10.1002/lsm.1900110302.
25. Sood AK, et al. Human papillomavirus DNA in LEEP plume. Infect Dis Obstet Gynecol. 1994;2(4):167–70. https://doi.org/10.1155/S1064744994000591.
26. Kwak HD, et al. Detecting hepatitis B virus in surgical smoke emitted during laparoscopic surgery. Occup Environ Med. 2016;73(12):857–63.
27. Gloster HM Jr, Roenigk RK. Risk of acquiring human papillomavirus from the plume produced by the carbon dioxide laser in the treatment of warts. J Am Acad Dermatol. 1995;32(3):436–41. https://doi.org/10.1016/0190-9622(95)90065-9.
28. Bigony L. Risks associated with exposure to surgical smoke plume: a review of the literature. AORN J. 2007;86(6):1013–20. https://doi.org/10.1016/j.aorn.2007.07.005.
29. Limchantra IV, Fong Y, Melstrom KA. Surgical smoke exposure in operating room personnel: a review. JAMA Surg. 2019;154(10):960–7. https://doi.org/10.1001/jamasurg.2019.2515.
30. Gianella M, Hahnloser D, Rey JM, Sigrist MW. Quantitative chemical analysis of surgical smoke generated during laparoscopic surgery with a vessel-sealing device. Surg Innov. 2014;21(2):170–9. https://doi.org/10.1177/1553350613492025.
31. https://www.cdc.gov/coronavirus/2019-ncov/hcp/clinical-guidance-management-patients.html
32. https://www.who.int/publications-detail/clinical-management-of-severe-acute-respiratory-infection-when-novel-coronavirus-(ncov)-infection-is-suspected
33. Sartelli M, Chichom-Mefire A, Labricciosa FM, Hardcastle T, Abu-Zidan FM, Adesunkanmi AK, Ansaloni L, Bala M, Balogh ZJ, Beltrán MA, Ben-Ishay O, Biffl WL, Birindelli A, Cainzos MA, Catalini G, Ceresoli M, Che Jusoh A, Chiara O, Coccolini F, Coimbra R, Cortese F, Demetrashvili Z, Di Saverio S, Diaz JJ, Egiev VN, Ferrada P, Fraga GP, Ghnnam WM, Lee JG, Gomes CA, Hecker A, Herzog T, Kim JI, Inaba K, Isik A, Karamarkovic A, Kashuk J, Khokha V, Kirkpatrick AW, Kluger Y, Koike K, Kong VY, Leppaniemi A, Machain GM, Maier RV, Marwah S, McFarlane ME, Montori G, Moore EE, Negoi I, Olaoye I, Omari AH, Ordonez CA, Pereira BM, Pereira Júnior GA, Pupelis G, Reis T, Sakakhushev B, Sato N, Segovia Lohse HA, Shelat VG, Søreide K, Uhl W, Ulrych J, Van Goor H, Velmahos GC, Yuan KC, Wani I, Weber DG, Zachariah SK, Catena F. The management of intra-abdominal infections from a global perspective: 2017 WSES guidelines for management of intra-abdominal infections. World J Emerg Surg. 2017;12:29. https://doi.org/10.1186/s13017-017-0141-6. Erratum in: World J Emerg Surg. 2017;12:36.
34. De Simone B, Sartelli M, Coccolini F, Ball CG, Brambillasca P, Chiarugi M, Campanile FC, Nita G, Corbella D, Leppaniemi A, Boschini E, Moore EE, Biffl W, Peitzmann A, Kluger Y, Sugrue M, Fraga G, Di Saverio S, Weber D, Sakakushev B, Chiara O, Abu-Zidan FM, Ten Broek R, Kirkpatrick AW, Wani I, Coimbra R, Baiocchi GL, Kelly MD, Ansaloni L, Catena F. Intraoperative surgical site infection control and prevention: a position paper and future addendum to WSES intra-abdominal infections guidelines. World J Emerg Surg. 2020;15(1):10. https://doi.org/10.1186/s13017-020-0288-4. Erratum in: World J Emerg Surg. 2021;16(1):18.
35. Obi AT, Barnes GD, Napolitano LM, Henke PK, Wakefield TW. Venous thrombosis epidemiology, pathophysiology, and anticoagulant therapies and trials in severe acute respiratory syndrome coronavirus 2 infection. J Vasc Surg Venous Lymphat Disord. 2021;9(1):23–35. https://doi.org/10.1016/j.jvsv.2020.08.030. Epub 2020 Sep 8.
36. Carfora V, Spiniello G, Ricciolino R, et al. Anticoagulant treatment in COVID-19: a narrative review. J Thromb Thrombolysis. 2021;51:642–8. https://doi.org/10.1007/s11239-020-02242-0.
37. Temesgen ZM, DeSimone DC, Mahmood M, Libertin CR, Varatharaj Palraj BR, Berbari EF. Health care after the COVID-19 pandemic and the influence of telemedicine. Mayo Clin Proc. 2020;95(9S):S66–8. https://doi.org/10.1016/j.mayocp.2020.06.052. Epub 2020 Jul 27.

38. Hakim AA, Kellish AS, Atabek U, Spitz FR, Hong YK. Implications for the use of telehealth in surgical patients during the COVID-19 pandemic. Am J Surg. 2020;220(1):48–9. https://doi.org/10.1016/j.amjsurg.2020.04.026. Epub 2020 Apr 21.

39. Turolla A, Rossettini G, Viceconti A, Palese A, Geri T. Musculoskeletal physical therapy during the COVID-19 pandemic: is telerehabilitation the answer? Phys Ther. 2020;100(8):1260–4. https://doi.org/10.1093/ptj/pzaa093.

Principles of Management of Surgical Complications

32

Nikolaos Pararas, Anastasia Pikouli, Konstantinos Nastos, and Emmanouil Pikoulis

32.1 Introduction

> **Learning Goals**
> - To manage the risk of complication
> - Prevention and risk assessment
> - Early recognition of postoperative complication
> - Appropriate and timely management

More than 230 million surgical operations are performed globally annually, according to data from the World Health Organization (WHO) [1]. In developed countries, the surgical mortality estimate is between 0.5% and 0.8%, with a complication rate of 3–17% of the cases [1]; these figures are reported to be even higher in developing countries [2]. When evaluating only emergency and urgent procedures, these rates rise and, although there are not many reported studies in this context, the mortality rate is reported to be about ten times higher [3, 4]. This may be explained by the lack of time to execute a complete or even satisfactory preoperative evaluation and a consequent risk assessment of these patients. Numerous challenges are present when performing non-elective emergency surgical procedures; the perioperative care of these high-risk patients appears to have considerable deficiencies. Outcomes are variable and generate an enormous health cost through the prolonged hospital stay and the use of intensive care and other hospital resources.

While there are several specific initiatives and patient pathways for single operations, there is a lack of an overall strategy for the care of all these patients at higher risk of complications and even death.

This high-risk group consists of 12–15% of all surgical cases but contributes to 80% or more of postoperative complications and deaths. A practical, efficient, and timely approach to preventing and managing complications is mandatory in the emergency setting of surgery.

32.2 Classification of Complications

All emergency operations carry a risk, and the complication can be categorized as being general, because of undergoing any surgical procedure or as specific to the specific operation being performed. They may be further divided by time of onset to (a) immediate (within the first 24 h of surgery), (b) early (within 30 days or during the inpatient episode), or (c) late (after

N. Pararas (✉) · A. Pikouli · K. Nastos · E. Pikoulis
3d Department of Surgery, Attikon General Hospital, National & Kapodistrian University of Athens (NKUA), Faculty of Medicine, Athens, Greece
e-mail: mpikoul@med.uoa.gr

Table 32.1 Surgical and non-surgical complications in the postoperative period

Postoperative day	1	2	3	4	5+
Pain	Wound pain				
Infection		Wound infection			Tissue infection
Gastrointestinal				Anastomotic leak/fistula	
	Vomiting/nausea/	Ileus/	Abdominal	compartment	syndrome
Respiratory	Atelectasis		Pulmonary embolism/	Lung infection	
Cardiovascular	Myocardial Infarction	Atrial Fibrillation	Hemorrhage	Hypovolemia	
Urinary		Acute	kidney	Injury	
	Retention				

30 days). In Table 32.1, the time order of onset of some common general postoperative complications is summarized.

32.2.1 Management of the Risk of the Complications

The most important in managing any surgical complication remains is (a) the prevention and risk assessment, (b) early recognition, and (c) appropriate and timed management.

32.2.1.1 Prevention and Risk Assessment

The preoperative assessment of comorbidities and pre-morbid function allows the surgeons to predict possible risks for patients undergoing any surgical intervention. The surgical team can then institute risk-reducing measures to minimize specific complications.

This part involves the chance to optimize comorbid conditions and their management along with the initiation of specific prophylactic measures, such as the choice of anesthetic technique or the use of antibiotics. This phase cannot always be applied in an emergency setting.

An additional measure to reduce operative complications is the implementation of the World Health Organization (WHO) Surgical Safety checklist. This has been demonstrated to reduce surgical morbidity by 30% and mortality by almost 50% by identifying, eliminating, and preventing errors [3].

32.2.1.2 Early Recognition

Early detection and a well-timed intervention are key factors to reduce the morbidity of postoperative complications, and this depends on the alertness of clinicians, with attention given to detail. Most hospitals promote the use of Early Warning Scores (EWS) to identify and respond to patients present in the emergency setting. The scores that reach a certain threshold will initiate a call for urgent clinician review.

32.2.1.3 Appropriate and Timely Management of Complications

After early recognition, it is crucial to implement appropriate management strategies to significantly reduce morbidity or even mortality. This might involve medical or surgical therapies and may refer the patient to other specialties or even transfer to a higher level of care.

32.2.2 Common Surgical Complications in the Emergency Setting

32.2.2.1 Hemorrhage

Perioperative bleeding that results in cardiovascular instability is associated with poor prognosis and has a high incidence of morbidity or even mortality [4]. Hypovolemia can be largely avoided, and therefore prophylactic and early resuscitative measures should be applied to lessen or avoid the physiological upset.

Types of hemorrhage include (a) the primary hemorrhage, which is intra-operative bleeding, or a continuation of intra-operative bleeding noticed after surgery and usually occurs because of inadequate hemostasis. (b) reactionary hemorrhage refers to bleeding that occurs immediately postoperatively (within 24 h, typically 4–6 h) because of patient warming, vasodilation, and increasing blood pressure during recovery from anesthesia. (c) secondary hemorrhage that typically presents 7–14 days following the operation and usually results from local infection.

32.2.2.2 Prevention

Usually, in the elective setting, the patient's risk of bleeding should be carefully assessed preoperatively, including a review of his medications such as anticoagulants, or antiplatelet agents, and their indications. It is usually safe to stop these drugs during the perioperative period depending on the risk of the specific operation; nonetheless, it is often best to obtain specialist advice from hematology or cardiology. Sometimes in the emergency setting, there is no time to do so. Some patients may also present with pre-existing anemia due to comorbidity, dietary insufficiency, or the acute pathology that necessitates the operation. In the emergency, setting blood should be drawn for crossmatching and group. This should be completed within enough time to address any potential difficulties created by the detection of unusual antibodies unless the patient's pathology dictates otherwise.

The planning phase must also include arrangements for the use of cell-salvage machines where available if a significant blood loss is anticipated. The use of the meticulous surgical technique is crucial, to avoid unnecessary blood loss intraoperatively, and difficulties when encountered should be communicated to the operating room and anesthesia team. Preoperative dehydration should be avoided by the appropriate use of intravenous fluids when required.

32.2.2.3 Diagnosis

The primary hemorrhage must be identified intraoperatively at the time of operation, controlled, and dealt with appropriately. The reactionary or secondary hemorrhage could be identified postoperatively in the form of an external bleed (blood in drains or active bleeding) or internal bleed (patient is pallor, confused and oliguric, tachycardic, hypotensive, with low serum hemoglobin).

32.2.3 Management

The control of significant hemorrhage requires adequate venous access, with simultaneous control of the bleeding source and the administration of appropriate volume replacement and blood products.

32.2.4 Postoperative Pain

Immediate postoperative pain is a significant cause of morbidity, with around 40% of patients experiencing moderate-to-severe pain on the same day of surgery [5]. The pain could be acute, being related to the immediate postoperative surgical period, or might become chronic if it extends beyond the expected healing time (typically more than three months). The untreated pain can result in respiratory compromise (diaphragmatic splinting, atelectasis, sputum retention, and infection), tachycardia, hypertension, paralytic ileus, urinary retention, immobility, low mood, and more complications [5, 6].

32.2.4.1 Prevention

Preventing the development of pain is always more effective than treating the already established pain. Perioperative plans for analgesia should consider the nature and time length of the procedure, as well as the planned incision. Another key to the successful management of postoperative pain is to consider patient factors such as age, anxiety, and pre-existing pain, which have been shown to be predictors of postoperative symptoms. Pre-emptive analgesia should be multimodal, and parenteral or oral analgesics can be augmented by the application of a local anesthetic, applied as either a local or regional block.

32.2.4.2 Diagnosis
Pain is subjective and reported by the patient, though the use of a verbal scale or visual analog score can help quantification.

32.2.4.3 Management
The management of acute pain should be accomplished according to the WHO analgesic ladder. Starting with simple analgesia and then escalating by including compound preparations, NSAIDs, and opioids. The routes of administration that might be utilized to achieve a satisfactory level of pain relief are numerous. Similarly, the use of patient-controlled analgesia (PCA) should be considered. Multimodal therapy is the best method to achieve a satisfactory outcome, and when available, a pain management team should be involved in guiding the patient's care and taking pain management decisions.

32.2.5 Fever

Fever is frequent in the first few days after major operations and can pose a diagnostic challenge for the care team. While the definition of fever is variable, many use 38 °C as the threshold, although this can be hospital and unit-specific [7–9]. Early postoperative fever is often caused by the inflammatory stimulus of tissue damage and exposure to foreign materials during surgery and resolves spontaneously over a few days. Some call this "physiologic" fever. Hence, early postoperative fever occurring in the first three days after surgery usually requires no further diagnostic evaluation and workup other than reviewing the patient's history and medications and performing a focused physical examination [10–13].

Starting on postoperative day four and onward, the infections that are related to the surgical procedure are more common. The differential diagnosis should also include non-infectious conditions, some of which can be life-threatening. A correct diagnosis with immediate initiation of appropriate therapy can be lifesaving. Infections are most commonly in the superficial or deep surgical site, the urinary tract, or the lungs. Non-infectious causes may include drug fever, inflammatory reactions, and deep vein thrombosis. It is significant to consider a broad differential and not presume that fever is due to infection. It is also of great importance to emphasize that the presence of a fever varies for many conditions, and its absence does not eliminate the probability of a condition being present. Fever as a symptom of infection may be reduced or absent in immunocompromised patients, including those receiving chemotherapy, glucocorticoids, and post-transplant immunosuppression. Patients who are older, frail, cachectic, or have chronic renal failure may also have an altered fever response to infection.

32.2.6 Respiratory Complications

Respiratory complications are frequent and are often related to inadequate postoperative analgesia, a pre-existing lung disease (such as chronic obstructive pulmonary disease (COPD)), or a combination of both causes. Basal atelectasis is the most frequent cause of low oxygen saturation and low fever in the first 12–24 h after surgery, and this is the critical window in which targeted interventions can prevent any infectious complications.

32.2.6.1 Prevention
Optimization of pre-existing lung disease is important, while most of the time impossible in the emergency setting. These patients with severe respiratory problems are better managed in combination with a respiratory specialist. An active chest infection is usually a contraindication to elective procedures, but not in emergency ones. A valuable measure for patients undergoing major chest or abdominal surgery, when applicable, is preoperative physiotherapy. The physiotherapist should teach the patients deep breathing exercises as well as techniques for effective expectoration of secretions that can be supported by the routine use of incentive spirometry devices and saline or bronchodilator nebulizers. Another

essential measure is adequate analgesia, and patients should be taught strategies to minimize the impact of their incision on the respiratory function by the application of postural maneuvers and additional support.

32.2.6.2 Diagnosis

Tachypnoea or productive cough can be the signs of a respiratory infection, and these can be accompanied by dullness to percussion and reduced air entry on auscultation. A patient's observation chart review could confirm reduced oxygen saturations and increased respiratory rates. Imaging of the chest will help differentiate consolidation, collapse, or effusions, and blood tests can show increased inflammatory markers.

Management

Chest physiotherapy should be introduced, if not already applied, alongside supplemental oxygen, and analgesia should be optimized. Alveolar collapse should respond to deep breathing, though positive pressure ventilation (non-invasive or invasive) might be required for refractory cases. For infections (raised inflammatory markers with consolidation on imaging), sputum and blood cultures should be sent to guide ongoing treatment with broad-spectrum antibiotics. Most of the patients with respiratory complications will benefit from nebulized saline, bronchodilators, and significant effusions that may require percutaneous drainage. However, despite all the efforts, some patients will deteriorate rapidly due to respiratory complications, and early involvement of a critical care specialist in this group of patients is essential. A low threshold of suspicion should be maintained for pulmonary embolism in these patients, and a CT pulmonary angiogram (CTPA) should be arranged.

32.2.7 Venous Thromboembolism

Virchow's Triad describes the three factors whose consequence is venous thrombosis: reduced venous flow/stasis (e.g., immobility), endothelial damage (e.g., smoking), and hypercoagulability (e.g., heritable coagulopathies). A thrombus usually develops within the deep venous systems of the leg (DVT). Nevertheless, it can as well migrate proximally or dislodge and travel within the venous system (embolism) and potentially cause occlusion of pulmonary vessels (pulmonary embolism). In 2005, for example, there were 25,000 deaths in the UK from hospital-acquired thromboembolic disorders. Therefore, national guidelines now exist for its prevention and treatment [14]. Prophylactic measures should, therefore, be universally adopted in surgical patients and be aimed at reducing venous stasis, promoting early ambulation, and using prophylactic doses of anticoagulation agents [14, 15].

32.2.7.1 Prevention

The National Institute for Health and Care Excellence (NICE) developed guidelines for surgical patients that are as follows:

- ensure adequate hydration during the perioperative period
- use regional anesthesia above general anesthesia where possible
- promote early ambulation after surgery
- at admission, all patients should undergo formal risk assessment, and venous thromboembolism (VTE) prophylaxis should be administered where indicated
- patients' risk of bleeding or developing VTE should be further assessed after 24 h
- in patients without contraindication, start mechanical VTE prophylaxis.
- Apply graduated elastic compression stockings or foot impulse devices with intermittent pneumatic calf compression
- for patients who have had major surgery in the abdomen or pelvis, VTE prophylaxis should be prescribed for 28 days postoperatively

32.2.7.2 Diagnosis

DVT of the lower limb:

- Mild fever could be present
- Dilatation of superficial veins
- Unilateral calf swelling and tenderness
- Erythema of the skin

Investigation:

- Duplex Ultrasound
- Venography

Pulmonary Embolism:

- Tachycardia
- Tachypnoea and decreased oxygen saturation
- Pleuritic-type chest pain
- Hemoptysis
- Circulatory collapse or cardiac arrest

Investigation:

- ECG: Sinus tachycardia, right heart strain (S1Q3T3 pattern)
- Chest radiograph: wedge-infarct
- Type 1 respiratory failure on arterial blood gasses
- CT pulmonary angiogram (CTPA) is the golden standard

32.2.7.3 Management

The treatment should start by administering oxygen to the patient, starting a therapeutic dose of heparin, if safe, and continuing with mechanical compression devices. If the clinical suspicion is high, then the first anticoagulant dose should be given while we arrange for further investigations. Fibrinolytic agents can be considered for cases of extensive DVT or life-threatening PE, but they are contraindicated in cases of recent surgery. Alternatively, a radiological or surgical thrombectomy or embolectomy might be necessary. In the existence of an extensive DVT or when multiple embolic episodes have been encountered, a filter could be placed radiologically in the inferior vena cava to reduce the risk of a major PE. After the acute episode, the exact cause of the DVT/PE should be carefully investigated. Then, a risk/benefit evaluation should be performed for the prescription of prolonged oral anticoagulation. A patient who experienced a first thromboembolic event due to reversible risk factors, such as immobilization, surgery, or trauma, should be discharged on warfarin therapy for at least three months; while patients who have recurrent VTE or pre-existing irreversible risk factors, such as known thrombophilia, should be placed on long-term anticoagulation. However, this decision should be made in collaboration with a hematologist.

32.2.8 Surgical Site Infections (SSIs)

They are defined as infections that occur at the site of an operation within 30 days from surgery if no foreign body or implant is left within the patient during surgery or within one year of an operation if a foreign body or an implant is left in situ [1]. Fifteen percent of hospital-related infections are accounted for SSIs and are related to significant morbidity and mortality [16]. In the literature, each SSI accumulates excess costs and can increase hospital length of stay by up to 7 days [17, 18]. Patients who develop SSIs are twice as likely to die following a surgical procedure and, if discharged, they have a five-fold increased chance of being re-admitted [18]. The incidence of wound infections is associated with the type of operation being performed: clean operations have an infection rate of <1%, contaminated procedures (e.g., appendicectomy) 15–20%, and infected procedures (e.g., Hartmann's procedure for bowel perforation) 40%.[19] Two-thirds of all SSIs are related to the wound, and the remaining one-third are confined to the organ space [20]. The organisms that cause such infections usually originate from the patients' normal skin or bowel flora. Less commonly, bacterial contamination may occur from an exogenous source, such as from contamination by airborne pathogens, operating room staff, non-sterile instruments, or prostheses [3].

Prevention

Numerous modifiable risk factors exist to avoid an SSI.

- Preoperatively:
- Patient factors:
- Control hyperglycemia
- Treat existing bacterial infection (MRSA screening)
- Optimize nutrition
- Intraoperatively:
- Surgical factors:
- hair removal (Clipping, not shaving)
- Aseptic technique
- Meticulous surgical technique
- Minimize the operating time
- Avoid or correct hypothermia by using warming devices
- Antibiotic prophylaxis where and when appropriate
- Utilization of drains and sutures to avoid fluid collections (when necessary) like hematoma, seroma
- Minimize Operating Room "traffic."
- Postoperative:
- infection control and strict hygiene discipline and hand hygiene
- Isolation of infected patients, the clean ward environment
- Regular wound inspections
- Early removal of sutures, clips, and drains
- Avoid unnecessary administration of antibiotics
- Minimize hospital length of stay.

32.2.9 Antibiotic Prophylaxis

The administration of prophylactic antibiotics can significantly reduce the incidence of an SSI, and there is good evidence in the international literature to support their use for various emergency operations such as emergency gastrointestinal, vascular, oropharyngeal, open heart, craniotomies, and obstetric and gynecological procedures, even in orthopedic prosthesis placement and spinal operations. The antibiotics should be administered at the time of induction of anesthesia, and a second dose should follow intraoperatively for procedures expected to last for more than 4 h. The choice of antibiotic agents will be based on the most likely pathogens for each procedure and will be guided by local protocols. In the WHO Guidelines for Safe Surgery 2009, current recommendations of agents for prophylaxis can be found [3].

32.2.9.1 Diagnosis

An established superficial SSI may cause swelling, redness, heat, pain, purulent wound discharge, or even wound dehiscence. A deeper infection might be more challenging to diagnose but may result in irritation or pain of local structures, such as the diaphragm in subphrenic collections, and both can cause systemic clinical signs of sepsis (tachycardia, tachypnoea, high fever, and malaise). For deeper infections, clinical suspicion is often accompanied by confirming laboratory or radiological findings.

32.2.9.2 Management

Targeted therapy is the key to management, with source control, drainage of collections (surgical or radiological), and the administration of appropriate empiric antibiotics as early as possible following collection of relevant culture samples.

32.3 Conclusion

In conclusion, improved results when dealing with postoperative complications depend primarily on two aspects: firstly, the early recognition of patients at high risk, which allows the implementation of individualized care; and secondly, early treatment of complications, which indicates prompt intervention and thus reduces the morbidity and the mortality of these patients. Finally, recognizing failures in the surgical patient care process is vital so that improvements can be suggested in different moments of the perioperative period to ameliorate the quality of patient care and eventually have better outcomes.

Do and Dont's
- Always check patients during post-operative course for potential complication.
- Evaluate patients in the light of preoperative potential favoring factors for complications.
- Do not under- or overestimate complication risk.
- Do not apply one-size-fits-all in preventing and treating post-operative complications.

Take-Home Messages
- The complication rate in emergency operations can be ten times higher than the elective ones; low threshold on patient's postoperative symptoms for complications.
- Early detection and a well-timed intervention are essential factors to reduce the morbidity of the postoperative complications.
- After recognizing a complication, it is crucial to implement immediate appropriate management strategies to significantly reduce morbidity or even mortality.

Questions
1. At what time after surgery "early" complications are found?
   A. **Within 30 days**
   B. Within 40 days
   C. Within 45 days
   D. Within 60
2. After how many days post-surgery an anastomotic leak is suspected?
   A. 1
   B. 2
   C. **4**
   D. 7
3. After how many days post-surgery a pulmonary embolism is suspected?
   A. 1
   B. **3**
   C. 0
   D. 2
4. By how much the implementation of the World Health Organization (WHO) Surgical Safety checklist reduces the surgical morbidity?
   A. 10%
   B. 20%
   C. **30%**
   D. 50%
5. How many days after an emergency surgery secondary hemorrhage presents?
   A. 1–2
   B. 3–5
   C. 5–7
   D. **7–14**
6. What is the most common cause of a secondary bleeding?
   A. **Local infection**
   B. Anticoagulants
   C. Vasodilation
   D. Inadequate hemostasis
7. What is the most common reason for early, day 1, postoperative fever?
   A. Pneumonia
   B. Urinary Tract Infection
   C. Wound Infection
   D. **Exposure to foreign material during surgery**
8. Which of the following is the investigation of choice to diagnose a lower limb DVT?
   A. X-Ray
   B. Ultrasound
   C. **Duplex Ultrasound**
   D. Computerized Tomography
9. Which one of the following symptoms CANNOT be found in pulmonary embolism?
   A. tachycardia
   B. **bradycardia**
   C. tachypnea
   D. hemoptysis

10. What is the incidence of wound infection in an infected procedure (e.g., Hartmann's)?
    A. 10%
    B. 20%
    C. 30%
    D. **40%**

References

1. Gawande AA, Thomas EJ, Zinner MJ, Brennan TA. The incidence and nature of surgical adverse events in Colorado and Utah in 1992. Surgery. 1999;126:66–75.
2. Kable AK, Gibberd RW, Spigelman AD. Adverse events in surgical patients in Australia. Int J Qual Health Care. 2002;14:269–76.
3. Weiser TG, Regenbogen SE, Thompson KD, et al. An estimation of the global volume of surgery. Lancet. 2008;372:139–44.
4. World Health Organisation. WHO guidelines for safe surgery 2009: safe surgery saves lives. Switzerland: World Health Organisation; 2009.
5. Gawande AA, Kwaan MR, Regenbogen SE, Lipsitz SA, Zinner MJ. An Apgar score for surgery. J Amer Coll Surg. 2007;204:201–8.
6. Wu CL, Raja SN. Treatment of acute postoperative pain. Lancet. 2011;377:2215–25.
7. Australian and New Zealand College of Anaesthetics and Faculty of Pain Medicine. Acute pain management: scientific evidence. 3rd ed. Australia: Australian and New Zealand College of Anaesthetics and Faculty of Pain Medicine; 2010.
8. Garibaldi RA, Brodine S, Matsumiya S, Coleman M. Evidence for the non-infectious etiology of early postoperative fever. Infect Control. 1985;6:273.
9. Galicier C, Richet H. A prospective study of postoperative fever in a general surgery department. Infect Control. 1985;6:487.
10. Crompton JG, Crompton PD, Matzinger P. Does atelectasis cause fever after surgery? Putting a damper on dogma. JAMA Surg. 2019;154:375.
11. Livelli FD Jr, Johnson RA, McEnany MT, et al. Unexplained in-hospital fever following cardiac surgery. Natural history, relationship to the postpericardiotomy syndrome, and a prospective study of therapy with indomethacin versus placebo. Circulation. 1978;57:968.
12. Hobar PC, Masson JA, Herrera R, et al. Fever after craniofacial surgery in infants under 24 months of age. Plast Reconstr Surg. 1998;102:32.
13. Guinn S, Castro FP Jr, Garcia R, Barrack RL. Fever following total knee arthroplasty. Am J Knee Surg. 1999;12:161.
14. Ghosh S, Charity RM, Haidar SG, Singh BK. Pyrexia following total knee replacement. Knee. 2006;13:324.
15. National Institute for Health and Clinical Excellence. Venous thromboembolism: reducing the risk. London: National Institute for Healthand Clinical Excellence; 2010.
16. National Institute for Health and Clinical Excellence. Venous thromboembolic diseases: the management of venous thromboembolic diseases and the role of thrombophilia testing. London: National Institute for Health and Clinical Excellence; 2010.
17. Coello R, Charlett A, Wilson J, Ward V, Pearson A, Borriello P. Adverse impact of surgical site infections in English hospitals. J Hosp Infect. 2005;60:93–103.
18. Kirkland KB, Briggs JP, Trivette SL, Wilkinson WE, Sexton DJ. The impact of surgical-site infections in the 1990s: attributable mortality, excess length of hospitalization, and extra costs. Infect Control Hosp Epidemiol. 1999;20:725–30.
19. Ellis H, Calne R, Watson C. General surgery: lecture notes. Chichester: Wiley-Blackwell; 2011.
20. Horan TC, Culver DH, Gaynes RP, Jarvis WR, Edwards JR, Reid CR. Nosocomial infections in surgical patients in the United States, January 1986 June; 1992.

Iatrogenic Complications of Digestive Endoscopy

Aleix Martínez-Pérez, Carmen Payá-Llorente, and Nicola de'Angelis

Learning Goals
- To know the incidence, risk factors, and etiologies of the different iatrogenic endoscopic complications, together with its implications in the timing and setting of presentation.
- To understand the key points to guide the clinical decisions regarding the patient's management after the diagnosis.
- To differentiate the spectrum of surgical alternatives for iatrogenic endoscopic perforations, its current indications, and limitations.

33.1 Introduction

33.1.1 Epidemiology

Iatrogenic bowel perforations during a colonoscopy (IPC) are the most dreadful complication of the procedure. IPC are associated with high morbidity and mortality rates. Its overall incidence has been estimated at 5.8 per 10,000 colonoscopies [1]. The maximum acceptable incidence of IPC at diagnostic colonoscopies should not exceed 0.1% [1–3]. The sigmoid colon is the most frequent site of perforation (up to 65%), followed by the cecum, the ascending, the transverse, and the descending colon. Although the vast majority of colonoscopy perforations are intra-peritoneal, extra-peritoneal or combined forms have been also described [4].

Upper digestive endoscopy (UDE) is a commonly performed procedure, which is generally associated with a low incidence of complications. Adverse events, including iatrogenic perforations, are developed in 1 in 2500–11,000 procedures [5]. Esophageal iatrogenic perforations are the most frequent, they occur during both diagnostic and therapeutic procedures. They may involve any level of the organ and constitute the commonest cause of esophageal perforation. Endoscopic retrograde cholangiopancreatography (ERCP) is a complex procedure used to diagnose and treat different pancreato-biliary disorders. ERCP is considered a safe and effec-

A. Martínez-Pérez (✉)
Department of General and Digestive Surgery, Hospital Universitario Doctor Peset, Valencia, Spain

Faculty of Health Sciences, Valencian International University (VIU), Valencia, Spain

C. Payá-Llorente
Department of General and Digestive Surgery, Hospital Universitario Doctor Peset, Valencia, Spain

N. de'Angelis
Unit of Colorectal and Digestive Surgery, DIGEST Department, Beaujon University Hospital, AP-HP, University of Paris Cité, Clichy, France

tive technique, but complication rates are around 10% [6]. The most common are pancreatitis, cholangitis, bleeding, and perforation. The risk of perforation by ERCP is not despicable (0,6%), and this adverse event is linked with high morbidity and mortality [7].

33.1.2 Pathophysiology

Table 33.1 shows the main risk factors for IPC. Older, female, or low-BMI patients are more prone to present this complication. A greater risk is expected for therapeutic over diagnostic procedures. Polypectomies can result in perforations especially if multiple, sessile, or large polyps are resected. Higher rates have been also found after the performance of advanced excision techniques such as argon plasma coagulation, endoscopic mucosal resection (EMR), or endoscopic submucosal dissection (ESD) [8]. Stenting of benign or neoplastic strictures and balloon dilatation is associated with IPC incidences of up to 10% [9]. IPC mainly follows two main pathways: (1) direct mechanical trauma, or (2) barotrauma secondary to excessive pneumatic distension (Table 33.2). Indirect traumatisms are infrequent and produced because of the bowing or stretching in the distal parts of the colon. The presence of redundant colon, diverticula, or adhesions from previous surgeries increases the risk of mechanical trauma [10]. Perforations due to over-insufflation are usually located at the cecal walls, where larger bowel diameter and a thinner muscular layer are present. Thermal injuries produced at therapeutic endoscopies could be followed by colonic wall ischemia, which can result in delayed perforations (up to 24–72 h after the index procedure) [11].

Perforations secondary to diagnostic explorations are usually located at the cervical or upper thoracic esophagus. Conversely, those secondary to a sudden increase in the intra-luminal pressure (i.e., Mallory–Weiss Syndrome) are more frequently diagnosed at the lower third of the organ. Perforations at non-therapeutic UDE are less frequent. The risk factors for its development include esophageal strictures, malignancies, or the presence of diverticula (Table 33.1). Upper gastrointestinal dilatation procedures for complex strictures (i.e., caustic) carry a higher risk

Table 33.1 Risk factors for iatrogenic perforations during digestive endoscopy

Colonoscopy	Upper digestive endoscopy
Patient	**Diagnostic**
• Age (from 65 years)	• Anterior cervical osteophytes
• Female gender	• Esophageal stricture or web
• Low BMI	• Malignancy
• Previous abdominal surgery	• Cervical rib
• Comorbidity	• Zenker's diverticulum
– Crohn's disease	• Duodenal diverticulum
– Diverticulosis	**Stricture dilatation**
– Bevacizumab therapy	• Complex (multiple/long/tortuous)
Operator's experience and center volume	• Malignant
Clinical setting	• Achalasia
• Intestinal obstruction	**Foreign body removal**
• ICU admission	• Past history of foreign body removal
Therapeutic colonoscopy	• Irregular, sharp objects
• Polypectomy, if:	• Delay >24h
– Polyps >20 mm	**ERCP**
– Sessile polyps	• Therapeutic:
Multiple polyps	– Sphincterotomy, balloon dilatation
• APC, EMR, ESD	– Guidewires, baskets, stents, injections
• Stenting	• Altered anatomy (i.e., Billroth type II).
• Balloon dilatation	• Oddi's sphincter dysfunction
	Other
	• ESD, SEMS
	• Sclerotherapy for variceal hemostasis

Table 33.2 Pathogenic pathways for iatrogenic perforations during colonoscopy

	Direct trauma	Barotrauma
Incidence	More frequent	Less frequent
Mechanism	Direct mechanical harm by the endoscope	Pneumatic distension
Cause	Instrumental insertion Endoscope movements (retroflexion, torsion).	Over-insufflation
Predisposing factors	Redundant colon Diverticulum Adhesions from prior surgery	Thinner colonic walls
Perforation features	Larger Sigmoid colon	Linear Cecum

for perforation than those for esophageal rings or peptic ulcers. Gastric perforations during endoscopic mucosal resection (EMR) have been described as larger lesions that can be resected in the stomach. ERCP-related perforation usually occurs after therapeutic maneuvers such as sphincterotomy, papillary balloon dilatation, or when cannulating the Oddi's sphincter with guidewires, baskets, or stents. Other risk factors for pare surgically altered anatomy (e.g., Billroth type II reconstruction) or Oddi's sphincter disfunction [12]. The Stapfer et al. classification divides ERCP perforations into four types in descending order of severity (Table 33.3) [13].

Table 33.3 Stapfer's classification of ERCP-related perforations

Type	Description and Mechanism of Injury	Frequency
I	Duodenal wall perforation (by the duodenoscope)	17%
II	Retroperitoneal duodenal perforation (secondary to periampullary injury).	58%
III	Bile duct or pancreatic duct perforation (by instrumentation, stone extraction, or stenting)	13%
IV	Retroperitoneal gas alone (by excessive insufflation)	10%

33.1.3 Other Complications of Digestive Endoscopy

33.1.3.1 Bleeding

Its incidence in diagnostic endoscopy is less than 1%, bleeding is associated with therapeutic procedures such as polypectomy, EMR, or ESD [14, 15]. Resuscitation and endoscopic hemostasis are the first therapeutic steps (Fig. 33.1a). Surgery is only indicated when endoscopic treatment fails. In such cases, intraoperative endoscopy could allow to find where the bleeding is. Percutaneous angiography with selective embolization can be performed in colonoscopy perforations before surgery, and also in the gastroduodenal artery in cases of ERCP-related bleeding not controllable endoscopically. If the bleeding was previously localized, a segmental colonic resection can be performed, otherwise an extended resection (e.g., subtotal colectomy) is unavoidable. Post-ERCP hemorrhage surgical treatment options to be considered are the ligation of the gastroduodenal artery or suturing the ampulla through a duodenotomy.

33.1.3.2 Small Bowel Perforation

The incidence of small bowel perforation is 0.4% [16]. Endoscopic closure can be only applied if

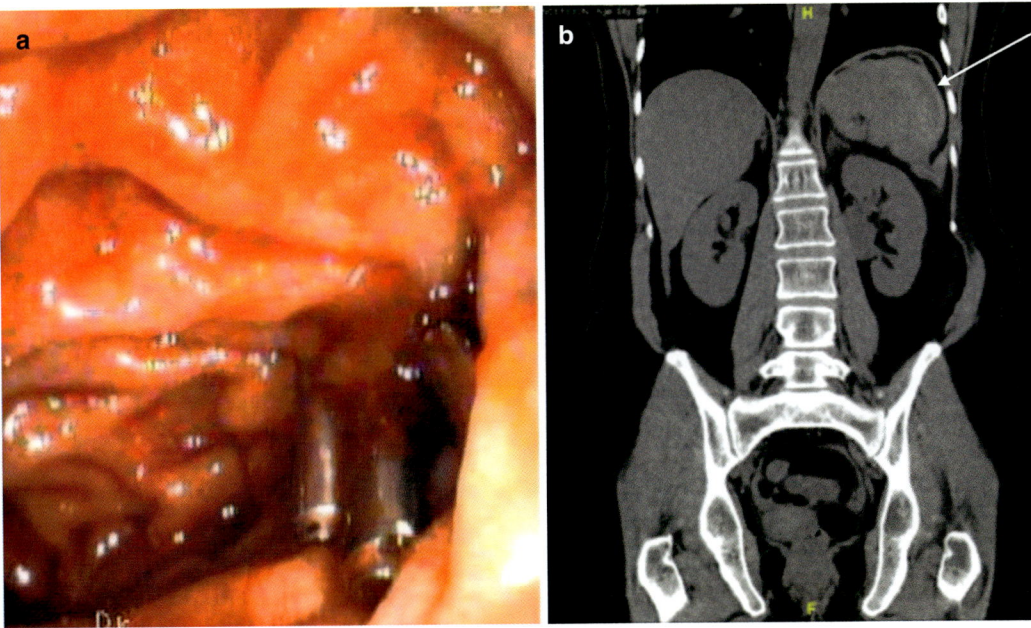

Fig. 33.1 (a) Hemorrhage treated with endo-clips during UDE; (b) Splenic hematoma after colonoscopy (white arrow)

detected during the index endoscopy. Otherwise, surgical resection or repair is necessary.

33.1.3.3 Endoscopic Stents and Instruments

Endoscopic stenting is linked with adverse events, such as improper positioning, perforation, or stent migration. Tracheal compression leading to aspiration and respiratory compromise has been described. A retained guidewire or impacted baskets are specific complications of ERCP. Endoscopic retrieval is the first therapeutic option, whereas surgery is indicated after its failure.

33.1.3.4 Adverse Events of Percutaneous Endoscopic Enteral Access

The overall rate of adverse events related to percutaneous endoscopic gastrostomy (PEG) is 13% [17]. Severe PEG-related adverse events are aspiration, pneumonia, pneumoperitoneum, hemorrhage, perforation, buried bumper syndrome, infections (e.g., necrotizing fasciitis), colocutaneous fistula, and peristomal leakage. The buried bumper syndrome consists of an ischemic necrosis of the gastric wall secondary to excessive traction of the fixation system. Direct percutaneous endoscopic jejunostomy and percutaneous endoscopic gastrostomy with jejunal extension allow post-pyloric feeding. These techniques are associated with occlusion and proximal migration of the jejunal extension.

33.1.3.5 Cardiopulmonary Adverse Events

Its incidence is about 1.4% and they include hypoxemia, aspiration pneumonia, respiratory arrest, myocardial infarction, arrhythmias, stroke, and shock [18]. Patients' age, higher ASA grade, and previous cardiopulmonary disease increase the likelihood of these adverse events [18]. Aspiration is particularly associated with patients with advanced age, intestinal obstruction, or massive upper gastrointestinal bleeding.

33.1.3.6 Infectious Adverse Events

Cases of infection with hepatitis B and C, or bacterial infections have been described as secondary to the contamination of the equipment. The translocation of microorganisms produces transient bacteriemia in approximately 4% of colonoscopies or UDE. This risk is increased if therapeutic techniques such as sclerotherapy or dilatation are performed [19]. The incidence of endocarditis is extremely low.

33.1.3.7 Other Adverse Events

Thromboembolic events, gas explosion, splenic injury (Fig. 33.1b), acute appendicitis, diverticulitis, subcutaneous emphysema, intraabdominal hemorrhage, and entrapment of the endoscope are other uncommon adverse events reported in the literature.

33.2 Diagnosis

33.2.1 Clinical Presentation

33.2.1.1 Colonoscopy Perforations

More than 50% of the perforations are immediately identified by the operator during the colonoscopy, by direct visualization of the parietal defect or the intra-abdominal structures [20]. However, an important number of IPC are detected after the procedure. In this scenario, the diagnosis of IPC needs the support of clinical, biochemical, and radiological explorations [21]. The delay in the diagnosis of IPC, and also the time interval between the diagnosis and the definitive treatment, are crucial for the patient's prognosis.

The symptoms of an IPC highly depend on the size, the cause, and the location of the perforation. The nature and degree of intra-peritoneal contamination also impact on the clinical presentation. In the majority (90%) of the patients, the symptoms will start within the first 48 h after the endoscopy. In the case of covered perforations with abscess formation, the diagnosis can be delayed by several days. The most common symptoms of IPC are abdominal pain and distension. They are usually associated with guarding or rebound tenderness, tachycardia, fever, or bleeding. Few patients (<5%) will remain completely asymptomatic. Extra-peritoneal perforations, which are remarkably less frequent, can be diagnosed as a result of subcutaneous emphysema, pneumo-retroperitoneum, or pneumo-mediastinum.

33.2.1.2 Upper Digestive Endoscopy Perforations

The clinical and biochemical presentation during the early period after the perforation is poorly specific. Pain is the most frequent symptom of esophageal perforations. It is usually accompanied by dyspnea, tachycardia, fever, and leukocytosis. Cervical perforations usually produce neck and chest pain, and also subcutaneous emphysema, hoarseness, or dysphagia. In thoracic perforations, the chest pain can be referred to the abdominal area, and associated dyspnea. Acute abdominal pain is more common in perforations of the gastro-esophageal junction (EGJ) and below this area. In Stapfer's I perforations, the clinical symptoms are commonly recognized (e.g., abdominal pain, fever, tachycardia, subcutaneous emphysema, rebound tenderness, or generalized abdominal wall rigidity in advanced cases). In the other types of ERCP-related perforations, the clinical symptoms are often vague.

33.2.2 Diagnostic Tests

33.2.2.1 Colonoscopy Perforations

If IPC is suspected after the procedure, the minimum biochemical markers to be requested are the white blood cell (WBC) count and the C-reactive protein (CRP). When a delayed presentation of IPC is suspected, the increasing levels of the pro-calcitonin (PCT) marker can be useful to support the suspicion [3]. The diagnosis of ICP should be confirmed with the demonstration of extra-colonic free air (Fig. 33.2). Thoracic and abdominal X-rays can detect free peritoneal air with a high positive predictive value (PPV), but they are unable to detect intra-abdominal free fluid [22]. Ultrasound can be used in children or during pregnancy. CT scan is more accurate to detect free air, it can be found at: (1) the mesenteric, retroperitoneal, or mediastinal areas; (2) the abdominal, chest, or neck walls; (3) inside the mesenteric and portal venous systems. Double-contrast CT (intravenous + rectal) has been used when IPC without diffuse peritonitis is suspected, as it allows to diagnose contained perforations which may be suitable to successfully undergo non-operative management [23].

33.2.2.2 Upper Digestive Endoscopy Perforations

Plain chest X-ray allows to identify indirect signs of esophageal perforation, such as free air at the soft tissues of the neck, subcutaneous emphysema, pleural effusion, mediastinal widening, pneumomediastinum, hydrothorax, or pneumothorax. Pneumoperitoneum can be found in the perforations located below the EGJ. Those radiologic findings may not be present shortly after the perforation occurs. Contrast-enhanced computed tomography (CT) is the imaging examination of choice in patients with suspicion of perforation. CT scan with oral water-soluble contrast has a high sensitivity to identify the site of perforation and small amounts of air or fluid. If the clinical suspicion of perforation persists after this exploration, the use of barium contrast can be justified to discard small defects [24]. Stapfer's types II and III ERCP-related perforations are usually diagnosed during the endoscopy, when extravasation of the contrast agent from the biliary tree is evidenced (Fig. 33.3). Stapfer's type I lesions are usually lateral and may therefore remain initially undiagnosed. In delayed presentations, increased levels of leukocytes and CRP can be detected [25].

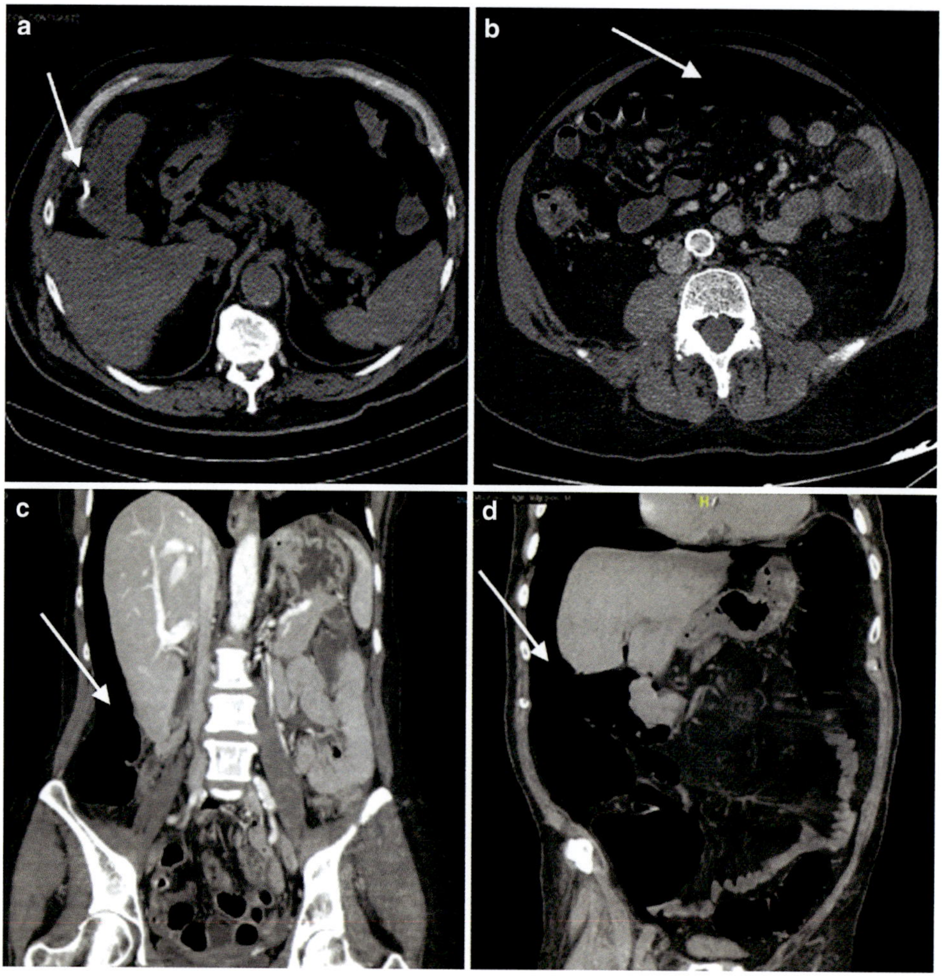

Fig. 33.2 CT images of colonoscopy-related perforations (**a**) Endoclip located in the hepatic flexure (white arrow). (**b–d**) Pneumoperitoneum after colonoscopy

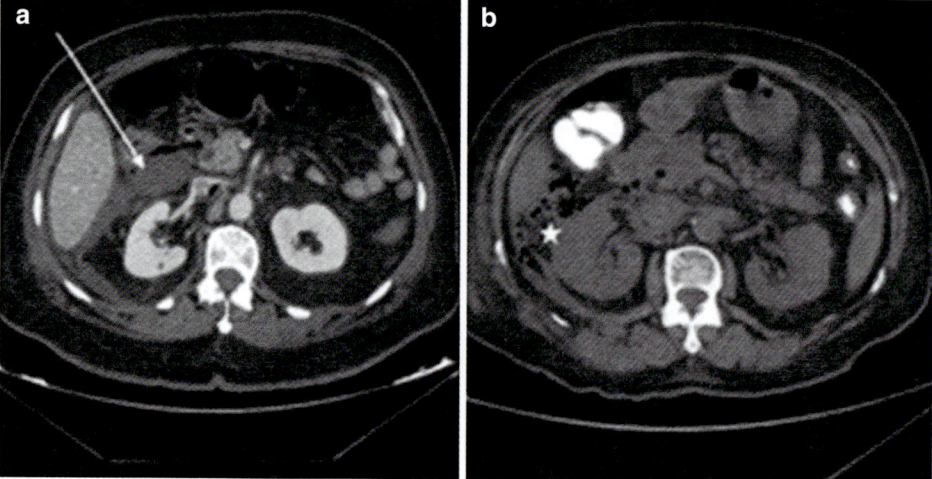

Fig. 33.3 CT images of ERCP-related perforations (**a**) Stapfer's type II perforation showing retroperitoneal fluid collection and pneumoperitoneum (white arrow). (**b**) Stapfer's type IV perforation with only retroperitoneal air (white star)

Differential Diagnosis

Colonoscopy Perforations

The post-polypectomy coagulation syndrome mimics IPC. It is produced by a full-thickness electrical burn during polypectomy, with serosal irritation. The symptoms start usually 1–5 days after the endoscopy. This is typically an intense abdominal pain that can be accompanied by localized peritoneal irritation, fever, or leukocytosis. Remarkably, CT imaging will not reveal free air (remember that imaging studies are always indicated when IPC is suspected to confirm the diagnosis). The treatment of choice for the post-polypectomy syndrome is conservative.

Upper Digestive Endoscopy Perforations

When an esophageal perforation is suspected, a CT scan allows to perform the differential diagnosis of the disease, ruling out other pathologies such as esophageal mural hematoma or aortic dissection. Asymptomatic pneumomediastinum can be detected by CT after 31% of the endoscopic submucosal dissections (ESD) performed in the esophagus [26]. Similarly, the detection of retroperitoneal air, which is visualized by CT in 29% of asymptomatic patients 24 h after an ERCP, does not correlate with the degree of injury or the final need for surgery [27]. Acute pancreatitis is the most common serious complication after ERCP (3.5%), while cholangitis (1.4%) and cholecystitis (0.5%) are less common % [7]. All of them produce could produce symptoms mimicking gastric or duodenal perforations. Their diagnosis and treatment are based on the same principles as in a non-iatrogenic scenario [28, 29].

33.3 Treatment

33.3.1 Medical Treatment

33.3.1.1 Colonoscopy Perforations

Once IPC is diagnosed, the decision between surgery or non-surgical alternatives relies upon the type of injury, the patient's clinical status, and the underlying colonic pathology (Fig. 33.4). In selected cases with localized pain, absence of fever or free fluids at radiological explorations, and hemodynamic stability, conservative medical treatment can be initially considered [3]. This approach can be used also in IPC diagnosis and successfully treated during the index procedure (Fig. 33.5a). The conservative treatment is based on the repeated observation of the clinical and radiologic features every 3–6 h. Patients receive bowel rest, intravenous fluids and broad-spectrum antibiotics, and a close follow-up. If the clinical conditions worsen, or signs of sepsis or diffuse peritonitis appear, the surgical treatment should not be delayed. In selected cases, the drainage of the free air can mitigate the pain and improve respiratory function [30]. The consecutive assessment of the patient's vital signs should be accompanied by at least WBC, CRP, and PCT laboratory tests. CT scan is the technique of choice to confirm the diagnosis in cases with clinical deterioration, and before hospital discharge after a clinically successful conservative treatment. All the patients with ICP require antimicrobial therapy covering Gram-negative bacteria and anaerobes. As they are considered at risk of venous thromboembolism, antithrombotic prophylaxis is generally recommended during hospitalization.

33.3.1.2 Upper Digestive Endoscopy Perforations

Endoscopic closure is the first approach for perforations discovered during the primary procedure. Different endo-luminal therapies as endoscopic

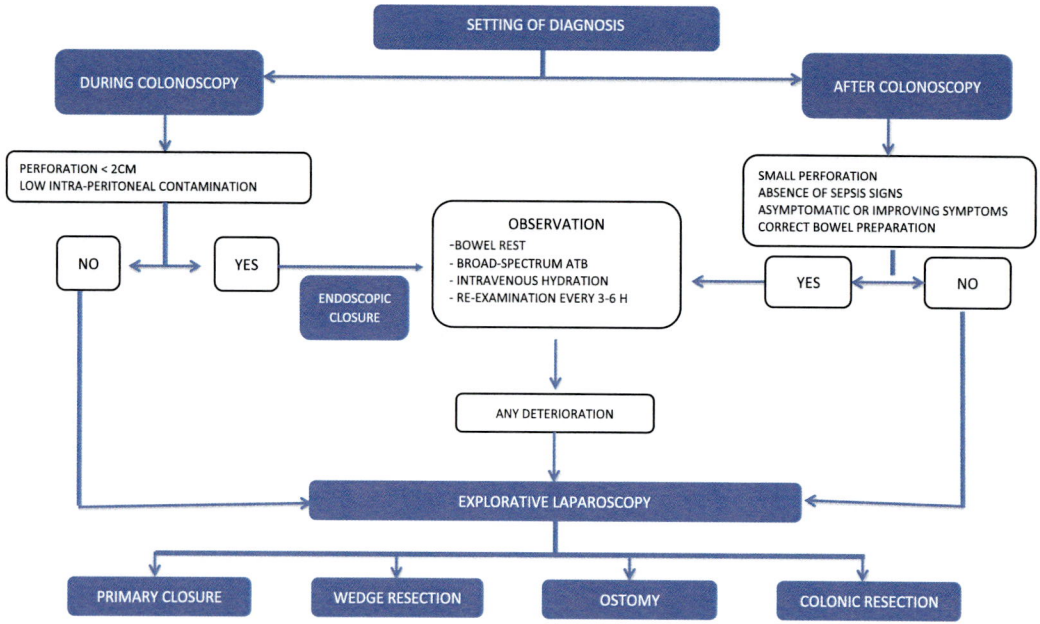

Fig. 33.4 Management of iatrogenic perforations during colonoscopy

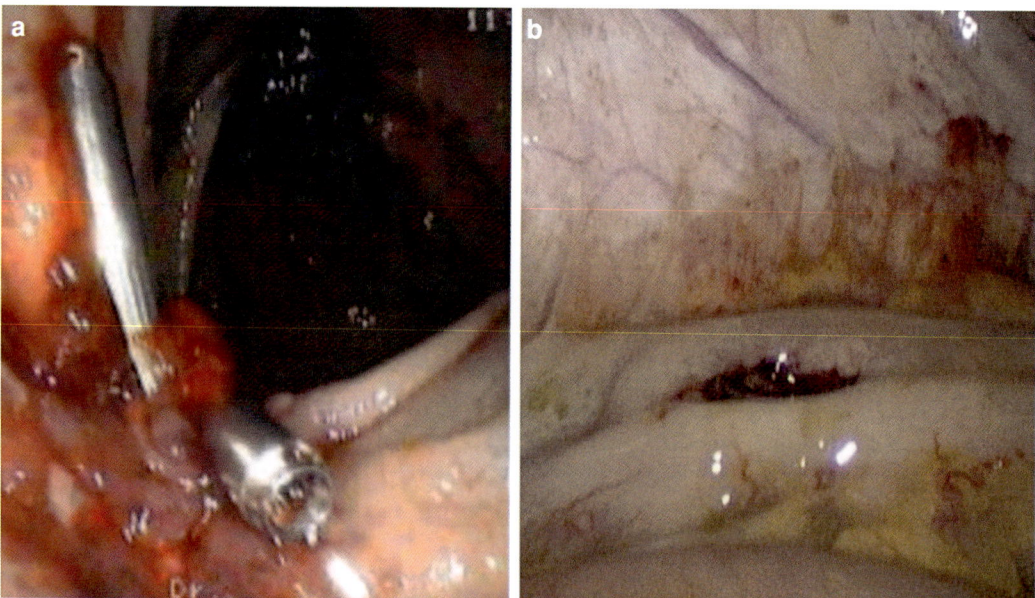

Fig. 33.5 (a) Endoscopic closure with endo-clips of iatrogenic colonoscopy perforation. (b) Endoscopy-related sigmoid perforation evidenced during explorative laparoscopy

clipping (through- or over-the-scope), insertion of metal stents, or endo-luminal vacuum therapies, have demonstrated their effectiveness in these situations. In case of perforations diagnosed after the procedure, the decision between surgical or conservative treatments is based on a combination of factors englobing: (1) the location, type, and mechanism of injury; (2) the delay from initial endoscopy and the patient's general status; and (3) the existence of underlying diseases.

Similar to colonoscopy-related perforations, conservative management is based on bowel rest, intravenous hydration, broad-spectrum antibiotics, and close clinical surveillance [31]. Generally, conservative management can be considered in stable patients presenting small and contained wall disruptions with minimal contamination. Proton pump inhibitor therapy should be administered [32]. Especially in ERCP-related perforations, nasogastric/nasoduodenal tube placement or percutaneous biliary drainage could decrease the volume of fluids loading the perforation. In Stapfer's type I perforations, if the perforation is detected during the endoscopy, an endoscopic closure may be performed, otherwise, surgery is mandatory. In Stapfer's types II–III perforations, the initial treatment is non-operative, as the perforations are usually contained in the retroperitoneal space. Moreover, in the cases with delayed diagnosis, a repeated ERCP to insert a biliary stent could be also an option in clinically stable patients. Stapfer's type IV perforations only need observation (Fig. 33.6). Parenteral nutrition should be considered patients in which a prolonged bowel is expected.

In case of esophageal perforations, the criteria developed by Altorjay et al. (Table 33.4) can be followed to select suitable patients for conservative management [33]. The Pittsburgh group perforation severity score can be useful in these situations, as patients with scores lesser than 3 would benefit from non-surgical treatments [34]. Similar to perforations diagnosed and treated during the endoscopy, early and ade-

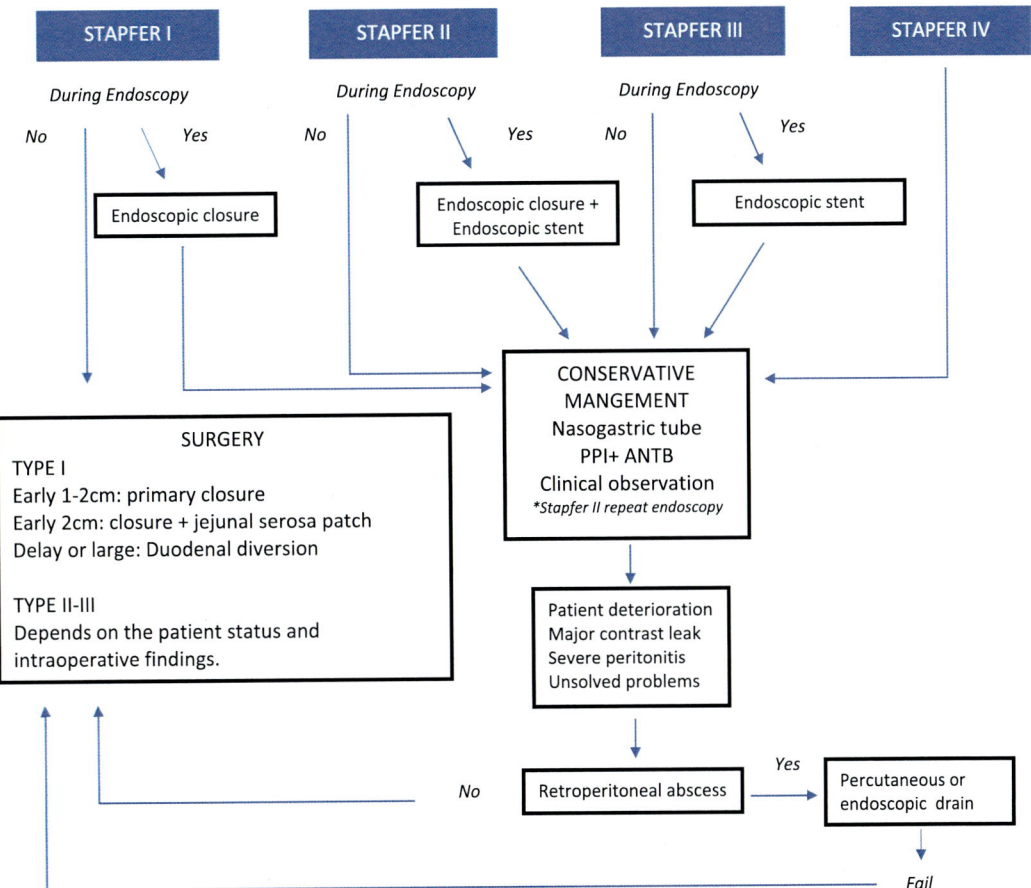

Fig. 33.6 Decision algorithm for CPRE-related perforations

Table 33.4 Criteria for conservative management of esophageal perforations

Altorjay	Pittsburgh perforation severity score	
	Variable	Score
Consider non-operative management if:		
– Early perforation and/or encapsulated extravasation	Age >75 years	1
	Tachycardia	1
– Minimal symptoms	Leukocytosis	1
– No signs of sepsis	Pleural effusion	1
– Absence of malignancy or esophageal obstructive disease	Fever (>38.5°)	2
	Non-contained leak	2
– Availability of adequate diagnostic and therapeutic techniques and surgical skills	Respiratory compromise	2
	Timing <24 h	2
	Hypotension	3
	Cancer	3

quate nutritional support is mandatory. In all cases undergoing non-operative management, other invasive procedures can be added to achieve local source control (e.g., percutaneous drainage of pleural, mediastinal, or retroperitoneal collections) [31].

33.3.2 Surgical Treatment

33.3.2.1 Colonoscopy Perforations

Surgical intervention should be preferentially considered if concomitant colonic diseases requiring surgery (e.g., neoplasms) exist, also in immunosuppressed or transplanted patients [3]. Different surgical procedures for the management of ICP have been described. They include the primary closure of the defect, a colonic lateral resection englobing the perforation site, a colostomy by exteriorizing the perforation, or a standard colonic resection. The final decision is mainly empirical and should be made after inspection of the whole abdominal cavity. It depends on (a) the size, location, and etiology of the ICP; (b) the viability of surrounding colon and mesocolon; (c) the degree and time of evolution of peritonitis; (d) the patient's general status and the presence of comorbidities; (e) the quality of the colonic preparation; (f) the presence of residual lesions not resected during the initial colonoscopy [35].

Explorative laparoscopy is the ideal first-line approach for the surgical management of ICP (Fig. 33.5b). The laparoscopic approach provides better outcomes in terms of postoperative complications and length of hospital stay than conventional laparotomy [35]. A primary suture of the perforation could be feasible when the tissues appear healthy and well-perfused. A wedge resection can be performed if an excessive narrowing of the colonic lumen is prevented. In the rest of the cases, a colonic resection may be the best option. In case of delayed surgeries, or in patients with severe comorbidities or poor clinical status, exteriorizing the perforation via a colostomy, or a primary resection with staged anastomosis could be considered. Abdominal drain placement is justified in case of delayed surgery, poor bowel preparation, or high peritoneal contamination.

33.3.2.2 Upper Digestive Endoscopy Perforations

Surgery is indicated in all patients who are not suitable for conservative management. An adequate exposition of the surgical field to properly identify the perforation is mandatory. Explorative laparoscopy/thoracoscopy would be the first step in the surgical procedure depending on the surgeon's skills and available technological resources. Surgery should include sepsis control with local debridement and drainage of collections. The primary closure of the defect could be attempted, if feasible. To leave proper drainage of the area, and to assure adequate nutritional enteral support (e.g., nasogastric tube, decompressive gastrostomy, surgical jejunostomy, and central venous catheterization) are critical steps during the surgical procedure [32].

At cervical perforations, the esophagus is usually accessed by a left lateral incision following the anterior border of the sternocleidomastoid muscle. In large perforations (e.g., >50%) drainage alone and/or esophagostomy should be considered. Thoracotomy is usually required for thoracic perforations, although an abdominal transhiatal approach can be used in selected cases. If direct repair is not feasible the remaining options are esophageal diversion, resection, or exclusion. Perforations at the abdominal esophagus, as gastric perforations, usually require surgery. The use of a buttress for cervical (e.g., sternocleidomastoid, or digastric muscles) or thoracic (e.g., intercostal muscle and pericardium) perforations can be justified. To perform a fundoplication is feasible to cover GEJ and gastric perforations, or in thoracic ones, if they are approached transhiatally.

The surgical treatment of UDE iatrogenic perforations sometimes requires the performance of additional surgical maneuvers, especially in cases of ERCP-related perforation, as cholecystectomy, common bile duct exploration, or biliary diversion. Surgical treatment of Stapfer's type I duodenal perforations depends on the delay from the initial procedure and the size of the perforation. Small perforations (up to 2 cm), which are diagnosed early, can be treated with primary closure (i.e., debridement of devitalized tissue and transversal closure in one or two layers). A jejunal serosal patch can be added in these situations. In patients with a delayed diagnosis or presenting large perforations, duodenal diversion with pyloric exclusion should be performed. The procedure includes a primary duodenal repair, the closure of the pylorus with a running suture trough a gastrotomy or by stapling, and a gastrojejunostomy. A lateral duodenostomy or a retrograde duodenostomy (i.e., from the distal jejunal site) can be added to the previous. In Stapfer's types II–III perforations, surgery is only indicated in patients not responding to conservative management, or in those presenting major contrast leaks, diffuse peritonitis, or retroperitoneal fluid collections not suitable for percutaneous drainage. In cases in which an early diagnosis is made, retroperitoneal washout and adequate drainage could be sufficient. To perform a primary closure through a small transverse duodenotomy or a sphincteroplasty are the other surgical alternatives. Delayed surgeries are often associated with significant contamination; therefore, a pyloric exclusion or a duodenal/biliary drainage would be the most adequate option.

33.3.3 Prognosis

33.3.3.1 Colonoscopy Perforations

Depending on the delay in the IPC management and the pre-existing pathologies, the related mortality can be as high as 25% [36]. The adequate choice of the ideal surgical procedure for each patient is pivotal to mitigating the odds of important postoperative morbidity. Surveillance endoscopy is indicated within 3–6 months postoperatively if the primary colonoscopy was incomplete or non-resected polyps remain in place.

33.3.3.2 Upper Digestive Endoscopy Perforations

Esophageal perforations are associated with considerable mortality (12%), which is higher in those located in the abdomen (i.e., cervical 5.9%, thoracic 10.9%, and intra-abdominal 13.2%). In absence of treatment, the contamination of the adjacent spaces rapidly flows into severe sepsis and organ failure. A high degree of clinical suspicion is critical for the patient's behavior. The delay in receiving the definitive treatment is the key factor for the patient's survival. Delays greater than 24 h are associated with mortality rates of over 20% [37]. Therefore, the surgical intervention should be undertaken as soon as possible after the decision is made. Duodenal perforations Stapfer's type I are associated with an overall mortality of 20% [38]. Despite the majority of the patients with type II perforations do not require surgery initially (<5%), those who finally operated present also high mortality rates [39]. Stapfer's type III and IV have a good prognosis with non-operative treatments.

> **Dos and Don'ts**
>
> - Computed tomography is the imaging technique of choice to confirm the clinical suspicion of endoscopy-related perforations.
> - Conservative management can be considered in selected cases of colonic or esophageal perforations presenting small and contained wall disruptions with minimal contamination.
> - Conservative management is the treatment of choice for Stapfer's types II–IV ERCP-related perforations.

- The conservative management is based on fasting, intravenous hydration, broad-spectrum antibiotics, and close clinical surveillance. Proton pump inhibitor therapy should be administered in patients with upper gastrointestinal perforations.
- Early and adequate nutritional support is also mandatory.
- In cases not suitable for conservative management, or after its failure, surgery should be performed with the minimum delay.
- Explorative laparoscopy/thoracoscopy could be the first-line surgical approach depending on the surgeon's skills and available technological resources.
- Endoscopic treatment is the technique of choice in cases of bleeding. Selective angioembolization or surgery is employed when it fails.

Take-Home Messages
- Early diagnosis is critical for the patient's behavior. The clinical and biochemical presentation during the early period could be poorly specific. A high degree of suspicion is mandatory.
- Thoracic/abdominal computed tomography is the gold standard exploration to confirm after the procedure the clinical suspicion of endoscopy-related perforations.
- After the diagnosis of iatrogenic endoscopic perforations, conservative management can be considered in selected patients. This approach requires close clinical observation and repeated imaging and biochemical tests.
- Primary suture, wedge resection, ostomy creation, and colonic resection, are the different options for the surgical treatment of IPC. The final choice is made after a careful inspection of the abdomen and is based on the perforation features, the patient's general status, the surgeon's experience, and the availability of the surgical resources.
- Duodenal wall perforations after ERCP (Stapfer's type I) require of surgery if not detected during the endoscopy. Periampullary duodenal perforation (Stapfer's type II) and bile duct and pancreatic perforation (Stapfer's type III) can be managed non-operatively. Retroperitoneal free air alone (Stapfer's type IV) does not need treatment.

10 Test Questions (4 Options)

1. Which is the maximum recommended incidence of iatrogenic perforations during diagnostic colonoscopy?
   A. 1%
   B. 0.01%
   C. **0.1%**
   D. 10%
2. One of the following does not confer a higher risk for colonoscopy perforation.
   A. Placement of metal stent for malignant obstruction
   B. **Male sex**
   C. Low BMI
   D. Repeated dilatation for benign stricture
3. One of the following sentences is false regarding endoscopic perforations.
   A. The most frequent etiology of esophageal perforations is iatrogenic.
   B. **Colonoscopy perforations due to barotrauma are usually located at the splenic flexure.**
   C. Dilatation of esophageal caustic strictures is associated with a higher risk of perforation.
   D. The sigmoid colon is the most frequent site of colonic perforation.

4. The choice between the different surgical alternatives for IPC relies on:
   A. The size, location, and etiology of the ICP.
   B. The degree of peritonitis and the patient's general status.
   C. The presence of non-resected colonic lesions.
   D. **All the previous.**
5. When operating IPC:
   A. A colonic resection is recommended when the tissues appear healthy and well-perfused.
   B. A wedge resection can be performed disregarding the narrowing of the intestinal lumen.
   C. **In delayed surgeries, exteriorizing the perforation via a colostomy, or a primary resection with staged anastomosis could be considered.**
   D. Primary suture is always an acceptable choice.
6. Regarding iatrogenic perforations during upper gastrointestinal endoscopy:
   A. Those located in the abdominal esophagus or the stomach can be usually managed by a conservative approach.
   B. The use of a buttress is never recommended.
   C. Direct repair should be always attempted.
   D. **If direct repair is not feasible the remaining options are esophageal diversion, resection, or exclusion.**
7. One of the following supports the non-operative management of a perforation located at the cervical esophagus:
   A. **Encapsulated perforation**
   B. Delayed perforation.
   C. Signs of sepsis.
   D. Unresected adenocarcinoma of the GEJ.
8. One of the following is false regarding iatrogenic perforations during ERCP:
   A. Stapfer's type I is uncommonly diagnosed during the procedure.
   B. **In Stapfer's type IV retroperitoneal air can be associated with retroperitoneal abscess.**
   C. In Stapfer's type II a repeated ERCP to insert a biliary stent can be used in stable patients.
   D. Non-operative management in Stapfer's type III is successful in 95% of patients.
9. One of the following sentences is false:
   A. A pyloric exclusion is an option in Stapfer's type II and III perforations.
   B. The laparoscopic approach is limited to early diagnosis and expert surgeons for ERCP perforations.
   C. **Common bile duct exploration is never indicated in the management of ERCP perforation.**
   D. The risk of mortality after ERCP-related perforation is around 10%.
10. Which one of the following related adverse events is not characteristic of patients undergoing percutaneous gastrostomy?
    A. Buried bumper syndrome
    B. **Intestinal obstruction**
    C. Pneumoperitoneum
    D. Necrotizing fasciitis

References

1. Rex DK, Schoenfeld PS, Cohen J, Pike IM, Adler DG, Fennerty MB, et al. Quality indicators for colonoscopy. Am J Gastroenterol. 2015;110(1):72–90.
2. Rembacken B, Hassan C, Riemann JF, Chilton A, Rutter M, Dumonceau JM, et al. Quality in screening colonoscopy: position statement of the European Society of Gastrointestinal Endoscopy (ESGE). Endoscopy. 2012;44(10):957–68.

3. de'Angelis N, Di Saverio S, Chiara O, Sartelli M, Martinez-Perez A, Patrizi F, et al. 2017 WSES guidelines for the management of iatrogenic colonoscopy perforation. World J Emerg Surg. 2018;13:5.
4. Dehal A, Tessier DJ. Intraperitoneal and extraperitoneal colonic perforation following diagnostic colonoscopy. JSLS. 2014;18(1):136–41.
5. Committee ASoP, Ben-Menachem T, Decker GA, Early DS, Evans J, Fanelli RD, et al. Adverse events of upper GI endoscopy. Gastrointest Endosc. 2012;76(4):707–18.
6. Cotton PB, Lehman G, Vennes J, Geenen JE, Russell RC, Meyers WC, et al. Endoscopic sphincterotomy complications and their management: an attempt at consensus. Gastrointest Endosc. 1991;37(3):383–93.
7. Andriulli A, Loperfido S, Napolitano G, Niro G, Valvano MR, Spirito F, et al. Incidence rates of post-ERCP complications: a systematic survey of prospective studies. Am J Gastroenterol. 2007;102(8):1781–8.
8. Heldwein W, Dollhopf M, Rosch T, Meining A, Schmidtsdorff G, Hasford J, et al. The Munich Polypectomy Study (MUPS): prospective analysis of complications and risk factors in 4000 colonic snare polypectomies. Endoscopy. 2005;37(11):1116–22.
9. van Halsema EE, van Hooft JE, Small AJ, Baron TH, Garcia-Cano J, Cheon JH, et al. Perforation in colorectal stenting: a meta-analysis and a search for risk factors. Gastrointest Endosc. 2014;79(6):970–82 e7; quiz 83 e2, 83 e5.
10. Garcia Martinez MT, Ruano Poblador A, Galan Raposo L, Gay Fernandez AM, Casal Nunez JE. Perforation after colonoscopy: our 16-year experience. Rev Esp Enferm Dig. 2007;99(10):588–92.
11. Samalavicius NE, Kazanavicius D, Lunevicius R, Poskus T, Valantinas J, Stanaitis J, et al. Incidence, risk, management, and outcomes of iatrogenic full-thickness large bowel injury associated with 56,882 colonoscopies in 14 Lithuanian hospitals. Surg Endosc. 2013;27(5):1628–35.
12. Enns R, Eloubeidi MA, Mergener K, Jowell PS, Branch MS, Pappas TM, et al. ERCP-related perforations: risk factors and management. Endoscopy. 2002;34(4):293–8.
13. Stapfer M, Selby RR, Stain SC, Katkhouda N, Parekh D, Jabbour N, et al. Management of duodenal perforation after endoscopic retrograde cholangiopancreatography and sphincterotomy. Ann Surg. 2000;232(2):191–8.
14. Tsuji Y, Ohata K, Ito T, Chiba H, Ohya T, Gunji T, et al. Risk factors for bleeding after endoscopic submucosal dissection for gastric lesions. World J Gastroenterol. 2010;16(23):2913–7.
15. Ko CW, Dominitz JA. Complications of colonoscopy: magnitude and management. Gastrointest Endosc Clin N Am. 2010;20(4):659–71.
16. Gerson LB, Tokar J, Chiorean M, Lo S, Decker GA, Cave D, et al. Complications associated with double balloon enteroscopy at nine US centers. Clin Gastroenterol Hepatol. 2009;7(11):1177–82.e3.
17. Lee C, Im JP, Kim JW, Kim SE, Ryu DY, Cha JM, et al. Risk factors for complications and mortality of percutaneous endoscopic gastrostomy: a multicenter, retrospective study. Surg Endosc. 2013;27(10):3806–15.
18. Sharma VK, Nguyen CC, Crowell MD, Lieberman DA, de Garmo P, Fleischer DE. A national study of cardiopulmonary unplanned events after GI endoscopy. Gastrointest Endosc. 2007;66(1):27–34.
19. Nelson DB. Infectious disease complications of GI endoscopy: Part I, endogenous infections. Gastrointest Endosc. 2003;57(4):546–56.
20. Iqbal CW, Cullinane DC, Schiller HJ, Sawyer MD, Zietlow SP, Farley DR. Surgical management and outcomes of 165 colonoscopic perforations from a single institution. Arch Surg. 2008;143(7):701–6; discussion 6-7.
21. Yang SK, Xiao L, Zhang H, Xu XX, Song PA, Liu FY, et al. Significance of serum procalcitonin as biomarker for detection of bacterial peritonitis: a systematic review and meta-analysis. BMC Infect Dis. 2014;14:452.
22. Iqbal CW, Chun YS, Farley DR. Colonoscopic perforations: a retrospective review. J Gastrointest Surg. 2005;9(9):1229–35: discussion 36.
23. Shanmuganathan K, Mirvis SE, Chiu WC, Killeen KL, Scalea TM. Triple-contrast helical CT in penetrating torso trauma: a prospective study to determine peritoneal violation and the need for laparotomy. AJR Am J Roentgenol. 2001;177(6):1247–56.
24. Ivatury RR, Moore FA, Biffl W, Leppeniemi A, Ansaloni L, Catena F, et al. Oesophageal injuries: position paper, WSES, 2013. World J Emerg Surg. 2014;9(1):9.
25. Chandrasekhara V, Khashab MA, Muthusamy VR, Acosta RD, Agrawal D, Bruining DH, et al. Adverse events associated with ERCP. Gastrointest Endosc. 2017;85(1):32–47.
26. Tamiya Y, Nakahara K, Kominato K, Serikawa O, Watanabe Y, Tateishi H, et al. Pneumomediastinum is a frequent but minor complication during esophageal endoscopic submucosal dissection. Endoscopy. 2010;42(1):8–14.
27. Genzlinger JL, McPhee MS, Fisher JK, Jacob KM, Helzberg JH. Significance of retroperitoneal air after endoscopic retrograde cholangiopancreatography with sphincterotomy. Am J Gastroenterol. 1999;94(5):1267–70.
28. Okamoto K, Suzuki K, Takada T, Strasberg SM, Asbun HJ, Endo I, et al. Tokyo Guidelines 2018: flowchart for the management of acute cholecystitis. J Hepato-Biliary-Pancreatic Sci. 2018;25(1):55–72.
29. Miura F, Okamoto K, Takada T, Strasberg SM, Asbun HJ, Pitt HA, et al. Tokyo Guidelines 2018: initial management of acute biliary infection and flowchart for acute cholangitis. J Hepato-Biliary-Pancreatic Sci. 2018;25(1):31–40.
30. Broeders E, Al-Taher M, Peeters K, Bouvy N. Verres needle desufflation as an effective treatment option for colonic perforation after colonoscopy. Surg Laparosc Endosc Percutan Tech. 2015;25(2):e61–4.

31. Vogel SB, Rout WR, Martin TD, Abbitt PL. Esophageal perforation in adults: aggressive, conservative treatment lowers morbidity and mortality. Ann Surg. 2005;241(6):1016–21; discussion 21-3.
32. Chirica M, Kelly MD, Siboni S, Aiolfi A, Riva CG, Asti E, et al. Esophageal emergencies: WSES guidelines. World J Emerg Surg. 2019;14:26.
33. Altorjay A, Kiss J, Voros A, Bohak A. Nonoperative management of esophageal perforations. Is it justified? Ann Surg. 1997;225(4):415–21.
34. Schweigert M, Sousa HS, Solymosi N, Yankulov A, Fernandez MJ, Beattie R, et al. Spotlight on esophageal perforation: A multinational study using the Pittsburgh esophageal perforation severity scoring system. J Thorac Cardiovasc Surg. 2016;151(4):1002–9.
35. Martinez-Perez A, de'Angelis N, Brunetti F, Le Baleur Y, Paya-Llorente C, Memeo R, et al. Laparoscopic vs. open surgery for the treatment of iatrogenic colonoscopic perforations: a systematic review and meta-analysis. World J Emerg Surg. 2017;12:8.
36. Teoh AY, Poon CM, Lee JF, Leong HT, Ng SS, Sung JJ, et al. Outcomes and predictors of mortality and stoma formation in surgical management of colonoscopic perforations: a multicenter review. Arch Surg. 2009;144(1):9–13.
37. Biancari F, D'Andrea V, Paone R, Di Marco C, Savino G, Koivukangas V, et al. Current treatment and outcome of esophageal perforations in adults: systematic review and meta-analysis of 75 studies. World J Surg. 2013;37(5):1051–9.
38. Paspatis GA, Arvanitakis M, Dumonceau JM, Barthet M, Saunders B, Turino SY, et al. Diagnosis and management of iatrogenic endoscopic perforations: European Society of Gastrointestinal Endoscopy (ESGE) Position Statement—Update 2020. Endoscopy. 2020;52(9):792–810.
39. Vezakis A, Fragulidis G, Polydorou A. Endoscopic retrograde cholangiopancreatography-related perforations: diagnosis and management. World J Gastrointest Endosc. 2015;7(14):1135–41.

Further Reading [1]

Ben-Menachem T, Decker GA, Early DS, Evans J, Fanelli RD, Fisher DA, et al. Adverse events of upper GI endoscopy. Gastrointest Endosc. 2012;76(4):707–18.

Chandrasekhara V, Khashab MA, Muthusamy VR, Acosta RD, Agrawal D, Bruining DH, et al. Adverse events associated with ERCP. Gastrointest Endosc. 2017;85(1):32–47.

Chirica M, Kelly MD, Siboni S, Aiolfi A, Riva CG, Asti E, et al. Esophageal emergencies: WSES guidelines. World J Emerg Surg. 2019;14:26.

de'Angelis N, Di Saverio S, Chiara O, Sartelli M, Martinez-Perez A, Patrizi F, et al. WSES guidelines for the management of iatrogenic colonoscopy perforation. World J Emerg Surg. 2017;2018(13):5.

Dumonceau JM, Kapral C, Aabakken L, Papanikolaou IS, Tringali A, Vanbiervliet G, et al. ERCP-related adverse events: European Society of Gastrointestinal Endoscopy (ESGE) Guideline. Endoscopy. 2020;52(2):127–49.

Fisher DA, Maple JT, Ben-Menachem T, Cash BD, Decker GA, Early DS, et al. Complications of colonoscopy. Gastrointest Endosc. 2011;74(4):745–52.

Paspatis GA, Arvanitakis M, Dumonceau JM, Barthet M, Saunders B, Turino SY, et al. Diagnosis and management of iatrogenic endoscopic perforations: European Society of Gastrointestinal Endoscopy (ESGE) Position Statement—Update 2020. Endoscopy. 2020;52(9):792–810.

---

[1] Highlight here the most important publications related to the chapter content (i.e., Guidelines).

End-of-Life Care, Including the Role of Intensive Care in Tissue and Organ Donation

34

Christopher James Doig and Kevin J. Solverson

Learning Goals
- Review principles behind OTD as part of quality EOL care in the ICU.
- Understand neurological determination of death from historical to current perspectives.
- Review the underlying concept of donation after cardiac death with special attention to novel data regarding the resumption of cardiocirculatory activity in WWLSI.

C. J. Doig (✉)
Departments of Critical Care Medicine, Cumming School of Medicine, University of Calgary, Calgary, Canada

Department of Medicine, Cumming School of Medicine, University of Calgary, Calgary, Canada

Department of Community Health Sciences, Cumming School of Medicine, University of Calgary, Calgary, Canada
e-mail: cdoig@ucalgary.ca

K. J. Solverson
Departments of Critical Care Medicine, Cumming School of Medicine, University of Calgary, Calgary, Canada

Department of Medicine, Cumming School of Medicine, University of Calgary, Calgary, Canada

Division of Pulmonary Medicine, Cumming School of Medicine, University of Calgary, Calgary, Canada
e-mail: kevin.solverson@ahs.ca

This is a difficult time to write a chapter on end-of-life (EOL) care in the intensive care unit (ICU). Since March 2020, when the World Health Organization declared the infection related to SARs CoV-2 virus (COVID-19) as a pandemic, acute care health systems, including ICU have managed a high number of patients with respiratory failure. The demand for ICU care, the number of patients on ventilators, and the ability to cope, is a reminder of the worldwide infection from polio in the 1950s, and its role in the genesis of ICUs [1]. Before the introduction of ventilatory support, polio resulted in large numbers of healthy individuals developing neuromuscular respiratory failure and dying. ICUs (sometimes called respiratory units) were developed as a consolidated place to manage these patients. In parallel, improved pre- and intra-operative resuscitation of hemorrhagic shock and surgical techniques for traumatic injuries (learnt from military conflicts) led to the operative survival of individuals that would otherwise have died [2]. Patients dying at night because of deterioration attributed to an inability to monitor vital signs continuously led to the 'shock ward' at LA County/USC Medical Center [3]. The genesis of ICU admitting desperately ill patients then, and now, is that some don't survive: EOL care is integral to ICU care.

Advancements in organ and tissue transplantation came from an understanding of the biology of immunosuppression and the refinement of surgical techniques such that organ replacement is the preferred approach to end-stage organ failure. EOL care and death as a source of organs and tissue for transplantation are inexorably linked. This chapter will discuss aspects of EOL care in the ICU, and the importance of the ICU in organ and tissue donation (OTD).

Worldwide consensus on principles of EOL care for the critically ill has been published [4]. Humanistic medical care should respond to the population and environment where it is practiced. Our perspective is informed by working in an academic centre, with neurocritical care, trauma, transplant recipients, and general multisystem patients. We treat individuals from diverse ethno-cultural and religious backgrounds, including a large indigenous population—these groups have experienced unconscious bias or systemic racism which includes in the health care system. Health care in Canada is publicly funded, and funding ICUs in response to supply or demand should not overtly affect treatment decisions. With these disclosures, we hope, the broad principles covered are not unique to our environment.

34.1 End-of-Life Care in ICU

Many patients admitted to ICU die. Despite a preference to die at home, one Canadian study found 87% of deaths occurred in the hospital [5]. Almost 20% of these occurred in ICUs, varying from 15 to 27% depending on the hospital. One in four to one in six ICU patients (particularly tertiary (referral) or in academic health centres) die prior to discharge: this is often a surprise to families and practitioners unfamiliar with ICU [6]. The dying process usually follows one of three paths: first is the physiologically unstable patient admitted to ICU—these patients receive active resuscitation, become unsupportable, and die soon after admission; second is the ICU patient with multisystem (occasionally single) organ failure such that ongoing interventions will not prevent death—these individuals commonly die after a decision to withhold or withdraw life-sustaining interventions (WWLSI); finally, some patients have a primary brain injury and are determined dead based on specific neurological criteria (neurological determination of death (NDD), frequently known as 'brain death') [7]. The remainder of the chapter will focus on these last processes.

WWLSI is contemplated when a patient lacks the probability of surviving or when current/planned treatments/interventions and prognosis are not aligned with their previously expressed goals. EOL care and WWLSI decisions should always be approached with integrity, humility, and compassion [8–10]. Implicit in a WWLSI decision is the anticipation of death, and a change in EOL care goals from survival to comfort. In this context: (1) WWLSI is considered distinct and separate from medically assisted death or euthanasia, and (2) traditional western biomedical ethics do not distinguish between withholding and withdrawal [11]. This perspective may not be normative in some jurisdictions as withdrawal of LSI may not be permitted, or in some sociocultural contexts withholding of LSI may not be accepted. There may be a psychological distinction where the moral agency involved in withdrawing LSI (an act) is perceived differently than withholding LSI (no act is done).

Whenever possible, communications regarding goals of care (GOC) including EOL care should be prior to ICU admission. Advanced care planning should happen with all persons (for example through advanced directives or 'living wills') but particularly with individuals admitted to the hospital, with a chronic condition, or of advancing age. Unfortunately, these discussions often do not occur or are not documented prior to ICU admission [12]. Sometimes, the severity of illness and interventions may preclude discussions with the patient. Therefore, decisions will need to be made with or by a proxy or surrogate. A proxy or surrogate should be the individual(s) who best understand(s) the wishes of the patient and can provide a substituted decision [13]. The proxy or surrogate is usually a family member, however, whom the patient considers as 'family' may be broader than simply linked by birth [14]. Poor experiences with the health care system including systemic discrimination, medical error or treatment complications, conflict between patient/family and the healthcare team or within either of these parties and explicit or implicit conduct which suggests a lack of respect may complicate discussions and decisions [15, 16]. Inherent information asymmetry in the healthcare provider: patient relationship contributes to a disproportionate power imbalance favouring the health care team.

Communication skills should be developed broadly across training programs, including as part of undergraduate medical education [17, 18]. There should be an emphasis for ICU practitioners on competency training and feedback in specific EOL communication skills [19, 20]. There is no one 'right-way' in EOL care, and attention to process and information communicated is required [21]. Patient and surrogate preferences in decision-making are not singular, with most preferring a shared decision-making process with the physician (health care team) or autonomously after hearing the opinion of the physician [22].

ICU care should adopt patient and family-centred care whereby the health care team partners with the patient/family to deliver personalized care respectful and responsive to their needs, including communication, at the forefront [23, 24]. In our ICUs, we use protocolized processes of care, including measured quality indicators, which begin at ICU admission. All patients have a GOC designation at the time of ICU admission. Family members are introduced to the ICU within 20 min of ICU admission, and the first visit is permitted if possible (this includes family presence during active resuscitation). We do not restrict hours of access for family visits. Families are encouraged to attend and participate in daily clinical rounds, including presenting their perspectives and asking questions. Multidisciplinary family meetings occur separately from daily rounds for comprehensive updates. Translational language services and remote connectivity with video streaming are arranged as needed. Cultural and spiritual practices are supported (e.g. smudging ceremonies for indigenous persons). Prior to EOL discussions, a second opinion from another critical care physician is obtained. Private rooms are used, and patients transitioned to EOL care, have an indicator (a white rose emblem on the door) to inform other health care providers to maintain a quiet, dignified, and respectful environment. Finally, all individuals are offered the opportunity for organ/tissue donation.

34.2 Organ and Tissue Donation

34.2.1 Brain Death and Organ Donation

At the time of death, offering the opportunity for donation is part of respectful EOL care. Attention often focuses on organ donation, but tissue donation saves lives, and improves the quality of life (think a burn victim who benefits from a biological wound dressing with allograft tissue, or the return of sight after a successful corneal transplant). It is the opportunity to donate that should be the focus, not if or what is donated.

Neurological injury is common in all ICUs, and it is necessary that critical care physicians have the competency to determine NDD. Proximate causes of brain injury leading to NDD have changed [25, 26]. In a population sample (rather than a sample drawn from a specific type of ICU), the most common causes of NDD were hypoxic–ischemic (anoxic) brain injury (approximately 50%), followed by traumatic brain injury (25%), intracranial haemorrhage (10%), subarachnoid haemorrhage (8%), and ischemic stroke (3%). The incidence of NDD from anoxic injury increased from 1.1 to 3.1 per million population, whereas the incidence of NDD from traumatic brain injury decreased from 4.4 to less than 3 per million population.

The seminal criteria for the determination of brain death are attributed to the Ad Hoc Committee of the Harvard Medical School [27]. NDD is accepted worldwide, albeit, with some jurisdictions having unique specific requirements [28–31]. General requirements for NDD include: (1) an established aetiology, (2) the absence of confounding factors, (3) the absence of awareness (usually determined by the absence of response to painful and other stimuli), (4) absent brainstem reflexes, and (5) absent visible respiratory effort despite a normal stimulus (raised partial pressure of arterial carbon dioxide) [32]. Some criteria vary slightly between jurisdictions such as the number of times and interval between assessments, who can perform and the training required for an NDD, whether ancillary investigations are needed, if families can refuse to accept NDD, and specific details of confounding factors (e.g. core body temperature). The use of ancillary tests, usual imaging of cerebral blood flow, also varies. Often ancillary tests are relied on when confounding features or physiologic instability preclude complete clinical assessment. Each imaging modality has benefits, limitations, and a variable evidence base [33].

In many jurisdictions, even with 'presumed consent' legislation, consent or authorization is obtained from the family. As there is an inherent power imbalance in the provider:family relationship, thoughtful and careful discussions with accurate information are necessary for any family decision to be correct within their framework of beliefs [34, 35]. A poorly executed discussion may result in psychological harm to families, and relevant to OTD, may not preserve an opportunity for donation. Despite the widespread societal acceptance of donation, not all individuals will consent or authorize donation [36]. There has been debate as to whether the discussion about organ donation should involve a 'nudge' to influence a family to proceed with donation [37, 38]. ICU must respect and provide the same level of care and bereavement support to patients and families regardless of decisions to proceed or not with organ donation acknowledging the request and decision may have lasting effects [39]. We separate the discussion of death from the organ donation request. In our process, we inform the family that death has occurred, and ensure bereavement and spiritual support. After an interval, we inform about the donation possibility, explore if the patient had communicated their wishes, and seek assent from organ donation coordinators to attend and obtain formal consent. The coordinators review in detail the processes of management, including expected duration, until organ recovery occurs.

From the interval of NDD and consent, to organ recovery, the ICU's role is to maintain optimal physiologic organ function. All NDD donors will require ventilatory and often circulatory support, with the maintenance of fluid and electrolyte balance [40]. ICU physicians as experts in physiologic support, through participation in organ donor management, increase the number and function of transplantable organs [41]. The first consensus guidelines, a Canadian collaboration of ICU and transplant professionals, was published in 2006, and others have followed [42–45]. The updated Canadian guidelines used a formal 'Grading of Recommendations Assessments, Development, and Evaluation' methodology, including multidisciplinary health professionals with varied clinical expertise and patient partners. The guidelines contain a total of 1: 'strong recommendation', 30: 'conditional recommendations', 1: 'good practice', and 4: 'no recommendations' [43, 46]. The 4 recommendations thought to have the most impact on clinical practice were: (1) no routine administration of thyroid hormone, (2) against routine coronary angiography, (3) to maintain donor core body temperature in the range of 34–35 degrees centigrade, and (4) to use a lung protective ventilation strategy. The full recommendations are available in a supplement published with their report.

34.3 Donation After Cardiac Death

Donation after cardiac death (DCD) has expanded the source of organs for transplant, and recipients of DCD organs have long-term graft function comparable to organs from NDD donors [47]. Most programs with DCD organ procurement focus on 'controlled' donation: donation that follows consensual WWLSI, the practice common in ICUs [32]. 'Uncontrolled' DCD usually follows the unsuccessful cardiac arrest in the community/emergency department, is uncommon in ICU, and will not be discussed further.

'Re-emergence' of DCD followed the report of the 'Pittsburgh Protocol', and, recovery of organs from DCD has since become commonplace in many countries [48]. There is a distinction between donors following NDD, and DCD: in the former, death determination occurs and then the patient becomes a 'potential donor'; in the latter, individuals became potential donors before they die. The distinction of when a patient is considered a 'potential donor' is relevant. With DCD, individuals should only be considered potential donors following consensual decisions on WWLSI, and this should precede, be distinct, and preclude prior involvement of organ donor procurement organizations. As stated in an alternative way, expertise in WWLSI resides within critical care, and decisions to approach families about WWLSI should be by ICU clinicians who are independent of transplant proceedings including immediate responsibility of caring for potential transplant recipients [49]. Otherwise, there is a risk that families or other health care professionals may perceive decisions on prognosis, and recommendations of WWLSI as influenced by organ donation potential [50]. Maintenance of the trust of families is requisite, particularly for neurological injury [51]. In a Canadian study which examined EOL care decisions in neurologically injured patients, there was significant variability in the duration of treatment prior to WWLSI [52]. Other research identified variability in the extremes of care considered appropriate in common ICU scenarios [53]. Variability in prognosis and WWLSI should be minimized and research continues to be needed to examine decision-making in determining prognosis. If not, trust in both critical care and donation practices could suffer from the perception described nearly 60 years ago "it seems inevitable that the fact that someone else is waiting for this patient's kidney must to some extent influence the decision" [54]. In our centre, we follow a local guideline on DCD practice, similar to subsequently published national recommendations [55]. The first step of this guideline is the necessity of a consensual decision in the multidisciplinary care team that WWLSI is appropriate, and this must include the participation of current consultants, and a second formal opinion, prior to discussions with the family.

There have been other ethical and pragmatic concerns described in the process of DCD [56]. Care must be situated within the local environment, including DCD processes of care [57]. The process of death in DCD changes. WWLSI in most ICU patients is in a quiet location, with time for grieving both leading up to, and following, the moment of death. In DCD processes must minimize 'warm ischemia' to recovered organs i.e. the time between low blood oxygen and low blood pressure/absent circulation. In some centres when DCD recovery is planned, WWLSI occurs in an operating room with the donor separated from their family. Alternatively, WWLSI occurs in the ICU with family present, but rapidly after death donors are transported to the operating room. In either circumstance, a period of 'no-touch' by the health care team of 2–5 min, ostensibly to follow the 'dead-donor rule' ensures that the donor is 'truly dead' prior to organ recovery [58]. The duration to ensure that circulation has irreversibly stopped has created controversy. In a recent study, Dhanani and others enrolled over 600 ICU patients and studied physiologic activity associated with WWLSI [59]. These authors found that bedside ICU providers recognized only 1% of episodes of a resumption of circulation, whereas a retrospective analysis of arterial and ECG waveform data demonstrated resumption occurred in 14% of patients. However, no resumption of circulation occurred after an interval of approximately 4.5 min. These results support a minimum of a 5-min interval (no touch) following death determination death prior to beginning any procedure related to organ recovery.

There are other aspects of NDD and DCD in the published literature. To be fully informed, we encourage exploring some of these concerns [60–63].

34.4 Conclusion

The need for high-quality critical care, and to provide care for patients at EOL will remain linked. ICU providers must be aware and assess how their patients' ethnocultural and religious backgrounds impact EOL care. Trust between patients/families and the healthcare team is crucial and results from demonstrating high-quality patient and family-centred care and effective and empathetic communication. Knowledge of local requirements in death determination, medical management of the donor, and DCD is critical to minimize unnecessary variability and improve outcomes. It is a privilege to care for patients and their families at EOL, and with this comes the responsibility to ensure optimal care.

Do and Dont's

Do:
- Practice excellence in patient-family-centred care particularly at end-of-life.
- Focus on the importance of communication and understanding of patient/family perspective.
- Consider the option of organ and tissue donation as part of quality end-of-life care
- Provide the opportunity of OTD to patients/families in a compassionate manner.
- Do follow relevant (inter)national guidelines for your hospital/region/country/health system.

Don't:
- Think that OTD is unique to neurocritical care or trauma centres.
- Jump to 'early' conclusions and avoid negative bias regarding prognosis.
- Violate the 'dead-donor' rule.

Take-Home Messages
- Organ and tissue donation is a part of quality ICU-based end-of-life care. Critical care has an important role in determining prognosis (and therefore eligibility to donate), building trust through demonstrating excellence in patient family-centred care, and providing humanistic care through empathetic and compassionate communication. Not all individuals may donate, but it is important to respect the autonomy and wishes of those who have chosen to donate organs or tissues to help others.

Multiple Choice Questions

1. Recent research on patient preferences demonstrates that individuals wish to die:
   A. In the hospital after receipt of intensive interventions.
   B. Following the administration of medications to hasten their death.
   C. Only after 24 h of observation in the hospital.
   D. **At home, in the presence of family.**

2. Deaths of patients in hospital:
   A. Usually follow an emergency surgical procedure.
   B. Are often after a prolonged period of hospitalization.
   C. **One in four hospital deaths may occur in an ICU.**
   D. Are a result of medical intervention in countries which support medical assistance in dying.

3. The most common precipitating medical event resulting in death as determined by neurological criteria is:
   A. **Hypoxic–ischemic brain injury.**
   B. Traumatic brain injury.
   C. Ischemic cerebrovascular accidents (strokes).
   D. Non-traumatic brain haemorrhage.

4. Organs recovered from donors who have died from cardiocirculatory criteria:
   A. Remain a rare source of organs.
   B. **Requires evidence of permanent cessation of spontaneous circulatory function.**

C. Was first introduced as a practice in the past 20 years.

D. Potential donors should be considered as any individual at the time of their admission to ICU.

5. Recent research on the monitoring of cardiocirculatory physiology in the ICU has demonstrated:

A. Loss of cardiac and circulatory activity occurs rapidly following WWLSI.

B. **Auto-resuscitation (spontaneous return of circulation) did not occur after 5 min of observation.**

C. Any return of pulse and blood pressure is quickly and accurately recognized by ICU providers.

D. The resumption of any cardiac or circulatory activity is a very rare event following WWLSI in ICU.

References

1. Wunsch H. The outbreak that invented intensive care. Nature. 2020. https://www.nature-com/articles/d41586-020-01019-y. Accessed 29 April 2021.
2. Woodard SC. The story of the mobile army surgical hospital. Military Med. 2003;168:503–13.
3. Kelly FE, Fong K, Hirsch N, Nolan JP. Intensive care medicine is 60 years old: the history and future of the intensive care unit. Clin Med (London). 2014;14:376–9.
4. Sprung CL, Truog RD, Curtis JR, et al. Seeking worldwide professional consensus on the principles of end-of-life care for the critically ill. Am J Respir Crit Care Med. 2014;190:855–66.
5. Heyland DK, Lavery JV, Tranmer JE, Shortt SE, Taylor SJ. Dying in Canada: is it an institutionalized, technologically supported experience? J Palliat Care. 2000;16(Suppl):S10–6.
6. Azoulay E, Chevret S, Leleu G, et al. Half the families of intensive care unit patients experience inadequate communication with physicians. Crit Care Med. 2000;28:3044–9.
7. Prendergast TJ, Claessens MT, Luce JM. A national survey of end-of-life care for critically ill patients. Am J Resp Crit Care Med. 1998;158:1163–7.
8. Solverson KJ, Roze des Ordons AL, Doig CJ. Withholding and withdrawing life support: difficult decisions around care at the end of life. Can J Anaesth. 2017;65:9–13.
9. Roze des Ordons AL, MacIsaac L, Everson J, Hui J, Ellaway RH. A pattern of compassion in intensive care and palliative care contexts. BMC Palliat Care. 2019;18:15. https://doi.org/10.1186/s12904-019-0402-0.
10. Berlinger N, Jennings B, Wolf SM. The hastings center guidelines for decisions on life-sustaining treatment and care near the end of life: revised and expanded second edition. Oxford, UK: Oxford University Press; 2013.
11. Bandrauk N, Downar J. Paunovic B on behalf of the Canadian Critical Care Society Ethics Committee. Withholding and withdrawing of life-sustaining treatment: the Canadian Critical Care Society position paper. Can J Anaesth. 2018;65:105–22.
12. Frank C, Heyland DK, Chen B, Farquhar D, Myers K, Iwaasa K. Determining resuscitation preferences of elderly inpatients: a review of the literature. CMAJ. 2003;169:795–9.
13. Torke AM, Sachs GA, Helft PR, et al. Scope and outcomes of surrogate decision making among hospitalized older adults. JAMA Intern Med. 2014;174:370–7.
14. Brown SM, Rozenblum R, Aboumatar H, et al. Defining patient and family engagement in the intensive care unit. Am J Respir Crit Care Med. 2015;191:358–60.
15. Abbott KH, Sago JG, Breen CM, Abernathy AP, Tulsky JA. Families looking back: one year after discussion of withdrawal or withholding of life-sustaining support. Crit Care Med. 2001;29:197–201.
16. Schuster RA, Hong SY, Arnold RM, White DB. Investigating conflicts in ICUs—is the clinicians' perspective enough? Crit Care Med. 2014;42:328–35.
17. Roze des Ordons A, Kassam A, Simon J. Goals of care conversations teaching in residency—a cross-sectional survey of postgraduate program directors. BMC Med Educ. 2017;17:6. https://doi.org/10.1186/s12909-016-0839-2.
18. Bush SH, Roze des Ordons A, Chary S, Boyle AB. The development and validation of updated palliative and end-of-life care competencies for medical undergraduates in Canada. J Palliat Med. 2019;22:1498–500.
19. Roze des Ordons AL, Doig CJ, Couillard P, Lord J. From communication skills to skillful communication: a longitudinal curriculum for critical care medicine fellows. Acad Med. 2017;92:501–5.
20. Wessman BT, Sona C, Schallom M. Improving caregivers' perceptions regarding patient goals of care/end-of-life issues for the multidisciplinary critical care team. J Int Care Med. 2017;32:68–76.
21. Heyland DK, Cook DJ, Rocker GM, et al. Decision-making in the ICU: perspectives of the substitute decision-maker. Int Care Med. 2003;29:75–82.
22. Heyland DK, Tranmer J, O'Callaghan CJ, Gafni A. The seriously ill hospitalized patient: preferred role in end-of-life decision making? J Crit Care. 2003;18:3–10.

23. Davidson JE, Aslakson RA, Long AC, et al. Guidelines for family-centred care in the neonatal, pediatric, and adult ICU. Crit Care Med. 2017;45:103–28.
24. Seaman JB, Arnold RM, Scheunemann LP, et al. An integrated framework for effective and efficient communication with families in the adult intensive care unit. Ann Am Thorac Soc. 2017;14:1015–20.
25. Kramer AH, Baht R, Doig CJ. Time trends in organ donation after neurologic determination of death: a cohort study. CMAJ Open. 2017;5. https://doi.org/10.9778/cmajo.20160093.
26. Kramer AH, Hornby K, Doig CJ, et al. Deceased organ donation potential in Canada: a review of consecutive deaths in Alberta. Can J Anaesth. 2019;66:1347–55.
27. Ad Hoc Committee of the Harvard Medical School. A definition of irreversible coma. JAMA. 1968;205:337–40.
28. Greer DM, Shemie SD, Lewis A, et al. Determination of brain death/death by neurologic criteria. The World Brain Death Project. JAMA. 2020;324:1078–97.
29. Lewis A, Bakkar A, Kreiger-Benson E, et al. Determination of death by neurologic criteria around the world. Neurology. 2020;95:e299–309.
30. Wahlster S, Wijdicks EFM, Patel PV, et al. Brain death declaration: practices and perceptions worldwide. Neurology. 2015;84:1870–9.
31. Wijdicks EF. Brain death worldwide: accepted fact, but no global consensus in diagnostic criteria. Neurology. 2002;58:20–5.
32. Citerio G, Cypel M, Dobb GJ, et al. Organ donation in adults: a critical care perspective. Int Care Med. 2016;42:305–15.
33. Kramer AH. Ancillary testing in brain death. Semin Neurol. 2015;35:125–38.
34. Kentish-Barnes N, Siminoff LA, Walker W, et al. A narrative review of family members' experience of organ donation request after brain death in the critical care setting. Int Care Med. 2019;45:331–42.
35. Zheng K, Sutherland S, Cardinal P, et al. Patient-centered and family-centered care of critically ill patients who are potential organ donors: a qualitative study protocol of family member perspectives. BMJ Open. 2020;10:e037527. https://doi.org/10.1136/bmjopen-2020-037527.
36. Morgan SE, Harrison TR, Afifi WA, Long SD, Stephenson MT. In their own words: the reasons why people will (not) sign an organ donor card. Health Communication. 2008;23:23–33.
37. Whyte KP, Selinger E, Caplan AL, Sadowski J. Nudge, nudge or shove, shove—the right way for nudges to increase the supply of donated cadaver organs. Am J Bioethics. 12:32–9.
38. Potts M, Verheijde JL, Rady MY. When a nudge becomes a shove. Am J Bioethics. 2012;12:40–2.
39. Manzari ZS, Mohammadi E, Heydari A, Sharbaf HRA, Azizi JM, Khaleghi E. Exploring families' experiences of an organ donation request after brain death. Nurs Ethics. 2012;19:654–65.
40. Al-Khafaji A, Murugan R, Kellum JA. What's new in organ donation: better care of the dead for the living. Int Care Med. 2013;39:2031–3.
41. Singbartl K, Murugan R, Kaynar AM, et al. Intensivist-led management of brain-dead donors is associated with an increase in organ recovery for transplantation. Am J Transplant. 2011;11:1517–21.
42. Shemie SD, Ross H, Pagliarello J, et al. Organ donor management in Canada: recommendations of the forum on medical management to optimize donor organ potential. CMAJ. 2006;174:S13–32.
43. Ball IM, Hornby L, Rochwerg B, et al. Management of the neurologically deceased organ donor: A Canadian clinical practice guideline. CMAJ. 2020;192:E361–9.
44. Kotloff RM, Blosser S, Fulda GJ, et al. Management of the potential organ donor in the ICU: Society of Critical Care Medicine/American College of Chest Physicians/Association of Organ Procurement Organizations Consensus Statement. Crit Care Med. 2015;43:1291–325.
45. Pandit RA, Zirpe KG, Gurav SK, et al. Management of potential organ donor: Indian Society of Critical Care Medicine: position statement. Indian J Crit Care Med. 2017;21:303–16.
46. GRADE; www.gradeworkinggroup.org
47. Smith M, Dominguez-Gil B, Greer DM, Manara AR, Souter MJ. Organ donation after circulatory death: current status and future potential. Int Care Med. 2019;45:310–21.
48. Ethical, psychosocial, and public policy implications of procuring organs from non-heart-beating cadavers. Arnold RM, Youngner SJ, guest editors. Kennedy Institute of Ethics Journal Volume 3, 1993. Johns Hopkins University Press, Baltimore.
49. Shemie S, Baker AJ, Knoll G, et al. Donation after cardiocirculatory death in Canada. CMAJ. 2006;175:S1–24.
50. van Haren FMP, Carter A, Cavazzoni E, et al. Conflicts of interest in the context of end of life care for potential organ donors in Australia. J Crit Care. 2020;59:166–71.
51. Bastami S, Matthes O, Krones T, Biller-Andorno N. Systematic review of attitudes toward donation after cardiac death among health care providers and the general public. Crit Care Med. 2013;41:897–905.
52. Turgeon AF, Lauzier F, Simard JF, et al. Mortality associated with withdrawal of life-sustaining therapy for patients with severe traumatic brain injury: a Canadian multicentre cohort study. CMAJ. 2011;183:1581–8.
53. Cook DJ, Guyatt GH, Jaeschke R, et al. Determinants in Canadian health care workers of the decision to withdraw life support from the critically ill. JAMA. 1995;273:703–8.
54. Woodruff MFA. Ethical problems in organ transplantation. BMJ. 1964:1457–60.
55. Healey A, Hartwick M, Downar J, et al. Improving quality of withdrawal of life-sustaining measures in

organ donation: a framework and implementation toolkit. Can J Anaesth. 2020;67:1549–56.
56. Gries CJ, White DB, Truog RD, et al. Ethical and policy considerations in organ donation after circulatory determination of death. Am J Resp Crit Care Med. 2013;188:103–9.
57. Cooper J. Organs and organisations: situating ethics in organ donation after circulatory death in the UK. Soc Sci Med. 2018;209:104–10.
58. Robertson J. The dead donor rule. Hast Center Rep. 1999;29:6–14.
59. Dhanani S, Hornby L, van Beinum A, et al. Resumption of cardiac activity after withdrawal of life-sustaining measures. New Engl J Med. 2021;384:345–52.
60. Rady MY, Verheijde JL. Scientific and ethical challenges in end-of-life organ donation. Crit Care Med. 2015;43:e526.
61. Joffe A. Are recent defences of the brain death concept adequate? Bioethics. 2010;24:47–53.
62. Joffe A. Confusion about brain death. Nat Rev Neurosci. 2006;7:590. https://doi.org/10.1038/nrn1789-c1.
63. Glannon W. The moral insignificance of death in organ donation. Camb Q Healthc Ethics. 2013;22:192–202.

Futility of Care and Palliative Care

35

Paolo Malacarne and Silvia Pini

35.1 Introduction

> **Learning Goals**
> - Futile is a medical treatment that at a particular time for a specific patient reasonably unlikely to reach the" goal of care" appreciated as a benefit from the patient.
> - In emergency surgery, the patient's high rate of frailty and/or the severity of acute illness associated with high-risk surgery are the most important triggers in order to ask the question of surgical futility.
> - Concurrent palliative care must be integrated into the context of surgical reasoning.

Improved technology, surgical and critical care techniques have given medicine the ability to prolong life in the direst circumstances [1], even when there is no hope for successful treatment of their underlying pathology [2].

The availability of increasingly effective treatments, even lifesaving surgical procedures, is not, in itself, a reason for their unlimited and extensive use: is there a limit to medical treatment?

The medicine's obligation to preserve life cannot be put forward to scrupulous attention to associated morbidity, pain, suffering, and loss of functional status that limit this medicine's obligation itself and must be known by physicians and shared with patients and families.

Any medical or surgical treatment must be aimed at a "goal of care", according to principles of biomedical ethics such as respect for autonomy, nonmaleficence, beneficence, and justice [3].

35.2 The Medical Futility

The concept of medical futility was introduced in late 1980 [2, 4] and it has been a continuous topic of discussion in medicine for several decades [1], with so many "rises and falls" [2, 5] that some authors have abandoned the concept of futility all together as an unhelpful term [1].

The initial definition of futility proposed by Schneiderman [4] is "any effort to achieve a result that is possible but that the reasoning or the experience suggests that it is highly improbable and that cannot be systematically produced."

According to this definition any medical or surgical treatment that reasonably unlikely reaches the "goal of care" is "futile."

P. Malacarne (✉) · S. Pini
Anesthesia and Intensive Care Unit, Azienda Ospedaliera Universitaria Pisana, Pisa, Italy

In order to assess the futility of a specific treatment the first step that must be done is to specify "the goal of therapy" of that specific treatment.

The futility is not, indeed, a "free-floating" concept but it is linked to a specific goal [6], and the goal of medicine is not to preserve organ function or to restore physiological parameters but to treat and improve the health of a person as a whole [7].

The second step is to evaluate the difference between the effect obtained from the treatment and the benefit appreciated by the patient (effective treatments, if not beneficial, may still be futile).

From this point of view, medical futility may be defined as any treatment that is unlike to produce any significant benefit for the patient or that the patient has the capacity to appreciate as a benefit [8].

There are several attempts to interpret medical futility and consequently numerous definitions and terms:

Physiologic futility: any treatment that is expected not to produce its desired physiologic purpose (such as restoring arterial blood pressure) has to be considered as physiologically futile.

It is important to consider that certain treatments, although effective at causing a measurable physiologic change, may not help patients achieve their "goal of care," thereby remaining futile treatments [9]: even the physiologic effects are no benefits unless the patient has the capacity to appreciate them as benefits [10]. Although an intervention may have an anatomic, physiologic, or biochemical effect on a patient, it must improve the patient as a whole to avoid being designated as futile [1].

Quantitative futility: in its first definition [4], it is a treatment that in the last 100 cases has been useless. In this case, based on personal experience, experiences shared with colleagues, and considerations of reported empirical data, the physician may define treatment as futile. This statement is not an absolute certainty: the question is similar to the statistical evaluation of significance: how many times do we have to fail before we agree to call treatment as futile? 1%, or 3% or 5%? It is reasonable to decide a threshold below which to accept the possibility of error, even if the error can have dire consequences [10]. Another widespread definition is that futile is a treatment that has a chance of producing the desired effect low or poor, less than a predefined percentage [2].

Qualitative futility: The treatment provided is likely to result in an unacceptable quality of life perceived by the patient [1, 2] and his effect will not be appreciated as a benefit. The patient's current or projected condition will result in an intolerable inability to engage in or derive pleasure from life [11]. To identify universally acceptable quality outcomes is impossible therefore qualitative futility is the most controversial type of futility.

Imminent demise futility: any treatment that will not change the imminent death, (except any treatment aimed at alleviating sufferance).

Compassionate futility: any treatment without the chance of being efficacious in relation to the accepted goal but performed as an act of compassion and care toward the patients and/or their families [3].

Futility may appear as an elusive, theoretical concept but when it is discussed at the bed of the patient shows all its concreteness: futility, indeed, refers to a particular intervention at a particular time for a specific patient. The same intervention that is futile for a patient might not be futile for another patient or for the same patient in another phase of his illness.

In the process to define futility, there are two main actors: the patient (and/or his family) that must define a successful outcome as a clinical benefit that aligns with his self-defined goal of care, and the physician that must determine the level of certainty that that outcome will occur [12].

Between the patient's self-defined goal of care and the physician's determination of the level of certainty to achieve that goal there is not a sharp border but a window of negotiation that must be opened balancing the effectiveness (determined by physicians), benefits (subjective and determined by the patients) and burdens (determined by both) of the treatment [13].

35.3 Futility and Emergency Surgery

The concept of futility is an incredibly controversial topic in surgery [1, 8, 11, 12, 14–18] due to many factors:

- There is no standard definition of acceptable risk, an acceptable threshold of risk, or high-risk surgery [16].
- The patient may tolerate an operation but not a post-operative complication [14]: patients who receive surgery often survive the initial treatment, but often suffer from severe complications due to comorbidity and frailty [14],
- Some major operations indicated, but not always appropriated, may not prolong life but instead may increase additional pain, [12, 18] and the patient's suffering at the end of their life [15],
- An operation may even precipitate death [16],
- Surgery requires the consent of multiple agents: patient, surgeon, anesthetist and intensivist, and routinely requires balancing the ethical principles of beneficence, nonmaleficence, respect for the autonomy of the patient, and distributive justice [1],

In emergency surgery the decision to define treatment as futile is even more complex due to several peculiarities:

1. Emergency surgery may often be performed as a lifesaving procedure as a delay in surgery can reduce the overall outcome [14]. Unfortunately too often there is not enough time to implement the correct procedures that characterize a good medical-patient relationship.
2. Emergency surgery is often practiced on high-risk patients due to frailty, comorbidities, and severe derangement of physiological parameters and the physicians involved may not correctly know the real pre-operative quality of life of the patient: how bad are the comorbidities. Which is the stage of failure?
3. There is high pressure to operate by families in order to "Do everything": due to external pressure and prognostic uncertainty, some providers err on the side of operative intervention despite suspected futility [17].
4. It is necessary, especially for emergency surgery, that all the actors involved have expressed their consent to the procedure (patient/families, surgeon, and anesthetist).
5. We have several tools to calculate the risk of surgical treatment (risk calculator of ACS-NSQIP [19], the score of frailty [14], Charlson Index, ASA, NELA, P-POSSUM [15], and the decision-making process is, obviously, facilitated by an accurate risk estimation, which should be shared between the surgeon, the anesthetist and the patient [19]. In emergency surgery, the limited time available makes it difficult to use the risk-assessment tools.

A definition of futility useful to evaluate the quality and the appropriateness of a treatment done has been proposed thanks to a post hoc analysis: futile is an operation performed on patients that had an extreme risk of mortality (beyond 75%) and that died within 48 h of their operation [16]; another definition is related to patients who died within 72 h of surgery [15].

When a large number of risk factors occur (such as high age, high ASA grade, high frailty score, and high numbers of organ failure) they could be used to inform patients and their families of the risk of surgery and they could result in a decision for palliative care [20].

Patients and families that are involved in the surgical decision-making process need to be guided by an expert physician due to a lack of medical knowledge and to an emotional condition that can obscure rational thinking.

Furthermore in order to achieve informed consent, surgeons should take charge of this situation and accept more responsibility to define treatment as futile and should become more conservative in offering high-risk/low-benefit procedures [12].

Surgery may not be in the patient's best interest and a comfortable and dignified death is the most appropriate available goal in these circumstances [11].

35.4 Challenges, Contrasts, and Their Resolution

Two are the principal critical issues concerning futility:

- The absence of laboratory tests or clinical criteria for accurate and certain definitions.
- The possible different opinions among the subjects involved.

The judgment of futility is based on a probabilistic assessment, not certainty, of failure to reach the goal: what is the threshold of probability of making mistakes that we are ready to accept and how much should the probability of success for treatment or the quality of life be in order to consider the treatment futile [2]?

There is no consensus in empirically determining the threshold for a physician's judgment that further treatment would be futile [4].

The problem that arises is the uncertainty of prognosis which can lead to a kind of paralysis of action: prognostic paralysis [20].

In presence of different opinions about the goal of therapy and/or the futility, who has the right authority and competence to determine futility: the physician, patient, or family members? [2].

It is necessary to develop a process to resolve disputes, conflicts, and legitimate disagreement over futility [4]. The first and most important step is to improve the communication between physicians, patient, and their families, perhaps making use of the contribution of professional and or ethic consultant, gaining valuable time for good communication: but many of these solutions are useful in election situations are difficult or impossible to implement in emergency surgery.

A good communication process is especially needed in case of legitimate disagreement/ disparity between the patient's priorities and surgical possibilities. In these cases, it is necessary to manage emotions and correctly relate to unrealistic and unreasonable expectations of the patients and their families, accurately present viable alternatives, in primis palliative care, in a way that the patients and their families do not perceive as abandonment by the physician. Often "Everything be done" means "Do not abandon me".

Several questions are matter of discussion in this context:

1. Why to choose to pursue surgery with a 95% chance of painful death instead of selecting comfort care with a 100% chance of a comfortable death [12]?
2. When both outcomes involve death, why is it difficult to appreciate the true burden of added pain due to surgery [12]?
3. Why in the case of high-risk treatment may the attention of the patients and their family be "captured" by the word "death" (if we don't proceed he dies, if we proceed he has a high probability to die) and they might not be able to focus their attention on the real burden of the added pain due to surgery?
4. Do everything (on an instinctive level death is never the answer and humans want to play the odds even when unfavorable): is survival with significant pain and suffering often still considered better than death [12]?
5. Is life-saving the first goal of medicine?

35.5 Ethical Foundation and Ethical Implication of Futility

The ethical lawfulness of medical futility is based on the possibility of reasonably and plausibly arguing according to the four principles of biomedical ethics [3]: respect for autonomy, nonmaleficence, beneficence, and justice.

The first ethical challenge of futility's question was that human life cannot be decided only by physicians, but the patients and their families also have the right to take part in the decision-making process: the "goal of care" and the "goal of therapy", to which the decision of futility is linked, are clearly worded on the basis of respect of patient's autonomy, in order to providing care that is respectful of and responsive to individual patient preferences, needs, wishes and values and ensuring that patient values guide all clinical decision (voce biblio 1 di 8).

The physician must actively take part in decision-making, functioning as a clinical and moral agent [3, 12]. At present, a binary approach is often offered to patients or their families in terms of death or survival: however, survival will be probably complicated for high-risk patients with the impaired long-term quality of life [15]: that condition may be perceived even worse than death [16]. Rather than leaving this difficult decision to the patient and/or his/her family, surgeons should accept more responsibility for defining futility and be more conservative in offering high-risk/low-benefit procedures [12].

The futile treatment turns against almost all the principles of ethical lawfulness:

1. Nonmaleficence because it generates suffering and pain.
2. Beneficence because its effect will not be perceived as beneficial by the patient.
3. Distributive justice because it consumes resources no more available for other patients.

Only treatments that improve patients' comfort and minimize the suffering of both patients and their families, which are equally as important as those aimed at saving patients' lives, are ethically lawful [7].

From an ethical point of view, there is a well-defined concept that justifies the decision of medical futility:

- the proportionality of treatments in term of balance between burdens and benefits
- the equivalence between withholding and withdrawing of treatments, though lifesaving.
- it is profoundly different to kill vs letting and or allowing to die.

The first consequence of ethical lawfulness of the decision of futility is that the physician is not obliged to perform a futile treatment, even if technically lifesaving: medical professionals have no ethical obligation to provide a futile treatment [5].

35.6 Palliative Care in Emergency Surgery

Palliative care [4, 21] is a multidisciplinary specialty that aims to relieve suffering and to maintain the highest supported quality of life for patients and to support their families. The American College of Surgeons and other scientific societies emphasized the need to provide palliative care alongside life-prolonging and curative surgical treatment [22–28].

The surgeon must think of a palliative option if the surgery may be not resolutive of disease; in this case, there are several possibilities:

- a surgery employed with curative intention but with residual disease, associated with palliative care
- a surgical procedure used with the primary intention of improving quality of life and relieving symptoms, associated with palliative care
- to give up surgery and proceed with palliative care, even if the patient and family members have expectations: the surgeon must balance this expectation with the futility of intervention and the sufferings caused by the intervention.

Palliative care in surgery may be defined as a surgical or medical procedure used with the primary intention of improving quality of life or relieving symptoms caused by advanced disease.

The effectiveness of palliative care in surgery is therefore judged by the presence and durability of patient-reported symptom resolution.

These situations are frequent in seriously ill oncologic or non-oncologic patients with severe comorbidities and frailty that come in an emergency (e.g., in presence of intestinal perforation, occlusion, ischemia, and infarction).

If surgical quality is valued solely on survival duration, this incentivizes surgeons to prolong life, not to improve it, and can impede the integration of palliative care: instead, we must integrate palliative care principles into rescue-oriented surgical culture.

In order to identify surgical patients who would benefit from a palliative care specialist's consultation, the surgeon can be helped by a series of "triggers" as in primis high-frailty rate [14] and high-risk surgery [15]: too often the wrong mental association between palliative care and hospice leads to delay the palliative treatments, which instead must be concurrent with the other standard treatments.

A patient with an advanced disease who after surgery presents signs and symptoms of clinical failure has to be promptly directed to a palliative care process.

Data suggest that disease-directed care, rather than palliative care, does not prolong life and may in fact cause a worse quality of life in patients

Why does it seem easier to target palliative care for the medical patient than the potential surgical patient?

Surgical patients are less likely to be referred to palliative care than patients with chronic medical conditions, and many surgical patients do not receive palliative care.

A common fallacy prevalent in surgical culture is for surgical intervention and palliation to be regarded as mutually exclusive or sequential strategies in the trajectory of surgical illness. Modern surgeons play a complex role as both providers and gatekeepers in meeting the palliative needs of their patients. Surgical palliative care is ideally delivered by surgical teams as a component of routine surgical care and includes management of physical and psychosocial symptoms, basic communication about prognosis and treatment options, and identification of patient goals and values. In this direction, we must implement Preoperative Advanced care planning and improve the communication between surgeons, patients, and their family members. A critical issue is a careful communication with the patient and, where possible, carers and relatives, as well as other specialists and healthcare professionals involved in the team.

Meeting the palliative care needs of elderly surgical patients requires early recognition, advanced care planning, and multidisciplinary interventions that align patients' goals with possible outcomes.

Palliative care is not a defeat for the surgeon, and surgery should not be the default modality for patients with extremely poor survival due to baseline serious illness or acute surgical conditions.

Any surgical procedure undertaken to relieve symptoms and to enhance the quality of life, with little or no bearing on the overall survival of the patient, constitute a part of "Palliative Surgery." In this perspective, surgery comprises a potentially viable option of palliation, not just the mere operative procedure.

Surgical palliation actually must imply a broad repertoire of approaches and challenges, all at the same degree of importance, including operations, endoscopic interventions, communication, teamwork, psychological competence, social intelligence, and the recognition of spiritual aspects of life. This should not be an outsourced enterprise for a group of "holistic" or "caring surgeons", but it should be seen as a part of the practice and responsibility of every surgeon.

An effective and quality palliative surgery requires assessment of optimal timing and selection of suitable operative procedure(s) with minimal perioperative morbidity and mortality.

For surgeons, a professional duty should be to contribute to the care of patients with palliative care by taking responsibility and collaborating with other health professionals to deliver palliative care of a high standard.

Among the many priorities in the context of surgery palliative care [23], the choice of outcomes that matter to the patient, better communication (the time of communication is an integral part of "optimal surgical timing") and the integration of palliative care principles and practices into routine surgical practice is certainly the most urgent fields to be implemented. In emergency surgery, the urgency of time cannot be an excuse for evading what is no less important than good surgical technique.

Dos and Don'ts

- The goal of care must be discussed and agreed with the patient and/or his family.
- The concurrent palliative care must be integrated into the practice of emergency surgery.
- The time of communication during the decision-making process must be adequate and considered as an integral part of care.
- The palliative surgery and palliative care should not be considered surgery failure.
- The palliative care should not be considered care delegated to specialists other than surgeons.

Take-Home Messages

- The availability of increasingly effective treatments, even life-saving surgical procedures, is not, in itself, a reason for their unlimited and extensive use.
- Any surgical treatment must be aimed at a goal of care according to principles of biomedical ethics: respect for autonomy, non-maleficence, beneficence, and justice.
- If the effect and efficacy of surgical treatment are not appreciated as a benefit for the patient, this treatment is futile.
- The most important cause of contrast between doctors and patients about the goal of care is bad and incorrect communication.
- The palliative care is not a defeat for the surgeon: palliative care must be integrated into the principles and practice of emergency surgery.

Multiple Choice Questions (4 answers) (the first is the correct answeer)

1. What is a medical futility?
   A. any medical or surgical treatment which reasonably unlikely reaches the "goal of care"
   B. any medical or surgical treatment which does not satisfy the doctor
   C. any medical or surgical treatment which has more risk than benefit
   D. any medical or surgical treatment which has too high costs
2. What is a palliative care?
   A. multidisciplinary specialty that aims to relieve suffering and to maintain the highest supported quality of life for patients and to support their families
   B. the treatments that are done in the last days of life
   C. the care practice only in hospice
   D. the alternative treatments to surgery
3. What is a palliative surgery?
   A. a surgical procedure used with the primary intention of improving quality of life and relieving symptoms, associated with palliative care
   B. an unsuccessful surgical treatment
   C. a surgical treatment not explained to the patient
   D. a surgical treatment other than envisaged by the surgeon
4. What is the surgical futility?
   A. a surgical treatment which not reached the goal of care
   B. a surgical treatment that does not satisfy the surgeon
   C. a surgical treatment that causes sufferance
   D. a surgical treatment not agreed with the patient

References

1. Grant SB, Modi PK, Singer EA. Futility and the care of surgical patients: ethical dilemmas. World J Surg. 2014;38:1631–7.
2. Aghabarary M, Nayeri ND. Medical futility and its challenges: a review study. J Med Ethics Hist Med. 2016;9:11.
3. Beauchamp TL, Childress JF. Principles of biomedical ethics. 7th ed. Oxford University Press; 2013.
4. Schneiderman LJ, Jecker NS, Jonsen AR. Medical futility: its meaning and ethical implication. Ann Int Med. 1990;112:949–54.
5. Helft PR, Siegler M, Lantos J. The rise and fall of the futility movement. NEJM. 2000;343:293–5.
6. Sokol DK. The slipperiness of futility BMJ. 2009;338:1418.
7. Saric L, Prkic I, Jukic M. Futile treatment-a review. Bioethical Inquiry. 2017;14:329–37.
8. Maerz LL, Mosenthal AC, Miller RS, et al. Futility and the acute care surgeon. J Trauma Acute Care Surg. 2015;78:1216–9.
9. Goede M, Wheeler M. Advances directives, living wills and futility in perioperative care. Surg Clin N Am. 2015;95:443–51.
10. Schneiderman LJ. Defining medical futility and improving medical care. Bioeth Inquiry. 2011;8:123–31.
11. Jones JW, Mc Culloigh LB. Futility and surgical intervention. J Vasc Surg. 2002;35:1305.
12. Hatchimonji JS, Sisti DA, Martin ND. Surgical futility and patient-centered care: the effects of human nature in decision making. Bull Am Coll Surg. 2016;101:20–3.
13. Pellegrino, Edmund D. Decisions at the End of Life-The Abuse of the Concept of Futility. Practical Bioethics. 2005;1(3):3–6.
14. Soreide K, Desserud K. Emergency surgery in the elderly: the balance between function, frailty, fatality and futility. Scand J Trauma Resusc Emerg Med. 2015;23:10.
15. Aggarwal G, Broughton KJ, Williams L, et al. Early Postoperative death in patients undergoing emergency high-risk surgery: toward a better understanding of patients for whom surgery may not be beneficial. J Clin Med. 2020;9:1288.
16. Chiu AS, Jean RA, Resion B, et al. Early postoperative death in extreme-risk patients: a perspective on surgical futility. Surgery. 2019;166:380–5.
17. Morris RS, Ruck J, Conca-Cheng AM, Smith TJ, et al. Shared decision making in acute surgical illness: the surgeon's perspective J Am Coll Surg 2018;226:784-795
18. Cooper Z. Indicated But Not Always Appropriate: Surgery in Terminally Ill Patients With Abdominal Catastrophe. Ann Surg. 2018;268(1):e4. https://doi.org/10.1097/SLA.0000000000002777.
19. Scotton G, Del Zotto G, Bernardi L. Is the ACS-NSQIP Risk Calculator accurate in predicting Adverse postoperative outcomes in the emergency setting ? An Italian single-center preliminary study. World J Surg. 2020;44:3710–9.
20. Desserud KF, Veen T, Soreide K. Emergency general surgery in the geriatric patient. BJS. 2016;103:52–61.
21. Lilley EJ, Khan KT, Johnston FM, et al. Palliative care intervention for surgical patients. A systematic review. JAMA. 2016;151:172–83.
22. Soreide J. Palliative surgical care. BJS. 2010;97:970–1.
23. Lilley EJ, Cooper Z, Schwarze ML, et al. Palliative care in syrgery: definiting the research priorities. Ann Surg. 2018;267:66–72.
24. Miller P. Surgical palliative care-where are we in 2020 ? Am Surg. 2020;86:1436–40.
25. Dunn GP. Surgery, palliative care and the American College of Surgeons. Am Pall Med. 2015;4:5–9.
26. Sigman M, Miller P. Practicing primary palliative care: a call for action. Bull Am Coll Surg. 2019. https://bulletin.facs.org/2019/11/practicing-primary-palliative-care-a-call-to-action/. Last access March 2023.
27. Aziz H, Lunde J, Barraco R, et al. Evidence-basd review of trauma center care and routine palliative care process for geriatric trauma patients; a collaboration from the American Association for the Surgery of Trauma Geriatric Trauma Committee, and the Eastearn Association for the Surgery of Trauma Guidelines Committee. J Trauma Acute Care Surg. 2019;86:737–43.
28. Simpkin A, Schwartzstein RM. Tolerating uncertainly—the next medical revolution. NEJM. 2016;375:1713–5.

Communication in Emergency General Surgery

36

Evika Karamagioli

36.1 Introduction

> **Learning Goals** *(Listing the Chapter Core Messages)*
> - Analyze the relevance of non-technical skills with an emphasis on good communication in the emergency surgery practice outcomes.
> - Present the need for introducing and practicing communication verbal and nonverbal tools and processes as part of patient safety protocols.
> - Demonstrate the need for training on communication skills for all members of surgical teams in the case of emergency surgery.

According to the international bibliography effective and efficient quality care does not only result from the technical interaction between the surgeon and the patient in the operating room. Instead, it lies on a series of complex reciprocal interactions between surgeon, patient, medical team, equipment, and the hospital along with a procession of parameters that have to do with the sociopolitical and cultural environment in question [1, 2].

As it is expected in the case of emergency surgeries directly linked to manmade and natural disasters, crisis, and mass casualties, considering the specific conditions (in the forms of all types of burdens, that is, resources, processes, etc.) that influence the whole healthcare system, human factors interdependencies and interactions share a dominant part on the final outcome.

Under this context non-technical competences including leadership, teamwork, task management, critical thinking, decision making, and situational awareness defined as personal, cognitive, and social resource skills complement to technical skills, provide a safe and efficient task performance in case of medical emergencies, both inside and outside hospital units and OR.

Effective and efficient communication is a key component of successful leadership and teamwork and an essential parameter within emergency medicine surgical teams when dealing with emergency situations, disasters, and crisis. Whereas problematic communication including omissions, misinterpretations, and conflicts arising, can result in adverse surgical events and postoperative malpractice claims, on the other hand, good communication processes and practices underpin efficient collaboration, joint coordination of work, andhelping to construct a mutual awareness of the situation [3].

E. Karamagioli (✉)
MSc Global Health—Disaster Medicine, School of Medicine, National and Kapodistrian University of Athens (NKUA), Athens, Greece

Challenges and breakdowns in communication between operating room (OR) team members are related to adverse surgical events and postoperative malpractice claims, as well as the way that medical information and orders are transferred, performed, and documented to be acknowledged as key elements impacting on patient's safety [4, 5].

This chapter discusses why and how communication is linked to the performance of medical emergency surgical teams, representing an integral part of their surgical outcomes, proposes tools, and processes that could be used for its improvement.

36.2 Communication as a Key Component of Teamwork in the OR

36.2.1 What Does Communication in the Perioperative Environment Entails?

The perioperative environment with an emphasis on the OR is a dynamic, highly technical, and stressful environment, where fast-paced is driven by pressing time constraints, as well as extraordinarily complex procedures, foster medical errors, which can potentially contribute to negative outcomes [6].

The human factor in the sense of surgeon and emergency surgical teams per se may be a proper challenge in the operating room, since, in a high-reliability operating room, teamwork entails mutual performance monitoring, team leadership, backup behavior, flexibility, team orientation, mutual trust, along with shared mental models. All these components will not be attended barely for effective and efficient communication [7].

Emergency surgical teams are personified by interdisciplinarity, and interdependency, while operative and post-operative management of patients requires dealing with changes and uncertainties in the daily surgical program, and a strong focus on time and resource consumption. What makes surgical processes prone to medical errors can be detected in the number of steps and people involved, as well as the fact that the essential interventions for healing are frequently invasive and also complicate. Nevertheless, when strong congruent operative teams are in place and mutual goals are agreed upon, communication among members of the team can actually become one of its strengths. The involvement of more than one discipline and the individual requires concrete, understandable, culturally sensitive, and contextually relevant communication.

Examples and cases of communication failures can be detected between care providers during surgical care, and between transition points during 'hand-offs' or 'handovers'. Information shared at these transition points is required to facilitate the continuity of information and patient care, and to prevent medical errors [8–10].

36.2.2 External and Internal Determinants Causing Gaps in Communication

With operating rooms recognized as complex environments, in which distractions, interruptions, and disruptions (DIDs) are frequent [11], the causes of interpersonal communication breakdown that emergency surgeons and their teams experience during their everyday practice are multiple.

What is needed or what is missing most of the time, according to the international bibliography, are the skills and the abilities to engage in teamwork, to understand the complexity of the clinical situation, to make appropriate decisions, and to act efficiently [12] as defined in Picture 36.1.

Multiple determinants have been recognized for prohibiting surgical team members from interacting efficiently while exchanging essential information in the operating room, as well as throughout the overall management of surgical patients. Determinants of communication can involve factors at individual, team, task, and organizational or environmental levels [7].

The failure in communication and the communication gaps are more likely in the surgical context and could be associated with external factors related to the organization of the healthcare unit, as well as the processes that are implemented such as noise, low voice volume, distance, time, or even the lack of visual cues, such as when masks cover facial expressions, lack of privacy, frequent interruptions, limited time, 24-h clinical care, staff shortages, few resources, unpredictability, overcrowding, and never-ending patient intakes [13]. In addition, medical staff in the ED work with many complicated situations, such as death, violence, rape, acute illness, and accidents, which affect their emotional statement, as well as create communication gaps due to the nature of their existence.

At the same time, the internal factors that generate communication gaps, are related to the personal characteristics of the members of the surgical teams and the other healthcare professionals that are directly and indirectly involved (such as surgeons, anesthesiologists, nurses, technicians, internists, radiologists, pathologists, etc.). These internal factors are detected in the cross-cultural differences in communication, illustrated by language barriers, different

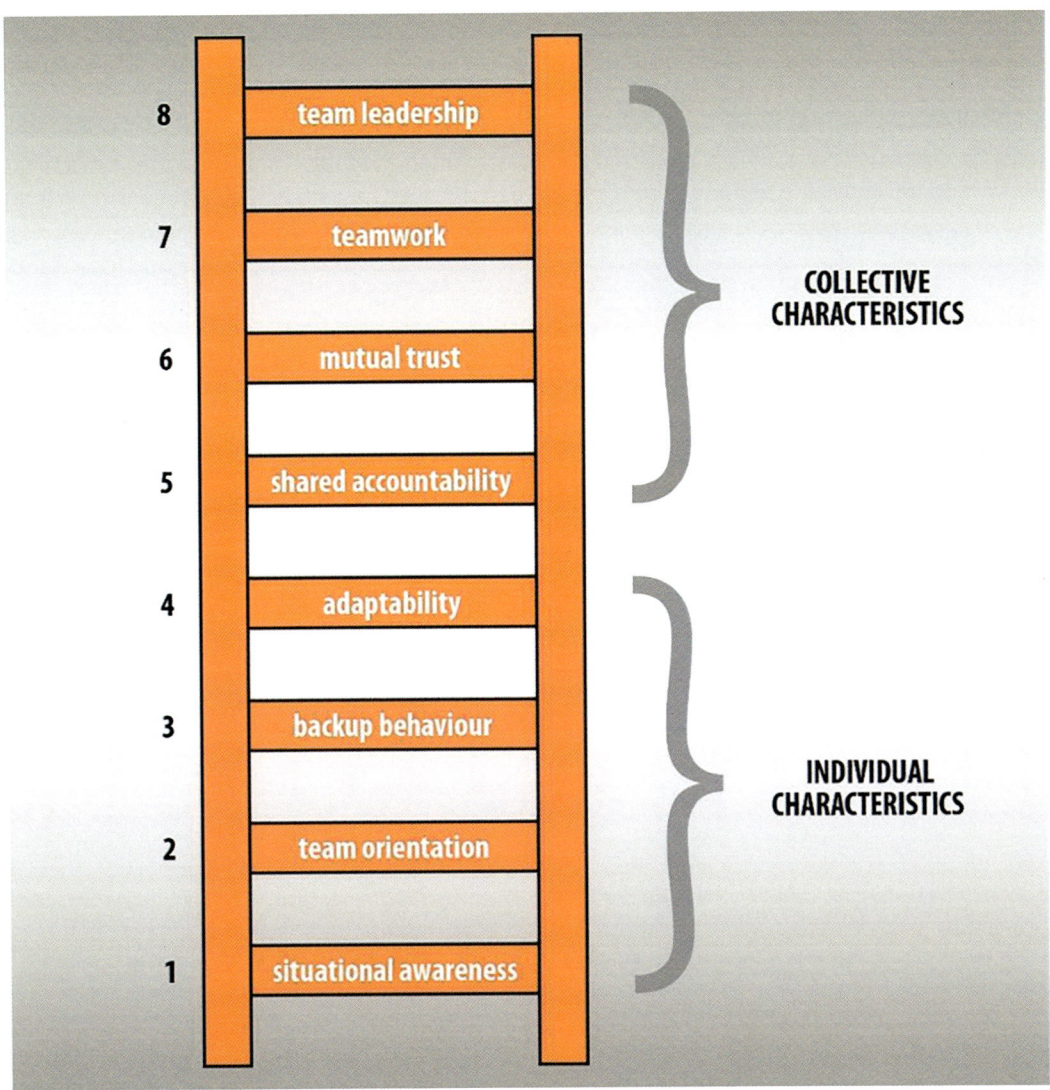

Picture 36.1 Effective interaction in the OR ladder

linguistic behaviors, sociopragmatic failure, past experiences, a variety of organizational cultures, as well as the relationships of everyone involved.

Reported barriers to effective team communication include also human characteristics and behavioral patterns such as non-listening behaviors, cross-communication, aggressiveness, poor or not handover, not following patient directives, dependency on leadership, along with non-respecting behavior toward the patient. Multiple conversations between subgroups of staff were also noted as an impediment. A lack of closed-loop communication is also considered as a key barrier to effective team communication.

36.3 Introducing a Comprehensive Communication Model

36.3.1 Ten Proposals for Breaking the Communication Gap

An efficient and effective communication encourages the members of an interprofessional team to fortify their shared mental model, enhancing team's situational awareness and cooperation, and reducing risks to patient safety. The interdependent activities of healthcare professionals in the operating room are inextricably linked with precise and adequate information sharing, which leads to an efficient coordination and cooperation toward a common understanding of intentions and actions for a shared goal of safe and efficient surgery. Once communication collapse, information will disappear, and the team's shared mental model would deteriorate [7, 14].

Four of the most common scenarios, where communication fades are (a) when the operating room staff fails to receive available information, (b) the poor communication or misunderstandings between staff members, (c) the surgical staff members fail to share their concerns, and (d) the surgical staff members dismiss the concerns of other staff members.

In practical terms therefore indicative communication improvement golden rules (as shown in Picture 36.2) should:

- Create a shared mind model of the patient's situation, and allow personnel from differing backgrounds to understand both the clinical and logistical implications of the case. It ensures that team members are familiar with one another's roles and responsibilities; that they are able to anticipate the needs of other team members and that have a high level of adaptive capacity.
- Incorporate briefing and debriefing of 10 min rule as standardized communication and interaction, teamwork, and situational awareness procedure.
- Introduce participatory models of communication checklist so as to ensure that interactions and interrelations are captured and that the theatre team are all on the same page and share a sense of shared accountability for the outcome of the procedure.
- Introduce concrete guidelines for the call-out (when, what, and how) during the perioperative phase.
- Encourage close loom communication by introducing a standardized protocol. In times of high-stress communication often shifts from an explicit to a tacit form without the team being aware of it. This leads to missed information and poor outcomes [15].
- Introduce concrete guidelines for the call-out (when, what, and how) during the perioperative phase.
- Training on non-technical skills with real life simulations insisting on being aware of roles, effectively communicating and interacting, entails trust and respect, show adaptability to the resources and fluid structure with an emphasis on both verbal and nonverbal communication.
- Incorporate social media platforms and technological tools as mechanisms of interaction.
- Adopt an overcommunication strategy as it helps promote discipline, accountability, and strategic direction in the team.

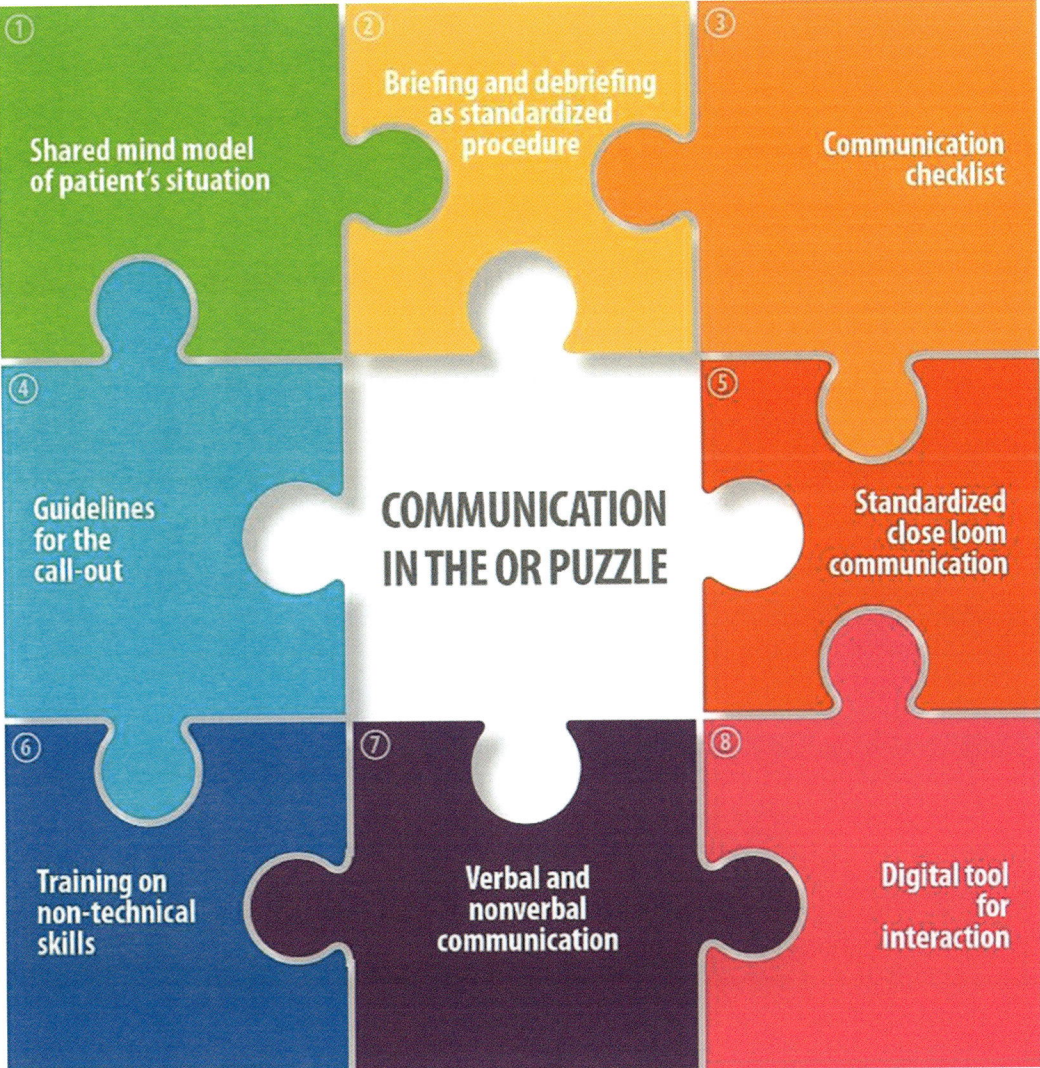

Picture 36.2 Effective communication guidelines

36.3.2 The Role of Digital Technology and Digital Media

Instantaneous access to information through digital technology and digital media has allowed information technology to enhance the access to healthcare, by improving the quality and reducing the cost. In an acute trauma setting digital technology and media are substantially easy to use, improving significantly the means of communication among the members of the trauma team. Additionally, by providing precise and reliable information of patients' status through pictures and videos in real time, they ameliorate physician's response, as well as patients' management.

Digital technology and media have also proven utility in patient follow-up and as valuable teaching tools. Although strict rules need to be used to govern the use of smartphones in order to secure the safety and secrecy of patient information, the regulations must allow easy integration of smartphone technology into the current practices [16].

36.3.3 The COVID Experience or How Nonverbal Communication Counts Equally

The COVID-19 pandemic caused -among other- great challenges in healthcare provider's self-care and consequently the standard of patient safety. Since the early days of the pandemic, with surgical theaters being converted into additional ICUs to support critically ill patients, the emergency surgeons assumed the responsibility to manage infected and non-infected patients and work safely to limit the spread of the virus in healthcare facilities and to decrease morbidity and mortality rate, which may result from delay diagnosis and treatment of surgical patients [17]. The operation process for COVID-19 patients is not only resource-consuming but also stressful for surgeons. Under these harsh circumstances, the safety of patients' and healthcare workers is of paramount importance that could be assured through logistical preparedness, careful organization cooperation, and sound communication of the team during the perioperative period [18]. Nevertheless, the operating procedure is acutely exposed to ineffective and negative communication events, due to the presence of PPE, since some forms of PPE may impair and compromise the transfer of information between surgical staff in the operating room. These conditions accrete emotional stress in the operating room, as well as enable miscommunication. At these moments, verbal communication through the use of hand signals is considered as a powerful strategy to complement the quality of care provided to the surgical patient, even in the era of COVID-19 [19]. The value of the potential use of nonverbal message is to convey meaningful information was considered of value event before the pandemic as a remedy to reduce voice levels in the OR non-verbal communication must also be taken into consideration since it represents more than 65 % of the communication [20].

36.4 Conclusion

Health professionals in emergency surgical teams perform surgical procedures in a context of variable complexity, characterized by frequent changes and uncertainties in their daily surgical program, a high degree of interdependency among team members, and a strong focus on time and resource consumption. Within surgical teams dealing with emergency medical situations efficient communication through modern or traditional methods is inextricably linked to positive patient experience.

Efficient and effective communication encourages the members of an interprofessional team to fortify their shared mental model, enhancing the team's situational awareness and cooperation, and reducing risks to patient safety. Digital technology has gradually improved the access to healthcare by instantaneous access to information, improving the means of communication among the members of the trauma team. Under unprecedented situations, such as the COVID-19 pandemic, non-verbal communication is considered as a powerful strategy to complement the quality of care provided to the surgical patient.

Dos and Don'ts
- Creating a shared mind model for the emergency surgery team.
- Use structured and standardized tools and processes and methods for both verbal and nonverbal communication among the emergency surgical teams.
- Invest in briefing and debriefing even in emergency surgery.
- Invest in non-technical skills training emphasizing teamwork.
- Incorporate new technologies and digital media in the communication facilitators.
- Exercise the use of pragmatic overcommunication.

Take-Home Messages
- Surgery alone is not enough to ensure quality care.
- Effective interprofessional Communication is linked to the performance of emergency surgery teams.
- Both verbal and non-verbal communication count.
- Communication is linked to leadership and teamwork.
- Standardized communication processes and tools can shorten communication gaps.

Multiple Choice Questions

1. Problematic communication in the case of surgical teams can cause
   A. omissions and misinterpretations
   B. conflicts among members of the surgical teams
   C. none of the above
   D. all of the above (correct answer)

2. Which of the following prohibits good communication in the emergency surgery practice
   A. the introduction of relevant checklists
   B. the use of non-verbal cues
   C. none of the above (correct answer)
   D. all of the above

3. Non-technical skills with an emphasis on good communication in the emergency surgery practice include the following
   A. team leadership and teamwork and team orientation
   B. flexibility and mutual trust
   C. none of the above
   D. all of the above (correct answer)

4. The most common scenario where communication fades is
   A. when the operating room staff fails to receive available information (correct answer)
   B. when staff use close loop communication
   C. when the handover is complete
   D. when the team members share their concerns

5. The use of digital technology can improve communication as
   A. It improves access to information
   B. It improves patients management
   C. none of the above
   D. all of the above (correct answer)

6. Communication among surgical team members is not as important as the communication between surgeon and patient
   A. Yes it is (correct answer)
   B. No it is not
   C. It is only in emergency cases
   D. It is only in everyday cases

7. Effective communication in the OR depends
   A. on the way the surgical teams exchange information and interact
   B. not only on the way the surgical team exchange information and interact but also on the way the surgical team exchange information and interact with other healthcare professionals involved (correct answer)
   C. on the way surgeons only communicate and interact
   D. none of the above

8. Which of the following is an essential mechanism in order to ensure effective communication?
   A. briefing and debriefing of 10 min rule as a standardized procedure
   B. guidelines for the call-out (when, what, how) during the perioperative phase
   C. all of the above involved (correct answer)
   D. none of the above

9. COVID-19 due to the need of using PPE has
   A. caused added extra burden in communication processes in the OR
   B. shown the need to invest in the use of non-verbal communication
   C. all of the above involved (correct answer)
   D. none of the above

10. Structured and standardized tools and processes and methods for both verbal and nonverbal communication among the emergency surgical teams
    A. Can cause delays and mix-ups
    B. Can be a burden for the surgical teams
    C. all of the above involved
    D. none of the above (correct answer)

References

1. Vincent C, Amalberti R. Safer healthcare: strategy for the real world. 1st ed. Springer Open; 2016.
2. Shorrock ST, Williams C. Human factors and ergonomics in practice: improving system performance and human well-being in the real world. 1st ed. CRC Press; 2017.
3. Flowerdew L, Brown R, Vincent C, Woloshynowych M. Development and validation of a tool to assess emergency physicians' nontechnical skills. Ann Emerg Med. 2012;59:376–85.
4. Columbus A, Castillo-Angeles M, Berry W, Haide A, Salim A, Havens JM. An evidence-based intraoperative communication tool for emergency general surgery: a pilot study. J Surg Res. 2018;228:281–9.
5. Amaniyan S, Faldaas BO, Logan PA, Vaismoradi M. Learning from patient safety incidents in the emergency department: a systematic review. J Emerg Medicine. 2020;58(2):234–44.
6. Penprase B, Elstun L, Ferguson C, Schaper M, Tiller C. Preoperative communication to improve safety: a literature review. Nurs Manage. 2010;41(11):18–24; quiz 24-5. https://doi.org/10.1097/01.NUMA.0000390370.89205.74.
7. Etherington N, Wu M, Cheng-Boivin O, et al. Interprofessional communication in the operating room: a narrative review to advance research and practice. Can J Anesth/J Can Anesth. 2019;66:1251–60.
8. Morris AM, Hoke N. Communication is key in the continuum of care. OR Nurse. 2015;9:14–9.
9. Johnson F, Logsdon P, Fournier K, et al. Switch for safety: perioperative hand-off tools. Aorn J. 2013;98:494–507.
10. Espin S, Indar A, Gross M, et al. Processes and tools to improve teamwork and communication in surgical settings: a narrative review. BMJ Open Qual. 2020;9:e000937.
11. Mcmullan R, Urwin R, Gates P, Sunderland N, Johanna N, Westbrook I. Are operating room distractions, interruptions and disruptions associated with performance and patient safety? A systematic review and meta-analysis. Int J Qual Health Care. 2021;33.(2)
12. Tørring B, Gittell JH, Laursen M, et al. Communication and relationship dynamics in surgical teams in the operating room: an ethnographic study. BMC Health Serv Res. 2019;19:528.
13. Hull L, Arora S, Aggarwal R, Darzi A, Vincent C, Sevdalis N. The impact of nontechnical skills on technical performance in surgery: a systematic review. J Am Coll Surg. 2012;214(2):214–30.
14. Green B, Oeppen RS, Smith DW, Brennan PA. Challenging hierarchy in healthcare teams—ways to flatten gradients to improve teamwork and patient care. Br J Oral Maxillofac Surg. 2017;55:449–53.
15. Maini A, Buck A, editors. Emergency trauma management course, participant manual. First edition. PDF version 1.2. Melbourne, Australia; 2013.
16. Karpeh MS Jr, Bryczkowski S. Digital communications and social media use in surgery: how to maximize communication in the digital age. Innov Surg Sci. 2017;2(3):153–7. https://doi.org/10.1515/iss-2017-0019.
17. De Simone B, Chouillard E, Sartelli M, et al. The management of surgical patients in the emergency setting during COVID-19 pandemic: the WSES position paper. World J Emerg Surg. 2021;16:14.
18. Bhattacharjee HK, Chaliyadan S, Verma E, Kumaran K, Bhargava P, Singh A, Maitra S, Parshad R. Emergency Surgery during COVID-19: lessons learned. Surg J (New York, NY). 2020;6(3):e167–70. https://doi.org/10.1055/s-0040-1716335.
19. Duan X, Sun H, He Y, Yang J, Li X, Taparia K, Zheng B. Personal protective equipment in COVID-19. J Occup Environ Med. 2021;63(3):221–5.
20. Tiferes J, Hussein AA, Bisantz A, Higginbotham DJ, Sharif M, Kozlowski J, et al. Are gestures worth a thousand words? Verbal and nonverbal communication during robot-assisted surgery. Appl Ergon. 2019;78:251–62.

Further Reading

Anonymous (n.d.) (highlight here the most important publications related to the chapter content (i.e., Guidelines)

Etherington N, Wu M, Cheng-Boivin O, et al. Interprofessional communication in the operating room: a narrative review to advance research and practice. Can J Anesth/J Can Anesth. 2019;66:1251–60.

WHO Surgical Safety Checklist. https://www.who.int/patientsafety/topics/safe-surgery/checklist/en/

37

Patient Safety and Risk Management

Boris E. Sakakushev

37.1 Introduction

> **Learning Goals**
> - What is Patient Safety in medicine, surgery and emergency general surgery?
> - What is risk assessment and management and how are they implemented to assure better quality and patient safety in surgery?
> - How does Covid 19 pandemic changes everyday emergency surgery practice and what are we going to expect in the future?

37.1.1 Patient Safety

Patient safety is a global health issue receiving rapidly increasing attention. Patient safety is the absence of avoidable harm inflicted on the patient through the actions and/or negligence of employees or through flaws in the healthcare system [1].

PS is a new healthcare discipline that emphasizes the reporting, analysis, and prevention of medical errors which often lead to adverse healthcare events. Recognizing that healthcare errors impact one in every 10 patients around the world, the WHO calls patient safety an endemic concern [2].

In 1919 WHO announced that 134 million adverse events occur each year due to unsafe care in hospitals in low- and middle-income countries, contributing to 2.6 million deaths. More than 15% of hospital expenses can be attributed to treating patient safety failures. WHO outlined that 4 out of 10 patients are harmed in the primary and ambulatory care, where 80% of harm in these settings can be avoided and concluded that "No one should be harmed in healthcare".

The death rate per year from iatrogenic injury and error varies from 44,000 to 98,000, exceeding the number of deaths in auto accidents in USA, similarly autopsy series suggest 15% error rate in the practice of medicine [3].

On the first-ever World Patient Safety Day on 17 September 2019, WHO launched a global campaign to create awareness of global social, economic and medical significance of patient safety and urge people to show their commitment to making healthcare safer [4]. This date was established by the 72nd World Health Assembly in May 2019, following adoption of resolution WHA72.6 on 'Global action on patient safety'. The resolution recognizes PS as a global health priority and promotes the objectives of World Patient Safety Day, namely to increase public

B. E. Sakakushev (✉)
Research Institute at Medical University of Plovdiv (RIMU), First Clinic of General Surgery, UMHAT St. George, Plovdiv, Bulgaria
e-mail: Boris.Sakakushev@mu-plovdiv.bg

awareness and engagement, enhance global understanding, and spur global solidarity and action to progress patient safety.

The World Health Organization defines patient safety as 'the absence of preventable harm to a patient during the process of health care' and the discipline of patient safety as 'the coordinated efforts to prevent harm, caused by the process of health care itself, from occurring to patients' [5].

"Patient safety is a key component of the human right to a healthy life and universal access to health services" [6].

Defined as 'the prevention of harm to patients' (Kohn et al. 2000) or as 'the prevention of errors and adverse effects to patients associated with health care' (WHO 2016), PS is inextricably linked to the identification and classification of categories such as 'adverse events', 'clinical incidents', 'adverse effects', 'harm' and 'medical error'. PS is dependent on the possibility of easily transforming vulnerable clinical situations or adverse patient effects into well-defined and delineated incidents that can be codified, classified, reported, counted and managed. As such, an organizing tool in the appearance of countable risk objects (Hilgartner 1992) has been introduced into healthcare with the safety programme [7]. Introduction of patient safety technology into healthcare is likely to cause rearrangements of roles, responsibilities, and earlier practices of both more formalized and invisible or informal character.

Patient safety has been the essence of medical ethics credo since Hippocrates "primum non nocere", do not harm, currently focusing on avoiding medical errors.

The principles of PS state that the discipline of Patient Safety acknowledges that risk is inherent in medicine and error is inherent in human condition. Wrong-site and wrong-patient surgeries happen not because of incompetent surgeons, but because of unreliable processes of patient identification and surgical site marking.

The first principle of PS discipline proposes that the fertile ground for medical errors is the "soil" of the healthcare delivery system and not the "seed" of the clinician.

The second states that the safer care is a function of good teams, nor good individuals acting alone, rejecting the notion of "I" in favor of "we".

The third fundamental principle of PS is "Just Culture", based on three premises—first—to learn from adverse events and therefore to report them; second—to shift the focus away from blaming and punishing the clinician, who is not exempt from human error; and third is balance between the "no-blame" approach and learning trough reporting with appropriate accountability, assessing judiciously human errors [8].

Quality and patient safety are integral aspects of modern healthcare. In recent years, we have seen a significant increase in the number of meaningful quality improvement and patient safety efforts across the globe, as a result of the recognition that:

1. Medical errors are a potentially preventable source of patient morbidity and mortality
2. Faulty systems, rather than negligent individuals, are often responsible for safety mishaps and suboptimal quality of care
3. Thoughtful efforts to improve quality of care and safeguard patient safety can simultaneously improve patient outcomes while decreasing healthcare costs, thus significantly improving the value of care provided [9].

Back in 2006 Stevenson et al., in their pilot study have outlined that suboptimal quality of care and adverse events are often perceived to be the result of system failure, for which a novel approach for evaluating quality of care is needed, implementing interventions designed to increase the awareness and responsibility of individual members of staff. Today changing organization, roles and management, still minimal evidence of their efficacy in improving quality of care is to be found [10].

Moving the focus from patient to the providers and environment has revealed failed practices and poor communication as the key elements that led to patient injury and harm, after system problems and therefore requiring systemic solutions [8].

"Experience is merely the name men gave to their mistakes."

37 Patient Safety and Risk Management

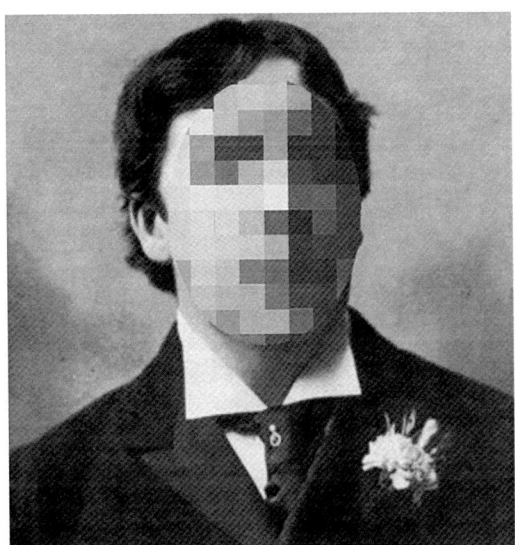

Fig. 37.1 Oscar Wilde 1854–1900

Errors are to be expected in health care and may be classified as being the result of commission, omission or inition (Fig. 37.1).

An error of inition is a failure of effort or will and is a failure of professionalism. Adverse events occur in around 10% of surgical patients and may be even more common in emergency surgery. There is little formal teaching on surgical error in surgical education and training programmes despite their frequency [11].

Cognitive errors are the result of some 30 cognitive biases, the most important of which are availability, confirmation, framing, attribution, search satisfying, hindsight, authority and anchoring biases [3].

Diagnostic error may result in irrevocable harm, therefore it is dangerous and expensive. Physicians rely on instinctual thinking, which leads to errors in judgment and decision-making. Metacognition will help us understand and resolve the root cause of preventable cognitive errors in medicine. Diagnostic errors occur at a rate of 10—15% and are the most common reason for malpractice litigation, representing the most costly malpractice category. Diagnostic errors occur with "familiar" diagnoses and result in a significant rate of preventable mortality. Most diagnostic errors are attributable to a cognitive lapse on the part of the physician.

Technical errors are a common cause of surgical adverse events and include direct manual errors, errors in judgment, and errors due to lack of knowledge. Lack of specialization or expertise in a particular procedure, low volume, communication breakdown, and physician fatigue can contribute to technical errors [3].

Common issues related to PS are retained surgical items and wrong site Surgery (WSS) [8]. Retained surgical items and unretrieved device fragments in the operating room (OR), for instance, being system problems, can be prevented by multistakeholder use of reliable OR practices and effective communication techniques. Wrong Site Surgery (WSS) generally concerns surgical procedures performed on the wrong side, laterally, of the correct patient, but in fact it encompasses the only field of surgical errors, including performing wrong operations on wrong patients, or correct operations on wrong level or patient site. This results in significant harm for the patient, family, caregivers and institution.

Retained surgical items (RSI) still represent the most frequently encountered sentinel event in OR worldwide. A retained surgical sharp (RSS) is a never event and is defined as a lost sharp (needle, blade, instrument, guidewire, metal fragment) that is not recovered prior to the patient leaving the operating room.

The term "Never Event", as defined by the National Quality Forum, is a medical error that should never occur, usually is preventable and results in significant patient harm. These must be reported to the patient as well as to the hospital incident committee.

A "near-miss" sharp (NMS) is an intraoperative event where there is a lost surgical sharp, that is recovered prior to the patient leaving the operating room. Both NMS and RSS events are difficult to quantify and their reporting to the Joint Commission (JC) is voluntary, so that underreporting remains a reasonable concern. NMS are less likely voluntarily reported as the problem was rectified prior to the patient leaving the OR and therefore the degree of risk to the patient (and provider/hospital) has been significantly reduced.

Fig. 37.2 Reasons' Swiss cheese model [13]

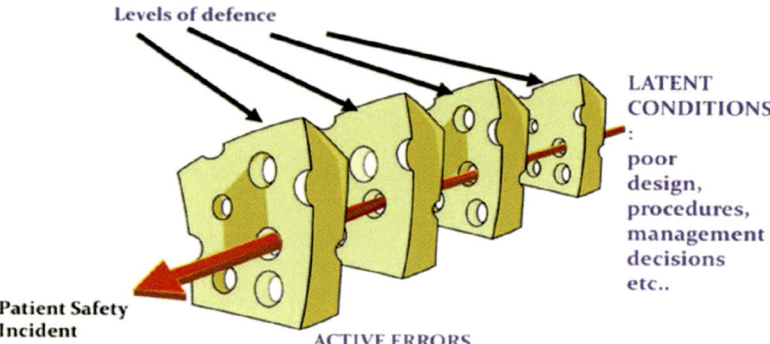

Avoidance of harm to patients can be achieved by blocking inevitable error and avoiding preventable error. However, error does occur in surgery and patients get injured. Assuming the statement of Corrigan et al. in 2000 "To Err is Human" the system nature of healthcare delivery has become broadly recognized. The process of quality measurement and error investigation foster quality and safety improvement and development of systems, more resistant to human error. This is the place for error disclosure systems, routinely underestimated and neglected, but really owing the potential for best error prevention and learning and culture tool. Creating and implementing a system of medical error disclosure will optimize the healthcare system, satisfy stakeholders and evolve and result in optimal, patient centered care delivery [8].

With underreporting of such incidents, it is unrealistic to expect aggressive development of new prevention and detection strategies, also because awareness about the issue of "near-miss" or retained surgical sharps remains limited [12].

There is a global consensus that a system approach is required to tackle patient safety. This is based on the work of British psychologist James Reason, who concluded that safety failures are almost never caused by isolated errors, with most accidents resulting from multiple, smaller errors in environments with serious underlying flaws. Reason described this as the 'Swiss Cheese Model' and advocated that organisations should identify the individual holes within their systems and make changes in order to both shrink the size of the holes and create enough overlap so that the holes do not align (Fig. 37.2) [13]. Reason used the terms active errors to describe errors made by individuals (which he argued are inevitable as no practitioners are able to practice perfectly) and latent errors to describe the failures of systems that allow the inevitable active errors to cause harm [13].

Activities to improve patient safety in health care systems include

1. Identify current issues regarding patient safety
2. Revise systems, education, and training to address known patient safety issues
3. Educate health care professionals about the importance of patient safety concepts. Establish a system of checks and balances to reduce medical errors. Ensure practical application of patient safety concepts (training)
4. Enhance patient interaction to reduce errors and repeat the process to address errors that persist [14].

PS and RM integral process, development and interaction substantially determine the patient management outcomes in medicine, surgery and especially in EGS.

37.1.2 Patient Safety in Surgery

Surgery accounts for a large number of medical errors because of the critical nature o operative interventions. In fact, in a report by Gawande and colleagues, 66% of al adverse events were found to be surgical in nature, most of which occurred in the OR. More than half of these were thought to be preventable. ORS are intricate, high-stress environments characterized by a broad array of technological tools and interdisciplinary personnel, accompanied by a unique set of team dynamics, where professionals from multiple specialties whose goals and training differ widely are required to work in a closely coordinated manner. This complex setting provides multiple opportunities for suboptimal communication, clashing motivations, and errors arising from cognitive biases, poor interpersonal skills, and substandard environmental factors, all independent of technical incompetence [15].

Weizer & al. identified 66 countries reporting surgical data between 2005 and 2013, estimating, that 312·9 million operations took place in 2012 with an intent to save life. This was an increase of 33·6% over 8 years, accounting for 1533 operations per 100 000 people [16]. Unfortunately, unsafe surgical care can cause substantial harm, leading to crude mortality rate after major surgery of 0.5–5% and complications after inpatient operations reaching 25% of patients. In developed countries, almost 50% of all adverse events in hospitalized patients are related to surgical care, where half of the cases in which surgery led to harm are considered preventable.

Tentative estimates suggest that one in ten patients suffers from an adverse event in hospital. In the US, nearly 100,000 people die from the consequences of mistreatment. The intensive care units record 1.7 medical errors per patient and day. The most affected disciplines are the operative disciplines, particularly general surgery [17].

Since the Institute of Medicine released its landmark patient safety report To Err Is Human, 21 years ago, the new report from medical liability insurer Coverys takes a close look at why patient safety is still far from optimal. The report examined 20,211 closed medical malpractice claims from 2010 to 2019 to provide risk managers, clinicians, and healthcare executives a unique view into factors that lead to claims, intending to proactively reduce conditions that result in patient harm and financial risk [18].

Around 200 million surgical procedures are performed globally every year. Even with a conservative low estimate of 1–2% average complication rate , at least 2–4 million patients annually will suffer harm from surgical care. These facts impose some intuitive questions:

- How many patients and their families have been involved in a transparent shared decision-making process of surgery?
- How many times other alternative treatments or conservative treatment have been proposed?
- How often patients have been encouraged to seek for second opinion?
- How many patients have undergone "unnecessary operations " and suffered "unnecessary" complications, including preventable death from unneeded treatment?

The answers remain elusive. Here is a "moment of truth" question for all surgeons. How likely are you to consider having a surgical procedure done on yourself that you would recommend to your patients? Being intrinsically biased to towards recommending unnecessary surgery, we as surgeons must embrace the concept of "shared decision making" as a core pilar in the partnership with our patients. Listening skills, empathy and compassion should no longer be considered optional humanistic virtues for surgeons, if we are truly dedicated and committed to providing appropriate and safe surgical care to our patients [19]. "Surgical care is inherently risky, and when things go wrong, is a common basis for malpractice claims," the report concluded. "Despite widely distributed guidance, checklists, team training, and simulation aimed at reducing their prevalence, events continue to occur involving retained foreign bodies, wrong site procedures, and less-than-optimal team performance."

The OR environment is often characterized as a tight, congested area with an array of wires, tubes, and lines, known as the "spaghetti syndrome. Consequently, movements by members of the surgical team are often obstructed; instruments and supplies may be difficult to access and maintain, and the risk of accidental disconnection of devices and human error increases. Poor lighting, suboptimal temperature, and excessive or unwanted noise have been shown to negatively affect surgical performance. Unnecessary noise may also hinder appropriate communication needed among the OR staff. [15].

Contemporary surgical practice is more sophisticated, efficient and effective than ever before, and yet the incidence of adverse events during surgical care is reported at approximately 15% of cases in retrospective series, and in reality is probably greater. The global burden of adverse incidents occurring in the operating theatre is staggering and stands comparison with the mortality sustained in armed conflict, representing the consequences of our well-intentioned but imprecisely executed actions in the operating theatre Adverse events are typically seeded from deficiencies in non-technical skills (i.e. cognitive and social skills that complement technical skills and contribute to safe and efficient task performance [20].

Adverse event rates for surgical conditions remain unacceptably high, despite multiple nationwide and global patient safety initiatives like the '100,000 Lives Campaign' (2005/2006) and subsequent '5 Million Lives Campaign' (2007/2008) by the Institute for Healthcare Improvement (IHI), the 'Surgical Care Improvement Project' (2006) and 'Universal Protocol' (2009) by the Joint Commission, and the WHO 'Safe Surgery Saves Lives' campaign accompanied by the global implementation of the WHO surgical safety checklist (2009) [14].

Non-technical errors are usually due to communication break down which can contribute to adverse events. Sentinel events are defined as an unexpected occurrence involving death or serious physical or physiological injury or the risk thereof [19].Patients can categorize unanticipated outcomes as malpractice, suggesting negligence or incompetence on the part of a professional. However for physicians and healthcare providers unanticipated outcomes and even some adverse events from the patient prospective are often viewed as known complications in practice.

Strategies to reduce surgical errors can be better decision making, operative planning and team performance for common operations, particularly in high risk circumstances like emergencies, reoperations and patients with difficult anatomy. Surgery itself is predisposed to adverse events by definition. Technical errors are the most important part in this field because they have a profound impact on complications and because they are preventable. They can be either attributable to direct intraoperative manual errors or to knowledge or judgement issues of surgical tactics. Different operations have different risks in terms of safety and result in different outcomes. The most common types of operations associated with technical errors are general or gastrointestinal, spine and gynecology surgery. Visceral injuries, like bowel injuries and haemorrhage, as well as retention of surgical materials are the most recurrent adverse events in abdominal surgery, often causing a high mortality rate and permanent disabilities [19].

Patient Safety Culture (PSC) is an important aspect for advancement in healthcare that embodies crucial patient care guidelines and processes for preventing adverse events in health care and include established safety values and knowledge of specific patient care protocols [8].

Surgery must adopt prevention based problem-solving approach, facing the possibility of technical error, such as improving anatomy knowledge, senior specialist consultation and collaboration, implementation and standardization of evidence based perioperative process of care and team training and simulations. Progress will also depend heavily on system analysis, education and the development of guidelines, and standards of practice and prevention. Transformation to a culture of safety is slow and challenging, especially for surgeons, due to fear of professional and legal consequences. Human error is inevitable and unavoidable. Surgeons should be able to study their errors in an open manner, use them as learning opportunities to improve health care and make every effort to decrease them [19].

Poor communication has been increasingly regarded as a causal factor in a large percentage of sentinel events within the healthcare system. The interplay between different members of the surgical team is yet another critical component of surgical performance. Studies have shown that teamwork factors alone account for 45% of variance in errors committed by surgeons [15]. The human factor methods of studying surgical patient safety include observational studies; surveys, interviews and focus groups; and retrospective review. Most popular human factor methods of improving surgical patient safety are checklists, briefings and team training, handoff protocols and interventions, focused on well-being.

One of the most challenging issues to improve patient safety is preventing wrong-site surgery, with 95 wrong-patient, wrong-site, or wrong-procedure sentinel events reported to The Joint Commission in 2017. The last published (2006–2009) VHA rate of in–operating room (in-OR) adverse events was 0.4 adverse events per 10,000 procedures [21].

Despite increased awareness of safety, errors routinely continue to occur in surgical care. Disruptions in the flow of an operation, such as teamwork and communication failures, contribute significantly to adverse events. Although it is apparent that some incidence of human error is unavoidable, there is evidence in medicine and other fields that systems can be better designed to prevent or detect errors before a patient is harmed. The complexity of factors leading to surgical errors requires collaboration between surgeons and human factors experts to carry out the proper prospective and observational studies. Only when we are guided by this valid and real-world data can useful interventions be identified and implemented. Improving the design of equipment, the order, allocation, and definition of surgical tasks, the design of the surgical environment, and the organization of services and support around the maintenance and improvement of surgical flow could all yield improvements in surgical performance and eventually caregiver and patient outcomes [15].

In recent years studies of process failures, communication, teamwork, interruptions and distractions have now identified multiple vulnerabilities implicit within systems of surgical care [22].

The increasing share of surgical care as an essential component of health care worldwide will continue to rise with the escalation of traumatic injuries incidences, cancers and cardiovascular disease, not rarely being the only choice of therapy.

37.1.3 Patient Safety in Emergency General Surgery

The American Association for the Surgery of Trauma and the American College of Surgeons Committee on Trauma defined emergency general surgery (EGS) as a field in 2003. EGS constitutes 7%, approximately 3 million, of all hospital annual admissions of patients in the United States where 850,000 EGS operations. The following seven procedures—partial colectomy, small bowel resection, cholecystectomy, peptic ulcer disease, lysis of adhesions, appendectomy, and laparotomy account for 80% of the operative EGS burden. EGS patients are a unique subset of patients with higher rates and risks of postoperative complications, mortality, readmissions, and care discontinuity. Approximately 50% of the patients undergoing emergency general surgery develop postoperative complications and 15% are readmitted to the hospital within 30 days of their index operation [23].

The American Association for the Surgery of Trauma (AAST) was the first to develop a formal definition of emergency general surgery (EGS) in 2013 [24]. The EGS patient was conceptually defined as "any patient (inpatient or emergency department) requiring an emergency surgical evaluation (operative or non-operative) for diseases within the realm of general surgery as defined by the American Board of Surgery".

Emergency general surgery was clearly defined, separate from trauma surgery and other general surgical specialties, for the first time in 2003 by the American Association for the Surgery of Trauma (AAST) and the American College of Surgeons Committee on Trauma [25].

Over the past 10 years, acute care surgery has become widely accepted as a distinct surgical specialty and practice paradigm, encompassing 3 areas of surgical practice: trauma surgery, emergency general surgery, and surgical critical care. In the USA, the incidence and prevalence of EGS conditions exceed that of other common, highly studied public health problems, including newly diagnosed cancers and new onset diabetes. More than 3 million patients are admitted annually to US hospitals with EGS conditions, representing over 7% of all US hospitalizations. Moreover, there are over 850,000 EGS operations performed annually in the USA [26, 27].

Recent studies have shown that EGS patients are at uniquely higher risk for medical errors and complications following surgery, with EGS patients up to eight times more likely to die compared to patients undergoing the same procedure electively [28, 29].

Hospital admissions for Emergency General Surgery (EGS) have increased 28% since 2001, with over 27 million admissions annually, representing more hospital admissions per year than the sum of all new diagnoses of cancer or diabetes. (1) Patients who undergo EGS procedures are up to 8 times more likely to die, than those undergoing the same procedure electively. (2) EGS admissions and costs are projected to increase 45% to $41.20 billion annually by 2060 using US Census projections [30].

Emergency General Surgery accounts for 11% of all hospital admissions yet represents the majority (50%) of all surgical mortality in the United States. Therefore, improving healthcare outcomes in the United States will require addressing optimal care and outcomes in EGS [31].

Emergency surgery deals with the sickest patients with often unexpected conditions, in an environment which has availability of treatment facilities on a "first come—first served basis" rather than a triaged system within many hospitals. The relative inconsistency of the emergency team and "short notice" aspect to the work, places it at the forefront of risk from surgical error.

The elevated mortality rates of emergency surgery are attributable to risks from the nature of the illness, to the level of staff experience and the time and timing of interventions, with an incomplete information base contributing to variable outcomes. It is still a deficient area of supervision of training surgeons, team members preparation and familiarity as well as awareness and importance of human factors in emergency surgery which is on an early stage of acceptance within the profession.

The prevalence and severity of EGS-driven hospitalizations present a significant public health cost burden. The total estimated cost of EGS hospitalizations in 2010 was $28.4 billion, and this is expected to nearly double by 2060 [32].

Patients undergoing emergency general surgery (EGS) procedures are up to eight times more likely to die than patients undergoing the same procedures electively. This excess mortality is often attributed to nonmodifiable patient factors including comorbidities and physiologic derangements at presentation, leaving few targets for quality improvement. Patients from 303 hospitals, representing 153,544 admissions, 2008–2011, at hospitals with lower risk-adjusted trauma mortality show 33% lower risk of mortality after admission for EGS procedures. The structures and processes that improve trauma mortality may also improve EGS mortality. Emergency general surgery–specific systems measures and process measures are needed to better understand drivers of variation in quality of EGS outcomes [31].

Evidence of a "weekend effect" is limited in emergency general surgery (EGS). Analyzing 438,110 EGS patients from The National Inpatient Sample (NIS) data, January 2014–September 2015, of whom 103,450 underwent weekend operation, Hatchimonji et al. discovered a weekend effect on mortality (OR 1.22; 95%CI 1.02–1.46) and an interactive effect between weekend operation and teaching status on complications (teaching OR 1.22; 95%CI 1.15–1.29; interaction OR 1.13; 95%CI 1.03–1.25) [33].

Delivery of thromboprophylactic treatment on an emergency general surgery admissions according to guidelines resulted in 61% reduction in radiologically detected clinical episodes of thromboembolism 2 months after admission demonstrating that the quality improvement process results in in major sustainable development in thromboprophylaxis [34].

Anonymous incident reporting and validation of incident reports could provide useful input for the design of an effective tool to govern patient safety in emergency medical service organisations and hospital-based emergency departments. As emergency care organisations are lacking evidence-based and feasible tools to govern patient safety within their structure, established strategies from other high-risk sectors like aviation is needed to be evaluated in emergency care settings, using an experimental design with valid outcome measures to strengthen the evidence base [35].

"The only surgeons without complications are retired or liars." [6].

Emergency general surgery is characterized by an exceptionally high level of variability, which can be subcategorized as patient-variability (acute physiology and comorbidities) and system-variability (operating room resources and workforce)q Patient-variability and system-variability, with focus on multidisciplinary communication as a modifier, represent potential domains for quality improvement in this field [36].

EGS continues to grow and consolidate as an area of practice constituting a significant portion of urgent and emergent care the healthcare system, development of accurate, validated severity measures will allow for planning for the optimum care of these patients as we move forward [37].

The principles of a consultant-led, patient-centered surgical management, continuity of care and specificity of expertise in managing surgical patients' complications and readmissions are particularly valuable and advisable in the field of Acute Care Surgery. Applying them in the management of the emergency surgical patients both in the perioperative period, will improve the outcomes and guarantee patient safety [38].

37.1.4 Risk and Patient Safety

Patient safety program introduce risks, closely connected to the highly principle-based nature of the current paradigm, its strong standardization claims, its 'measure-and-manage' strategies and its blame-free ethos. These are the risks that could be determined as the self-inflicted plagues of the program [7]. The notion of risk is used to determine when threats, dangers, vulnerabilities, or problems are constituted as measurable risk objects, most often through probability measures, while striving to account for and manage them. Risk should be understood as unwanted potential consequences, as a situation that involves 'the possibility of loss, injury, or other adverse or unwelcome circumstance' (Oxford English Dictionary). The accountability claim attributed to the risk label should be held in mind in discussions on how, when managing some risk via certain types of risk management tools, new areas of concern arise that must equally be attended to and accounted for; they are the risk of risk management.

Second order risk is a concept that draws attention to possible redistributions of focus from the concrete clinical situation, or from what could be determined as first-order safety issues, to second-order processes, such as the implementation and maintenance of the technologies themselves. Such redistributions show themselves as specific side effects of quality and safety technologies such as reporting and classification systems, medical information systems or specific safety technologies and procedures [7].

Although standardization risk is perhaps the dominant organizing principle of contemporary safety management, it is at the same time the most criticized part of PS program, as it is said to undermine the complexity and situated status of risk, healthcare practices and clinical work. Standardization is supported by the program's failsafe systems approach, stating that safety is best ensured by creating systems that reduce variation and make it as hard as possible for healthcare professionals to make mistakes.

37.2 Diagnosis

37.2.1 Risk Assessment

Risk assessment is a structural and systematic procedure that depends on the correct identification of the hazards and an appropriate estimation of the risks arising from them, with a view to making inter-risk comparisons for the purposes of their control or avoidance. Risk assessment in a numerical manner will help hospitals to assess their safety status and prioritize their action plan in view of their resources [39].

Proactive risk assessments were used to systematically identify and prioritize hazards in surgical wards and allowed interventions to be recommended [40].

Risk assessments and outcome predictions for EGS patients are aided by validated scoring systems including Charlson age-comorbidity index (CACI), Emergency Surgery Score (ESS), and the Physiological and Operative Severity Score for the enumeration of Mortality and Morbidity (POSSUM). In addition, the AAST has developed a grading system for reporting anatomic severity of multiple EGS conditions. Further, the American College of Surgeons National Surgical Quality Improvement Program (NSQIP) universal Surgical Risk Calculator is available online and through smartphone apps [24].

Surgeon can have a major impact on assessing risk and that a reduction in risk can have a significant impact on reducing patient safety incidents, complaints and litigation. Correct and accurate assessment of the death and complication risk in every patient and its integration into the consent process with supporting documentation can radically reduce complaints and litigation, both areas that surgeons find most painful [41].

Disclosing and reporting of medical errors is a basic tenet for improving patient safety. Implementing Quality Assurance Protocols, like this of Denver Health is aimed to lower the threshold of reporting all perceived complications, "near-misses", and "no-harm events", mandating a standardized peer-review of all reported occurrences in a "real-time" fashion, and relies on three cornerstones: anonymous "real-time" reporting of any suspected adverse occurrence, including "near miss" and "no harm" events; peer-review of each reported event at a weekly QA conference, using a standardized case review form; and corrective action is defined for each reviewed case [42]. Within two years of implementation of this QA process, the median rate of reported occurrences increased more than sixfold from 1.7 to 11.1 per 100 surgical procedures, the overall complication rate for the entire Department of Orthopaedics at Denver Health increased fivefold, from 1.4% to 6.7%. The reported 5-fold increase in complications within the department likely reflects the improved open and more honest reporting format and critical peer-review of each reported occurrence, rather than a decreased quality of care.

The thorough reporting and peer-review of surgical errors creates a new dilemma for the practicing surgeon: an increased quality of reporting leads to an increased complication rate, thus affecting the individual surgeon's professional track record and the respective institution's ranking among peers. Until legislation provides legal protection for medical error disclosure and analysis, we continue to rely on the limited and anecdotal reporting of medical errors and surgical complications in the peer-reviewed biomedical literature [43].

The Surgical Risk Preoperative Assessment System is a parsimonious, universal surgical risk calculator integrated into electronic health record used for populating clinical decision support tools to lessen the burden on the busy surgeon [44].

Individualized preoperative risk assessment of adverse outcomes for patients undergoing surgical procedures has the potential to improve the processes of informed consent and shared decision making, guide perioperative care, and ultimately reduce occurrence of postoperative complications [45].

Proactive risk assessments were used to systematically identify and prioritize hazards in surgical wards and allowed interventions to be recommended. The 5 most hazardous processes prioritized for modified health care failure mode are hand hygiene, isolation of infection, vital signs, medication delivery, and hand off. Of 190 failures within these processes, 50 (26%) are considered hazardous and did not have effective control measures in place [40].

Surgical Risk Preoperative Assessment System (SURPAS) was designed as a user-friendly tool to provide accurate risk assessment based on eight preoperatively available predictor variables. It provides individualized preoperative risk assessment for eight different 30-day postoperative adverse outcomes: mortality, overall morbidity, and six complication clusters (infectious, transfusion and cardiac, renal, pulmonary, venous thromboembolic, and neurological complications). SURPAS provides accurate risk assessments based on eight preoperatively available predictor variables, four of which are operative characteristics (work, Relative Value Unit, inpatient/outpatient operation, primary surgeon specialty, and emergency operation status) and four of which are patient characteristics-ASA class, functional health status, age, and sepsis within 48 h of surgery. SURPAS has proved the potential to enhance the informed consent and shared decision making, processes, guide perioperative care, and ideally, ultimately reduce occurrence of postoperative complications [46].

New strategies to improve patient safety in surgery include the implementation of defined surgical safety checklists, standardized "readbacks" to improve communication in perioperative services, and medical team training programs [47].

Progressive refinements to SURPAS improve the accuracy of the models,

and facilitate its easier use and implementation, predisposing future prospective external validation studies [48].

The quality of trauma care is assessed by the Performance Improvement and Patient Safety (PIPS) Program, based on trauma records and severity indexes. Several severity scoring systems are available; some are universally accepted and reviewed periodically in order to improve their accuracy. These include the Trauma and Injury Severity Score (TRISS) implemented in 1992, a tool well suited for the evaluation of the quality of care and to propose improvements in trauma care. The TRISS comprises the Revised Trauma Score (RTS) and Injury Severity Score (ISS) indexes as well as the trauma type (blunt or penetrating) and the patient age. The ISS does not consider more than one lesion in each body region in its calculation, which may underestimate the severity. The updated ISS, the New Injury and Severity Score (NISS), considered the three most serious injuries in calculating the severity of the trauma, regardless of the body region affected, thus seeking to increase the sensitivity of the index, as trauma patients can present multiple severe injuries in the same body region. New Trauma and Injury Severity Score (NTRISS)-like, TRISS SpO_2, and NTRISS-like SpO_2. The first new variation (NTRISS-like) combines the physiological BMR parameters of the GCS, systolic blood pressure (SBP), and the anatomical variable of the NISS. The second and third variations include SpO_2. In the TRISS SpO_2, the RTS is replaced by GCS and SBP values and SpO_2 score; in the NTRISS-like SpO_2, the value assigned to SpO_2 was added to the NTRISS-like index. All these given the clinical significance and ease of obtaining information from their components, seem to be good options to estimate the survival probability of trauma victims [49].

The Emergency Surgery Score (ESS) was recently developed and retrospectively validated as an accurate mortality risk calculator for emergency general surgery. The multicenter prospective observational study of The Association for the Surgery of Trauma, April 2018–June 2019, with 19 centers enrolled, with 1649 patients (aged >18 years) undergoing emergency laparotomy show 30-day mortality and complication rates 14.8% and 53.3%; 57.0% of patients required ICU admission. ESS gradually and accurately predicted 30-day mortality; 3.5%, 50.0%, and 85.7% of patients with ESS of 3, 12, and 17 died after surgery. ESS accurately predicted complications; 21.0%, 57.1%; and 88.9% of patients with ESS of 1, 6, and 13 developed postoperative complications [50]. Therefore ESS is useful for perioperative patient and family counseling, triaging patients to the intensive care unit, and benchmarking the quality of emergency general surgery care.

In broader UK practice for emergency laparotomies (some of which are not high-risk), both a consultant surgeon and consultant anaesthetist are present for 83% of operations performed during daytime hours on a weekday. However, for operations performed after midnight, where the predicted risk of death is more than twice as high as it is for daytime cases [51].

Analyzing 124,335 emergency general surgery patients from 2007 to 2017 Gaitanidis et al. Found out that Emergency Surgery Score, a validated risk calculator, accurately predicts mortality and morbidity in the elderly EGS patient [52].

Emergency Surgery Score can prove useful for (1) perioperative patient and family counseling, (2) triaging patients to the intensive care unit, and (3) benchmarking the quality of emergency general surgery care [50].

Risk stratification tools (RST) facilitate a meaningful comparison of surgical outcomes between surgeons, hospitals and healthcare systems [54]. In the emergency setting we differentiate trauma scoring systems, critical care scoring systems, surgical risk stratification tools and Track and trigger systems [53].

The ideal RST for EGS will meet six criteria for the generalized EGS patient population:

1. Accurately quantify morbidity and mortality risk in the EGS population.
2. Use readily obtainable objective data.
3. Be applicable early prior to a surgical intervention.
4. Be applicable in non-operative cases.
5. Can be used for auditing purposes.
6. Application that facilitates use in clinical practice.

Surgical RST, used to predict perioperative morbidity and mortality, fall under two general categories: physiologic scores and risk prediction models and are explicitly designed for use in the perioperative setting.

The American Society of Anesthesiologists Physical Status Grading (ASA-PS) was introduced in 1941 as a preoperative grading of the physical status of patients, and was subsequently modified in 1963. There are five grades based on the presence or absence of mild to serious life-threatening systemic disease, with an additional classification of E designated for emergency surgery.

The American College of Surgeons National Surgical Quality Improvement Programme (ACS-NSQIP) database was used to develop a web-based tool to estimate the surgical risk of most operations. The resulting Universal Surgical Risk Calculator tool requires 21 preoperative factors (demographics, comorbidities, procedure), using regression models to predict mortality as well as six postoperative complications based on the preoperative risk factors.

The Charlson Comorbidity Index (CCI) was originally developed to facilitate classification of risk of death extrapolated from comorbidities, to be used in longitudinal studies. Charlson Age-Comorbidity Index (CACI) combines 19 medical conditions weighted 1–6, with age weighted 1 for every decade past 40 years.

The Emergency Surgery Acuity Score is a preoperative risk stratification system that predicts perioperative mortality in emergency surgery patients. It captures both patient comorbidities and the acute physiology at presentation. The ESAS includes 3 demographic variables, 10 comorbidities and 9 laboratory variables. Based on the relative impact of these 22 predictors, using weighted averages, a score is derived that ranges from 0 to 29 points.

Like ESAS, the Physiological Emergency Surgery Acuity Score (PESAS), was derived from sequential analyses of ACS-NSQIP and composed of 10 physiologic points linked to advanced clinical acuity and postoperative mortality.

The Physiological and Operative Severity Score for the Enumeration of Mortality and Morbidity (POSSUM) was devised in 1996 in the UK as a simple scoring system that could be used in surgical audit and is a 12 factor, four grade, physiological score (ranging from 12 through 88) plus a 6-factor operative severity score (ranging from 6 through 44).

The Perioperative Mortality Risk Score (PMRS) is a risk score for 30-day postoperative mortality derived from a study of surgical patients aged 70 years or older.

The Surgical Apgar Score (SAS) is a 10-point score based on the lowest heart rate, lowest mean arterial pressure and estimated blood loss intraoperatively

The original Surgical Mortality Score (SMS) is a risk stratification model for in-hospital mortality for patients undergoing surgical procedures developed across a range of surgical specialties in England.

The Surgical Outcome Risk Tool (SORT) is a preoperative risk prediction tool for death within 30 days of surgery in adults.

The Surgical Risk Scale was developed as an alternative system for comparative audit that used easily collected clinical data independent of the surgeon. The Surgical Risk Scale has three components: the Confidential Enquiry into Perioperative Deaths grade (categorized as elective, scheduled, urgent and emergency), the ASA-PS grade and the British United Provident Association (BUPA) operative grade (categorized as major, intermediate, major, major plus and complex major)

The Surgical Risk Score is an ASA-PS-based model to predict mortality based on preoperative data alone. It was formulated using data of all types of operations excluding cardiac surgeries and caesarian section. This score includes ASA-PS status, age, type of surgery (elective, urgent emergency) and degree of surgery (minor, moderate or major as described by the modified Johns Hopkins surgical severity score).

Track and trigger systems are defined as scoring systems that rely on periodic or interval measurements of data points (afferent information) with predetermined action plans (efferent action) when certain data or scoring thresholds are reached. Such systems are geared towards early identification of, and subsequent team-based response to, changes in patient physiologic status linked to adverse in-hospital outcomes.

In this vulnerable EGS patients, evidence-based RST that accurately predict individual risk will facilitate decision making, enhance informed consent and permit the comparison of outcomes in patient groups that share similar comorbidity profiles. Such an RST must incorporate information regarding an individual patients acute and chronic physiology through readily accessible data points, and expeditious use must be feasible. While valuable in the setting of acute injury, trauma scoring systems do not comprehensively evaluate the comorbid conditions inherent to the EGS population and are therefore not ideal for use in EGS.

The ACS-NSQIP surgical risk calculator incorporates a comprehensive body of preoperative data and accounts for the specific planned procedure. It has been previously validated in the EGS population and has shown broad statistical reliability [53].

Teamwork in the operating theatre is becoming increasingly recognized as a major factor in clinical outcomes. Self-assessment of teamwork is influenced by professional differences and most robust self-assessment tool is the Safety Attitudes Questionnaire (SAQ), while the most robust observational tool is the Non-Technical Skills (NOTECHS) system [54].

37.3 Treatment

37.3.1 Risk Management and PS

Risk Management is the setting-up of organizational instruments, methods and actions that enable the measurement or estimation of medical risk and subsequently evolve strategies to handle it [55].

Risk Management requires an integrated view of the risk-error problem, requiring a coordinated, multi-disciplinary approach that will ensure complementary measures and shared objectives of the proposed actions understood by all the players within the existing hospital structures. Assuring better safety aims at destroying traditional opportunism for new concepts of risk management in especially esteemed professionals and create solid pillars for optimal collaboration of medical specialists especially surgeons. Risk management and patient safety professionals are engaged in a close working relationship, which may be characterized by smooth integration, wary cooperation, or conflict.

The processes and outcome goals for risk management and patient safety are: identify, analyze, mitigate, and prevent clinical risk, with the overall objective of improving clinical outcomes throughout the organization. The process is multidisciplinary and collaborative. Data sources include patient and caregiver concerns; voluntarily submitted patient incident reports; sentinel and significant events; coded information such as the DRG-triggered hospital-acquired conditions; claims; write-offs due to service or potential errors; risk and quality assessments; literature and evidence-based practice; and external alerts from national and international sources [56].

Patient safety is everyone's responsibility and requires a team effort. Risk management and quality management must work together for the cause of patient safety.

37.3.2 Risk Management in Health Care

Risk management in health care emerged as a result of the malpractice crisis of the 1970s. Professionals with clinical experience were hired with the hope that they could identify the systemic problems in specific clinical fields, like surgery, engage clinicians and educate them about the need to modify specific behaviors, and work collaboratively with others on the clinical and administrative teams to help design environments that would be more conducive to the delivery of safe care. Although at times successful—for example, the dramatic changes in safety associated with the delivery of surgery and the enhancement of patient quality in that specialty—generally the hard work did not pay off [57].

Historically, one of the most significant sources of risk management was the patient incident or the lawsuit that often followed. Even proactive risk management activities often were instituted only after a problem, or a provider was identified as high risk. When an adverse event was reported it was the top priority to meet with all parties involved in the treatment of the patient, record the information, and counsel them not to repeat the information to anyone else. Risk managers were primarily focused on managing the adverse events. Medical errors are inherent in the work of healthcare providers, where most often they are result of a complex interplay of multiple factors; while rarely they are due to the carelessness or misconduct of single individuals.

There are three axioms, or rules for approaching patient safety management with a pragmatic attitude in concrete clinical situations [7]:

1. Take point of departure in the clinical situation.
2. Be cautious about ideals of risk elimination through system optimization.
3. Preserve the importance of training, habits, and experiences.

They summarize the attitude to patient safety management and are supported by the presented pragmatic alternatives to mainstream safety thinking. Present safety management efforts should preserve the importance of training, habits and experiences.

Risk management in healthcare comprises the clinical and administrative systems, processes, and reports employed to detect, monitor, assess, mitigate, and prevent risks [58]. By employing risk management, healthcare organizations proactively and systematically safeguard patient safety as well as the organization's assets, market share, accreditation, reimbursement levels, brand value, and community standing. Deployment of healthcare risk management has traditionally focused on the important role of *patient safety* and the reduction of medical errors that jeopardize an organization's ability to achieve its mission and protect against financial liability. But with the expanding role of healthcare technologies, increased cybersecurity concerns, the fast pace of medical science, and the industry's ever-changing regulatory, legal, political, and reimbursement climate, healthcare risk management has become more complex over time. Maintaining high clinical quality will increasingly impact financial performance towards a greater emphasis on value and outcomes. Hospitals and other healthcare systems are expanding their risk management programs to ones that are increasingly proactive and view risk through the much broader lens of the entire healthcare ecosystem.

To expand the role of risk management across the organization, hospitals and other healthcare facilities are adopting a more holistic approach called Enterprise Risk Management (ERM) which includes traditional aspects of risk management like patient safety and medical liability and encompasses eight risk domains [58].

ERM in healthcare promotes a comprehensive framework for making risk management decisions which maximize value protection and creation by managing risk and uncertainty and their connections to total value. It uses technology to synchronize risk mitigation efforts across the entire organization and remove risk associated with siloed departments or business units. Additionally, data analytics are embedded to support decision-making, departmental cohesiveness, risk prioritization, and resource allocation.

Successful teamwork in RM includes four domains. The first—team climate consists of critical leadership, existence of communication environment and staff briefing. The second—planning incorporates critical in threat management, SOP briefings, plans, workload assignments and contingency management. The third—execution requires to be critical in error management monitor, cross check, workload management and vigilance. The final forth domain advocates review, modify for undesired state management, evaluation of plans, inquiry and assertiveness. The high functioning team needs open lines of communication and an accurate shared mental model of the current state of affairs [19]

The *role of the healthcare risk manager* is to oversee and facilitate the ERM framework, proactively identify risks, estimate potential consequences, develop, respond and execute containment plans when adverse and unforeseen situations transpire. Current responsibilities of the healthcare risk manager include communicating with stakeholders, documenting and reporting on risk and adverse circumstances, and creating processes, policies, and procedures for responding to and managing risk and uncertainty and finally monitor the *shifting landscape* of the healthcare risk continuum.

Performing risk management in healthcare, risk managers need to identify, quantify and prioritize risk; investigate and report sentinel events; perform compliance reporting; capture and learn from near misses and good catches; think beyond the obvious to uncover latent failures; deploy proven analysis models for incident investigation; invest in a robust risk management information system and find the right balance of risk financing/transfer/retention.

Healthcare organizations need to have an established and on-going risk management plan being the guiding document for how an organization strategically identifies, manages and mitigates risk. Healthcare risk management plans communicate the purpose, scope, and objectives of the organization's risk management protocol as well as define the roles and responsibilities of the risk manager and other staff involved in risk mitigation.

The fundamental components of healthcare risk management plans consist of education, training, patient & family grievances, purpose, goals, & metrics, reporting protocols, communication, contingency, response & mitigation plans. The healthcare risk management plan needs to be a living document that is frequently updated and improved based on emerging risks, lessons learned, new information, and changes in the healthcare system and practice of medicine.

With more than 5000 members American Society for Healthcare Risk Management (ASHRM) promotes effective and innovative risk management strategies and professional leadership through education, recognition, advocacy, publications, networking, and interactions with leading health care organizations and government agencies. ASHRM initiatives focus on developing and implementing safe and effective patient care practices, preserving financial resources, and maintaining safe working environments [59]."The medical culture that silently taught the ABCs as Accuse, Blame, and Criticize is fading. Rising in its place is a safety culture emphasizing blameless reporting, successful systems, knowledge, respect, confidentiality, and trust."

Only an integrated management of medical risk will bring about changes in clinical practice, promote an increase in health care awareness that is ever closer to both patient and operator, and contribute indirectly to a decrease in the cost of health services, thus ultimately facilitating the allocation of resources to interventions directed to the development of safe and efficient health organizations and facilities. What needs to change is the way in which risk management is orientated. The team should constructs a root cause analysis of systems and structures in advance of those risks actually materializing, so embedding a risk management discipline into the fabric of healthcare operations and corporate and strategic planning.

Hazards and risks are often misinterpreted as one term, while actually they are not the same. A hazard is something with the potential to cause harm, whereas a risk is the likelihood that illness, injury, or even death might result because of the hazard. Risk management comprises five basic steps: identifying hazards, assessing and prioritizing risks, deciding on control measures, implementing control measures, and monitoring and reviewing.

The risk manager needs to be more fully engaged in providing leadership to the organization that will enable it to make sound business decisions that balance fiscal accountability with quality of patient care and error reduction. The risk management process has to create a high reliability organization is grounded on the principles of reduction in variability through standardization of equipment and procedures, consistent clear leadership committed to safety and excellence, and an open non-punitive reporting culture. What is needed is intranet (or web based) reporting, and paging a risk manager, performance improvement of the staff and train them to identify potential problems and patient safety issues when doing prospective or retrospective audits. The risk manager has to protect sensitive information to ensure patient confidentiality and to keep specific information gathered for a specific purpose out of the hands of those who might use it inappropriately or incorrectly for other purposes but, on the other, He must decide what to share and with whom, and to assist the organization in designing a managerial policy, so that a true picture of risk and benefit can be appreciated. Risk managers should attempt to chart a new future. Risk managers must be part of a team that constructs a root cause analysis of systems and structures in advance of those risks actually materializing, thus embedding a risk management discipline into the fabric of healthcare operations and corporate and strategic planning.

Risk management needs to be more fully engaged in providing leadership to the organization to enable it to make sound business decisions that balance fiscal accountability with quality of patient care and error reduction.

The creation of a high reliability organization is fundamental to patient safety. It is important to develop a common taxonomy around error reporting so that consistency is maintained both in identifying the event and summarizing the causal factors contributing to it. Risk managers who accept change and think of new ways to embed risk management principles into their organizations to help create meaningful and sustainable change will prosper. Those who don't should get out now. They are destined to fail and to fail their organizations.

Most healthcare risk managers look forward to the opportunities ahead and are dedicated to managing their organization's risk and enhancing patient safety. Those risk managers who accept change and think of new ways to embed risk management principles into their organizations to help create meaningful and sustainable change will prosper. Those who don't should get out now. They are destined to fail and to fail their organizations.

37.3.3 Risk Management in Surgery and Emergency General Surgery

Adverse event rates for surgical conditions remain unacceptably high, despite multiple nationwide and global patient safety initiatives like the '100,000 Lives Campaign' (2005/2006) and subsequent '5 Million Lives Campaign'

(2007/2008) by the Institute for Healthcare Improvement (IHI), the 'Surgical Care Improvement Project' (2006) and 'Universal Protocol' (2009) by the Joint Commission, and the WHO 'Safe Surgery Saves Lives' campaign accompanied by the global implementation of the WHO surgical safety checklist (2009) [14].

A culture of surgical safety requires devotion of the leadership to the safety mission, including dedicated time, focus, and financial investment. Beyond the organizational leadership, there should be a committee on patient safety and advisory boards, which include supervisors, middle managers, risk managers, safety officers, quality improvement officers, physician staff, nursing staff, and other clinical staff, and this committee should focus on the culture of the health care system as a whole. Teaching in medical schools and residency should be designed to reflect the importance of safety culture within health care and surgery. Specific tools, such as checklists, pre-briefs, debriefs, executive walk rounds, and event reporting systems can help to create a culture of patient safety, but no individual tool will work in isolation [15].

Nearly one-third of patients having an emergency laparotomy in the UK do not have their risk documented preoperatively. The 30-day mortality for this undocumented group was found to be 7.1% in the 2017 NELA report. Patients for whom risk was not determined were less likely to be assessed preoperatively by a consultant surgeon and were less likely to go to critical care postoperatively,15 suggesting that the failure to assess risk results in some high-risk patients not receiving potentially protective interventions [51].

> "Measure twice, cut once. This is more important in surgery than in carpentry" [6].

The risk of error can be minimized by good situational awareness, matching perception to reality, and, during treatment, reassessing the patient, team and plan. It is important to recognize and acknowledge an error when it occurs and then to respond appropriately without shaming or blaming. Classification of surgical error promotes understanding of how the error was generated, and utilizes a language that encourages reflection, reporting and response by surgeons and their teams, however, the individual surgeon still needs to reflect on their own contribution and performance [11].

When physicians are sued for "medical malpractice" today, they are actually sued for negligence. In the legal sense negligence is defined as "a failure to exercise the care that a reasonable prudent person would exercise in like circumstances". The concept of legal negligence consists of 4 factors—duty, breach of duty, causation and damages [19]. Active efforts at risk management can decrease the incidence of medical liability suits and improve the defense of the suits that occur. Risk management focuses on the patient at risk and actively manages the case so that communication is improved and documentation of the case is appropriate. Physicians should notify the risk management department within their practice and hospital, whenever they become concerned that a particular patient's care results in an unexpected outcome that could lead to litigation.

Examples of risk management initiatives are the Colorado Physician Insurance Company (COPIC), which instituted the "3Rs Program" standing for "Recognize, Respond, and Resolve. The American Academy of Orthopedic Surgeons (AAOS) has promoted the Team Strategies & Tools to Enhance Performance and Patient Safety (Team-STEPPS) program seeking to improve communication between healthcare workers, better define team roles and responsibilities, resolve interpersonal conflicts and provide techniques to eliminate barriers to quality and safety [19].

Active efforts at improving patient safety and communication within patients are integral to successful risk management. Combining these efforts with programs like COPIC and 3Rs can dramatically improve patient satisfaction and resolution of unexpected medical events. Physicians and hospitals should aggressively employ these tactics is an effort to improve the patient's overall care and positively affect the patient's experience. Successful risk management is not typically an attempt simply to close down and "circle the wagons".

WHO,s global and regional initiatives to address surgical safety, like Safe Surgery Saves Lives defines set of standards on four areas in which dramatic improvements could be made in the safety of surgical care: surgical site infection prevention, safe anaesthesia, safe surgical teams and measurement of surgical services. The WHO Surgical Safety Checklist aims to decrease errors and adverse events, and increase teamwork and communication in surgery [5].

The 19-item checklist is now used by a majority of surgical providers around the world, resulting in significant reduction of morbidity and mortality. Factors for it successful implementation concern issues like staff engagement, leadership, multidisciplinarity, coaching, discussion, education, training, feedback and local adaptation.

The SAFROS Project was funded by the European Commission and aims to understand patient safety in robotic surgery through the development of technologies and procedures to assist surgeons. and to explore whether safe robotic surgery can improve the level of patient safety currently achievable by traditional surgery.

The WHO Global Initiative for Emergency and Essential Surgical Care (GIEESC) is a global forum of health providers that share knowledge, advise policy formation and develop educational resources to reduce the burden of death and disability from conditions that could be treated through surgery. Strengthening emergency and essential surgical care it empowers healthcare systems by multidisciplinary and multisectoral effort. The WHO has had major success in surgery through the Global Patient Safety Initiative, Surgical Safety Checklist, and Infection Prevention and Control with the recently published WHO Global Guidelines for the prevention of Surgical Site Infections, which needs a multidisciplinary team and a multi-modal approach to move the guidelines into practice.

The WHO Surgical Safety Checklist has become a high-profile symbol for patient safety efforts in surgery, showing its positive effects on teamwork, communication, and patient outcomes [60].

Institutional cultural norms and infrequent communication between the team members in the operating room can compromise a patient's safety in the operating room. Implementation of the World Health Organization Surgical Safety Checklist (WHO SSC) has improved multidisciplinary communication practices and reduced morbidity and mortality in surgical settings. The role of the checklist is to improve the completion of critical tasks, which have the potential of increasing risk or be life threatening if missed, at points where the detection of missed task is still possible. The WHO Surgical Safety Checklist has three components—the first part occurs before the induction of anesthesia and is initiated by the anesthesia team and includes confirmation of the patient's identity, procedure, and consent and site marking. The second part occurs before skin incision and is initiated by the surgery team. It focuses on introduction of all team members by name and role, patient's identity, procedure and site of incision, and prophylactic antibiotics. The surgery [23].

The WHO SCC includes the following steps—Before induction of anesthesia, Before skin incision and Before patient leaves the operating room. The SURPASS preoperative and postoperative checklist includes admission to ward, recovery room or ICU, ward boarding and discharge. Combining the surgery checklists has a more significant impact on patient safety and clinical outcomes than adhering to a single checklist [61].

The usage of the World Health Organization Surgical Safety Checklist and the Surgical Patient Safety System (SURPASS) checklist is beneficial for patients, indicates research on 9000 surgical procedures, outlining that joint use of the WHO SCC and the SURPASS was associated with fewer complications, fewer reoperations, fewer hospital readmissions thus improving processes of care and patient safety [62].

Performing a realist synthesis to examine the implementation and sustained use of checklist protocols in surgery Gillespie et al. found out that the sustained use of surgical checklists is discipline-specific and more successful when medical staff are actively participating and leading the implementation process. Second, involving clinicians in tailoring the checklist to the nuances of their context and encouraging them to reflect on and evaluate the implementation process enable greater participation and ownership. In implementing surgical checklists, the weakest link in the chain appears to include leadership, tailoring, and reflection on the process. Focusing on yielding more data on checklist implementation, is better than undertaking process evaluations and designing studies across multiple healthcare settings and then collecting data on how implementation varied across contexts [63].

> "The checklist only works if the front line team actually uses it" [6].

Checklists should not be a solitary measure of the reliability of our safety environment but a method by which we can foster accountability and ensure the most basic steps to improve patient care are accomplished. Sustained use of checklists requires difficult cultural change and organizational efforts [19].

Checklists liberate the surgeon's mind from the task of remembering routine obligate procedures and need to be employed. Checklists are not a panacea however against all forms of individual or team error [3].

To achieve an optimal level of patient safety in the OR, checklist should be performed, strictly applied by the hospital administration and modified in personal work practices to ameliorate the level of patient safety in surgery. Development of a risk management program for patient safety in the OR with defined roles, monitoring, evaluation, analysis, and continuous improvement is a must [2]. The checklist should be implemented as part of the daily surgical routine as an organized document which should contain:

1. The patient's identity, site of surgery, and the name of the procedure in order to minimize the percentage of errors of identification.
2. Checking the patient presurgical condition and surgical site marking should be a routine procedure in order to minimize the possibility of wrong site surgery.
3. The surgical consent of the patient, increasing the level of communication between the surgeons and the patients discussing their conditions and the possible outcomes of the surgeries.
4. Assessing the possibility of blood loss
5. Organized discussions of the surgical team before surgeries
6. Application and monitoring of a clear prophylactic antibiotics policy
7. Development of a risk management program for patient safety in the OR with defined roles, monitoring, evaluation, analysis, and continuous improvement.

Checklists result in significantly improved standardization, evidence-based management of postoperative complications, and quality of ward rounds, thereafter representing low-cost intervention to reduce rates of failure to rescue and to improve patient care [38].

A recent survey of 846 operating room staff and surgeons from 138 hospitals in China show widespread acceptance of WHO Surgical Safety Checklist (SSC) and its value in improving patient safety. The overall compliance of 79.8% and overall adverse events rate of 2.7% demonstrates that the WHO SSC remains a powerful tool for surgical patient safety in China. Cultural changes in nursing assertiveness and surgeon-led teamwork and checklist ownership are the key elements for improving compliance, which monitoring is ensured by standardised audits [64].

The introduction of checklists to support the performance of surgical teams is associated with significant decreases in patient mortality and improvements in communication and teamwork. The degree to which checklists can support surgical teams relies on a structured implementation strategy coordinated by experienced sponsors and executed by local teams. Previous experiences implementing checklists through population-level quality improvement programs have demonstrated the critical elements to effective implementation of checklists [15].

Patient Safety tools provided by NHS Improvement include a National Reporting and Learning System (NRLS) for reporting Serious

Incidents, as well as a National Patient Safety Alerting System (NPSAS), which enables the dissemination of patient safety alerts to healthcare providers via a central alerting system [13].

Evidence-based surgical safety tools should focus on encouraging the use of huddle strategies focused on modifiable factors unique to the EGS surgical subspecialty. The EGS communication tool can work as an adjunct to the WHO SCC and potentially improve intraoperative communication and PS in EGS patients. The communication tool created in Brigham and Women Hospital, Boston MA, and Harvard Medical School, which consists of three phases: (1) identification of modifiable huddle points, (2) pilot testing, and (3) implementation of the tool in the OR, has been institutionally successfully implemented into all operating rooms. Before the surgical incision, alongside with the WHO SCC, the EGS team acknowledges if the case is classified as an EGS procedure and verbalizes the anticipated postoperative disposition of the patient. All team members are encouraged to call a team huddle to discuss any concerns at any time [23].

Effective communication is one of the most critical safety aspects in patient safety in surgery [3]. Structured communication is a critical technical tool for patient safety in surgery. Promising new strategies of standardized communication in health care include written checklists and standardized verbal communication strategies, including 'readbacks', and perioperative briefings/debriefings, in alignment with crew resource management programs from professional aviation. Despite the global implementation of surgical safety checklists in the past decade, general compliance appears poor, and serious preventable adverse events continue to occur.

On July1 2004, The United States Joint Commission published the Universal Protocol, designed to eliminate wrong site, side procedure, patient surgery. It consisted of three parts [3, 19]:

1. Patient verification of the procedure to be performed.
2. Surgical site marking
3. A time-out before starting surgery.

Surgeons need to be aware of the areas of high risk by using accurate interpersonal communication and perform preoperative briefings to confirm the correct patients, site, operation, medicine, labs and equipment needed for a successful surgery, as well as use checklists and postoperative reviews. The surgeon as a team leader can help change the underlying tone of surgical experience by embracing these patient-centered tools [19].

Preventive strategies like The Universal Protocol consist of verification, site marking and "time out", fulfilled by a collaborative team approach. The Universal Protocol is a mandatory safety standard designed to eliminate wrong procedures by preoperative verification, site marking, and "time out" process to confirm the correct patient, procedure, site/side before any operation. Good teamwork, communication and redundant systems are the only way to reduce WSS. Institutions that have implemented medical team training programs and checklists, briefings and debriefings have substantially reduced the rate of WSS and overall surgical mortality [8].

Large cohort studies indicate that complication rates are approximately 15% for EGS patients requiring surgery, where wound-related complications are most common, followed by pulmonary issues. Mortality rates are relatively low, around 1.5% across multiple large studies, and have declined over time despite increasing volume, where postoperative stroke, major bleeding, and acute myocardial infarction present the highest risks for death [24].

The Lancet Commission on Global Surgery proposed the perioperative mortality rate (POMR) as one of the six key indicators of the strength of a country's surgical system. To improve the usefulness of POMR as a safety benchmark, standard reporting items should be included with any POMR estimate. Choosing a basket of procedures for which POMR is tracked may offer institutions and countries the standardisation required to meaningfully compare surgical outcomes across contexts and improve population health outcomes [65]. Perioperative mortality rates (POMR) though frequently reported in low-income and middle-income country lacks standardised approach for reporting and risk stratification, resulting in wide variation in POMR across procedures and specialties. A quality assessment checklist for surgical mortality studies could improve mortality reporting and facilitate benchmarking across sites and countries.

As Standard Operating Procedure (SOP) non-compliance has been a prominent reported cause of incidents reporting of non-compliance with SOPs associated with human failure by professionals themselves is an important area for improvement. Shortcomings in communication, mistakes, and forgetting are important targets for improvement to reduce perioperative incidents. Acknowledgement of the risk of human attitude, behaviour and failure are a prerequisite and a challenge for the development of tools to improve guideline adherence and effective communication, in order to improve perioperative patient safety [66].

Medication reconciliation in trauma is highly inaccurate and puts patients at risk for adverse events and poor clinical outcomes, therefore tools and techniques to improve its accuracy in patient population is needed [67].

Healthcare-Failure-Mode-Effects-Analysis (HFMEA) is a methodology which allows for hazardous process failures to be prospectively identified when managing deteriorating patients, assessing surgical competence and safe postoperative care and solutions to be recommended. Observations on surgical wards in 3 London hospitals with 100% response, discovered that outdated communication technology, understaffing, and hierarchical barriers were identified as root failure causes of escalation of care process in surgery. The expert consensus group recommended defined escalation protocols, human factors education, enhanced communication technology, and improved clinical supervision as basic risk management tools [68].

The current objective for safety in surgical practice integrates training, education, research, and delivery of clinical care requiring cooperation among the responsible institutions. The classification of the safe behaviours relevant to surgery, Non-Technical Surgical Skills for Surgeons, has made a major contribution to surgeons, educators, and curriculum developers appreciating the importance, content, and teaching of patient safety, for better understanding of operating team members social behaviours and cognitive skills needed to ensure safe and efficient surgical performance [20].

Efforts to reduce the high mortality and morbidity in EGS should include standardized EGS definitions, EGS severity assessment, risk-adjusted outcomes using a national EGS registry, inclusion of operative and nonoperative care, and development of standardized EGS patient care using evidence-based guidelines and bundles [30].

Success in patient safety depends on several factors that include identification, revision of systems, education, and training to address known patient safety issues. Medical educators and mentors must understand and practice the culture of patient safety so the new generation of surgeons will incorporate the same values intuitively by mimicking the leadership [14].

More complete understanding of task shifting, as a strategy to expand the surgical workforce, will strengthen strategic planning of surgical providers where shortages in the global surgical workforce lead to lack of access to surgical care of billions people worldwide [69].

Although there is an overall decrease in the number and severity of incorrect surgical procedures telling people to follow the policy is not enough to prevent incorrect surgery. The tools for risk management could be application of specialty-specific safety measures, continued leadership support and peer-to-peer communication, mindfully conducting time-outs, using standardized procedures, universal protocol, and human factors engineering to work toward eliminating incorrect surgical adverse events [21].

Solutions to reduce cognitive biases and enhance risk management are not very apparent like other areas of patient safety. Simple strategies include feedback and follow up, increase perception, making expertise more available," time out" to decrease reliance on memory, awareness of fatigue, stress, burnout and following guidelines. More advanced strategies are control of biases, computer based decision support system, simulation, game training and metacognition and cognitive forcing [3].

Recent publications emphasize the fact that our current patient safety protocols are indeed not safe in protecting our patients from suffering unintended and preventable harm [70].

Current approach for improving safety culture and engaging frontline clinicians to identify and mitigate defects in care delivery is The Johns Hopkins University, Comprehensive Unit-based Safety Program (CUSP), which discusses the scope and prevalence of perioperative harm, causes of error in healthcare, and perioperative never events. It analyzes safe practices, cognitive workload, fatigue, and the effects of noise in the OR, outlining risk management tools like dynamics of surgical teams, safer perioperative team communication, and the culture of safety [71].

The structured approach to quality and safety with integrated system of care, including a physician model, and commitment to transparency, bolstered by a strong health information technology infrastructure, demonstrates that excellent care quality and patient safety can be successfully advanced within healthcare institutions even when challenged by limited resources and socially disadvantaged and complex patients [42].

Although standardization is a common tool used in any field requiring consistent, high quality outcomes, it has not been a term widely used in surgery, or medicine overall, until 2000 when the Institute of Medicine published "To Err is Human: Building a safer Healthcare System." In this publication, the lack of standardization in health care was highlighted; "standardization and simplification are two fundamental human factors principles that are widely used in safe industries and widely ignored in health care." The lack of standardization is due to the fact that every specialty is different and that each patient is unique. The exposure of errors in health care brought new light to the fact that standardization is a critical component of providing effective and safe patient care. The accelerated transition to the electronic health record (EHR) has forced standardization of care, even on the unwilling clinician. The Affordable Care Act or "Obama Care" included significant financial incentives for hospitals to adopt EHR. Around the same time, checklists, although always used, were highlighted as effective tools to improve communication and teamwork, standardizing care along the way [15]. The literature supports standardized, evidence-based care to improve patient safety in the surgical setting, including checklists and ERP. Patient complexity and hospital setting can represent barriers to implanting standardized practices, but they can be overcome with thoughtful strategies. The electronic health record is a valuable tool for standardization and patient safety, but careful attention to development and implementation of order sets and pathways is required. When partnered with changes in culture, checklists and enhanced recovery programs increase standardization and reduce surgical morbidity and mortality. Culture, patient complexity, and rotating trainees can represent challenges to standardization, but can be mitigated with thoughtful strategies [15].

Accountability is another issue which can foster risk management of PS in EGS. which is defined as the responsibility of an individual provider or practitioner (e.g. physician or provider) in the care that he/she does or does not provide for an individual patient. Accountability is poorly wielded as a tool to improve health care delivery and quality [3].

37.3.4 COVID 19 and Patient Safety in Emergency General Surgery

On 29thof May, 2021, WHO reported for 169,118,995 confirmed cases of COVID-19, including 3,519,175 deaths worldwide, thus revealing the huge challenges and risks facing health workers globally, working in stressful environments making them more prone to errors which can lead to patient harm [72].

Health systems and healthcare workers all around the world, including emergency surgery teams, have met serious difficulties due to the rapid spread of COVID-19 [73].

Guidelines have recommended postponing, and even cancelling, all elective and semi-elective interventions, but little guidance has been provided "by surgeons for surgeons" concerning the emergency surgeries and interventions for general surgery and trauma patients [74].

Several reports on EGS patients with Covid 19 suggest that though the number of emergency surgeries performed have been reduced by half, emergency and non-postponable surgical interventions should be managed without delay and can be carried out safely in a COVID-19 pandemic [75].

Healthcare providers have always been the professionals most exposed to the risk of contracting to any kind of infection due to the nature of their profession. Elective interventions have been postponed to give care of patients with COVID-19. However, some interventions cannot be delayed, such as trauma surgery, acute abdomen, and emergency endoscopies. To maintain the sustainability of the healthcare system, the protection of healthcare providers should be the top priority. On the other hand, patients, who need emergency healthcare, should also be provided with appropriate treatment. Surgeons should act appropriately when an intervention is inevitable during the COVID-19 pandemic and choose a treatment method appropriately in the circumstances to protect themselves and their patients as much as possible [76].

Recognizing the global disastrous impact of Covid19 The World Society of Emergency Surgery educational board (WSES) conceived a position paper with the purpose of providing recommendations for the management of surgical patients in emergency setting under COVID-19 pandemic for the safety of the patient and healthcare workers based on available evidences and experienced surgeons' opinion. After performing a systematic review and meta-analysis the group of experts Deliberately and consecutively presented statements and 11 recommendations concerning Covid-19 patients in terms of diagnosis, preoperative screening, treatment/prophylaxis, indications for surgery according to TACIS, profound and exquisite safe measures for the surgeon and patient, close and specific for both surgical disease and Covid -19 prophylaxis and treatment until discharge. The aim is to provide an evidence-based guidelines for emergency surgeons to perform safe surgery during this pandemic to limit the diffusion of the SARSCoV-2 infection and to decrease mortality rate related to COVID-19 surgical patients. The basic steps are presurgical ward screening multidisciplinary management of COVID-19 surgical patients and protective measures for the staff and safety of the patient in the operating room if an immediate surgical procedure is mandatory [77].

The COVID-19 pandemic is a reminder that besides our core duty to care, we also have duties to improve and to learn, re-evaluate strategies that have harmed patients, families, so as to improve care. When the pandemic is finally over, we should be able to look back and conclude that critical care is stronger than ever before [78].

37.3.5 Future of Emergency General Surgery and Patient Safety

As the prevalence of injuries and non-communicable diseases increases, the provision of effective surgical care will become an increasingly important priority to reduce death and disability. In the global trend towards standardisation of curricula and competency-based training a cross-nationally coordinated strategy will be important to address the burden of surgical disease [79].

> "Patient safety is a core attitude and thus needs to be introduced early and then reinforced throughout postgraduate education and continuing professional development." (*Stefan Lindgren, President of the World Federation for Medical Education*)

Patient safety should be regarded as a new basic science for health professions education. Major reforms will be needed to incorporate patient safety into the curricula of professional schools, training programs, develop competencies and changing behavior.

The new curriculum should include capabilities for providing patient-centered care, working in interdisciplinary teams, using evidence-based practices, and applying quality improvement concepts. Students should be able to see individual safety problems with system lenses, identify and test potential solutions. A major barrier is the prevailing culture of shame, blame,

and denial about medical errors. The new curriculum shall create a culture of safety, allow optimal learning and give students opportunities to practice their new skills in real world settings [80].

The WSES process of building up a common training and educational program to promote EGS formation consisted of: formulating key steps; implementation of the National Delegate Project for refining the WSES guidelines, position papers, and consensus conferences according to each country's needs; performing many courses around the world; establishing key performance indicators (KPIs) for quality assessment of systems performance in both process and clinical outcomes; and set up the WIRES project (WSES International Registry of Emergency General Surgery to evaluate results on a macrodata basis and to give index allowing stratifying, evaluating, and improving the outcomes. All these activities inevitably will positively influence the global improvement of patient safety in the field of EGS [81].

Efforts to reduce the high mortality and morbidity in EGS should include standardized EGS definitions, EGS severity assessment, risk-adjusted outcomes using EGS registry, inclusion of operative and nonoperative care, and development of standardized EGS patient care using evidence-based guidelines and bundles [30].

Future risks for diagnostic and communication errors could emerge from new technology, novel procedures, and current events like the coronavirus pandemic, the growing use of urgent care, electronic health records, telehealth, and robotics.

In the era of new and ever-evolving technology we should determine how we can best utilize this information to help us become better acute care surgeons rather than letting the technology drive how we care for our patients [25].

Always ensure that benefits outweigh harms, and if there is uncertainty use your judgement and involve the patient in decision making [82].

Innovations, building research and evaluation will help us arrive more quickly to the goal of making patients safer.

Dos for PS and RM
- PS is currently recognized and highly assessed element of global healthcare.
- PS is extremely relevant and demanding for EGS.
- PS and RM are the pillars and bridges to quality achievement and improvement in EGS.
- Wider implementation into surgical practice of RM tools for PS like checklists, protocols and programs fosters easier formulation of consensus statements, guidelines and recommendations to finally reach standardization of care in EGS.

Don'ts for PS and RM
- PS and RM in EGS are still underestimated issues for the improvement of care quality.
- Error reporting and analysis are currently misunderstood basic tools for improving PS in EGS.
- Insufficient awareness and implementation of RM tools for PS in EGS is a major drawback for improving quality of care in this field.
- There is lack of enough body of scientific evidence on PS & RM in EGS to convince surgeons and decision makers for their utmost importance in quality assurance in this area.

Take-Home Messages

- PS and RM mutually are profoundly related and dependent categories in healthcare.
- PS and RM integral process, development and interaction substantially determine the patient management outcomes in medicine, surgery and especially in EGS.
- To perform effective risk management of patient safety in emergency general surgery we need protocolized and standardized pathways based on consensus statements, guidelines and recommendations.
- Recognizing the value of a culture of safety and accountability, providers must take performance measures for accountability.
- Innovations, building research and evaluation will help us arrive more quickly to the goal of making patients safer.

Multiple Choice Questions

1. The World Health Organization defines patient safety as:
   A. Uneventful treatment of patient in the healthcare system
   B. Successful medical management of every patient.
   C. **The absence of preventable harm to a patient during the process of health care**
   D. Optimal outcome in every patients' medical treatment
2. In 1919 WHO announced that adverse events occurring each year, due to unsafe care in hospitals in low- and middle-income countries account for:
   A. 134,000
   B. 1.34 million
   C. 13.4 million
   D. **134 million**
3. Patients undergoing emergency general surgery (EGS) procedures are more likely to die than patients undergoing the same procedures electively up to:
   A. up to two times
   B. up to five times
   C. **up to eight times**
   D. up to 12 times
4. Risk management in health care emerged as a result of:
   A. appeal for healthcare reform globally in the 1960s
   B. **the malpractice crisis of the 1970s**
   C. demand for multidisciplinary medical approach in 1980s
   D. profound technological advancement in medicine in 1990s.
5. Responsibilities of the healthcare risk manager include:
   A. communicating with stakeholders, documenting and reporting on risk and adverse circumstances,
   B. creating processes, policies, and procedures for responding to and managing risk and uncertainty
   C. monitor the **shifting landscape** of the healthcare risk continuum
   D. **A + B + C**
6. The WHO Surgical Safety Checklist consists of:
   A. 9 items
   B. 15 items
   C. **19 items**
   D. 25 items
7. Errors in health care may be classified as being the result of:
   A. **commission, omission or inition**
   B. cognitive and technical errors
   C. diagnostic and management errors
   D. A + B + C
8. The current objective for safety in surgical practice integrates:
   A. training and education,
   B. delivery of clinical care requiring cooperation among the responsible institutions

C. training and research,
D. **A + B + C**
9. Errors in medicine and surgery usually are result of:
    A. individual error
    B. institutional error
    C. **systemic error**
    D. team error
10. In developed countries, almost …% of all adverse events in hospitalized patients are related to surgical care, where half of the cases in which surgery led to harm are considered preventable
    A. 20%
    B. 30%
    C. 40%
    D. **50%**

References

1. Wagner C, Van der Wal G. Voor een goed begrip, bevordering patiëntveiligheid vraagt om heldere definities. Medisch Contact. 2005;60:1888–91.
2. Sayed A, Zayed M, El Qareh M, al. Patient safety in the operating room at a governmental hospital. J Egypt Public Health Assoc. 2013;88(2):85–9. https://doi.org/10.1097/01.EPX.0000430955.28520.e5.
3. Stahel P, Mauffrey C. Patient safety in surgery. London: Springer-Verlag; 2014. https://doi.org/10.1007/978-1-4471-4369-7-3.
4. WHO. World-patient-safety-day https://www.who.int/campaigns/world-patient-safety-day/2019
5. WHO. Patient safety. http://www.who.int/patientsafety/about/en, https://www.who.int/patientsafety/topics/safe-surgery/checklist/en/
6. Wu A, Bellandi T, Buckle P, al. Patient safety pearls. J Patient Safety Risk Manag. 2019;24(6):221–3. https://doi.org/10.1177/2516043519895121.
7. Pedersen KZ. Organizing patient safety: failsafe fantasies and pragmatic practices. Palgrave Macmillan. Health, Technology and Society; 2018. https://doi.org/10.1057/978-1-137-53786-7/.
8. Agrawal A. Patient Safety. A case-based comprehensive guide. Springer; 2014, ISBN: 978-1-4614-7418-0. https://doi.org/10.1007/978-1-4614-7419-7.
9. Bohnen JD, Anderson GA, Kaafarani HMA. Quality and patient safety indicators in trauma and emergency surgery: national and global considerations. Curr Trauma Rep. 2018;4:9–24.
10. Stevenson KS, Gibson SC, MacDonald D, et al. Measurement of process as quality control in the management of acute surgical emergencies. Br J Surg. 2007;94(3):376–81. https://doi.org/10.1002/bjs.5620.
11. Watters DA, Truskett PG. Reducing errors in emergency surgery. ANZ J Surg. 2013;83(6):434–7. https://doi.org/10.1111/ans.12194.
12. Weprin SA, Meyer D, Li R, et al. Incidence and OR team awareness of "near-miss" and retained surgical sharps: a national survey on United States operating rooms. Patient Saf Surg. 2021;15:14. https://doi.org/10.1186/s13037-021-00287-5.
13. Agency for Healthcare Research and Quality. Patient safety primer: systems approach; 2015. https://psnet.ahrq.gov/primers/primer/21/systems-approach
14. Kim FJ, da Silva RD, Gustafson D, et al. Current issues in patient safety in surgery: a review. Patient Saf Surg. 2015;9:26. https://doi.org/10.1186/s13037-015-0067-4/.
15. Zheng F. Patient safety. Surg Clin North Am. 2021;101(1):i. https://doi.org/10.1016/S0039-6109(20)30141-9.
16. Weiser TG, Haynes AB, Molina G, et al. Estimate of the global volume of surgery in 2012: an assessment supporting improved health outcomes. Lancet. 2015;385(Suppl 2):S11. https://doi.org/10.1016/S0140-6736(15)60806-6.
17. Imhof M. Malpractice in surgery safety culture and quality management in the Hospital De Gruyter; 2013. ISBN-13: 978-3110271324. doi: https://doi.org/10.1515/9783110271607
18. Palmer J. Report: after 20 years, why isn't patient safety better? PSQH December 2, 2020. https://www.psqh.com/analysis/report-after-20-years-why-isnt-patient-safety-better/?
19. Stahel P. Surgical patient safety. A case based approach; 2017. ISBN-10: 0071842632
20. Youngson GG, Flin R. Patient safety in surgery: non-technical aspects of safe surgical performance. Patient Safety Surg. 2010;4:4. https://doi.org/10.1186/1754-9493-4-4.
21. Neily J, Soncrant C, Mills PD, et al. Assessment of incorrect surgical procedures within and outside the operating room: a follow-up study from US Veterans Health Administration Medical Centers. JAMA Netw Open. 2018;1(7):e185147. Published 2018 Nov 2. https://doi.org/10.1001/jamanetworkopen.2018.5147.
22. Nagpal K, Vats A, Lamb B, et all. Information transfer and communication in surgery: a systematic review. Ann Surg 2010;252:225–239
23. Cohen T, Ley E, Gewertz B. Human factors in surgery. Enhancing safety and flow in patient care. Springer Nature Switzerland AG; 2020. ISBN: 978-3-030-53126-3. https://doi.org/10.1007/978-3-030-53127-0.
24. Brown C, Inaba K, Martin M, Salim A. Emergency general surgery (EGS) a practical approach. Springer International Publishing; 2019. ISBN: 978-3-319-96285-6. https://doi.org/10.1007/978-3-319-96286-3.
25. Lyu H, Najjar P, Havens J. Past, present, and future of Emergency General Surgery in the USA. Acute Med Surg. 2018;5:119–22. https://doi.org/10.1002/ams2.327.

26. Becher RD, Davis KA, Rotondo MF, et al. Ongoing evolution of emergency general surgery as a surgical subspecialty. JACS. 2018;226(2):194–200. https://doi.org/10.1016/j.jamcollsurg.2017.10.014.
27. Gale SC, Shafi S, Dombrovskiy VY, et al. The public health burden of emergency general surgery in the United States: a 10 year analysis of the Nationwide Inpatient Sample-2001-2010. J Trauma Acute Care Surg. 2014;77:202–8.
28. Kwan TL, Lai F, Lam CM, et al. Population-based information on emergency colorectal surgery and evaluation on effect of operative volume on mortality. World J Surg. 2008;32(2077–82):14.
29. Havens JM, Peetz AB, Do WS, et al. The excess morbidity and mortality of emergency general surgery. J Trauma Acute Care Surg. 2015;78:306–11.
30. Havens J, Neiman, Pooja U, Campbell B, et al. The future of emergency general surgery. Ann Surg. 2019;270(2):221–2. https://doi.org/10.1097/SLA.0000000000003183.
31. Scott JW, Tsai TC, Neiman PU, et al. Lower emergency general surgery (EGS) mortality among hospitals with higher-quality trauma care. J Trauma Acute Care Surg. 2018;84:433–40.
32. Ogola GO, Gale SC, Haider A, Shafi S. The financial burden of emergency general surgery: National estimates 2010 to 2060. J Trauma Acute Care Surg. 2015;79:444. https://doi.org/10.1097/TA.0000000000000787.
33. Hatchimonji JS, Kaufman EJ, Sharoky CE, Ma LW, Holena DN. A 'weekend effect' in operative emergency general surgery. Am J Surg. 2020;220(1):237–9. https://doi.org/10.1016/j.amjsurg.2019.11.024.
34. Kreckler S, Morgan R. Catchpole K.etal.Effective prevention of thromboembolic complications in emergency surgery patients using a quality improvement approach. BMJ Qual Safety. 2013;22:916–22.
35. Hesselink G, Berben S, Beune T, et al. Improving the governance of patient safety in emergency care: a systematic review of interventions. BMJ Open. 2016;6:e009837. https://doi.org/10.1136/bmjopen-2015-009837.
36. Columbus A, Morris M, Lilley E, et al. Critical differences between elective and emergency surgery: identifying domains for quality improvement in emergency general surgery. Surgery. 2018;163(4):832–8.
37. Miller PR. Defining burden and severity of disease for emergency general surgery. Trauma Surg Acute Care Open. 2017;2:e000089. https://doi.org/10.1136/tsaco-2017-000089.
38. Di Saverio S, Tugnoli G, Catena F, et al. Surgeon accountability for patient safety in the Acute Care Surgery paradigm: a critical appraisal and need of having a focused knowledge of the patient and a specific subspecialty experience. Patient Saf Surg. 2015;13(9):38. https://doi.org/10.1186/s13037-015-0084-3.
39. Sadhra S, Rampal K. Basic concepts and developments in health: risk assessment and management. In: Sadhra SS, Rampal KG, editors. Occupational health risk assessment and management. 4th ed. Oxford: Blackwell Science Ltd; 1999. p. 2–3.
40. Anderson O, Brodie A, Vincent CA, al. A systematic proactive risk assessment of hazards in surgical wards. Ann Surg. 2012;255(6):1086–92. https://doi.org/10.1097/SLA.0b013e31824f5f36.
41. Copeland G. Assessing and reducing risk in the general surgical patient: preoperative and perioperative factors. Clinical Risk. 2005;11(5):185–9. https://doi.org/10.1258/1356262054825885.
42. Mehler PS, Colwell CB, Stahel PF. A structured approach to improving patient safety: lessons from a public safety-net system. Patient Saf Surg. 2011;5(1):32.
43. Gallagher TH, Studdert D, Levinson W. Disclosing harmful medical errors to patients. N Engl J Med. 2007;356:2713–9. https://doi.org/10.1056/NEJMra070568.
44. Meguid RA, Bronsert MR, Hammermeister KE, et al. The surgical risk preoperative assessment system: determining which predictor variables can be automatically obtained from the electronic health record. J Patient Safety Risk Management. 2019;24(6):230–7. https://doi.org/10.1177/2516043519876489.
45. Hammermeister KE, Henderson WG, Bronsert MR, al. Bringing quantitative risk assessment closer to the patient and surgeon. A novel approach to improve outcomes. Ann Surg. 2016;263:1039–41.
46. Lambert-Kerzner A, Ford KL, Hammermeister KE, et al. Assessment of attitudes towards future implementation of the "Surgical Risk Preoperative Assessment System" (SURPAS) tool: a pilot survey among patients, surgeons, and hospital administrators. Patient Saf Surg. 2018;12:12. https://doi.org/10.1186/s13037-018-0159-z.
47. de Vries EN, Prins HA, Boermeester MA, SURPASS Collaborative Group. Effect of a comprehensive surgical safety system on patient outcomes. N Engl J Med. 2010;363:1928–37. https://doi.org/10.1056/NEJMsa0911535.
48. Henderson WG, Bronsert MR, Hammermeister KE, Lambert-Kerzner A, Meguid RA. Refining the predictive variables in the "Surgical Risk Preoperative Assessment System" (SURPAS): a descriptive analysis. Patient Saf Surg. 2019;13:28. https://doi.org/10.1186/s13037-019-0208-2.
49. Domingues CA, Coimbra R, Poggetti RS, Nogueira LS, de Sousa RMC. New Trauma and Injury Severity Score (TRISS) adjustments for survival prediction. World J Emerg Surg. 2018;13:12. https://doi.org/10.1186/s13017-018-0171-8.
50. Kaafarani HMA, et al. Prospective validation of the Emergency Surgery Score in emergency general surgery: an Eastern Association for the Surgery of Trauma multicenter study. J Trauma Acute Care Surg. 2020;89(1):118–24. https://doi.org/10.1097/TA.0000000000002658.
51. Lees N., Peden C., Dhesi J.& al. The Royal College of Surgeons of England Working Group on the perioperative care of the high-risk general surgical patient.

The high-risk general surgical patient: raising the standard. updated recommendations on the perioperative care of the high-risk general surgical patient; 2018. ©The Royal College of Surgeons of England
52. Gaitanidis A, Mikdad S, Breen K, et al. The Emergency Surgery Score (ESS) accurately predicts outcomes in elderly patients undergoing emergency general surgery. Am J Surg. 2020;220(4):1052–7. https://doi.org/10.1016/j.amjsurg.2020.02.017. Epub 2020 Feb 17.
53. Havens JM, Columbus AB, Seshadri AJ, et al. Risk stratification tools in emergency general surgery. Trauma Surg Acute Care Open. 2018;3(1):e000160. https://doi.org/10.1136/tsaco-2017-000160.
54. Li N, Marshall D, Sykes M, al. Systematic review of methods for quantifying teamwork in the operating theatre. BJS Open. 2018;2(2):42–51. https://doi.org/10.1002/bjs5.40.
55. Messano GA, Spaziani E, Turchetta F, et al. Risk management in surgery. G Chir. 2013;34(7-8):231–7. https://doi.org/10.11138/gchir/2013.34.7.231.
56. Rapala, Kathryn and Leonhardt, Kathryn, Risk management & patient safety: focus on the patient and the rest falls into place (2009). College of Nursing Faculty Research and Publications. 828. https://epublications.marquette.edu/nursing_fac/828
57. Kuhn AM, Youngberg BJ. The need for risk management to evolve to assure a culture of safety. BMJ Qual Safety. 2002;11:158–62.
58. What is risk management in healthcare? NEJM Catalyst; April 25, 2018. https://catalyst.nejm.org/doi/full/10.1056/CAT.18.0197/
59. Carroll R. Risk management handbook for health care organizations, Student Edition American Society for Healthcare Risk Management (ASHRM). ISBN: 978-0-470-30017-6, April 2009 Jossey-Bass.
60. Perry W, Kelley E. Checklists, global health and surgery: a five-year checkup of the WHO Surgical Safety checklist programme. Clinical Risk. 2014;20(3):59–63. https://doi.org/10.1177/1356262214535734.
61. Cheney C. Combine surgery checklists to boost patient safety and clinical outcomes. Health Leaders Media; 2020.
62. Storesund A, Haugen AS, Flaatten H, et al. Clinical efficacy of combined surgical patient safety system and the world health organization's checklists in surgery: a nonrandomized clinical trial. JAMA Surg. 2020;155(7):562–70. https://doi.org/10.1001/jamasurg.2020.0989.
63. Gillespie BM, Marshall A. Implementation of safety checklists in surgery: a realist synthesis of evidence. Implement Sci. 2015;10:137. https://doi.org/10.1186/s13012-015-0319-9.
64. Tan J, Ngwayi JR, Ding Z, et al. Attitudes and compliance with the WHO surgical safety checklist: a survey among surgeons and operating room staff in 138 hospitals in China. Patient Saf Surg. 2021;15:3. https://doi.org/10.1186/s13037-020-00276-0.
65. Ng-Kamstra JS, Arya S, Greenberg SLM, et al. Perioperative mortality rates in low-income and middle-income countries: a systematic review and meta-analysis. BMJ Glob Health. 2018;3(3):e000810. https://doi.org/10.1136/bmjgh-2018-000810.
66. Heideveld-Chevalking AJ, Calsbeek H, Damen J, et al. The impact of a standardized incident reporting system in the perioperative setting: a single center experience on 2563 'near-misses' and adverse events. Patient Saf Surg. 2014;8:46. https://doi.org/10.1186/s13037-014-0046-1.
67. DeAntonio JH, Nguyen T, Chenault G, al. Medications and patient safety in the trauma setting: a systematic review. World J Emerg Surg. 2019;14:5. https://doi.org/10.1186/s13017-019-0225-6.
68. Johnston M, Arora S, Anderson O, King D, Behar N, Darzi A. Escalation of care in surgery: a systematic risk assessment to prevent avoidable harm in hospitalized patients. Ann Surg. 2015;261(5):831–8. https://doi.org/10.1097/SLA.0000000000000762.
69. Federspiel F, Mukhopadhyay S, Milsom P, et al. Global surgical and anaesthetic task shifting: a systematic literature review and survey. Lancet. 2015;385(Suppl 2):S46. https://doi.org/10.1016/S0140-6736(15)60841-8.
70. Landrigan CP, Parry GJ, Bones CB, et al. Temporal trends in rates of patient harm resulting from medical care. N Engl J Med. 2010;363:2124–34. https://doi.org/10.1056/NEJMsa1004404.
71. Sanchez J. Handbook of perioperative and procedural patient safety. Elsevier Publishing; 2020. ISBN: 9780323661799.
72. https://covid19.who.int; https://www.who.int/campaigns/world-patient-safety-day/2020
73. Flemming S, Hankir M, Ernestus R-I, et al. Surgery in times of COVID-19—recommendations for hospital and patient management. Langenbecks Arch Surg. 2020;405:359–64.
74. Kamer E, Çolak T. What to do when a patient infected with COVID-19 needs an operation: a pre-surgery, peri-surgery and post-surgery guide. Turk J Colorectal Dis. 2020;30:1–8.
75. Sert O, Kayaoglu S. Performing general surgery emergencies safely during COVID-19 outbreak. J Anesthesia Intensive Care Emerg Pain Med. 2021;17(1):20–5. https://doi.org/10.22514/sv.2020.16.0077.
76. Gok AFK, Eryilmaz M, Ozmen MM, Alimoglu O, Ertekin C, Kurtoglu MH. Recommendations for trauma and emergency general surgery practice during COVID-19 pandemic. Turk J Trauma Emerg Surg. 2020;26(3):335–42. https://doi.org/10.14744/tjtes.2020.79954/.
77. Simone D, et al. The management of surgical patients in the emergency setting during COVID-19 pandemic: the WSES position paper. World J Emerg Surg. 2021;16 https://doi.org/10.1186/s13017-021-00349-0.
78. Arabi YM, Azoulay E, Al-Dorzi HM, et al. How the COVID-19 pandemic will change the future of critical care. Intensive Care Med. 2021;47(3):282–91. https://doi.org/10.1007/s00134-021-06352-y.

79. Zerhouni YA, Abu-Bonsrah N, Mehes M, et al. General surgery education: a systematic review of training worldwide. Lancet. 2015;385(Suppl 2):S39. https://doi.org/10.1016/S0140-6736(15)60834-0.
80. Wu A, Busch I. Patient safety: a new basic science for professional education. GMS. J Med Educ. 2019;36(2):Doc21. https://doi.org/10.3205/zma001229.
81. Coccolini F, Kluger Y, Catena F, al. WSES worldwide emergency general surgery formation and evaluation project. World J Emerg Surg. 2018;13:13. https://doi.org/10.1186/s13017-018-0174-5.
82. Justin Morgenstern, "Stop saying "First, do no harm"", First10EM blog, July 20, 2020.

38. Quality Evaluation in Emergency General Surgery

Michael Sugrue, Randal Parlour, Brendan Skelly, and Angus Watson

38.1 Introduction

A major challenge for health services worldwide is dealing with variations in emergency general surgery care (EGS) [1–3]. Frequently the care delivered to EGS patients is considered to be sub-optimal [4, 5]. Patients with emergency surgical conditions need prompt attention, early diagnosis, and excellence in treatment to ensure good outcomes. To achieve these goals, a system with adequate planning, resourcing, and monitoring has to be in place. There is abundant local, national, and international evidence that clinical decision-making in EGS, while improving, is frequently sub-optimal [6] and this impacts negatively upon the quality and safety of care and patient outcomes. EGS patients are characterised by extremely demanding intraoperative and perioperative complexities, which are exacerbated by a paucity of evidence-based guidelines, pathways and quality metrics [7, 8]. This chapter outlines areas in EGS care to lay a foundation for improving patient outcomes, enhancing the quality and safety of patient care.

> **Learning Goals**
> - This chapter will outline the concept of achieving quality care in EGS and highlight the value of key outcomes and performance indicators.

38.2 Context: Defining the Problem

It has been reported previously that EGS, and its associated burden, account for more than half of the surgical workload across the NHS [9, 10] and half of all surgical mortality within the United States [11]. This is compounded by inefficient triage of patients presenting with abdominal pain; wide variability in diagnostic pathology testing rates between clinical teams and wide variability in outcome rates following emergency surgery. This marked variation in outcomes and the provision of care is exacerbated by the high-risk nature of the speciality. Saunders et al. (2012) found that mortality for emergency laparotomy ranged from 3.6 to 41.7 per cent in 35 NHS hospitals, while a report from the National Emergency Laparotomy Audit (NELA), published in 2015, found stark variation in compliance with key standards, such as early input by senior clinicians, timely antibiotic therapy and documentation of risk of death [6, 12]. NELA identified the overall mortality rate for emergency laparotomy as 15% and this has now fallen to under 10% [13]. In a review by Watson et al. [14], it was indicated that in more than 1 in 10 cases, patients with a high-risk diagnosis, who underwent a major EGS procedure during the study period, died in the hospital within 30 days of their surgical intervention making an EGS laparotomy one of the most lethal procedures to have in the hospital. The rates of mortality and complications are almost five times greater than those for elective procedures. Gale et al, in a 10-year study across acute hospitals within the United States, found EGS activity accounted for 7%–11% of hospital admissions [15]. Patients requiring emergency surgical care are frequently the sickest, are older people and have significant co-morbidities and poorer outcomes. There are approximately 150,000 emergency surgery patients admitted annually in Ireland [16], and close to 14 million in the European Union.

The global burden of death and disability associated with emergency general surgical conditions is considerably higher than that for contrasting health conditions which attract significantly increased attention and investment. For example, the annual number of deaths from the top 11 emergency surgical conditions (over 1 million) is considerably higher than the number of maternal deaths globally (250,000).

38.3 Towards Quality EGS Care

The barriers to achieving high-quality, safe and effective EGS care across health systems require many different linked disciplines to come together. Within the United States previous indications implied that specific national quality targets for EGS were being realised [1]. Unfortunately, there appears to be a lack of adoption of agreed-on criteria for the optimal care of EGS patients across a majority of acute hospitals and extensive variation regarding the processes of care [17]. These barriers can be primarily classified as related to both organisational and provider-level factors. For instance, issues aligned to inflexible hospital infrastructures and/or the presence or absence of a dedicated surgical team. These factors impact negatively upon intended improvements in accessibility, quality and cost-effectiveness of EGS care.

Additional significant components, recognised by Daniel and colleagues (2019), have the capacity to heighten risk and increase the likelihood that patients will be in receipt of suboptimal care. These comprise lack of access to advanced imaging; absence of proactive EGS quality initiatives; lack of dedicated operating theatre time for unscheduled cases; surgeons not being freed of elective responsibilities while covering EGS services. An examination of empirical literature reveals a composite of alternative constituent features which also have the potential to play a critical role. Lim et al. [18] and Chana et al. [10] propose that the prompt availability of both a consultant surgeon and operating theatre can reduce both patient length of stay and potential complications for EGS conditions.

A further study [19], employing a retrospective cohort analysis of 69,490 EGS patients admitted between 2007 and 2012, examined variation in outcomes for EGS patients in Australia, the United Kingdom and the United States. In particular, the authors focused on hospital-level and patient-level variables and how these may impact both patient outcomes and the delivery of high-quality care. In particular, Chana and colleagues identified the role played by hospital structures in establishing and maintaining variations in care. This revealed a number of domains within which EGS care could be enhanced, including intensive care unit capacity and consultant workload. Advances in these domains alone resulted in significant improvements in patient mortality and underline the multi-disciplinary nature of EGS care. These findings are supported by further work undertaken within the UK [20]. Significant improvements that can impact positively upon the quality of care delivery have also been demonstrated through the adoption of a quality-driven and team-oriented approach [21].

A number of contemporary and pivotal strategic reports relating to EGS care have been reported in many countries; Ireland [16, 22, 23]; United Kingdom [14, 24, 25]; Great Britain and Ireland [26]; United States [27] giving insight into the ongoing challenges and limitations across the scope of EGS and have emphasised the need for improvements in the delivery of the quality and safety of EGS care whilst also outlining possible mechanisms through which this transformation can be achieved. They also refer to the overriding need to enhance the patient experience of EGS care.

In a review of the standards of emergency surgical service provision [24], the authors highlight the current lack of data for benchmarking to improve the quality of care. This stands in sharp contrast to a range of elective procedures where audit results indicate year-on-year improvements. The report further identifies the need and opportunity to both agree on optimal pathways and to develop quality indicators and performance measures for patients requiring unscheduled surgical care. Unfortunately, EGS care currently is often perceived as unscheduled but in fact, is 'very scheduled' with large numbers of admissions occurring with regular precision often in the evening and at night time.

In 2017 Donegal Clinical Research Academy in conjunction with WSES held the first global summit on performance outcomes in EGS [28]. This summit established a solid foundation for

Table 38.1 Keys to effective EGS quality systems

Designation of emergency surgical services
Leadership: Directors of EGS and ASU
Quality Patient care metrics 1/4 reported.
Emergency Surgical Teams and Support Staff
Training/Education in EGS and PROMS
Patient follow-up, benchmarking and quality initiatives
Incentivise higher-value healthcare
Comprehensive research programs
Patient and Family Partnerships

performance indicators in clinical and systems delivery in EGS care. Watson et al. [14] also advocated the systematic use of protocols and pathways in EGS. Interestingly, they also propound the introduction of new roles in EGS such as advanced nurse practitioners which, they indicate, can make a significant impact on the quality of care delivered to EGS patients.

Li Hsee and colleagues in Auckland, have made tremendous progress in advancing care in EGS with the use of Acute Surgical Units and quality indicators. Hsee and colleagues, in their white paper at the Donegal Summit in 2016, identify key aspects of an EGS system (Table 38.1) [28, 29].

38.3.1 Leadership

Clinical leadership in emergency surgery is paramount and needs to be identified early on. The appointment should be a well-respected surgeon who has a clear understanding of the acute surgical process and a commitment to quality surgical care. Clinical governance is achieved through the support and partnership of surgical colleagues, senior hospital management and often the institutional chief executive. An appointed steering group may be beneficial to advocate for the resources of an emergency surgical service.

38.3.2 Patient Care

There should be a balance between elective and emergency surgical streams. Patient-centred care often requires a separation of emergency surgical patient care from elective settings. Emergency surgical resources need to be protected and ring-fenced to that effect. A clear acute surgical pathway from admission to discharge must be recognized and developed. Timely access to investigations, diagnostic and pathology services contribute to the efficiency of emergency service. Where possible a dedicated operating room and sessions must be made available to the emergency surgical service. Emergency surgical care is led by consultant surgeons to provide timely and accurate decision-making and treatment. There is a potential to decrease healthcare costs by reducing unnecessary investigations. Emergency surgical cases, where clinically appropriate, should be scheduled during standard hours. The aim is to reduce unnecessary surgery after hours and overnight. There is evidence that prolonged hours increase the risk of serious errors that can lead to patient harm and death. A multi-disciplinary approach to the overall care of the patient is vital. This would include nurse specialists and allied health providers.

38.3.3 Emergency Surgical Team and Supporting Staff

While there is no set team structure, emergency surgical team design depends on the cohort of patients, case mix and resources available. Appropriately trained and competent healthcare professionals are required to provide the service. The consultant surgeon should not have other commitments while managing the emergency surgical service. It is ideal for surgical trainees to gain competency in the management of emergency surgical patients. It is also valuable to involve nursing colleagues. A multi-disciplinary radiology meeting dedicated to emergency surgical service will provide education and improve patient care. Sufficient administrative support must be employed to facilitate the team.

38.3.4 Training

While the aim is to improve surgical patient care, there is an opportunity to provide training for emergency surgeons. This allows surgical fellows and senior residents to obtain concentrated expertise in the acute and emergency aspects of surgery. As an emergency surgical service is a consultant-led service, it facilitates the supervision of residents, interns and medical students. It is also an invaluable field for training in surgical nursing and emergency anaesthesiology. Accreditation is required in emergency surgical training. The world-leading Emergency Abdominal Surgery course (EASC) established in 2012 has now 3 levels of courses including medical student, trainee/junior consultant and consultant courses. With over 2000 trained in 12 countries, EASC provides an excellent platform for emergency abdominal surgery (www.easccourse.com) [30]. The European Society of Trauma and Emergency Surgery's (ESTES) Emergency Surgery Course (ECS) offers a practical 2-day course in a broad range of EGS conditions. Many surgical colleges have already incorporated emergency surgical training into their curriculum. Studies have shown certified emergency programs improve outcomes in patients undergoing emergency surgery.

Chief residents and Senior registrars in the Unit should be encouraged to undertake **European Board of Surgery Qualification in Emergency Surgery.** This two-stage quality validation process consists of an eligibility assessment and an examination leading to the award of the title 'Fellow of the European Board of Surgery in Emergency Surgery—F.E.B.S./EmSurg'. A UEMS fellowship (F.E.B.S.) would offer a high-level validated quality-controlled process reflecting knowledge and skills in emergency surgery. Suggested standards in optimal education and training are shown in Table 38.2

38.3.5 Patient Follow-Up, Benchmarking and Quality Initiatives

Follow-up for patients post-discharge from the emergency surgical service is an integral part of emergency surgical care. Monitoring includes factors such as histology, wound reviews and

38.4 EGS Registry

Internationally, trauma registries have played a significant role during the past fifty years in enhancing trauma care delivery [7]. The evolution of an extensive and systematic National Trauma Data Bank (NTDB) allowed benchmarking and created an appreciation of risk-adjusted outcomes. Surgical Colleges including RCSI [16, 23] have acknowledged the impact of models of care and clinical registries in improving the delivery of surgical care. However, there is an underlying requirement for relevant urgent transformation of EGS services focusing in particular upon the implementation of multi-disciplinary clinical care pathways; data generation to demonstrate the variation between surgical specialities and their outcomes; rapid access to diagnostic services; and accurate EGS information systems, audits of process and clinical outcomes, including patient-reported outcomes.

In a recent examination of the past, present, and future of Emergency General Surgery in the USA, Lyu et al. [31] outlined the significance of prospectively collected clinical data in order to suitably risk-adjust for the disparate EGS patient population. The provision of high-quality and safe EGS care is a complex matter impacted by multifarious elements [32].

Evans et al. [33] have previously defined a clinical registry as a system for the acquisition of a defined minimum data set from patients who experience a specific procedure or therapy; are diagnosed with a disease; or use a healthcare resource. An example of the Letterkenny University hospital minimum data set is shown in Fig. 38.1.

Larsson et al. [34] have argued for a more expansive definition that acknowledges clinical registries as significant institutional catalysts for interventions to enhance outcomes over time. This recognises the role played by these registries in the analysis of variation in care delivery, and based upon this, the identification and adoption of 'best practice'. Key outcome and performance indicators should be an integral part of a registry and EGS system and examples are shown in Table 38.3.

Table 38.2 Key standards in training in emergency surgery care

Setting goals for education culture and environment
Governance and resource management-keeping costs to a minimum
Facilitating Learners either through real or virtual platforms
Supporting surgical trainers
Supporting a multidisciplinary teamwork approach as per EASC Courses
Curricula development accreditation and performance assessment
Innovation and skills development as with ESTES ESC
Access to learning opportunities in all aspects of emergency surgery
Accreditation of education and competency assessment
Feedback analysis

further patient assessments. Participation in departmental mortality and morbidity audits is essential. Data collection and interval reviews of key performance indicators are also valuable. Surgical services should benchmark common measures for service and patient care improvement. Patient participation in EGS service planning and feedback is essential. This can be facilitated through PROMS and PREMS whilst currently, the Association of Surgeons of Ireland Great Britain and DCRA are establishing a patient advocacy group.

38.3.6 Designation of Emergency Surgical Services

An increasing number of tertiary care hospitals are utilising a dedicated emergency surgical service with sub-speciality support. In urban and rural settings, the regionalisation of acute care has been supported. Its aim is not only to provide optimal care for the patients in the speciality but also to support for outlying community hospitals where complex surgical conditions can be transferred. It is a safety net for the improvement of emergency surgical patient care. While regionalisation and designation policies are complex with multiple competing issues, careful planning and evaluations are required. A localized policy and regional escalation plan are necessary to facilitate communication and resource utilisation.

Fig. 38.1 An example of an EGS registry minimum data set

Minimum Data Set					
Demographics					
Database no					
Unique ID					
Age					Text box
Gender					DD
Consultant Surgeon					DD
Residence pre admission					DD
Presenting Complaint					DD
Provisional Diagnosis					DD
Include in study					DD
Emergency Department					
Date					DD
Referred by					DD
Registered Time					DD
Triage Time					DD
Time Referred					DD
Time Seen					DD
Emergency Department Observations					
Pulse	/min	SpO2		%	BP mmHg
RR	/min	Temp		C	
Co-Morbidities					
	Anti-Coags				DD
Admission Lab Value Information					
WCC	DD	Hb	DD	CRP	DD
Amylase	DD	GGT	DD	Creat	DD
INR	DD	Base Excess/Deficit	DD	Lactate	DD
Imaging					
CXR					DD
PFA					DD
US	DD	Booked	DD	Performed DD	Reported DD
CT	DD	Booked	DD	Performed DD	Reported DD
MRI	DD	Booked	DD	Performed DD	Reported DD
Disposition					
Moved to	DD	Date	DD	Time	DD
Antibiotics			DD		
Surgery			DD		
Surgery					
Date Booked	DD		Time Booked		DD
Date of Surgery	DD		Time of Induction		DD
ASA Score					DD

Surgeon	DD
Procedure	DD
Findings	Text Box
Post-Op	
Destination	DD
Complications	DD
Complication Classisification/Clavien-Dindo	DD
Final Diagnosis	DD
Discharge Date	DD

Data from surgical registries may serve multiple purposes including improving the quality of healthcare, and enhancement of patient safety. The increasing sophistication and analytic capabilities of clinical registries and databases contribute considerably in all of these domains due to their use of accurate, credible, risk-adjusted, and concurrent clinical data which is acquired for these specific purposes.

We can improve healthcare through clinical registries by monitoring the quality of care, benchmarking performance, describing variations in patterns of treatment, and conducting research [35]. Registries have had a major impact upon health service research [36]; health outcomes [37]; adherence to clinical guidelines [38]; cost of care delivery [34]; improving healthcare processes and providing details of patient-reported outcomes [39].

Table 38.3 Key outcome indicator for all conditions

	Target
Small Bowel Obstruction	
1. Enrolment of the patient on the SBO pathway in ED	100%
2. Complicated SBO* seen by consultant <2 h of surgical review	90%
3. Complicated SBO having CT abdomen <4 h of surgical review.	80%
4. Gastrograffin given <24 h of admission for SBO	90%
5. Persistent SBO operated <4 days have elapsed,	90%
6. Complicated obstruction with peritonitis/strangulated hernia have surgery <4 h from surgical referral.	90%
7. Patients post laparotomy admitted to HDU/ICU.	90%
8. Laparotomy closure wound/suture ratio measured	90%
9. In-hospital wound complications <10%.	100%
10. Plain abdominal X-ray not performed	80%
Appendicitis	
Acute Appendicitis histologically confirmed	>90%
Laparoscopic approach used	>90%
Conversion to open surgery	<10%
Postoperative complications <30 days	<10%
Readmission rates 30 days post-discharge	<5%
Cholecystitis	
The abdominal US should be completed within 24 h of admission	90%
Patients admitted with acute cholecystitis should undergo cholecystectomy <3 days of admission	60%
Re-admission <90 days with recurrent cholecystitis	10%
No hospital bile leak	98
Re-admission <30 days post either cholecystectomy, cholecystostomy or ERCP	10%

Parlour et al. [40] advocate that an EGS registry, which they have developed in Ireland with EU interregional support, will promote transparency and allow quality outcome development and analysis.

In a systematic review of the impact of clinical registries on the quality of patient care and clinical outcomes, Hoque et al. [35] found limited evidence of studies that evaluated registries as an intervention to improve healthcare quality. Stey et al. [41] undertook a distinct systematic review that focused on surgical registries and how they may be used to improve the quality of surgical care. The review included eighteen registries that were consistent with the study inclusion criteria. Similar to Hoque et al. [35] there was reported evidence from multiple studies which indicated that surgical care had been improved by registry participation.

Despite any acknowledged limitations the registry concept continues to attract attention as a crucial means for improving both quality and outcomes related to the delivery of surgical care. This viewpoint is emphasised by Sedrakyan et al. [42] within a Lancet commentary that linked surgical registries with advancements in the quality of care delivery. Surgical registries facilitate access to comprehensive data on procedures, practices, and outcomes that enable an appreciation of how suboptimal outcomes may be ameliorated. Sedrakyan et al. [42] outline key characteristics of an effective surgical registry which include the need for continuous data collection, data infrastructure, establishing quality indicators, and outcome feedback to practitioners to enable improvements in healthcare.

Similarly, Larsson et al. [34] have also previously affirmed the impact of clinical registries on systematic quality improvement whilst also reducing total healthcare costs for a specific condition. This supports accountability within surgical teams by locating the responsibility for improved quality firmly in their domain and focusing attention on the common goal of improved value in healthcare. Establishing a robust emergency surgical registry can facilitate collaboration with both national and international partners that will augment research and quality improvement endeavours. The WIRES project (WSES International Registry of Emergency General Surgery) is an example of this and has been established to enable access for EGS surgeons to register their activity and to develop a worldwide register of surgical emergencies [43]. This will provide an opportunity for the evaluation of macro data facilitating stratification, evaluation and improvement of outcomes.

38.5 Emergency Surgery Outcomes Advancement Project (eSOAP)

The challenges confronting EGS services in the Republic of Ireland, Northern Ireland and Scotland are coherent with those highlighted previously in England [14]. Essentially these are relative to concerns around training, workforce and operational issues. These are central to variation in outcomes that have been identified across EGS and have been amplified by both the Health Service Executive/Royal College of Surgeons in Ireland [16] and the Nuffield Trust/Royal College of Surgeons of England [14].

Watson [14] has once again raised the fundamental necessity to address matters relating to the quality of EGS care. An example from the National Emergency Laparotomy Audit [6] is propounded which identified that almost 50% of patients admitted across England and Wales with peritonitis and requiring surgery, had yet to receive the first dose of antibiotics after 3.5 h.

Parlour and colleagues in Northern Ireland and Scotland commenced the Emergency Surgery Outcome Advancement Project (eSOAP) in late 2018 as part of a Centre for Personalised Medicine, Clinical Decision Making and Patient Safety (CPM), supported by the European Union's PEACE IV Programme, managed by the Special EU Programmes Body (SEUPB). This project has identified how to improve many aspects in the care of Appendicitis, Cholecystitis, Colorectal Surgery and EGS care generally [44–47].

38.6 Conclusion

There is an established requirement to generate quality care systems that includes a clear plan, with designated leadership, and with published transparent national (and in time global) plans for EGS. There is a need to legislate certain minimum standards of care including outcome indicators. NELA recently advocated involving local clinical teams, using EGS registry data, with regular reports and web tools, to monitor EGS performance and patient outcomes. Benchmarked data can be used to raise concerns or challenge apparent gaps in care pathways. Commissioners of care, executive and senior leadership teams are responsible for providing adequate resources, financial investment and infrastructure targeted to enable the development of quality EGS care. To save lives we need to act—we owe it to our patients and their families.

> **Take-Home Messages**
> To be a great surgeon or provider of EGS care your patients should receive high-quality care with optimal outcomes. Using key outcome indicators and performance analysis is an essential part of this.

> **Questions**
> 1. KPI are
>   A. **Key Performance Indicators**
>   B. Key Products Indicators
>   C. Key Performance Insights
>   D. Kinetics Performance Indicators
> 2. In acute appendicitis KPI are
>   A. Number of appendectomies
>   B. **% of the Normal appendix in a pathology report**
>   C. Number of US
>   D. Number of CT scans
> 3. The timing of early cholecystectomy is
>   A. **A KPI**
>   B. Unuseful
>   C. Delayed
>   D. Within 24 h
> 4. The use of a registry
>   A. Is mandatory
>   B. **Is part of a quality improvement strategy**
>   C. Is unuseful
>   D. Is outdated
> 5. KPIs are
>   A. **Useful for any clinical activity**
>   B. Unuseful
>   C. Useful only for appendicitis cholecystitis
>   D. Cost related

References

1. Santry HP, Madore JC, Collins CE, Ayturk MD, Velmahos GC, Britt LD, et al. Variations in Implementation of acute care surgery: results from a national survey of university-affiliated hospitals. J Trauma Acute Care Surg. 2015;78(1):60–7.
2. Tan BH, Mytton J, Al-Khyatt W, Aquina CT, Evison F, Fleming FJ, Griffiths E, Vohra RS. A comparison of mortality following emergency laparotomy between populations from New York state and England. Ann Surg. 2017;266(2):280–6.
3. Aggarwal G, Peden CJ, Mohammed MA, Pullyblank A, Williams B, Stephens T, et al. Evaluation of the collaborative use of an evidence-based care bundle in emergency laparotomy. JAMA Surg. 2019; https://doi.org/10.1001/jamasurg.2019.0145.
4. Royal Australasian College of Surgeons. The case for the separation of elective and emergency surgery [Internet]. RACS; 2011 [Cited 29 March 2016]. http://www.surgeons.org/media/college-advocacy/.
5. Shafi S. Pursuing quality—Emergency General Surgery Quality Improvement Program (EQIP); 2015. https://www.mdedge.com/surgery/article/101812/pursuing-quality-emergency-general-surgery-quality-improvement-program-eqip
6. NELA Project Team. First patient report of the National Emergency Laparotomy Audit. London: RCoA; 2015. ISBN: 978-1-900936-12-5.
7. Becher RD, Meredith JW, Chang MC, et al. Creation and implementation of an emergency general surgery registry modelled after the National Trauma Data Bank. J Am Coll Surg. 2012;214:156–63.
8. Parlour R, Johnson A, Loughlin P, Watson A, Sugrue M, Drake A. Time for metrics in emergency surgical care - the role of an emergency surgery registry. Anaesthesiol Intensive Ther. 2019;51(4):306–15. https://doi.org/10.5114/ait.2019.87360.
9. Behar N, King D. Proposal for a new specialty: emergency general surgery. http://careers.bmj.com/careers/advice/view-article.html?id=20007882; 2012.
10. Chana P, Burns EM, Arora S, et al. A systematic review of the impact of dedicated emergency surgical services on patient outcomes. Ann Surg. 2016;263:20–7.
11. Scott JW, Olufajo OA, Brat GA, et al. Use of national burden to define operative emergency general surgery. JAMA Surg. 2016;151(6):e160480. https://doi.org/10.1001/jamasurg.2016.0480.
12. Saunders DI, Murray D, Pichel AC, Varley S, Peden CJ, Network UKEL. Variations in mortality after emergency laparotomy: the first report of the UK Emergency Laparotomy Network. Br J Anaesth. 2012;109(3):368–75.
13. NELA Project Team. Sixth patient report of the National Emergency Laparotomy Audit. London: RCoA; 2020. ISBN: 978-1-900936-24-8.
14. Watson R, Crump H, Imison C, Currie C, Gaskins M. Emergency general surgery: challenges and opportunities. Research Report. Nuffield Trust; 2016.
15. Gale SC, Shafi S, Dombrovskiy VY, Arumugam D, Crystal JS. The public health burden of emergency general surgery in the United States: a 10-year analysis of the Nationwide Inpatient Sample–2001 to 2010. J Trauma Acute Care Surg. 2014;77:202–8.
16. Royal College of Surgeons in Ireland (RCSI). Model of care for acute surgery and the national policy and procedure for safe surgery. Royal College of Surgeons in Ireland; 2013. http://www.rcsi.ie/files/surgery/docs/20131030121710_RCSI_Model_of_Care_for_Acute_S.pdf
17. Daniel VT, Ingraham AM, Khubchandani JA, Ayturk D, Kiefe CI, Santry HP. Variations in the delivery of emergency general surgery care in the era of acute care Surgery. Joint Commission J Qual Patient Saf. 2019;45(1):14–23.
18. Lim DW, Ozegovic D, Khadaroo RG, et al. NELA project team. First patient report of the National Emergency Laparotomy Audit. RCoA London, 2015. World J Surg. 2013;37(2266) https://doi.org/10.1007/s00268-013-2118-2.
19. Chana P, Joy M, Casey N, Chang D, Burns EM, Arora S, Darzi AW, Faiz OD, Peden CJ. Cohort analysis of outcomes in 69 490 emergency general surgical admissions across an international benchmarking collaborative. BMJ Open. 2017;7(3):e014484. https://doi.org/10.1136/bmjopen-2016-014484.
20. Symons NR, Moorthy K, Almoudaris AM, Bottle A, Aylin P, Vincent CA, Faiz OD. Mortality in high-risk emergency general surgical admissions. Br J Surg. 2013;100:1318–25. https://doi.org/10.1002/bjs.9208.
21. Dijkink S, van der Wilden GM, Krijnen P, et al. Polytrauma patients in the Netherlands and the USA: a bi-institutional comparison of processes and outcomes of care. Injury. 2017;49:104.
22. Sugrue G, Conroy R, Sugrue M. Radiology & emergency surgery. In: Sugrue M, Catena F, Coccolini F, Kluger Y, Maier R, Moore E, editors. Resources for optimal care of emergency surgery. 1st ed. Springer International Publishing. (in press). ISBN: 978-3-030-49362-2.
23. Royal College of Surgeons in Ireland (RCSI). Surgical services 2020 and beyond. Royal College of Surgeons in Ireland; 2017. http://www.rcsi.ie/files/surgery/docs/20170419030935_1345%20Mealy%202017.pdf
24. Royal College of Surgeons of England (RCSE). Emergency surgery: standards for unscheduled surgical care. Guidance for providers, commissioners and service planners. The Royal College of Surgeons of England; 2011. www.rcseng.ac.uk/publications/docs/emergency-surgery-standards-for-unscheduledcare
25. Royal College of Surgeons of England (RCSE). Emergency surgery policy briefing. The Royal College of Surgeons of England; 2014.
26. Anderson I. The future of emergency surgery—a joint document. Association of Surgeons of Great Britain and Ireland; 2015. https://www.acpgbi.org.uk/content/uploads/2016/07/Future-of-EGS-joint-document_Iain-Anderson_140915.pdf

27. Institute of Medicine. IOM report: the future of emergency care in the United States health system. Acad Emerg Med. 2006;13:1081–5.
28. Sugrue M, Maier R, Moore EE, Boermeester M, Catena F, Coccolini F, et al. Proceedings of resources for optimal care of acute care and emergency surgery consensus summit Donegal Ireland. World J Emerg Surg. 2017;12:47.
29. Hsee L, Devaud M, Middleberg L, Jones W, Civil I. Acute surgical unit at Auckland City Hospital: a descriptive analysis. ANZ J Surg. 2012;82(9):588–91.
30. https://www.easccourse.com. Accessed 7 May 2021.
31. Lyu HG, Najjar P, Havens JM. Past, present, and future of Emergency General Surgery in the USA. Acute Med Surg. 2018;5(2):119–22. https://doi.org/10.1002/ams2.327.
32. Baggaley A, Robb L, Paterson-Brown S, et al. Improving the working environment for the delivery of safe surgical care in the UK: a qualitative cross sectional analysis. BMJ Open. 2019;9:e023476. https://doi.org/10.1136/bmjopen-2018-023476.
33. Evans SM, Scott IA, Johnson NP, et al. Development of clinical-quality registries in Australia: the way forward. Med J Aust. 2011;194:360–3.
34. Larsson S, Lawyer P, Garellick G, et al. Use of 13 disease registries in 5 countries demonstrates the potential to use outcome data to improve health care's value. Health Aff (Millwood). 2012;31:220–7. https://doi.org/10.1377/hlthaff.2011.0762.
35. Hoque DME, Kumari V, Hoque M, Ruseckaite R, Romero L, Evans SM. Impact of clinical registries on quality of patient care and clinical outcomes: a systematic review. PLoS One. 2017;12(9):e0183667.
36. Hickey GL, Grant SW, Cosgriff R, Dimarakis I, Pagano D, Kappetein AP, et al. Clinical registries: governance, management, analysis and applications. Eur J Cardio-Thorac Surg. 2013;
37. Gliklich RE, Dreyer NA, Leavy MB. Registries for evaluating patient outcomes: a user's guide. 3rd ed. Agency for Health Care Research and Quality; 2014.
38. Fonarow GC, Yancy CW, Heywood JT. Adherence to heart failure quality-of-care indicators in US hospitals: analysis of the ADHERE Registry. Arch Internal Med. 2005;165(13):1469–77. https://doi.org/10.1001/archinte.165.13.1469.
39. Breckenridge K, Bekker HL, Gibbons E. How to routinely collect data on patient-reported outcome and experience measures in renal registries in Europe: an expert consensus meeting. Nephrol Dial Transplant. 2015;30(10):1605–14.
40. Parlour R, Sugrue M, Skelly B and Watson A. Emergency general surgery: inaugural registry report. Emergency Surgery Outcomes Advancement Project; 2020. https://dcra.ie/images/Emergency-General-Surgery-Inaugural-Report.pdf. ISBN: 9780992610968.
41. Stey AM, Russell MM, Ko CY, et al. Clinical registries and quality measurement in surgery: a systematic review. Surgery. 2015;157:381–95. https://doi.org/10.1016/j.surg.2014.08.097.
42. Sedrakyan A, Campbell B, Graves S, Cronenwett JL. Surgical registries for advancing quality and device surveillance. Lancet. 2016;359:1358–60. https://doi.org/10.1016/S0140-6736(16)31402-7.
43. Coccolini F, Kluger Y, Ansaloni L, et al. WSES worldwide emergency general surgery formation and evaluation project. World J Emerg Surg. 2018;13:13.
44. Badrin AS, Maguire U, Johnston A, Bucholc M, Sugrue M. Unplanned reoperation and interventional radiology post appendicectomy: a metaanalysis. HSOA J Emerg Med Trauma Surg Care. 2020;2020(7):049. https://doi.org/10.24966/ETS-8798/100049.
45. Bailey K, Choynowski M, Kabir SM, Lawler J, Badrin A, Sugrue M. Meta-analysis of unplanned readmission to hospital post-appendectomy: an opportunity for a new benchmark. ANZ J Surg. 2019;89(11):1386–91.
46. Mc Geehan G, Edelduok IM, Bucholc M, Watson A, Bodnar Z, Johnston A, Sugrue M. Systematic review and meta-analysis of wound bundles in emergency midline laparotomy identifies that it is time for improvement. Life. 2021;11(2):138.
47. Lawler J, Choynowski M, Bailey K, Bucholc M, Johnston A, Sugrue M (2020) A meta-analysis of the impact of post-operative infective complications on oncological outcomes in colorectal cancer surgery. BJS Open 2020 Oct;4(5):737.

Part II

Head, Face and Neck

Head and Brain Trauma

Giacomo Bertolini, Luca Cattani, Corrado Iaccarino, Anna Fornaciari, and Edoardo Picetti

Learning Goals
The aim of this chapter is to provide concise and practical insights about the epidemiology, pathophysiology, imaging, neuromonitoring and management of severe traumatic brain injury patients.

39.1 Introduction

Traumatic brain injury (TBI), defined by the Centers for Disease Control and Prevention as a disruption in the normal brain function caused by a bump, blow, or jolt to the head, or penetrating head injury, is a major global health problem being the first injury-related cause of death and disability worldwide [1–4]. According to the Glasgow Coma Scale (GCS) score, TBI can be clinically classified as mild (GCS 13–15), moderate (GCS 9–12) and severe (GCS 3–8) [5]. Considering the burden of TBI on the global trauma care, every physician involved in the acute management of polytrauma patients needs to have a basic knowledge about brain injury. Therefore, the aim of this chapter is to provide concise and practical insights about the epidemiology, pathophysiology, imaging, neuromonitoring and management of severe TBI patients. The challenging and difficult scenario regarding the management of polytrauma patients with concomitant head injuries will also be discussed.

39.2 Epidemiology

Globally, the annual incidence rate of TBI is close to 369 cases per 100 000 people [1]. Mild, moderate and severe TBI account for the 81%, 11% and 8% of total injuries, respectively [6]. Two different trends can be observed in the high-income (HICs) and the low–middle-income countries (LMICs) in terms of primary causes and incidence. In the HICs, the 2016 annual incidence of TBI was of 298 cases per 100 000 people, which represents a 9.6% decrease with respect to the 1990–2016 period mainly, attributable to injury-prevention and educational programmes [1]. In HICs, an epidemiological shift

G. Bertolini
Department of Neurological Surgery, Parma University Hospital, Parma, Italy

Department of Biomedical and Neuromotor Sciences (DIBINEM), University of Bologna, Bologna, Italy

L. Cattani · A. Fornaciari · E. Picetti (✉)
Department of Anesthesia and Intensive Care, Parma University Hospital, Parma, Italy
e-mail: lcattani@ao.pr.it

C. Iaccarino
Department of Biomedical, Metabolic and Neural Sciences, University of Modena and Reggio Emilia, Modena and Reggio Emilia, Italy

© The Author(s), under exclusive license to Springer Nature Switzerland AG 2023
F. Coccolini, F. Catena (eds.), *Textbook of Emergency General Surgery*,
https://doi.org/10.1007/978-3-031-22599-4_39

has been detected over this period, with the major causes of TBI being increasingly fall-related (especially in elderly patients) and not traffic-related [7–9]. Conversely, in the LMICs, the TBI incidence has been increasing up to 33% over the last decades, with many traffic-related cases that involve young patients [1, 6, 9].

39.3 Pathophysiology

Following a TBI, we can observe two phases: the primary injury and the (delayed) secondary injury [10–13]. The primary injury, inflicted at the time of the trauma, is caused by external physical forces of variable magnitude applied to the head (primary insult). These can result in skull fractures, hematomas, contusions and axonal injury [10–13]. The most effective intervention for the primary injury is the prevention of the primary insult, which can be pursued with different strategies (i.e., in case of road traffic accidents with the utilization of seat belts or helmets, speed regulation, etc.) [12]. The secondary injury, resulting from the activation of different molecular and cellular pathways by the first insult, evolves over time and is characterized by changes in axonal ionic permeability, release of excitatory neurotransmitters, mitochondrial dysfunction, energy failure, necrosis and apoptosis [10–14]. These processes are also associated with the development of cytotoxic (cellular energy failure) and vasogenic [blood–brain barrier (BBB) dysfunction] brain edema [14]. The magnitude of the secondary injury is closely associated with the neurological outcome (the greater is the magnitude, the worse is the outcome) [10–14]. Until now, no specific drugs are available in daily clinical practice to specifically target the above-mentioned pathologic pathways. Moreover, after a TBI, several secondary insults (i.e., hypotension, hypoxia, intracranial hypertension, seizures, fever, etc.) can exacerbate the secondary injury [12, 13]. In this context, the main objective of the neurocritical care is to prevent secondary insults to the injured brain.

39.3.1 Intracranial Pressure and Cerebral Perfusion Pressure

The intracranial pressure (ICP), which is generally less than 10 mmHg in physiological condition, is related to the volume of the three intracranial components: brain parenchyma (80%), blood (10%) and cerebrospinal fluid (CSF) (10%) [15–17]. These are contained inside a rigid box (the skull) and an increase in the volume of one of the three compartments, if not associated with a compensatory reduction of the others, leads to an increase in the ICP (the "Monroe-Kelly" doctrine) [15, 16]. As the volume of one of these compartments change, or an additional compartment is introduced, subsequent variations will occur according to the exponential pressure–volume relationship and the cerebral compliance (Fig. 39.1). Under physiological circumstances, an initial volume increase following a TBI is well-tolerated as at first the CSF, and then, the cerebral blood compartments are able to behave as buffer systems with a null or minimum effect on the ICP. However, after a critical point, the CSF displacement into the spinal subarachnoid space and the vascular compression exhausts their compensatory capacity. In this case, any further increase in the cranial volume, even minimal, coincides with an exponential increase in the ICP [15, 16]. The main causes of post-traumatic intracranial hypertension (ICP > 20–22 mmHg) are intracranial blood collections [i.e., acute subdural hematoma (SDH), acute epidural hematoma (EDH), etc.] and cerebral edema [12, 15–17]. Increases in ICP are associated with a reduction in cerebral perfusion pressure [CPP = mean arterial pressure (MAP)—ICP] with a consequent risk of ischemic injury [15, 16]. CPP in an adult patient after severe head injury should be maintained between 60 and 70 mmHg according to the autoregulatory status of the patient [17]. Precisely, cerebral pressure autoregulation (Fig. 39.2) is the ability of the cerebral vasculature to maintain a constant cerebral blood flow (CBF) over a range of systemic blood pressures (MAP 50–150 mmHg) [18]. The autoregulatory curve generally shifts

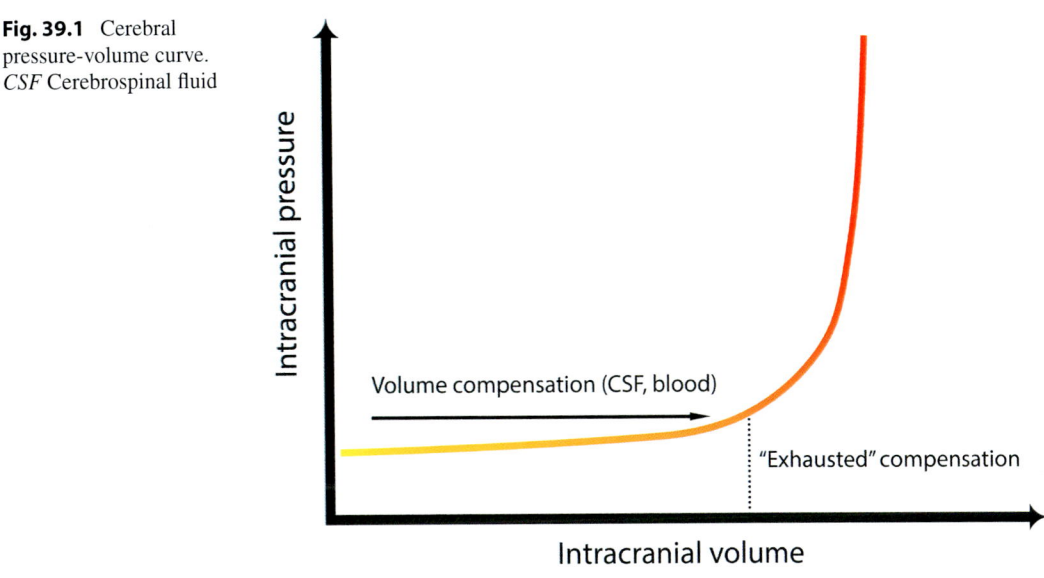

Fig. 39.1 Cerebral pressure-volume curve. *CSF* Cerebrospinal fluid

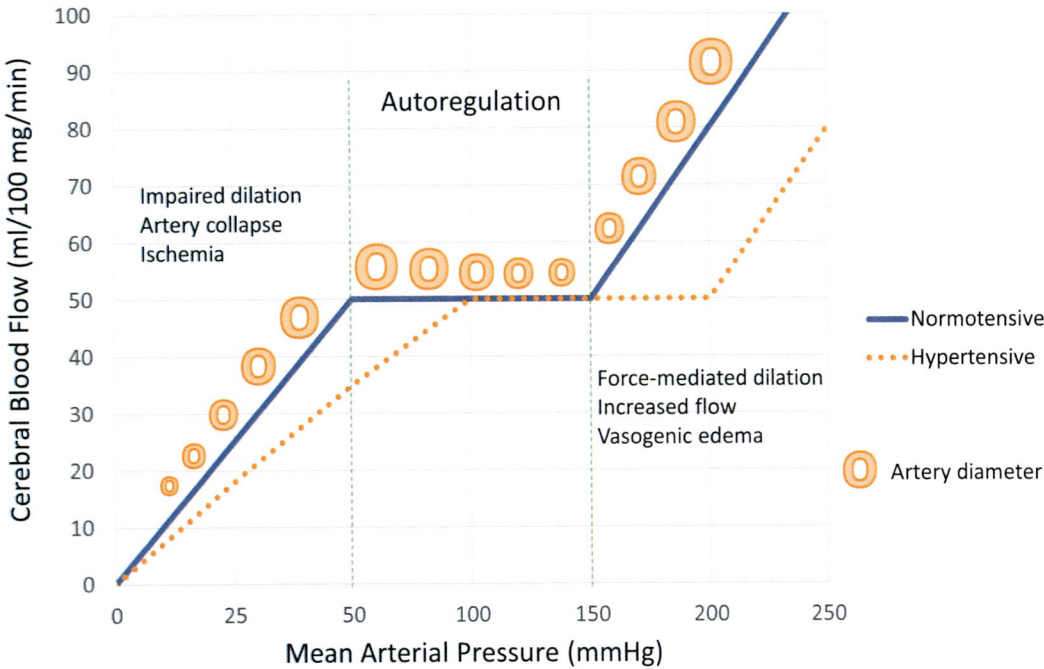

Fig. 39.2 Cerebral pressure autoregulation curve

to the right in case of chronic arterial hypertension [18]. When MAP decreases, cerebral vessels dilate to maintain CBF until they become maximally dilated. A further reduction in MAP results in CBF reduction. Contrarily, cerebral vessels constrict in response to a rise in MAP until maximum vasoconstriction is attained. At high MAP, exceeding the autoregulatory range, cerebral vessels passively dilate with a resultant increase in CBF. Considering the above, in patients with intact cerebral pressure autoregulation, an increase in MAP is associated with a reduction in ICP. The contrary (↑MAP – ↑ICP) is observed when autoregulation is lost. The latter condition is associated with an unfavorable neurological outcome in TBI [18].

39.4 Diagnosis

39.4.1 Imaging

The brain computed tomography (CT) can be considered as the most important radiological examination in the evaluation of a patient with head injury, because (especially in the acute phase) it provides us with fundamental information regarding therapy (medical and/or surgical) and monitoring (i.e., indications for ICP monitoring) [19, 20]. In particular, brain CT is widely and rapidly accessible especially in case of brain injuries requiring neurosurgical consultation (i.e., hematoma) [19, 20]. The brain CT angiography can be useful for screening patients at risk of blunt cerebrovascular injuries (i.e., arterial dissection) (Table 39.1) [19–21]. Conversely, magnetic resonance imaging (MRI) can be useful in the evaluation of brainstem and white matter axonal injuries, but considering its limited availability and longer imaging time, it is rarely utilized in the acute phase of TBI [19, 20]. The most frequent post-traumatic brain lesions are reported in Fig. 39.3.

39.4.1.1 Skull Fractures

The presence of skull fractures should carefully be investigated in TBI patients being a source of direct damage or an indirect sign of possible underlying lesions [20]. A higher mortality risk was observed in patients suffering skull fractures in severe TBI [21]. Skull fractures are generally divided into two major groups: penetrating and non-penetrating [20]. Although penetrating fractures may be a source of direct injury, as bone fragments could disrupt and damage the underlying structures (brain, vessels and dura mater), also the non-penetrating fractures could have deleterious effects [19]. The linear non-penetrating fracture could involve vascular structures (i.e., dural venous sinuses or arterial vessels) or skull base foramina and provoke other pathologies, such as cerebral hematomas or venous thrombosis [20, 22].

39.4.1.2 Traumatic Subarachnoid Hemorrhage

Traumatic subarachnoid hemorrhage (tSAH), resulting from the disruption of small vessels within the subarachnoid space stretched at the time of impact, is detected with an incidence ranging from 41% to 61% in admission CT scan of TBI patients and is associated with poor neurological outcomes [23–26]. A greater amount of subarachnoid blood is an indicator of more severe initial brain damage, and it represents a risk factor for the progression of post-traumatic intracerebral hematoma and is associated with an increased risk of cerebral vasospasm [27–29].

39.4.1.3 Epidural Hematoma

EDH is a blood collection, typically biconvex, between the inner table of the skull and the external surface of the dura mater. It is frequently associated with a skull fracture involving the

Table 39.1 Screening criteria for blunt cerebrovascular injury according to the expanded Denver[a] criteria

Signs or symptoms of BCVI
• Potential arterial hemorrhage from neck, nose, or mouth
• Cervical bruit in patients < 50 years old
• Expanding cervical hematoma
• Focal neurologic deficit: TIA, hemipareisis, vertebrobasilar symptoms, Homer's syndrome
• Stroke on CT or MRI
• Neurologic deficit inconsistent with head CT
Risk factors for BCVI
• High-energy transfer mechanism
• Displaced mid-face fracture (Lefort II or III)
• Mandible fracture complex skull fracture/basilar skull fracture/occipital condyle fracture
• Cervical spine fracture, subluxation, or ligamentous injury at any level
• Severe TBI with and GCS < 6
• Near-hanging with anoxia
• Clothesline-type injury or seat belt abrasion with significant swelling, pain, or altered mental status
• Scalp degloving
• Blunt cardiac rupture
• Upper rib fractures

BCVI Blunt cerebrovascular injury, *TIA* Transient ischemic attack, *CT* Computed tomography, *MRI* Magnetic resonance imaging, *TBI* Traumatic brain injury, *GCS* Glasgow coma scale

[a] Geddes AE, Burlew CC, Wagenaar AE, Biffl WL, Johnson JL, Pieracci FM, Campion EM, Moore EE. Expanded screening criteria for blunt cerebrovascular injury: a bigger impact than anticipated. Am J Surg. 2016; 212(6): 1167–1174

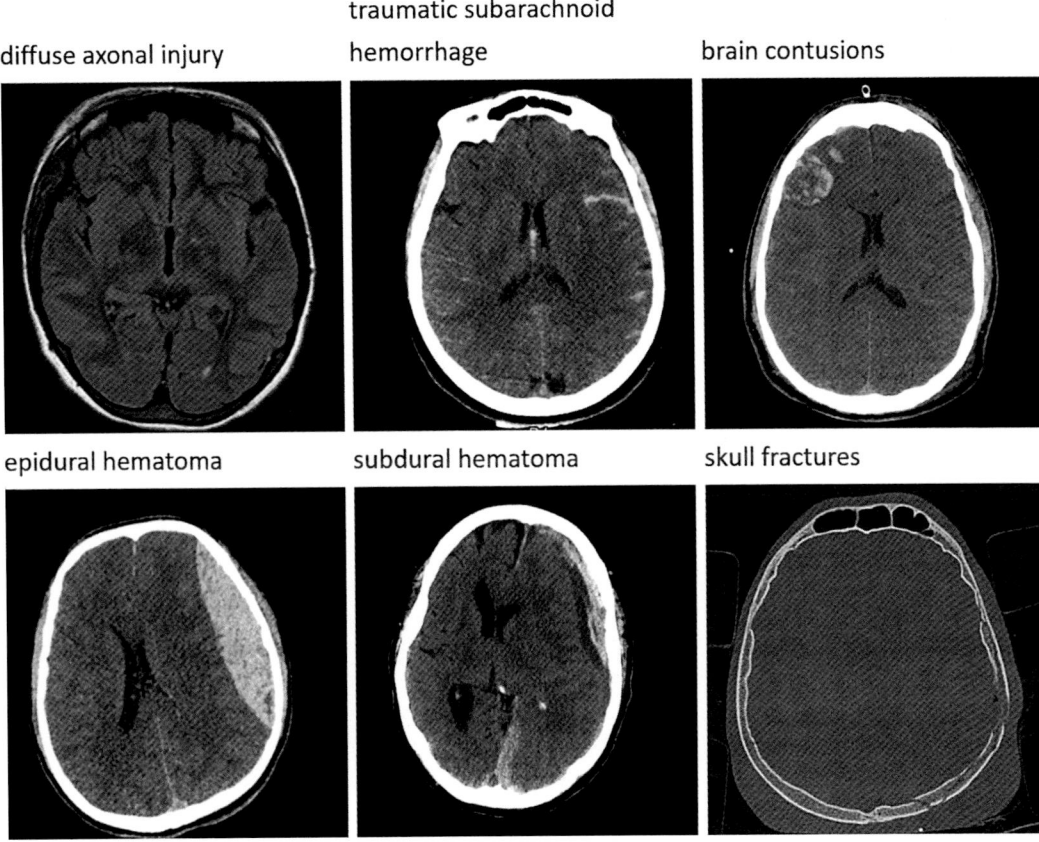

Fig. 39.3 Post-traumatic brain lesions frequently observed in clinical practice

course of arterial or venous structures (usually the middle meningeal artery) [20]. EDH, frequently observed after a TBI, represents a potential life-threatening situation being associated with a sudden increase of the ICP and consequent neurological deterioration [20]. However, if promptly recognized and treated, EDH shows a favourable and better outcome compared to other intracranial injuries, such as brain contusions, tSAH, and acute SDH [26, 30].

39.4.1.4 Subdural Hematoma

SDH is a blood collection among the dura and arachnoid membrane ("crescent moon-shaped") generally due to the stretching, tearing, or rupture of vascular structures (i.e., bridging veins or cortical arteries) subsequent to a TBI. It represents another frequently encountered radiological finding after head injury often associated with underlying parenchymal lesions [19]. Acute SDH, among TBI-related mass effect lesions, represents the subgroup characterized by the worst prognosis [26, 30]. Acute SDH is a neurosurgical emergency, for which a reduction in mortality was observed if the hematoma is removed within 4 h from injury [31]. A significant improvement in the survival rate for the surgically treated patients was observed over the last 20 years (from 59% to 73%), based on the Trauma Audit and Research Network database [32]. Age, GCS, pupil reactivity and the Injury Severity Score at the admission were the variables independently associated with survival in the multivariate analysis [32].

39.4.1.5 Brain Contusions

Brain contusions represent one of the most common findings associated with TBI. They are characterized by hyperdense (hemorrhage) and hypodense (edema) components and are the consequence of the mechanical impact between the brain parenchyma and the skull [20]. Cerebral contusions, generally located in the frontobasal and temporal lobe, are worthy of clinical and radiological monitoring due to high risk of evolution in the first hours after the trauma [28, 33]. Controversy exists concerning the association between radiological and clinical evolution of brain contusions. In particular, most reported radiological risk factors for brain contusion progression are initial large size, tSAH, SDH, increased midline shift and basal cisterns compression [28, 34].

39.4.1.6 Diffuse Axonal Injury

Diffuse axonal injury (DAI) is characterized by small hemorrhagic lesions in white matter tracts generally caused by shearing forces related to an acceleration/deceleration injury with a rotational component [20]. CT scan is characterized by a low sensitivity for this type of lesions (petechial hemorrhage), usually underestimating the real impact on the brain. For this reason, the radiological reference standard examination for DAI evaluation is MRI [20]. DAI features could be found in up to 72% of MRI in TBI patients [35]. In pure severe DAI (without other cerebral lesions), in general, a discrepancy between the poor clinical status (coma) and the CT scan (absence of gross alterations) is observed [20]. DAI lesions typically occur at the interfaces of gray and white matter in the cerebral hemispheres, the body/splenium of the corpus callosum, midbrain, and upper pons [20].

Three grades of DAI have been described according to the anatomical location of the histopathological axonal injury [34]. Axonal injuries were detected in the lobar subcortical white matter in grade 1, in the corpus callosum in grade 2, and in the brainstem in grade 3 lesions [36].

Brainstem lesions are generally associated with an unfavourable neurological outcome. [35, 36]

39.4.2 Neuromonitoring

The goal of neuromonitoring is to prevent or minimize secondary insults to the injured brain and to guide therapeutic interventions [12, 13, 37]. Several monitoring techniques are available for clinical use allowing also measuring multiple parameters simultaneously (multimodal neuromonitoring). In this way, a more comprehensive picture of the brain pathophysiology and its response to treatment is possible [37]. We will mainly focus on three monitoring techniques: (1) neurological examination, (2) ICP monitoring and (3) brain tissue oxygenation monitoring ($PbtO_2$).

39.4.2.1 Neurological Examination

Basic clinical examination, generally including GCS assessment (Fig. 39.4) coupled with investigation of pupil diameter and reactivity to light, is of paramount importance to identify neurological deterioration and potential need for surgical interventions [12, 38]. A complete GCS evaluation can be affected by tracheal intubation and/or facial injuries hindering verbal response and eye opening, respectively. In this regard, motor response is the most easily evaluable component of the GCS [12, 38]. Neurological evaluation is difficult to obtain in deeply sedated patients for ICP control; in this setting and with ICP monitoring, the "wake-up" test (sedation hold) to obtain a reliable neurological evaluation could be dangerous [39]. Pupillary evaluation (diameter and reactivity to light) is important [12, 40, 41]; in fact, a dilated unreactive pupil is generally related to the compression of the third cranial nerve due to midline shift and uncal herniation. This condition is frequently observed in TBI patients with an ipsilateral enlarging mass (i.e., SDH, EDH, etc.) requiring urgent neurosurgical intervention [41]. Dilated and non-reactive pupils (in the absence of toxicological causes) are a signs of severe brain damage [41].

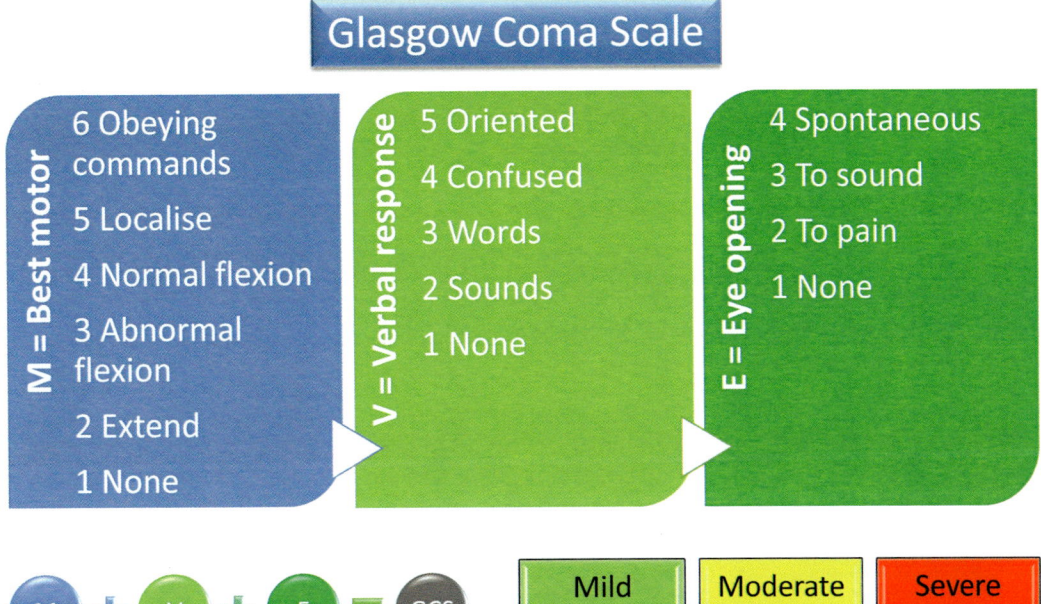

Fig. 39.4 Glasgow coma scale. GCS = Glasgow coma scale

39.4.2.2 ICP Monitoring

Intracranial hypertension and low CPP are dangerous secondary insults for the injured brain and are associated with increased mortality and disability [42–45]. Precisely, these insults need to be considered in terms of intensity and duration ("dose effect") [43–45]. Invasive ICP monitoring is recommended (level IIb) by the Brain Trauma Foundation (BTF) guidelines for the management of TBI patients, "to reduce in-hospital and 2-week post-injury mortality" [17]. However, specific indications regarding which patients should be monitored have not been reported, due to lack of evidence-based data [17, 46]. Invasive ICP monitoring is very useful in daily clinical practice for timely estimation and management of intracranial hypertension and CPP [12]. Nevertheless, two consensus conferences recommend ICP to be monitored in all salvageable comatose patients with radiological signs of intracranial hypertension, and not to be monitored in patients with minimal intracranial pathology (i.e., DAI and small petechiae) [47, 48]. Recommendations from the Milan consensus conference on ICP monitoring in TBI patients [47] are reported in Fig. 39.5.

To support an accurate CPP estimation, the Neuroanaesthesia and Critical Care Society of Great Britain and Ireland and the Society of British Neurological Surgeons recommend to place and level the arterial transducer (for invasive blood pressure monitoring) at the height of the tragus, for invasive blood pressure monitoring [49]. This operation (leveling and zeroing) needs to be repeated after any change in head elevation. The MAP utilized for CPP calculation (CPP = MAP − ICP) should be the one existing at the level of the mid cranial fossa (tragus). When the head is elevated above the heart, the arterial blood pressure in the brain is reduced considering both the angle of elevation and the distance from the right atrium. In daily clinical practice worldwide, brain-injured patients are managed with different degrees of head elevation. For this reason, the leveling of the arterial transducer is critical for the correct MAP measurement and CPP calculation.

ICP monitoring can be performed with different probes [15] (Fig. 39.6):

- fiberoptic intraparenchymal
- intraventricular
- subdural (actually less used).

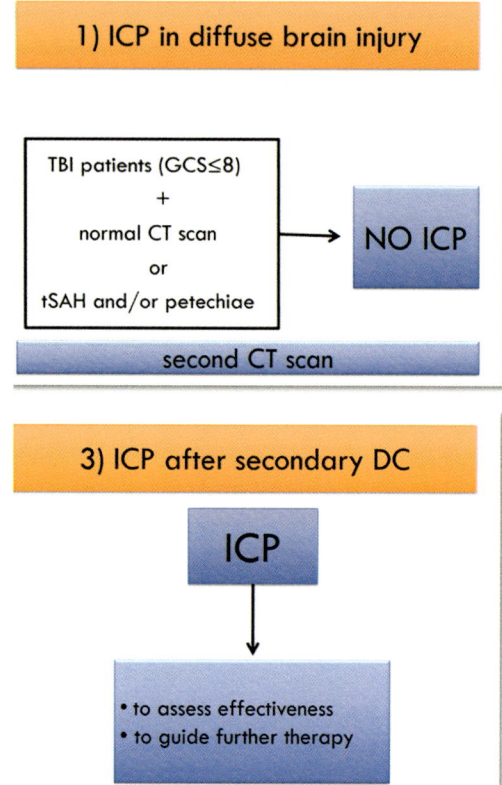
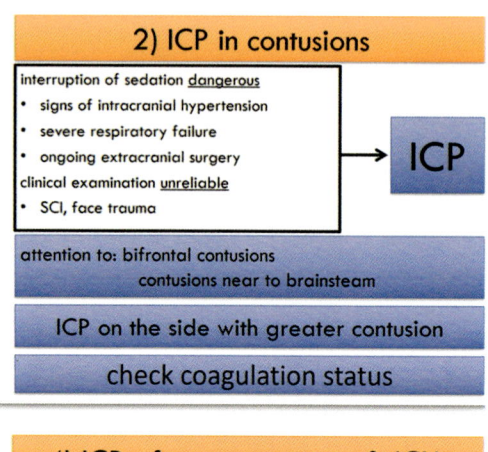
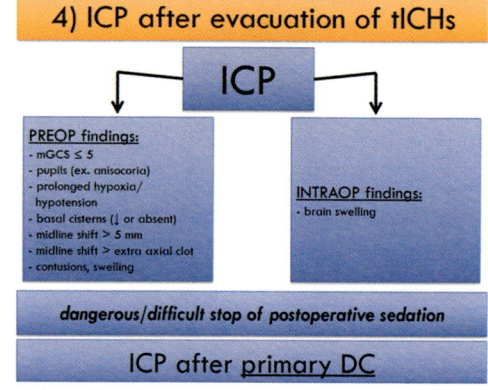

Fig. 39.5 Recommendations from the Milan consensus conference on intracranial pressure monitoring in traumatic brain injury patients. *ICP* Intracranial pressure, *TBI* Traumatic brain injury, *GCS* Glasgow coma scale, *tSAH* Traumatic subarachnoid hemorrhage, *DC* Decompressive craniectomy, *SCI* Spinal cord injury, *tICH* Traumatic intracerebral hematoma, *POSTOP* Postoperative

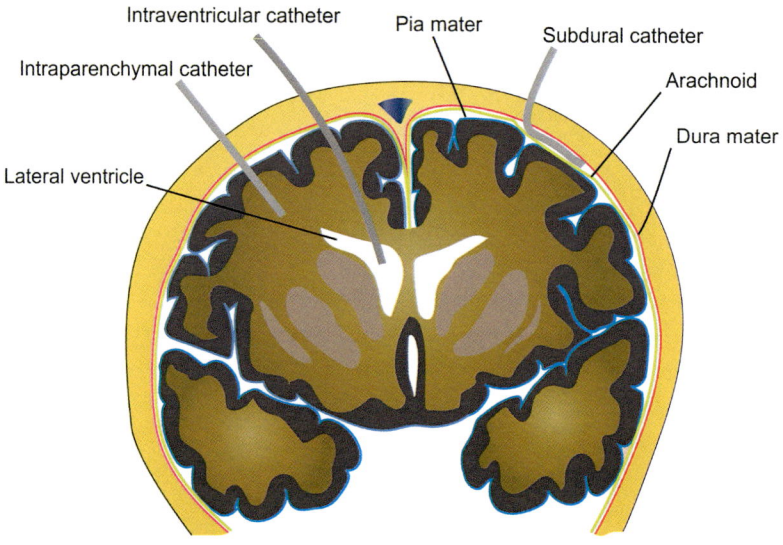

Fig. 39.6 Probes for intracranial pressure monitoring

Before inserting a catheter for ICP monitoring, it is necessary to correct all coagulation abnormalities to minimize bleeding complications [47]. To reduce the risks of infection, the catheters should not be left in place more than 2 weeks [15].

The fiberoptic intraparenchymal catheter is less invasive than the intraventricular one, easier to insert and associated with fewer complications (i.e., hemorrhagic, infectious) [50]. It is generally positioned in the non-dominant hemisphere (usually the right) after a skin incision of about 1 cm (landmarks: 10 cm from the root of the nose on the mid-pupillary line, from here 3 cm on the right to avoid the sagittal sinus). The fiberoptic sensor is inserted at a depth of about 1.5 cm from the skull [51].

External ventricular drain (EVD) is historically considered the "gold standard" for the ICP monitoring. It also plays a therapeutic action through the drainage of the CSF. EVD is not easy to position in case of major changes in the normal shape of the ventricular system [50]. Its positioning, with respect to the fiberoptic intraparenchymal probe, requires: a skin incision of about 3 cm, the puncture of the dura mater and the insertion for no more than 6–7 cm toward the contralateral medial canthus [52].

39.4.2.3 Brain Tissue Oxygenation Monitoring

Because the brain has very limited oxygen and glucose reserves, it is crucial to maintain a CBF adequate to its metabolic demand after TBI [10–12, 37]. Brain hypoxia has been observed after TBI (also in the absence of intracranial hypertension) and is associated with poor neurological outcome [53–55]. Because ICP and CPP do not always reflect tissue oxygenation in the injured brain, $PbtO_2$ can provide fundamental information, especially in the acute phase, when the risk of secondary brain injury is higher. For invasive brain tissue oxygenation monitoring, a probe is inserted in the subcortical white matter under examination (generally in the apparently normal brain tissue but in some case also in a peri-hematoma region). The probe is able to monitor the partial pressure of oxygen in the extracellular fluid of brain tissue in a very small region (near 1 mm^3) around the catheter tip [56]. Data deriving from a recent study suggest to maintain a $PbtO_2$ >20 mmHg [56]. Several multicenter randomized trials are ongoing to better elucidate the role of brain tissue oxygenation monitoring (in addition to ICP monitoring) after TBI [57]. A management algorithm for adult patients with both brain oxygen and ICP monitoring has been developed by the Seattle International Severe TBI Consensus Conference [58]. In this regard, the most frequent interventions utilized to optimize $PbtO_2$ (>20 mmHg) are normobaric hyperoxia, CPP augmentation and red blood cell transfusions [58].

39.5 Treatment

Intracranial hypertension and low CPP, being associated with poor neurological outcome, are conditions that require a rapid evaluation and treatment [42–45]. The first step in the management of severe salvageable TBI patients is to recognize the presence of intracranial lesions requiring urgent neurosurgical intervention (i.e., SDH, EDH, etc.); the use of medical therapy alone can be very dangerous for patients presenting with an emergent surgical lesion [12, 59]. The latest surgical TBI guidelines of the BTF published in 2006 [60–64] are summarized in Table 39.2.

For the management of intracranial hypertension, a staircase approach is generally utilized, where the therapy intensity level is increased step by step, introducing gradually more aggressive interventions which are generally associated with greater risks/adverse effects when no response is observed [12, 59, 65].

Two algorithms for the management of adult severe TBI patients have been recently published deriving from a consensus of 42 international neurotrauma experts utilizing a Delphi approach [58, 66]. The content of these two algorithms, one for patients with ICP monitoring alone and the other for patients with simultaneous ICP and $PbtO_2$ monitoring, is summarized in Fig. 39.7.

Table 39.2 Summary of the Brain Trauma Foundation guidelines regarding the surgical management of the traumatic brain injury patients (2006)

Acute epidural hematoma (EDH)	Acute Subdural hematoma (SDH)	Traumatic parenchymal lesions	Depressed cranial fractures
• **evacuation:** – >30 mL (regardless of GCS) – (immediately) patient with GCS <9 and anisocoria • **non-operative management** (neurological examination and serial CT scans) if <30 mL (with thickness <15 mm and midline shift <5 mm) and GCS >9 without focal deficits	• **evacuation:** – (immediately) thickness >10 mm or midline shift >5 mm (regardless of GCS) – [in patients with GCS <9, thickness <10 mm and midline shift <5 mm] in case of GCS reduction by 2 points respect to the admission and/or pupillary abnormalities (i.e. anisocoria) and/or ICP >20 mmHg	• **surgery (evacuation and/or decompression):** – [a] neurological deterioration referable to the increase in lesion size [b] intracranial hypertension refractory to maximal medical therapy [c] mass effect on CT scan – patients with GCS 6–8 with frontal or temporal contusions >20 mL with midline shift >5 mm and/or compression of the basal cisterns on CT scan – any lesion >50 mL	• **surgery:** open compound depressed cranial fractures greater than the thickness of the cranium • **non-operative management:** open compounddepressed cranial fractures in the absence of: dural penetration, significant intracranial hematoma, depression >10 mm, frontal sinus involvement, gross cosmetic deformity, wound infection, pneumocephalus, or great wound contamination

GCS Glasgow coma scale, *CT* Computed tomography, *ICP* Intracranial pressure

39.5.1 CSF Drainage with EVD

The EVD, when already available for ICP monitoring, can be utilized for CSF drainage and intracranial hypertension management [64]. In this regard, some aspects must be kept in mind when using this device [50, 67, 68]. Excessive CSF drainage may increase the risk of intracranial bleeding. In addition, unless a double-reading catheter (fluid coupled + fiberoptic) is used, ICP monitoring is not possible during CSF drainage which makes intracranial hypertension episodes undetectable.

39.5.2 Osmotherapy

Hyperosmolar agents [i.e., intravenous (IV) mannitol 0.25–1 g/kg or hypertonic saline 3% 100–250 mL every 4–8 h] are effective in the control of ICP through various mechanisms, such as a reduction in blood viscosity [cerebral vasoconstriction → ↓ cerebral blood volume (CBV)—short lived effect] and an increase in plasma osmolarity (long lasting effect) [69]. This last effect depends on the integrity of the BBB and is based on the removal of water from the normal brain tissue. In clinical practice, because mannitol has a diuretic effect, it should not be used in case of hypovolemia; in this case, hypertonic saline might be a most reasonable choice [59]. It is recommended to avoid a serum Na >155 mEq/lt or an osmolarity >320 mEq/lt to minimize the risk of renal failure [66].

39.5.3 Hyperventilation

Low arterial carbon dioxide levels ($PaCO_2$), generally induced by an increase in mechanical minute ventilation, result in CSF alkalosis leading to a cerebral vasoconstriction with concurrent reduction in CBF, CBV and then of ICP [70, 71]. These effects are temporary with a duration of approximately 24 h. Moreover, hyperventilation is associated with the risk of development of cerebral ischemia [70–72]. In this regard, an additional monitoring for the detection of cerebral ischemia (i.e., jugular venous oximetry and brain tissue oxygenation) is suggested [58]. Profound hypocapnia ($PaCO_2$ 25 mmHg) is not recommended as a prophylactic maneuver [17], but it could be utilized as a temporary measure associated with other therapies when treating a

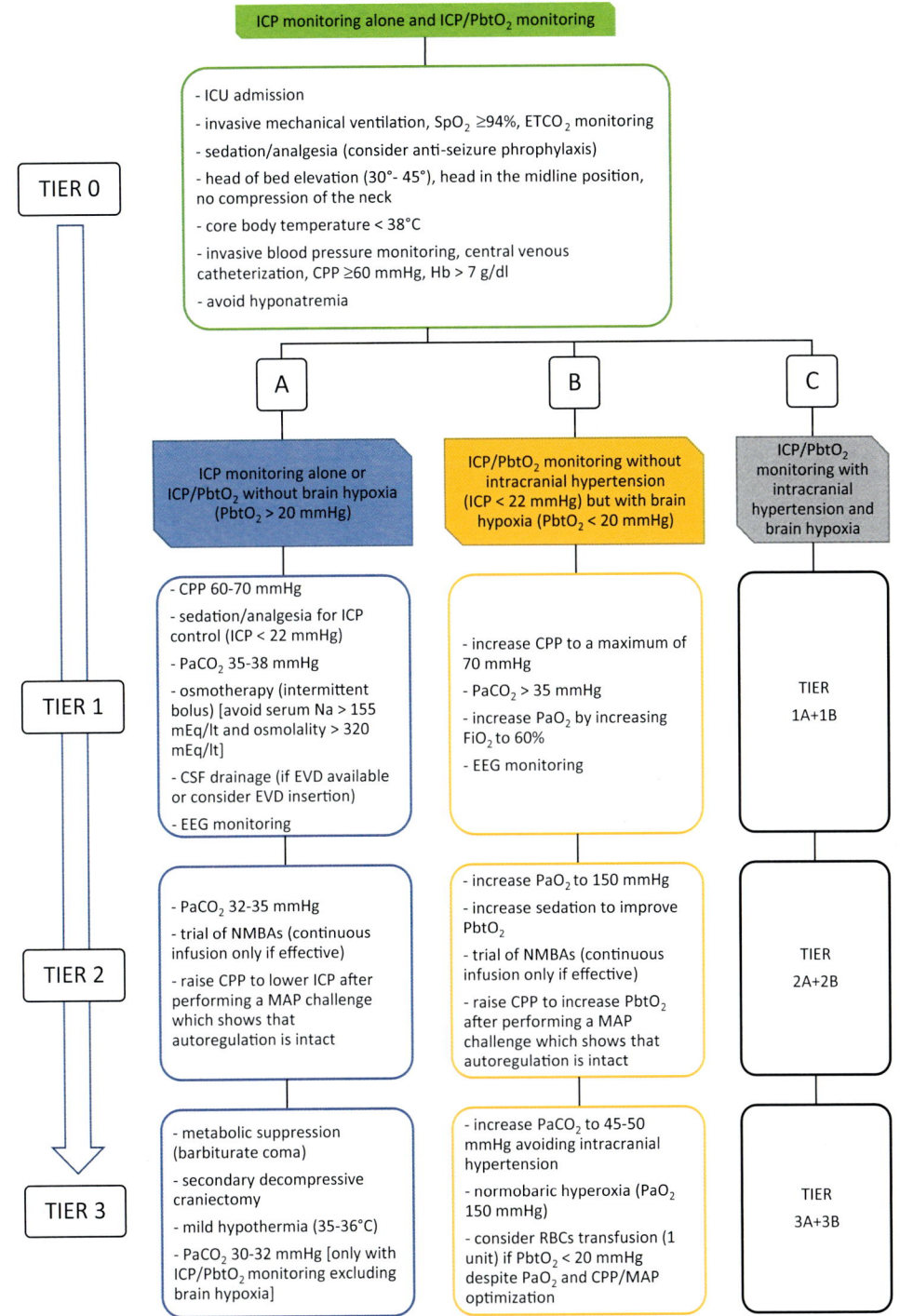

Fig. 39.7 Summary of the Seattle International Severe Traumatic Brain Injury Consensus Conference. *ICP* Intracranial pressure, *PbtO₂* Brain tissue oxygenation, *ICU* Intensive care unit, *SpO₂* Peripheral oxygen saturation, *ETCO₂* End-tidal carbon dioxide, *CPP* Cerebral perfusion pressure, *Hb* Hemoglobin, *PaCO₂* Arterial partial pressure of carbon dioxide, *Na* Sodium, *PaO₂* Arterial partial pressure of oxygen, *FiO₂* Inspiratory oxygen fraction, *CSF* Cerebrospinal fluid, *EVD* External ventricular drain, *EEG* Electroencephalogram, *NMBA* Neuromuscular blocking agent, *MAP* Mean arterial pressure, *RBC* Red blood cell

patient with brain herniation waiting an emergency neurosurgical procedure (i.e., SDH evacuation) [59, 71].

39.5.4 Metabolic Suppression (Barbiturate Coma)

Barbiturates [i.e., IV Pentobarbital loading dose: 30–40 mg/kg over 4 h and maintenance 2–3.5 mg/kg/h or IV Thiopental loading dose 3 mg/kg bolus followed by 10–20 mg/kg over 1 h and maintenance 3–5 mg/kg/h; consider weaning from Thiopental after 24–48 h of ICP control: initially consider reduction of 500 mg/12 h and after, looking at the ICP, more rapid (dosage halved every 12 h)] are effective in the control of intracranial hypertension, because they reduce cerebral metabolism and CBF [59, 65]. Although electroencephalogram or bispectral index can be utilized to monitor cerebral electrical activity/depth of anesthesia, barbiturate dosage should be titrated to ICP control [59]. Considering their dangerous side effects (arterial hypotension, dyskalemia, immunosuppression, ileus, adrenal insufficiency, etc.), barbiturates are reserved for refractory intracranial hypertension after the failure of other therapies [59, 65]. During barbiturate coma, pupillary light reflex can disappear and nutrition requirements can be reduced [59].

39.5.5 Hypothermia

Mild hypothermia (32–25 °C) has been utilized for neuroprotection and ICP control in several trials [73]. Hypothermia exerts its effects through various mechanisms, such as a reduction in: (1) cerebral metabolism (↓ CBF, CBV and ICP), (2) BBB permeability, (3) free radicals/excitotoxic substances/pro-inflammatory cytokines production, (3) apoptosis and (4) epileptic activity and cortical depolarization [74, 75]. Despite its effectiveness on ICP control, hypothermia was associated with worse neurologic outcome in clinical trials [73, 76]. As barbiturate coma, hypothermia is reserved to patients with refractory intracranial hypertension, being associated with different important side effects (hypovolemia, electrolytes disturbances, coagulation abnormalities, immunosuppression, hyperglycemia, pressure ulcers, etc.) [74, 75].

39.5.6 Decompressive Craniectomy

Decompressive craniectomy (DC) is a surgical procedure that consists in removing a part of the skull and opening the dura by increasing its size (duroplasty) [77, 78]. In this way, the skull is converted from a closed box to an open box able to accommodate brain swelling [77, 78]. DC can be primary (not ICP driven—refers to leaving a bone flap out after evacuating an intracranial mass lesion) and secondary (ICP driven—typically used as last-tier therapy for patients with refractory intracranial hypertension despite maximal medical therapy) [77, 78]. Despite secondary DC being effective in ICP control, recent trials have shown differences in neurological outcome [79, 80]. In the DC in Patients with Severe TBI trial, DC (bifrontal for patients with diffuse brain injury) decreased ICP and intensive care unit stay but was associated with more unfavorable neurological outcomes [79]. In the Randomized Evaluation of Surgery with Craniectomy for Uncontrollable Elevation of ICP trial, DC (mainly unilateral) resulted in lower mortality but higher rates of vegetative state, lower severe disability, and upper severe disability [80]. A better profile was observed in patients aged ≤40 years [78]. DC is associated with several complications (central nervous system and wound infections, cerebral hematomas, CSF disturbances, etc.) and, as other "extreme" therapies (i.e., hypothermia, barbiturate coma), should be reserved for selected patients with refractory IH [81].

Some technical considerations for the DC [80–83] are (Fig. 39.8):

1. several types of skin incision are proposed for a DC. The more proposed classic trauma flap question-mark incision, without involving the external ear, but with some complication related to the risk of damage the superficial temporal artery (STA) and the need to divide the temporal muscle. The "n-type" and the "T-type" (or Kempe) incisions are both formed by two perpendicular incisions and

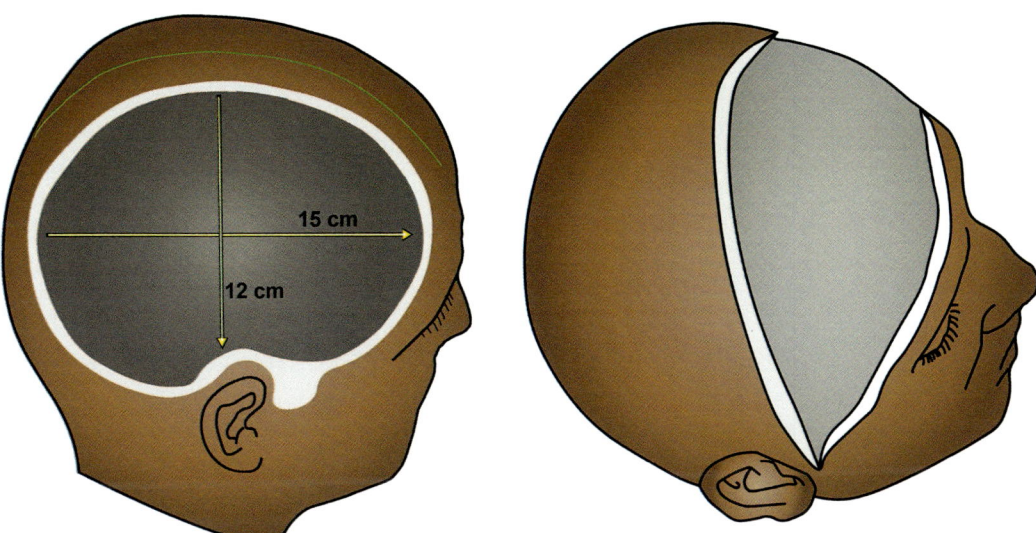

Fig. 39.8 Technical considerations regarding decompressive craniectomy

suggested to avoid to split the temporal muscle, but with some risk of complications connected with the angulated portion of the skin incision and the potential injury of STA. More recently has been proposed a modified question-mark incision, ending behind the ear. The advantage is the absence of risk to damage the STA and the possibility to detach from the bone the preserved temporal muscle with significantly reduced cranioplasty failure rates [84]. Nevertheless, the not-splitted Temporal Muscle did not allow an easy removal of the basal temporal portion of the bone flap that is a fundamental aspect of the decompressive role of DC. An unadequate dimension and basal extension of DC can be associated with a worst outcome. This aspect still needs to be explored in the latter proposed incision.

2. DC is one of the new topic of the 4th Edition of the BTF Guidelines for the management of severe TBI. A large frontotemporoparietal DC (not less than 12 × 15 cm or 15 cm diameter) is reported as a recommendation of level II A over a small frontotemporoparietal DC being associated with reduced mortality and improved neurologic outcomes in patients with severe TBI. The dimensions of the bone flap should incorporate the removal of the bone from the floor of the middle cranial fossa (this applies to both bifrontal and unilateral DCs)

3. the dura must be open and a plastic (duroplasty) must be made, generally with biocompatible material, to increase its size. A watertight closure seems to be not so mandatory. A recent randomized controlled study comparing watertight duraplasty versus not watertight duraplasty showed in the not watertight duraplasty group no higher incidence of surgical complications and a decreased surgical time [85].

Do's
- to recognize the presence of intracranial lesions requiring urgent neurosurgical intervention
- for the management of intracranial hypertension use a staircase approach
- hyperosmolar agents are effective in the control of ICP
- profound hypocapnia could be utilized as a temporary measure associated with other therapies when treating a patient with brain herniation waiting an emergency neurosurgical procedure
- considering their dangerous side effects barbiturates, hypothermia and DC are reserved for refractory intracranial hypertension after the failure of other therapies

> **Don'ts**
> - the use of medical therapy alone can be very dangerous for patients presenting with an emergent surgical lesion
> - profound hypocapnia is not recommended as a prophylactic maneuver
> - small frontotemporoparietal DC (less than 12 × 15 cm or 15 cm diameter)

39.6 Traumatic Brain Injury in Polytrauma Patients

The acute phase of TBI patients with polytrauma is a challenging condition to manage. In polytrauma trauma patients, exsanguination is the most frequent cause of early death, while the TBI is the most common cause of delayed mortality and disability [86]. Furthermore, TBI is frequently associated with extracranial hemorrhage that is known to worsen the outcome by exacerbating secondary insults, such as intracranial hypertension and arterial hypotension with cerebral hypoperfusion [87]. In the 2019, the World Society of Emergency Surgery decided to organize an international consensus conference regarding the monitoring and management of severe adult TBI polytrauma patients during the first 24 h after injury [88]. Forty experts (emergency surgeons, neurosurgeons, and intensivists) participated in the online consensus process performed with a modified Delphi approach. The 16 recommendations generated and the related algorithm are shown in Table 39.3 and in Fig. 39.9, respectively.

Table 39.3 Summary of the World Society of Emergency Surgery consensus conference guidelines on monitoring and management of severe adult traumatic brain injury patients with polytrauma in the first 24 h[a]

Number	Recommendation	Agreement (%)
1	All exsanguinating patients (life-threatening hemorrhage) require immediate intervention (surgery and/or interventional radiology) for bleeding control.	100
2	Patients without life-threatening hemorrhage or following measures to obtain bleeding control (in case of life-threatening hemorrhage) require urgent neurological evaluation [pupils + Glasgow Coma Scale motor score (if feasible), and brain computed tomography (CT) scan] to determine the severity of brain damage (life-threatening or not).	100
3	After control of life-threatening hemorrhage is established, all salvageable patients with life-threatening brain lesions require urgent neurosurgical consultation and intervention.	100
4	Patients (without or after control of life-threatening hemorrhage) at risk for intracranial hypertension (IH) (without a life-threatening intracranial mass lesion or after emergency neurosurgery) require intracranial pressure (ICP) monitoring regardless of the need of emergency extra-cranial surgery (EES)	97.5
5	We recommend maintaining systolic blood pressure (SBP) >100 mmHg or mean arterial pressure (MAP) >80 mmHg during interventions for life-threatening hemorrhage or emergency neurosurgery. In cases of difficult intraoperative bleeding control, lower value may be tolerated for the shortest possible time.	82.5

Table 39.3 (continued)

Number	Recommendation	Agreement (%)
6	We recommend red blood cell (RBC) transfusion for hemoglobin (Hb) level <7 g/dL during interventions for life-threatening hemorrhage or emergency neurosurgery. Higher threshold for RBC transfusions may be used in patients "at risk" (i.e., the elderly and/or patients with limited cardiovascular reserve due to pre-existing heart disease).	97.5
7	We recommend maintaining an arterial partial pressure of oxygen (PaO_2) level between 60 and 100 mmHg during interventions for life-threatening hemorrhage or emergency neurosurgery.	95
8	We recommend maintaining an arterial partial pressure of carbon dioxide ($PaCO_2$) level between 35 and 40 mmHg during interventions for life-threatening hemorrhage or emergency neurosurgery.	97.5
9	In cases of cerebral herniation, awaiting or during emergency neurosurgery, we recommend the use of osmotherapy and/or hypocapnia (temporarily).	90
10	In cases requiring intervention for life-threatening systemic hemorrhage, we recommend, at a minimum, the maintenance of a platelet (PLT) count > 50.000/mm3. In cases requiring emergency neurosurgery (including ICP probe insertion), a higher value is advisable.	100
11	We recommend maintaining a prothrombin time (PT)/activated partial thromboplastin time (aPTT) value of <1.5 normal control during interventions for life-threatening hemorrhage or emergency neurosurgery (including ICP probe insertion).	92.5
12	We recommend, if available, that Point-of-Care (POC) tests [e.g., thromboelastography (TEG) and rotational thromboelastometry ROTEM] be utilized to assess and optimize coagulation function during interventions for life-threatening hemorrhage or emergency neurosurgery (including ICP probe insertion).	90
13	During massive transfusion protocol initiation, we recommend the transfusion of RBCs/plasma/PLTs at a ratio of 1/1/1. Afterwards, this ratio may be modified according to laboratory values.	92.5
14	We recommend maintaining a cerebral perfusion pressure (CPP) ≥60 mmHg when ICP monitoring becomes available. This value should be adjusted (individualized) based on neuromonitoring data and the cerebral autoregulation status of the individual patient.	95
15	In the absence of possibilities to target the underlying pathophysiologic mechanism of IH, we recommend a stepwise approach, where the level of therapy, in patients with elevated ICP, is increased step by step, reserving more aggressive interventions, which are generally associated with greater risks/adverse effects, for situations when no response is observed.	97.5
16	We recommend the development of protocols, in conjunction with local resources and practices, to encourage the implementation of a simultaneous multisystem surgery (SMS) [including radiologic interventional procedures] in patients requiring both intervention for life-threatening hemorrhage and emergency neurosurgery for life-threatening brain damage.	100

[a]Picetti E, Rossi S, Abu-Zidan FM, Ansaloni L, Armonda R, Baiocchi GL, Bala M, Balogh ZJ, Berardino M, Biffl WL, Bouzat P, Buki A, Ceresoli M, Chesnut RM, Chiara O, Citerio G, Coccolini F, Coimbra R, Di Saverio S, Fraga GP, Gupta D, Helbok R, Hutchinson PJ, Kirkpatrick AW, Kinoshita T, Kluger Y, Leppaniemi A, Maas AIR, Maier RV, Minardi F, Moore EE, Myburgh JA, Okonkwo DO, Otomo Y, Rizoli S, Rubiano AM, Sahuquillo J, Sartelli M, Scalea TM, Servadei F, Stahel PF, Stocchetti N, Taccone FS, Tonetti T, Velmahos G, Weber D, Catena F. WSES consensus conference guidelines: monitoring and management of severe adult traumatic brain injury patients with polytrauma in the first 24 hours. World J Emerg Surg. 2019 Nov 29; 14: 53

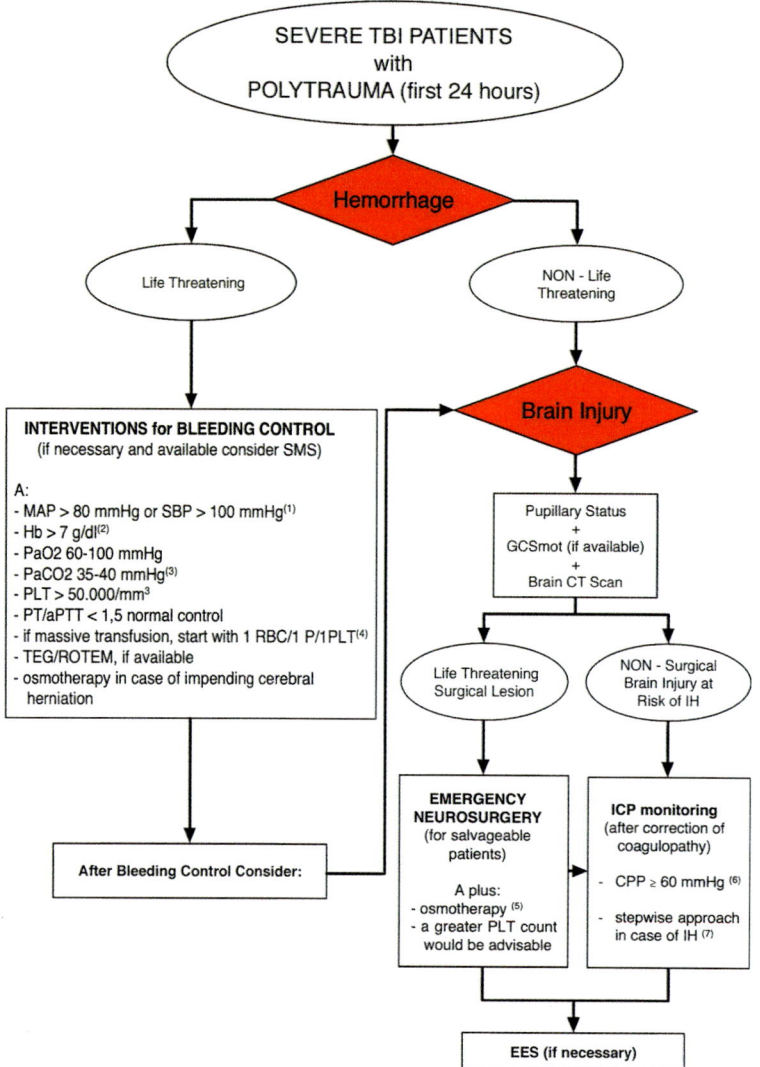

Fig. 39.9 Algorithm of the World Society of Emergency Surgery consensus conference guidelines on monitoring and management of severe adult traumatic brain injury patients with polytrauma in the first 24 h*

*Picetti E, Rossi S, Abu-Zidan FM, Ansaloni L, Armonda R, Baiocchi GL, Bala M, Balogh ZJ, Berardino M, Biffl WL, Bouzat P, Buki A, Ceresoli M, Chesnut RM, Chiara O, Citerio G, Coccolini F, Coimbra R, Di Saverio S, Fraga GP, Gupta D, Helbok R, Hutchinson PJ, Kirkpatrick AW, Kinoshita T, Kluger Y, Leppaniemi A, Maas AIR, Maier RV, Minardi F, Moore EE, Myburgh JA, Okonkwo DO, Otomo Y, Rizoli S, Rubiano AM, Sahuquillo J, Sartelli M, Scalea TM, Servadei F, Stahel PF, Stocchetti N, Taccone FS, Tonetti T, Velmahos G, Weber D, Catena F. WSES consensus conference guidelines: monitoring and management of severe adult traumatic brain injury patients with polytrauma in the first 24 h. World J Emerg Surg. 2019 Nov 29; 14: 53

(1) Lower values could be tolerated, for the shortest possible time, in case of difficult intraoperative bleeding control. (2) Higher threshold could be used in patients "at risk" (i.e., elderly and/or with limited cardiovascular reserve because of pre-existing heart disease). (3) Lower values, temporarily, only in case of impending cerebral herniation. (4) Afterward, this ratio can be modified according to laboratory values. (5) Not only in case of impending cerebral herniation but also for cerebral edema control. (6) This value should be adjusted (individualized) considering neuromonitoring data and cerebral autoregulation status. (7) This approach is recommended in the absence of possibilities to target the underlying pathophysiologic mechanism of IH. Abbreviations: *SMS* Systemic multisystem surgery (including radiologic interventional procedures), *CT* Computed tomography, *GCS* Glasgow Coma Scale (mot = motor part of GCS), *MAP* Mean arterial pressure, *SBP* Systolic blood pressure, *Hb* Hemoglobin, *PaO2* Arterial partial pressure of oxygen, *PaCO2* Arterial partial pressure of carbon dioxide, *RBC* Red blood cell, *P* Plasma, *PLT* Platelet, *PT* Prothrombin time, *aPTT* Activated partial thromboplastin time, *TEG* Thromboelastography, *ROTEM* Rotational thromboelastometry, *ICP* Intracranial pressure, *CPP* Cerebral perfusion pressure, *IH* Intracranial hypertension, *EES* Extracranial emergency surgery

Take Home Messages
- TBI is a major global health problem being the first injury-related cause of death and disability worldwide.
- Considering the burden of TBI on the global trauma care, every physician involved in the acute management of polytrauma patients need to have a basic knowledge about brain injury.
- Increases in ICP are associated with a reduction in cerebral perfusion pressure with a consequent risk of ischemic injury and unfavourable neurological outcome.
- Brain CT can be considered as the most important radiological examination in the evaluation of a patient with head injury, because (especially in the acute phase) it provides us with fundamental information regarding therapy (medical and/or surgical) and monitoring (i.e., indications for ICP monitoring).
- Invasive ICP monitoring is very useful in daily clinical practice for timely estimation and management of intracranial hypertension and CPP.
- The first step in the management of severe salvageable TBI patients is to recognize the presence of intracranial lesions requiring urgent neurosurgical intervention (i.e., SDH, EDH, etc.); the use of medical therapy alone can be very dangerous for patients presenting with an emergent surgical lesion.
- For the management of intracranial hypertension, a staircase approach is generally utilized, where the therapy intensity level is increased step by step, introducing gradually more aggressive interventions which are generally associated with greater risks/adverse effects when no response is observed.

Multiple Choice Questions
1. TBI can be clinically classified as:
   A. severe, very severe and moderate
   B. moderate, very moderate and severe
   C. mild, moderate and severe
   D. mild, very mild and severe
   correct answer: C.
2. The primary injury after TBI:
   A. is inflicted at the time of the trauma and is caused by external physical forces of variable magnitude applied to the head (primary insult)
   B. results from the activation of different molecular and cellular pathways
   C. does not exist
   D. none of the above
   correct answer: A.
3. The secondary injury after TBI:
   A. does not exist
   B. is inflicted at the time of the trauma and is caused by external physical forces of variable magnitude applied to the head (primary insult)
   C. results from the activation of different molecular and cellular pathways by the first insult and evolves over time
   D. none of the above
   correct answer: C.
4. Traditionally, secondary insults that can exacerbate the secondary injury are:
   A. polyuria
   B. hypotension and hypoxia
   C. hypokalemia
   D. hyperkalemia
   correct answer: B.
5. The CPP is the difference between:
   A. the systolic arterial pressure and the ICP
   B. the MAP and the ICP

C. the diastolic arterial pressure and the ICP
D. none of the above
correct answer: B.

6. Brain contusions are characterized by:
   A. hyperdense (hemorrhage) and hypodense (edema) components
   B. only a hyperdense part (hemorrhage)
   C. only a hypodense part (edema)
   D. none of the above
   correct answer: A.

7. Basic clinical neurological evaluation in severe TBI patients generally includes:
   A. the GCS and the pupillary evaluation
   B. the GCS only
   C. the pupillary evaluation only
   D. none of the above
   correct answer: A.

8. The probes generally utilized for ICP monitoring are:
   A. intraventricular and lumbar
   B. fiberoptic intraparenchymal and lumbar
   C. intraventricular, fiberoptic intraparenchymal and subdural
   D. subdural and fiberoptic intraparenchymal
   correct answer: C.

9. Osmotic agents are:
   A. nicardipine and olanzapine
   B. mannitol and hypertonic saline
   C. nimodipine and nicardipine
   D. olanzapine and ranitidine
   correct answer: B.

10. Barbiturate coma is utilized for the management of elevated ICP as:
    (a) tier 3 therapy
    (b) tier 1 therapy
    (c) basic therapy
    (d) none of the above
    correct answer: A.

References

1. GBD 2016 Traumatic Brain Injury and Spinal Cord Injury Collaborators. Global, regional, and national burden of traumatic brain injury and spinal cord injury, 1990-2016: a systematic analysis for the Global Burden of Disease Study 2016. Lancet Neurol. 2019;18(1):56–87.
2. GBD 2016 Neurology Collaborators. Global, regional, and national burden of neurological disorders, 1990-2016: a systematic analysis for the Global Burden of Disease Study 2016. Lancet Neurol. 2019;18(5):459–80.
3. Centers for Disease Control and Prevention. Page last reviewed: August 28, 2020 https://www.cdc.gov/traumaticbraininjury/index.html (accessed Apr 10, 2021).
4. Rubiano AM, Carney N, Chesnut R, Puyana JC. Global neurotrauma research challenges and opportunities. Nature. 2015;527(7578):S193–7.
5. Maas AI, Stocchetti N, Bullock R. Moderate and severe traumatic brain injury in adults. Lancet Neurol. 2008;7(8):728–41.
6. Dewan MC, Rattani A, Gupta S, Baticulon RE, Hung YC, Punchak M, Agrawal A, Adeleye AO, Shrime MG, Rubiano AM, Rosenfeld JV, Park KB. Estimating the global incidence of traumatic brain injury. J Neurosurg. 2018;1:1–18. https://doi.org/10.3171/2017.10.JNS17352. Epub ahead of print.
7. Peeters W, van den Brande R, Polinder S, Brazinova A, Steyerberg EW, Lingsma HF, Maas AI. Epidemiology of traumatic brain injury in Europe. Acta Neurochir (Wien). 2015;157(10):1683–96.
8. Majdan M, Plancikova D, Brazinova A, Rusnak M, Nieboer D, Feigin V, Maas A. Epidemiology of traumatic brain injuries in Europe: a cross-sectional analysis. Lancet Public Health. 2016;1(2):e76–83.
9. Iaccarino C, Carretta A, Nicolosi F, Morselli C. Epidemiology of severe traumatic brain injury. J Neurosurg Sci. 2018;62(5):535–41. https://doi.org/10.23736/S0390-5616.18.04532-0.
10. Kinoshita K. Traumatic brain injury: pathophysiology for neurocritical care. J Intensive Care. 2016;4:29.
11. Blennow K, Brody DL, Kochanek PM, Levin H, McKee A, Ribbers GM, Yaffe K, Zetterberg H. Traumatic brain injuries. Nat Rev Dis Primers. 2016;2:16,084.
12. Stocchetti N, Carbonara M, Citerio G, Ercole A, Skrifvars MB, Smielewski P, Zoerle T, Menon DK. Severe traumatic brain injury: targeted management in the intensive care unit. Lancet Neurol. 2017;16(6):452–64.
13. Maas AIR, Menon DK, Adelson PD, Andelic N, Bell MJ, Belli A, Bragge P, Brazinova A, Büki A, Chesnut RM, Citerio G, Coburn M, Cooper DJ, Crowder AT,

Czeiter E, Czosnyka M, Diaz-Arrastia R, Dreier JP, Duhaime AC, Ercole A, van Essen TA, Feigin VL, Gao G, Giacino J, Gonzalez-Lara LE, Gruen RL, Gupta D, Hartings JA, Hill S, Jiang JY, Ketharanathan N, Kompanje EJO, Lanyon L, Laureys S, Lecky F, Levin H, Lingsma HF, Maegele M, Majdan M, Manley G, Marsteller J, Mascia L, McFadyen C, Mondello S, Newcombe V, Palotie A, Parizel PM, Peul W, Piercy J, Polinder S, Puybasset L, Rasmussen TE, Rossaint R, Smielewski P, Söderberg J, Stanworth SJ, Stein MB, von Steinbüchel N, Stewart W, Steyerberg EW, Stocchetti N, Synnot A, Te Ao B, Tenovuo O, Theadom A, Tibboel D, Videtta W, Wang KKW, Williams WH, Wilson L, Yaffe K. InTBIR Participants and Investigators. Traumatic brain injury: integrated approaches to improve prevention, clinical care, and research. Lancet Neurol. 2017;16(12):987–1048.
14. Ng SY, Lee AYW. Traumatic brain injuries: pathophysiology and potential therapeutic targets. Front Cell Neurosci. 2019;(13):528.
15. Smith M. Monitoring intracranial pressure in traumatic brain injury. Anesth Analg. 2008;106(1):240–8.
16. Tonetti T, Biondini S, Minardi F, Rossi S, Picetti E. Definition and pathomechanism of the intracranial compartment syndrome. In: Coccolini F, Malbrain MLNG, Kirkpatrick AW, et al. Compartment syndrome. 1st ed. Springer Nature Switzerland 2021; 7-16.
17. Carney N, Totten AM, O'Reilly C, Ullman JS, Hawryluk GW, Bell MJ, Bratton SL, Chesnut R, Harris OA, Kissoon N, Rubiano AM, Shutter L, Tasker RC, Vavilala MS, Wilberger J, Wright DW, Ghajar J. Guidelines for the management of severe traumatic brain injury, fourth edition. Neurosurgery. 2017;80(1):6–15.
18. Rangel-Castilla L, Gasco J, Nauta HJ, Okonkwo DO, Robertson CS. Cerebral pressure autoregulation in traumatic brain injury. Neurosurg Focus. 2008;25(4):E7.
19. Mutch CA, Talbott JF, Gean A. Imaging evaluation of acute traumatic brain injury. Neurosurg Clin N Am. 2016;27(4):409–39.
20. Schweitzer AD, Niogi SN, Whitlow CT, Tsiouris AJ. Traumatic brain injury: imaging patterns and complications. Radiographics. 2019;39(6):1571–95.
21. Geddes AE, Burlew CC, Wagenaar AE, Biffl WL, Johnson JL, Pieracci FM, Campion EM, Moore EE. Expanded screening criteria for blunt cerebrovascular injury: a bigger impact than anticipated. Am J Surg. 2016;212(6):1167–74.
22. Bokhari R, You E, Bakhaidar M, Bajunaid K, Lasry O, Zeiler FA, Marcoux J, Baeesa S. Dural venous sinus thrombosis in patients presenting with blunt traumatic brain injuries and skull fractures: a systematic review and meta-analysis. World Neurosurg. 2020;142:495–505.
23. Servadei F, Murray GD, Teasdale GM, Dearden M, Iannotti F, Lapierre F, Maas AJ, Karimi A, Ohman J, Persson L, Stocchetti N, Trojanowski T, Unterberg A. Traumatic subarachnoid hemorrhage: demographic and clinical study of 750 patients from the European brain injury consortium survey of head injuries. Neurosurgery. 2002;50(2):261–7.
24. Mattioli C, Beretta L, Gerevini S, Veglia F, Citerio G, Cormio M, Stocchetti N. Traumatic subarachnoid hemorrhage on the computerized tomography scan obtained at admission: a multicenter assessment of the accuracy of diagnosis and the potential impact on patient outcome. J Neurosurg. 2003;98(1):37–42.
25. MRC CRASH Trial Collaborators, Perel P, Arango M, Clayton T, Edwards P, Komolafe E, Poccock S, Roberts I, Shakur H, Steyerberg E, Yutthakasemsunt S. Predicting outcome after traumatic brain injury: practical prognostic models based on large cohort of international patients. BMJ. 2008;336:425–9.
26. Murray GD, Butcher I, McHugh GS, Lu J, Mushkudiani NA, Maas AI, Marmarou A, Steyerberg EW. Multivariable prognostic analysis in traumatic brain injury: results from the IMPACT study. J Neurotrauma. 2007;24:329–37.
27. Servadei F, Picetti E. Traumatic subarachnoid hemorrhage. World Neurosurg. 2014;82(5):e597–8.
28. Chang EF, Meeker M, Holland MC. Acute traumatic intraparenchymal hemorrhage: risk factors for progression in the early post-injury period. Neurosurgery. 2006;58(4):647–56.
29. Al-Mufti F, Amuluru K, Changa A, Lander M, Patel N, Wajswol E, Al-Marsoummi S, Alzubaidi B, Singh IP, Nuoman R, Gandhi C. Traumatic brain injury and intracranial hemorrhage-induced cerebral vasospasm: a systematic review. Neurosurg Focus. 2017;43(5):E14.
30. Maas AI, Steyerberg EW, Butcher I, Dammers R, Lu J, Marmarou A, Mushkudiani NA, McHugh GS, Murray GD. Prognostic value of computerized tomography scan characteristics in traumatic brain injury: results from the IMPACT study. J Neurotrauma. 2007;24(2):303–14.
31. Seelig JM, Becker DP, Miller JD, Greenberg RP, Ward JD, Choi SC. Traumatic acute subdural hematoma: major mortality reduction in comatose patients treated within four hours. N Engl J Med. 1981;304(25):1511–8.
32. Fountain DM, Kolias AG, Lecky FE, Bouamra O, Lawrence T, Adams H, Bond SJ, Hutchinson PJ. Survival trends after surgery for acute subdural hematoma in adults over a 20-year period. Ann Surg. 2017;265(3):590–6.
33. Alahmadi H, Vachhrajani S, Cusimano MD. The natural history of brain contusion: an analysis of radiological and clinical progression. J Neurosurg. 2010;112(5):1139–45.
34. Iaccarino C, Schiavi P, Picetti E, Goldoni M, Cerasti D, Caspani M, Servadei F. Patients with brain contusions: predictors of outcome and relationship between radiological and clinical evolution. J Neurosurg. 2014;120(4):908–18. https://doi.org/10.3171/2013.12.JNS131090. Epub 2014 Feb 7.
35. Skandsen T, Kvistad KA, Solheim O, Strand IH, Folvik M, Vik A. Prevalence and impact of dif-

36. Adams JH, Doyle D, Ford I, Gennarelli TA, Graham DI, McLellan DR. Diffuse axonal injury in head injury: definition, diagnosis and grading. Histopathology. 1989;15(1):49–59.
37. Smith M. Multimodality neuromonitoring in adult traumatic brain injury: a narrative review. Anesthesiology. 2018;128(2):401–15.
38. Teasdale G, Maas A, Lecky F, Manley G, Stocchetti N, Murray G. The Glasgow coma scale at 40 years: standing the test of time. Lancet Neurol. 2014;13(8):844–54.
39. Helbok R, Kurtz P, Schmidt MJ, Stuart MR, Fernandez L, Connolly SE, Lee K, Schmutzhard E, Mayer SA, Claassen J, Badjatia N. Effects of the neurological wake-up test on clinical examination, intracranial pressure, brain metabolism and brain tissue oxygenation in severely brain-injured patients. Crit Care. 2012;16(6):R226.

35. fuse axonal injury in patients with moderate and severe head injury: a cohort study of early magnetic resonance imaging findings and 1-year outcome. J Neurosurg. 2010;113(3):556–63.

40. Marmarou A, Lu J, Butcher I, McHugh GS, Murray GD, Steyerberg EW, Mushkudiani NA, Choi S, Maas AI. Prognostic value of the Glasgow Coma Scale and pupil reactivity in traumatic brain injury assessed prehospital and on enrollment: an IMPACT analysis. J Neurotrauma. 2007;24(2):270–80.
41. Adoni A, McNett M. The pupillary response in traumatic brain injury: a guide for trauma nurses. J Trauma Nurs. 2007;14(4):191–6.
42. Marmarou A, Eisenberg HM, Foulkes MA, Marshall LF, Jane JA. Impact of ICP instability and hypotension on outcome in patients with severe head trauma. J Neurosurg. 1991;75(1S):S59–66.
43. Vik A, Nag T, Fredriksli OA, Skandsen T, Moen KG, Schirmer-Mikalsen K, Manley GT. Relationship of "dose" of intracranial hypertension to outcome in severe traumatic brain injury. J Neurosurg. 2008;109(4):678–84.
44. Güiza F, Depreitere B, Piper I, Citerio G, Chambers I, Jones PA, Lo TY, Enblad P, Nillson P, Feyen B, Jorens P, Maas A, Schuhmann MU, Donald R, Moss L, Van den Berghe G, Meyfroidt G. Visualizing the pressure and time burden of intracranial hypertension in adult and paediatric traumatic brain injury. Intensive Care Med. 2015;41(6):1067–76.
45. Güiza F, Meyfroidt G, Piper I, Citerio G, Chambers I, Enblad P, Nillson P, Feyen B, Jorens P, Maas A, Schuhmann MU, Donald R, Moss L, Van den Berghe G, Depreitere B. Cerebral perfusion pressure insults and associations with outcome in adult traumatic brain injury. J Neurotrauma. 2017;34(16):2425–31.
46. Picetti E, Iaccarino C, Servadei F. Letter: guidelines for the management of severe traumatic brain injury fourth edition. Neurosurgery. 2017;81(1):E2.
47. Stocchetti N, Picetti E, Berardino M, Buki A, Chesnut RM, Fountas KN, Horn P, Hutchinson PJ, Iaccarino C, Kolias AG, Koskinen LO, Latronico N, Maas AI, Payen JF, Rosenthal G, Sahuquillo J, Signoretti S, Soustiel JF, Servadei F. Clinical applications of intracranial pressure monitoring in traumatic brain injury: report of the Milan consensus conference. Acta Neurochir (Wien). 2014;156(8):1615–22.
48. Chesnut R, Videtta W, Vespa P, Le Roux P. Participants in the International Multidisciplinary Consensus Conference on Multimodality Monitoring. Intracranial pressure monitoring: fundamental considerations and rationale for monitoring. Neurocrit Care. 2014;21(Suppl 2):S64–84.
49. Thomas E, NACCS, Czosnyka M, Hutchinson P, SBNS. Calculation of cerebral perfusion pressure in the management of traumatic brain injury: joint position statement by the councils of the Neuroanaesthesia and Critical Care Society of Great Britain and Ireland (NACCS) and the Society of British Neurological Surgeons (SBNS). Br J Anaesth. 2015;115(4):487–8.
50. Servadei F, Picetti E. Intracranial pressure monitoring and outcome in traumatic brain injury: the probe does matter? World Neurosurg. 2015;83(5):732–3.
51. Marcus HJ, Wilson MH. Insertion of an intracranial pressure monitor. N Engl J Med. 2015;373(22):e25.
52. Dossani RH, Patra DP, Terrell DL, Willis B. Placement of an external ventricular drain. N Engl J Med. 2021;384(2):e3.
53. van den Brink WA, van Santbrink H, Steyerberg EW, Avezaat CJ, Suazo JA, Hogesteeger C, Jansen WJ, Kloos LM, Vermeulen J, Maas AI. Brain oxygen tension in severe head injury. Neurosurgery. 2000;46(4):868–76; discussion 876-8.
54. Longhi L, Pagan F, Valeriani V, Magnoni S, Zanier ER, Conte V, Branca V, Stocchetti N. Monitoring brain tissue oxygen tension in brain-injured patients reveals hypoxic episodes in normal-appearing and in peri-focal tissue. Intensive Care Med. 2007;33(12):2136–42.
55. Oddo M, Levine JM, Mackenzie L, Frangos S, Feihl F, Kasner SE, Katsnelson M, Pukenas B, Macmurtrie E, Maloney-Wilensky E, Kofke WA, LeRoux PD. Brain hypoxia is associated with short-term outcome after severe traumatic brain injury independently of intracranial hypertension and low cerebral perfusion pressure. Neurosurgery. 2011;69(5):1037–45; discussion 1045.
56. Okonkwo DO, Shutter LA, Moore C, Temkin NR, Puccio AM, Madden CJ, Andaluz N, Chesnut RM, Bullock MR, Grant GA, McGregor J, Weaver M, Jallo J, LeRoux PD, Moberg D, Barber J, Lazaridis C, Diaz-Arrastia RR. Brain oxygen optimization in severe traumatic brain injury phase-II: a phase II randomized trial. Crit Care Med. 2017;45(11):1907–14.
57. Leach MR, Shutter LA. How much oxygen for the injured brain—can invasive parenchymal catheters help? Curr Opin Crit Care. 2021;27(2):95–102.
58. Chesnut R, Aguilera S, Buki A, Bulger E, Citerio G, Cooper DJ, Arrastia RD, Diringer M, Figaji A, Gao G, Geocadin R, Ghajar J, Harris O, Hoffer A, Hutchinson P, Joseph M, Kitagawa R, Manley G, Mayer S, Menon DK, Meyfroidt G, Michael DB, Oddo M, Okonkwo D, Patel M, Robertson C, Rosenfeld JV, Rubiano

AM, Sahuquillo J, Servadei F, Shutter L, Stein D, Stocchetti N, Taccone FS, Timmons S, Tsai E, Ullman JS, Vespa P, Videtta W, Wright DW, Zammit C, Hawryluk GWJ. A management algorithm for adult patients with both brain oxygen and intracranial pressure monitoring: the Seattle International Severe Traumatic Brain Injury Consensus Conference (SIBICC). Intensive Care Med. 2020;46(5):919–29.
59. Picetti E, Rossi S, Ottochian M, Stein DM. Brain injury in the ACS patient: nuts and bolts of neuromonitoring and management. In: Picetti E, Pereira BM, Razek T, et al. editors. Intensive care for emergency surgeons. 1st ed. Springer Nature Switzerland 2019; 89-112.
60. Bullock MR, Chesnut R, Ghajar J, Gordon D, Hartl R, Newell DW, Servadei F, Walters BC, Wilberger J. Surgical Management of Traumatic Brain Injury Author Group. Surgical management of acute epidural hematomas. Neurosurgery. 2006;58(3 Suppl):S7–15.
61. Bullock MR, Chesnut R, Ghajar J, Gordon D, Hartl R, Newell DW, Servadei F, Walters BC, Wilberger J. Surgical Management of Traumatic Brain Injury Author Group. Surgical management of acute subdural hematomas. Neurosurgery. 2006;58(3 Suppl):S16–24.
62. Bullock MR, Chesnut R, Ghajar J, Gordon D, Hartl R, Newell DW, Servadei F, Walters BC, Wilberger J. Surgical Management of Traumatic Brain Injury Author Group. Surgical management of traumatic parenchymal lesions. Neurosurgery. 2006;58(3 Suppl):S25–46.
63. Bullock MR, Chesnut R, Ghajar J, Gordon D, Hartl R, Newell DW, Servadei F, Walters BC, Wilberger J. Surgical Management of Traumatic Brain Injury Author Group. Surgical management of posterior fossa mass lesions. Neurosurgery. 2006;58(3 Suppl):S47–55.
64. Bullock MR, Chesnut R, Ghajar J, Gordon D, Hartl R, Newell DW, Servadei F, Walters BC, Wilberger J. Surgical Management of Traumatic Brain Injury Author Group. Surgical management of depressed cranial fractures. Neurosurgery. 2006;58(3 Suppl):S56–60.
65. Stocchetti N, Maas AI. Traumatic intracranial hypertension. N Engl J Med. 2014;370(22):2121–30.
66. Hawryluk GWJ, Aguilera S, Buki A, Bulger E, Citerio G, Cooper DJ, Arrastia RD, Diringer M, Figaji A, Gao G, Geocadin R, Ghajar J, Harris O, Hoffer A, Hutchinson P, Joseph M, Kitagawa R, Manley G, Mayer S, Menon DK, Meyfroidt G, Michael DB, Oddo M, Okonkwo D, Patel M, Robertson C, Rosenfeld JV, Rubiano AM, Sahuquillo J, Servadei F, Shutter L, Stein D, Stocchetti N, Taccone FS, Timmons S, Tsai E, Ullman JS, Vespa P, Videtta W, Wright DW, Zammit C, Chesnut RM. A management algorithm for patients with intracranial pressure monitoring: the Seattle International Severe Traumatic Brain Injury Consensus Conference (SIBICC). Intensive Care Med. 2019;45(12):1783–94.
67. Fried HI, Nathan BR, Rowe AS, Zabramski JM, Andaluz N, Bhimraj A, Guanci MM, Seder DB, Singh JM. The insertion and management of external ventricular drains: an evidence-based consensus statement: a statement for healthcare professionals from the neurocritical care society. Neurocrit Care. 2016;24(1):61–81.
68. Lele AV, Hoefnagel AL, Schloemerkemper N, Wyler DA, Chaikittisilpa N, Vavilala MS, Naik BI, Williams JH, Venkat Raghavan L, Koerner IP, Representing SNACC Task Force for Developing Guidelines for Perioperative Management of External Ventricular and Lumbar Drains. Perioperative management of adult patients with external ventricular and lumbar drains: guidelines from the Society for Neuroscience in Anesthesiology and Critical Care. J Neurosurg Anesthesiol. 2017;29(3):191–210.
69. Ropper AH. Hyperosmolar therapy for raised intracranial pressure. N Engl J Med. 2012;367(8):746–52.
70. Laffey JG, Kavanagh BP. Hypocapnia. N Engl J Med. 2002;347(1):43–53.
71. Stocchetti N, Maas AI, Chieregato A, van der Plas AA. Hyperventilation in head injury: a review. Chest. 2005;127(5):1812–27.
72. Coles JP, Fryer TD, Coleman MR, Smielewski P, Gupta AK, Minhas PS, Aigbirhio F, Chatfield DA, Williams GB, Boniface S, Carpenter TA, Clark JC, Pickard JD, Menon DK. Hyperventilation following head injury: effect on ischemic burden and cerebral oxidative metabolism. Crit Care Med. 2007;35(2):568–78.
73. Ahmed AI, Bullock MR, Dietrich WD. Hypothermia in traumatic brain injury. Neurosurg Clin N Am. 2016;27(4):489–97.
74. Polderman KH. Induced hypothermia and fever control for prevention and treatment of neurological injuries. Lancet. 2008;371(9628):1955–69.
75. Polderman KH, Herold I. Therapeutic hypothermia and controlled normothermia in the intensive care unit: practical considerations, side effects, and cooling methods. Crit Care Med. 2009;37(3):1101–20.
76. Andrews PJ, Sinclair HL, Rodriguez A, Harris BA, Battison CG, Rhodes JK, Murray GD. Eurotherm3235 Trial Collaborators. Hypothermia for intracranial hypertension after traumatic brain injury. N Engl J Med. 2015;373(25):2403–12.
77. Servadei F, Compagnone C, Sahuquillo J. The role of surgery in traumatic brain injury. Curr Opin Crit Care. 2007;13(2):163–8.
78. Kolias AG, Kirkpatrick PJ, Hutchinson PJ. Decompressive craniectomy: past, present and future. Nat Rev Neurol. 2013;9(7):405–15.
79. Cooper DJ, Rosenfeld JV, Murray L, Arabi YM, Davies AR, D'Urso P, Kossmann T, Ponsford J, Seppelt I, Reilly P, Wolfe R, DECRA Trial Investigators, Australian and New Zealand Intensive Care Society Clinical Trials Group. Decompressive craniectomy in diffuse traumatic brain injury. N Engl J Med. 2011;364(16):1493–502.

80. Hutchinson PJ, Kolias AG, Timofeev IS, Corteen EA, Czosnyka M, Timothy J, Anderson I, Bulters DO, Belli A, Eynon CA, Wadley J, Mendelow AD, Mitchell PM, Wilson MH, Critchley G, Sahuquillo J, Unterberg A, Servadei F, Teasdale GM, Pickard JD, Menon DK, Murray GD, Kirkpatrick PJ, RESCUEicp Trial Collaborators. Trial of decompressive craniectomy for traumatic intracranial hypertension. N Engl J Med. 2016;375(12):1119–30.
81. Kurland DB, Khaladj-Ghom A, Stokum JA, Carusillo B, Karimy JK, Gerzanich V, Sahuquillo J, Simard JM. Complications associated with decompressive craniectomy: a systematic review. Neurocrit Care. 2015;23(2):292–304.
82. Hutchinson PJ, Kolias AG, Tajsic T, Adeleye A, Aklilu AT, Apriawan T, Bajamal AH, Barthélemy EJ, Devi BI, Bhat D, Bulters D, Chesnut R, Citerio G, Cooper DJ, Czosnyka M, Edem I, El-Ghandour NMF, Figaji A, Fountas KN, Gallagher C, Hawryluk GWJ, Iaccarino C, Joseph M, Khan T, Laeke T, Levchenko O, Liu B, Liu W, Maas A, Manley GT, Manson P, Mazzeo AT, Menon DK, Michael DB, Muehlschlegel S, Okonkwo DO, Park KB, Rosenfeld JV, Rosseau G, Rubiano AM, Shabani HK, Stocchetti N, Timmons SD, Timofeev I, Uff C, Ullman JS, Valadka A, Waran V, Wells A, Wilson MH, Servadei F. Consensus statement from the international consensus meeting on the role of decompressive craniectomy in the management of traumatic brain injury: consensus statement. Acta Neurochir (Wien). 2019;161(7):1261–74.
83. Hawryluk GWJ, Rubiano AM, Totten AM, O'Reilly C, Ullman JS, Bratton SL, Chesnut R, Harris OA, Kissoon N, Shutter L, Tasker RC, Vavilala MS, Wilberger J, Wright DW, Lumba-Brown A, Ghajar J. Guidelines for the management of severe traumatic brain injury: 2020 update of the decompressive craniectomy recommendations. Neurosurgery. 2020;87(3):427–34.
84. Veldeman M, Daleiden L, Hamou H, Höllig A, Clusmann H. An altered posterior question-mark incision is associated with a reduced infection rate of cranioplasty after decompressive hemicraniectomy. J Neurosurg. 2020;24:1–9. https://doi.org/10.3171/2020.2.JNS193335. Epub ahead of print.
85. Vieira E, Guimarães TC, Faquini IV, Silva JL, Saboia T, Andrade RVCL, Gemir TL, Neri VC, Almeida NS, Azevedo-Filho HRC. Randomized controlled study comparing 2 surgical techniques for decompressive craniectomy: with watertight duraplasty and without watertight duraplasty. J Neurosurg. 2018;129(4):1017–23. https://doi.org/10.3171/2017.4.JNS152954. Epub 2017 Nov 17.
86. Callcut RA, Kornblith LZ, Conroy AS, Robles AJ, Meizoso JP, Namias N, Meyer DE, Haymaker A, Truitt MS, Agrawal V, Haan JM, Lightwine KL, Porter JM, San Roman JL, Biffl WL, Hayashi MS, Sise MJ, Badiee J, Recinos G, Inaba K, Schroeppel TJ, Callaghan E, Dunn JA, Godin S, McIntyre RC Jr, Peltz ED, O'Neill PJ, Diven CF, Scifres AM, Switzer EE, West MA, Storrs S, Cullinane DC, Cordova JF, Moore EE, Moore HB, Privette AR, Eriksson EA, Cohen MJ, Western Trauma Association Multicenter Study Group. The why and how our trauma patients die: a prospective Multicenter Western Trauma Association study. J Trauma Acute Care Surg. 2019;86(5):864–70.
87. Galvagno SM Jr, Fox EE, Appana SN, Baraniuk S, Bosarge PL, Bulger EM, Callcut RA, Cotton BA, Goodman M, Inaba K, O'Keeffe T, Schreiber MA, Wade CE, Scalea TM, Holcomb JB, Stein DM, PROPPR Study Group. Outcomes after concomitant traumatic brain injury and hemorrhagic shock: A secondary analysis from the Pragmatic, Randomized Optimal Platelets and Plasma Ratios trial. J Trauma Acute Care Surg. 2017;83(4):668–74.
88. Picetti E, Rossi S, Abu-Zidan FM, Ansaloni L, Armonda R, Baiocchi GL, Bala M, Balogh ZJ, Berardino M, Biffl WL, Bouzat P, Buki A, Ceresoli M, Chesnut RM, Chiara O, Citerio G, Coccolini F, Coimbra R, Di Saverio S, Fraga GP, Gupta D, Helbok R, Hutchinson PJ, Kirkpatrick AW, Kinoshita T, Kluger Y, Leppaniemi A, Maas AIR, Maier RV, Minardi F, Moore EE, Myburgh JA, Okonkwo DO, Otomo Y, Rizoli S, Rubiano AM, Sahuquillo J, Sartelli M, Scalea TM, Servadei F, Stahel PF, Stocchetti N, Taccone FS, Tonetti T, Velmahos G, Weber D, Catena F. WSES consensus conference guidelines: monitoring and management of severe adult traumatic brain injury patients with polytrauma in the first 24 hours. World J Emerg Surg. 2019;14:53.

Suggested References

Adoni A, McNett M. The pupillary response in traumatic brain injury: a guide for trauma nurses. J Trauma Nurs. 2007;14(4):191–6.

Callcut RA, Kornblith LZ, Conroy AS, Robles AJ, Meizoso JP, Namias N, Meyer DE, Haymaker A, Truitt MS, Agrawal V, Haan JM, Lightwine KL, Porter JM, San Roman JL, Biffl WL, Hayashi MS, Sise MJ, Badiee J, Recinos G, Inaba K, Schroeppel TJ, Callaghan E, Dunn JA, Godin S, McIntyre RC Jr, Peltz ED, O'Neill PJ, Diven CF, Scifres AM, Switzer EE, West MA, Storrs S, Cullinane DC, Cordova JF, Moore EE, Moore HB, Privette AR, Eriksson EA, Cohen MJ, Western Trauma Association Multicenter Study Group. The why and how our trauma patients die: A prospective Multicenter Western Trauma Association study. J Trauma Acute Care Surg. 2019;86(5):864–70.

Chesnut R, Aguilera S, Buki A, Bulger E, Citerio G, Cooper DJ, Arrastia RD, Diringer M, Figaji A, Gao G, Geocadin R, Ghajar J, Harris O, Hoffer A, Hutchinson P, Joseph M, Kitagawa R, Manley G, Mayer S, Menon DK, Meyfroidt G, Michael DB, Oddo M, Okonkwo D, Patel M, Robertson C, Rosenfeld JV, Rubiano AM, Sahuquillo J, Servadei F, Shutter L, Stein D, Stocchetti N, Taccone FS, Timmons S, Tsai E, Ullman JS, Vespa P, Videtta W, Wright DW, Zammit C, Hawryluk

GWJ. A management algorithm for adult patients with both brain oxygen and intracranial pressure monitoring: the Seattle International Severe Traumatic Brain Injury Consensus Conference (SIBICC). Intensive Care Med. 2020;46(5):919–29.

Chesnut R, Videtta W, Vespa P, Le Roux P. Participants in the international multidisciplinary consensus conference on multimodality monitoring. Intracranial pressure monitoring: fundamental considerations and rationale for monitoring. Neurocrit Care. 2014;21(Suppl 2):S64–84.

Güiza F, Depreitere B, Piper I, Citerio G, Chambers I, Jones PA, Lo TY, Enblad P, Nillson P, Feyen B, Jorens P, Maas A, Schuhmann MU, Donald R, Moss L, Van den Berghe G, Meyfroidt G. Visualizing the pressure and time burden of intracranial hypertension in adult and paediatric traumatic brain injury. Intensive Care Med. 2015;41(6):1067–76.

Güiza F, Meyfroidt G, Piper I, Citerio G, Chambers I, Enblad P, Nillson P, Feyen B, Jorens P, Maas A, Schuhmann MU, Donald R, Moss L, Van den Berghe G, Depreitere B. Cerebral perfusion pressure insults and associations with outcome in adult traumatic brain injury. J Neurotrauma. 2017;34(16):2425–31.

Hawryluk GWJ, Aguilera S, Buki A, Bulger E, Citerio G, Cooper DJ, Arrastia RD, Diringer M, Figaji A, Gao G, Geocadin R, Ghajar J, Harris O, Hoffer A, Hutchinson P, Joseph M, Kitagawa R, Manley G, Mayer S, Menon DK, Meyfroidt G, Michael DB, Oddo M, Okonkwo D, Patel M, Robertson C, Rosenfeld JV, Rubiano AM, Sahuquillo J, Servadei F, Shutter L, Stein D, Stocchetti N, Taccone FS, Timmons S, Tsai E, Ullman JS, Vespa P, Videtta W, Wright DW, Zammit C, Chesnut RM. A management algorithm for patients with intracranial pressure monitoring: the Seattle International Severe Traumatic Brain Injury Consensus Conference (SIBICC). Intensive Care Med. 2019;45(12):1783–94.

Hutchinson PJ, Kolias AG, Tajsic T, Adeleye A, Aklilu AT, Apriawan T, Bajamal AH, Barthélemy EJ, Devi BI, Bhat D, Bulters D, Chesnut R, Citerio G, Cooper DJ, Czosnyka M, Edem I, El-Ghandour NMF, Figaji A, Fountas KN, Gallagher C, Hawryluk GWJ, Iaccarino C, Joseph M, Khan T, Laeke T, Levchenko O, Liu B, Liu W, Maas A, Manley GT, Manson P, Mazzeo AT, Menon DK, Michael DB, Muehlschlegel S, Okonkwo DO, Park KB, Rosenfeld JV, Rosseau G, Rubiano AM, Shabani HK, Stocchetti N, Timmons SD, Timofeev I, Uff C, Ullman JS, Valadka A, Waran V, Wells A, Wilson MH, Servadei F. Consensus statement from the international consensus meeting on the role of decompressive craniectomy in the management of traumatic brain injury : consensus statement. Acta Neurochir (Wien). 2019;161(7):1261–74.

Iaccarino C, Schiavi P, Picetti E, Goldoni M, Cerasti D, Caspani M, Servadei F. Patients with brain contusions: predictors of outcome and relationship between radiological and clinical evolution. J Neurosurg. 2014;120(4):908–18. https://doi.org/10.3171/2013.12.JNS131090. Epub 2014 Feb 7.

Kolias AG, Kirkpatrick PJ, Hutchinson PJ. Decompressive craniectomy: past, present and future. Nat Rev Neurol. 2013;9(7):405–15.

Leach MR, Shutter LA. How much oxygen for the injured brain—can invasive parenchymal catheters help? Curr Opin Crit Care. 2021;27(2):95–102.

Lele AV, Hoefnagel AL, Schloemerkemper N, Wyler DA, Chaikittisilpa N, Vavilala MS, Naik BI, Williams JH, Venkat Raghavan L, Koerner IP, Representing SNACC Task Force for Developing Guidelines for Perioperative Management of External Ventricular and Lumbar Drains. Perioperative management of adult patients with external ventricular and lumbar drains: guidelines from the society for neuroscience in anesthesiology and critical care. J Neurosurg Anesthesiol. 2017;29(3):191–210.

Maas AIR, Menon DK, Adelson PD, Andelic N, Bell MJ, Belli A, Bragge P, Brazinova A, Büki A, Chesnut RM, Citerio G, Coburn M, Cooper DJ, Crowder AT, Czeiter E, Czosnyka M, Diaz-Arrastia R, Dreier JP, Duhaime AC, Ercole A, van Essen TA, Feigin VL, Gao G, Giacino J, Gonzalez-Lara LE, Gruen RL, Gupta D, Hartings JA, Hill S, Jiang JY, Ketharanathan N, Kompanje EJO, Lanyon L, Laureys S, Lecky F, Levin H, Lingsma HF, Maegele M, Majdan M, Manley G, Marsteller J, Mascia L, McFadyen C, Mondello S, Newcombe V, Palotie A, Parizel PM, Peul W, Piercy J, Polinder S, Puybasset L, Rasmussen TE, Rossaint R, Smielewski P, Söderberg J, Stanworth SJ, Stein MB, von Steinbüchel N, Stewart W, Steyerberg EW, Stocchetti N, Synnot A, Te Ao B, Tenovuo O, Theadom A, Tibboel D, Videtta W, Wang KKW, Williams WH, Wilson L, Yaffe K. InTBIR Participants and Investigators. Traumatic brain injury: integrated approaches to improve prevention, clinical care, and research. Lancet Neurol. 2017;16(12):987–1048.

Picetti E, Rossi S, Abu-Zidan FM, Ansaloni L, Armonda R, Baiocchi GL, Bala M, Balogh ZJ, Berardino M, Biffl WL, Bouzat P, Buki A, Ceresoli M, Chesnut RM, Chiara O, Citerio G, Coccolini F, Coimbra R, Di Saverio S, Fraga GP, Gupta D, Helbok R, Hutchinson PJ, Kirkpatrick AW, Kinoshita T, Kluger Y, Leppaniemi A, Maas AIR, Maier RV, Minardi F, Moore EE, Myburgh JA, Okonkwo DO, Otomo Y, Rizoli S, Rubiano AM, Sahuquillo J, Sartelli M, Scalea TM, Servadei F, Stahel PF, Stocchetti N, Taccone FS, Tonetti T, Velmahos G, Weber D, Catena F. WSES consensus conference guidelines: monitoring and management of severe adult traumatic brain injury patients with polytrauma in the first 24 hours. World J Emerg Surg. 2019 Nov;29(14):53.

Picetti E, Rossi S, Ottochian M, Stein DM. Brain injury in the ACS patient: nuts and bolts of neuromonitoring and management. In: Picetti E, Pereira BM, Razek T, et al. Intensive care for emergency surgeons. 1st ed. Springer Nature Switzerland 2019; 89-112.

Smith M. Multimodality neuromonitoring in adult traumatic brain injury: a narrative review. Anesthesiology. 2018;128(2):401–15.

Stocchetti N, Maas AI. Traumatic intracranial hypertension. N Engl J Med. 2014;370(22):2121–30.

Stocchetti N, Carbonara M, Citerio G, Ercole A, Skrifvars MB, Smielewski P, Zoerle T, Menon DK. Severe traumatic brain injury: targeted management in the intensive care unit. Lancet Neurol. 2017;16(6):452–64.

Stocchetti N, Picetti E, Berardino M, Buki A, Chesnut RM, Fountas KN, Horn P, Hutchinson PJ, Iaccarino C, Kolias AG, Koskinen LO, Latronico N, Maas AI, Payen JF, Rosenthal G, Sahuquillo J, Signoretti S, Soustiel JF, Servadei F. Clinical applications of intracranial pressure monitoring in traumatic brain injury: report of the Milan consensus conference. Acta Neurochir (Wien). 2014;156(8):1615–22.

Teasdale G, Maas A, Lecky F, Manley G, Stocchetti N, Murray G. The Glasgow Coma Scale at 40 years: standing the test of time. Lancet Neurol. 2014;13(8):844–54.

Thomas E, NACCS, Czosnyka M, Hutchinson P, SBNS. Calculation of cerebral perfusion pressure in the management of traumatic brain injury: joint position statement by the councils of the Neuroanaesthesia and Critical Care Society of Great Britain and Ireland (NACCS) and the Society of British Neurological Surgeons (SBNS). Br J Anaesth. 2015;115(4):487–8.

Tonetti T, Biondini S, Minardi F, Rossi S, Picetti E. Definition and pathomechanism of the intracranial compartment syndrome. In: Coccolini F, Malbrain MLNG, Kirkpatrick AW, et al. Compartment syndrome. 1st ed. Springer Nature Switzerland 2021; 7-16.

Vik A, Nag T, Fredriksli OA, Skandsen T, Moen KG, Schirmer-Mikalsen K, Manley GT. Relationship of "dose" of intracranial hypertension to outcome in severe traumatic brain injury. J Neurosurg. 2008;109(4):678–84.

Emergency Surgical Access to the Neck

40

Iván Trostchansky and Fernando Machado

40.1 Introduction and Learning Goals

Emergency surgical access to the neck may be a challenging task in many situations when a time-based decision process is required. The presence of an injury involving any of the several vital anatomical structures in this region can be associated with significant morbidity and mortality.

Surgical access may be also necessary to deal with an infectious process involving anatomical spaces. In both cases (trauma or infection), full anatomical comprehension and specific technical knowledge are necessary to adequately accomplish this objective.

By reading this chapter, you will be able to:

- become familiar with a priority-guided surgical approach to penetrating neck injuries
- choose the optimal surgical access to the neck
- know the main technical aspects of cervical emergency exploration

---

I. Trostchansky
Emergency Department, Hospital de Clínicas—School of Medicine UdelaR, Montevideo, Uruguay

Emergency Department, Hospital de Clínicas, Montevideo, Uruguay

F. Machado (✉)
Emergency Department, Hospital de Clínicas—School of Medicine UdelaR, Montevideo, Uruguay
e-mail: fmachado@fmed.edu.uy

40.2 Surgical Anatomy of the Neck

The neck is a crossroad region of important visceral, vascular and nervous structures arranged in the limited space between the head, the thorax and the upper limbs. Its lower limit is the upper border of the clavicles and the sternal manubrium in front, the scapula and the seventh cervical vertebral body at the back. The neck's upper limit is defined by the lower border of the mandible in front and to the sides, ascending to the external occipital protuberance and superior occipital line posteriorly.

The cervical spine protects the spinal cord, and the brachial plexus originates from it.

The nape region is arranged in four muscular planes that support and extend the head. These muscular planes are surrounded by the cervical fascia that is divided into two sheets: superficial fascia and deep fascia. The latter is divided into three leaves: superficial, medium and deep. Between these fasciae and muscles, the neck spaces are delimited (Fig. 40.1).

The deep muscular plane is wrapped by the deep layer of the deep cervical fascia. Over the middle line are the prevertebral muscles and laterally the scalenes muscles with the phrenic nerve descending over the anterior scalene muscle. This muscle separates the subclavian vein from the artery.

© The Author(s), under exclusive license to Springer Nature Switzerland AG 2023
F. Coccolini, F. Catena (eds.), *Textbook of Emergency General Surgery*,
https://doi.org/10.1007/978-3-031-22599-4_40

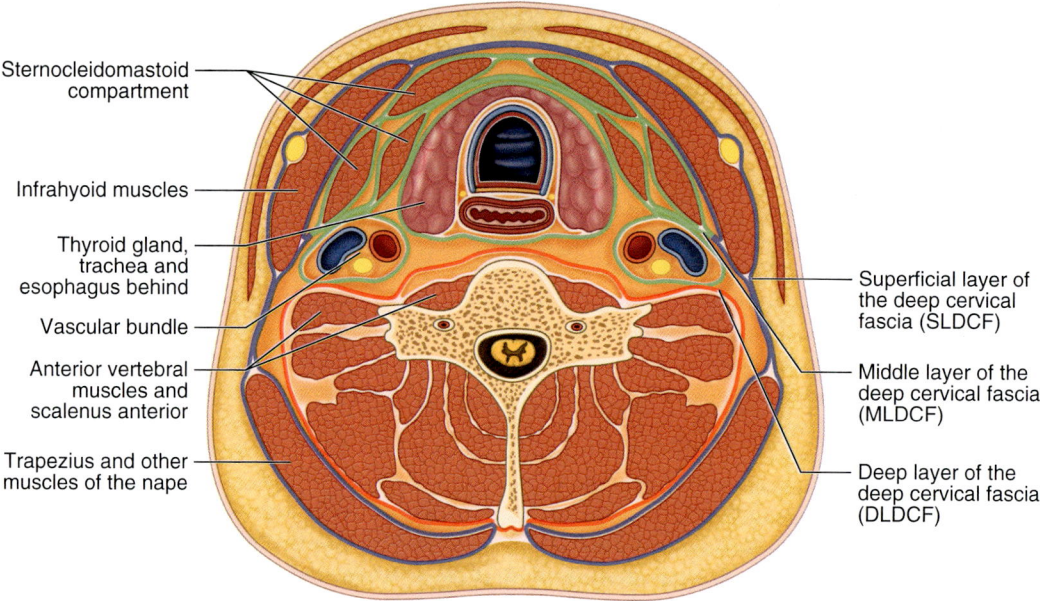

Fig. 40.1 Cross section of the neck with fasciae and spaces. (1) Superficial layer of the deep cervical fascia (SLDCF). (2) Middle layer of the deep cervical fascia. (3) Deep layer of the deep cervical fascia. (4) Sternocleidomastoid compartment. (5) Infrahyoid muscles. (6) Thyroid gland, trachea and esophagus behind. (7) Vascular bundle. (8) Anterior vertebral muscles and scalenus anterior. (9) Trapezius and other muscles of the nape

The intermediate muscular plane is composed of the infrahyoid muscles. They are involved by the middle layer of the deep cervical fascia that surrounds the thyroid gland, the trachea and the esophagus. The sternohyoid and omohyoid muscles can be useful for making a flap to isolate esophageal and tracheal repairs to prevent fistula formation.

The sternocleidomastoid muscles (SCM) are covered by the superficial layer of the deep cervical fascia (SLDCF). The SCM is highly important as a landmark in surgical access to the neck. The anterior border of the muscle is key to access the carotid bundle and the aerodigestive tract. The internal jugular vein is located deep in relation to the muscle.

In the surface, just beneath the dermis, the platysma muscle is surrounded by the superficial layer of the cervical fascia. All injuries that go through this thin superficial muscle are defined as penetrating.

The aerodigestive tract in the midline and the neurovascular bundles (carotid arteries, internal jugular veins and pneumogastric nerve) on both sides are among the muscles and their fasciae. The brachial plexus and subclavian vessels run from the cervical spine and thorax through the upper limb, supported by the first rib. The subclavian artery and the subclavian vein are difficult to access for bleeding control all along their extension.

A clear knowledge of the surface anatomy with its landmarks is essential to plan surgical procedures. However, it should be noted that these anatomical landmarks may be distorted in the presence of an expanding hematoma difficulting the correct siting of surgical incisions (Fig. 40.2).

The anatomical division of the neck in a triangle-based conception is not useful in trauma [1]. Considering three overlapping zones as Monson et al. [2] proposed in 1969 and Roon and

40 Emergency Surgical Access to the Neck

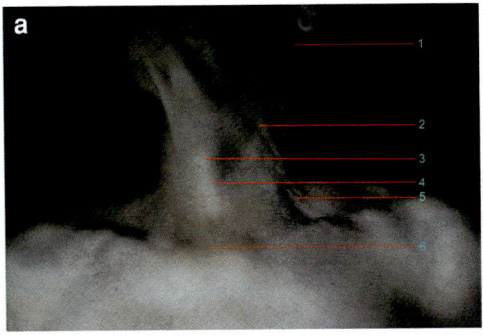 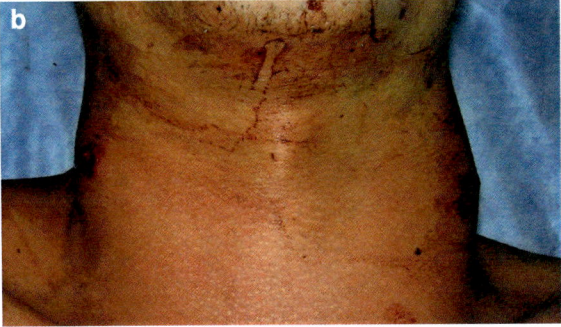

Fig. 40.2 (a) Surface anatomy of the neck. (1) Angle of the mandible. (2) Anterior border of sternocleidomastoid muscle with the external jugular vein crossing in the surface. (3) Adam's apple. (4) Cricothyroid membrane. (5) Platysma's fibers under the skin. (6) Suprasternal notch. (b) Superficial landmarks are difficult to find in the presence of a cervical hematoma. This patient suffered a side-to-side gunshot wound to the neck

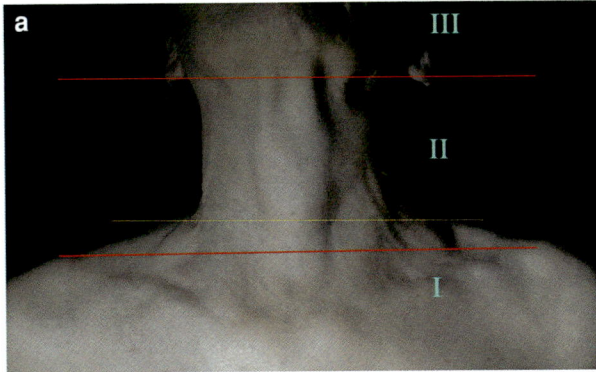 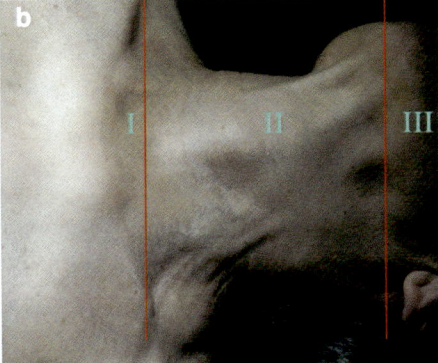

Fig. 40.3 (a) Three zones of the neck (Monson). The yellow line indicates the Zone I extension to the level of the cricoid cartilage (Roon and Christensen). (b) In operative position, the narrowest surgical field of Zones I and III are clearly shown

Christensen slightly modified later in 1979 has proved more useful [3].

Monson's Zone I accurately describe the zone of the base of the neck and thoracic outlet. Zone II is the largest one, reaching into the mandible angle, where zone III begins, to continue upward into the base of the skull (Fig. 40.3).

40.2.1 Arteries

Four arteries rise from the base of the neck and the upper mediastinum to the skull and face: two in an anterior position (common carotid arteries) and two in a deep position (vertebral arteries).

40.2.1.1 Carotid Arteries

The left common carotid artery originates directly from the aortic arch in the mediastinum, while the right one originates from the innominate trunk, together with the right subclavian artery. Both of them join the lateral aspect of the esophagus and laryngotracheal axis and ascend in medial position in relation to the internal jugular vein. The internal jugular vein lies immediately beneath the SCM. The pneumogastric nerve descends in the posterior angle between both vascular structures.

To obtain a good access to the carotid artery, it is necessary to ligate and cut the facial vein and, usually, the middle thyroid vein.

Common carotid arteries split into external and internal carotids just beneath the mandibular angle, at the upper portion of Zone II.

40.2.1.2 Subclavian Artery

The subclavian artery originates from the innominate artery on the right and directly from the aortic arch on the left, thus providing an intrathoracic path that enables clamping it through a high left thoracotomy.

40.2.1.3 Vertebral Artery

Vertebral arteries are the first branch of the subclavian arteries. These are located deep in their position, ahead of the seventh cervical vertebra and behind the common carotid artery (section V1 of the vertebral artery), where the surgical approach is extremely difficult. The artery ascends through the foramina of the transverse processes of the upper six cervical vertebrae, where it is inaccessible to direct surgical domain (section V2).

40.2.2 Larynx and Trachea

The larynx is placed in the upper section of the airway in the neck, corresponding along its vertical extension to the bodies of fourth, fifth and sixth cervical vertebrae. The larynx is a triangular box shaped structure with a prominent vertical ridge (Adam's apple). This is one of the most important landmarks in the neck's superficial anatomy.

Between the thyroid cartilage (superiorly) and the arch of the cricoid cartilage (inferiorly), the "conus elasticus" (cricothyroid membrane), with the middle cricothyroid ligament is located. Emergency surgical access to the airway is usually done through this thick central part of the membrane.

The cervical trachea is a cartilaginous and membranous tube flattened posteriorly and closely related to the esophagus behind. For this reason, associated injuries are not uncommon. These structures are closely related to the thyroid gland and the carotid vascular bundles on both sides.

The thyroid isthmus is a well-vascularized structure that crosses over the third or fourth tracheal ring, where the trachea is deeper into the neck and more difficult to access.

The brachiocephalic artery lies over the anterior tracheal wall at the suprasternal notch in up to 33,4% of patients [4]. These are all reasons why the emergency surgical access to the trachea may be challenging in an actively bleeding patient with an expanding cervical hematoma.

40.2.3 Pharynx and Esophagus

Behind the larynx, the constrictor inferior of the pharynx arises from both sides of cricoid and thyroid cartilages in a close relationship with the carotid vascular bundle.

The cervical portion of the esophagus begins opposite the sixth cervical vertebra at the inferior border of the cricoid cartilage. It descends in the midline toward the thoracic outlet behind, and slightly to the left of the trachea.

The retropharyngeal and retroesophageal spaces are in continuity. They are in front of the prevertebral muscles communicating directly with the upper mediastinum, where infectious processes can spread.

The thick mucous lining of the esophagus is the most important layer to correctly identify and repair in cases, where an esophageal perforation is recognized.

40.3 Indications of Surgical Access to the Neck

40.3.1 Conditions

The indications of an emergency surgical access to the neck may be for:

- neck injury (usually penetrating) with hard signs of bleeding or visceral involvement

- maxillofacial injury with an upper airway obstruction
- a neck infectious process

40.3.2 Diagnosis

Clinical judgement is the most important tool in the decision-making process, mainly in the search and recognition of hard signs of injury (see later).

Complementary evaluation by imagenology and/or endoscopy studies should be always clinically oriented.

An active search for a hidden injury is necessary if only soft signs are present. A neck CT scan or an angio CT may be first line studies to decide among surgical exploration or a minimally invasive approach. Additional testing may be necessary to discard unrecognized injuries (bronchoscopy, esophagoscopy, esophagram, etc.).

40.3.3 When to Operate the Above-Mentioned Conditions

40.3.3.1 Trauma

Trauma is the commonest indication for emergency neck surgery, usually in the setting of penetrating trauma. Surgical exploration because of blunt trauma is uncommon, and may be just necessary during follow-up, as an elective procedure.

The therapeutic approach to neck penetrating injuries has evolved with the advance and development of imaging techniques. Since Fogelman and Stewart in 1956 [5], all neck penetrating injuries used to be considered an indication for systematic neck exploration. This approach was followed by a high rate of unnecessary explorations (50%). Therefore, a selective approach (known also as Zone Approach) has been considered the best practice based on the next topics:

- clinical presentation: presence (or absence) of hard signs of airway/visceral/vascular injury. Hard signs are defined as suspected vascular, airway or digestive injuries with immediate potential for becoming life-threatening, see Table 40.1

Table 40.1 Schematic clinical presentation of neck injuries

Airway hard signs	Airway soft signs
Upper airway obstruction	Stridor[a]
Bubbling wound	Hoarseness[a]
Massive subcutaneous emphysema	Mild emphysema
Vascular hard signs	**Vascular soft signs**
Pulsatile Bleeding or Expanding Hematoma	Absence of common carotid pulse without neurologic deficit
Hematemesis/ Hemoptysis[b]	Palpable Thrill, audible fremitus[c]
Shock otherwise unexplained	Non-Expansive Hematoma
Neurological hard signs	**Digestive soft signs**
Evolving stroke/ neurologic deficit	Difficulty or pain when swallowing (Esophagus)

[a]CT-scan has replaced bronchoscopy in the OR for the assessment of patients with stridor and hoarseness. Around 85% of airway injuries present hard signs
[b]Possible consequence of an associated carotid injury
[c]Hard signs in other classifications, usually may be evaluated through Angio CT scan to define therapeutic approach

- the zone involved (I–II–III)
- logistic considerations based on hospital resources (CT scan, angiography, endoscopy)

The gold rules are:

- All superficial injuries to the platysma muscle are not penetrating, and the patient may be discharged.
- The presence of at least one hard sign is an indication for emergency surgical exploration. Fig. 40.4.

The "no zone" approach has been proposed by some authors in recent years. This conception is based on the lack of correlation found between the area involved and the injured organ or structure (zone approach).

The type of weapon, the trajectory of the bullet in gunshot wounds, and the patient's clinical condition (presence or not of hard signs) will help the surgeon to decide on the next therapeutic step [6–8].

In the presence of severe facial injuries, or distortion of the upper airway anatomy, or any

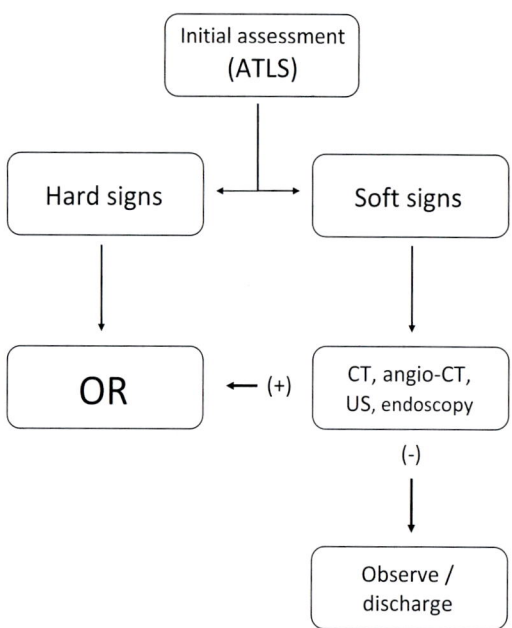

Fig. 40.4 Clinical guided decisions in penetrating neck trauma

and eventually an air–fluid level at the retropharyngeal space (Minnigerode's sign).

40.4 Management

40.4.1 General Strategies in Trauma

Upon the arrival of a patient presenting a neck injury, two essential points must be considered:

1. evaluation of the airways' patency
2. presence or absence of active bleeding.

In the presence of hard signs, ensuring airway patency in the trauma bay should be the only reason to delay the patient's transfer to the operating room (OR).

Verifying the anatomical integrity of the airway is of the utmost importance. In the presence of an expanding hematoma, an endotracheal intubation is warranted, eventually with fiberoptic aid.

Once the airway is patent, in the presence of an active bleeding, the operator should take a series of orderly measures to gain, at least, transient bleeding control.

A compressive maneuver over the wound trying to stop a venous bleeding may be appropriate for the initial management.

When the bleeding is not manageable by compressive measures, it originates in an arterial injury, or is a limited size wound (such as gunshot wounds), a Foley catheter or an N° 3 or N° 4 Fogarty balloon may be placed through the wound. The balloon is then filled with saline and pulled outward to compress the bleeding vessel.

Given the difficult surgical access to Zone III injuries, this technique is recommended in this situation. If the bleeding is controlled, the wound is closed over the catheter and the patient conducted to the OR.

The surgeon should always be prepared to change or enlarge or combine different surgical incisions. This is particularly true to gain access to proximal and distal control in vascular injuries.

In the operation room, remember:

other scenario leading to a "can't intubate, can't oxygenate" (CICO) situation, emergent surgical access to the airway is mandatory, either by a cricothyrotomy or by a tracheostomy [9–15].

40.3.3.2 Infection

The presence of a suppurative process in any of the anatomical neck spaces, regardless of its etiology, is an indication for surgical exploration and provided that a minimally invasive approach is not possible.

The CT scan is the first option to fully evaluate the neck, evenly extended to the thorax.

Ultrasonography (US) can be a useful tool for the initial screening whenever there are diagnostic doubts on the nature of a new onset swelling. It has a great value when an US-guided puncture is necessary to obtain a microbiological sample and even to guide the best place for the surgical incision if a CT scan is not available.

In low-income countries, where hospitals may not have many resources, a neck X-ray may show the presence of emphysema in the deeper spaces, the forward push of the airway in the lateral view

40 Emergency Surgical Access to the Neck

- be sure to have a vascular surgical set of instruments
- place the patient in a supine position with both arms extended
- the head should be in hyperextension and oriented opposite to the surgical access
- obtain two large peripheral intravenous lines
- if a subclavian vein injury is suspected, the line should be placed on the opposite side
- prepare and drape the surgical field from jaw to knees

40.4.2 Anterior Approach to the Sternocleidomastoid Muscle (ASCM)

40.4.2.1 Indication
- It is the classical approach for penetrating neck trauma, since it grants access to Zone II, the largest and the most frequently affected zone.
- It offers a wide exposure of the neck's structures (carotid and its bifurcation, vertebral arteries in V1 sector, internal jugular vein and aerodigestive tract).
- It may be combined with other maneuvers.
- If bilateral zone II injuries are identified, two approaches are possible:
  - U-shaped incision, whose vertical sides are ASCM approaches joined by an inferior horizontal cervical incision
  - a high transverse cervicotomy

40.4.2.2 Position
- Supine position with a small roll under the shoulders for neck hyperextension and face rotated to the other side
- If cervical spine status is unknown, we do not recommend hyperextending the neck.
- Cervical immobilization is only necessary if there is suspicion of injury to the cervical spine.
- As a rule, low energy penetrating cervical trauma (stab wound) does not associate with unstable cervical fractures [13].

40.4.2.3 Technical Aspects
- The incision must be placed along the anterior border of the SCM (Fig. 40.5).
- It may be extended from the sternal notch to the mastoid.
- Branches of the facial nerve run near the mandibular angle. To avoid injuring them, it is advisable to curve the incision back when approaching the mastoid.
- After the fascial plane is open, the internal jugular vein is the first structure beneath the muscle.
- Crucial next step: identification and ligation of the facial vein are necessary to give access to the common carotid artery and the visceral space as well.
- Gaining access to the aerodigestive tract requires lateralization of the neurovascular bundle. The surgeon should be observant of the laryngeal nerve's relationships.
- To access the anterior aspect of the trachea, it may be necessary to divide the thyroid's isthmus.

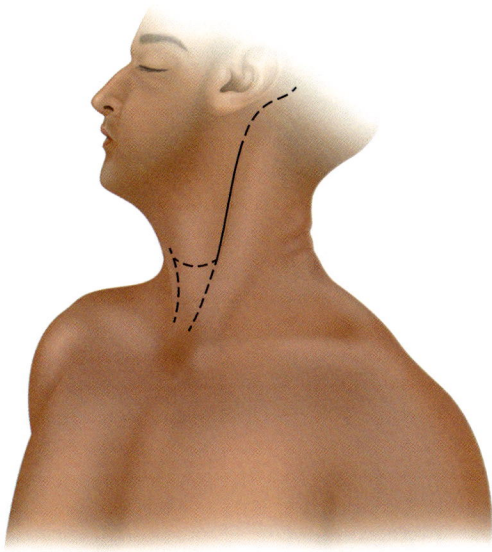

Fig. 40.5 Anterior approach to the sternocleidomastoid muscle with possible extensions (dotted lines)

- To access the esophagus, it is necessary to cut the omohyoideus muscle and the middle thyroid vein.
- For high located injuries, in Zones II and III borders, endovascular control with a Fogarty catheter is recommended. It should be inserted upward through an arteriotomy in the proximal common carotid artery. If the hospital lacks, the necessary resources to deal with these difficult access injuries, performing a subluxation or a partial resection of the mandible ramus may be helpful.

40.4.3 Supraclavicular Approach

40.4.3.1 Indication
- The supraclavicular approach may be the surgeon's first option for Zone I vascular injuries.
- An associated high thoracotomy through the third intercostal space in the left side should be considered to gain control of the intrathoracic portion of the vessel. This option is always safer and leads to lower morbidity than a trapdoor approach.

40.4.3.2 Position
- Same as ASCM

40.4.3.3 Technical Aspects
- An incision is made 1–2 cm over and parallel to the clavicle (Fig. 40.6).
- The clavicular head of the SCM must be sectioned to open the inner part of the region.
- The subclavian vein is then exposed.
- For a better control of the subclavian artery, you can cut the scalenus anterior muscle.

40.4.4 Sternotomy

40.4.4.1 Indication
- It provides an optimal access to the heart and vascular structures of the upper mediastinum.

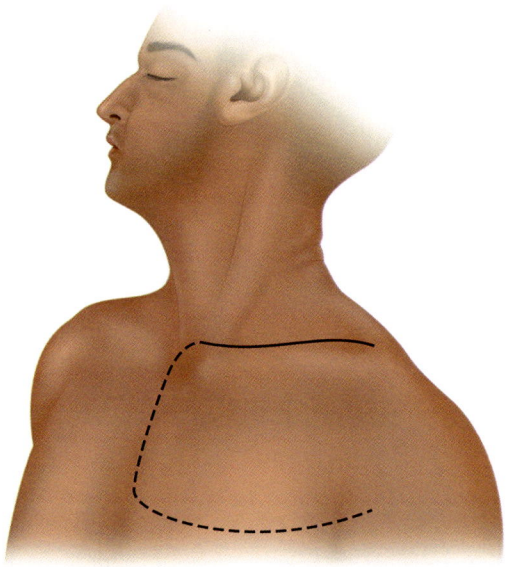

Fig. 40.6 Supraclavicular incision with possible extension through a partial sternotomy and an associated thoracotomy (trapdoor, in dotted lines)

- It may be used as an extension of the SA or the ASCM, for proximal vascular control or to control associated visceral injuries in the thoracic outlet, if needed (Fig. 40.7).

40.4.4.2 Position
- Dorsal Decubitus Position

40.4.4.3 Technical Aspects
- Interclavicular ligament's section.
- Blunt dissection behind the sternum along its full length, to separate the left innominate vein and pericardium from the bone.
- Sternum section with a sternal saw (best option) or a Lebsche sternum knife.
- The sternotomy may be partially performed through the manubrium of the sternum with an extension to any of both sides as a "trapdoor" incision, leading to a good exposition of the upper mediastinum (Fig. 40.6). However, the surgeon must bear in mind this is a more painful and morbid approach

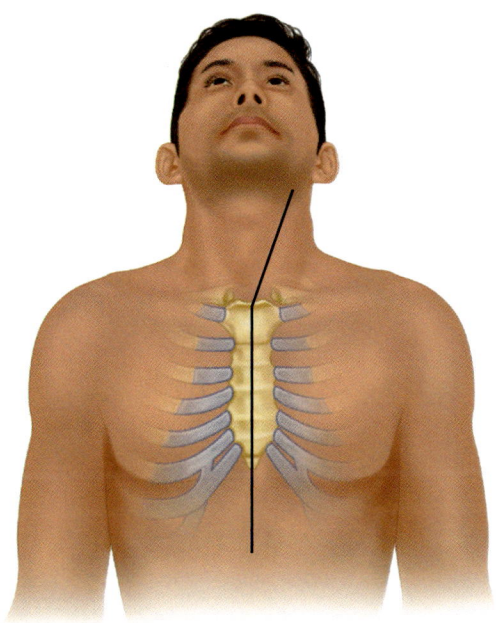 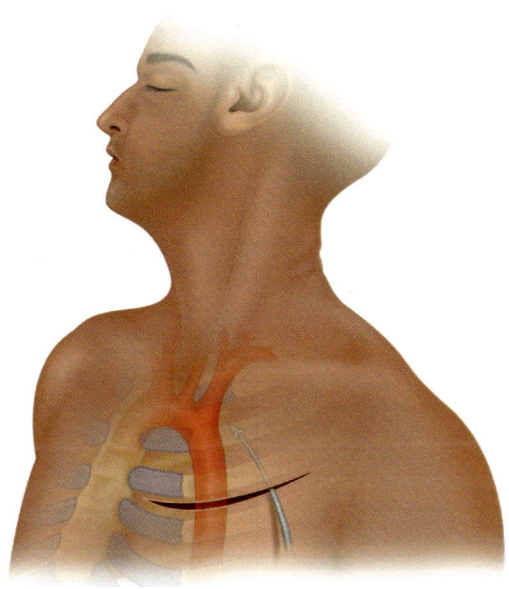

Fig. 40.7 Sternotomy as an extension of an ASCM

Fig. 40.8 High left thoracotomy (through the third intercostal space) to gain control to the intrathoracic segment of the subclavian artery

40.4.5 Anterior Thoracotomy

40.4.5.1 Indications

- The surgeon should consider performing a thoracotomy whenever a patient presents a Zone I penetrating injury with an active bleeding and of probable thoracic origin (innominate vein, left subclavian artery) or an associated aerodigestive injury not accessible for repair from a neck approach.
- If the left subclavian artery is the source of the bleeding, a high left thoracotomy through the third space may be the best option (Fig. 40.8).
- A sternotomy or a right thoracotomy should be considered as alternative options in the case of right-sided injuries.

Table 40.2 summarizes the different approaches in relation to the suspected injury

Table 40.2 Approaches in emergency surgical access to the neck

Approach	Indications	Tips
ASCM[a]	Zone II injuries when common carotid, internal jugular vein, tracheal or esophageal injuries are suspected	Do not hesitate to extend the incision whenever necessary. Always ligate and cut the facial vein.
Supraclavicular	Zone I injuries, or if a subclavian artery injury is suspected.	Do not neglect the phrenic nerve and seek to protect it.
Sternotomy	Zone I injuries in an hemodynamically stable patient or as an extension of ASCM or supraclavicular approaches	Be mindful of the left innominate vein

[a]Anterior approach to the sternocleidomastoid muscle

40.5 Simplified Approach to Particular Neck Injuries

40.5.1 Airway

Clinical signs of airway injury include hoarseness, stridor, dyspnea, subcutaneous emphysema (in the absence of pneumothorax), bubbling from the wound and large volume hemoptysis, [13, 14] Table 40.1.

If an injury is suspected, an endoscopic assessment of the airway should be performed whenever possible, including bronchoscopy prior to surgical exploration, if the patient's clinical situation allows it [11, 13, 14].

40.5.1.1 Cricothyroidotomy
- Cricothyroidotomy should be the first option unless the larynx is too injured to prevent it.
- Adam's apple is the principal initial landmark to guide the maneuver.
- The different techniques are grouped into anatomical–surgical (open: conventional and rapid four-step technique) and puncture (percutaneous and needle).
- A surgeon's goal is to be trained in any of them, given the lack of high-level evidence favoring one over the other [16].

Open Cricothyroidotomy
- The head and neck should be in hyperextension (if a cervical spine injury has been discarded).
- Disinfect the area.
- Identify Adam's apple or laryngeal prominence.
- Immobilize the larynx with the left hand (right-handed).
- Identify the cricothyroid space.
- Make a vertical incision (less bleeding and allows the incision to be extended with better exposure).
- Identify the cricothyroid membrane.
- Make a transverse incision using an N° 11 blade, parallel to the superior border of the cricoid cartilage to avoid a vocal cords' injury (the incision should be the size of the small finger's tip).
- Use a small speculum or a hemostat to keep the orifice open.
- Insert an orotracheal intubation tube N° 6 or a tracheostomy tube.
- Connect the tube to a mechanical ventilation device or a resuscitation bag.
- Confirm correct positioning (chest movements, auscultation, capnography, O_2 Sat).
- Fix the tube properly.

Percutaneous Puncture
- Multiple kits are available for this procedure.
- A Seldinger-type technique is used to guide their insertion into the tracheal tube.
- Other systems, such as laparoscopic trocars, provide color marks that guide the trocar's passage through the skin, the cricothyroid membrane, and, finally, the posterior aspect of the larynx [15].

Needle Cricothyroidotomy
- This is a transient oxygenation technique that does not warrant ventilation and allows to prepare a better access to the airway to avoid life-threatening hypoxia.
- The tracheal lumen is accessed by means of a percutaneous puncture with an N° 14 needle through the cricothyroid membrane.

40.5.1.2 Tracheostomy
Tracheostomy may be a life-saving procedure in laryngeal injuries, while arrangements for a specialist consultation for proper laryngeal management are made.

- An emergency tracheostomy may be indicated in some situations:
  - Laryngeal tears and fractures
  - Limited wounds of the cervical trachea (not open to the outside). Once repaired, it may be advisable to perform a tracheostomy distal to the suture at the end of the procedure.
- In the case of a widely open wound on the anterior aspect of the trachea (e.g., slaughter wound), introducing an intubation tube directly through the orifice may be a life-saving maneuver. The tube may be eventually

guided by an introducer, such as an Eichmann spark plug. In these circumstances, extreme care must be taken to avoid an excessive introduction, since the airway is being accessed below the larynx, and not from the mouth.

40.5.2 Surgical Access to the Esophagus

To access the esophagus, the neck should be approached through a left ASCM incision whenever an esophageal injury is diagnosed or suspected, except when the lesion is clearly on the right side.

If the exploration will be bilateral due to other associated injuries, previously mentioned combined approaches may be used [17].

Primary repair of the injured esophagus usually can be performed, and it should be the first objective if:

- it is not a destructive injury.
- the injury is not greater than 50% of the esophagus's circumference.
- the repair is performed within the first 12 h after the injury occurs (Grade 1C) [18].

If a primary repair is decided, it is advisable to respect the following principles:

- Achieving an excellent exposure
- Preserving recurrent nerve
- Debriding as much non-viable tissue
- Observing the entire length of the injury and identifying the full extent of the mucosal lesion
- Closuring the injury in one or two layers without tension with absorbable 3.0 suture
- Drainage is always placed
- Avoiding contact between the esophagus's repair and the carotid artery [17–19].

If a primary esophageal repair is not possible, a lateral esophagostomy or a terminal cervical esophagostomy should be the course of action. The first option is preferable, since it avoids the need for reconstruction [17, 18]. (Grade 2A)

A nutritional plan must be ensured. The placement of a feeding tube through the esophagus if a repair was done, or a gastrostomy in the second case, is essential [17].

40.5.3 Arteries and Veins

The general recommendations to deal with a vascular injury are the following [20]:

1. Gain proximal and distal control before entering the hematoma
2. Avoid long and unnecessary dissections
3. Ensure good exposure
4. Be mindful of the patient's physiological situation
5. Make early damage control decisions (shunts)
6. Control bleeding with proximal and distal clamping or balloons before inserting the shunt
7. Administer heparin (50 U/mL) proximal and distal to the injury
8. Perform an arteriography whenever the patient is stable
9. Remember venous repairs are not mandatory

40.5.3.1 Surgical Access to Carotid and Jugular Vein Injuries

Carotid Injuries

Penetrating carotid injuries occurs in 4.9–6% of penetrating neck trauma [20, 21].

In many hospitals, the approach to patients with hard signs is generally performed without angiography. This is, of course, not the case at specialized centers with hybrid ORs, where combined endovascular approaches are possible [22].

An exception to direct surgical management is the patient who present with a pulseless carotid or a palpable thrill/murmur without neurological deficit. These signs are considered hard signs. However, in these circumstances, the management may be troublesome, since direct surgical exploration is not indicated. An angio-CT scan is preferred to rule out thrombosis (in the absence of pulse) and a venous-artery fistula (thrill/murmur) [19].

Once surgical exploration provides evidence of a carotid injury, fixing this lesion is the preferred approach over ligation. This is true for both, the common and the internal carotid artery, mainly in patients with no neurological deficit prior to surgery who are expected to have better chances of survival and less neurological impairment [13, 22].

There is a long-standing debate about the best course of action for patients that present with neurological signs. Since it might be difficult to know whether the neurological deficit is due to hypoxia or substance consumption, it has been recommend repairing the injury in those patients with GCS of 9 or higher. As 75% of patients with GCS of 8 or below will not improve, both ligation or repair are acceptable options [19].

If a small lesion or a lateral defect is present, a suture should be performed with a 6-0 polypropylene. For larger injuries, or side-to-side defects, the repair may be done utilizing a venous patch (internal saphenous), an allogenic biological tissue or polytetrafluoroethylene prosthesis [23, 24].

For larger injuries, resection plus anastomosis with interposition of the internal saphenous or prosthesis may be necessary. In situations where damage control techniques are indicated, intraluminal shunts can be placed mainly in ICA [25]. Ligation may be accepted as a last resource.

Carotid external injuries may be ligated.

Vein Injuries

Surgery is not always required in venous injuries. The system's low pressure favors its spontaneous occlusion [13, 25].

Internal jugular vein injuries can lead to a large hematoma that is usually explored. In this situation, the vein may be repaired or even ligated. This decision depends on the circumstances. The only exception is bilateral internal jugular vein injury. In this situation, one of the veins must be repaired at least to prevent cerebral oedema [25].

In patients without neurological impairment or GCS of 9 or higher, the surgeon should always attempt to fix the artery.

It is always important to interpose a well-vascularized muscle flap (digastric, omohyoid or sternocleidomastoid flap) between a vascular repair and a visceral suture, such as an esophageal repair, to prevent an arterial rupture if a digestive fistula develops [25].

40.5.3.2 Surgical Access to Vertebral Artery Injuries

Bleeding originating in the vertebral artery is always a deep bleeding, next to the vertebral bodies. These injuries are extremely difficult to deal with. Ligating the artery before entering the transverse processes of cervical vertebrae is an option. Once inside the foramen transversarium, applying pressure with bone wax may be the only successful approach to gain bleeding control [20].

40.5.4 Infections Surgical Therapy

The infection of the deep spaces of the neck may be dental in origin, secondary to a peritonsillar tissue infection, secondary to pharyngeal or esophageal perforation or be a traumatic evolutive consequence.

The different deep neck spaces are delimited by fasciae planes, as shown in Fig. 40.1. The most important are the lateral pharyngeal, the retropharyngeal, the submandibular, and the pretracheal spaces [26, 27].

A localized swelling with inflammatory signs may be observed in the neck or in the midline of the posterior pharyngeal wall, depending on the location of the primary process.

The diagnosis is usually confirmed with a CT scan, and the proper drainage incision should be guided by imaging as well as clinical presentation.

In summary, the management of these patients includes:

- always checking the airway is patent (a tracheostomy may be necessary)
- administering antibiotic therapy
- inserting a drain (see Table 40.3)

Table 40.3 Different approaches to drainage in deep cervical spaces infections

Neck's space	Technical topics
Submandibular	Extraoral approach: 4 cm behind the mandible angle in the declining part of the abscess to minimize scarring Intraoral
Lateral to the pharynx	Extraoral: ASCM[a] or like submandibular
Retropharyngeal space	Extraoral: ASCM[a] Intraoral drainage of the abscess

[a]Anterior approach to the sternocleidomastoid muscle

Dos and Don'ts
Airway

Do
- Correct identification of anatomical landmarks.
- Consider cricothyroidotomy as the first choice to gain emergency surgical access to the airway whenever possible.

Don't
- Perform a skin horizontal incision for cricothyroidotomy.

Initial Bleeding Control

Do
- Quickly control bleeding.

Don't
- Delay the decision to take the patient to the OR.

ASCM

Do
- Ligate the facial vein to obtain adequate access. Always.
- Remember to do proximal and distal control in vascular injuries

Don't
- Operate without vascular instruments.
- Forget the recurrent nerve during dissection or moving the aerodigestive tract.

Supraclavicular Access

Do
- Remember to protect the phrenic nerve. Always.

Don't
- Resect the clavicle's head.

Sternotomy

Do
- Request a sternum saw. If that is not an option, ask for a Lebsche knife instead.

Don't
- Injure the venous innominate trunk while performing the sternotomy.

Vascular

Do
- You can ligate venous injuries
- Make early damage control decisions

Don't
- Maneuver without good injury exposition
- Try vascular repair without proximal and distal control

Esophagus

Do
- Approach cervical esophageal injuries through a left ASCM incision

Don't
- Neglect to preserve the recurrent nerve

Take-Home Messages

- The patient must be transferred to the OR whenever hard signs are present.
- Emergency surgical access to the airway must be done in the 'can't intubate, can't oxygenate' scenario (CICO).
- The ASCM approach is the most frequently used, and the most versatile approach for the treatment of cervical injuries.
- Low energy blunt trauma in patients without neurological impairment is not commonly associated with a cervical spine injury.
- Removing the inferior insertion of anterior scalene muscle may grant a better access to the subclavian artery
- A sternotomy provides optimal exposition of the heart and large vessels.
- In patients without neurological impairment or with nine or higher points in GCS, the surgeon should always attempt to fix a carotid artery injury.
- A well-irrigated muscle flap must be interposed whenever a vascular and an aerodigestive repair are simultaneously performed.
- Vertebral artery bleeding at the V2 portion (intervertebral channel) may be controlled by applying pressure with wax bone
- If an esophagus injury exists, try primary repair whenever possible. If the primary repair is not possible, perform a lateral esophagostomy.
- Always ensure the patient's nutritional contribution.

Questions and Answers

1. The Zone Approach concept considers:
   A. **the clinical presentation, the zone involved and logistics**
   B. the clinical presentation and the zone involved
   C. just the clinical presentation
   D. just the zone involved
2. The presence of hard signs in the initial assessment:
   A. **is usually an indication for an emergency surgical resolution and the patient should be transferred to the OR**
   B. is an indication for the patient to be transferred immediately to the ICU (Intensive Care Unit)
   C. should always be followed by an emergency CT scan to guide the next therapeutic decisions
   D. is always an indication for the surgeon to stop the treatment in the Emergency Department and transfer the patient to angiography
3. A surgeon treating a patient in a CICO situation (can't intubate can't oxygenate):
   A. should try to intubate the patient once again
   B. **must obtain an immediate surgical access to the airway**
   C. should choose a technique regardless of their own expertise
   D. favor a tracheostomy as first option because of its technical simplicity
4. In relation to cricothyroidotomy, it is true to consider that:
   A. a skin transverse incision is always favored because of its simplicity
   B. ventilating a patient through a needle puncture of the cricothyroid membrane at least for 15 min should be possible
   C. **the Adam's apple is the most important anatomical landmark to begin performing the technique.**
   D. the vocal cords are located distant enough to not be a concern
5. When treating a patient with an active bleeding in the neck:
   A. compression maneuvers are generally useless and should never be done

B. given the small space where they develop, Zone III bleedings are usually easily controlled
C. **an expansive hematoma is an indication for orotracheal intubation**
D. in the case of hemodynamic deterioration, emergency surgery should be postponed in favor of an adequate reposition

6. In relation to the anterior access to the sternocleidomastoid muscle (ASCM), the following considerations are relevant:
   A. **it should be the surgeon's first option to approach zone II injuries in general**
   B. it is difficult to combine with other surgical approaches to the neck.
   C. the inferior thyroid artery ligation is always the key maneuver to open the region more widely.
   D. the recurrent laryngeal nerve should always be identified and dissected to avoid injuring it.

7. In an emergency supraclavicular access to the neck the surgeon should consider that:
   A. the phrenic nerve under the sternocleidomastoid muscle must be identified and preserved
   B. given its small caliber, the vertebral artery is always an easy to control vascular structure
   C. **the subclavian artery can be reached through either a complementary high left thoracic incision or a trapdoor incision**
   D. an extension through a sternotomy provides an excellent exposition of the thoracic esophagus, should this be necessary

8. In the setting of vascular injuries in the neck, it is true that:
   A. proximal and distal control of a subclavian artery may usually be done through an ASCM approach
   B. the presence of a neurological impairment is an indication for an emergency fixation of all common carotid artery injuries
   C. all internal jugular vein injuries must be repaired
   D. **zone III injuries ideally should be assessed before a surgical exploration is decided to better deal with vascular injuries at this level**

9. In a cervical esophageal injury, it is of the highest importance:
   A. to repair the muscular layer, as this is the strongest layer in this region of the esophagus
   B. **to interpose a well-vascularized muscular flap between the esophagus and the other structures**
   C. not to drain the neck in these circumstances given the high rate of drain-related morbidity)
   D. to look for associated cervical spine injuries almost always present

10. In the setting of a deep neck infection, it is important to keep in mind that:
    A. these may spread to the upper mediastinum only through the posterior retroesophageal space
    B. these may spread to the upper mediastinum only through the paratracheal space
    C. **these may be drained through several approaches, usually guided by a CT scan**
    D. the incision is usually centered by the most fluctuating zone, independently of the CT scan findings

References

1. Fernandez Russo GAH. Anatomía Clínica y Quirúrgica del Cuello. Rev Arg Anat Onl. 2012;3(suppl. 3):7–113.
2. Monson DO, Saletta JD, Freeark RJ. Carotid vertebral trauma. J Trauma. 1969;9:987.
3. Roon AJ, Christensen N. Evaluation and treatment of penetrating cervical injuries. J Trauma. 1979;19:391.
4. Weightman WM, Gibbs NM. Prevalence of major vessels anterior to the trachea at sites of potential front-of-neck emergency airway access in adults. Br J Anaesth. 2018;121(5):1166–72. https://doi.org/10.1016/j.bja.2018.07.013. Epub 2018 Aug 22.
5. Fogelman MJ, Stewart RD. Penetrating wounds of the neck. Am J Surg. 1956;91(4):581–93; discussion, 593-6. https://doi.org/10.1016/0002-9610(56)90289-6.
6. Shiroff AM, Gale SC, Martin ND, Marchalik D, Petrov D, Ahmed HM, Rotondo MF, Gracias VH. Penetrating neck trauma: a review of management strategies and discussion of the 'No Zone' approach. Am Surg. 2013;79(1):23–9. https://doi.org/10.1177/000313481307900113.
7. Prichayudh S, Choadrachata-anun J, Sriussadaporn S, Pak-art R, Sriussadaporn S, Kritayakirana K, Samorn P. Selective management of penetrating neck injuries using "no zone" approach. Injury. 2015;46(9):1720–5. https://doi.org/10.1016/j.injury.2015.06.019. Epub 2015 Jun 16.
8. Madsen AS, Bruce JL, Oosthuizen GV, Bekker W, Smith M, Manchev V, Laing GL, Clarke DL. Correlation between the level of the external wound and the internal injury in penetrating neck injury does not favor an initial zonal management approach. BJS Open. 2020;4(4):704–13. https://doi.org/10.1002/bjs5.50282. Epub 2020 Jun 11.
9. Tallon JM, Ahmed JM, Sealy B. Airway management in penetrating neck trauma at a Canadian tertiary trauma center. CJEM. 2007;9:101–4.
10. Van Waes OJ, Cheriex KC, Navsaria PH, et al. Management of penetrating neck injuries. Br J Surg. 2012;99(Suppl 1):149–54.
11. Lee WT, Eliashar R, Eliachar I. Acute external laryngotracheal trauma: diagnosis and management. Ear Nose Throat J. 2006;85:179–84.
12. Sperry JL, Moore EE, Coimbra R, Croce M, Davis JW, Karmy-Jones R, McIntyre RC Jr, Moore FA, Malhotra A, Shatz DV, Biffl WL. Western Trauma Association critical decisions in trauma: penetrating neck trauma. J Trauma Acute Care Surg. 2013;75(6):936–40. https://doi.org/10.1097/TA.0b013e31829e20e3.
13. Nowicki JL, Stew B, Ooi E. Penetrating neck injuries: a guide to evaluation and management. Ann R Coll Surg Engl. 2018;100, 6(1):–11. https://doi.org/10.1308/rcsann.2017.0191. Epub 2017 Oct 19.
14. Burgess CA, Dale OT, Almeyda R, Corbridge RJ. An evidence based review of the assessment and management of penetrating neck trauma. Clin Otolaryngol. 2012;37(1):44–52. https://doi.org/10.1111/j.1749-4486.2011.02422.x.
15. Helm M, Gries A, Mutzbauer T. Surgical approach in difficult airway management. Best Pract Res Clin Anaesthesiol. 2005;19(4):623–40. https://doi.org/10.1016/j.bpa.2005.06.002.
16. Bribriesco A, Patterson GA. Cricothyroid approach for emergency access to the airway. Thorac Surg Clin. 2018;28(3):435–40. https://doi.org/10.1016/j.thorsurg.2018.04.009.
17. Petrone P, Kassimi K, Jiménez-Gómez M, Betancourt A, Axelrad A, Marini CP. Management of esophageal injuries secondary to trauma. Injury. 2017;48(8):1735–42. https://doi.org/10.1016/j.injury.2017.06.012. Epub 2017 Jun 19.
18. Chirica M, Kelly MD, Siboni S, Aiolfi A, Riva CG, Asti E, Ferrari D, Leppäniemi A, Ten Broek RPG, Brichon PY, Kluger Y, Fraga GP, Frey G, Andreollo NA, Coccolini F, Frattini C, Moore EE, Chiara O, Di Saverio S, Sartelli M, Weber D, Ansaloni L, Biffl W, Corte H, Wani I, Baiocchi G, Cattan P, Catena F, Bonavina L. Esophageal emergencies: WSES guidelines. World J Emerg Surg. 2019;(14):26. https://doi.org/10.1186/s13017-019-0245-2.
19. Feliciano DV. Penetrating cervical trauma. "Current Concepts in Penetrating Trauma", IATSIC Symposium, International Surgical Society, Helsinki, Finland, August 25–29, 2013. World J Surg. 2015;39(6):1363–72. https://doi.org/10.1007/s00268-014-2919-y.
20. Pereira BM, Chiara O, Ramponi F, Weber DG, Cimbanassi S, De Simone B, Musicki K, Meirelles GV, Catena F, Ansaloni L, Coccolini F, Sartelli M, Di Saverio S, Bendinelli C, Fraga GP. WSES position paper on vascular emergency surgery. World J Emerg Surg. 2015;(10):49. https://doi.org/10.1186/s13017-015-0037-2.
21. Navsaria P, Omoshoro-Jones J, Nicol A. An analysis of 32 surgically managed penetrating carotid artery injuries. Eur J Vasc Endovasc Surg. 2002;24(4):349–55.
22. Lee TS, Ducic Y, Gordin E, Stroman D. Management of carotid artery trauma. Craniomaxillofac Trauma Reconstr. 2014 Sep;7(3):175–89. https://doi.org/10.1055/s-0034-1372521.
23. Feliciano DV. Management of penetrating injuries to carotid artery. World J Surg. 2001;25(8):1028–35. https://doi.org/10.1007/s00268-001-0055-y. Erratum in: World J Surg 2002;26(2):284.
24. Brown MF, Graham JM, Feliciano DV, Mattox KL, Beall AC Jr, De Bakey ME. Carotid artery injuries. Am J Surg. 1982;144(6):748–53. https://doi.org/10.1016/0002-9610(82)90563-3.

25. Kumar SR, Weaver FA, Yellin AE. Cervical vascular injuries: carotid and jugular venous injuries. Surg Clin North Am. 2001;81(6):1331–44, xii–xiii. https://doi.org/10.1016/s0039-6109(01)80010-4.
26. Osborn TM, Assael LA, Bell RB. Deep space neck infection: principles of surgical management. Oral Maxillofac Surg Clin North Am. 2008;20(3):353–65. https://doi.org/10.1016/j.coms.2008.04.002.
27. Maharaj S, Ahmed S, Pillay P. Deep neck space infections: a case series and review of the literature. Clin Med Insights Ear Nose Throat. 2019;(12):1179550619871274. https://doi.org/10.1177/1179550619871274.

Face and Neck Infections

41

Alfons Mogedas, Mireia Pascua, and Xavier Guirao

41.1 Introduction

Learning Goals
- To understand in a very comprehensive view the pathophysiology of the main type of face and neck infection.
- To give a clear-cut approach of clinical and diagnostic aspects of FNI.
- To better assess the severity in those situations that need early adequate management.
- Principles in designing adequate empirical antibiotic treatment.
- To clarify aspects of focus control: where and how.

41.1.1 Epidemiology

Severe FNI encompasses a low percentage of patients admitted to the emergency department or at the intensive care unit in developed countries. Nevertheless, people from lower-middle incomes countries, the elderly and child, are still groups at risk of severe FNI. Otherwise, FNI in pediatric and young people (7–18 years) [1] are at risk of peritonsillar abscess-related FNI, and both communities encompass a large proportion of FNI attended at emergency room departments [2]. In addition, in patients from 21 to 50 years, odontogenic infections predominate [3–6].

The main risk factors associated with the FNI are alcohol abuse [1], diabetes mellitus [3, 5] and previous radiotherapy treatment [7]. In addition, branchial and thyroglossal cysts may be the initial infectious focus promoting severe latero-cervical or retropharyngeal infections [8, 9]. Otherwise, head and neck and maxillofacial units are very active at the operative room and postoperative surgical site infections are now more frequently documented. It has been shown a surgical site infection rate in between 21% and 41% [10–12] in patients submitted to major head and neck surgical procedures, mainly after free-flap or vascularized bone reconstruction. Such excess of SSI purports an increase in hospital costs up to 17,000 euros and an increase in length of hospital stay of 8 days [10].

Diagnosis delay and inappropriate FNI management may induce complicated FNI. Such delay has been associated with a high rate of

A. Mogedas
Unit of Maxilofacial Surgery, Parc Tauli, Hospital Universitari, Sabadell, Spain

M. Pascua
Unit of Endocrine Surgery, Department of General Surgery, Hospital Universitari de Bellvitge, L'Hospitalet de Llobregat, Spain

X. Guirao (✉)
Unit of Endocrine, Head and Neck Surgery, Department of General Surgery, Parc Tauli, Hospital Universitari, Sabadell, Spain

morbidity and mortality. For instance, after deep FNI, it has been documented complications, such as septic shock, mediastinal abscess and paravertebral osteomyelitis with a mortality rate ranging from 7.7% to 11% [1, 13]. More severe FNI such as necrotizing fasciitis or Lemierre's syndrome purports a much dismal prognosis with a mortality rate in between 18% and 25% [14, 15].

41.1.2 Etiology

We can split the etiology section in first, where the infection initiates and spread afterward to produce FNI and second, the main pathogens involved.

41.1.2.1 Origin of FNI: Primary Focus of Infection

Despite progressive improvement of dental care, odontogenic focus is still the predominant primary focus in FNI, mainly in low–middle-income countries [3–6, 16–18]. In another studies, dental focus is the second most frequent infectious origin right after oropharyngeal infection [1, 16, 19], being tonsillitis the predominant seminal infection of FNI in pediatric population [1, 19]. Additional primary focus has been documented after infected adenopathy [19], congenital cysts [1, 8] of the neck, skin of the ear [20], or in some countries, complicated sialadenitis [17].

41.1.2.2 Microbiology

Microbiome of the Head and Neck Mucosal Spaces

It is has been shown that head and neck microbiome is site specific and may change under some circumstances. For instance, oral microbiome is the second body site (just after colon) with the highest bacterial diversity. Firmicutes, Bacteroidetes and Proteobacteria are the predominant phyla of oropharyngeal cavity [21]. In addition, *Pseudomonaceae* and *Streptococcaceae* are the predominant families of bacteria at the middle ear and tonsil, respectively [21]. Furthermore, *Fusobacterium necrophorum* is part of the normal microbiota of the oropharynx and the gastrointestinal tract and does not normally invade mucosa.

Nevertheless, viral or bacterial co-infections may promote invasion at the peritonsillar area [22]. In addition, the ratio of anaerobic/aerobic in saliva is 10:1, and these bacteria are always present in normal or in pathologic conditions [23].

Microbiology in Face and Neck Infections

Theoretically, the microorganisms responsible for the specific FNI derive from the microbiome population previously exposed. The reason behind the phenotype expression from components of head and neck microbiome to a elicited pathogens FNI remains unknown. Nevertheless, there is quite relevant bench of work, showing that the involved microorganisms in those accepted clinical entities of FNI are in close relationship with the responsible primary infectious focus. For instance, deep bilateral submandibular infection (Ludwig's angina) is produced from a disseminated initial odontogenic focus. Then, mixed flora encompassing Gram-positive, Gram-negative and Gram-positive anaerobe bacteria [23] are the core-microorganisms that should be taken in to the account [3, 4, 9, 11, 13, 24]. It should be noted that core pathogens may vary depending on additional variables. For instance, it is quite surprising that in Taiwan, *Klebsiella pneumoniae* is the more frequent pathogen involved in deep neck infections [3]. In addition, observational studies have documented a progressive shift from the formerly most frequent pathogen, such as *Streptococcus pyogenes* to *Streptococcus viridans* [4]. Although Group A β-hemolytic *Streptococcus pyogenes* has been classically involved in severe type II necrotizing fasciitis, other Gram-positive bacteria (Group *Streptococcus viridans* or *Staphylococcus aureus*) with or without additional mixed Gram-negative bacteria (*Klebsiella pneumoniae* or *Pseudomonas aeruginosa*) are also able to produce such severe infection [7, 15]. Although *Fusobacterium necrophorum* is the pathogen more frequently isolated in patients with severe FNI with additional vascular and septic metastatic foci (Lemierre's syndrome) [22, 25, 26], additional bacteria species may also be involved [26].

Pathogens with some antibiotic-resistant phenotype (MRSA, *Enterobacter* spp., *Enterococcus* spp.) may appear in patients with nosocomial postoperative acquired infection [12, 16] or in those treated with immunosuppressive drugs. *Staphylococcus aureus* has been isolated from complicated branchial cleft cysts [8] and in FNI coming from suppurative thyroiditis [27]. Furthermore, tuberculous [1] and non-tuberculous [28] mycobacterium should be keep in mind in those FNI with primarily negative cultures or recurrent/persistent infections.

In Table 41.1, accepted clinical entities and possible-related pathogens are displayed.

41.1.3 Classification

FNI display a wide range of clinical presentations due to the complex anatomy. The existence of different compartments limited by superficial and deep cervical fascia purports connections between anatomical spaces allowing the infection to spread to additional compartments and cavities far away from the primary source of infection. Experimental studies by insufflating pressurized air in fresh cadavers elegantly

Table 41.1 Pathogens involved and empirical antibiotic treatment of the FNI, according to the initial suspected clinical diagnosis

	Main pathogens	Antibiotic	
			Allergy to β-lactam
Deep neck submandibular infection (Ludwig angina)	*S. viridans, Prevotella spp, Porphyromonas Fusobacterium spp. Peptostreptococcus spp.*	Amoxicillin[a] and clavulanic acid 2 g–0.5 g/8 h iv	Clindamycin (300–900 mg/6–8 h) **or** Vancomycin[b] (15–20 mg/kg/8–12 h i.v) + Metronidazole 0.5 g/6h
Associated risk factors			
Traumatism	**and** *S. aureus +/− S. epidermidis*[c]	Amoxicillin and clavulanic acid 2g–0.5 g/8 h iv	Clindamycin (300–900 mg/6–8 h) **or** Vancomycin (15–20 mg/kg/8–12 h i.v) + Metronidazole 0.5 g/6 h
Immunosuppression (diabetes, renal insufficiency, cirrhosis, corticoids)	**and** Gram negative bacteria, *Pseudomonas spp, Klebsiella pneumoniae, E. coli*	Piperacillin–Tazobactam 4 g/6-h iv **or** Imipenem 1 g/6 h iv **or** Meropenem 1 g/8 h iv	Clindamycin (300–900 mg/6–8 h) + Metronidazole (0.5 g/6 h) + [4]Amikacin[d] (20 mg/kg/d)
Lemièrre syndrome	*Fusobacterium necrophorum, Streptococcus spp, Staphylococcus aureus, Pseudomonas spp and Enterococcus spp*	Piperacillin–Tazobactam[e] 4 g/6-h iv **or** Imipenem 1 g/6 h iv **or** Meropenem 1 g/8 h iv	Clindamycin (300–900 mg/6–8 h) + Metronidazole (0.5 g/6 h) + Amikacin[d] (20 mg/kg/d)
Necrotizing fasciitis	*Streptococcus* group A beta-hemolyticus, *Staphylococcus aureus* with or without with *Enterobacteriacea* or *Pseudomonas aeruginosa*	Piperacillin–Tazobactam[f] 4 g/6-h iv **or** Imipenem 1 g/6 h iv **or** Meropenem 1 g/8 h	Clindamycin (300–900 mg/6–8 h) + Metronidazole (0.5 g/6 h) + Amikacin[d] (20 mg/kg/d)
Acute bacterial parotitis	*Staphyloccocus aureus Streptococcus viridans Fusobacrerium* spp. *Prevotella* spp. *Porphyromonas* spp *Peptostreptococcus* spp. and *E. coli* and additional enterobacteracea	Amoxicillin[g] and clavulanic acid 2–0.2 g/8 h iv **or** Piperacillin–Tazobactam[g] 4 g0.5 g/6-h iv	Clindamycin (300–900 mg/6–8 h) or Linezolid 600 mg/12 h iv + Ciprofloxacin[h] 400 mg/8–12 h
Acute bacterial thyroiditis	*Staphylococcus aureus Streptococcus spp.*	Amoxicillin and clavulanic acid 2.2 g/8 h iv **or** Ertapenem 1g/12–24h iv	Cefazolin 1–2g/8h iv +/- Clindamycin 600mg/8h iv

(continued)

Table 41.1 (continued)

	Main pathogens	Antibiotic	
			Allergy to β-lactam
Cervical cysts infection	Staphylococcus aureus Parvimonas micra Prevotella intermedia	Amoxicillin and clavulanic acid 2 g/8 h iv **or** Piperacillin–Tazobactam 4 g/6-h iv	Clindamycin 300–450/8 h **or** Meropenem 1 g/8 h
Necrotizing external otitis	Pseudomonas aeruginosa Staphylococcus aureus	Ceftazidime 2 g/8 h iv **or** Piperacillin–Tazobactam 4 g/6 h iv	Ciprofloxacin 500 mg/12 h or Levofloxacin 500 mg/24 h

[a]*Notes:* Penicillin G-Na (4MU/4–6 h iv) (in combination with metronidazole) may eventually be given to adjust empirical antibiotic treatment after microbiological results and antibiogram is known. *Streptococcus mitis* group (*Streptococcus viridans* group) displays penicillin resistance and intermediate resistance in 10% and 20%, respectively. More than 50% are also resistant to clindamycin and macrolides (Mensa)

[b]In those circumstances of an increased volume of distribution is suspected (severe sepsis or septic shock) consider an initial load dose of 20–23 mg/kg

[c]When methicillin resistance *Staphylococcus aureus* is suspected, either Vancomycin or Linezolid (600 mg/12 h iv) should be added to the empirical antibiotic treatment

[d]Amikacin 20 mg/kg/d may be administered in as a single dose adjusted for lean body weight. Higher dose (30 mg/kg/d iv) might eventually be given when high volume of distribution is suspected (severe sepsis or septic shock)

[e]Because de severity of the infection, broad-spectrum antibiotic therapy should be given. Having pathogens being identified and antibiogram performed, adjusting empirical antibiotic treatment to Penicillin plus Metronidazole is advised if the microorganisms are sensitive to these compounds

[f]Because de severity of the infection, broad-spectrum antibiotic therapy should be given. If Group A beta-haemolytic *Streptococcus pyogenes* is identified (or suspected after Gram-stain results), Penicillin G-Na 4MU/4–6 h iv and Clindamycin 600–900 mg/6–8 h iv or Linezolid 600 mg/12 h iv, is preferred

[g]In patients at risk for methicillin-resistant *Staphylococcus aureus* infection, Linezolid 600 mg/12 h iv/oral or Tedizolid 200 mg/d or Daptomycin 8 mg/kg/d iv or Vancomycin 15–20 mg/kg/8–12 h iv, should be empirically added

[h]In patients with severe sepsis or septic shock, consider an initial dose of 600–800 mg and 400–600 mg iv afterward. In paediatric patients consider antibiotic alternatives

demonstrated how the initial infection of the maxillofacial area and the oral cavity spreads to the superior mediastinum [29] (Fig. 41.1a, b). Then, to better understand the extension and the main initially infectious focus of the different clinically apparent FNI, clinicians and surgeons should be familiar with face and neck anatomical and fascial compartments [30, 31]. Table 41.2 shows the main FNI and their relationship among the involved anatomical spaces and the primary focus of infection and symptoms.

41.1.4 Pathophysiology

41.1.4.1 Odontogenic Infection Source

Protracted caries, gingivitis and periodontitis may evolve invading the dental pulp cavity promoting periapical abscess. Infection may progress through the medullary and cortical bone toward the periosteum and spread to those least resistance tissues and may even fistulate to the skin. The final location of the infection will be determined by the position and length of the affected tooth root and the cortical perforation site, and second, by the anatomical arrangement of the muscles and aponeurosis adjacent to the maxillae (Fig. 41.2). Distant spread occurs through lymphatic drainage that encompasses the submaxillary cell lymph nodes producing cervical lymphadenitis and abscess later on.

41.1.4.2 Tonsil Infection Source

It is thought that either localized inflammation or direct viral/bacterial invasion into the superficial oropharyngeal mucosa, the infection is running down the nasopharynx [32]. Spread from peritonsillar abscess is the most common origin of deep neck infection in adults. The pathophysiology is

41 Face and Neck Infections

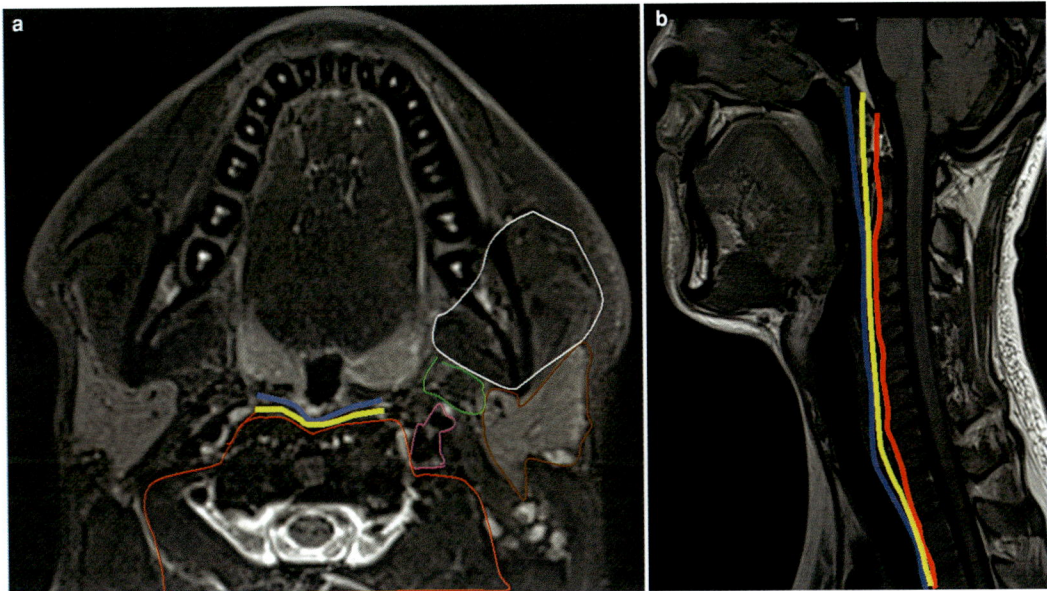

Fig. 41.1 (**a**) MRI axial section. Parotid space (brown), Masticator space (white), Pharyngeal mucosal space (yellow), Parapharyngeal space (green), Carotid space (Pink), Perivertebral space (red), Retropharyngeal space (blue), Danger space (yellow). (**b**) Sagittal section MRI: retropharyngeal space (blue), dangerous space (yellow) and perivertebral space (red)

Table 41.2 Relationship among anatomical spaces, primary focus of infection and symptoms of the main types of face and neck infections

Type of face and neck infection	Primary focus of infections	Anatomical spaces involved if progression	Symptoms
Suprahyoid			
Masticator space infection	Odontogenic	Sublingual Buccal Parotid Parapharyngeal	Trismus Mandibular pain
Parotid space infection/abscess	Acute/chronic sialadenitis Reactive/Necrotizing lymphadenopathy	Masticator Parapharyngeal Carotid sheath	Tumour and oedema at the parotid region
Submandibular/sublingual infection (Ludwig angina)	Odontogenic infection Peritonsillar abscess Sialadenitis Diving ranula Suppurative lymphadenopathy Epiglottitis Trauma	Parapharyngeal Retropharyngeal	Trismus Dysphagia Neck swelling Stridor Double tongue sign
Supra and Infrahyoid (whole length)			
Carotid space: Lemierre Syndrome	Peritonsillar abscess Cervical adenitis	Septic metastasis (lung)	Neck fullness Trismus Lateral neck pain Severe sepsis

(continued)

Table 41.2 (continued)

Type of face and neck infection	Primary focus of infections	Anatomical spaces involved if progression	Symptoms
Retropharyngeal abscess/phlegmon	Nasopharynx Middle ear Sinuses	Danger space Mediastinum	Fever Malaise Neck swelling Stridor
Perivertebral space	Pyogenic vertebral osteomyelitis	Neural foramina Epidural space	Fever and severe neurologic symptoms
Posterior cervical space infection/abscess	Suppurative lymphadenopathy	Parapharyngeal	Deep lateral neck infection/abscess symptoms
Infrahyoid			
Visceral space	Laryngitis Infected laryngocele Tracheobronchitis Suppurative thyroiditis Neck cyst infections	Carotid sheath Retropharyngeal Mediastinum	Specific symptoms of the viscera involved

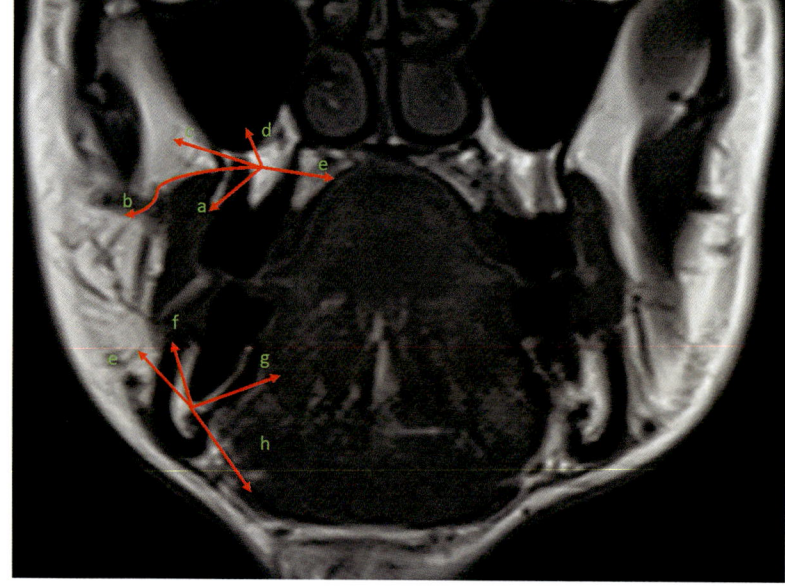

Fig. 41.2 Axial view of MRI image section to explain the pathophysiology of the spread patterns in odontogenic elicited face and neck infections. Upper teeth: (**a**) Vestible, (**b**) Buccal space, (**c**) Temporal, infratemporal, (**d**) Maxillary sinus, (**e**) Palate. Inferior teeth: (**e**) Buccal space, (**f**) Vestible, (**g**) Sublingual space, (**h**) Submandibular space

not yet certain, but it is suspected to be a complication of bacterial tonsillar cellulitis.

41.1.4.3 Cervical Adenitis

Suppurative adenitis usually comes from a cervical-infected node that undergone liquefaction necrosis. Pediatric patients are at high risk. This clinical picture decreases with the age of the patient, although suppurative adenitis is increasing in older patients. The most frequent cause of lymph node enlargement (and further node infection) is respiratory viruses, AIDS and bacteria (*Staphylococcus aureus* and Group A *Streptococcus*). In cat-scratch disease related to *Bartonella hensalae* infection is a very common cause of enlarged cervical lymph nodes in children. In this situation, roughly, 10% of patients develop fluctuant lymph nodes that require drainage [2].

41.2 Diagnosis

41.2.1 Clinical Presentation

The primary source of the infection may determine the clinical presentation. A patient with fever, neck tumefaction complaining of cervicalgia, the diagnosis of deep neck infection should be seriously considered [5]. Sometimes, a localized inflammatory tumor nearby an specific area (parotid, laterocervical or ear, see Fig. 41.3a–c) will facilitate a straightforward diagnosis and treatment. Otherwise, more subtle symptoms such as dysphagia, dysphonia, or sialorrhea [17] should expeditiously lead to an oral–pharyngeal exam. Trismus is a common finding, but may be lacking in patients with pure peritonsillar abscess without parapharyngeal space involvement [33]. Nevertheless, we must to keep in mind that some patients may require urgent care for stridor and respiratory failure and/or septic shock in a patient with less apparent neck clinical inflammation [13] in patients with Ludwig angina or cervical necrotizing (and crepitant) fasciitis.

41.2.2 Tests

41.2.2.1 Laboratory and Microbiological Tests

Vital signs, white-cell count and coagulation parameters will be useful to classify the degree of sepsis [34] and to correctly manage these patients with suspected FNI early on (Fig. 41.4). Biological inflammatory markers such as C-reactive protein and procalcitonin may be useful in those patients with less apparent clinical signs or in those with inadequate urgent myeloid response. In addition, two consecutive blood cultures should be drawn before starting antibiotic treatment, and if possible, adequate sample of pus at the inflammatory site should be obtained before antibiotic treatment and the definitive drainage would be carried out and expeditiously sent for microbiological culture [23]. Swab for sampling pus from the cavity must be avoided if possible. Take enough sample material trough fine-needle aspiration sterile method instead.

41.2.2.2 Diagnostic Imaging Tests

Although adequate anamnesis and clinical exam should be performed right away, clinical assessment underestimates the extent of deep neck infection in a roughly 70% of patients [13], and in only 50% of patients, the anatomical space involved is correctly diagnosed [35]. Then, diagnostic imaging test should be performed in an otherwise stable patient.

Ultrasound

Ultrasound (US) is transportable to the patient site and is also useful for US-guided fine-needle aspiration. US is particularly useful in children or in pregnant women by avoiding radiation [36], to diagnose peritonsillar or upper parapharyngeal infections and is better than CT-scan in differentiating abscess from cellulitis [33].

Contrast Enhanced CT-Scan (CECT)

Since the early 90s, CECT is routinely used to confirm, classify and guide the best strategy to deal with deep FNI [1, 3, 4, 13, 16, 19, 36–38]. It has been documented that CECT has a sensitiv-

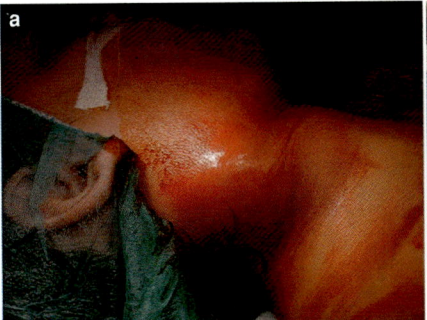
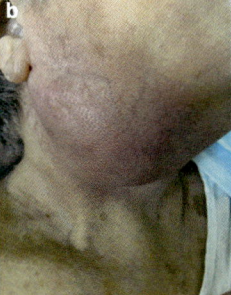
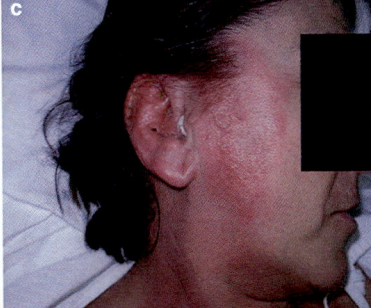

Fig. 41.3 (**a**) Laterocervical abscess in a pediatric patient. (**b**) Parotid abscess. (**c**) External otitis

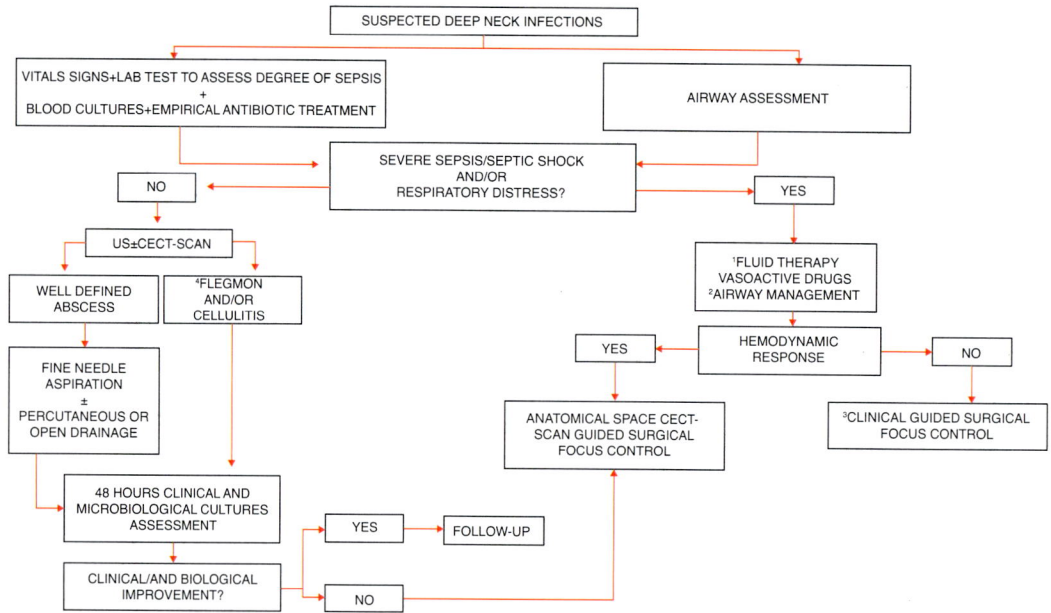

Fig. 41.4 Suggested algorithm in the management of FNI
US Ultrasonogram exam. Consider ultrasonogram exam in pediatric patients and in low-middle severe cases of neck infections
CECT–SCAN Contrast enhanced CT-scan
There are scanty data that pediatric patients may respond to the antibiotic treatment alone
1 Survival Sepsis Campaign principles (Rhodes 2017)
2 Close observation, video-laryngoscopy or fiberoptic-guided oral intubation in awake patient or open tracheostomy under local anesthesia. Emergent tracheostomy should be prevented as much as possible
3 Clinical-guided surgical focus control should be considered (without CECT–SCAN) if necrotizing fasciitis of the neck is suspected
4 If edema is surrounding airway space, short course of corticosteroids may improve dysphagia and trismus and may shorten length of the stay

ity and specificity of 95% and 98%, respectively [16]. In addition, CECT is universally recommended as a first choice of imaging test, even in pediatric population [1] when infection of submandibular, parapharyngeal or retropharyngeal spaces is suspected [13, 17] or to anticipate an impending airway obstruction [19, 37].

Magnetic Resonance Imaging (MRI)

Use of MRI gives improved soft-tissue definition over CECT without the use of radiation. MRI angiography is better than CECT in the diagnosis of vascular complications of deep FNI, such as internal jugular vein thrombosis, carotid erosion or with impending rupture. MRI should also be used when central nervous system involvement is suspected [33].

Furthermore, by not using iodinated contrast enhancement, MRI may carry an additional advantage for patients who have impaired renal function or have a previous history of reactions to iodinated contrast agents [36]. Conversely, because the image acquisition takes longer, this technique may not be suitable for pediatric patients or in those patients with septic shock.

Differential Diagnosis
The absence of local and systemic inflammatory signs and symptoms will definitively exclude FNI. Under these circumstances, most probably, we will be in front of inflammatory or tumoral lymph nodes, non-complicated cervical cysts, salivary gland neoplasms or cervical endocrine benign of malign tumors. Very rarely, low grade inflammatory FNI such as chronic or recurrent cervical abscess may be produced by tuberculous and non-tuberculous *Mycobacterium*.

41.3 Treatment

41.3.1 Medical Treatment

The bottom line of the treatment of FNI encompasses control of airway, severity of sepsis assessment, early empirical antibiotic treatment and infectious focus control. In addition, patients with severe sepsis or septic shock will follow the recommendations of the survival sepsis campaign [34].

41.3.1.1 Antibiotic Treatment

After blood cultures have been drawn, empirical antibiotic treatment should begin as soon as possible, taking in to the account the expected microorganisms for each specific clinical entity, the initial focus of infection, the host' risk factors for bacterial resistance and possible antibiotic adverse events. In selected cases, where phlegmonous inflammation predominates in an otherwise stable patient, antibiotic treatment alone may suffice [17].

Table 41.2 displays the accepted clinical entities, the main core pathogens involved and the recommended empirical antibiotic treatment [39]. Overall, the rule of thumb for a severe septic patient or for an overwhelming FNI is: Hits hard first by giving broad spectrum antibiotic, covering for possible multi-drug resistant bacteria and de-escalate later on in view of the microbiological and susceptibility results [25]. The rational for this strategy relies on the evidence that inadequate empirical antibiotic treatment has been associated with a worse outcome [40]. Furthermore, anaerobes microorganisms should always be covered both at the very beginning and the process throughout, mainly in those patients with a suspected initial oropharyngeal infection [23, 41].

41.3.1.2 Assessment and Control of Airway

Stridor and obstruction of the patient's airway and acute respiratory failure are a dismal complication of advanced FNI. Risk for airway obstruction (AO) should be assessed early on in the overall management of FNI (Fig. 41.4). Observational studies have documented that around 10% of patients observed AO [16]. Furthermore, open tracheostomy has been performed in between 4.2% and 28% of patients with severe FNI [3, 13, 16, 42, 43]. Risk factors for AO and need for open tracheostomy are multiple compartment infection, retropharyngeal abscess, Ludwig angina [3, 4] and *Klebsiella pneumoniae* infection [43]. Although emergent tracheostomy under local anesthesia has been advocated [13, 33], it might be better to anticipate and avoid such dramatic situation. Then, in patients at risk, we must to try first performing airway control with flexible fibrobroncoscopy (or videolaryngoscopy as an alternative)-guided oral intubation in awake patient. Surgical cricothyroidotomy recently emerged during COVID-19 pandemic might be a better option than an emergent tracheostomy under local anesthesia

41.3.1.3 Additional Co-adjuvant Medical Treatments

Corticosteroids

Corticosteroids have been always considered a two edges sword when administered as a co-adjuvant therapy in septic patients. Theoretical benefit of steroids treatment such as inhibition of a disproportionate inflammatory response has been always counterbalanced by a decrease in the immune response and an increased risk of superinfection.

Severe FNI displays edema and inflammation that may quickly surround critical neck structures such the airway and carotid sheath. To prevent AO, head and neck surgeons use to give a short course of corticosteroids therapy along with antibiotic treatment. Low-to-moderate level of scientific evidence supports such behavior. Randomized controlled trial in patients with peritonsillar abscess demonstrated in dexamethasone group, a lower pain scores and earlier oral intake and return to the normal activities, without an excess of adverse events [44]. Also recently published meta-analysis support the concept that a short course of corticosteroids as a co-adjuvant therapy may help for a quicker recovery and protects against AO [45].

Anticoagulation

Anticoagulation remains controversial in the management of thrombotic complications from head and neck infections and further research is required to establish evidence to reach a consensus on the antithrombotic therapy. In patients with Lemierre's syndrome, it has been suggested that anticoagulation therapy should be started when patients show a poor clinical response, those with intracranial thrombosis and in those patients, where predisposing thrombophilia has been substantiated [25].

41.3.2 Focus Control of Infection

Focus control is the mainstay of the treatment of FNI and open surgical debridement is performed in between 69% and 87% of patients [3, 17, 19]. Strategy and type of access will be highly dependent on the severity of FNI, localization, extension and the pathogenic stage observed at the diagnostic imaging test. Overall, we must to perform early open surgical debridement in those patients with FNI, where a well-defined abscess larger than 3 cm has been documented, in severe sepsis or septic shock patients, when FNI encompasses two or more anatomical spaces and in descending infections [16]. General surgeon should be competent for the initial surgical management of severe FNI. Nevertheless, head and neck and maxillofacial surgeons should provide technical support when needed.

Optimal surgical approach should be performed trough the shorter way to reach the infected cavity and with fully knowledge of the relevant anatomical structures to avoid intraoperative bleeding and/or nervous injury. Fine-needle aspiration might be of some help to delineate the best place to made the incision (Fig. 41.5).

Percutaneous Abscess Drainage Observational studies have documented that in selected patients (hemodynamic stability, moderate severity of sepsis and relatively small volume abscess), percutaneous US-guided drainage may be an alternative method to the classical open surgical

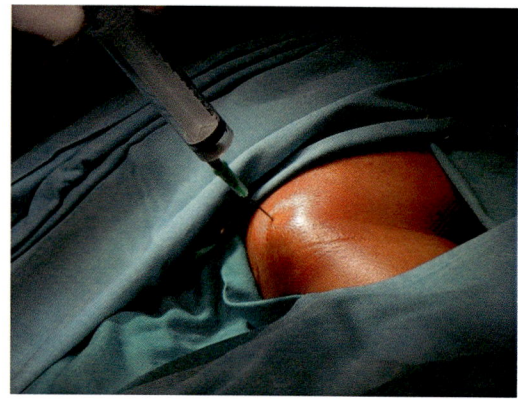

Fig. 41.5 Laterocervical abscess in a pediatric patient. Fine-needle aspiration allows for first, enough sample material for microbiologic culture. And second, to guide open extraoral focus control

access [46, 47]. In addition, fine-needle aspiration to void the whole abscess may also be trayed in some patients [3, 13]. Nevertheless, close follow-up is needed to early detect therapeutic failure [13] (Fig. 41.4).

Strategy and basic surgical technique for specific face and neck spaces follows.

41.3.2.1 Abscess of Canine, Buccal, Vestibular and Palatal Spaces

The involvement of the vestibule or the palate spaces produces localized and painful swelling, usually in relation to the infected tooth. In most cases, the infections that affect these spaces originate from an odontogenic focus. In the canine space, the incision is placed in the fundus of the vestibule. Patients usually present swelling in the canine fossa and edema may extend to the ipsilateral lower eyelid. The eye may be closed if the infection grows uncontrollably. Caution must be taken not to injure the angular vein and infraorbital nerve (Fig. 41.6).

When buccal space is involved, we are able to see a swelling in the cheek area. Then, incision should be placed at the posterior area of the jugal mucosa and blunt dissection is made toward the buccinator muscle. Caution should be exercised not to injure the facial vessels, branches of the

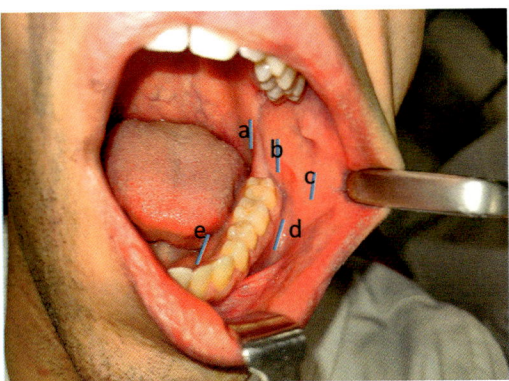

Fig. 41.6 Intraoral approaches to the: (**a**) Retropharyngeal space, (**b**) Masticator spaces, (**c**) Buccal space, (**d**) Vestible, (**e**) Floor of the mouth

facial nerve and the Stenon's duct. Oral surgical approach is performed through an intraoral incision using local anesthesia, such as articaine hydrochloride (72.9 mg) and epinephrine (0.018 mg).

The extraoral approach to drain these facial spaces is reserved for those cases in which adequate drainage cannot be achieved by oral approach, making a 2–3 cm incision through the mandibular body to avoid damaging the marginal branch of the facial nerve (Fig. 41.7). Some patients may benefit from combined approach [3].

41.3.2.2 Masticator Space Abscess

Masticator space infection usually comes after the third molar infection. These patients usually present with jaw pain and trismus. In protracted infection, facial edema and dysphagia may appear. Extension to the temporal area follows when after complicated infections of posterior molar of maxilla. Early diagnosis and treatment should be done to avoid orbital extension and optical neuritis.

An intraoral approach at the retromolar trigone is appropriate for draining abscesses medial to the ramus of the mandible (Fig. 41.6). The extraoral approach is used for draining abscesses lateral to the mandibular ramus and is performed through an incision 3 cm below the mandibular ridge (to avoid injuring the marginal branch of the facial nerve) and posterior to the submaxillary gland. General anesthesia is recommended. Caution should be taken not to injure the facial artery and vein (Fig. 41.7). In addition, extraoral approach is mandatory when trismus is present and the patient is unable to collaborate. Superficial and deep temporal space are approached through the Guillies incision, 2.5 cm superior and anterior to the helix]taking care to avoid temporal vessels. This approach is used for infections that extend to the infra-temporal fossa, lateral to the zygomatic arch [48] (Fig. 41.7).

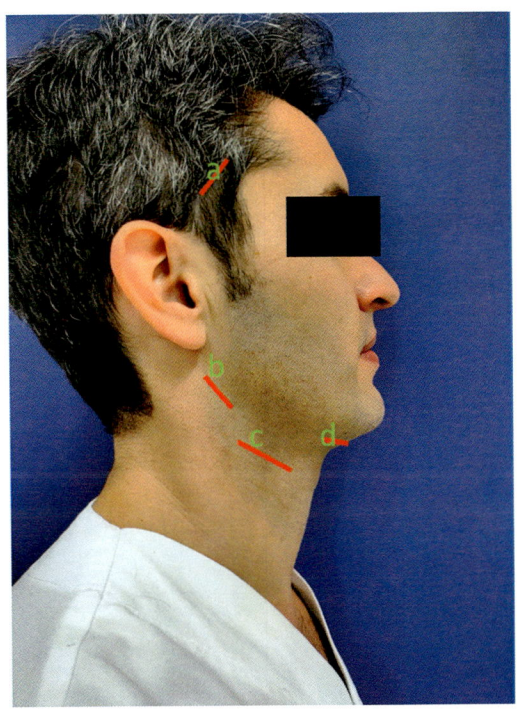

Fig. 41.7 Extraoral approaches to the head and neck spaces. (**a**) Guilles approach, (**b**) Retromandibular approach, (**c**) Submandibular approach and (**d**) Submental approach

41.3.2.3 Parotid Space

An external, retromandibular approach is used to drain a parotid space abscess. A blunt dissection should be performed in order to avoid facial nerve branches and the retromandibular vein. Again, fine-needle aspirations helps to take adequate material for microbiologic culture and to guide external incision [48].

41.3.2.4 Debridement of the Floor of the Mouth: Ludwig Angina

Debridement of the floor of the mouth may be done by intraoral or extraoral incision. Intraoral drainage is feasible only those patients with uncomplicated infections limited to the sublingual compartment and near the lingual mandibular cortical. Key anatomical structures that should be preserved are the Wharton's duct and the lingual nerve.

The external approach is performed through an incision made approximately 3–4 cm below the inferior border of the mandible following the cervical Langer's lines and posterior to the submandibular gland following by careful blunt dissection through the platysma and mylohyoid muscle (Fig. 41.7). Bilateral approach is frequently needed. Sometimes, a submental incision is also needed to reach the anterior part of the floor of the mouth. If this is done, special caution must be taken in avoiding anterior jugular veins injury. Blunt or finger dissection is then used in a superior–medial direction to enter the submandibular space. Care should be taken to dissect toward the lingual aspect of the mandible in the area of the posterior molars to avoid the facial vessels. It is sometimes unavoidable penetrate trough the oral mucosa when teeth are extracted concomitantly. However, in the authors' experience, such event has not led to an oro-cutaneous fistula [42, 49]. In pediatric patients, a more conservative approach is first advised.

Surgical drains should always be left in place. We often use red rubber catheters in addition to Penrose drains to irrigate the space. Nevertheless, observational studies have demonstrated that drain irrigation can be time-consuming, uncomfortable to the patient and also may have the potential to seed skin flora deep into a fascial space [36]. In addition, The use of non-irrigating drains appears to be equally efficacious as irrigating drains in the management of severe odontogenic infection [50].

41.3.2.5 Debridement of Central Compartment of the Neck.

Postoperative surgical site infections after thyroid or parathyroid surgery are seldom reported. In addition, isolated clinical cases of cervical infections form necrotic thyroid nodules have been documented. Nevertheless, early diagnosis and treatment are critical to prevent a more severe and descending infection. Central neck compartment abscess may be approached through a Kocher's incision and after minimal sub-platysma dissection is made, the space between sternocleidomastoid and pre-thyroid muscles is open it (back door approach). Careful blunt dissection will prevent carotid sheath structures injury (Fig. 41.8a, b).

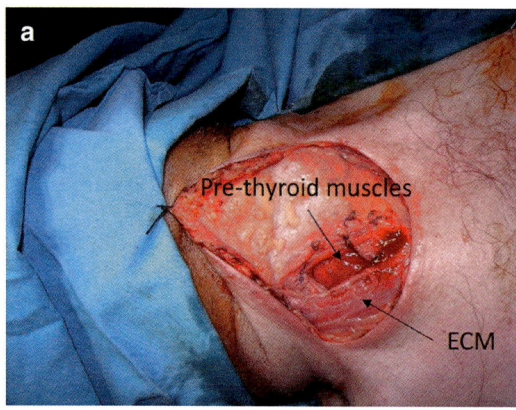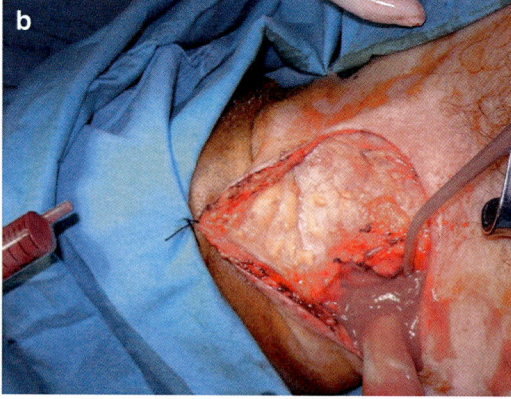

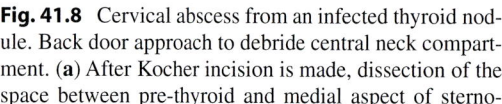

Fig. 41.8 Cervical abscess from an infected thyroid nodule. Back door approach to debride central neck compartment. (**a**) After Kocher incision is made, dissection of the space between pre-thyroid and medial aspect of sternocleidomastoid muscle is performed. (**b**) Blunt dissection allows for a safe debridement avoiding relevant anatomical structures to the carotid sheath

Dos and Don'ts

Dos

- Assess severity and patient's airway before moving forward to radiology department
- If a patient with severe FNI initiates progressive respiratory distress, do not panic. Raise the head of the patient's bed, give high FiO_2 and corticosteroids. Then, assess with the anesthesiologist to perform fiberbronchoscopy-guided intubation in awake patient, with a thin (5–6 mm), well-lubricated orotraqueal tube. In meantime, prepare percutaneous cricothyroidotomy kit.
- Before surgical or radiological debridement is performed, plan when and how you will take adequate sample for microbiology cultures.
- If you are not confident with an specific neck surgical approach, talk with head and neck colleague to assist you. You will learn from him!

Don'ts

- Do not underestimate oral infection in a diabetic or immunosuppressed patient
- Do not wait for additional test to confirm sepsis. If clinical and physical exam suggests that deep neck infection is ongoing, immediate antibiotic treatment is needed.
- Do not perform tracheostomy with local anesthesia as first initial step to control FNI patient's airway.
- Avoid tiny surgical debridement with local anesthesia at the emergency surgical department. Take the patient at the OR and discuss with the anesthesiologist the best comprehensive approach instead.
- Do not wait to take patient at the OR if severe FNI is confirmed.

Take Home Messages

- Pain in the neck, fever and trismus: Has this patient risk for airway obstruction?
- I'm sure that this patient with an inflammatory latero-cervical mass has a huge neck abscess. We better of order a contrast enhanced CT-scan. Is this patient stable enough to perform such image technique test?
- This diabetic patient with fever and submandibular painful edema complaints some dysphagia without an evident stridor. Are you sure that we are not dealing with Ludwig angina and the airway obstruction in on the way?
- Patient with ultrasonogram demonstrated latero-cervical abscess is at the operating room, draped and we are ready to perform open debridement. Let us go to open it as soon as possible. Keep in mind to perform fine-needle aspiration first, localize the abscess, take enough sample material and made the incision afterward.
- We are dealing with a patient with severe necrotizing cervical fasciitis. Microbiologist informs that Gram stain from the already debride greyish tissue debridement is positive for Gram positive chain cocci: this patients has Type II necrotizing fasciitis due to Group A beta-hemolytic *Streptococcus pyogenes*, being the best antibiotic treatment high doses of penicillin and clindamycin.

Multiple Choice Test Questions

1. Which of the following are considered risk factors for face and neck infections
   A. Sex
   B. Hypercholesterolemia
   C. Hypertension
   D. Diabetes mellitus

Correct answer: D

2. The reason behind that diabetic patients are prone to complicated FNI is…
   A. Hyperosmolar milieu facilitates microorganisms growth
   B. Reactive hyperinsulinemia increases inappropriate inflammatory response
   C. The phagocytic and killing functions of neutrophil phagocytosis are impaired
   D. Desiccation because polyuria may facilitate soft tissue infections

   Correct answer: C

3. Overall, what is the main initial infection focus of FNI in adult patients?
   A. Odontogenic
   B. Tonsillar
   C. Cervical cysts
   D. Parotid tumor

   Correct answer: A

4. What is the main initial infection focus of FNI in pediatric patients?
   A. Odontogenic
   B. Tonsillar
   C. Cervical cysts
   D. Parotid tumor

   Correct answer: B

5. *Klebsiella pneumoniae* is the main microorganism involved in FNI in which country?
   A. Spain
   B. Italy
   C. Russia
   D. Taiwan

   Correct answer: D

6. Which of the following conditions is not a complication of protracted FNI
   A. Descending mediastinitis
   B. Postoperative pancreatitis
   C. Epidural abscess
   D. Thrombophlebitis of internal jugular vein (Lemierre's syndrome)

   Correct answer: B

7. 7 A 72-year-old woman with known type 2 diabetes mellitus, rheumatoid arthritis, and hypothyroidism presented to a local hospital emergency room via ambulance due to upper respiratory symptoms for the previous 2 days. On examination, the patient was afebrile, tachycardic (110–120 beats per minute), and tachypneic. Mild to moderate submandibular and neck edema was noted, greater on the left than on the right. Her oral examination revealed no apparent odontogenic source for the presumed abscess. Her white blood cell count was $33.0 \times 10^9/L$ with 18% bands, lactic acid was 2.7 mmol/L, and CRP was 205 mg/L and procalcitonin was 6.77 ng/m. What is the most adequate initial management:
   A. Most probably, this patient has a deep FNI and we need a contrast enhanced CT-scan to decide the best surgical strategy
   B. Apyrexia excludes severe sepsis. We must assess for cardiac failure
   C. The patient is at high risk for airway obstruction and respiratory arrest. After blood cultures, broad spectrum antibiotics and corticosteroids are given and fiberoptic-guided oral intubation in awake patients should be performed right away.
   D. Impending airway obstruction is on the way. Surgical tracheostomy under local anesthesia should be done right now.

   Correct answer: C

8. Surgical resident on call is required to assess a patient admitted to the surgical ward complaining of fever and painful tumor in to the right cheek. The patient had been operated on for a recurrent benign small bowel obstruction and is nothing per mouth, under TPN and with nasogastric tube. Physical exam reveals painful and inflammatory round tumor at the right preauricular area.
   A. Most probably, this patient has external malignant otitis. Antipseudomonal antibiotic should be given and CT scan ordered.

B. We suspect of FNI from odontogenic origin. Page to maxillofacial colleague right away.
C. This patient is at risk for acute purulent parotitis. After blood cultures, broad spectrum antibiotics covering for *Staphylococcus aureus* should be given. Ultrasonogram may help to diagnose parotid abscess that may ultimately require adequate drainage.
D. This patient has a clear acute postoperative parotitis. Fine-needle aspiration should be performed to discard parotid abscess.

Correct answer: C

9. We are dealing with a patient at the operating room with severe and quickly progressive deep FNI. Microbiologist informs that Gram stain from the already debrided greyish tissue is positive for Gram positive arranged in chains cocci. Then,

A. We are dealing with type II cervical necrotizing fasciitis due to *Streptococcus pyogenes*. We must to clean and excise all necrotic tissue preserving relevant vascular and neural structures. The best antibiotic treatment includes high doses of penicillin and clindamycin.
B. Clostridial myonecrosis should be suspected. Wide cervical muscles should be excised and hyperbaric oxygen treatment initiated.
C. Because the absence of pus, the prognosis of infection is much better. Gram-positive cocci may be related to a contaminated sample.
D. We are in front of latero-cervical abscess probably due to *Staphylococcus aureus* infection. We must to debride only well-defined abscess and anti-staphylococcus antibiotic prescribed.

Correct answer: A

10. Which of the following microorganisms has been mainly related to Lemierre's syndrome?
    A. *Mycobacterium fortuitum*
    B. *Fusobacterium necrophorum*
    C. *Streptococcus pyogenes*
    D. *Streptococcus viridans*

Correct answer: B

References

1. Huang CM, Huang FL, Chien YL, Chen PY. Deep neck infections in children. J Microbiol Immunol Infect. 2017;50(5):627–33.
2. McKellop JA, Bou-Assaly W, Mukherji SK. Emergency head & neck imaging: infections and inflammatory processes. Neuroimaging Clin N Am. 2010;20(4):651–61.
3. Huang TT, Liu TC, Chen PR, Tseng FY, Yeh TH, Chen YS. Deep neck infection: analysis of 185 cases. Head Neck. 2004;26(10):854–60.
4. Parhiscar A, Har-El G. Deep neck abscess: a retrospective review of 210 cases. Ann Otol Rhinol Laryngol. 2001;110(11):1051–4.
5. Priyamvada S, Motwani G. A study on deep neck space infections. Indian J Otolaryngol Head Neck Surg. 2019;71(Suppl 1):912–7.
6. Stalfors J, Adielsson A, Ebenfelt A, Nethander G, Westin T. Deep neck space infections remain a surgical challenge. A study of 72 patients. Acta Otolaryngol. 2004;124(10):1191–6.
7. Mortimore S, Thorp M. Cervical necrotizing fasciitis and radiotherapy: a report of two cases. J Laryngol Otol. 1998;112(3):298–300.
8. Bullock R, Soares DP, James M. An infected branchial cyst complicated by retropharyngeal abscess, cervical osteomyelitis and atlanto-axial subluxation. BMJ Case Rep. 2010;2010
9. Montgomery GL, Ballantine TV, Kleiman MB, Wright JC, Reynolds J. Ruptured branchial cleft cyst presenting as acute thyroid infection. Clin Pediatr (Phila). 1982;21(6):380–3.
10. Penel N, Lefebvre JL, Cazin JL, Clisant S, Neu JC, Dervaux B, et al. Additional direct medical costs associated with nosocomial infections after head and neck cancer surgery: a hospital-perspective analysis. Int J Oral Maxillofac Surg. 2008;37(2):135–9.
11. Kamizono K, Sakuraba M, Nagamatsu S, Miyamoto S, Hayashi R. Statistical analysis of surgical site infection after head and neck reconstructive surgery. Ann Surg Oncol. 2014;21(5):1700–5.

12. Karakida K, Aoki T, Ota Y, Yamazaki H, Otsuru M, Takahashi M, et al. Analysis of risk factors for surgical-site infections in 276 oral cancer surgeries with microvascular free-flap reconstructions at a single university hospital. J Infect Chemother. 2010;16(5):334–9.
13. Crespo AN, Chone CT, Fonseca AS, Montenegro MC, Pereira R, Milani JA. Clinical versus computed tomography evaluation in the diagnosis and management of deep neck infection. Sao Paulo Med J. 2004;122(6):259–63.
14. Tung-Yiu W, Jehn-Shyun H, Ching-Hung C, Hung-An C. Cervical necrotizing fasciitis of odontogenic origin: a report of 11 cases. J Oral Maxillofac Surg. 2000;58(12):1347–52; discussion 53.
15. Lin C, Yeh FL, Lin JT, Ma H, Hwang CH, Shen BH, et al. Necrotizing fasciitis of the head and neck: an analysis of 47 cases. Plast Reconstr Surg. 2001;107(7):1684–93.
16. Boscolo-Rizzo P, Marchiori C, Montolli F, Vaglia A, Da Mosto MC. Deep neck infections: a constant challenge. ORL J Otorhinolaryngol Relat Spec. 2006;68(5):259–65.
17. Bottin R, Marioni G, Rinaldi R, Boninsegna M, Salvadori L, Staffieri A. Deep neck infection: a present-day complication. A retrospective review of 83 cases (1998-2001). Eur Arch Otorhinolaryngol. 2003;260(10):576–9.
18. da Silva Junior AF, de Magalhaes Rocha GS, da Silva Neves de Araujo CF, Franco A, Silva RF. Deep neck infection after third molar extraction: a case report. J Dent Res Dent Clin Dent Prospects. 2017;11(3):166-169.
19. Côrte FC, Firmino-Machado J, Moura CP, Spratley J, Santos M. Acute pediatric neck infections: Outcomes in a seven-year series. Int J Pediatr Otorhinolaryngol. 2017;99:128–34.
20. Carlton DA, Perez EE, Smouha EE. Malignant external otitis: the shifting treatment paradigm. Am J Otolaryngol. 2018;39(1):41–5.
21. Hong P, Liu CM, Nordstrom L, Lalwani AK. The role of the human microbiome in otolaryngology-head and neck surgery: a contemporary review. Laryngoscope. 2014;124(6):1352–7.
22. Hagelskjaer Kristensen L, Prag J. Human necrobacillosis, with emphasis on Lemierre's syndrome. Clin Infect Dis. 2000;31(2):524–32.
23. Brook I. Anaerobic bacteria in upper respiratory tract and other head and neck infections. Ann Otol Rhinol Laryngol. 2002;111(5 Pt 1):430–40.
24. Cordesmeyer R, Kauffmann P, Markus T, Sommer C, Eiffert H, Bremmer F, et al. Bacterial and histopathological findings in deep head and neck infections: a retrospective analysis. Oral Surg Oral Med Oral Pathol Oral Radiol. 2017;124(1):11–5.
25. Campo F, Fusconi M, Ciotti M, Diso D, Greco A, Cattaneo CG, et al. Antibiotic and anticoagulation therapy in Lemierre's syndrome: case report and review. J Chemother. 2019;31(1):42–8.
26. Karkos PD, Karkanevatos A, Panagea S, Dingle A, Davies JE. Lemierre's syndrome: how a sore throat can end in disaster. Eur J Emerg Med. 2004;11(4):228–30.
27. Chainchel Singh MK, Vijayanathan A. Idiopathic thyroid abscess—a rare occurrence. Eur Endocrinol. 2019;15(1):42–3.
28. Ferzli GS, Thakkar P, Goldstein NA, Chernichenko N. Third branchial cleft cyst with mycobacterium infection. OTO Open. 2017;1(2):2473974x17705832.
29. Kitamura S. Anatomy of the fasciae and fascial spaces of the maxillofacial and the anterior neck regions. Anat Sci Int. 2018;93(1):1–13.
30. Hansen BW, Ryndin S, Mullen KM. Infections of deep neck spaces. Semin Ultrasound CT MR. 2020;41(1):74–84.
31. Kubal WS. Face and neck infections: what the emergency radiologist needs to know. Radiol Clin North Am. 2015;53(4):827–46. ix
32. Li RM, Kiemeney M. Infections of the neck. Emerg Med Clin North Am. 2019;37(1):95–107.
33. Osborn TM, Assael LA, Bell RB. Deep space neck infection: principles of surgical management. Oral Maxillofac Surg Clin North Am. 2008;20(3):353–65.
34. Rhodes A, Evans LE, Alhazzani W, Levy MM, Antonelli M, Ferrer R, et al. Surviving sepsis campaign: international guidelines for management of sepsis and septic shock: 2016. Crit Care Med. 2017;45(3):486–552.
35. Wang B, Gao BL, Xu GP, Xiang C. Images of deep neck space infection and the clinical significance. Acta Radiol. 2014;55(8):945–51.
36. Taub D, Yampolsky A, Diecidue R, Gold L. Controversies in the management of oral and maxillofacial infections. Oral Maxillofac Surg Clin North Am. 2017;29(4):465–73.
37. Lee MH, Carmichael RA, Read-Fuller AM, Reddy LV. Fatal deep neck infection and respiratory arrest. Proc (Bayl Univ Med Cent). 2019;32(1):67–9.
38. Skitarelic N, Mladina R, Morovic M, Skitarelic N. Cervical necrotizing fasciitis: sources and outcomes. Infection. 2003;31(1):39–44.
39. Mensa J, Soriano A, Garcia-Sanchez JE, Letang E, López-Suñe E, Marco F, et al. Guia Mensa. Terapeutica Antimicrobiana. Versión electrónica. GARMENMED. SCP. Last update March 2023.
40. Yang SW, Lee MH, Lee YS, Huang SH, Chen TA, Fang TJ. Analysis of life-threatening complications of deep neck abscess and the impact of empiric antibiotics. ORL J Otorhinolaryngol Relat Spec. 2008;70(4):249–56.
41. Zirk M, Zoeller JE, Peters F, Ringendahl L, Buller J, Kreppel M. Cefazolin versus ampicillin/sulbactam as an empiric antibiosis in severe odontogenic neck infection descending from the lower jaw-retrospective analysis of 350 cases. Clin Oral Investig. 2021;25(2):563–70.
42. Bross-Soriano D, Arrieta-Gomez JR, Prado-Calleros H, Schimelmitz-Idi J, Jorba-Basave S. Management of Ludwig's angina with small neck incisions: 18

43. Chang CM, Lu FH, Guo HR, Ko WC. Klebsiella pneumoniae fascial space infections of the head and neck in Taiwan: emphasis on diabetic patients and repetitive infections. J Infect. 2005;50(1):34–40.
44. Chau JK, Seikaly HR, Harris JR, Villa-Roel C, Brick C, Rowe BH. Corticosteroids in peritonsillar abscess treatment: a blinded placebo-controlled clinical trial. Laryngoscope. 2014;124(1):97–103.
45. Kent S, Hennedige A, McDonald C, Henry A, Dawoud B, Kulkarni R, et al. Systematic review of the role of corticosteroids in cervicofacial infections. Br J Oral Maxillofac Surg. 2019;57(3):196–206.
46. Biron VL, Kurien G, Dziegielewski P, Barber B, Seikaly H. Surgical vs ultrasound-guided drainage of deep neck space abscesses: a randomized controlled trial: surgical vs ultrasound drainage. J Otolaryngol Head Neck Surg. 2013;42:18.
47. Dabirmoghaddam P, Mohseni A, Navvabi Z, Sharifi A, Bastaninezhad S, Safaei A. Is ultrasonography-guided drainage a safe and effective alternative to incision and drainage for deep neck space abscesses? J Laryngol Otol. 2017;131(3):259–63.
48. Vieira F, Allen SM, Stocks RM, Thompson JW. Deep neck infection. Otolaryngol Clin North Am. 2008;41(3):459–83. vii
49. Barakate MS, Jensen MJ, Hemli JM, Graham AR. Ludwig's angina: report of a case and review of management issues. Ann Otol Rhinol Laryngol. 2001;110(5 Pt 1):453–6.
50. Bouloux GF, Wallace J, Xue W. Irrigating drains for severe odontogenic infections do not improve outcome. J Oral Maxillofac Surg. 2013;71(1):42–6.

Further Reading

Hansen BW, Ryndin S, Mullen KM. Infections of deep neck spaces. Semin Ultrasound CT MR. 2020;41(1):74–84.

Trauma to the Face

42

Kerry P. Latham and Mark W. Bowyer

42.1 Introduction

Learning Goals
- Understand facial injury indications for airway and bleeding control
- Describe indications for repair of facial injuries in the first 24 h from injury as well as those that may wait.
- Understand evidence-based timing and management of facial trauma.

42.1.1 Epidemiology

The National Trauma Data Bank (NTDB) helps provide demographic information and mechanism of injury information [1, 2]. Approximately 11% of all trauma admissions have a facial fracture [1, 2]. Traumatic brain injuries are associated 39% of the time [1]. Five percent of pediatric trauma patient admissions have facial fractures [2, 3]. Up to five percent of patients with a facial fracture will also have a cervical spine injury. The NTDB does not capture all facial traumas but likely captures the most severe trauma with concomitant injuries and a resultant increased morbidity and mortality compared to the Nationwide Emergency Department Sample [1, 2].

42.1.2 Etiology

In the United States, the majority of patients that present to trauma centers with facial fractures have fractures that result from blunt trauma, most frequently from motor vehicle collisions. Motor Vehicle Collisions and pedestrian struck by vehicle are most prevalent in the young and young adult and decrease with age as falls rise with increasing age [2, 4]. Gunshot wounds and interpersonal violence (being struck in the face) are the mechanisms with the highest rates of mandible fracture while stabbings and falls having the lowest [2, 4]. In children the most common mechanisms of injury were; motor vehicle collision (55.1%), violence (11.8%), and falls (8.6%) [3].

Facial injury patterns and mechanism of injury vary by gender and age. There is an increase in proportion of midface and orbit fractures with increasing age [2] The rate of fractures requiring repair peaks for individuals between ages 18 and 40 and decreases with age [1, 2] Facial bones thin with age and are, therefore, more vulnerable to fracture from lower energy mechanisms of injury, and thus, the fracture patterns seen in the aged are less likely to warrant the need for repair.

K. P. Latham · M. W. Bowyer (✉)
Department of Surgery, Uniformed Services University and the Walter Reed National Military Medical Center, Bethesda, MD, USA
e-mail: mark.bowyer@usuhs.edu

The proportion of pediatric patients with facial fractures increases substantially with age [2, 3]. Young children have developing sinuses and their skulls are large compared to their face. The craniofacial skeleton grows and develops in a top-down sequence with the skull being largely grown by age three, orbits by age ten, midface by early teen years, and the mandible in early adulthood. The face is largely protected in a young child in primary dentition with few sinuses. A toddler does not yet have a frontal sinus seen on imaging and their maxillary sinuses are filled with secondary dentition that has not errupted. The skull to face ration is a newborn is 8:1 and 2:1 in an adult. In toddlers, the skull is more likely to be injured than the face. Mandible fractures are more common in teenagers. As the face grows, sinuses develop, and secondary dentition comes in, facial fractures increase. The activities also change as children grow leading to changes in injury patterns. As children grow older, they engage in sports and more unsupervised activities that can result in trauma. Children with facial fractures have higher injury severity scores, longer hospital stays, more ICU and ventilator days, as well as higher hospital charges [3]. Children with facial fractures, compared to those without have more severe associated injury to the head and chest, with higher overall mortality [3].

42.1.3 Classification

The clinical management of facial fractures is greatly enhanced by the use of multidetector computed tomography (CT), as it provides significant detail allowing for better classification of the injuries. The facial skeleton is formed by six paired (lacrimal, palatine, maxilla, zygoma, nasal, inferior nasal concha) and two unpaired bones (vomer, and mandible), and as such facial fractures are often described (by radiologists) as to how they relate to structures like orbits or sinuses [5]. Historically, midface facial fractures were described by the classification system developed by Rene Le Fort in 1901, as shown in Fig. 42.1. The Le Fort system was conceptualized when low-speed trauma was predominant and more importance is now placed on the maxillary occlusion bearing segments of the face made up of four vertical and four horizontal buttresses [5]. Modern Facial Surgeons classify facial fractures

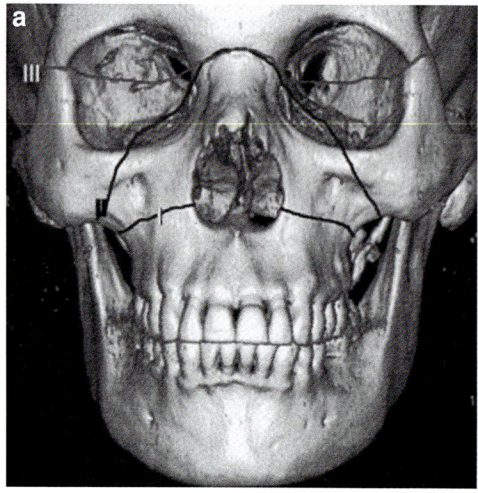 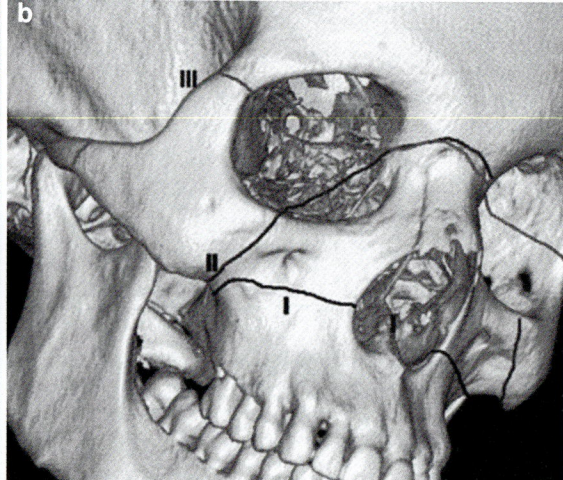

Fig. 42.1 Original Le Fort classification of midface fracture. Type I is a horizontal fracture involving the alveolar ridge; Type II, a pyramidal shaped fracture of the nasofrontal suture; and Type III, a horizontal craniofacial dislocation. (**a**) frontal view of 3D reconstruction of skull and face demonstrating Le Fort I, II and III lines of fracture. (**b**) oblique view to demonstrate intraorbital view of Le Fort II and III fracture lines Reproduced without change from Gómez Roselló, E. *et al.*; *Insights Imaging* 11, 49 (2020) [5] under the terms of the Creative Commons Attribution 4.0 International License (http://creativecommons.org/licenses/by/4.0/)

Table 42.1 Patterns and classifications of facial fractures. Reproduced with formatting changes from Gómez Roselló, E. et al.; Insights Imaging 11, 49 (2020) [5] under the terms of the Creative Commons Attribution 4.0 International License (http://creativecommons.org/licenses/by/4.0/)

Multiple buttresses fracture Pterygoid process	Le Fort YES	I, The anterior margin of the nasal fossa II, the inferior orbital rim III, the zygomatic arch	
	Le Fort NO	Medial: Naso-orbito-ethmoidal complex- (Markowitz and Manson) classification	Type I—medial canthal tendon is intact and connected to a single large fracture fragment
			Type II—the fracture is comminuted, and the medial canthal tendon is attached to a single bone fragment
			Type III—comminution extends to the medial canthal tendon insertion site on the anterior medial orbital wall at the level of the lacrimal fossa, with resultant tendon avulsion.
One/few buttresses fracture		Lateral: Zygomaticomaxillary complex Mandible → characterized by location Orbital "blow out" fracture Frontal sinus fractures Alveolar process or nasal bone	

into the following regions; cranio-orbital, naso-orbital ethmoid, midface, mandible and panface. Of patients presenting to a trauma center after a motor vehicle collision, 11% are diagnosed with a facial fracture with the following prevalence of classification: nasal fracture (5.6%), midface (3.8%), other (3.2%), orbital (2.6%), mandible (2.2%), and panfacial fractures (0.8%) [4]. In children, the most common facial fractures were mandible (32.7%), nasal (30.2%), and maxillary/zygoma (28.6%) [3]. To confuse matters further even more, some facial surgeons describe the location of fractures by portioning the face into upper, middle, and lower thirds. Table 42.1 provides a more practical classification schema that may help to better understand the patterns of facial fractures.

In review of the NTDB, facial fracture repair is independently affected by sex, age, race and insurance type [2]. A decrease odds of early repair was associated with female, non-white, and uninsured status [2]. Aside from mandible fractures, the majority of facial fractures are not repaired at the index admission. Fifteen percent of those injured with a firearm have a craniofacial injury. Cranial injuries are an independent risk factor for poor outcome, such as increased inpatient mortality [6].

42.2 Diagnosis

42.2.1 Clinical Presentation

When possible, it is best to obtain a history and physical exam to include assessment of cranial nerves, sensation, vision, occlusion, and patient's pain and symptoms [7]. Severe facial trauma including mandible and midface fractures can lead to severe swelling that can compromise the airway. Establishing a secure airway is a priority. The patient may be uneasy laying down on their back for assessment in the trauma bay due to bleeding or swelling. Awake fiberoptic airway or crichothyroidotomy may be required. A secure airway and sedation may be required before head and neck specialists arrive for consultation, so the trauma team's history and physical exam of the conscious patient are important.

42.2.2 Tests

A history and physical exam are critical to the understanding injuries and functional impact. Vision, sensation, motor function and occlusion are important to assess [7]. For patients with facial fractures, it is important to keep in mind the structures that might be affected by fracture and the resultant clinical findings or possible complications that might result (Table 42.2). Fine cut CT of the face with 3D reconstructions provide the majority of the information required for operative decision making with regard to fracture reduction and fixation. Plain films are technically demanding for the diagnostic imaging technician and many views require C-spine clearance prior to the exam. CT scans can be performed rapidly with ease of positioning and consistent technical quality. The ideal image is from vertex to menton.

42.3 Treatment

42.3.1 Medical Treatment

Up to 5% of patients with facial trauma may have an associated cervical spine injury. Until the C-spine can be cleared radiologically and clinically, strict precautions must be ensured during the perioperative period. Moving the patient for transport and surgical positioning are critical times for the care team to coordinate maintaining C-spine precautions. When possible, it is best to clear the C-spine prior to repair of facial fractures to improve the ease of surgery.

Evidence-based guidelines dictate best practices for antibiotic use with facial trauma. Perioperative antibiotics are indicated for surgery. Post-procedure antibiotics are indicated for open fractures of the mandible [8–10]. No significant infection reduction is seen after 72 h of antibiotics as treatment for mandible fracture [8–10]. Additional antibiotics may be indicated for specific wounds, such as animal bites. Dog bites are the most common animal bite. In adults, defensive wounds to the extremities (86%) are most common followed by wounds to the head and neck (23%) [11]. In toddlers, the majority (65%) of dog injuries are in the head and neck region [12]. The nose, lips, and cheeks comprise the "central target area" and are the most common structures damaged in cases of facial dog bites [12]. Dog bites can be crushing injuries, and so, facial fractures of the central face should also be ruled out [12]. Avulsed tissue can be used as a graft after washing and debridement, as the face is very vascular and may support at least partial revascularization. There are more than one hundred types of bacteria associated with dog bites, including: *Pasteurella*, *Staphylococcus*, and *Streptococcus* [11]. Appropriate wound care includes wash out, antibiotics, prophylaxis for tetanus and consideration for rabies. Rabies vaccination should be confirmed as up to date after a dog bite. Rabies immunoglobin should be injected on the day of

Table 42.2 Structures potentially affected by facial fractures and the resultant findings and complications. Reproduced with minimal change from Gómez Roselló, E. *et al.; Insights Imaging* 11, 49 (2020) [5] under the terms of the Creative Commons Attribution 4.0 International License (http://creativecommons.org/licenses/by/4.0/)

Affected structures	Possible findings/complications
Intra-orbital contents	Blindness, ophthalmoplegia and diplopia, increased orbital volume with exophthalmos
Nerve foramina	Orbital apex (CN I) → unilateral blindness; Superior orbital fissure—(CN III, CN IV, CN V1, and CN VI) → ophthalmoplegia, diplopia, ptosis; Mandibular canal (branch of CN V3) → anesthesia of the ipsilateral lower lip, chin, anterior tongue, and mandibular teeth. (CN = cranial nerve)
Temporalis muscle impingement	Trismus
Teeth	Dental fracture, avulsion, devitalization, malocclusion, soft-tissue infection, airway aspiration
Drainage canals impairment	Frontal recess, sphenoethmoidal recess or ostiomeatal complex → mucocele Lacrimal duct → dacryocystitis
Medial canthal tendon	Telecanthus
Cribriform plate	Leakage of cerebrospinal fluid
Multiple middle face or condylar fractures	Blunt carotid artery injury
Posterior extension	Blunt carotid artery injury, skull base nerve foramina affectation

the bite, in and around the wound as well as at the depth of the wound when rabies is a possibility.

Patients with significant burns to the face should be transferred to a burn center. In the initial medical response and stabilization securing an airway, assessing the burns and wound care are a priority. Indications for intubation include a Glasgow coma scale of 8 or less, symptomatic inhalation injury, deep facial burns, and burns exceeding 40% of total body surface area. Inhalation injury should be considered and evaluated when facial burns are present [13]. Clinical signs of inhalation injury include voice changes, perioral soot, hypoxia, singed nasal hairs, and shortness of breath. Bronchoscopy is useful to evaluate for tracheal and bronchial burn and lavage can be performed to remove debris. Patients diagnosed with inhalation injury benefit from aerosolized heparin mixed with albuterol [13]. Every patient with facial burns should have a thorough eye exam, and if available, consult an ophthalmologist. Shave and debride the face, to evaluate the wounds fully and allow for proper wound care. Apply mafenide acetate (Sulfamylon®) cream twice a day to ear burns to avoid chondritis [13]. Pressure from endotracheal tube ties can lead to facial necrosis as the face continues to swell after the burn [13]. To secure endotracheal tubes, circum-mandibular wire or suture or wiring or suturing the dentition can secure the airway that avoids pressure and allows for wound care.

42.3.2 Treatment

The need for urgent airway control or urgent bleeding control for isolated facial injuries is rare with gunshot wounds to the face being a leading cause [14, 15]. In general, bleeding of the face responds to nasal and oral packing and pressure. Blood vessels of the face are generally small caliber and occlude quickly with pressure and packing, even when named vessels are transected. The vast blood supply to the face allows significant blood loss from the face and scalp prior to cessation of bleeding. Vascular perfusion redundancy allows for resilient tissue perfusion despite traumatic disruption in blood supply. If hemorrhage does not respond to pressure or packing, angiographic embolization is a successful tool [14]. Urgent exploration and fracture stabilization are also indicated for persistent bleeding not responsive to packing when embolization is not available [14]. A common sense algorithm for managing facial trauma is presented in Fig. 42.2.

Aside from urgent airway, bleeding, ocular or neurotrauma emergencies facial injuries can be delayed until after more urgent injuries have been addressed. When patients have facial fractures in combination with neuro or ocular trauma that require emergent surgery, collaborative multi-disciplinary surgeries are indicated. This is particularly of note for cranial injuries requiring intervention where associated orbital and midface injuries also require surgery. These interventions may share common approaches and benefit from a team approach as after a major neurosurgery the patient may be limited in return to OR for non-urgent matters. Involving the head and neck trauma team when there is concomitant neuro and ocular trauma enhances teamwork and improves efficiency of care for the trauma patient.

Large tissue avulsions in need of delicate cleaning and repair are most appropriately done in the OR when the size is large as debridement and anesthesia are more difficult at the bedside in the trauma bay. Day of injury repair is also indicated when the patient would benefit from general anesthesia and the superior lighting and equipment the operating room affords. For example, patients who require facial nerve of lacrimal system exploration and repair are generally best treated in the operating room at the time of the complex laceration closure. Often, a superior wash out and debridement can be performed in the operating room particularly with major tissue avulsions or an animal mauling.

The majority of facial fractures can be definitively addressed more than 24 h after injury without an increase in morbidity [17, 18]. Fractures can be very painful when there is motion during activities of daily living and basic functions. This is notable for mandible fractures where eating, speaking and performing oral hygiene can be painful due to the bony motion caused by the

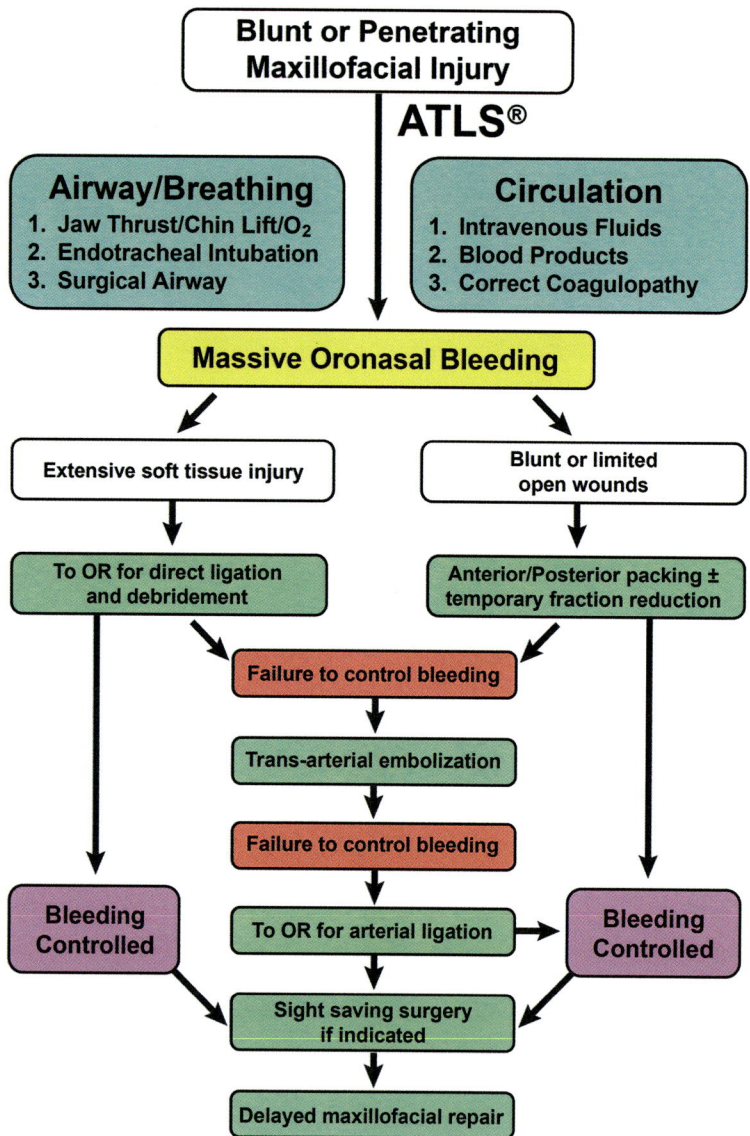

Fig. 42.2 Algorithm for managing maxillofacial trauma. Adapted from Tuckett et al. [16] with permission

muscles of mastication. It is not surprising that mandible fractures are the facial fracture that most reliably requires repair and are generally repaired at that admission. Severe concomitant extremity injuries were also associated with increase rate of repair, again likely due to energy of the mechanism of injury and displacement [2]. For ease of reduction most fractures that require fixation are addressed by 2 weeks. Earlier attention for a significantly impacted fracture may avoid difficulty with reduction and early bony healing caused by impaction. Isolated orbit fractures that require an implant repair are most likely to be addressed at another setting or more distant time frame from the initial injury [2].

Lacerations and other open wounds to the face require proper care and technique to achieve an acceptable cosmetic result and decrease rates of infection. Initial wound care of a facial wound is the same as applied to a wound anywhere on the body. The wound should be fully cleansed and examined throughout. All foreign bodies, debris, and dried blood should be removed. The choice of anesthetic and its method of delivery depend on the location of the wound, the mechanism of injury, and the practitioner's comfort level with various techniques, including local administration, regional nerve blocks, and topical anesthetics [19]. Wound closure can be achieved using sutures, staples, or tissue adhesive. Suture choice is based on the location and size of the wound (Table 42.3). When sutures are placed on facial skin, they should be positioned 1–2 mm from the skin edge and approximately 3 mm apart, which is closer than in other sites on the body. This technique allows better tissue approximation and improved cosmetic outcomes [20]. Complex injuries to the lids, nose, lips, and ears are best managed by facial specialty consultants in a delayed fashion once life threatening is treated.

42.3.3 Prognosis

Mortality after sustaining facial fractures is due to associated injuries, such as brain injury or other life-threatening injuries. Although mortality from facial trauma is rare, significant trauma can significantly impair quality of life with loss of vision, malocclusion, very different facial appearance, inability to smile or blink, oral incompetence, unintelligible speech, difficulty eating [2, 12]. Reconstruction after severe facial trauma is often staged and requires a long-term team approach. High energy ballistic wounds are among the most devastating.

> **Dos and Don'ts**
> - Do—consider a prophylaxis to prevent complications—tetanus, rabies (indicated bites), and antibiotics.
> - Do—involve facial trauma team members in the treatment plan early to optimize opportunities for operative collaboration and treatment plan prioritization and efficiency
> - Do—perform a history and physical exam
> - Don't under estimate the potential swelling from facial trauma (particularly ballistic injuries) that can lead to airway compromise.

Table 42.3 Optimal suture material for facial wounds by location. Adapted from Sabatino and Moskovitz [19] with permission

Site of injury	Suture size	Optimal material (good alternative)
Cheek, forehead, nose skin	5-0, 6-0	Nylon, prolene (cat gut or chromic for pediatric patients or patients who will not return for removal)
Ear skin	4-0	Nylon (chromic)
Eyelid skin	6-0, 7-0	Nylon (chromic)
Frontalis muscle	3-0, 4-0	Vicryl (chromic)
Galea	3-0, 4-0	Vicryl (chromic)
Lip or intraoral mucosa	4-0	Chromic (Vicryl)
Lip muscle	4-0	Vicryl (chromic)
Nasal mucosa	6-0	Nylon (chromic)
Subcutaneous tissue	4-0, 5-0	Vicryl (chromic)
		Prolene can be substituted whenever nylon is recommended

> **Take-Home Messages**
> - The face is very vascular but despite the potential for significant blood loss ongoing bleeding can most commonly be managed with packing and pressure
> - Facial lacerations require careful attention to wound care and suture selection to achieve optimal cosmetic results
> - Involve head and neck trauma surgeons in the care plan early
> - The majority of facial injuries can be addressed after 24 h with exceptions including combined neurotrauma and certain complex facial laceration.

Questions

1. Massive Facial Bleeding should first be managed with:
   A. Angiography and Embolization
   B. Ligation of Bleeding Vessel
   C. **Packing and Pressure**
   D. Ligation External Carotid Arteries
2. The need for urgent airway due to facial trauma is most commonly associated with
   A. **Gunshot wound**
   B. Dog bite
   C. Mandible fracture
   D. NOE fracture
3. When treating a patient in the first 4 h after a dog bite wash out the wound and consider antibiotics, tetanus, and..
   A. **RIG**
   B. aggressive debridement
   C. delayed primary closure
   D. infectious disease consult
4. The recommended timeline to repair most facial fractures is:
   A. the first 8 h
   B. the first 24 h
   C. **the first 2 weeks**
   D. 6 weeks
5. The isolated fractured facial bone that is generally repaired early or that admission is:
   A. nasal bone fracture
   B. orbital fracture
   C. **mandible fracture**
   D. zygomatic-maxillary fracture
6. The initial step to control massive oronasal hemorrhage caused by blunt trauma is:
   A. **anterior and posterior packing of the nose**
   B. urgent transfer to operating room for direct ligation
   C. application of intranasal laser coagulation
   D. angioembolization
7. The best choice of suture for an injury to the nasal mucosa is.
   A. 4-0 Vicryl
   B. 5-0 Nylon
   C. **5-0 Chromic**
   D. 4-0 Prolene
8. Which of the following best describes the facial skeleton?
   A. It is formed by four paired and five unpaired bones
   B. It is comprised of five vertical and four horizontal buttresses
   C. It is comprised of four vertical and five horizontal buttresses
   D. **It is formed by six paired and two unpaired bones**
9. Clinical signs of inhalation injury include all of the following EXCEPT?
   A. Voice changes
   B. **Blisters on the lips**
   C. Perioral soot
   D. Singed nasal hairs
10. The most common facial fractures in children is?
    A. Maxilla
    B. Nasal
    C. Zygoma
    D. **Mandible**

Acknowledgements

Disclaimer: The contents of this presentation are the sole responsibility of the author(s) and do not necessarily reflect the views, opinions or policies of Uniformed Services University of the Health Sciences (USUHS), the Department of Defense (DoD) or the Departments of the Army, Navy, or Air Force. Mention of trade names, commercial products, or organizations does not imply endorsement by the U.S. Government. None of the authors have additional disclosures or conflicts of interest.

References

1. CDC. National estimates of nonfatal injuries treated in hospital emergency departments—United States, 2000. MMWR. 2001;50:340–6.

2. Wasicek PJ, Gebran SG, Ngaage LM, Liang Y, Ottochian M, Morrison JJ, Nam AJ. Contemporary characterization of injury patterns, initial management, and disparities in treatment of facial fractures using the National Trauma Data Bank. J Craniofac Surg. 2019;30(7):2052–6.
3. Imahara SD, Hopper RA, Wang J, et al. Patterns and outcomes of pediatric facial fractures in the united states: a survey of the National Trauma Data Bank. J Am Coll Surg. 2008;207:710–6.
4. Hyman DA, Saha S, Nayar HS, et al. Patterns of facial fractures and protective device use in motor vehicle collisions from 2007 to 2012. JAMA Facial Plast Surg. 2016;18:455–46.
5. Gómez Roselló E, Quiles Granado AM, Artajona Garcia M, Juanpere Martí S, Laguillo Sala G, Beltrán Mármol B, Pedraza GS. Facial fractures: classification and highlights for a useful report. Insights Imaging. 2020;11(1):49.
6. Allareddy V, Nalliah R, Lee MK, et al. Impact of facial fractures and intracranial injuries on hospitalization outcomes following firearm injuries. JAMA Otolaryngol Head Neck Surg. 2014;140:303–11.
7. Truong TA. Facial trauma: initial assessment and evaluation of traumatic facial injuries. In Seminars in plastic surgery, Vol. 31, No. 2, p. 69. Thieme Medical Publishers; (2017, May).
8. Morrow BT, Samson TD, Schubert W, Mackay DR. Evidence-based medicine: mandible fractures. Plastic Reconstr Surg. 2014;134(6):1381–90.
9. Doerr TD. Evidence-based facial fracture management. Facial Plastic Surg Clin. 2015;23(3):335–45.
10. Lucca M, Shastri K, McKenzie W, Kraus J, Finkelman M, Wein R. Comparison of treatment outcomes associated with early versus late treatment of mandible fractures: a retrospective chart review and analysis. J Oral Maxillofac Surg. 2010;68(10):2484–8.
11. Dhillon J, Hoopes J, Epp T. Scoping decades of dog evidence: a scoping review of dog bite-related sequelae. Can J Public Health. 2019;110(3):364–75. https://doi.org/10.17269/s41997-018-0145-3.
12. Tu AH, Girotto JA, Singh N, Dufresne CR, Robertson BC, Seyfer AE, et al. Facial fractures from dog bite injuries. Plastic Reconstr Surg. 2002;109(4):1259–65.
13. https://jts.amedd.army.mil/assets/docs/cpgs/Burn_Care_11_May_2016_ID12.pdf
14. Orthopoulos G, Sideris A, Velmahos E, Troulis M. Gunshot wounds to the face: emergency interventions and outcomes. World J Surg. 2013;37(10):2348–2352.2.
15. Abramowicz S, Allareddy V, Rampa S, et al. Facial fractures in patients with firearm injuries: profile and outcomes. J Oral Maxillofac Surg. 2017;75:2170–6.
16. Tuckett JW, Lynham A, Lee GA, Perry M, Harrington U. Maxillofacial trauma in the emergency department: a review. Surgeon. 2014;12(2):106–14.
17. Barker DA, Oo KK, Allak A, Park SS. Timing for repair of mandible fractures. Laryngoscope. 2011;121:1160–3.
18. Biller JA, Pletcher SD, Goldberg AN, Murr AH. Complications and the time to repair of mandible fractures. Laryngoscope. 2005;115:769–72.
19. Sabatino F, Moskovitz JB. Facial wound management. Emerg Med Clin North Am. 2013;31(2):529–38.
20. Semer NB. Practical plastic surgery for non-surgeons. Philadelphia: Haley and Belfus; 2001. p. 145–59.

Further Reading

Doerr TD. Evidence-based facial fracture management. Facial Plastic Surg Clin. 2015;23(3):335–45.

Sabatino F, Moskovitz JB. Facial wound management. Emerg Med Clin North Am. 2013;31(2):529–38.

Semer NB. Practical plastic surgery for non-surgeons. Philadelphia: Haley and Belfus; 2001. p. 145–59.

Tuckett JW, Lynham A, Lee GA, Perry M, Harrington U. Maxillofacial trauma in the emergency department: a review. Surgeon. 2014 Apr;12(2):106–14.

Traumatic Neck Injuries

43

Rathnayaka M. Kalpanee D. Gunasingha
and Mark W. Bowyer

43.1 Introduction

> **Learning Goals**
> - Describe the types of injuries that blunt and penetrating neck trauma can cause.
> - Discuss the diagnosis of the different types of neck injury.
> - Review the surgical and non-surgical options for neck trauma.
> - Understand the treatment of blunt cerebrovascular injury (BCVI).

43.1.1 Epidemiology

The neck contains critical aerodigestive and neurovascular structures, and any trauma to the area has the capability to cause significant injury. A survey of the 2011 Nationwide Emergency Department Sample showed that 4.1% of all emergency department visits were primarily related to injury of the head and neck region [1]. The majority of patients involved were men (56.8%). Falls (38.9%) and blunt trauma (26.2%) were the most common mechanisms; penetrating trauma accounted for 2.9% of injuries [1]. Ninety-seven percent of the patients were treated and discharged, but 2.7% of the patients were admitted for further treatment and 0.1% died [1]. Mortality rates have been shown to be lower in blunt neck trauma (4.9%) versus penetrating trauma (6.0%) [2]. The 2016 National Trauma Data Bank showed that while neck injury was involved in 2.29% of incidents, serious injuries (AIS ≥3) of the neck had the highest case fatality rate (17.4) [3, 4]. Penetrating neck injuries have a mortality rate of 10%, with the most common immediate cause of death being from vascular injury, and the most common cause of delayed mortality was from unrecognized esophageal injury [5]. Overall, mortality from head and neck trauma is related to age, gunshot wound (GSW) as mechanism, higher ISS, and presence of shock at presentation [6].

43.1.2 Etiology

Neck injury can be the result of blunt trauma or penetrating trauma [5]. Blunt trauma can be due to motor vehicle collisions (MVC), falls, injuries during recreational activities (sports, horseback riding), strangulation, and near-hanging. Penetrating trauma can be due to a stabbing, blast injury, or from a GSW. The mechanism of the injury is important in considering what injuries might be present. In blunt trauma, there is a

R. M. K. D. Gunasingha · M. W. Bowyer (✉)
Department of Surgery, Uniformed Services University and the Walter Reed National Military Medical Center, Bethesda, MD, USA
e-mail: mark.bowyer@usuhs.edu

chance of delayed presentation to medical care. Symptoms, such as neck pain, may seem insignificant at the time of injury, but serious consequences, such as vocal fold paresis or aphonia, may be the end result [7].

43.1.3 Classification

43.1.3.1 Anatomy

It is important to understand the anatomic relationships within the neck to determine which structures could have been injured. Knowledge of the triangles of the neck (Fig. 43.1) and their contents (Fig. 43.2) is useful to help postulate possible injuries and the subsequent workup and treatment required. The anterior and lateral areas of the neck are most susceptible to injury. The anterior and posterior triangles of the neck are separated by the sternocleidomastoid. The posterior triangle is bordered by the sternocleidomastoid anteriorly, the trapezius posteriorly, and the clavicle inferiorly. The external jugular vein and the accessory nerve pass through this triangle. The cervical plexus and trunks of the brachial plexus cross the floor of the posterior

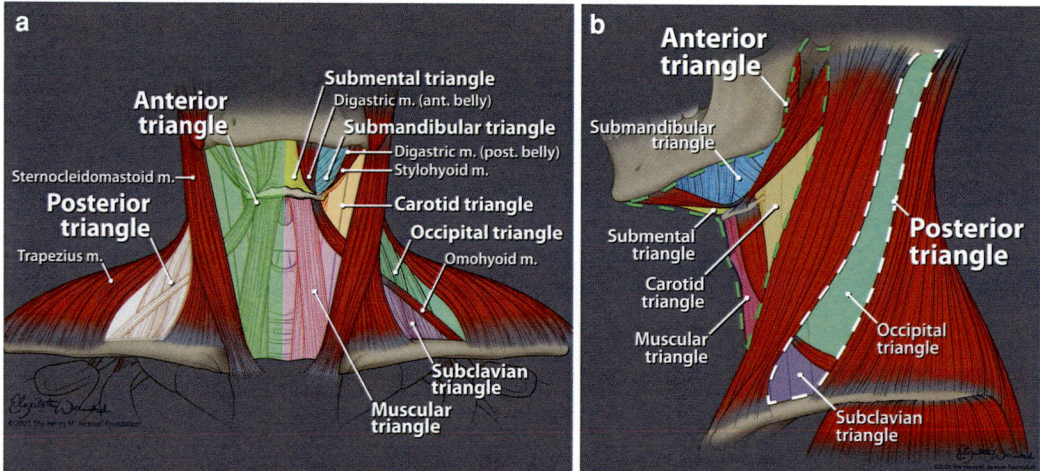

Fig. 43.1 (**a**) Anterior view of the anatomical triangles of the neck. (**b**) Lateral view of the anatomical triangles of the neck. Courtesy of the Henry M. Jackson Foundation for the Advancement of Military Medicine

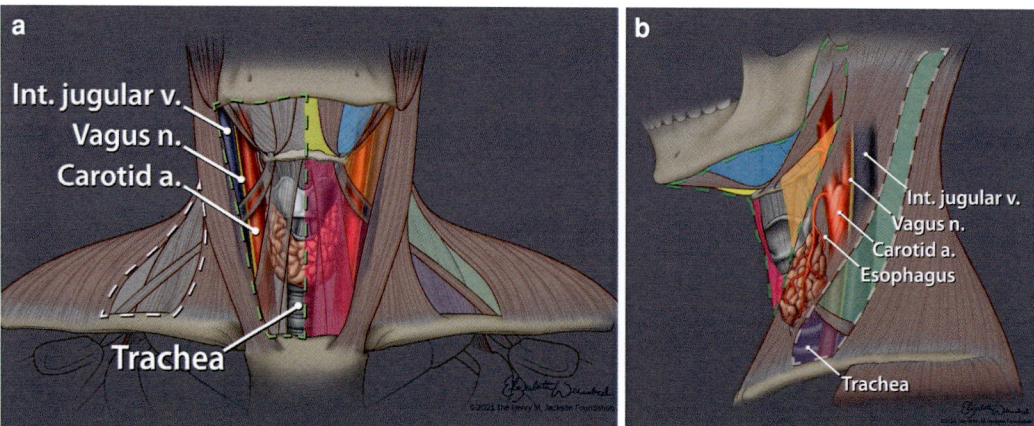

Fig. 43.2 (**a**) Anterior view of the neurovascular and aerodigestive structues of the neck. (**b**) Lateral view of the neurovascular and aerodigestive structues of the neck. Courtesy of the Henry M. Jackson Foundation for the Advancement of Military Medicine

triangle along with the distal part of the subclavian artery. While the posterior triangle has some important neurovascular components, the anterior triangle contains the most vital structures (Fig. 43.3). The anterior triangle of the neck is bordered by the midline of the neck medially, the mandible superiorly, and the anterior border of the sternocleidomastoid laterally. The common carotid artery (CA), vagus nerve, and internal jugular veins (IJV) run vertically in this area, and the facial artery and vein pass into the submandibular triangle. Important nerves include the hypoglossal and vagus nerves. The thyroid lies midline in the muscular triangle.

The neck can be further divided into three zones (Fig. 43.4), which can be helpful in determining the treatment and management of penetrating neck trauma [8]. Zone 1 is between the clavicles and the cricoid cartilage. This zone contains the great vessels, aortic arch, distal trachea, esophagus, lung apices, and cervical nerve roots. Zone 2 is from the cricoid cartilage to the angle of the mandible. The zone contains closely packed vital structures, such as carotids and vertebral arteries, IJV, trachea, and esophagus. Finally, Zone 3 is from the angle of the mandible to the skull base and is consequently difficult to reach surgically. It contains salivary glands, distal common carotid and internal carotid arteries, and cranial nerves.

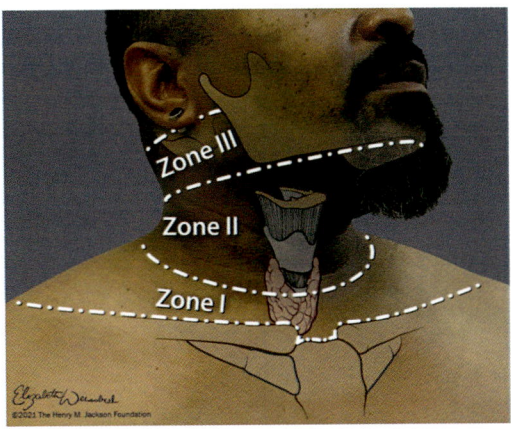

Fig. 43.4 Zones of the neck as seen obliquely. Zone 1 is between the clavicles and cricoid cartilage; Zone 2 is between the cricoid and the angle of the mandible; and Zone 3 is from the angle of the mandible to the skull base. Courtesy of the Henry M. Jackson Foundation for the Advancement of Military Medicine

43.1.4 Pathophysiology

Penetrating trauma is mainly caused by firearms and sharp objects that have crossed the platysma. Worldwide, stabbing is the most common mechanism, but in the United States, GSW are more common [9]. Stabbings cause injuries that are localized, and structures at risk are in the path of the weapon. However, it is difficult to determine the depth of the wound from the superficial appearance, and these wounds should not be probed or explored outside of an operating room [10]. Patients who are stabbed are less likely than those with GSWs to have cervical spine and CA injuries [11]. The damage caused by GSWs is related to the velocity of the projectile [12]. Vascular injuries in penetrating trauma can cause life-threatening hemorrhage in addition to thrombosis and are a major source of morbidity [5].

Blunt trauma is from a physical blow or a direct force to the neck, with MVC being the most common cause. Before seatbelts and other safety improvements in cars, in a crash, an unbelted driver would move forward with an extended anterior neck that was a target for the wheel, dashboard, or windshield [13]. With the introduction and widespread use of seatbelts, laryngotracheal injury due to MVC has decreased [13].

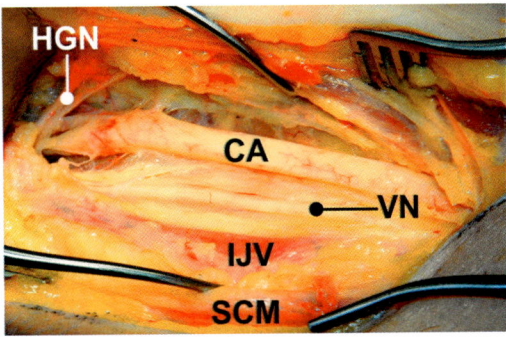

Fig. 43.3 Exposure of the contents of the anterior triangle of the right side of the neck. The head is to the left and the omohyoid muscle and facial vein have been divided to expose the vagus nerve (VN) between the common carotid artery and the internal jugular vein, with the sternocleidomastoid muscle seen retrated laterally and the hypoglossal nerve seen caudally

Injuries from sports and recreational activities, such as horseback riding, can also cause significant laryngotracheal injury [7, 14–16]. Near-hanging or strangulation is an infrequent cause of blunt neck trauma, but in addition to direct compression of the neck, injury to the cervical spine and spinal cord as well as cerebral hypoxia from vascular obstruction must be considered [5, 17]. In blunt trauma, vascular injuries are caused by shear forces. A patient who has excessive movement of the cervical spine or who meets the expanded Denver Criteria (Table 43.1) should be screened for BCVI, an infrequent, but high morbidity, injury [18–20].

43.2 Diagnosis

All patients should be evaluated in a standardized fashion with a thorough understanding of the history and mechanism of the trauma. The primary survey of airway, breathing, and circulation should be assessed rapidly. In injuries to the neck, all three of these are at risk. Temporizing measures and definitive treatment will be discussed in the treatment section.

43.2.1 Clinical Presentation (Symptoms + Physical Findings)

43.2.1.1 Laryngotracheal Injuries
Laryngotracheal injuries require a high degree of suspicion. Mainly caused by blunt trauma, patients may present with hoarseness, cough, and/or dyspnea [21]. Disruption in the airway above the glottis may cause cervical emphysema or progressive airway obstruction [21]. With severe disruption, patients may present with stridor, necessitating early, rapid intervention [5]. Bubbles in the soft tissue or continued air leak from a chest tube should also raise suspicion for airway injury[13].

43.2.1.2 Esophageal Injuries
Penetrating esophageal injuries can be occult with no obvious physical findings or symptoms. This delay of treating occult injuries leads to a high morbidity and mortality, usually from infections complications, such as mediastinitis [21–23]. When detected within 24 h, over 90% survive [21]. Odynophagia, drooling, and hematemesis could be seen with esophageal injury [24]. Dysphagia and crepitus after blunt trauma can indicate esophageal rupture [21].

43.2.1.3 Vascular Injuries
Hemorrhage causes 50% of the deaths from penetrating neck injuries [12, 21, 25]. The classic "Hard signs" of vascular injury indicate a high risk for vascular involvement [21]. These include bruit or thrill, expanding or pulsatile hematoma, pulsatile or severe hemorrhage, or pulse defect. Patients with hard signs should undergo operative exploration immediately. "Soft signs" of vascular injury in the neck include a history of significant hemorrhage, stable hematoma, or neurological defect. If the patient is not in extremis,

Table 43.1 Expanded Denver Health Medical Center Blunt Carotid Vascular Injury screening guidelines. Computed tomography angiography is indicated if one or more screening criteria are present. Adapted from Geddes, et al, 2016 [20] with permission

The expanded Denver health screening criteria for BCVI	
Risk factors for BCVI (*High-energy transfer mechanism with*):	Signs/symptoms of BCVI
Le Fort II or III Fracture	
Mandible Fracture	Arterial Hemorrhage from neck/nose/mouth
Complex skull fracture	Cervical bruit in patients <50 years
Severe traumatic brain injury (TBI) w GCS <6	Expanding cervical hematoma
Fracture or ligamentous injury of cervical spine	Focal neurological deficit: – TIA, hemiparesis
Near hanging with anoxic injury	– vertebrobasilar symptoms – Horners syndrome
Seat belt abrasion across neck	
TBI with thoracic injury	
Scalp degloving	Neurologic deficit inconsistent with CT
Thoracic vascular injury	Stroke on CT or MRI
Blunt cardiac rupture	
Upper rib fracture	

then the patient should undergo further diagnostic evaluation to determine if intervention is needed. Furthermore, imaging is important in diagnosing blunt vascular injury. One study found that 60% of patients with blunt cervical injury had injuries that were not suspected on initial evaluation [26]. One-fourth of these patients will develop signs of an ischemic stroke within the first 24 h [21]. The expanded Denver criteria are helpful in screening which patients should be screened for BCVI with computed tomography (CT)–angiography. While BCVI is rare, these expanded criteria (Table 43.1) have shown a significant increase in the identification of these injuries and, thus, initiation of early treatment [20].

43.2.1.4 Cervical Spine Injuries

There are three columns of the cervical spine, and to have an unstable fracture, two of them must be fractured. A stabbing is highly unlikely to cause an unstable fracture. A GSW that transverses the spine could cause an unstable fracture, but these patients nearly always present with neurological symptoms [21]. Blunt trauma causes most cervical spine trauma. These patients are likely to have on a cervical collar on presentation. If patients require endotracheal intubation, in-line cervical traction is safe with an assistant [21].

A CT of the neck should be done if there is any concern for cervical spine injury. If the patient's physical exam is abnormal, and the CT neck is normal, a neck magnetic resonance imaging (MRI) should be obtained [27]. Appropriate spine specialists should be consulted if there is a cervical spine fracture, ligamentous injury, or spinal cord injury [27]. If there are no abnormalities, the cervical collar can be safely removed [27].

43.2.2 Tests (Labs, Imaging)

It must by emphasized that any unstable patient should undergo surgical exploration. Neck injury and the presence of hemorrhagic shock, evolving stroke, expanding hematoma, or unstable airway should mandate transfer of the patient to the operating room without further imaging, other than a quick chest X-ray, and primary trauma work-up.

In the absence of surgical emergency, patients should be evaluated with standard labs, imaging, and diagnostic evaluation. Standard trauma labs, such as complete blood count, basic metabolic panel, and type and cross for blood, should be drawn as soon as possible. If the patient is hemodynamically stable, the next step should be imaging if there is violation of the platysma muscle or other suspicion of injury.

Multi-detector CT (MDCT), 16-channel or higher, is the imaging study of choice. Free air in the neck is suggestive for a laryngotracheal or esophageal injury [21, 28]. If imaging is normal, but there is still a high degree of suspicion for a laryngotracheal or an esophageal injury, bronchoscopy and endoscopy should be completed in the operating room in the event that injury requiring operative intervention is found. Cervical spine fractures can also be assessed. When MDCT is done with intravenous contrast, sensitivity of identifying a vascular injury is around 90% [21, 29]. A 4-vessel cerebral angiogram is the gold standard, but due to its invasiveness and the high degree of accuracy with MDCT, an angiogram should be done only if high suspicion for vascular injury remains.

43.3 Treatment

Management of neck injuries will be mainly dependent on the zone of injury as described previously. A hemodynamically unstable patient with a penetrating injury to the neck, violating the platysma, warrants surgical exploration. The airway must be secured and adequate ventilation assured prior to further evaluation, as up to 10% of patients with penetrating neck injury can have airway compromise [5]. Early endotracheal intubation is recommended, if possible [21]. If unable to quickly and easily intubate, providers should proceed to advanced airway techniques or a cricothyrotomy. Hemorrhage through a penetrating neck wound can be temporized with digital compression or a Foley catheter balloon (Fig. 43.5) until definitive control is achieved in the operating room [30].

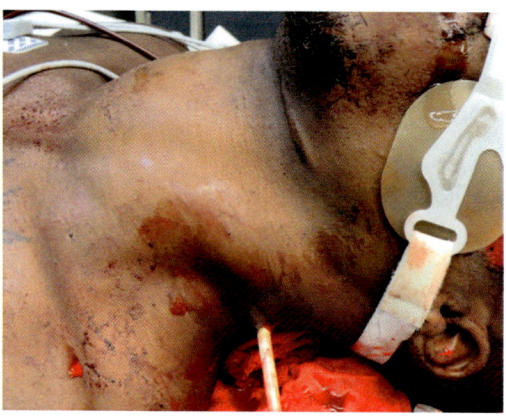

Fig. 43.5 Temporary control of exsanguinating hemorrhage from a gunshot wound to the posterior triangle of the left neck with a Foley catheter balloon

43.3.1 Medical Treatment (Interventional Radiology Included)

Patients with normal imaging and low suspicion for occult injury after a thorough physical exam can be discharged with as necessary follow-up. If there is suspicion for occult injury, the patient should be monitored for changes for at least 24 h [8]. Non-operative management in penetrating neck injuries has increased over the years, and if patients are appropriately selected, there is no effect on mortality [10, 11]. Additional studies, such as a gastrograffin or thin barium swallow study, can help identify small esophageal injuries. Laryngoscopy can aid in identifying injuries to the larynx. If the patient has only minor airway symptoms and a minor hematoma, observation with humidified oxygen with voice rest with possible steroids and/or antibiotics is sufficient for initial management [13, 21]. With more edema, a larger hematoma, minor mucosal disruption without exposed cartilage, or non-displaced fractures, patients will require serial examinations, as these injuries can worsen with time [13, 21, 31, 32].

If endovascular expertise is available, Zone 1 or Zone 3 vascular injuries may be amenable to endovascular treatment. Covered stents have been successfully used in Zone 1 injuries [8]. Zone 3 vascular injuries are difficult to reach operatively. Endovascular techniques should be tried initially, with coiling or embolization of a vessel (Fig. 43.6) if it can be sacrificed or a covered stent if patency is needed [33]. Vertebral artery injuries are relatively uncommon, but present challenges to access. Embolization of the proximal vertebral artery is the treatment of choice [34]. If unsuccessful, the vertebral artery should be ligated at its origin at the subclavian and the foramen closed with bone wax [10, 34].

BCVI is primarily managed with antiplatelet and anticoagulation medications. Figure 43.7 shows an algorithmic approach to a commonsense approach to manage the different grades of BCVI (as defined in the figure caption). Endovascular treatment should be attempted on grade V injuries that are surgically inaccessible [35]. Up to 80% of BCVIs will resolve with or without anticoagulation, but grade III and IV injuries are unlikely to resolve and require close follow-up with possible intervention [19, 35].

43.3.2 Surgical Treatment (Open and MIS Techniques)

43.3.2.1 Laryngotracheal Injuries

It is important to consult and expert in otolaryngology early in order to achieve the best outcomes in laryngeal injuries [32, 36]. The main goals include securing the airway and reconstructing the larynx, with restoration of voice and swallowing being long-term goals [31]. Fracture of the hyoid bone can be treated conservatively with pain management and voice rest. Stents can be placed to prevent adhesions from extensive mucosal trauma and to prevent stenosis [13, 31]. Non-displaced fractures of the thyroid cartilage and the cricoid cartilage should be treated with supportive measurements, such as voice rest and anti-reflux medications. Displaced fractures of the thyroid require open reduction and fixation with a mini-plate and displaced fractures of the cricoid need wire fixation and stent placement [13, 31].

Patients with tracheal transection rarely survive to make it to the hospital [13]. For those tracheal injuries that do, obtaining an airway

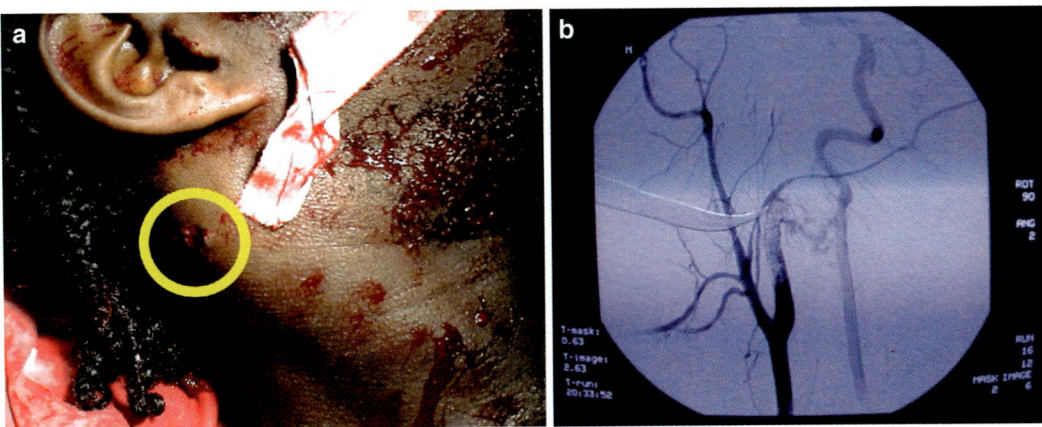

Fig. 43.6 (a) A gunshot wound to zone 3 of the right neck. (b) Management of zone 3 injury with endovascular coiling

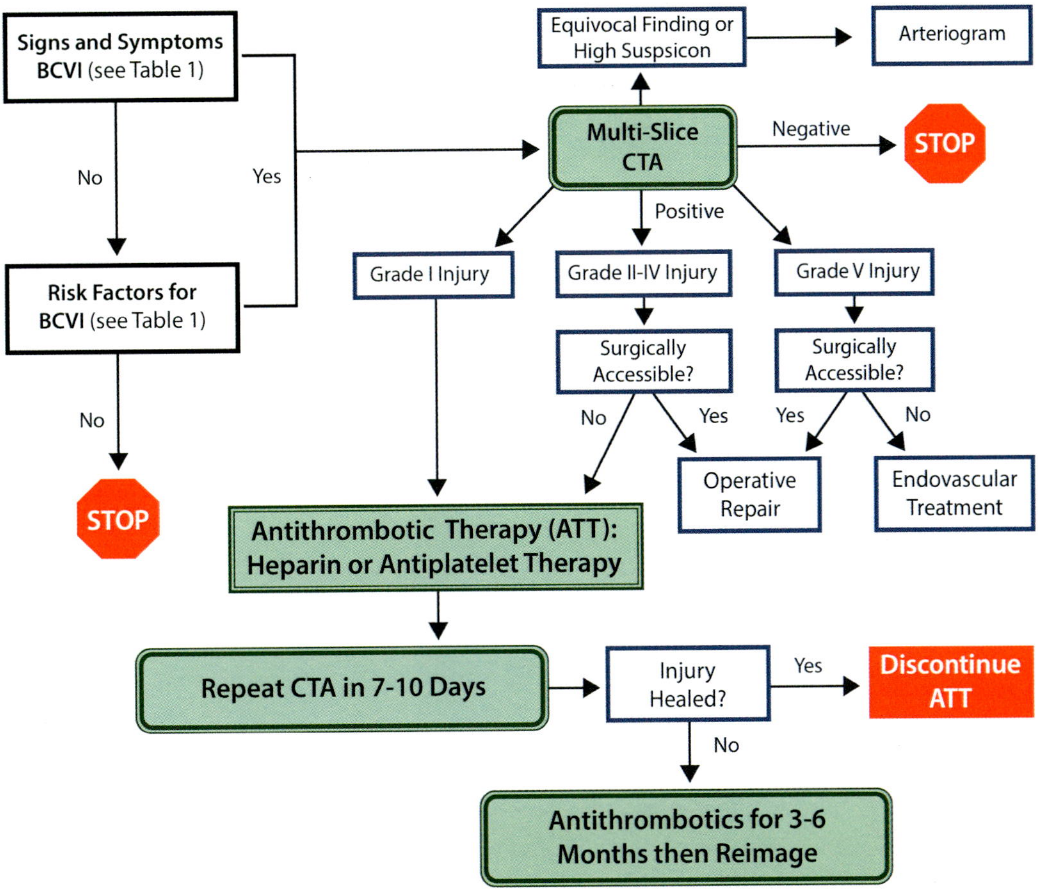

Fig. 43.7 Algorithmic approach to the diagnosis and management of blunt carotid vascular injury. CT angiogram should be done with at least a 64 channel multidetector row machine. Grade I injury = luminal irregularity or dissection with <25% luminal narrowing; Grade II = dissection, or intramural hematoma with >25% luminal narrowing; Grade III = pseudoaneurysm; Grade IV = occlusion; and Grade V = transection with free extravasation. Adapted from Geddes, et al. with permission [20]

distal to the injury is of primary importance. A collar incision is best for cervical tracheal injuries (Zone 2), and an extension into an upper median sternotomy will give better exposure for the proximal intrathoracic tracheal injuries (Zone 1) [13]. A right posterolateral thoracotomy will allow better exposure for the distal intrathoracic trachea and the posterior membranous aspect of the trachea [13, 16]. The tracheal edges should be debrided to healthy tissue and then repaired in an interrupted, end-to-end fashion with absorbable suture, taking care to avoid the blood supply on the lateral aspects [13, 37]. The repair should be buttressed with a healthy muscle pedicle flap.

43.3.2.2 Esophageal Injuries

Esophageal injuries in the neck should be primarily repaired unless the patient is in extremis, disruption is greater than 50% of the circumference, or there is a plan for delayed surgical exploration. In these cases, wide drainage or a cervical esophagostomy should be used. A left-sided incision along the anterior border of the sternocleidomastoid or a collar incision provides good exposure to the cervical esophagus [38, 39]. Once the esophagus is isolated and the injury notes, the tissue should be debrided until the edges are healthy and closed in a single or double layer fashion with absorbable sutures [38]. A feeding tube should be passed under visualization at this time to prevent any disruption of the repair [39]. Muscle flaps from the sternocleidomastoid, strap, or omohyoid can be used to buttress the closure and a drain placed in the area prior to skin closure can help with easy and early identification of a leak [38]. Drains can be removed 5–7 days post-operatively.

43.3.2.3 Vascular Injuries

Surgical management of vascular injuries differs based on the zone of injury. Zone 1 injuries present risk to the great vessels. Subsequent repair may necessitate cardiothoracic surgery. The best approach is through a median sternotomy or anterolateral thoracotomy. If more proximal control is necessary, the incision can be extended along the anterior sternocleidomastoid or clavicle. As mentioned previously, endovascular techniques have been shown to be successful in repairing Zone 1 injuries. Zone 2 injuries can be easily accessed through an anterior sternocleidomastoid incision (Fig. 43.3). Jugular veins can be ligated without much consequence, whereas every attempt should be made to repair CA, since outcomes better compared with ligation [25, 40]. Either an interrupted, transverse arteriorrhaphy, or continuous vein or polytetrafluoroethylene (PTFE) patch angioplasty with polypropylene suture can be used for the repair [25]. Less commonly, interposition vein or PTFE grafts may be needed to bridge a large segmental defect [40]. Zone 3 injuries are difficult to access surgically, so endovascular approaches are primarily used as discussed above. However, in the instance of continuous hemorrhage, a Fogarty balloon can be passed from a cut down on the common carotid distally into the internal carotid or blindly (if hemorrhage is rapid) and inflated to cease the hemorrhage [40]. If this measure fails, multiple anterior and posterior operative approaches have been described [40].

43.3.3 Prognosis

While neck trauma is relatively uncommon, it carries one of the highest mortalities. Zone 1 injuries carry the highest risk of death, while Zone 2 injuries have the best prognosis [5]. Complications for these patients after surgery are also important to take into consideration. In patients with laryngotracheal injuries, follow-up is necessary until resolution of normal voice [32]. These patients may have long-term morbidities, such as issues with swallowing that could put them at risk for aspiration and infections. Those that survive near-hangings or suffocation attempts may die from other pulmonary or hypoxic complications. Vascular injuries present short-term and long-term complications. In the short term, blunt or penetrating injuries to the carotid or vertebral vessels may cause an ischemic stroke. The rate of stroke can be decreased up to 75% with antiplatelet or anticoagulation therapy in BCVI [21]. In the long term, these same vessels may develop stenosis and put the patient at risk of stroke. Fistula tracts can form between areas of injury and repair. Therefore, patients should have regular follow-up with someone aware of their injury history.

> **Dos and Don'ts**
> - Do—complete a primary and secondary assessment on a patient with neck trauma.
> - Do—identify the potential injured structures within the neck using diagnostic imaging or endoscopic procedures in a stable patient.
> - Do—consider BCVI in patients with excessive extension of the cervical spine or who meet the expanded Denver criteria.
> - Don't—go to surgical exploration immediately for all Zone 2 injuries.
> - Don't—forget that long-term complications may need future interventions.

> **Take-Home Messages**
> - Neck trauma can cause severe morbidity and has high mortality.
> - A systematic approach guided by anatomical considerations should be used in the evaluation of any patient with neck trauma.
> - Unstable patients with neck injury should be taken emergently to the operating room
> - Diagnostic imaging and/or endoscopic procedures can aid in identifying injured structures.
> - Injuries found on work-up should guide surgical versus non-surgical approach.

Questions

1. A 34-year-old man presents to the trauma bay with a gunshot wound above the clavicles and below the cricoid cartilage. He is hypotensive and tachycardic. What intervention should take place?
   A. **A median sternotomy with as needed neck or clavicular extension and repair**
   B. Endovascular embolization
   C. Diagnostic imaging work-up
   D. An incision along the border of the anterior sternocleidomastoid and repair

   A is the correct answer. This injury is in Zone 1 with the greatest risk of injury to the great vessels. A median sternotomy is the correct approach with as needed extensions for vascular control or other injuries. Diagnostic imaging would be inappropriate in an unstable patient. Endovascular embolization is more appropriate for Zone 3 injuries and an anterior sternocleidomastoid incision is the best approach for a Zone 2 injury.

2. A 25-year-old man presents with a Zone 2 stab wound that appears to have violated the platysma. He is able to speak, breathing without difficulty, and normotensive. He does acknowledge hoarseness. What is the next step in his evaluation?
   A. Operative exploration
   B. Endoscopy
   C. **Multi-detector CT scan with intravenous contrast**
   D. Observation

   C is the correct answer. This patient is stable and can undergo an imaging work-up prior to more invasive endoscopic procedures. Operative exploration is not the next step since he is stable; if an injury is found on imaging, the patient can proceed to the operating room. Since the patient has platysmal violation and hoarseness, he should not be simply observed.

3. A 50-year-old woman is in a high-speed motor vehicle accident. She is found to have a bruising from her seat belt across her neck, and she has a mandibular fracture. CT with intravenous contrast reveals a grade 1 blunt cerebrovascular injury of the left carotid that is not surgically accessible. What is the next step?
   A. Endovascular treatment
   B. Endovascular embolization
   C. Operative ligation
   D. **Start antiplatelet therapy**

   D is the correct answer. This patient has a grade 1 BCVI of the left carotid. Grade 1 injuries usually resolve without intervention. Antiplatelet therapy with reimaging is the therapy of choice. Endovascular or operative treatment is premature. Ligation should be avoided for carotid injuries; this would greatly increase the risk of stroke.

4. A 43-year-old woman presents with a knife wound to the back of her neck. The wound is along the posterior border of her sternocleidomastoid. Which nerve is at risk of being injured?
   A. Vagus nerve
   B. **Accessory nerve**
   C. Facial nerve
   D. Hypoglossal nerve

   B is the correct answer. The accessory nerve in the major nerve in the posterior triangle, whose border starts at the posterior border of the sternocleidomastoid. The vagus, facial, and hypoglossal nerve are not in the posterior triangle.

5. A 16-year-old girl is brought in after a near-hanging. She had a GCS of 6 at the scene and is currently being masked. She has a cervical collar in place. During the primary assessment, which of the following interventions should take place first?
   A. Operative intervention for laryngeal trauma
   B. Cricothyroidotomy
   C. **Endotracheal intubation**
   D. CT imaging

   C is the correct answer. This patient has a GCS below 8 and does not have a secure airway. While this patient has a high risk of having a cervical spine injury, she needs to have her airway secured during the primary assessment. Patients with cervical spine injury can be intubated with in-line stabilization with an assistant and minimal movement. CT imaging and operative intervention are inappropriate at this stage. The patient does not need a cricothyroidotomy at this time.

6. A 15-year-old boy is brought in to the emergency room with 2 days of hoarseness. He states that he was hit in the neck during a hockey game. He denies trouble breathing or swallowing. He has tenderness in his neck anteriorly. In addition to consulting the specialists, what is the next best step?
   A. **CT scan**
   B. Nasolarynoscopy
   C. Observation
   D. Discharge

   A is the correct answer. Hoarseness after a neck injury is concerning for a laryngotracheal injury. Observation and discharge right away would be inappropriate. CT scan would be the first step to injury any injuries in the neck. It can be followed by nasolarynoscopy, which is invasive.

7. A 40-year-old man presents with a stab wound from a hunting knife. He is hypotensive and tachycaridic. His airway is secured, and after appropriate evaluation, the patient is taken to the operating room. Which vessel is in the posterior triangle of the neck?

A. **Subclavian artery**
B. Vertebral artery
C. Internal jugular vein
D. Carotid artery

A is the correct answer. The distal subclavian artery lies deep in the posterior triangle of the neck. Penetrating injury can cause damage to this vessel and subsequent hemorrhage. The vertebral artery, internal jugular vein, and carotid artery are not in the posterior triangle of the neck.

8. A 39-year-old patient presents to the emergency room with a gunshot wound to the neck. He is stable and undergoes imaging. He is noted to have no vascular injuries or aerodigestive injuries on the CT scan. An esophageal injury is still suspected this patient. What additional imaging study can be used to diagnosis an esophageal injury?
   A. **Gastrograffin swallow study**
   B. Thin barium swallow study
   C. CT scan with oral contrast
   D. MRI

   A is the correct answer. A CT scan can quickly identify vascular and aerodigestive injuries. However, some occult esophageal injuries might not be detected. MRI is incorrect and is too time intensive. Given the high morbidity and mortality from esophageal injuries, it is important to identify and fix them early. Gastrograffin, a water soluble contrast, can be used during a dynamic swallow study to identify any leaks. If it is negative, a thin barium swallow can then be done.

9. A 20-year-old woman presents with a gunshot wound after a domestic abuse incident. The wound is located above the angle of the mandible. There is concern for a carotid injury. What should the next step be?
   A. Open operative repair of carotid
   B. **Endovascular repair of carotid**
   C. Open ligation of carotid
   D. Antiplatelet agent

   B is the correct answer. This injury is in Zone 3 and should be dealt with using endovascular methods. Open approaches are difficult in Zone 3. There is no indication to give this patient an antiplatelet agent; that would be appropriate in a patient with certain types of BCVI.

10. A patient who sustained severe blunt neck trauma after a motor vehicle accident is discharged from the hospital. In addition to other injuries, the patient sustained a laryngotracheal injury and continues to have trouble swallowing and continues to have a hoarseness at discharge. What is important for long-term outcomes after the patient's laryngotracheal injury?
    A. Speech therapy
    B. Occupational therapy
    C. Follow-up with primary care physician
    D. **Follow-up till resolution of hoarseness**

    D is the correct answer. After laryngotracheal injury, it is important to ensure long-term follow. The patient may need future procedures to deal with complications of the injury. Speech therapy, occupational therapy, and regular primary care physician follow-up are critical for the patient's overall recovery from the trauma.

Acknowledgements The authors wish to thank Ms. Elizabeth N. Weissbrod, MA, CMI for her excellent illustrations created for this chapter.

Disclaimer: The contents of this presentation are the sole responsibility of the author(s) and do not necessarily reflect the views, opinions, or policies of Uniformed Services University of the Health Sciences, the Department of Defense, or the Departments of the Army, Navy, or Air Force. Mention of trade names, commercial products, or organizations does not imply endorsement by the U.S. Government. None of the authors have additional disclosures or conflicts of interest.

References

1. Sethi RKV, Kozin ED, Fagenholz PJ, Lee DJ, Shrime MG, Gray ST. Epidemiological survey of head and neck injuries and trauma in the United States. Otolaryngol Head Neck Surg (United States). 2014;151:776–84.
2. Forner D, Noel CW, Guttman MP, Haas B, Enepekides D, Rigby MH, et al. Blunt versus penetrating neck trauma: a retrospective cohort study. Laryngoscope. 2021;131:E1109–16.
3. Blitzer DN, Ottochian M, O'Connor J, Feliciano DV, Morrison JJ, DuBose JJ, Scalea TM. Penetrating injury to the carotid artery: characterizing presentation and outcomes from the national trauma data bank. Ann Vasc Surg. 2020;67:192–9.
4. University of Alabama CIREN Center. Ranking the AIS body regions in regards to contribution to MVC-related mortality: A comparison of NASS and NTDB data. 2014 presentation to National Highwat Traffic Safety Administration. Accessed at https://www.nhtsa.gov/sites/nhtsa.gov/files/documents/uab_ciren_presentation_083114.pdf
5. Colwell C. Neck trauma. In: Koyfman A, Long B, editors. The emergency medicine trauma handbook. Cambridge: Cambridge University Press; 2019. p. 164–74.
6. Jesin M, Rashewsky S, Shapiro M, Tobler W, Agarwal S, Burke P, et al. Predictors of mortality, hospital utilization, and the role of race in outcomes in head and neck trauma. Oral Surg Oral Med Oral Pathol Oral Radiol. 2016;121:12–6.
7. Mendis D, Anderson JA. Blunt laryngeal trauma secondary to sporting injuries. J Laryngol Otol. 2017;131:728–35.
8. Sperry JL, Moore EE, Coimbra R, Croce M, Davis JW, Karmy-Jones R, et al. Western trauma association critical decisions in trauma: penetrating neck trauma. J Trauma Acute Care Surg. 2013;75:936–40.
9. Abdullahi H, Adamu A, Hasheem MG. Penetrating arrow injuries of the head-and-neck region: case series and review of literature. Niger Med J. 2020;61(5):276–80.
10. Kendall JL, Anglin D, Demetriades D. Penetrating neck trauma. Emerg Med Clin North Am. 1998;16:85–105.
11. Tatum JMMD, Barmparas GMD, Dhillon NKMD, Edu SMD, Margulies DRMD, Ley EJMD, Nicol AJMBCB, PhD NPH, MBChB. Penetrating pharyngoesophageal injury: practice patterns in the era of nonoperative management—a national trauma data bank review from 2007 to 2011. J Invest Surg. 2020;33(10):896–903.
12. Mahmoodie M, Sanei B, Moazeni-Bistgani M, Namgar M. Penetrating neck trauma: review of 192 cases. Arch Trauma Res. 2012;1:14–8.
13. Moonsamy P, Sachdeva UM, Morse CR. Management of laryngotracheal trauma. Ann Cardiothorac Surg. 2018;7:210–6.
14. Trofa DP, Park CN, Noticewala MS, Lynch TS, Ahmad CS, Popkin CA. The impact of body checking on youth ice hockey injuries. Orthop J Sports Med. 2017;5(12):2325967117741647.
15. Mutore K, Lim J, Fofana D, Torres-Reveron A, Skubic, J. Hear hoofbeats? Think head and neck trauma: a 10-year NTDB review of equestrian related trauma in the United States. MEDI 9331 Scholarly Activities Clinical Years. Vol. 9; 2020. https://scholarworks.utrgv.edu/som9331/9
16. Prokakis C, Koletsis EN, Dedeilias P, Fligou F, Filos K, Dougenis D. Airway trauma: a review on epidemiology, mechanisms of injury, diagnosis and treatment. J Cardiothorac Surg. 2014;9:117.
17. Schellenberg M, Inaba K, Warriner Z, Alfson D, Roman J, Van Velsen V, Lam L, Demetriades D. Near hangings: epidemiology, injuries, and investigations. J Trauma Acute Care Surg. 2019;86(3):454–7.
18. Cook A, Osler T, Gaudet M, Berne J, Norwood S. Blunt cerebrovascular injury is poorly predicted by modeling with other injuries: analysis of NTDB data. J Trauma. 2011;71(1):114–9.
19. George E, Khandelwal A, Potter C, Sodickson A, Mukundan S, Nunez D, Khurana B. Blunt traumatic vascular injuries of the head and neck in the ED. Emerg Radiol. 2019;26(1):75–85.
20. Geddes AE, Burlew CC, Wagenaar AE, Biffl WL, Johnson JL, Pieracci FM, Campion EM, Moore EE. Expanded screening criteria for blunt cerebrovascular injury: a bigger impact than anticipated. Am J Surg. 2016;212(6):1167–74.
21. Rathlev NK, Medzon R, Bracken ME. Evaluation and management of neck trauma. Emerg Med Clin North Am. 2007;25(3):679–94.
22. Demetriades D, Theodorou D, Cornwell E, Berne TV, Asensio J, Belzberg H, Velmahos G, Weaver F, Yellin A. Evaluation of penetrating injuries of the neck: prospective study of 223 patients. World J Surg. 1997;21(1):41–7; discussion 47-8.
23. Asensio JA, Berne J, Demetriades D, Murray J, Gomez H, Falabella A, Fox A, Velmahos G, Shoemaker W, Berne TV. Penetrating esophageal injuries: time interval of safety for preoperative evaluation—how long is safe? J Trauma. 1997;43(2):319–24.
24. Chagnon FP, Mulder DS. Laryngotracheal trauma. Chest Surg Clin N Am. 1996;6(4):733–48.
25. Nowicki JL, Stew B, Ooi E. Penetrating neck injuries: a guide to evaluation and management. Ann R Coll Surg Engl. 2018;100(1):6–11.
26. McKevitt EC, Kirkpatrick AW, Vertesi L, Granger R, Simons RK. Blunt vascular neck injuries: diagnosis and outcomes of extracranial vessel injury. J Trauma. 2002;53(3):472–6.
27. Ciesla DJ, Shatz DV, Moore EE, Sava J, Martin MJ, Brown CVR, Alam HB, Vercruysse GA, Brasel KJ, Inaba K, Western Trauma Association Critical Decisions in Trauma Committee. Western Trauma Association critical decisions in trauma: cervical spine clearance in trauma patients. J Trauma Acute Care Surg. 2020;88(2):352–4.

28. Shi J, Uyeda JW, Duran-Mendicuti A, Potter CA, Nunez DB. Multidetector CT of laryngeal injuries: principles of injury recognition. Radiographics. 2019;39(3):879–92.
29. Sliker CW. Blunt cerebrovascular injuries: imaging with multidetector CT angiography. Radiographics. 2008;28(6):1689–708; discussion 1709-10.
30. Navsaria P, Thoma M, Nicol A. Foley catheter balloon tamponade for life-threatening hemorrhage in penetrating neck trauma. World J Surg. 2006;30(7):1265–8.
31. Wasif M, Dhanani R, Ghaloo SK, Awan MS, Danish MH, Hussain HM, Pasha HA. Management of laryngotracheal trauma: a review of current trends and future directions. J Pak Med Assoc. 2020;70(Suppl 1):S60–4.
32. Parida PK, Kalaiarasi R, Alexander A. Management of laryngotracheal trauma: a five-year single institution experience. Iran J Otorhinolaryngol. 2018 Sep;30(100):283–90.
33. DuBose J, Recinos G, Teixeira PG, Inaba K, Demetriades D. Endovascular stenting for the treatment of traumatic internal carotid injuries: expanding experience. J Trauma. 2008;65(6):1561–6.
34. Roberts LH, Demetriades D. Vertebral artery injuries. Surg Clin North Am. 2001;81(6):1345–56.
35. Kim DY, Biffl W, Bokhari F, Brakenridge S, Chao E, Claridge JA, Fraser D, Jawa R, Kasotakis G, Kerwin A, Khan U, Kurek S, Plurad D, Robinson BRH, Stassen N, Tesoriero R, Yorkgitis B, Como JJ. Evaluation and management of blunt cerebrovascular injury: a practice management guideline from the Eastern Association for the Surgery of Trauma. J Trauma Acute Care Surg. 2020;88(6):875–87.
36. Mendelsohn AH, Sidell DR, Berke GS, John MS. Optimal timing of surgical intervention following adult laryngeal trauma. Laryngoscope. 2011;121(10):2122–7.
37. Kelly JP, Webb WR, Moulder PV, Moustouakas NM, Lirtzman M. Management of airway trauma. II: Combined injuries of the trachea and esophagus. Ann Thorac Surg. 1987;43(2):160–3.
38. Sudarshan M, Cassivi SD. Management of traumatic esophageal injuries. J Thorac Dis. 2019;11(Suppl 2):S172–6.
39. Chirica M, Kelly MD, Siboni S, Aiolfi A, Riva CG, Asti E, et al. Esophageal emergencies: WSES guidelines. World J Emerg Surg. 2019;14:26.
40. Feliciano DV. Management of penetrating injuries to carotid artery. World J Surg. 2001;25(8):1028–35.

Further Reading

Alao T, Waseem M. Neck Trauma. 2021 Feb 10. In: StatPearls [Internet]. Treasure Island, FL: StatPearls Publishing; 2021 Jan.

Bromberg WJ, Collier BC, Diebel LN, Dwyer KM, Holevar MR, Jacobs DG, Kurek SJ, Schreiber MA, Shapiro ML, Vogel TR. Blunt cerebrovascular injury practice management guidelines: the Eastern Association for the Surgery of Trauma. J Trauma. 2010;68(2):471–7.

Chandrananth ML, Zhang A, Voutier CR, Skandarajah A, Thomson BNJ, Shakerian R, Read DJ. 'No zone' approach to the management of stable penetrating neck injuries: a systematic review. ANZ J Surg. 2021;91:1083–90.

Farley LS, Schlicksup KE. Tracheal Injury. 2020 Aug 10. In: StatPearls [Internet]. Treasure Island, FL: StatPearls Publishing; 2021 Jan.

Nowicki JL, Stew B, Ooi E. Penetrating neck injuries: a guide to evaluation and management. Ann R Coll Surg Engl. 2018;100(1):6–11.

Santiago-Rosado LM, Sigmon DF, Lewison CS. Tracheal trauma. 2020 Jul 10. In: StatPearls [Internet]. Treasure Island, FL: StatPearls Publishing; 2021 Jan.

Sperry JL, Moore EE, Coimbra R, Croce M, Davis JW, Karmy-Jones R, McIntyre RC Jr, Moore FA, Malhotra A, Shatz DV, Biffl WL. Western Trauma Association critical decisions in trauma: penetrating neck trauma. J Trauma Acute Care Surg. 2013;75(6):936–40.

Management of Neck Surgery Complications

44

Giovanna Di Meo, Alessandro Pasculli, and Mario Testini

Abbreviations

BRLNP	Bilateral recurrent laryngeal nerve palsy
CL	Chyle leak
CT	Computed tomography
IONM	Intraoperative nerve monitoring
MMN	Marginal mandibular nerve
ND	Neck dissection
PG	Parathyroid gland
PH	Postoperative haematoma
PNX	Pneumothorax
RLN	Recurrent laryngeal nerve
RLNP	Recurrent laryngeal nerve palsy
SAN	Spinal accessory nerve
URLNP	Unilateral recurrent laryngeal nerve palsy
VF	Vocal fold

> **Learning Goals**
> - Providing a comprehensive knowledge of the neck surgery sequelae, with the description of epidemiology, etiology, pathophysiology and clinical features of each complication.
> - Giving the basis of the diagnostic intra-operative and post-operative assessment, describing the risks to avoid, the alarming symptoms and signs and guiding the clinical decisions in the lab tests and imaging.
> - Depicting the treatment approaches, which can be intraoperative and post-operative, medical and surgical.

44.1 Introduction

44.1.1 Epidemiology

Neck surgery complications may widely vary from immediately life-threatening scenario that could be solved with proper treatment, often without sequelae, to rather minor complications that promptly manifest themselves and affect the patient's quality of life.

Though the morbidity of each complication is relatively rare (e.g., permanent recurrent nerve

G. Di Meo · A. Pasculli · M. Testini (✉)
Department of Precision and Regenerative Medicine and Ionian Area, Unit of Academic General Surgery "V. Bonomo", University of Bari, Polyclinic Hospital, Bari, Italy
e-mail: mario.testini@uniba.it

injury), in reviewing the total incidence of neck surgery complications as a whole, we record a significant rise. Moreover, the rarity of each complication is closely related to the surgical volume and experience.

44.1.2 Classification

- Inferior laryngeal nerve injury
- Spinal accessory nerve injury
- Marginal mandibular branch of the facial nerve injury
- Phrenic and vagus nerve injuries
- Hypoparathyroidism
- Chyle leak
- Postoperative haematoma
- Major vessels injury
- Tracheomalacia
- Pneumothorax
- Laryngotracheal complex injuries
- Cervical oesophagus injuries
- Seroma and wound infection

44.2 Inferior Laryngeal Nerve Injury

44.2.1 Epidemiology

The incidence of inferior or recurrent laryngeal nerve (RLN) palsy (RLNP) varies from 0% to 4% and has been related to the extent of thyroidectomy, the presence of Graves' disease, thyroid carcinoma and the need for reoperation [1]. Most cases of RLNP are transient, while less than 1% of cases are permanent. Bilateral RLNP (BRLNP) may also occur to a much rarer extent as one out of 1000 cases in specialized thyroid units [2]. RLNP, bearing the most serious consequences in thyroid surgery, is accordingly the most common cause of medical malpractice [3].

44.2.2 Etiology

Vocal fold (VF) paralysis is reported preoperatively in 2–4% of cases. Since clinical assessment of voice quality does not correlate with its objective evaluation, preoperative laryngoscopy is always recommended for all patients before thyroid surgery [4, 5].

Causes of intraoperative recurrent laryngeal nerve (RLN) injury include section (mistaken surgical technique), ligature without transection, mistake during hemostasis and dissection manoeuvres, stretch/traction during thyroid lobe medialization, excessive aspiration near the RLN, compression, contusion and pressure damage, thermal or electrical injury by hemostatic devices, and ischemic damage due to an excessive RLN dissection. Indeed, extensive resections, thyroid malignancy, paratracheal lymph node dissection, substernal goitre and recurrent goitre have been identified as significant independent risk factors for RLNP [6].

Non-surgical causes of RLN damage are difficult tracheal intubation, neuritis caused by scar tissue, viral neuritis, neuromuscular diseases, cerebrovascular accidents, and diabetic RLN neuropathy.

44.2.3 Pathophysiology

Routinely nerve injury is classified into three types according to Sunderland's classification. Neuropraxia is a simple contusion of a nerve with temporary block of axonal transmission, without anatomical modifications of perineurium, endoneurium or axons. It is the most common lesion and is associated with a return to normal function over weeks to months. Axonotmesis is the second type of injury, and it is characterized by a significant anatomical disruption/interruption of the axon followed by regeneration that takes a prolonged time. Neurotmesis is the last type of lesion caused by a complete anatomical disruption of the nerve with no chance of spontaneous repair as it requires surgical correction [7, 8].

Intraoperative routine visual identification and exposure of RLN is the gold standard for RLN management, reducing significantly RLNP rates. However, anatomical RLN lesions are only exceptional reasons for post-operative VF palsy, and intraoperative nerve monitoring (IONM) gives the surgeon additional protection for the RLN integrity. IONM aids early and definite localization of RLN to prevent visual misidentification, avoid excessive traction, identify extralaryngeal branches, anatomical variation, distored RLN, and, furthermore, contribute to the confirmation and dissection of RLN [1, 4].

44.2.4 Diagnosis

44.2.4.1 Clinical Presentation

The event causes impairment in one-to-three situations: the voice, the swallowing or the ventilation.

Unilateral RLNP (URLNP) causes insufficient laryngeal closure during swallowing, cough and phonation, and may cause dyspnea during exertion (due to the absence of normal inspiratory abduction of the paralyzed VF). Aspiration related to URLNP can be severe and poorly tolerated, especially in patients with compromised pulmonary function [1]. The glottal air leak during phonation causes a breathy, bitonal or rough voice. Moreover, these patients experience an increased vocal effort, laryngeal spasms with a decrease in communication effectiveness, leading to a decrease in voice-related quality of life [5]. Nevertheless, the voice can completely recover in URLNP even without complete remobilization of the paralyzed VF.

In the case of BRLNP, voice quality is usually good, while the paramedian position of the VFs may jeopardize airway patency. BRLNP often causes dyspnea at rest or exertion that may require a tracheotomy, while aspiration is rare. However, BRLNP might be lethal because of respiratory failure or negative pressure pulmonary oedema acutely requiring a tracheotomy to improve the size of the glottic space and subsequent surgery. Post-operative extubation failure is an uncommon but devastating complication characterized by the need for the reinstitution of ventilatory support within 72 h of planned endotracheal tube removal [4]. The obstructive aetiology of this condition is mainly secondary to thyroid surgery complications, such as BRLNP, above all, tracheomalacia and neck haematoma.

44.2.4.2 Tests

Assessment of RLN function during surgery through IONM could be crucial to prevent and predict post-operative RLNP. On the other hand, post-operative laryngoscopy is the only reliable measure of VF function (deviation and mobility).

44.2.5 Treatment

44.2.5.1 Medical Treatment

Patients should be referred to specialized laryngologists to optimize the management of both transient and permanent RLNP. Patients who experience post-operative extubation failure may require reintubation, and the use of video laryngoscopes (Glidescope) may be a helpful aid during the procedure.

44.2.5.2 Surgical Treatment

In case of failed reintubation, an emergency tracheotomy may be necessary, while an elective and temporary one could be the treatment of choice in patients with dyspnoea at rest. If breathing issues do not recover in BRLNP laryngeal surgery (partial arytenoidectomy, posterior cordotomy or VF lateralization) may be necessary to improve breathing and/or decannulate patients with a temporary tracheotomy.

44.2.6 Prognosis

RLNP is considered the worst one among thyroid surgery complications both for its potential impact on the immediate patient recovery after surgery and for the consequences on her/his future quality of life.

44.3 Spinal Accessory Nerve Injury

44.3.1 Epidemiology

The reported frequency of post-operative spinal accessory nerve (SAN)-related morbidity is 46.7% for radical neck dissections (ND), 42.5% for selective ND and 25% for modified ND [9].

44.3.2 Etiology

SAN is usually encountered during ND of levels II and V, minimally invasive lymph node biopsies and tumour resections in its close proximity, where it comes to lie near the internal jugular vein. SAN dissection and any degree of traction pose a risk of iatrogenic damage resulting in shoulder dysfunction and pain known as "shoulder syndrome" [10–12].

44.3.3 Pathophysiology

SAN injury results in trapezius and sternocleidomastoid muscles atrophy, leading to shoulder functional impairment and scapulothoracic joint instability. Consequent shoulder girdle's weakness leads to muscular overuse of the remaining functional muscles. Therefore, this imbalance often causes severe pain exacerbated by physical activity. In general, modified nerve-sparing dissections are followed by a significant but temporary and reversible phase of shoulder dysfunction, while radical ND is followed by profound and permanent trapezius muscle weakness and denervation. IONM could aid nerve identification and preservation; tracking changes indeed are significantly related to shoulder complaints [9, 11].

44.3.4 Diagnosis

44.3.4.1 Clinical Presentation

The initial clinical manifestation of SAN damage is nuchal and shoulder pain caused by trapezius muscle paralysis and the levator scapulae muscle overuse, followed by shoulder motion restriction and dropping and winging of the scapula, eventually becoming a disabling condition. Furthermore, secondary periarthritis may lead to a 'frozen shoulder'. The onset of symptoms and the diagnosis often are not readily appreciated neither by the primary surgeon nor by the treating physician and occurs months after injury.

44.3.4.2 Tests

Electromyography and nerve conduction studies could allow early detection of SAN injuries.

44.3.5 Treatment

44.3.5.1 Medical Treatment

Physical therapy interventions are the usual first approach for patients with "shoulder syndrome". These conservative treatments include proximal scapular stabilization exercise, proprioceptive neuromuscular facilitation, neuromuscular electrical stimulation, shoulder strengthening exercises, and pool exercises.

44.3.5.2 Surgical Treatment

If the SAN lesion is recognized intraoperatively, nerve reconstruction through tension-free direct repair must be performed immediately. In the case of "shoulder syndrome" with a late onset, where the physiotherapy or other conservative treatments have failed, the aim ideally should be direct repair (tension-free end-to-end anastomosis). However, the delay between injury and nerve reconstruction, or the resection of a nerve segment, or its damage with electrocautery, often make the direct reconstruction not feasible; hence, secondary reconstructive procedures using various nerve transfers are needed. Finally, after surgery, a substantial motor re-education is required [11].

44.4 Mandibular Branch of the Facial Nerve Injury

44.4.1 Epidemiology

The reported prevalence of marginal mandibular nerve (MMN) injury ranges from 11% to as high as 43%, depending on parameters utilized and including different types of ND. During the immediate post-operative period, functional deficits are reported in 28.7% of patients and persistent palsy in 16% of cases [13].

44.4.2 Etiology

The MMN may be injured during ND, principally of level Ib in 18–21% of cases, and more rarely of level IIa in 1.26% of cases, during surgery for both benign and malignant parotid gland tumours as well as in any surgical procedure near the angle of the mandible and the submandibular triangle [14].

44.4.3 Pathophysiology

MMN is a branch of the facial nerve, which innervates the muscles of the lower part of the face and lower lip. Complete nerve neurotmesis or transient neuropraxia could be related to nerve stretching, devascularisation or conduction block due to diathermy current [15]. Temporary MMN dysfunction had a recovery time ranging from 3–6 months.

44.4.4 Diagnosis

It is advantageous to visualize and/or monitor the nerve function during the operation to make the intraoperative diagnosis of injury; otherwise, the post-operative clinical pattern will testify the nerve damage.

44.4.4.1 Clinical Presentation

The loss of innervation to the lower lip depressors may result in asymmetry of the smile because of the unopposed action of elevator muscles. The patient is unable to move the lower lip downward or laterally or to evert the vermilion border on the affected side, producing an elevation of the lower lip on the paralyzed side during smiling and talking, fewer of the teeth are visible on the affected side, and the lower lip appears flattened and inwardly rotated. The asymmetry is most apparent when the patient cries, defined as the 'asymmetric crying facies [13–15].

44.4.4.2 Tests

Electromyography test allows to determine the degree and the stage of muscles denervation and may help predict the expected outcome of a specific deficit [13, 15].

44.4.5 Treatment

In case of an incomplete paralysis or of a surely spared nerve during surgery, no irreversible procedure should be undertaken less than 12 months from the time of injury because of the potential spontaneous recovery. On the contrary, if nerve integrity is uncertain or loss of response to electrical stimulation has been demonstrated re-exploration should be performed.

44.4.5.1 Surgical Treatment

Techniques to rehabilitate patients with depressor complex deficits and lower lip asymmetry may be distinguished in two broad categories: dynamic and static procedures.

The first ones aim at rehabilitating focal depressors deficit and include single-stage direct neurotization using cross-facial nerve grafting, single-step procedures without the need for nerve graft (such as the mini-hypoglossal or the platysma motor nerve transfer), and platysma or digastric muscle transfers.

On the other hand, static procedures represent the most frequently employed techniques when addressing depressors deficit aiming to create an overall symmetry at rest when smiling by reducing the action of the contralateral depressor musculature or producing static downward forces in the affected lower lip. This approach includes chemodenervation using botulinum toxin injections to the contralateral depressor muscles (the most frequently employed), surgical myectomy of the depressor muscles, and selective MMN neurectomy. Finally, fascial slings (fascia lata or palmaris longus tendon) and tightening techniques (e.g., wedge resections, orbicularis oris muscle transposition, or Z-plasty) represent an alternative in cases of chemodenervation unsuccess [13].

44.5 Phrenic and Vagus Nerve Injuries

The frequency of unilateral phrenic nerve damage is about 8%; it can be an incidental finding following ND and can occur anywhere along its course. Most unilateral phrenic nerve injuries are usually transient or found to have no clinical significance. However, a small percentage of them could experience unilateral elevation of the diaphragm, lung atelectasis, pulmonary infiltrates and possible impairment of the respiratory function. Bilateral phrenic nerve paralysis has been reported with consequent respiratory failure.

The vagus nerve may be injured when the internal jugular vein is ligated during ND. If the damage occurs below the no-dose ganglion, it results in unilateral VF paralysis; if it occurs above, there is also dysphagia and aspiration. Unless co-morbid cardiac conditions exist, no significant cardiac complication should occur. Similarly, a unilateral vagus transection or damage should have little effect on the gastrointestinal tract [10].

44.6 Hypoparathyroidism

44.6.1 Epidemiology

Hypocalcemia is defined as serum adjusted Ca <200 mmol/L or 8 mg/dL. Post-operative hypocalcaemia is one of the most common complications after total thyroidectomy. The median incidence of transient and permanent hypocalcaemia, as recently reported in a meta-analysis, is 27 (19–38) and 1 (0–3)%, respectively [16, 17].

44.6.2 Etiology

Biochemical and clinical predictors of post-thyroidectomy hypocalcaemia have been identified, as perioperative PTH, post-operative changes in calcium, female sex, Graves' disease, thyroid cancer, central lymph node dissection, reoperations, large or substernal goitres, need for parathyroid autotransplantation and inadvertent excision of parathyroid glands (PGs) [16].

44.6.3 Pathophysiology

Even though the cause of post-operative hypocalcemia is multifactorial, one of the most important causes surely is PGs' inadequate or compromised blood supply (acute parathyroid insufficiency). PG's visual identification together with the estimation of their perfusion and viability could not be enough to assess parathyroid function. PGs' autofluorescence and indocyanine green fluorescence angiography are a currently widely used strategy to evaluate the PGs' real-time function during thyroid surgery [18, 19].

44.6.4 Diagnosis

44.6.4.1 Clinical Presentation

Hypocalcemia can present as an asymptomatic laboratory finding or as a severe, life-threatening condition (Table 44.1). The hallmark of

Table 44.1 Clinical features associated with hypocalcaemia

Neuromuscular irritability
• Chvostek's sign
• Trousseau's sign
• Paresthesias
• Tetany
• Seizures (focal, petit mal, grand mal)
• Muscle cramps
• Muscle weakness
• Laryngospasm
• Bronchospasm
Neurological signs and symptoms
• Extrapyramidal signs due to calcification of basal ganglia
• Calcification of cerebral cortex or cerebellum
• Personality disturbances
• Irritability
• Impaired intellectual ability
• Nonspecific EEG changes
• Increased intracranial pressure
• Parkinsonism
• Choreoathetosis
• Dystonic spasms

Table 44.1 (continued)

Neuromuscular irritability
Mental status
• Confusion
• Disorientation
• Psychosis
• Fatigue
• Anxiety
• Poor memory
• Reduced concentration
Ectodermal changes
• Dry skin
• Coarse hair
• Brittle nails
• Alopecia
• Enamel hypoplasia
• Shortened premolar roots
• Thickened lamina dura
• Delayed tooth eruption
• Increased dental caries
• Atopic eczema
• Exfoliative dermatitis
• Psoriasis
• Impetigo herpetiformis
Smooth muscle involvement
• Dysphagia
• Abdominal pain
• Biliary colic
• Dyspnea
• Wheezing
Ophthalmologic manifestations
• Subcapsular cataracts
• Papilledema
Cardiac
• Prolonged QT interval on EKG
• Congestive heart failure
• Cardiomyopathy

Adapted from Schafer AL and Shoback D: Hypocalcemia: definition, etiology, pathogenesis, diagnosis and management. Primer on the Metabolic Bone Diseases and Disorders of Mineral Metabolism, C. J. Rosen (ed), John Wiley and Sons, Eighth Edition. pp 572–578, 2013.

acute hypocalcemia is neuromuscular irritability varying from numbness and tingling in the fingertips, toes, and the perioral region to carpal spasm or tetany. Clinically, neuromuscular irritability can be demonstrated by eliciting Chvostek's or Trousseau's signs. Cardiac manifestations of hypocalcemia could be QT prolongation, T-waves abnormality or a pattern of acute anteroseptal injury on EKG without infarction [17].

44.6.4.2 Tests
Serum-adjusted calcium and PTH are the main lab test in hypocalcemic patients, while magnesemia, 25 (OH) vitamin D level, phosphatemia, alkaline phosphatase and nitrogen-level monitoring and correction could help the treatment of severe hypocalcemia.

44.6.5 Treatment

44.6.5.1 Medical Treatment
The decision to treat and how to treat hypocalcemia depends on its severity, symptoms, and rapidity with which hypocalcemia develops.

In patients with mild hypocalcemia whose symptoms are not life-threatening checking, other laboratory tests as PTH and vitamin D levels are useful. The consulting endocrinologist may choose to prescribe oral repletion with calcium and vitamin D for outpatient therapy.

In case of symptomatic or severe hypocalcemia, with cardiac arrhythmias or tetany, IV replacement is recommended, and hospitalization in an intensive care unit or specialized unit with access to cardiac monitoring and rapid ionized calcium determinations is ideal for optimal management and safety. Supportive treatment (i.e., IV fluid replacement, oxygen, and monitoring) often is required prior to directed treatment of hypocalcemia. Doses of 100–300 mg of elemental calcium in 50–100 mL of 5% dextrose in water should be given over 5–10 min. This dosage raises the ionized level to 0.5–1.5 mmol and should last 1–2 h. Caution should be used when giving calcium chloride intravenously, and it delivers higher amounts of calcium and is advantageous when rapid correction is needed. However, it should be administered via central venous access, also needing an arterial line for frequent measurement of ionized calcium [17].

44.7 Chyle Leak

44.7.1 Epidemiology

Chyle leak (CL) is an uncommon but serious complication of head and neck surgery ranging from 1 to 2.5% and approximately 1–4% of at-risk surgical cases [20].

44.7.2 Etiology

CL most often occurs after ND on the left side, but right-sided CL have been reported according to some authors with an almost equal incidence [21].

44.7.3 Pathophysiology

CL may be identified intraoperatively or postoperatively. Because of its proximity to the internal jugular vein and its thin vessel wall, the thoracic duct and its branches are particularly susceptible to inadvertent injury during dissection. Care should be taken to identify promptly any doubt CL during surgery and systematically fixing it with nonabsorbable ligatures, clips or electric haemostatic devices [10].

44.7.4 Diagnosis

44.7.4.1 Clinical Presentation
The CL may not be evident intraoperatively, and on post-operative day 1 or 2 (rarely later) a sudden high increase in drain output, especially following resumption of feedings that contain fat, raise suspicion of a CL. On neck examination, it could be evident erythema, lymphedema, a palpable fluid collection in the supraclavicular region, or the drain output would have a creamy or milky appearance. CLs are usually classified according to output as low (<500 mL/day) or high (>500 mL/day). The daily chyle flow through the thoracic duct ranges between 2 and 4 L transporting a large part of total body protein [21]. Therefore, it is evident that a CL may lead to serious protein loss and consequent malnutrition, immune compromise, electrolyte abnormalities, hypoalbuminaemia, and infection. Moreover, CL can lead to a topical damage of the surrounding tissues if untreated, as the overlying skin necrosis and major vessels damage [20].

44.7.4.2 Tests
CL is easily clinically diagnosed; however, the biochemical assay may offer a more specific measure. A drain fluid with a triglyceride level greater than 100 mg/dL or the presence of serum triglyceride or chylomicrons confirms the diagnosis.

44.7.5 Treatment

Both medical and surgical options exist for the post-operative management of CLs depending on drain output, patient performance status, available institutional expertise, and surgeon preference. Even though low output CL generally respond successfully to conservative management, drain output alone cannot guide the treatment choice.

44.7.5.1 Medical Treatment
In most cases, conservative measures effectively lead to the CL resolution in 2–4 weeks or more. First, because chyle flow is propelled by physical activity, patients should be at bed rest with a head of bed elevation to 30–40°, and stool softeners should be administered to reduce intrathoracic and intra-abdominal pressure due to bowel movement. Second, restriction of oral intake completely or to a nonfat, low-fat, or medium-chain fatty acid diet plays a crucial role in the medical management of this complication. Due to the potentially high volume fluid shift with protein and electrolytes loss, the fluid balance, electrolytes, and albumin should be checked closely for dehydration and malnutrition monitoring, and IV fluids and parenteral nutrition should be administered. Moreover, the use of octreotide injections has been advocated because of its effect on lymphatic and splanchnic blood flow, chyle production via reduction of gastric, pancreatic, and intestinal secretions, consequently preventing lipid absorption. Wound care has its key

role in the management of CL. The application of pressure dressings is a traditional but controversial measure, while suction drainage, placed during surgery, favour evacuation and monitoring of extravasated chyle to valuate both severity of leak and treatment effectiveness. Negative wound pressure therapy has been used in CL; it helps to remove fluid and to shrink wound size but requires exposure of the wound bed. In addition, the use of topical sclerosing agents such as cyanoacrylate, fibrin glue or tetracycline at the time of surgery or postoperatively through drainage tubing or percutaneous injection could favour the fibrosis process and the leak closure; nevertheless, they could both potentially injure surrounding structures (i.e., phrenic nerve) and obliterate the surgical field making redo surgeries much more challenging [20, 22, 23].

44.7.5.2 Surgical Treatment

Surgical re-exploration should be considered when conservative management have either been exhausted or deemed ineffective. A case in point is a drain output ranging from >500 mL/day to >1000 mL/day within the first 4–5 days when a clear and prompt response to medical measures is absent. At the time of re-exploration, local inflammation can make the damaged lymphatic duct identification arduous. Manoeuvres that raise intrathoracic and intra-abdominal pressure, Trendelenberg position, fatty diet the day before surgery are some measures that could coadiuvate the surgeon to localize the leak site. The treatment of the leaking duct could vary from ligation, muscle flap, the use of sclerosing agents, adhesive agents, or mesh; a suction drain is placed afterward.

Rarely, when a CL is persistent after redo surgery or when re-exploration is not advisable because of anatomical alteration such as a microvascular free flap, interventional radiologic procedures, or distant management of a thoracic duct leak may be necessary. Percutaneous transabdominal cannulation of the thoracic duct with lymphography and selective distal embolization with coils or glue is a safe, minimally invasive technique for the treatment of persistent CL, with a reported success rate of 45–70%. Finally, for patients with failed surgical correction, thoracoscopic ligation of the thoracic duct at the supradiaphragmatic hiatus can be an effective procedure that excludes the thoracic duct proximally [20].

44.8 Postoperative Haematoma

44.8.1 Epidemiology

The reported incidence of post-operative haematoma (PH) after neck surgery, depending on the definition utilized, range from 0.3% to 4.2%. However, in most series, the risk of clinically significant haemorrhage after thyroid surgery is 1% or less [24].

44.8.2 Etiology

Several studies have attempted to identify risk factors of post-operative haemorrhage following thyroidectomy; nevertheless, many of them are underpowered to detect statistically significant differences because of the rarity of this complication. Potential risk factors may be classified into two broad categories: patient-related and surgery-related factors summarized in Table 44.2

Table 44.2 Risk factors for post-thyroidectomy bleeding

Risk factors for post-thyroidectomy bleeding	
Patient-related factors	**Surgery-related factors**
Demographics	**Extent of surgery**
Age (older)	(bilateral)
Gender (male)	**Reoperative surgery**
Co-morbid disease	**Intraoperative blood loss**
Bleeding disorder (haemophilia, von Willebrand's disease)	**Technique for access and closure**
Therapeutic anticoagulation (e.g., coumadin)	Division of strap muscles
Aspirin or other antiplatelet drugs	Longitudinal closure of strap muscles (anterior jugular vein injury)
Steroid use	**Anaesthesia-related**
Cirrhosis	Coughing or retching during extubation
Chronic renal failure	Post-operative nausea and vomiting
Thyroid pathology	Post-operative hypertension
Malignancy	
Hyperthyroidism	

Adapted from Williams, R.T.; Angelos, P. Postoperative Bleeding. Thyroid Surg. 2013, 199–207

[25]. Among the patient-related risk factors, older age and male gender increased this risk, with odds ratios of 1.04 and 1.90, respectively [26]. Other risk factors in this group include untreated high blood pressure, any bleeding diathesis, inherited or acquired, the presence of large metastatic nodes, malignant histology and hyperthyroidism may also increase the risk of PH [24, 26, 27]. Surgery-related risk factors include the extent of surgery (bilateral versus unilateral thyroidectomy), reoperative surgery, intraoperative bleeding, surgical techniques (i.e., strap muscles transection or resection injury to the anterior jugular veins), and anaesthesia-related factors (coughing or retching during extubation, postoperative coughing or vomiting, hypertension due to pain) [24, 26].

44.8.3 Pathophysiology

About 50–75% of PHs manifest within 6–8 h after surgery, while 80–97% occur within 24 h; a late presentation of neck haematoma (beyond the first 24 h following surgery) is rare but possible [28]. Numerous mechanisms could lead to haematoma formation, including slipping of a ligature on a major vessel, reopening of cauterized veins, retching during recovery, Valsalva manoeuvres during reversal of anaesthesia, increased blood pressure in the immediate post-operative period and oozing from the cut edge of the thyroid gland in partial thyroidectomies. Superficial bleeding usually causes a haematoma superficial to the strap muscles and a prominent ecchymosis that does not produce respiratory distress. PH deep to the strap muscles develops from a major vessel-like cricothyroid artery, superior or inferior thyroid arteries, or the cut surface of the thyroid and might result in respiratory distress. The strap muscles themselves seem to work as a barrier between the haematoma and the trachea or the larynx and pharynx's venous and lymphatic drainage system [24, 26, 27, 29]. Respiratory distress by a life-threatening airway obstruction could occur. Routine use of drains or pressure dressing has not significantly reduced re-operation or respiratory distress rate [24, 29].

Many strategies have been proposed to prevent post-operative bleeding in neck surgery or mitigate its effects. Many surgeons recommend a Valsalva manoeuvre performed by the anesthesiologist before closure to increase venous pressure and eventually highlight bleeding sources; others advocate re-evaluation of haemostasis once the shoulder roll has been removed and the neck flexed decreased tension on blood vessels that may uncover additional bleeding sites. Furthermore, the closure of the strap muscles has been suggested to be incomplete, so that a space 3–4 cm in length allows for decompression of the deep space of the neck into the superficial layer, theoretically resulting in earlier visible neck swelling, increasing the blood volume needed to produce respiratory failure and finally giving more time to secure the airways [28]. No effect on bleeding complications by drain placement has been demonstrated. None of these methods, indeed, has proven to decrease rates of post-operative haemorrhage. Achieving optimal haemostasis by a meticulous technique is the only successful strategy each surgeon should pursue. Many devices and agents can be used to get intraoperative haemostasis like the Harmonic™ Scalpel (Ethicon Endo-Surgery,Cincinnati, OH), electrothermal bipolar vessel sealing system (LigaSure™, Valleylab, Boulder, CO), oxidized regenerated cellulose (e.g., Surgicel™, Ethicon,), gelatin compressed sponge (e.g., Gelfoam™, Pfizer, New York), topical thrombin (e.g., Floseal™, Baxter Healthcare Corporation, Deerfield, IL) and fibrin sealants (e.g., Tisseel™, Baxter Healthcare Corporation) [30, 31].

44.8.4 Diagnosis

44.8.4.1 Clinical Presentation

Since post-thyroidectomy bleeding is potentially fatal, rapid diagnosis and management are imperative. Surgeons and medical staffs at the ward should pay particular attention to any signs and symptoms of bleeding during the 24 h postoperative period. Signs and symptoms include progressively enlarging anterior or lateral neck swelling, bloody wound drainage (10–15%), dyspnoea or stridor (~50%), neck pain or pressure (25–50%), dysphagia (6–20%), agitation/confusion and sweating (5%) [26]. If a drain was placed another sign might be a significant drain output, even though in the presence of drain blood clots, there may still be significant bleeding despite low or no drain output.

44.8.4.2 Tests

The diagnosis is essentially clinical; blood tests may prove anaemia.

44.8.5 Treatment

The keys to PH management include early detection, close observation, airway management, and surgical intervention (Fig. 44.1).

Emergency treatment requires immediate removal of surgical skin sutures for the evacuation of haematoma and airway assessment. Immediate intubation should be performed in the case of respiratory distress from airway obstruction. The goal of wound decompression at the bedside is to relieve severe respiratory distress, hypoxia and the resulting cardiovascular instability. A conservative approach may be considered in selected asymptomatic patients with minimal non-expanding haematoma as long as a close observation is guaranteed [27, 32]. Superficial haematoma most likely does not require surgical intervention. During the bedside management, the strap muscles might be opened as well; therefore, if a significant improvement is observed, the patient is urgently transferred to the operating room for re-exploration. Instead, if the respiratory distress persists, the airway must be secured before transfer either by endotracheal intubation if a laryngoscopy expert is readily available or by a surgical emergency tracheostomy. Surgical re-exploration aims to identify and control any bleeding sources, remove the haematoma and irrigate the wound, carefully trying not to injure the PGs or the RLNs.

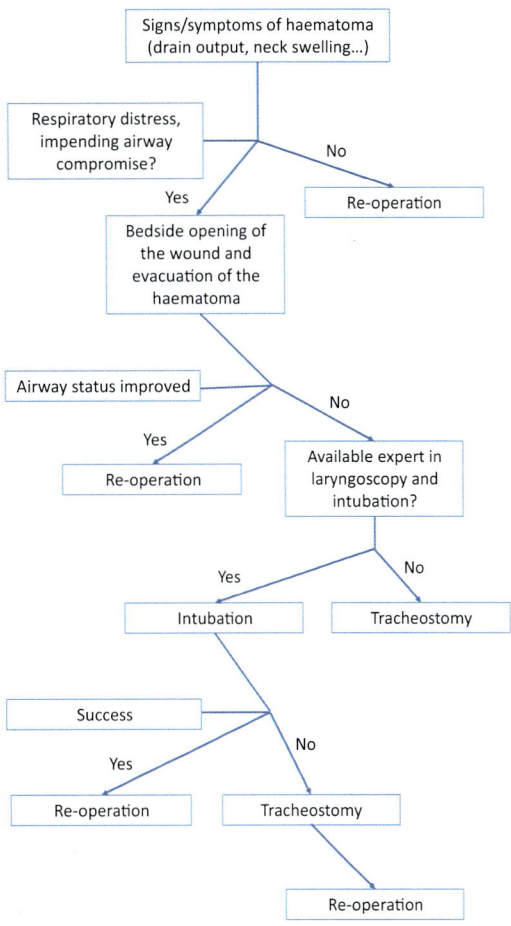

Fig. 44.1 Management algorithm for haematoma after thyroid surgery. Adapted from Miccoli, P.; Terris, D.J.; Minuto, N.M.; Seybt, M.W. Thyroid Surgery—Preventing and Managing Complications. 2013, 203

44.9 Major Vessels Injury

44.9.1 Epidemiology

The intraoperative haemorrhage from major vessels, such as common carotid artery, is rare during thyroid and parathyroid surgery, although it is increased during ND for cancer (Fig. 44.2).

44.9.2 Etiology

Thyroid surgery requires a deep knowledge of the normal anatomy and common anomalies of

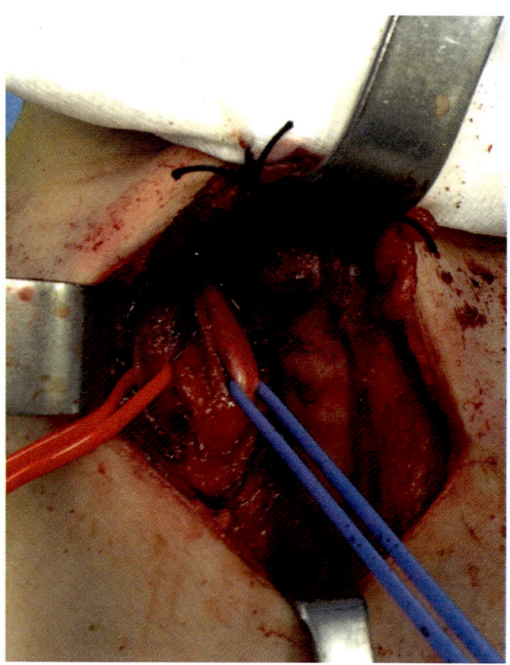

Fig. 44.2 Major vessels exposed after neck dissection

the neck vessels. Iatrogenic injuries to these organs can lead to very harmful complications, such as stroke, haemorrhagic shock, and embolism. Tortuous vessels in their normal places are the most common anatomic vascular anomaly. This situation is due to advanced age and atherosclerosis: the innominate artery, the right and left common carotid arteries, and the right subclavian artery are the vessels that are most prone to become tortuous.

The aberrant right subclavian artery, which often lies behind the oesophagus (80%), is the most common vascular variant of the neck vessels. Rarely, the aberrant right subclavian artery can be found between the trachea and the oesophagus (15%) or before the trachea (5%) [33]. A retro-oesophageal subclavian artery comes with an anomaly of the right RLN, which is named non-recurrent. Another variant is the origin from the innominate artery of the left common carotid artery found in 7–27% of patients [33]. This variant has no consequences on the course of the RLNs. Some anomalies affect the innominate artery, such as a left innominate artery or a retro-oesophageal one associated with a right aortic arch, or the high-riding innominate artery, that reaches the upper tracheal rings or the cricoid cartilage [34]. The neck extension during thyroid surgery can elevate even the normal innominate artery to a position immediately below the sternal notch. The intraoperative lesion of the innominate artery can lead to severe consequences, so it is essential to check the position of this artery by palpating its pulse during the division of the midline fascia between the strap muscles. Anomalies of the thyroid position are also associated with vascular variants: the ectopic mediastinal thyroid can receive the entire blood supply from thoracic vessels. The inferior thyroid arthery can be completely absent in other patients: 5% on the left and 2% on the right. In this case, the thyroid and PGs are supplied by branches originating from the left subclavian artery. The thyroidea ima artery is found in a small proportion of subjects: it arises directly from the aortic arch, and its bleeding is difficult to be dominated.

Risk factors for major vessel injuries are prior surgeries and radiation: the anatomic subversion should be expected with a careful study of the preoperative images. The internal jugular vein is the major neck vessel most exposed to injuries during ND, especially for level IV. Metastatic lymph nodes can displace the vein or be adherent to or invade it [35].

44.9.3 Pathophysiology

The tracheo-innominate fistula has particular pathophysiology: this is one of the most severe complications following thyroid surgery. The pathophysiology includes mechanical irritation from the endotracheal tube or longstanding surgical drain, infectious exposure, cancer infiltration. Risk factors are radiation treatment, steroid treatment, malnutrition, hypotension, and shock. The exposure of the vessel wall to air and tracheal secretion in case of tracheostomy or tracheal injury with subcutaneous emphysema, or even to saliva in case of pharyngeal would dehiscence after complex surgery, determines its erosion and the final step for the fistula formation [36].

Therefore, surgical planning is crucial: in case of suspected tracheal involvement due to thyroid malignancy, a plan to obtain immediate airway reconstruction is advisable. Reoperations are particularly risky for the disruption of the normal anatomic planes. The design of the skin incision and subsequent flaps should prevent wound complications that may put the major vessels at risk. In case of level V lymph nodal resection, with a potential sternocleidomastoid muscle sacrifice, the incision overlying the common carotid artery should be avoided. The ligation of the ima artery or any thyroid vessel coming from the mediastinum should be careful and accurate to avoid their retraction in the mediastinum. Exposure should always be carefully obtained to prevent vascular complications. Exposure does not need extended surgical incision, but it can also be granted through minimally invasive accesses.

44.9.4 Diagnosis

44.9.4.1 Clinical Presentation

Intraoperative venous bleeding tends to "fill the operating field", while an arterial one usually spills out of the wound and is pulsatile. Sometimes, severe venous bleeding can be confused with the arterial one, and this is particularly dangerous, even more, if coming from a vein below the clavicle or sternum, because the vein walls are thin and fragile and can easily tear during the attempts to control the haemorrhage.

The post-operative bleeding after thyroid, parathyroid, and, in general, any neck surgery can be life-threatening because of airway obstruction. This can be a consequence of an even small haematoma. Post-operative severe haemorrhages from major vessels are usually preceded by the sentinel bleed that can help prevent detrimental sequelae if promptly recognised [37]. This is the case of the rare injury of the common carotid artery.

44.9.4.2 Tests

The prevention of bleedings from major vessels of the neck starts from the preoperative study that has to consider any abnormal pulse in the neck at physical examination and any anomaly of the vascular anatomy at imaging studies. Pulsation in the central anterior low neck is a sign of a high-riding innominate artery. CT scan can identify a right retro esophageal subclavian artery. Further exams are the colour Doppler ultrasound, magnetic resonance angiography or even conventional angiography. After neck surgery, any bleeding from the wound or drain in the post-operative course should be seriously considered. The sentinel bleeding is a brisk and sudden haemorrhage that briefly stops that can anticipate a severe one from a tracheo-innominate fistula or the common carotid artery. Patients with histories of such bleeding should be hospitalized, if not already admitted, and undergo CT scan, to identify occult aneurysms, abscesses or fistulas, blood collections or air, or even active bleedings. Patients should then undergo tailored treatment, ranging from supportive fluids, antibiotics to surgery.

44.9.5 Treatment

44.9.5.1 Medical Treatment

The setting of a post-operative haemorrhage can be even dangerous without a strict management algorithm: the first goal is to grant and secure the maintenance of the airway. Oro-tracheal intubation or tracheostomy intubation should be obtained as soon as possible. The overinflation of the endotracheal tube's cuff can help control the bleeding from a tracheo-innominate fistula. Controlled mechanical ventilation, double intravenous access should be obtained, starting fluid resuscitation and requesting blood products. The overinflation of the endotracheal tube cuff after immediate intubation through a laryngectomy stoma or a tracheostomy is a temporary option to tamponade the bleeding from a trachea-innominate fistula. Finger pressure under the sternal notch or in the tracheal lumen if the airway is secured distally is other temporary options. Bedside packing after the opening of the wound is another possibility.

44.9.5.2 Surgical Treatment

The management of an intraoperative haemorrhage varies according to the injured vessel, but the first step to achieve is to maintain composure. Most of the intraoperative bleedings can be controlled with direct pressure from the surgeon's finger. Soon after the manual control of the bleeding, the surgeon should alert the operating room staff and anesthesiologist to request a vascular tray, gain large-bore intravenous accesses, request blood products or alert vascular or thoracic surgeons.

Once the great vessel injured is identified, it is important to obtain an adequate exposure for evaluation and repair, which is particularly true for the innominate artery and vein. These vessels can be exposed through one or more of the following steps, according to the level of the injury and the anatomy of the patient: the enlargement of the skin incision (collar incision with an inverted T extension), the enlargement of the division of the strap muscles, the division of the cervical thymus, a sternotomy or manubriotomy [36]. These steps should be adapted to the specific availability of the required instruments and the thoracic or vascular surgical team. Adequate suction and lighting are obvious requirements. The injured vessel should be isolated cephalad and caudal to the bleeding through circumferential dissection. The proximal control of the innominate artery is sometimes impossible without sternotomy: in this case, if the exposure of the lesion is adequate through the cervical incision, a direct attempt of repair is suggested without proximal control.

This dissection is complex and unsafe in the case of injuries to the innominate vein: in this case, a curved vascular clamp can be adopted, isolating the injured sector while allowing a partial flow. The vascular injury can be oversewn with non-resorbable stitches, such as polypropylene 5/0.

In case of extensive damage to the common carotid artery, it is possible to obtain a vein graft from the external or internal jugular vein. The risk of stroke is low if the repair is rapidly obtained.

The control of the intraoperative injury of the internal jugular vein can be achieved through the exposed general principles, usually without the sacrifice of the vein. Nevertheless, the vein can be sacrificed to remove bulky metastases or in case of injuries located deep in the neck, close to the branching from the innominate vein.

Transaxillary endoscopic or robotic approaches put the internal jugular vein at higher risk of injury, since the dissection proceeding from lateral to medial through the sternal and clavicular head of the sternocleidomastoid muscle can sometimes be too posterior. In case of a haemorrhage during transaxillary thyroidectomy, the internal jugular vein cannot be compressed. Debakey forceps can be used to tamponade the vein. Clip appliers are essential, but conversion is often required.

The treatment of a post-operative haemorrhage can be either surgical or angiographic. The endovascular techniques for large vessels injuries, with the deployment of coils or stents or the testing with balloon occlusion, are preferred, given that the patient is stable. The arterial stents are particularly indicated, since they allow the blood flow and reduce the incidence of stroke [37]. The surgical treatment can adopt different techniques determining the definitive interruption of the blood flow (clipping, ligation, and resection) or the blood flow maintenance.

The prevention of tracheo-innominate fistula, in case of tracheal injury with high running innominate artery, can be obtained thanks to the interposition of soft-tissue grafts (strap muscles, thymus, and sternocleidomastoid muscle). Rarely, a pedicled pectoralis muscle flap can be obtained, or even a microsurgical flap. The trachea-innominate fistula is often lethal, and even temporary control of the bleeding is rarely achieved. In the rare situation reaching the operatory room, definitive management requires a sternotomy. The trachea-innominate fistula is treated by ligation or graft repair of the innominate artery, the repair of the trachea with interposition of a soft-tissue graft like a sternocleidomastoid flap. An endovascular stent is another temporary option.

Post-operative bleeding from the common carotid artery is often dreadful. Risk factors are infection, dehiscence of the pharyngeal suture or pharyngocutaneous fistulas. Bedside would exploration is not recommended: after recognition, the patient should undergo aggressive airway control, fluid resuscitation, and immediate transfer to the operatory room or angiography service. A soft-tissue graft is advisable once the repair is obtained.

Both intraoperative and post-operative haemorrhage after neck surgery can be a complex scenario. An adequate preoperative study and intraoperative plan can minimize the risks and prevent the most severe sequelae.

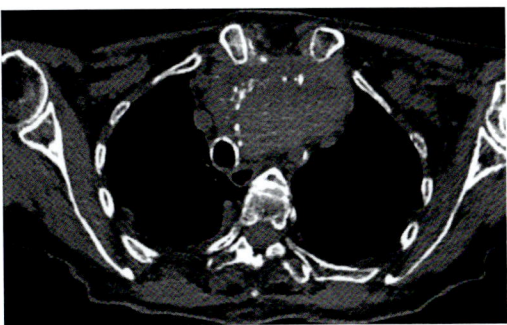

Fig. 44.3 Computed tomography scan of retrosternal prevascular goiter, with compression and dislocation of the trachea, oesophagus, supaortic trunks, innominate veins and superior vena cava

44.10 Tracheomalacia

44.10.1 Epidemiology

The incidence of tracheomalacia has been reported between 0.001% and 1.5%, especially following substernal goitre excision [38, 39]. It is noteworthy that some authors doubt its existence, and a number of large series failed to document any clear-cut case of tracheomalacia caused by a benign goitre [40].

44.10.2 Etiology

Tracheomalacia has been defined as an extreme degree of airway compression, where the trachea cross-sectional area is reduced to less than half. The risk of tracheomalacia seems to be increased in case of compressive goitre present for more than 5 years, bilateral, causing significant tracheal compression or occurring in elderly patients [40].

44.10.3 Pathophysiology

The longstanding goitre compression may completely destroy or considerably weaken tracheal rings resulting in poor support to the trachea (Fig. 44.3). Such an unsupported trachea is prone to collapse after thyroidectomy, resulting in post-operative respiratory obstruction [39, 40].

44.10.4 Diagnosis

44.10.4.1 Clinical Presentation

The main clinical feature is progressive hypoxaemia not responding to increasing fractionated inspired oxygen concentration (FiO_2). As soon as the tracheal diameter becomes less than 3.5 mm, signalling a critical functional obstruction, the stridor can be appreciated. Some criteria have been suggested to suspect tracheomalacia before extubation [40]:

- Soft and floppy trachea on palpation by the surgeon at the end of the procedure. However, because of the splinting effect of the endotracheal tube in situ, it may be difficult to appreciate a soft trachea. Accordingly, a gradual withdrawal of the tube for a short distance by the anesthesiologist may help the surgeon identify the tracheal wall's possible collapse.
- Obstruction to spontaneous respiration during gradual withdrawal of the endotracheal tube after thyroidectomy.
- Difficulty to overcome the endotracheal tube with the suction catheter during its gradual withdrawal.

After the closure of the wound, tracheomalacia can be suspected (a) if there is an absence of peritubal leak on deflation of endotracheal tube cuff, (b) absence of volume pressure loop on ventilator or (c) development of respiratory stridor along with a falling haemoglobin oxygen saturation (SpO_2) on pulse oximetry despite the administration of increasing FiO_2.

In addition, bilateral vocal cord paralysis or glottic/subglottic oedema should be ruled as a possible cause of stridor. It is also important to bear in mind that the collapse of a floppy trachea may not always be circumferential. The collapse of a portion of the lateral wall may occur, indeed, leading to respiratory obstruction in the postoperative period [40].

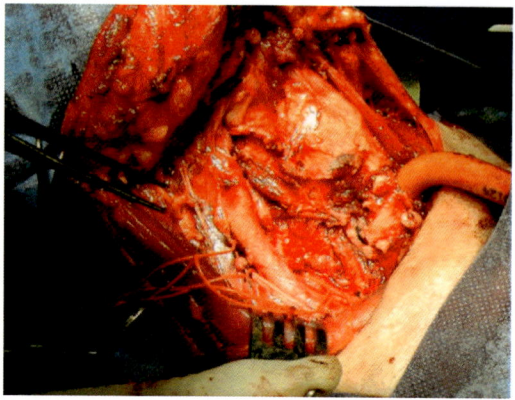

Fig. 44.4 Operating field after total thyroidectomy for massive metastases of renal carcinoma with tracheomalacia: a tracheostomy is performed at the end of the operation

44.10.4.2 Tests

Haemoglobin oxygen saturation (SpO_2) and laryngoscopy are useful to diagnose and monitor respiratory failure and rule out bilateral vocal cord paralysis or glottic/subglottic oedema, respectively.

44.10.5 Treatment

44.10.5.1 Surgical Treatment

When the diagnosis of tracheomalacia is posed, the treatment of choice is an early tracheostomy at the time of surgery, precisely identifying the most suitable tracheostomy site (Fig. 44.4). Early tracheostomy makes the trachea toilet and ventilatory care (e.g., suctioning) easier and provokes fibrosis of a soft trachea until it recovers from tracheomalacia. The tracheostomy tube is usually removed within 10 days in most patients. Other management methods for tracheomalacia include prolonged intubation, tracheopexy, tracheal resection, external splinting with Marlex mesh, and external miniplate fixation of tracheal cartilages and placement of a buttress or graft. Short-term intubation (for 48 h postoperatively) has been proposed as a splint before extubation. Nonetheless, a floppy trachea from a long-standing compression is hardly going to become a structurally competent one in such a short lapse of time [41].

44.11 Laryngotracheal Complex Injuries

Invasive thyroid cancer can put the laryngotracheal complex at risk of injuries during surgery. The surgeon should be experienced in adopting multiple approaches to the RLN and the laryngotracheal plane, reaching maximum infiltration areas after correctly identifying the nobile structures in ideal and uninvolved planes. The reoperations for recurrent thyroid disease show similar difficulties in identifying the correct planes.

During the preoperative workup, patients with vocal symptoms, recurrent disease, respiratory or swallowing anomalies, paralyzed or paretic vocal cord, evidence of infiltration of the larynx or trachea at laryngoscopy, or evidence of distal metastases, appropriate imaging of the laryngotracheal complex should be obtained.

The preoperative imaging study helps to plan a surgical strategy that foresees a potential reconstruction of the airway. Laryngoscopy, tracheoscopy and bronchoscopy are all required to clarify the extent of the airway invasion.

The involvement of the tracheal wall can be managed with a shave excision if superficial or a segmental or window resection if transmural. Shave resections carry a high risk of local recurrence, and therefore, it is recommended only for cases in which the involvement of the trachea is minimal [42–44]. Moreover, a circumferential involvement should be suspected based on the longitudinal extent of a tumour within the external wall or the lumen: in these situations, a segmental resection should be preferred to a window one. The surgical specimen of the tracheal resection should always be examined with frozen sections. The reconstruction of the trachea can be obtained with a sliding tracheoplasty for small windows. In case of resections involving less than one-third of the circumference of a few rings, a tracheotomy tube can be placed in the defect and removed after 3–4 days. If the resections involve approximately 50% of the circumference, more complex techniques are required, such as pectoralis or sternocleidomastoid myoperiosteal flaps. These reconstructions aim to prevent granulation on the mucosal aspect, which determines obstruction of the airway and supports the trachea wall during inspiration. An alternative technique consists of the following steps: at first, the skin of the neck is sutured to the trachea mucosa creating a stoma; after 3 weeks, when the stoma has healed, cartilage or titanium mesh is implanted in the subcutaneous tissue at the stomal edge through a circumferential incision, the tracheal wall is recreated by folding over the skin flap with the underlying cartilage or titanium, and the defect of the neck skin can be closed primarily or with a flap.

The segmental resection of the trachea is repaired through an end-to-end anastomosis, using interrupted stitches without tension. In cases of a few rings' resections, a mobilization of the trachea is sufficient to free the stumps from tension; in cases of more extensive resections, the mobilization of the laryngotracheal complex through the suprahyoid release is necessary. In sporadic cases, a hilar release can be applied to complete the reconstruction. The freeing of the trachea should anyway be cautious to avoid lesions to the RLNs and the vascularization. To keep the endotracheal tube in place after the operation for 1 day is advisable to avoid the immediate subcutaneous emphysema secondary to cough and Valsalva manoeuvres. To avoid undue early tension to the suture, due to hyperextension of the neck, a possible solution is the Grillo stitch, a suture that anchors the mentum to the chest that is maintained for 1 week.

The major concern after thyroid repair is the leak: a precise and strict technique with separate stitches circumferentially can minimize this risk. The air leak may cause infection, abscess, mediastinitis, and vessels' erosion.

The larynx can be invaded by thyroid cancer at the cricothyroid space or around the posterior aspect of the thyroid cartilage ala. In this case, the ala can be removed, given that cancer has not penetrated the pyriform sinus. In case of more extensive involvements, vertical hemilaryngectomy is suggested fashioning a temporary tracheostomy including the hemicricoid cartilage. Total laryngectomy is required when more than one-third of the cricoid cartilage or half of the laryngeal framework is involved [45]. To restore the laryngeal function is important to preserve an intact and mobile cricoarytenoid unit. Nevertheless, the necessity of adjuvant radiation therapy and the biological aggressiveness of the tumour should guide the decision to attempt an immediate reconstruction or not. The placement of a speaking valve and a tracheo-oesophageal puncture is an effective mean to control the disease and restore voice and swallowing, although with a permanent tracheostomy.

44.12 Pneumothorax

44.12.1 Epidemiology

Pneumothorax (PNX) can be spontaneous or traumatic; iatrogenic PNX is a subgroup of traumatic one [46]. PNX that manifests in the context of thyroid and parathyroid surgery is iatrogenic and overall rare, resulting from direct or indirect

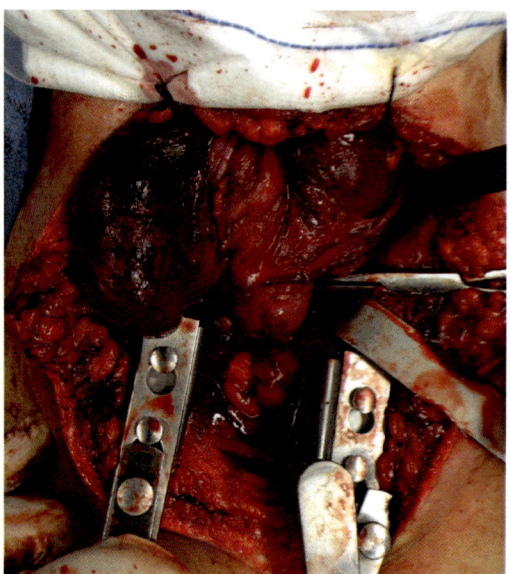

Fig. 44.5 Total thyroidectomy performed for a substernal goiter through a manubriotomy

injuries to the pleural sac. The main risk factors are substernal goitres, malignancies that invade the mediastinum, and extension of lymph nodes dissection below the clavicles (Fig. 44.5).

44.12.2 Etiology

During thyroid surgery, especially for substernal goitre or large malignancies with lymph nodes removal, the dissection can extend toward the pleural sac and superior mediastinum. In this case, the air or gas can directly access these spaces through direct lesion of the pleura with or without full-thickness perforations of the trachea or oesophagus, causing PNX with or without pneumomediastinum.

44.12.3 Pathophysiology

Tracheal injuries during thyroid surgery can determine an egress for air that can easily track down into the mediastinum: this lesion, without pleural injuries, is not in itself able to lead to PNX [47]. The risk of tracheal injury is maximum during the dissection of the thyroid isthmus and the freeing of the Zuckerkandl tubercles and is higher in case of extensive tracheal deformation. Tracheal perforations occur through the fibrous septations between rings. In the absence of pleural violation, a tracheal injury can cause only subcutaneous emphysema and pneumomediastinum, which often can heal spontaneously.

Oesophageal perforations may occur during surgery for thyroid malignancies because of anatomic disruption of the normal planes, resulting in leakage of air and fluids in the paratracheal region, potentially leading to pleural erosion and hydropneumothorax. Underlying lung diseases can also cause or facilitate this event, and this is the case of ND for metastatic thyroid carcinoma with lung metastases or positive pressure ventilation during general anaesthesia [48]. Indeed, the positive airway pressure from assisted ventilation can lead to alveolar rupture, and this is particularly common in patients with chronic obstructive lung disease or emphysema. Mechanical ventilation can determine the progression of a simple PNX to tension PNX, with risk of obstructive shock due to mediastinum displacement, contralateral lung compression and venous return drastic reduction.

44.12.4 Diagnosis

44.12.4.1 Clinical Presentation

Symptoms of PNX include pleuritic chest pain, palpitations and dyspnoea with shortness of breath. Signs are decreased ipsilateral chest excursion, diminished or absent breath sounds, and hyper-resonant percussion. These clinical manifestations might be subtle, while tachycardia, tachypnoea, and hypotension can suggest tension PNX, requiring immediate recognition and treatment. Arterial blood gas measurement is recommended if oxygen saturation falls below <92%: it usually reveals respiratory alkalosis. Hypercapnia is typically rare, assuming that the contralateral lung grants adequate ventilation. During general anaesthesia, PNX can manifest with tachycardia, hypotension, hypercapnia and hypoxia.

44.12.4.2 Tests

A computed tomography scan of the chest is the gold standard in the detection and measurement of PNXs, and it helps identify and describe the correct chest tube placement or underlying lung disease. Anyway, a chest radiograph in the upright posterior–anterior fashion is the first examination to be performed in case of suggestive clinical manifestations to identify the displacement of the visceral pleural line. Lateral and supine chest radiographs are less sensitive, while inspiratory and expiratory radiographs are equal. An essential limitation of a standard chest radiograph is the difficulty in measuring the size of the PNX.

44.12.5 Treatment

Most PNXs after thyroid surgery result from minor pleural injuries due to inadvertent electrocautery or blunt dissection. These situations grossly behave like primary spontaneous PNXs resulting from the rupture of pleural blebs. The course of these situations can vary from spontaneous and early sealing to ongoing air leak and progression. Moreover, these common situations must be distinguished from the rare ones depending on deep penetrating injuries of the pleura and the underlying lung.

Treatment should be subsequently framed, with approaches ranging from simple intercostal needle decompression to formal chest tube placement, always considering the risk of ongoing air leak and haemothorax. The therapeutic management should also be tailored to the patient characteristics, aiming to eliminate the air collection, favouring the pleural healing and preventing recurrences.

Observation, O_2 therapy, needle or catheter decompression, chest tube placement, persistent neck drains and thoracoscopy are all therapeutic options.

Dyspnoea and the size of the PNX are probably the main factors determining the strategy: the first prompts the indication for the operative treatment, regardless of size, the second indicates the timing of spontaneous resolution/reabsorption, that is based on a rate between 1.25% and 2.2% of the volume of the hemithorax per day.

44.12.5.1 Medical Treatment

Small PNXs can be described as follows: less than 15% of the hemithorax or less than 2–3 cm between the lung and the chest wall at chest radiograph [49]. Clinically stable patients with small PNX can be managed with observation and supplemental O_2 therapy. The discharge of these patients can be after 4–6 h of observation after a repeated chest radiograph, excluding progression of the PNX. Observation should be prolonged in patients living far from the emergency service or fragile patients with many comorbidities. Discharged patients should be aware of avoiding flying, diving, trips to a higher elevation and should be followed up after 48 h with a new chest radiograph and clinical evaluation.

44.12.5.2 Surgical Treatment

In case of PNX greater than 15% of the hemithorax or larger than 3 cm between the lung and the chest wall, or instability with tachycardia and hypoxia, or progressive PNX evident at chest radiographs, operative management is recommended. The treatment aims to prevent further damages, minimise the hospital stay, and re-expand the lung to prevent recurrences.

The choice among simple aspiration or chest tube placement as first-line treatment is debated. The decision making should take into account both devices and patients characteristics.

In case of aspiration, a 14–18 G needle is recommended; aspiration should cease after 2.5 L because of the high likelihood of air leak in this situation. Needle aspiration is less painful and equally efficacious as chest tube placement, but repeated aspiration is not recommended: a chest tube placement should be planned in case of failure of aspiration.

In case of tube placement as first line treatment, a small-bore catheter (<14 F) or a chest tube (16–22 F) should be considered. Both these devices can be attached to Heimlich valve or water seal device with or without suction [50].

The preferred place for simple aspiration is the second intercostal space in the midclavicular line.

Simple aspiration is feasible through commercial kits, usually made by a 14–18 G needle with a small-bore (7–14 F) catheter that is introduced in the pleural space. The air is manually aspirated after the needle removal, measuring the volume, syringe by syringe, evaluating the tactile resistance to aspiration. If there is no resistance after 2.5 L, an air leak is suspected, and further intervention should be considered.

After aspiration, the catheter can be immediately removed or attached to a water seal device or one-way valve, allowing for safe observation. Chest radiograph after 6 h should check for PNX progression.

The indicated place for the pleural drain is the fourth or fifth intercostal space in the middle or anterior axillary line, for larger devices, or the second intercostal space in the midclavicular line, for a small-bore catheter-directed toward the apex of the pleural space.

Small uncomplicated PNXs in stable patients are amenable for treatment with small chest tubes (<22 F) or catheters (<14 F). Larger PNXs, unstable patients, presence of air leak, and active intrathoracic haemorrhage are indications for larger tubes (≥24 F), allowing for a greater amount of air to flow through the device. The insertion procedure can be a classic Seldinger technique or a standard blunt dissection with Kelly forceps.

A water seal device without suction is recommended in case of air leaks and need for positive pressure ventilation. Suction should be, therefore, applied in case the lung fails to re-expand. Similarly, when the initial management requires a Heimlich valve, the switch to a water seal device with suction is recommended in re-expansion failure. In summary, suction is not routinely recommended, but the optimal pressure is between −10 to −20 cm H_2O.

Air leaks may originate from the lung or the drainage system and chest tube. After careful inspection of these devices, it is important to differentiate from broncho-pleural and alveolar–pleural fistulas. The first originates from an injury to a segmental, lobar or mainstem bronchus. The second originates from a lesion of the most distal airways. Alveolar–pleural fistulas are likely to seal spontaneously and are often visible during forced expiration. In case of persistent air leaks, after 14 days of observation, possible interventions are the one-way valve, infusion of autologous blood into the pleural space, pleurodesis, video-assisted thoracoscopy with oversewing of the fistula.

The most common complication of chest tube placement is malposition, which is associated with persistent PNX. This situation is clinically and radiologically suspected and confirmed through CT scan. The treatment is the repositioning or replacement. Other rare complications reported are lung injury, diaphragmatic perforation, subcutaneous placement, bleeding from an intercostal artery, recurrence, empyema, contralateral PNX, perforation of heart, abdominal organs, large vessels, cardiogenic shock, and pneumomediastinum.

The chest tube removal should be planned after radiologically proven resolution of the PNX. Moreover, the daily fluid output should be less than 100–200 mL/day. The removal steps should be first removing suction, then performing a trial with water seal, then final radiograph and removal. The clamping for 4–6 h before removal can help to identify small air leaks. In case of positive pressure ventilation, it is recommended to leave the chest tube in place until ventilation is required. The removal should be performed during a Valsalva manoeuvre, and a post-removal radiograph should be performed after 4–6 h.

Discharged patients should avoid diving, flying, high-elevation activities and should be educated about returning to the nearest emergency service in case of recurrent symptoms. The initial follow-up with chest radiograph should be planned after 1 week.

PNX after thyroid surgery is rare, but the surgeon should know its risks and be aware of its suggestive clinical signs and symptoms. The management should be tailored to the patient characteristics.

44.13 Injuries to the Cervical Oesophagus

The cervical oesophagus is exposed to infiltration by invasive thyroid and parathyroid cancer, but transmural involvement is rare. In addition, bening disease, if very large and extended posteriorly can put the oesophagus at risk during surgery.

Placing a bougie during thyroid or parathyroid surgery requiring oesophageal dissection can help identify the planes, dissect the musculature, and respect the submucosal. If a defect is created till the oesophageal mucosa, a primary repair is required, maintaining the bogie with an adequate caliper (38 F or larger). If primary repair is impossible, or the defect is diagnosed after surgery with severe contamination, adequate debridement and temporary drainage/diversion are required, with T-tube repair, oesophagostomy, oesophagectomy. The immediate reconstruction after oesophagectomy should be considered only in case of optimal surgical expertise and local and general patient conditions. In any case of primary repair, the suture should be covered with grafts from the pectoralis or the sternocleidomastoid muscles.

44.14 Seroma and Wound Infection

Seroma formation has been reported in 6–9% of neck surgeries and is more prevalent after ND, total thyroidectomy, and after surgery for substernal goitre.

Wound infections occur in 1–2% of cases, regardless of the extent of surgery, and may be secondary to PH. The management of these complications does not differ from other sites.

> **Dos and Don'ts**
> - Check for voice, swallowing issues or tremors after neck surgery.
> - Monitor the drain and the neck swelling in the first hours after neck surgery.
> - Avoid operating on patients with extensive neck malignancies without a panned strategy to manage vessels, trachea or oesophagus infiltration.
> - Avoid undertaking improvised bedside management of bleedings without planning the securing of the airway.

> **Take-Home Messages**
> - Laryngeal nerve injuries are rarely structural transections of the trunk: they are often consequences of excessive tractions and can be avoided thanks to intraoperative nerve monitor.
> - Hypocalcemia is one of the most common issues after thyroid surgery: most cases are transient and can be easily managed with medical therapy.
> - Laryngotracheal or oesophageal lesions during neck surgery are mostly due to malignancy: their management is often a careful intraoperative primary repair.
> - The accurate preoperative study helps prevent injuries to neck major vessels: the haemorrhage can be evident intraoperatively or postoperatively, with specific care to source control in the first case and airway management in the second.
> - Most PNX cases are caused by direct pleural lesion during neck surgery and can be managed with observation and O_2.

Questions

1. Criteria for intraoperative diagnosis of tracheomalacia:
   A. Soft and floppy trachea on palpation with the endotracheal tube in situ
   B. **Obstruction to spontaneous respiration during gradual withdrawal of the endotracheal tube after thyroidectomy**
   C. peritubal leak on deflation of endotracheal tube cuff
   D. easy overcoming of the endotracheal tube with the suction catheter during its gradual withdrawal

2. About Recurrent Laryngeal Nerve Palsy:
   A. Unilateral vocal cord palsy causes dyspnea at rest
   B. **Bilateral vocal cord palsy could cause post-operative extubation failure**
   C. Unilateral vocal cord palsy may require tracheotomy because of compromised swallowing
   D. Unilateral vocal cord palsy cannot recover without partial arytenoidectomy

3. About SAN injury:
   A. results in trapezius and sternocleidomastoid muscles atrophy
   B. symptoms and the diagnosis often occurs during firsts post-operative days
   C. **initial symptom is shoulder drop**
   D. electromyography allows diagnosis just months after injury

4. Which of the following is the major issue after a tracheal repair after tracheal resection for thyroid cancer?
   A. Stricture
   B. **Air leak**
   C. Dysphonia
   D. Necrosis

5. What is the correct management for an oesophageal injury diagnosed during thyroid cancer surgery?
   A. Cervical oesophagostomy
   B. Oesophagectomy
   C. **Primary repair with bogie**
   D. External drainage

6. Which of the following is the most common anomaly of the major vessels of the neck?
   A. **Aberrant right subclavian artery**
   B. Left innominate artery
   C. Innominate artery originating from the left common carotid artery
   D. Retro-oesophageal innominate artery

7. Which of the following are the cornerstones of intraoperative management of neck major vessels injuries during neck surgery?
   A. Packing and endovascular management
   B. **Composure, compression, anesthesiologic and specialistic alert and support, identification, exposure, proximal and distal control of the injured vessel, suture**
   C. Massive use of hemostatic agents before any attempt of isolating the injured vessel
   D. Compression and vascular surgery referral

8. What is the most common etiology of pneumothorax after neck surgery?
   A. **Inadvertent intraoperative direct lesion to the pleura**
   B. Alveolar rupture
   C. Tracheal perforation
   D. Oesophageal perforation

9. What is the correct management of a small pneumothorax in a stable patient after thyroid surgery?
   A. Observation
   B. O_2
   C. **Observation and O_2**
   D. Chest tube placement

> 10. What is the most common complication after chest tube placement for post-operative pneumothorax in thyroid surgery?
>   A. Hemothorax
>   B. Diaphragmatic lesions
>   C. Aortic/azygos vein lesions
>   **D. Chest tube displacement, diagnosed with CT scan**

References

1. Goldenberg D, Randolph GW, Holm TM, Pai SI, Shindo M, Quintanilla-Dieck L, et al. The recurrent laryngeal nerve [Internet]. Thyroid Surg. 2013:117–27. (Wiley Online Books). https://doi.org/10.1002/9781118444832.ch13.
2. Sarkis LM, Zaidi N, Norlén O, Delbridge LW, Sywak MS, Sidhu SB. Bilateral recurrent laryngeal nerve injury in a specialized thyroid surgery unit: would routine intraoperative neuromonitoring alter outcomes? ANZ J Surg. 2017;87(5):364–7.
3. Swonke ML, Shakibai N, Chaaban MR. Medical malpractice trends in thyroidectomies among general surgeons and otolaryngologists. OTO Open. 2020;4(2):2473974X20921141.
4. Shen WT, Kebebew E, Duh Q-Y, Clark OH. Predictors of airway complications after thyroidectomy for substernal goiter. Arch Surg [Internet]. 2004;139(6):656–60. https://doi.org/10.1001/archsurg.139.6.656.
5. Randolph GW, Kamani D. The importance of preoperative laryngoscopy in patients undergoing thyroidectomy: voice, vocal cord function, and the preoperative detection of invasive thyroid malignancy. Surgery. 2006;139(3):357–62.
6. Testini M, Gurrado A, Bellantone R, Brazzarola P, Cortese R, De Toma G, et al. Recurrent laryngeal nerve palsy and substernal goiter. An Italian multicenter study. J Visc Surg. 2014;151(3)
7. Gurrado A, Pasculli A, Pezzolla A, Di Meo G, Fiorella ML, Cortese R, et al. A method to repair the recurrent laryngeal nerve during thyroidectomy. Can J Surg. 2018;61(4)
8. Sunderland S. A classification of peripheral nerve injuries producing loss of function. Brain. 1951;74(4):491–516.
9. Popovski V, Benedetti A, Popovic-Monevska D, Grcev A, Stamatoski A, Zhivadinovik J. Spinal accessory nerve preservation in modified neck dissections: surgical and functional outcomes. Acta Otorhinolaryngol Ital organo Uff della Soc Ital di Otorinolaringol e Chir Cerv-facc. 2017;37(5):368–74.
10. Grant CS. Lesions following lateral neck dissection [Internet]. Thyroid Surg. 2013:169–77. (Wiley Online Books). https://doi.org/10.1002/9781118444832.ch19.
11. Mayer JA, Hruby LA, Salminger S, Bodner G, Aszmann OC. Reconstruction of the spinal accessory nerve with selective fascicular nerve transfer of the upper trunk. J Neurosurg Spine SPI [Internet]. 31(1):133–8. https://thejns.org/spine/view/journals/j-neurosurg-spine/31/1/article-p133.xml
12. Carr SD, Bowyer D, Cox G. Upper limb dysfunction following selective neck dissection: a retrospective questionnaire study. Head Neck. 2009;31(6):789–92.
13. Murthy SP, Paderno A, Balasubramanian D. Management of the marginal mandibular nerve during and after neck dissection. Curr Opin Otolaryngol Head Neck Surg. 2019;27(2):104–9.
14. Møller MN, Sørensen CH. Risk of marginal mandibular nerve injury in neck dissection. Eur Arch oto-rhino-laryngology Off J Eur Fed Oto-Rhino-Laryngological Soc Affil with Ger Soc Oto-Rhino-Laryngology - Head Neck Surg. 2012;269(2):601–5.
15. Chiesa Estomba C, Sistiaga Suárez J, González-García J, Larruscain-Sarasola E, Thomas Arrizabalaga I, Altuna MX. Marginal mandibular nerve injury during neck dissection of level IIa, and the influence of different types of dissection: diathermy versus cold knife. Otolaryngol Pol = Polish Otolaryngol. 2018;72(4):21–5.
16. Edafe O, Antakia R, Laskar N, Uttley L, Balasubramanian SP. Systematic review and meta-analysis of predictors of post-thyroidectomy hypocalcaemia. Br J Surg. 2014;101(4):307–20.
17. Shindo M. The parathyroid glands in thyroid surgery [Internet]. Thyroid Surg. 2013:137–43. (Wiley Online Books). https://doi.org/10.1002/9781118444832.ch15.
18. Vidal Fortuny J, Karenovics W, Triponez F, Sadowski SM. Intra-operative indocyanine green angiography of the parathyroid gland. World J Surg. 2016;40(10):2378–81.
19. Karampinis I, Di Meo G, Gerken A, Stasiunaitis V, Lammert A, Nowak K. Intraoperative indocyanine green fluorescence to assure vital parathyroids in thyroid resections. Zentralblatt fur Chir - Zeitschrift fur Allg Visz und Gefasschirurgie. 2018;143(4)
20. Delaney SW, Shi H, Shokrani A, Sinha UK. Management of chyle leak after head and neck surgery: review of current treatment strategies. Betka J, editor. Int J Otolaryngol [Internet]. 2017;2017:8362874. https://doi.org/10.1155/2017/8362874.
21. Roh J-L, Kim DH, Il PC. Prospective identification of chyle leakage in patients undergoing lateral neck dissection for metastatic thyroid cancer. Ann Surg Oncol. 2008;15(2):424–9.

22. Smoke A, Delegge MH. Chyle leaks: consensus on management? Nutr Clin Pract Off Publ Am Soc Parenter Enter Nutr. 2008;23(5):529–32.
23. Gregor RT. Management of chyle fistulization in association with neck dissection. Otolaryngol neck Surg Off J Am Acad Otolaryngol Neck Surg. 2000;122(3):434–9.
24. Godballe C, Madsen AR, Pedersen HB, Sørensen CH, Pedersen U, Frisch T, et al. Post-thyroidectomy hemorrhage: a national study of patients treated at the Danish departments of ENT Head and Neck Surgery. Eur Arch oto-rhino-laryngology Off J Eur Fed Oto-Rhino-Laryngological Soc Affil with Ger Soc Oto-Rhino-Laryngology - Head Neck Surg. 2009;266(12):1945–52.
25. Williams RT, Angelos P. Postoperative bleeding [Internet]. Thyroid Surg. 2013:199–207. (Wiley Online Books). https://doi.org/10.1002/9781118444832.ch22.
26. Burkey SH, van Heerden JA, Thompson GB, Grant CS, Schleck CD, Farley DR. Reexploration for symptomatic hematomas after cervical exploration. Surgery. 2001;130(6):914–20.
27. Rosato L, Avenia N, Bernante P, De Palma M, Gulino G, Nasi PG, et al. Complications of thyroid surgery: analysis of a multicentric study on 14,934 patients operated on in Italy over 5 years. World J Surg. 2004;28(3):271–6.
28. Samraj K, Gurusamy KS. Wound drains following thyroid surgery. Cochrane database Syst Rev. 2007;(4):CD006099.
29. Bergenfelz A, Jansson S, Kristoffersson A, Mårtensson H, Reihnér E, Wallin G, et al. Complications to thyroid surgery: results as reported in a database from a multicenter audit comprising 3,660 patients. Langenbeck's Arch Surg. 2008;393(5):667–73.
30. Testini M, Marzaioli R, Lissidini G, Lippolis A, Logoluso F, Gurrado A, et al. The effectiveness of FloSeal matrix hemostatic agent in thyroid surgery: a prospective, randomized, control study. Langenbeck's Arch Surg. 2009;394(5):837–42.
31. Testini M, Pasculli A, Di Meo G, Ferraro V, Logoluso F, Minerva F, et al. Advanced vessel sealing devices in total thyroidectomy for substernal goitre: a retrospective cohort study. Int J Surg. 2016;35
32. Reeve T, Thompson NW. Complications of thyroid surgery: how to avoid them, how to manage them, and observations on their possible effect on the whole patient. World J Surg. 2000;24(8):971–5.
33. Upadhyaya PK, Bertellotti R, Laeeq A, Sugimoto J. Beware of the aberrant innominate artery. Ann Thorac Surg. 2008;85(2):653–4.
34. Ozlugedik S, Ozcan M, Unal A, Yalcin F, Tezer MS. Surgical importance of highly located innominate artery in neck surgery. Am J Otolaryngol. 2005;26(5):330–2.
35. Franco I, Gurrado A, Lissidini G, Di Meo G, Pasculli A, Testini M. Floating left innominate vein neoplastic thrombus: a rare case of mediastinal extension of follicular thyroid carcinoma. Phlebology. 2015;30(2)
36. Allan JS, Wright CD. Tracheoinnominate fistula: diagnosis and management. Chest Surg Clin N Am. 2003;13(2):331–41.
37. Powitzky R, Vasan N, Krempl G, Medina J. Carotid blowout in patients with head and neck cancer. Ann Otol Rhinol Laryngol. 2010;119(7):476–84.
38. Mackle T, Meaney J, Timon C. Tracheoesophageal compression associated with substernal goitre. Correlation of symptoms with cross-sectional imaging findings. J Laryngol Otol. 2007;121(4):358–61.
39. Green WE, Shepperd HW, Stevenson HM, Wilson W. Tracheal collapse after thyroidectomy. Br J Surg. 1979;66(8):554–7.
40. Agarwal A, Mishra AK, Gupta SK, Arshad F, Agarwal A, Tripathi M, et al. High incidence of tracheomalacia in longstanding goiters: experience from an endemic goiter region. World J Surg. 2007;31(4):832–7.
41. Ozaki O, Sugino K, Mimura T, Ito K. Surgery for patients with thyroid carcinoma invading the trachea: circumferential sleeve resection followed by end-to-end anastomosis. Surgery. 1995;117(3):268–71.
42. McCarty TM, Kuhn JA, Williams WLJ, Ellenhorn JD, O'Brien JC, Preskitt JT, et al. Surgical management of thyroid cancer invading the airway. Ann Surg Oncol. 1997;4(5):403–8.
43. Honings J, Stephen AE, Marres HA, Gaissert HA. The management of thyroid carcinoma invading the larynx or trachea. Laryngoscope. 2010;120(4):682–9.
44. Nishida T, Nakao K, Hamaji M. Differentiated thyroid carcinoma with airway invasion: indication for tracheal resection based on the extent of cancer invasion. J Thorac Cardiovasc Surg. 1997;114(1):84–92.
45. McCaffrey TV, Lipton RJ. Thyroid carcinoma invading the upper aerodigestive system. Laryngoscope. 1990;100(8):824–30.
46. Sahn SA, Heffner JE. Spontaneous pneumothorax. N Engl J Med. 2000;342(12):868–74.
47. Noppen M, De Keukeleire T. Pneumothorax. Respiration. 2008;76(2):121–7.
48. Lee M-J, Kim E-K, Kim MJ, Kwak JY, Hong S, Park CS. Spontaneous pneumothorax in metastatic thyroid papillary carcinoma. J Clin Oncol Off J Am Soc Clin Oncol. 2007;25(18):2616–8.
49. MacDuff A, Arnold A, Harvey J. Management of spontaneous pneumothorax: British Thoracic Society Pleural Disease Guideline 2010. Thorax. 2010;65(Suppl 2):ii18–31.
50. Wakai A, O'Sullivan RG, McCabe G. Simple aspiration versus intercostal tube drainage for primary spontaneous pneumothorax in adults. Cochrane database Syst Rev. 2007;(1):CD004479.

Further Reading

Chirica M, Kelly MD, Siboni S, Aiolfi A, Riva CG, Asti E, et al. Esophageal emergencies: WSES guidelines World. J Emerg Surg. 2019;14:26. https://doi.org/10.1186/s13017-019-0245-2.

Part III

Thorax and Mediastinum

Emergency Surgical Access to the Thorax

Marc de Moya and Rebecca Mitchell

45.1 Introduction

> **Learning Goals**
> - Review the surgical anatomy of the thoracic cavity
> - Understand that injury pattern and patient stability dictates surgical incision priority
> - Describe each surgical approach to the thorax based on suspected injury

Unintentional injury is the third leading cause of death in the United States and is the leading cause of death in ages 1–44. In 2019, this was 173,040 deaths [1]. Approximately 25% of traumatic deaths are the result of an injury to the thorax. Thoracic injury is common in trauma; the incidence varies by mechanism with 40% of patients with penetrating trauma and 33% of patients with a blunt mechanism sustaining a thoracic injury. Up to 50% of unrestrained drivers involved in a motor vehicle crash sustain a thoracic injury and it is thought that up to 25% of driver deaths have a known thoracic injury [2]. The population-adjusted incidence of thoracic injury has been increasing every year. From 2007 to 2016, the incidence increased by 8% per year across all age groups, with the greatest incidence in people older than 85 years [3]. Most blunt thoracic injuries are managed non-operatively with a focus on pain control, but in those that do require surgical intervention, it is critical to understand the relative anatomy and surgical approach.

45.2 Diagnosis

There are a number of diagnoses that would warrant emergency access to the chest. These include vascular, pulmonary, cardiac, or esophageal injuries most commonly. The diagnosis of individual injuries is beyond the scope of this chapter as we focus on the surgical access to the chest.

45.3 Treatment

45.3.1 Anatomy of the Thorax

45.3.1.1 Thoracic Cavity

The thoracic cavity has three compartments—the mediastinum and right and left pleural cavities. The mediastinum is divided into the superior and inferior mediastinum. The inferior mediastinum is further divided into anterior, middle, and posterior.

The pleural cavities extend up into the neck, approximately 2 cm superior to the mid-clavicle. An injury in this area should lead to evaluation

M. de Moya (✉) · R. Mitchell
Medical College of Wisconsin, Milwaukee, WI, USA
e-mail: mdemoya@mcw.edu; rmitchell@mcw.edu

for hemopneumothorax. The inferior border of the pleural cavities is lined by the diaphragm. This varies by location—anteriorly in the midclavicular line at rib 8, in the midaxillary line at rib 10, and posteriorly at the T12 vertebra.

45.3.1.2 Thoracoabdominal Boundaries

The thoraco-abdominal regions include the overlap between the abdomen and the thorax. Any injury within this region should prompt attention to both cavities due to the high likelihood of both cavities being injured. Naturally, there are gunshot wounds that could traverse the chest from the lower abdomen, but the likelihood is less. All penetrating wound trajectories must be investigated to ensure that the full tract is known. It is the tract of the penetrating injury that will dictate the anatomical injuries.

The superior thoracoabdominal borders are the 4th intercostal space in the midclavicular line, the 6th intercostal space in the midaxillary line, and the 8th intercostal space in the scapular line. The inferior thoracoabdominal border is the costal margin. The flank is defined by the area between the anterior and posterior axillary lines from the costal margin to the iliac crest. The back is defined as the area from the costal margin to iliac crests between the posterior axillary lines.

45.3.1.3 Cardiac Box

The cardiac box is defined by anatomic landmarks—the superior border is the clavicle, lateral is the midclavicular line, and inferior is down to the costal margin. The same box can be drawn on the back, using the scapular spines as the lateral boundaries. The cardiac box has been used to identify those penetrating injuries that have a high likelihood of cardiac injury. However, with the ubiquitous use of ultrasound to evaluate the heart and pleural spaces, the boundaries of the box are unlikely to change management. For example, gunshot wounds can easily be outside the box and still cause a cardiac injury given the longer injury tract. Therefore, ALL thoracic penetrating injuries should have an extended FAST exam that includes the heart and pleural spaces [4].

45.3.1.4 Subclavian Artery Anatomy

The subclavian artery is divided into three parts relative to the anterior scalene muscle. The first portion is from the origin of the subclavian artery off the arch to the medial border of the anterior scalene muscle. The second portion is located posterior to the anterior scalene muscle. The third portion is lateral to the anterior scalene muscle until it becomes the axillary artery at the lateral border of the first rib. This anatomy becomes important when deciding on the surgical approach.

45.3.2 Surgical Incisions

45.3.2.1 Best Approach Incision for Anatomic Injury

If the patient decompensates in the trauma bay and loses signs of life, a rapid resuscitative thoracotomy is needed [5–9]. If the patient is physiologically compensating and there are signs of cardiac injury, an immediate trip to the operating room is required and a median sternotomy is the incision of choice. Otherwise, if mediastinal structures are involved an anterior thoracotomy may be the better approach with the side chosen for best exposure or bilateral anterolateral thoracotomies [10–13]. A posterolateral incision is not preferred in the immediate acute scenario due to required patient positioning and the possible need for abdominal access. (Table 45.1)

45.3.2.2 Finger or Tube Thoracostomy

A finger thoracostomy is often done emergently in the setting of hemodynamic instability and tension pneumothorax. In this situation, a scalpel is used to make an incision and enter the pleural cavity as fast as possible in the same 4–5th intercostal space in the mid-axillary line as you would for a chest tube [14, 15]. A finger is inserted to verify correct position, thus called a "finger thoracostomy". As soon as the pleural cavity is entered, the tension physiology should be relieved. A chest tube can then be placed as described next.

45 Emergency Surgical Access to the Thorax

Table 45.1 Injury and preferred surgical approach

Injury	Preferred surgical approach
Unknown/Emergent	Left 5th anterolateral thoracotomy with possible extension to bilateral as needed
Cardiac	Median sternotomy
Innominate/Proximal right subclavian artery	Median sternotomy
Proximal left subclavian artery	Left 3rd–4th anterolateral thoracotomy
Left mid subclavian artery	Supraclavicular or infraclavicular incision with resection or retraction of medial clavicle
Right mid subclavian artery	Sternotomy with infraclavicular extension
Distal subclavian artery	Infraclavicular incision
Right/Left pulmonary hilum	Right/left anterolateral thoracotomy
Carina or right mainstem bronchus	Right 4th posterolateral thoracotomy if no access to abdomen is needed; other option is right anterolateral thoracotomy with bump under right back to elevate right lateral chest wall by 30 degrees to gain better posterior access while maintaining patient supine for abdominal access.
Left mainstem bronchus	Left 5th posterolateral thoracotomy

Preparation:
- Secure the patient's arm above their head. The elbow should be bent at a 90-degree angle with the hand above the head. Using a soft wrist restraint can be helpful, otherwise use tape. The arm can also be secured extended out 90 degrees from the body. In the emergent setting, someone can hold the arm and secure it, while the surgeon performs the procedure.
- Prep and drape the chest wall in the standard sterile fashion. In the emergent setting of a finger thoracostomy, the area of the incision is quickly prepped and the incision is made.
- Draw up local anesthesia
- Clamp the external end of the chest tube

Steps of the Procedure:
- Identify the 4th intercostal space in the mid-axillary line. In a male patient, this is at approximately the level of the nipple and in a female, and it is two fingerbreadths cephalad to the inframammary fold. Ultimately, one should be in the triangle of safety: posterior border (latissimus dorsi), anterior border (pectoralis major), and nipple line. An alternative tip is to use the inferior margin of the axillary hairline. This also places you within the triangle of safety. The mid-to-anterior axillary line should be used in the axial plane. Anesthetize the area using local anesthesia, infiltrating into the dermis and down to the superior border of the 5th rib, injecting the periosteum. Avoid the inferior border of the rib, as this is where the neurovascular bundle lies.
- Make a 1.5–2 cm incision with a scalpel and carry this down through the subcutaneous tissues and incise the thoracic fascia. Use a Kelly clamp to penetrate through the intercostal muscle and pleura just over the rib, you should feel a pop when you enter into the pleural cavity. Spread the clamp to widen this opening and then remove the clamp with it still open to help widen the tract. Place your finger into the pleural cavity to verify correct location and rotate 360 degrees to feel for any adhesions. Take care to avoid self-injury when doing this in the presence of rib fractures.
- Place the chest tube through the thoracostomy with one clamp on the tip (optional) and one clamp on the back end of the tube to prevent blood coming out of the tube prior to attaching the collection canister. The tube should be directed posteriorly and toward the apex, while rotating the tube 360 degrees to avoid it becoming kinked and stuck in the fissure. The most important component is to ensure that it is in the pleural space. If you meet resistance while placing the tube, pull the tube back and repeat. Placing a Kelly clamp at the tip can help direct the chest tube into the thoracic cavity, but it is often easier to just insert the chest tube alone as it is stiff enough.

- Next, the authors recommend lavaging the chest with 1L of warmed saline as described by Kugler et al. 2017 [16, 17]. Then, attach the chest tube to the drainage system, suture the tube in place, and secure it with an occlusive dressing. Connect the drainage system to suction and band the connection site with a zip tie or tape the connection to prevent inadvertent disconnection. Obtain a post-procedure chest X-ray to verify placement and evaluate for evacuation of the hemo/pneumothorax.
- If the initial output from the chest tube is 1500 mL or more, the patient should be taken to the operating room for a thoracotomy with massive transfusion ongoing. If the initial output is less than this threshold, but the chest tube continues to drain 250 mL per hour for the next 3 h after placement, this ongoing bleeding should also be evaluated in the operating room [18].

> **Dos and Don'ts**
> - Do—Ensure you are in the triangle of safety
> - Do—Rotate the chest tube to decrease the chance of it getting kinked in the major fissure
> - Do—Give a dose of prophylactic antibiotics
> - Do Not—Clamp the end of the chest tube too close to where you connect to the collection device. This prevents you from connecting before you un-clamp the chest tube.

45.3.2.3 Left Anterolateral Thoracotomy (Resuscitative Thoracotomy)

In the setting of a patient losing signs of life in the trauma bay (or within 15 min prior to arrival in the setting of penetrating trauma), a left anterolateral thoracotomy (resuscitative thoracotomy) (Fig. 45.1) performed in the emergency room is the procedure of choice [19–21]. The use of endovascular balloon occlusion in these settings

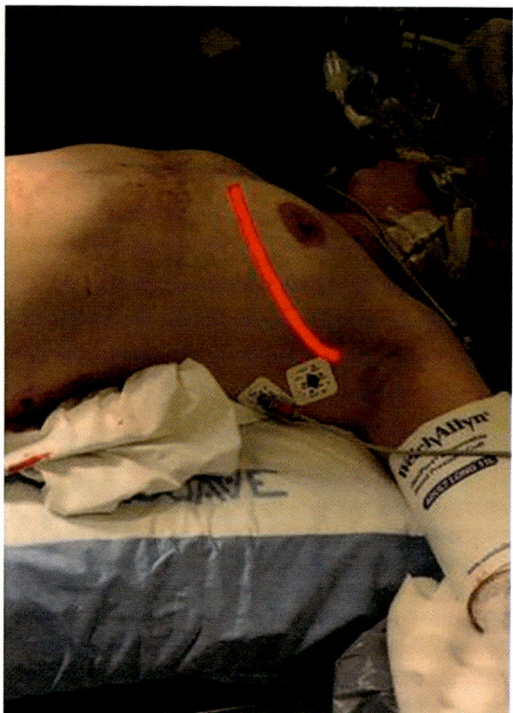

Fig. 45.1 Left anterolateral thoracotomy

has been considered by some but currently is not the standard of care and does not allow one to perform internal massage to supplement cardiac output or control bleeding in the chest. Suspicion should be high for a great vessel, cardiac, or aortic injury. External chest compressions may be initiated, while access is obtained and the instrument tray is opened; however, the effectiveness of external compression is poor in the face of profound hypovolemia. Therefore, no time should be wasted opening the chest [5, 6]. This incision allows for relieving cardiac tamponade, cross-clamping of the descending thoracic aorta in attempt to maintain perfusion to the brain and heart while allowing for open cardiac massage, and control of any bleeding in the thoracic cavity. Some have advocated to perform a simultaneous right-sided chest tube or finger thoracostomy; however, it is the authors' preference to simply enter the right chest immediately upon entering the left chest. This can be performed by retracting the pericardium posteriorly and bluntly entering the right-sided pleural space. This will diagnose any major hemorrhage on the right side or decompress any right-sided tension pneumothorax. If there is significant hemorrhage from the right side, then the decision to perform bilateral anterolateral thoracotomies (clam-shell thoracotomy) is made immediately.

The four main components of a resuscitative thoracotomy:

1. Incision to obtain access to the left thorax
2. Open the pericardium for either direct control of hemorrhage or internal cardiac massage
3. Cross-clamp the aorta
4. Control and cross-clamp the pulmonary hilum if needed

Preparation:
- Secure the patient's left arm over their head
- Prep and drape the entire chest
- Equipment:
  - Scalpel #20 or 10
  - 10" Mayo scissors
  - Finochietto retractor
  - Hemostats
  - 10" Metzenbaum scissors
  - Aortic clamp (Straight or Crawford type is preferred over Satinsky to ensure the tips are beyond the aorta for complete cross-clamp)
  - Satinsky clamp or a second Crawford clamp for possible pulmonary hilar clamping

Steps of the Procedure:
- Make an incision in the 4th or 5th intercostal space, along the superior border of the 5th or 6th rib in a curvilinear fashion along the course of the ribs. The easy anatomic landmark is to make an incision from the sternum to just under the nipple. In a woman, it is advised to lift the breast toward the head and make the incision in the infra-mammary fold. Extend the incision from the sternum medially, all the way down to the table laterally, following the rib. Use the scalpel to incise the skin, soft tissue, and pectoralis and serratus muscles. Transect the intercostal muscle and incise the pleura with heavy scissors, taking care not to injure the heart or lung. This should be opened from the sternum to the posterior extent of the wound. When done properly, the left internal mammary artery is divided and that can be dealt with later.
- Insert the Finochietto retractor with the crank of the handle closest to you or posterior. This allows you to extend the incision medially to the right thorax to perform bilateral thoracotomies without the crossbar in your way. Open the retractor until you can insert both hands into the chest cavity.
- Immediately push the pericardium posterior and bluntly force your hand in the avascular plane between the pericardium and sternum and open the right-sided pleura. If there is a significant amount of blood on the right side, immediately convert to a bilateral (clam-shell) anterolateral thoracotomy.
- Inspect the pericardium as you are pushing into the right side of the chest.
- If there is evidence of tamponade (hole in pericardium with hemorrhage or a purple blood filled pericardium), use a hemostat or toothed forceps to grasp the tense pericardium and elevate it. Use a Metzenbaum scissors to open the pericardium longitudinally anterior to the phrenic nerve, which also runs longitudinally. If the pericardium is too tense to grasp then make a small incision in it with the scalpel followed by the scissors. Take care to avoid injury to the myocardium. The pericardium must be opened beyond the apex and the base superiorly. The heart is then delivered out of the pericardium. The injury to the heart should be identified and controlled with direct finger pressure if able. Other techniques to control the hemorrhage include staples, vascular clamp, or foley balloon. However, if a cardiac injury is noted with hemopericardium, a clam-shell thoracotomy should be considered immediately to ensure full access to the right and left sides of the heart.
- If there is no evidence of tamponade or cardiac injury, gently retract the lung anteriorly and medially out of the way. Follow the posterior ribs back to the spine. The pleura

needs to be incised to gain access to the aorta. A small hole can be made with Metzenbaum scissors, either by cutting or using the tip of the scissors to bluntly penetrate into the pleura. Once a small hole is made, a finger can be used to easily make the hole bigger with blunt dissection. The aorta lies directly over the spine. After opening the pleura, bluntly pinch the aorta between your fingers to ensure that when the clamp is applied, you will be able to feel the right side of the aorta and ensure that the tips of the clamp are beyond the aorta. Take care not to injure the intercostal arteries coming off the aorta or the esophagus that lies anteriorly. Then, place the vascular clamp on the aorta.

- If there is a pulmonary hilar injury then one must divide the inferior pulmonary ligament taking care not to injure the inferior pulmonary vein. Once free from the ligament, the hilum can then be clamped with a vascular clamp, pinched with your fingers, or rotated 180 degrees to gain temporary control. When applying a vascular clamp, it is easier to apply coming from the inferior aspect and clamping parallel to the spine rather than perpendicular [22, 23].
- Continue massive transfusion to fill the heart while performing cardiac massage. If cardiac function returns, then proceed to the operating room to obtain more definitive control and continue resuscitation [24].

Dos and Don'ts
- Do—Extend skin incision from sternum to the stretcher
- Do—Initiate rapid blood transfusion simultaneously
- Do—Bluntly enter the right chest from the left side between the pericardium and the sternum
- Do-Not—delay the decision to perform a resuscitative thoracotomy
- Do-Not—compromise on your exposure (incision, opening up retractor widely, performing clam-shell if needed)

45.3.2.4 Bilateral Anterolateral Thoracotomy (Clam-Shell Thoracotomy)

If you perform a left anterolateral thoracotomy and, as mentioned above, you discover either blood coming from the right side of the chest or a cardiac injury, the incision can be extended to a bilateral/clamshell thoracotomy [25]. A right anterolateral thoracotomy is performed in the same interspace as the left (being careful not to go too low as the diaphragm is higher on the right side). The sternum is divided with a heavy scissors, Lebsche knife, or pneumatic saw. You now have access to the anterior heart, great vessels, and bilateral thoracic cavities. In making this incision, you will have divided both the right and left internal mammary arteries and you will need to identify and ligate all four ends before leaving the operating room.

45.3.2.5 Posterolateral Thoracotomy

A posterolateral thoracotomy is not performed in an emergent setting. For this incision, the patient is positioned in a lateral decubitus position which limits access to the contralateral chest and abdomen. For emergent operations, the patient should always be placed supine with their arms out. If there is concern for injury to a posterior mediastinal structure, it is reasonable to bump the ipsilateral side up a bit while maintaining the abdomen flat. This provides a bit more posterior access. In doing this, make sure that the ipsilateral arm is supported appropriately to avoid a stretch injury. The top leg should be extended at the knee and the bottom leg flexed at the knee with both joints padded with gel or pillows. The patient's torso is secured in position by a bean bag or rolls and tape placed across the hips to the table.

45.3.2.6 Pericardial Window

A pericardial window is performed when there is suspicion for an isolated penetrating cardiac injury with an equivocal FAST exam or a patient with long standing medical condition that may cause a chronic pericardial effusion. In addition, anyone being considered for a window must be hemodynamically stable; for those unstable, one should proceed directly to a median sternotomy. A pericardial window is performed in the operating room and one must be ready to immediately open the chest with a median sternotomy if an uncontrolled cardiac injury is diagnosed. If there is a small-to-moderate amount of sanguineous drainage but the patient remains hemodynamically normal, the pericardial sac can be irrigated with warm saline and a pericardial drain is placed and then observed for signs of ongoing bleeding. If there is continued bleeding, a median sternotomy should be performed. If the effluent is purely serous, this would rule out an injury, and no further intervention is necessary [26–28]. There are three different approaches to the pericardial window described below.

Preparation:
- In the operating room, the patient is placed with arms out at 90 degrees
- The patient is prepped and draped from the chin to knees bilaterally
- Equipment:
  - Scalpel #10
  - Metzenbaum scissors
  - Mayo scissors
  - Allis clamps
  - Narrow Richardson retractor

Steps of the Procedure:
- The subxiphoid approach—a midline incision is made over the xiphoid process. This is carried down through the subcutaneous tissues and the xiphoid process is cleared of surrounding fat. The xiphoid process is transected from the sternum using a heavy scissors. The sternum is elevated anteriorly, and the diaphragm displaced inferiorly as an extraperitoneal plane is created with blunt dissection using fingers just posterior to the sternum into the mediastinum. The pericardium is then grasped with two Allis clamps and incised vertically with scissors, taking care not to injure the heart.
- A second approach is transabdominal. This is used when the immediate concern for hemorrhage source was the abdomen and an exploratory laparotomy was performed. With the abdomen open, you can access the pericardium via an incision in the central tendon of the diaphragm. From the abdomen, one can easily visualize the pericardium moving deep to the tendinous portion of the diaphragm. Grasp this portion of the diaphragm with two Allis clamps and divide in between them until the pericardium is obvious. Then, the pericardium is grasped with Allis clamps and a small opening is made with the scissors.
- The left anterior Chamberlain approach is a mini-anterior thoracotomy made in the 5th intercostal space just to the left of the sternum. The incision is carried down to the pleura and a self-retaining retractor is applied to the overlying muscle. An opening is made in the pleura and the pericardium grasped with Allis clamps and incised.

45.3.2.7 Median Sternotomy

Median sternotomy is the incision of choice for an isolated injury to the anterior thorax or superior mediastinum with concern for injury to the heart or proximal great vessels [29, 30]. With multiple injuries and an unclear source of injury, an anterolateral thoracotomy should be used to allow for cross-clamping the aorta if needed. The median sternotomy allows access to the great vessels from the innominate to the left common carotid artery. The proximal left subclavian artery should be approached via a high left anterolateral thoracotomy as described in the next section. The median sternotomy can be extended with a lateral supra or infra-clavicular incision to obtain distal control of the subclavian artery or with a longitudinal cervical incision to obtain distal control of the carotid artery [31–34].

Preparation:
- In the operating room, the patient is placed with arms out at 90 degrees
- The patient is prepped and draped from the chin to knees bilaterally
- Equipment:
  - Scalpel #10
  - Pneumatic saw or Lebsche knife
  - Finochietto retractor

Steps of the Procedure:
- Skin incision is made from the sternal notch to the xiphoid process and carried down through the subcutaneous tissue. Using electrocautery to score the midline of the sternum can be helpful but is not necessary. Divide the interclavicular ligament with cautery or scissors and bluntly dissect just posterior to the manubrium at the sternal notch and xiphoid process. This will push the fat pad, thymus, and innominate vein posteriorly.
- Hold ventilation to avoid lung injury. Insert the saw at the sternal notch and lift anteriorly to raise the sternum away from the heart. Maintain the saw in the midline of the sternum to avoid transecting through the costal cartilage. A Lebsche knife can also be used.
- After cutting through the sternum, each person on either side of the patient places their fingers into the midline of the chest and pulls the sternum laterally to make enough space to place the Finochietto retractor. Place the Finochietto retractor and spread the sternum widely. When placing this retractor, make sure the handle is inferior to allow superior extension of the incision either over the clavicle, or a cervical extension longitudinally up the neck, if needed.
- If there is evidence of tamponade, the pericardial fat pad is retracted laterally to allow for midline longitudinal pericardiotomy, extending from the great vessels to the diaphragm.
- If the injury is to the subclavian vessels, a supra or infra-clavicular extension can be made from the median sternotomy either to the right or the left. Starting at the sternoclavicular junction, the incision is extended laterally superior to the clavicle, crosses over the mid-clavicle, and continues inferior to the clavicle until the deltopectoral groove. Further description is provided in the next section.
- If the injury is to the carotid vessels, a cervical extension can be made by extending the median sternotomy to create a longitudinal incision along anterior border of sternocleidomastoid muscle. This incision is carried down through the platysma and the sternocleidomastoid muscle is retracted laterally. The carotid sheath is then opened longitudinally to gain access to the vessels. The facial vein can be ligated to expose carotid bifurcation if necessary.

45.3.2.8 Left Subclavian Artery Injury

If a patient presents with a suspected injury to the left subclavian vessels with intrathoracic hemorrhage, the best incision for proximal control is an anterolateral thoracotomy in the 3rd or 4th interspace, above the level of the nipple [35]. This incision allows for packing or manual compression at the apex of the thorax to control the hemorrhage until proximal and distal control can be obtained. The proximal left subclavian artery is an intrathoracic structure as opposed to the proximal right subclavian artery which is a mediastinal structure. The take-off of the left subclavian artery is more posterior than one might think, and therefore, care is needed to not inadvertently clamp the left common carotid artery and mistake it for the subclavian.

Depending on the location of the injury, a clavicular incision with partial median sternotomy to connect to the thoracotomy incision has been described (trap-door incision). However, control of the proximal left subclavian artery can often be obtained through a median sternotomy. Therefore, the trap-door incision is unusual and not recommended. If the injury is directly behind the clavicle, the clavicle can be transected to aid in exposure. The incision may also need to be extended laterally and inferior to the clavicle to obtain appropriate distal exposure.

Preparation:
- In the operating room, the patient is placed with arms out at 90 degrees
- The patient is prepped and draped from the chin to knees bilaterally, making sure to include the ipsilateral axilla and shoulder as needed
- Equipment:
  - Vessel loops
  - Vascular clamps
  - Gigli saw

Steps of the Procedure:

- If the patient is requiring massive transfusion, perform an anterolateral thoracotomy in the left 3rd or 4th interspace, as described previously. Use a lap pad and hold manual pressure to control the bleeding at the apex.
- If the patient is stable and the injury location is favorable, it may be able to be repaired primarily through a clavicular incision. Starting at the sternoclavicular junction, the incision is extended laterally on the clavicle, crosses over the mid-clavicle, and continues inferior to the clavicle until the deltopectoral groove. The skin incision can be retracted either inferiorly or superiorly if made right over the clavicle, depending on the exposure needs. The incision is carried down through the muscular attachments to the clavicle—the platysma and sternocleidomastoid muscles superiorly and the pectoralis major and subclavius muscles inferiorly. The subclavian vein runs anterior and inferior to the subclavian artery, and just posterior to the clavicle. It is often adherent to the clavicle, do not injure it.
- The clavicle can be transected with a Gigli saw if needed to help with exposure. The medial and lateral pieces are retracted as needed. Another option is to disarticulate the clavicle from the sternoclavicular junction and retract the clavicle laterally. The final option is to resect the middle third of the clavicle if absolutely necessary.
- The anterior scalene muscle is then divided from its attachment on the first rib to expose the subclavian artery. Take care not to injure the phrenic nerve—it often appears diminutive and runs from lateral to medial over the anterior surface of the anterior scalene muscle. Obtain proximal and distal control of the artery using vessel loops or vascular clamps.
- Watch for a thoracic duct injury—it enters the distal subclavian vein superiorly, at the junction with the internal jugular vein.

45.3.2.9 Right Subclavian Artery Injury

The proximal right subclavian artery is a mediastinal structure, and therefore, proximal control is obtained via a median sternotomy [30]. Depending on the injury location, distal control may require supraclavicular extension as described previously. If the injury is to the distal right subclavian artery, this may be able to be managed through an infra-clavicular incision alone. The infra-clavicular incision is extended laterally to expose the distal subclavian or axillary arteries. When operating on the right subclavian artery, watch for the recurrent laryngeal nerve that wraps around the artery before ascending back through the neck. One may need to quickly gain access to the innominate artery via a median sternotomy if there is a more proximal right subclavian arterial injury.

> **Take-Home Messages**
> - Understanding the anatomy of the thoracic cavity
> - If the patient is decompensating in front of you and loses mentation despite resuscitation, the procedure of choice is a resuscitative thoracotomy. This can be extended to a bilateral thoracotomy if indicated.
> - Enter right chest from the left when performing a Resuscitative Thoracotomy
> - Median sternotomy is the incision of choice for an isolated injury to the anterior thorax or superior mediastinum with concern for injury to the heart or proximal great vessels.
> - Surgical access to the subclavian arteries is dependent on laterality and location of injury.
> - Do Not Compromise exposure
> - Do Not Delay hemorrhage control

Questions

1. The incision of choice for a left distal subclavian arterial injury is;
   A. Left sided neck incision
   B. **Left sided supra-clavicular incision**
   C. Median sternotomy
   D. Left anterolateral thoracotomy
2. The incision of choice for proximal control of the right subclavian artery is;
   A. Right sided neck incision
   B. Right sided infraclavicular incision
   C. Right sided supraclavicular incision
   D. **Median sternotomy**
3. The incision of choice for a cardiac injury is;
   A. **Median sternotomy**
   B. Left anterolateral thoracotomy
   C. Left posterolateral thoracotomy
   D. Right anterolateral thoracotomy
4. The initial priority when performing an operative exploration in an unstable patient is;
   A. Resuscitation with whole blood
   B. Resuscitation with fresh frozen plasma
   C. **Hemorrhage control**
   D. Contamination control
5. When performing a pericardotomy during a resuscitative thoracotomy what nerve structure must be identified and avoided;
   A. **Phrenic Nerve**
   B. Vagus Nerve
   C. Recurrent Laryngeal Nerve
   D. Anterior Vagal Trunk
6. What muscle must be divided in order to visualize the middle segment of the left subclavian artery via a left supra-clavicular incision?
   A. Sternocleidomastoid clavicular head
   B. Sternocleidomastoid sternal head
   C. **Anterior Scalene muscle**
   D. Posterior Scalene muscle
7. What vascular structure can be injured while dividing the inferior pulmonary ligament?
   A. Aorta
   B. Inferior vena cava when on the right side
   C. **Inferior pulmonary vein**
   D. Inferior pulmonary artery
8. What incision is contra-indicated in the emergent acute setting of a thoracoabdominal gun-shot wound?
   A. **Posterolateral thoracotomy**
   B. Anterolateral thoracotomy
   C. Median sternotomy
   D. Clam-shell thoracotomy
9. What structure must be incised in order to gain clear access to the aorta?
   A. Azygos vein
   B. Inferior pulmonary ligament
   C. **Parietal pleura**
   D. Interspinous ligament
10. How many minutes does one have prior to irreversible brain tissue damage to restore perfusion to the brain?
    A. 1
    B. 2
    C. **4**
    D. 6

References

1. Centers for Disease Control and Prevention. Web-based injury statistics query and reporting system (WISQARS) [Online]. (2003). National Center for Injury Prevention and Control, Centers for Disease Control and Prevention. www.cdc.gov/ncipc/wisqars.
2. Khandhar SJ, Johnson SB, Calhoon JH. Overview of thoracic trauma in the United States. Thorac Surg Clin. 2007;17(1):1–9. https://doi.org/10.1016/j.thorsurg.2007.02.004.
3. Ferrah N, Cameron P, Gabbe B, Fitzgerald M, Judson R, Marasco S, Kowalski T, Beck B. Ageing population has changed the nature of major thoracic injury. Emerg Med J. 2019;36(6):340–5. https://doi.org/10.1136/emermed-2018-207943. Epub 2019 Apr 2
4. Boulanger BR, Kearney PA, Tsuei B, Ochoa JB. The routine use of sonography in penetrating torso injury is beneficial. J Trauma. 2001;51(2):320–5. https://doi.org/10.1097/00005373-200108000-00015.

5. Seamon MJ, et al. An evidence-based approach to patient selection for emergency department thoracotomy. J Trauma Acute Care Surg. 2015;79(1):159–73. https://doi.org/10.1097/TA.0000000000000648.
6. Karmy-Jones R, Nathens A, Jurkovich GJ, et al. Urgent and emergent thoracotomy for penetrating chest trauma. J Trauma. 2004;56(3):664–8; discussion 668-9.
7. Siemens R, Polk HC Jr, Gray LA Jr, Fulton RL. Indications for thoracotomy following penetrating thoracic injury. J Trauma. 1977;17:493–500.
8. Mattox KL, Espada R, Beall AC Jr, Jordan GL Jr. Performing thoracotomy in the emergency center. JACEP. 1974;3:13–7.
9. Moore EE, Moore JB, Galloway AC, Eiseman B. Postinjury thoracotomy in the emergency department: a critical evaluation. Surgery. 1979;86:590–8.
10. Bodai BI, Smith JP, Blaisdell FW. The role of emergency thoracotomy in blunt trauma. J Trauma. 1982;22:487–91.
11. Branney SW, Moore EE, Feldhaus KM, Wolfe RE. Critical analysis of two decades of experience with postinjury emergency department thoracotomy in a regional trauma center. J Trauma. 1998;45:87–94.
12. Kish G, Kozloff L, Joseph WL, Adkins PC. Indications for early thoracotomy in the management of chest trauma. Ann Thorac Surg. 1976;22:23–8.
13. Millham FH, Grindlinger GA. Survival determinants in patients undergoing emergency room thoracotomy for penetrating chest injury. J Trauma. 1993;34:332–6.
14. Advanced Trauma Life Support. 10th ed. Student Course Manual. 2018. American College of Surgeons. ISBN78-0-9968262-3-5.
15. Oparah SS, Mandal AK. Operative management of penetrating wounds of the chest in civilian practice. Review of indications in 125 consecutive patients. J Thorac Cardiovasc Surg. 1979;77:162–8.
16. Kugler N, Carver TW, Milia D, Paul J. Thoracic irrigation prevents retained hemothorax: a prospective propensity scored analysis. JOTACS. 2017;83(6):1136–41.
17. Kugler N, Carver TW, Paul J. Thoracic irrigation prevents retained hemothorax: a pilot study. JSR. 2016;202(2):443–8.
18. Mowery NT, Gunter OL, Collier BR, Diaz JJ Jr, Haut E, Hildreth A, Holevar M, Mayberry J, Streid E. Practice management guidelines for management of hemothorax and occult pneumothorax. J Trauma. 2011;70(2):510–8.
19. Burlew CC, Moore EE, Moore FA, Coimbra R, McIntyre RC Jr, Davis JW, Sperry J, Biffl WL. Western Trauma Association critical decisions in trauma: resuscitative thoracotomy. J Trauma Acute Care Surg. 2012;73(6):1359–63; discussion 1363-1364.
20. Cogbill TH, Moore EE, Millikan JS, Cleveland HC. Rationale for selective application of emergency department thoracotomy in trauma. J Trauma. 1983;23:453–60.
21. Moore EE, Knudson MM, Burlew CC, et al. Defining the limits of resuscitative emergency department thoracotomy: a contemporary Western Trauma Association perspective. J Trauma. 2011;70:334–9.
22. Van Natta TL, Smith BR, Bricker SD, Putnam BA. Hilar control in penetrating chest trauma: a simplified approach to an underutilized maneuver. J Trauma. 2009;66(6):1564–9.
23. Thompson DA, Rowlands BJ, Walker WE, Kuykendall RC, Miller PW, Fischer RP. Urgent thoracotomy for pulmonary or tracheobronchial injury. J Trauma. 1988;28(3):276–80.
24. Seamon MJ, Shiroff AM, Franco M, Stawicki SP, Molina EJ, Gaughan JP, Reilly PM, Schwab CW, Pryor JP, Goldberg AJ. Emergency department thoracotomy for penetrating injuries of the heart and great vessels: an appraisal of 283 consecutive cases from two urban trauma centers. J Trauma. 2009;67:1250–7.
25. DuBose JJ, Morrison J, Moore LJ, Cannon JW, Seamon MJ, Inaba K, Fox CJ, Moore EE, Feliciano DV, Scalea T, AAST AORTA Study Group. Does clamshell thoracotomy better facilitate thoracic lifesaving procedures without increased complication compared with an anterolateral approach to resuscitative thoracotomy? results from the American association for the surgery of trauma aortic occlusion for resuscitation in trauma and acute care surgery registry. J Am Coll Surg. 2020;231(6):713–719.e1. https://doi.org/10.1016/j.jamcollsurg.2020.09.002. Epub 2020 Sep 16.
26. Thorson CM, Namias N, Van Haren RM, Guarch GA, Ginzburg E, Salerno TA, Schulman CI, Livingstone AS, Proctor KG. Does hemopericardium after chest trauma mandate sternotomy? J Trauma Acute Care Surg. 2012;72(6):1518–24; discussion 1524-1525.
27. Nicol AJ, Navsaria PH, Hommes M, Ball CG, Edu S, Kahn D. Sternotomy or drainage for a hemopericardium after penetrating trauma: a randomized controlled trial. Ann Surg. 2014;259(3):438–42.
28. Breaux EP, Dupont JB Jr, Albert HM, Bryant LR, Schechter FG. Cardiac tamponade following penetrating mediastinal injuries: improved survival with early pericardiocentesis. J Trauma. 1979;19(6):461–6.
29. Rhee PM, Foy H, Kaufmann C, Areola C, Boyle E, Maier RV, Jurkovich G. Penetrating cardiac injuries: a population-based study. J Trauma. 1998;45(2):366–70.
30. Beall AC Jr, Diethrich EB, Cooley DA, DeBakey ME. Surgical management of penetrating cardiovascular trauma. South Med J. 1967;60:698–704.
31. Reul GJ Jr, Beall AC Jr, Jordan GL Jr, Mattox KL. The early operative management of injuries to great vessels. Surgery. 1973;74:862–73.
32. O'Connor JV, Scalea TM. Penetrating thoracic great vessel injury: impact of admission hemodynamics and preoperative imaging. J Trauma. 2010;68(4):834–7.
33. Feliciano DV. Trauma to the aorta and major vessels. Chest Surg Clin N Am. 1997;7(2):305–23.
34. Demetriades D. Penetrating injuries to the thoracic great vessels. J Card Surg. 1997;12(2 Suppl):173–9; discussion 179-180.
35. Pate JW, Cole FH Jr, Walker WA, Fabian TC. Penetrating injuries of the aortic arch and its branches. Ann Thorac Surg. 1993;55(3):586–92.

Empyema 46

Linda C. Qu, Rahul Nayak, and Neil G. Parry

46.1 Introduction

Empyema is defined as infected pleural fluid or pus within the pleural space. The most common etiology for this disease is a complex effusion associated with bacterial pneumonia. However, emergency general surgeons and/or trauma surgeons would more commonly encounter these pleural infections as a complication from tube thoracostomy (TT) insertion or as a complication secondary to a retained traumatic hemothorax (Table 46.1). Data from the USA and UK would suggest that empyema affects up to 80,000 people annually combined and can carry a mortality rate up to 20% [1]. Early diagnosis and definitive management are essential to improve outcomes [2].

Traumatic hemothoraces and/or pneumothoraces are two of the most common injuries seen with thoracic trauma. Overall, 85% of all chest injuries requiring intervention can be managed with TT alone [3]. Although the mechanism of thoracic injury is an important determinant of the risk of thoracic infections (e.g., penetrating greater than blunt), TT alone is an independent risk factor for the development of empyema. Multiple series have demonstrated empyema rates of 3–10% associated with TT [4–7]. The

Table 46.1 Risk factors for empyema development

Patient factors	Immunosuppressive diseases/therapies Diabetes mellitus Chronic aspiration Malnutrition Bronchogenic carcinoma
Infectious	Bacterial pneumonia with parapneumonic effusion Mycobacterium tuberculosis
Post-traumatic (Pleural space contamination)	Tube thoracostomy Retained hemothorax Esophageal injury Diaphragmatic injury (especially with hollow viscus injury) Complicated subphrenic abscess

L. C. Qu
Division of General Surgery, Department of Surgery, Schulich School of Medicine and Dentistry, Western University, London, ON, Canada
e-mail: linda.qu@lhsc.on.ca

R. Nayak
Division of Thoracic Surgery, Department of Surgery, Schulich School of Medicine and Dentistry, Western University, London, ON, Canada
e-mail: rahul.nayak@lhsc.on.ca

N. G. Parry (✉)
Division of General Surgery, Department of Surgery, Schulich School of Medicine and Dentistry, Western University, London, ON, Canada

Division of Critical Care, Department of Medicine, Schulich School of Medicine and Dentistry, Western University, London, ON, Canada

Trauma Program, Victoria Hospital, London Health Sciences Center, London, ON, Canada
e-mail: neil.parry@lhsc.on.ca

reason for this is multifactorial but factors such as insertion technique, prolonged chest tube dwell time, underlying lung injury with pleural space contamination, diaphragm injury with associated bowel injury and retained hemothorax (RH) can all contribute to the risk of developing an empyema. In general, infections attributed to TT occur in two phases. The early phase is due to seeding of a hemothorax with contaminants introduced through the insertion process. The delayed phase is due to evolving intrathoracic processes resulting in contamination of the pleural space (e.g., pneumonia or RH) [8]. In fact, RH on its own, has been associated with empyema rates of up to 25% [9].

Retained hemothoraces have several broad definitions which have subsequently contributed to its diverse incidence and management options. Carrillo and Richardson defined it as retained blood in one-third of the pleural space 72 h after TT or clots of at least 500cc volume while DuBose and Inaba defined it as a heterogenous fluid collection (Hounsfield units 35–70) with evidence of pleural thickening as seen on computed tomography (CT) scan 14 days after TT [9–11]. The incidence of RH is estimated to be between 5% and 30% [12, 13].

> **Learning Goals (Listing the Chapter Core Messages)**
> - Identify risk factors associated with the development of empyema
> - Describe clinical presentation and diagnosis
> - Identify operative and non-operative management options

46.2 Diagnosis

Patients typically present with infectious symptoms (fever, tachycardia, malaise, and decreased appetite) associated with an acute respiratory illness (cough, dyspnea, and tachypnea) with associated pleural effusion (pleuritic chest pain and dyspnea). Clinical findings include decreased air entry, dullness to percussion and/or decreased expansion of the affected hemithorax. The presenting symptoms are related to the etiology and stage of empyema, degree of immunosuppression, and the virulence of the microorganisms involved. As such, some patients may present with a chronic constellation of symptoms, while others may present acutely septic.

Chest imaging is essential to evaluate the extent and complexity of the empyema. Chest radiographs with posterior–anterior (PA) and lateral projections are generally sufficient to delineate loculated fluid collections. The lateral projection can help demonstrate fluid pockets that may not readily be apparent in the PA projection (Fig. 46.1). They can also show basilar collections at the diaphragm (inverted D-shaped density) and decubitus films are very useful to determine if the fluid is loculated or free flowing. Bedside ultrasound is an excellent tool to diagnose and characterize complex pleural fluid collections. Typical findings may include echogenic debris within swirling fluid, thick pleural rind and/or septations within the fluid collection (Fig. 46.2). Ultrasound is also very useful to help guide aspiration or pleural drain insertion. However, IV contrast-enhanced CT remains the gold standard imaging modality to diagnose and characterize empyema. It provides the greatest information regarding pleural thickening, loculations and evidence of a trapped lung (Fig. 46.3). It may also help identify underlying neoplasms or retained foreign bodies that may be causing the empyema. Furthermore, it can differentiate between lung abscess and empyema [14].

Fluid aspiration remains the gold standard to diagnose empyema (Fig. 46.4). Empyema is confirmed if there is gross aspiration of pus, positive culture or gram stain, and/or altered biochemistry (pH <7.20, glucose <2.2 mmol/L or LDH >1000 IU/L; of which pH is the most important parameter). These effusions generally begin as simple exudative, parapneumonic fluid collections until they become progressively acidotic, infected and more complex (as demonstrated by an enlarging, loculated effusion with development of a thick exudate).

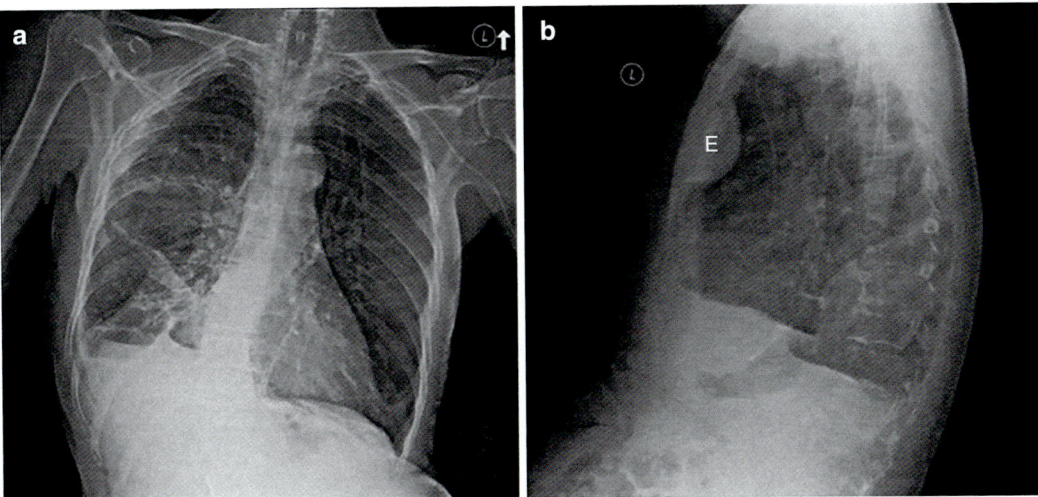

Fig. 46.1 (a) Posterior–anterior projection of chest X-ray in patient with loculated empyema. (b) Lateral projection demonstrating anterior loculated collection (E) not readily visible on PA view

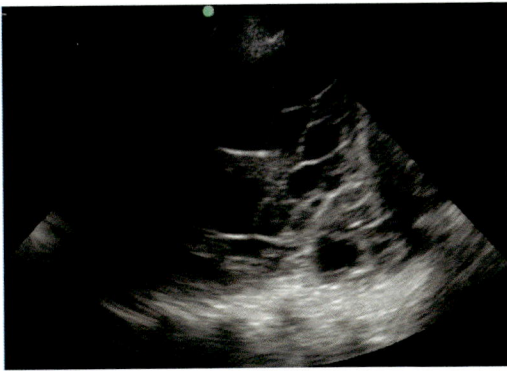

Fig. 46.2 Ultrasound of multi-loculated empyema (courtesy of Dr. Robert Arntfield)

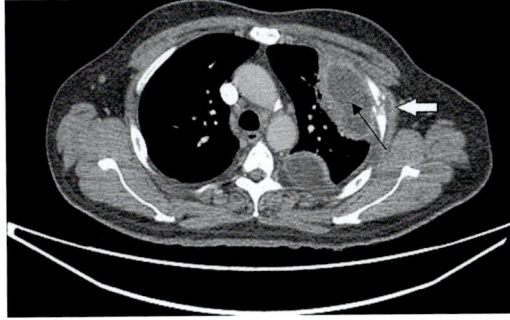

Fig. 46.3 Axial CT Chest with bony rib destruction (white arrow) secondary to empyema (black arrow)

1. Pus
2. Positive culture
3. Biochemistry
   - pH < 7.20
   - Glucose (< 2.2 mmol/l)
   - LDH > 1000 IU/l

Fig. 46.4 Diagnostic fluid aspirate

The development of empyema associated with pneumonia is classified into three stages reflecting the progression of the pleural disease from time of onset [15]. This staging system aids in predicting the clinical course and in guiding treatment options (Table 46.2).

However, the pathophysiology and evolution of a post-traumatic empyema differ from that described above. In the early phase, bacteria may be introduced into the chest from the initial trauma (i.e., penetrating injury) or may seed the pleural space after TT is performed.

In the delayed phase, an RH may develop. If left undrained, the RH can lead to the development of a fibrothorax, trapped lung, and/or empyema. Empyema as a complication from RH has

Table 46.2 Classification and treatment options for empyema

Stage[a]	Phase	Characteristics	Treatment options
I	Exudative	• Early/acute phase (0–2 weeks) • Exudative effusion • Free flowing effusion • Minimal septations present	• Tube thoracostomy[b] • VATS
II	Fibrinopurulent	• Transitional phase (2–6 weeks) • Extensive fibrin deposits (parietal ≫ visceral) • Thick fluid with multiple loculations • Lung may be collapsed but still expandable with adequate resolution of empyema	• VATS decortication[b] • Tube thoracostomy (+/− intrapleural fibrinolytics) • Open decortication
III	Organized	• Chronic phase (>6 weeks) • Extensive fibrin deposits over both parietal and visceral pleura with thick pleural peel • Lung becomes trapped/encased and unlikely to expand even with drainage of empyema	• VATS decortication • Open decortication • Chronic indwelling chest tube • Open thoracic Window

[a]Stages may overlap by 1 week; *VATS* Video-assisted thoracoscopic surgery
[b]Preferred approach

an incidence of 5–30%. This may be caused by a primary infection of the RH from contamination introduced into the pleural cavity or by secondary extension of an intrathoracic infection (e.g., pneumonia) with seeding of the RH [8, 16]. As such, early identification and treatment of RH can avoid these morbid complications.

46.3 Treatment

Management of an empyema begins with providing appropriate resuscitation, drawing blood cultures, optimizing nutrition, chest physiotherapy, and initiating venothromboembolic prophylaxis [1].

Appropriate antibiotics selection is of paramount importance. Empiric antibiotic therapy should cover community-acquired bacteria (mainly *Streptococcus spp.*, *Staphylococcus aureus*, *Eschericha coli*) and anaerobic organisms (*Bacteroides spp.*, *Peptostreptococcus spp.*, *Fusobacterium spp.*). A parenteral second- or third-generation cephalosporin (e.g., ceftriaxone) in combination with metronidazole or an aminopenicillin and beta-lactamase inhibitor combination (e.g., ampicillin/sulbactam) is recommended [17].

With hospital-acquired or postprocedural empyema, antibiotics should cover methicillin-resistant *Staphylococcus aureus* and *Pseudomonas aeruginosa* (e.g., vancomycin, ceftazidime, cefepime, piperacillin/tazobactam or imipenem).

When possible, antibiotic therapy should be tailored to the Gram stain and culture results. However, consideration should be given to empiric anaerobic coverage even when anaerobic cultures are negative. The duration of antibiotics is controversial, but a minimum of 2 weeks is recommended [17]. Ultimately, duration of antibiotics will depend on the organism, adequacy of source control, and clinical response.

Adequate, early drainage of the infected pleural fluid is fundamental to successful treatment. Thoracentesis alone is inadequate and not recommended [17]. TT is the initial treatment, to evacuate the infected pleural fluid with the goal of complete lung expansion to obliterate the infected space and allow for pleural surface apposition. Although large-bore TTs have been traditionally the norm, there is increasing evidence to suggest that small-bore percutaneous pleural catheters (≤14 French) have equivalent outcomes and can be used as first-line therapy in select patients [1]. The preference for small-bore tubes is becoming more widespread, as they are less painful, easy to insert and do not increase morbidity or mortality if patency is maintained [18, 19]. For multiloculated effusions, placement of small-bore catheters, often under image guidance, is recommended in patients that are not surgical candidates [17]. Although percutaneous drains are less traumatic, they often require multiple CT scans and can become easily blocked [20]. In later stages, when effusions are complex or purulent, a large bore TT may still be preferred as it allows the operator to place a finger in the chest and create a space to advance the chest tube.

Once a TT is placed, it should be connected to active suction (i.e., -20 cm H_2O) until the underlying lung demonstrates full expansion on imaging. The timing of chest tube removal has not been well-studied; however, low daily drainage (<100 mL/day) with no air leak is baseline parameters used to determine if the chest tube is ready to be removed.

Once initial resuscitation and chest tube placement is complete, further management is dependent on the stage of the empyema.

46.3.1 Stage 1 (Exudative)

This is the earliest stage of empyema and represents the first 2 weeks after symptom onset. In this stage, the infected fluid collection is not loculated and insertion of a pleural drain should suffice for management.

46.3.2 Stage 2 (Fibrinopurulent)

This stage represents the intermediate stage of the evolution of the empyema and occurs between 2 and 6 weeks from symptom onset. At this stage, there is significant fibrin deposition as the body attempts to contain the infection. Typical findings on CT or ultrasound demonstrate the development of septations and loculated effusions.

VATS decortication is the recommended approach for the fibrinopurulent phase and its success rate is directly dependent on the timing of referral [21]. The two main operative goals include: (1) debridement, which evacuates the infected material from the pleural space and (2) decortication, which peels off the organized cortex, obliterates the dead space and allows for lung re-expansion. The greater the delay in surgical intervention, the higher the likelihood of conversion to open thoracotomy. The conversion rates from VATS to open thoracotomy may be up to 50% [22]. Even when an empyema appears complex and chronic, a VATS first approach is preferred over thoracotomy as there is minimal morbidity associated with starting with VATS and converting to an open procedure as necessary.

The potential benefits of VATS include better postoperative pain control, shorter hospital stay, reduced pulmonary compromise, and decreased postoperative complications, including 30-day mortality [23, 24]. Potential contraindications to VATS include inability to tolerate one-lung ventilation and severe coagulopathy.

For patients who are not surgical candidates, the administration of intrapleural fibrinolytic therapy can be considered. Available agents for administration include tissue plasminogen activators (tPA), DNA dornase and streptokinase. The Multicenter Intrapleural Sepsis Trial 2 (MIST-2) demonstrated that using recombinant tissue plasminogen activator (TPA) and DNase compared to either single agent alone improved rates of resolution of empyema, reduced length of hospital stay and decreased the need for surgery at 3 months [25]. The favourable response rates demonstrated by this study have resulted in many centres utilizing this mode of treatment in surgical candidates as well. However, there have been no randomized trials comparing dual intrapleural fibrinolytic therapy to VATS decortications, but there have been several population-based studies demonstrating increased mortality with the use of non-operative therapy compared to operative management [26–28]. The current American Association of Thoracic Surgeons and British Thoracic Society guidelines do not recommend the routine use of fibrinolytics for stage 2 empyema [1, 17]. Indications and contraindications for decortication are listed in Table 46.3.

Table 46.3 Indications and contraindications for decortication

Indications	• Inadequately drained empyema • Chronic empyema • Clotted/organized hemothorax • Post-traumatic fibrothorax with evidence of lung entrapment • Lack of clinical resolution with non-operative management
Contraindications	• Bronchial stenosis • Extensive parenchymal disease in the affected hemithorax • Contralateral disease • Significant operative risk

46.3.3 Stage 3 (Organized)

This stage represents an organized phase that occurs 6 weeks or more from symptom onset. Patients present with chronic infectious and respiratory symptoms as well as chronic changes within the hemithorax, such as trapped lung and undrained collections. This is typically managed surgically requiring a staged approach with thoracotomy, the use of various muscle flaps (to obliterate persistent cavities) or even an open thoracic window (e.g., Clagett window). The management for this stage of empyema should involve a thoracic surgeon and is beyond the scope of this chapter.

46.4 Special Considerations

In the setting of retained hemothoraces, complete evacuation of the residual blood is key to prevent infectious complications. There is some data to suggest that VATS is superior to a second TT, as it been shown to decrease TT duration and the length of hospital stay [29]. Intrapleural fibrinolytics have been proposed as an alternative to VATS. However, the evidence for the efficacy of fibrinolytics is variable and of low quality [30–33]. Based on the available literature, the most recent Eastern Association for the Surgery of Trauma guidelines conditionally recommend VATS over intrapleural fibrinolytic therapy for RH to decrease rate of additional operative intervention and hospital length of stay [34]. It should be noted that fibrinolytics may still have a roll for patients with significant comorbidities who cannot undergo surgical intervention. Several studies have demonstrated that early VATS (<4 days) decreases the rate of conversion to thoracotomy, risk of empyema, need for additional procedure as well as hospital and intensive care unit length of stay [3, 35–39].

Another special situation is *empyema necessitans*, which occurs when the infection from the pleural space erodes through the chest wall and may present as a chest wall abscess (Fig. 46.3). This is generally managed with decortication and/or an open thoracic window.

> **Dos and Don'ts**
> - Initiate broad spectrum antibiotics early.
> - TT is the best initial step for evacuating early acute empyema but think twice before placing multiple chest tubes.
> - The role of intrapleural fibrinolytic therapy for stage 2 empyema remains controversial.
> - Early surgical intervention may lead to improved outcomes
> - A VATS first approach should be used in all cases of empyema

> **Take-Home Messages**
> - An organized approach to early diagnosis and definitive care are essential
> - VATS is the favoured approach for stage II empyema
> - Early VATS is recommended for RH

References

1. Davies HE, Davies RJO, Davies CWH, on behalf of the BTS Pleural Disease Guideline Group. Management of pleural infection in adults: British Thoracic Society pleural disease guideline 2010. Thorax. 2010;65(Suppl 2):ii41–53.
2. Finley C, Clifton J, FitzGerald JM, Yee J. Empyema: an increasing concern in Canada. Can Respir J. 2008;15(2):85–9.
3. Vassiliu P, Velmahos GC, Toutouzas KG. Timing, safety, and efficacy of thoracoscopic evacuation of undrained post-traumatic hemothorax. Am Surg. 2001;67(12):1165–9.
4. Eren S, Esme H, Sehitogullari A, Durkan A. The risk factors and management of posttraumatic empyema in trauma patients. Injury. 2008;39(1):44–9.
5. Aguilar MM. Posttraumatic empyema: risk factor analysis. Arch Surg. 1997;132(6):647.
6. Deneuville M. Morbidity of percutaneous tube thoracostomy in trauma patients. Eur J Cardiothorac Surg. 2002;22(5):673–8.
7. Helling TS, Gyles NR, Eisenstein CL, Soracco CA. Complications following blunt and penetrating injuries in 216 victims of chest trauma requiring tube thoracostomy. J Trauma Inj Infect Crit Care. 1989;29(10):1367–70.
8. Karmy-Jones R, Holevar M, Sullivan RJ, Fleisig A, Jurkovich GJ. Residual hemothorax after chest

tube placement correlates with increased risk of empyema following traumatic injury. Can Respir J. 2008;15(5):255–8.
9. DuBose J, Inaba K, Okoye O, Demetriades D, Scalea T, O'Connor J, et al. Development of posttraumatic empyema in patients with retained hemothorax: Results of a prospective, observational AAST study. J Trauma Acute Care Surg. 2012;73(3):752–7.
10. Carrillo EH, Richardson JD. Thoracoscopy in the management of hemothorax and retained blood after trauma. Curr Opin Pulm Med. 1998;4(4):243–6.
11. Casós SR, Richardson JD. Role of thoracoscopy in acute management of chest injury. Curr Opin Crit Care. 2006;12(6):584–9.
12. Cohen NS, Braig Z, Collins JN. Prevalence and management of posttraumatic retained hemothorax in a level 1 trauma center. Am Surg. 2018;84(9):e369–71.
13. Scott MF, Khodaverdian RA, Shaheen JL, Ney AL, Nygaard RM. Predictors of retained hemothorax after trauma and impact on patient outcomes. Eur J Trauma Emerg Surg. 2017;43(2):179–84.
14. Stark D, Federle M, Goodman P, Podrasky A, Webb W. Differentiating lung abscess and empyema: radiography and computed tomography. Am J Roentgenol. 1983;141(1):163–7.
15. Andrews N, Parker E, Shaw R, et al. Management of non-tuberculous empyema: a statement of the subcommittee on surgery from the American Thoracic Society. Am Rev Respir Dis. 1962;85:935–6.
16. Mandal AK, Thadepalli H, Mandal AK, Chettipalli U. Posttraumatic empyema thoracis: a 24-year experience at a major trauma center. J Trauma Inj Infect Crit Care. 1997;43(5):764–71.
17. Shen KR, Bribriesco A, Crabtree T, Denlinger C, Eby J, Eiken P, et al. The American Association for Thoracic Surgery consensus guidelines for the management of empyema. J Thorac Cardiovasc Surg. 2017;153(6):e129–46.
18. Rahman NM, Maskell NA, Davies CWH, Hedley EL, Nunn AJ, Gleeson FV, et al. The relationship between chest tube size and clinical outcome in pleural infection. Chest. 2010;137(3):536–43.
19. Filosso PL, Sandri A, Guerrera F, Ferraris A, Marchisio F, Bora G, et al. When size matters: changing opinion in the management of pleural space—the rise of small-bore pleural catheters. J Thorac Dis. 2016;8(7):E503–10.
20. Collop NA, Kim S, Sahn SA. Analysis of tube thoracostomy performed by pulmonologists at a teaching hospital. Chest. 1997;112(3):709–13.
21. Waller DA, Rengarajan A, Nicholson FHG, Rajesh PB. Delayed referral reduces the success of video-assisted thoracoscopic debridement for post-pneumonic empyema. Respir Med. 2001;95(10):836–40.
22. Landreneau RJ, Keenan RJ, Hazelrigg SR, Mack MJ, Naunheim KS. Thoracoscopy for empyema and hemothorax. Chest. 1996;109(1):18–24.
23. Farjah F, Backhus LM, Varghese TK, Mulligan MS, Cheng A, Alfonso-Cristancho R, et al. Ninety-day costs of video-assisted thoracic surgery versus open lobectomy for lung cancer. Ann Thorac Surg. 2014;98(1):191–6.
24. Chambers A, Routledge T, Dunning J, Scarci M. Is video-assisted thoracoscopic surgical decortication superior to open surgery in the management of adults with primary empyema? Interact Cardiovasc Thorac Surg. 2010;11(2):171–7.
25. Rahman NM, Maskell NA, West A, Teoh R, Arnold A, Mackinlay C, et al. Intrapleural use of tissue plasminogen activator and dnase in pleural infection. N Engl J Med. 2011;365(6):518–26.
26. Nayak R, Brogly SB, Lajkosz K, Lougheed MD, Petsikas D. Outcomes of operative and nonoperative treatment of thoracic empyema: a population-based study. Ann Thorac Surg. 2019;108(5):1456–63.
27. Semenkovich TR, Olsen MA, Puri V, Meyers BF, Kozower BD. Current state of empyema management. Ann Thorac Surg. 2018;105(6):1589–96.
28. Farjah F, Symons RG, Krishnadasan B, Wood DE, Flum DR. Management of pleural space infections: a population-based analysis. J Thorac Cardiovasc Surg. 2007;133(2):346–351.e1.
29. Meyer DM, Jessen ME, Wait MA, Estrera AS. Early evacuation of traumatic retained hemothoraces using thoracoscopy: a prospective, randomized trial. Ann Thorac Surg. 1997;64(5):1396–401.
30. Iuci I, Özçelik C, Ülkü R, Tuna A, Eren N. Intrapleural fibrinolytic treatment of traumatic clotted hemothorax. Chest. 1998;114(1):160–5.
31. Jerjes-Sanchez C, Ramirez-Rivera A, Elizalde JJ, Delgado R, Cicero R, Ibarra-Perez C, et al. Intrapleural fibrinolysis with streptokinase as an adjunctive treatment in hemothorax and empyema. Chest. 1996;109(6):1514–9.
32. Kimbrell BJ, Yamzon J, Petrone P, Asensio JA, Velmahos GC. Intrapleural thrombolysis for the management of undrained traumatic hemothorax: a prospective observational study. J Trauma Inj Infect Crit Care. 2007;62(5):1175–9.
33. Oğuzkaya F, Akçalı Y, Bilgin M. Videothoracoscopy versus intrapleural streptokinase for management of post traumatic retained haemothorax: a retrospective study of 65 cases. Injury. 2005;36(4):526–9.
34. Patel NJ, Dultz L, Ladhani HA, Cullinane DC, Klein E, McNickle AG, et al. Management of simple and retained hemothorax: a practice management guideline from the Eastern Association for the Surgery of Trauma. Am J Surg. 2021;221(5):873–84.

35. Abolhoda A. Diagnostic and therapeutic video assisted thoracic surgery (VATS) following chest trauma. Eur J Cardiothorac Surg. 1997;12(3):356–60.
36. Ahmed N, Chung R. Role of early thoracoscopy for management of penetrating wounds of the chest. Am Surg. 2010;76(11):1236–9.
37. Smith JW, Franklin GA, Harbrecht BG, Richardson JD. Early VATS For blunt chest trauma: a management technique underutilized by acute care surgeons. J Trauma Inj Infect Crit Care. 2011;71(1):102–7.
38. Lin H-L, Huang W-Y, Yang C, Chou S-M, Chiang H-I, Kuo L-C, et al. How early should VATS be performed for retained haemothorax in blunt chest trauma? Injury. 2014;45(9):1359–64.
39. Huang F-D, Yeh W-B, Chen S-S, Liu Y-Y, Lu I-Y, Chou Y-P, et al. Early management of retained hemothorax in blunt head and chest trauma. World J Surg. 2018;42(7):2061–6.

Further Reading

Davies HE, RJO D, Davies CWH, On Behalf of the BTS Pleural Disease Guideline Group. Management of pleural infection in adults: British Thoracic Society pleural disease guideline 2010. Thorax. 2010;65(Suppl 2):ii41–53.

Patel NJ, Dultz L, Ladhani HA, Cullinane DC, Klein E, McNickle AG, et al. Management of simple and retained hemothorax: a practice management guideline from the Eastern Association for the Surgery of Trauma. Am J Surg. 2021;221(5):873–84.

Shen KR, Bribriesco A, Crabtree T, Denlinger C, Eby J, Eiken P, et al. The American Association for Thoracic Surgery consensus guidelines for the management of empyema. J Thorac Cardiovasc Surg. 2017;153(6):e129–46.

Hemothorax and Pneumothorax

47

David A. Spain, Ara Ko, and Jamie Tung

47.1 Introduction

Pneumothorax and hemothorax are common emergency surgical problems encountered by the emergency general surgeon. The etiology may be secondary to traumatic causes or associated with medical pathology. Rapid diagnosis and appropriate initial treatment of these thoracic pathologies can be lifesaving in certain cases. Accordingly, these skills, as well as management of subsequent complications, should be within the emergency general surgeon's scope of practice.

> **Learning Goals**
> - How to diagnosis a hemothorax/pneumothorax
> - How to treat a hemothorax/pneumothorax
> - How to manage the complications of a hemothorax/pneumothorax

47.1.1 Epidemiology

Pneumothorax and hemothorax can be common sequelae of both traumatic and non-traumatic causes. As a significant global health problem, the incidence of non-traumatic pneumothorax is reported to be estimated 22.7 cases per 100,000 population annually in France [1], and up to 24 per 100,000 men and 9.8 per 100,000 women in England [2]. Chest trauma accounts for up to 25% of trauma-related deaths [3], with pneumothorax and/or hemothorax as common consequences of this type of injury. Studies have reported that blunt chest trauma results in pneumothorax and/or hemothorax rates ranging from 6.7% in those without any rib fractures, to up to 81.4% in those with more than two rib fractures [4, 5]. In addition, iatrogenic pneumothoraces are identified at a rate of up to 1.4% from invasive procedures [6], with the majority resulting from procedures, such as central venous catheters, thoracenteses, as well as barotrauma from mechanical ventilation [7]. As a frequently encountered surgical problem, the general surgeon should feel comfortable diagnosing, managing the initial incident as well as the complications that arise from this pathology.

D. A. Spain (✉) · A. Ko · J. Tung
Department of Surgery, Stanford University,
Stanford, CA, USA
e-mail: dspain@stanford.edu; arako@stanford.edu; jtungmd@stanford.edu

Table 47.1 Etiology and classification of pneumothorax and hemothorax

	Pneumothorax	Hemothorax
Non-Traumatic	Primary Pneumothorax – Subpleural blebs – Smoking – Genetic Secondary Pneumothorax – Airway disease – Infection – Interstitial lung disease – Malignancy – Rare conditions	– Coagulopathy – Infection – Malignancy – Pulmonary sequestration – Vascular rupture – Pulmonary vascular malformation
Traumatic	– Blunt injury – Penetrating injury – Iatrogenic/Procedure-related	

47.1.2 Etiology and Classification

The etiology of a pneumothorax and hemothorax can be generally categorized as non-traumatic and traumatic (Table 47.1).

47.1.2.1 Non-traumatic

A non-traumatic spontaneous pneumothorax occurs without apparent clinical lung disease (primary pneumothorax) or as a complication of underlying lung disease (secondary pneumothorax). Spontaneous primary pneumothorax has been associated with ruptured subpleural blebs, smoking, and genetic predispositions. Conditions that can result in a secondary pneumothorax include airway diseases (chronic obstructive pulmonary disease, asthma, and cystic fibrosis), pulmonary infections (necrotizing pneumonia, pneumocystis pneumonia, and COVID-19), interstitial lung diseases, neoplasia, and even rare conditions, such as thoracic endometriosis and lymphangioleiomyomatosis [8]. A non-traumatic hemothorax, though less common, can occur in the setting of coagulopathy, malignancy, infection, lung sequestration, vascular ruptures, and pulmonary vascular malformations [9].

47.1.2.2 Traumatic

Traumatic pneumothorax and/or hemothorax commonly occur as a consequence of blunt (motor vehicle collisions, motorcycle crashes, and falls) or penetrating chest injuries (gunshot wounds, stab wounds) [10]. Iatrogenic etiologies include any procedures that may potentially introduce air into the pleural space or cause hemorrhage from injury to thoracic organs or vessels. Iatrogenic pneumothorax has been seen with placement of subclavian or internal jugular central venous catheters, pacemakers, pulmonary needle biopsies, thoracenteses, thoracic/esophageal/diaphragm surgeries, and barotrauma in the setting of mechanical ventilation [11, 12]. Procedures most commonly associated with iatrogenic hemothorax are central line placements, needle biopsies, thoracenteses, and tube thoracostomies [13].

Regardless of the etiology, the same basic principles of management apply to most situations as they are explained by the same basic pathophysiology.

47.1.3 Pathophysiology

Understanding thoracic anatomy helps with comprehending the pathophysiology of hemothorax and pneumothorax. The structure of the human chest wall consists of intercostal muscles, 12 ribs on either side, the sternum, and costal cartilage. Under each rib lies the neurovascular bundle consisting of the intercostal artery, vein, and nerve. The inner chest wall is lined by parietal pleura, while the thoracic organs are covered by the visceral pleura. It is within this potential space between the parietal and visceral pleura, that air and/or blood can accumulate to cause a pneumothorax or hemothorax, with subsequent lung collapse and hypoxemia.

In a pneumothorax, air becomes trapped within the potential space as it leaks from injured lung parenchyma, tracheobronchial tree, or through an open chest wound or puncture. If air is introduced into the pleural space through a defect in the lung parenchyma or tracheobronchial tree, the pneumothorax can get larger upon application of positive pressure in the airway via endotracheal intubation and mechanical ventilation. In blunt trauma, sudden chest compression can abruptly increase alveolar pressure, causing rupture and escape of atmospheric air into the pleural space [14]. In penetrating chest injuries, an open chest wound ("sucking chest wound") can be the source of air into the pleural space, as the negative intrathoracic pressure with inspiration will bring atmospheric air into the thoracic cavity until there is equilibrium of the pressure gradient. In addition, if the soft tissue of the chest wall acts as a valve that allows air to be pulled into the pleural space but does not allow it to escape, a tension pneumothorax can result. Furthermore, violation of the parietal pleura along the inner chest wall may allow for leakage of air into subcutaneous tissues resulting in subcutaneous emphysema.

A hemothorax results from blood accumulation in the pleural space. It can occur due to injured lung parenchyma, rib fractures, injuries to intercostal vessels, or secondary to cardiac or great vessel injuries with an associated defect in visceral pleura.

Tension physiology can occur when intrathoracic pressure exerted by the pneumothorax or hemothorax overcomes venous return to the heart. On imaging, one may see tracheal deviation or mediastinal shifting to the contralateral hemithorax, as well as depression of the diaphragmatic contour. As this "mass effect" causes diminished venous return, hypotension ensues as decreased preload results in inadequate cardiac output.

47.2 Diagnosis

47.2.1 Clinical Presentation

The clinical presentation of a hemothorax or pneumothorax may be similar, and they may present concurrently. The patient may experience dyspnea, chest pain, tachypnea, tachycardia, hypoxia, and elevation of end-tidal CO_2. Should the patient have a tension component of the hemothorax or pneumothorax, there may also be hemodynamic instability as the increased intrathoracic pressure diminishes venous return. Clinical suspicion for a tension component is sufficient to proceed with needle or tube decompression, as awaiting confirmation with imaging may be fatal due to ongoing hemodynamic compromise.

On physical examination, patients may have decreased breath sounds on auscultation of the affected hemithorax. A dullness to percussion may be appreciated with a hemothorax, while tympany to percussion and/or subcutaneous emphysema may be present with a pneumothorax. Patients may also demonstrate unequal chest rise with breathing. Those with a tension component may also demonstrate tracheal deviation and jugular venous distention. Alternatively, it is also possible for patients to be asymptomatic, with the hemothorax or pneumothorax solely diagnosed on imaging.

47.2.2 Tests

Laboratory tests do not diagnose these intrathoracic pathologies, but some findings may help support diagnosis or guide management. For example, hypoxemia as demonstrated on a blood gas or a base deficit with a down-trending hematocrit may corroborate the suspicion of a clinically significant hemothorax requiring intervention with drainage and/or hemorrhage control.

Imaging can be the most beneficial in confirming the diagnosis of a pneumothorax or hemothorax. Initial evaluation may begin with an upright chest X-ray (CXR), demonstrating a distinct pleural line at a distance from the chest wall when suspicious for a pneumothorax. According to cadaver studies, accumulated pleural air volumes of 10–200 mL may be required to detect a pneumothorax on plain film depending on the view, with left lateral decubitus XRs being most sensitive (detected as low as 10–20 mL of air) and supine XRs being the least sensitive (over 200 mL of air) [15]. A pitfall in interpreting the CXR may be mistaking a skin fold for the pleural line. If the pneumothorax is associated with subcutaneous emphysema, radiolucent striations of the pectoralis muscle may be seen on plain film. A hemothorax may be identified with blunting of the costophrenic angle for which at least 175 mL of blood is needed to visualize on an upright CXR [16]. Another pitfall in misdiagnosis may occur when this obscuring of the costophrenic angle is not distinctly present due to obtaining a supine CXR rather than an upright film.

A large or tension hemothorax visualized on CXR may demonstrate ipsilateral opacification with shifting of the mediastinum to the contralateral hemithorax. This could be differentiated from a mucous plug causing a "white out" of the hemithorax, because in this case, the mediastinum would be shifted *toward* the ipsilateral hemithorax. Although a tension pneumothorax should be diagnosed clinically and rapidly treated with needle decompression or tube thoracostomy, if seen on CXR, it would also reveal shifting of the mediastinum to the contralateral side and may show a "deep sulcus sign" (Fig. 47.1).

Ultrasonography is another helpful imaging modality to evaluate pathology in the thorax. In the trauma setting, the Focused Assessment with Sonography in Trauma (FAST) was modified to include an "extended" portion (eFAST) with standard lung views to assess for pneumothorax and hemothorax. With the patient supine, an ultrasound probe is placed at the anterior lung field at approximately the 2nd to 4th intercostal space, mid-clavicular line.

Between two ribs, a white hyperechoic pleural line should be visualized with the appearance of lung sliding, which is the parietal and visceral pleura sliding over each other (Fig. 47.2). One may find a "lung-point sign" at the border of the pneumothorax, where there is a discontinuation of lung sliding. Depending on where this "lung-point sign" is identified (anterior mid-clavicular line, midaxillary line, posterior axillary line), the size of the pneumothorax can also be estimated from small to large, the more posterior it is detected [17].

Another ultrasound technique to demonstrate lung sliding uses the M-mode cursor, which detects motion over time. With the cursor over the pleural line, the top portion of the image shows the non-mobile chest wall as horizontal "waves" over the granular appearing image ("sand") which represents the lung sliding and motion under the pleural line (Fig. 47.3). This is appropriately named the "seashore sign." If there is no lung sliding, one would see an image resembling a "barcode," with the horizontal waves both above and below the pleural line to signify no motion. The presence of lung sliding can rule out a pneumothorax in that lung field. However, its absence could also be seen with pleural adhesions, atelectasis, mainstem intubation, acute respiratory distress syndrome (ARDS), and large pulmonary consolidations. Other normal reverberation artifacts produced by the visceral pleura include comet tails (B-lines) that look like a flashlight beaming downward, and its presence can also rule out a pneumothorax.

A hemothorax appears anechoic, as a black space, above the diaphragm on ultrasound. At least 20 mL of fluid accumulation is required for detection [18]. Although the diagnostic value of ultrasound may be operator dependent, its sensitivity of detecting a pneumothorax or hemothorax has been found to be higher than that of CXR with similar specificity [17, 19–21]. Of note, the utility of ultrasound is limited when subcutaneous emphysema does not allow for diffusion of the ultrasound beam through the chest wall, producing poor imaging.

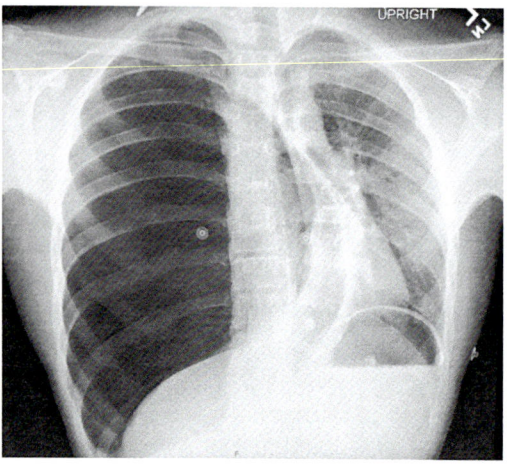

Fig. 47.1 CXR of a patient with a right-sided tension pneumothorax, mediastinal shift, and deep sulcus sign

Fig. 47.2 eFAST of the anterior lung field with a pleural line which would demonstrate lung sliding in real-time

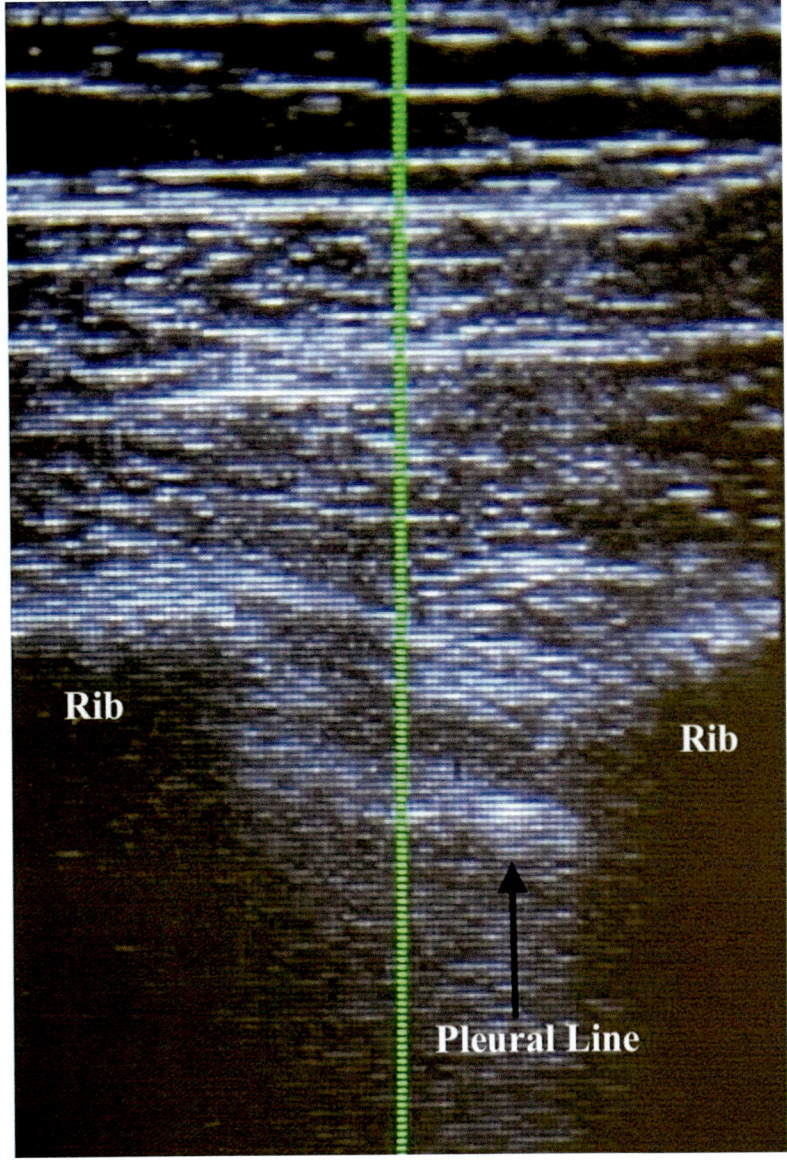

Computed tomography (CT) of the chest is considered the gold standard in evaluating for chest trauma. When a pneumothorax is not visualized on CXR but discovered on CT imaging, it is referred to as an occult pneumothorax and can be seen in up to 55% of chest injured patients [22]. Subcutaneous emphysema may be the only clinical predictor of occult pneumothorax [23]. Management may be based on symptoms or whether the patient is on positive pressure ventilation (PPV) due to concern for an expanding pneumothorax or development of a potential tension pneumothorax [24, 25].

In addition, a chest CT can detect as little as 2 mL of fluid in the thoracic cavity [16]. As opposed to ultrasound, which cannot differentiate simple pleural effusion from hemothorax, the density of fluid as evaluated by Hounsfield units (HU) on CT can help differentiate hemothorax from a hydrothorax or other simple pleural effusion. In general, 30–45 HU may represent liquid blood, while denser, clotted blood may be identified with a measurement of 50–90 HU [16].

Fig. 47.3 Lung ultrasound in M-mode demonstrating the "seashore sign"

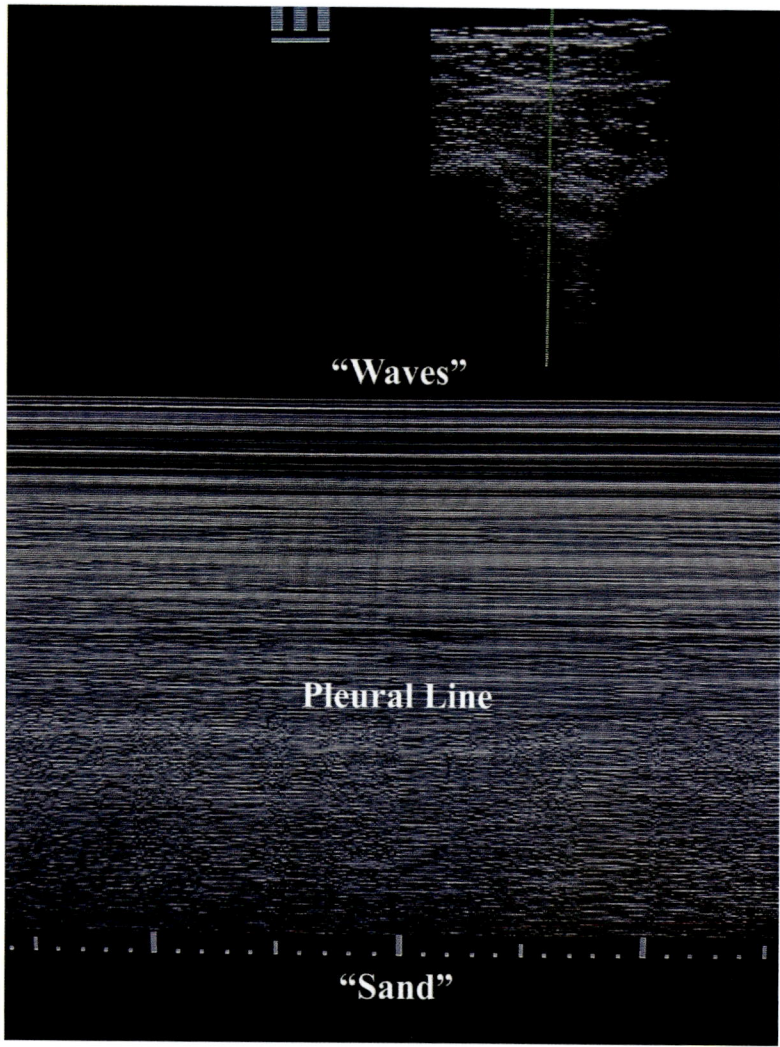

Differential Diagnosis

The differential diagnoses for hemothorax and pneumothorax include chest pathologies that may cause hypoxia, diminished breath sounds, and/or chest pain. When evaluating a patient with such signs and symptoms, one must consider the possible diagnoses or concomitant existence of the following: pneumonia, empyema, hydrothorax, transudative or exudative pleural effusions, pulmonary edema, rib fractures, ARDS, acute coronary syndrome, and thoracic aortic injury or dissection.

47.3 Treatment

47.3.1 Medical Treatment

After making the diagnosis of a hemothorax or a pneumothorax, the treatment algorithm may depend on its size as well as the clinical condition of the patient. Management will always include treatment of the patient's concomitant conditions and injuries. Outside of surgical treatment, management is generally limited to supportive therapy. If in the setting of trauma, correction of other injuries may need to take priority. Regardless, maintaining the oxygenation status of the patient will be required.

Regarding an open chest wound, immediate coverage of the site is the priority. Thus, coverage of an open chest wound is taught in many first aid classes to be applied in the prehospital setting. As a first step, using a gloved hand is recommended. An occlusive dressing is standard care, whether vented or unvented. There are a variety of commercial chest seals available including HyFin®, Asherman™, Bolin Chest Seal, or Halo chest seals. The authors do not have a particular recommendation or endorsement. If no commercial device is available, an occlusive dressing can be fashioned with any occlusive material such as a plastic sheet, bag, or packaging material along with an adhesive, such as dressing tape. However, as Kheirabadi and associates have found, a vented chest seal such as the Bolin Chest Seal may be preferred, as it is more likely to prevent a tension pneumothorax by allowing venting of the accumulated intrapleural air [26]. The Bolin Chest Seal compared similar to the Asherman™ chest seal, but was also the preferred product by Arnaud et al. given its propensity to better adhere to blood-soiled skin [27].

Traditionally, it was thought that supplemental oxygen could help resorb small pneumothoraces faster. Theoretically, increasing the partial pressure of oxygen to displace atmospheric air (primarily nitrogen) within the pneumothorax would allow the body to resorb it quicker [28]. However, it is debated whether the resolution rate is in fact increased. If a patient's oxygen saturation level is normal, extra oxygen is now thought to be unnecessary [29, 30].

Non-surgical treatment of a hemothorax is limited to resuscitation with blood products and correction of any coagulopathy, thus indirectly treating the hemothorax by preventing further blood loss into the chest cavity.

47.3.2 Surgical Treatment

47.3.2.1 Needle Decompression

In situations where a tension pneumothorax or hemothorax is suspected, immediate treatment in the form of needle decompression is performed. This is typically applied with the suspicion of a pneumothorax causing tension physiology. In theory, a tension hemothorax would also be alleviated with needle decompression. Needle decompression is preferred as a first line measure given its ease of employment, because it can be performed as an intermediate step, while a chest tube is being set up. Even in the hospital setting, it is still often faster to perform a needle decompression than to obtain and use a scalpel to create a finger or tube thoracostomy. It is also easy to perform in the pre-hospital setting and requires less training than a formal tube thoracostomy and is, therefore, taught to many care providers, whose training in chest tube placement would not be feasible [31].

The typical placement of a decompression needle (14 gauge, depth 1.5 inches) is in the 2nd intercostal space, just above the rib. This location is the authors' preference for several reasons. It is generally very easy to access the anterior chest as many patients are supine with their arms against their sides. Identification is rapid, as the clavicle can be a surrogate landmark for the 1st rib. In addition, the 2nd intercostal space should avoid most of the pectoralis muscle and most breast tissue. With a tension pneumothorax, needle decompression should release a rush of air, but may not be audible in a loud setting, such as the trauma bay.

There has been recent discussion and debate over whether the decompression needle in fact reaches the thoracic cavity in a significant portion of patients. This may either be because the patient has a thicker chest wall than usual, or the needle is not long enough. If there is concern that the needle did not enter the chest, another option is to perform a second needle decompression at the mid-axillary or anterior axillary line at the 4th or 5th intercostal space, as described in the updated Advanced Trauma Life Support guidelines to be used as the initial site of decompression [32]. The nipple or inframammary crease can be used as the anatomic landmark to help rapidly identify this level. However, the issues with an anterior 2nd intercostal decompression site can easily be overcome with a needle that is 6.5 cm (2.5 inches) long in order to achieve a 95% success rate [33, 34]. In fact, commercial decompression needles are often longer, such as the ARS® Decompression Needle at 8.9 cm (3.5 inches).

47.3.2.2 Tube Thoracostomy

After needle decompression of a tension pneumothorax or tension hemothorax, a formal tube thoracostomy is performed. In the setting of a pneumothorax or hemothorax without tension physiology, the placement of a chest tube is generally determined by the size and the patient's respiratory and clinical condition. An obvious pneumothorax on CXR may warrant placement of a chest tube [25].

However, in the case of an occult pneumothorax, there is ongoing debate over if and when to intervene with chest tube placement. Studies quote a range of 8% to over 50% of patients who fail conservative management and require tube thoracostomy for an expanding pneumothorax [35, 36]. Some report higher rates of overall complications for those who undergo chest tube placement versus observation for occult pneumothoraces [35]. Increased morbidity of chest tubes can be attributed to complications including improper chest tube positioning, vascular injury, post removal complications, increased hospital length of stay, infection, and pain. Given up to a 20% risk of chest tube complications, it is clinically acceptable to closely monitor an occult pneumothorax as long as the patient is not symptomatic or undergoing PPV [25]. A reasonable size is the 35 mm rule (as measured from the pleura to chest wall on CT chest) as a cutoff for occult pneumothoraces that require tube thoracostomy [37].

For those undergoing mechanical ventilation, two prospective studies offer differing recommendations. Enderson et al. randomized 40 trauma patients to observation versus tube thoracostomy and found 53% in the observation group who required PPV had progression of their pneumothorax, with 3 patients having tension physiology [36]. With a similar number of patients, Brasel and associates found that there was no significant difference in complications or emergent chest tube placements for respiratory decline between the groups, concluding that observation is safe [38]. However, the small sample sizes of these studies may limit the strength of recommendation and, therefore, ongoing discussion and investigation ensues (Clinical Trial NCT00530725). Given the conflicting evidence, utilization of the 35 mm rule seems reasonable even with patients undergoing positive pressure [39].

General clinical guidelines have previously recommended consideration of draining all traumatic hemothoraces, regardless of size. More recent studies have investigated when tube thoracostomy may not be required. There have been various measurement metrics to determine at what volume or size (as a surrogate of volume) a hemothorax should be drained. Not many CT scans will allow for volumetric measurements but measuring the thickness of the hemothorax on an axial CT image is a simple way to estimate the volume of blood and seems to correlate with requirement of drainage. A recent meta-analysis of occult hemothoraces also found that observation can fail in up to 23% of trauma patients. Greater than 300 mL of blood (similarly measured as a 1.5 cm pleural stripe) was a predictor of failure, thus warranting a chest tube [40, 41]. Furthermore, other investigations have found a higher risk for delayed hemothorax requiring intervention in the elderly trauma patient with certain rib fracture patterns, which could warrant closer monitoring or earlier intervention for these patients [42].

It is recommended that, if possible, a single intravenous dose of cefazolin 2 g be given prior to chest tube insertion. Infection rates related to chest tubes vary in the literature from 2% to 35%. The use of sterile technique of full body barrier drape, sterile gloves and gown, should also be adopted given the decrease in infection rates seen associated with this practice in placing central lines. It is only logical that an invasive surgical procedure warrants the same level of sterility [43]. This seems particularly true with penetrating wounds, where administration of antibiotics leads to decreased rates of empyema [44].

47.3.2.3 Chest Tube Size and Pigtail Catheters

It was traditionally taught that blood is more likely to clot in smaller bore chest tubes. However, an increasing body of literature suggests that a large tube may not be of any additional benefit and only confers more pain. If the blood in the pleural space is still in liquid form and has not coagulated, the tube size should not matter. If the blood has coagulated and is in a gelatinous state then again, the chest tube size will still not matter, as the hemothorax will not be evacuated despite a larger chest tube. Instead, the patient will require a video-assisted thoracoscopic surgery (VATS) or thoracotomy for evacuation at that point in time. Another described technique is a Yankauer-assisted evacuation often done in addition or in place of a VATS to help suction the clot out of the chest [45, 46]. The caveat to placing a smaller bore chest tube is that, in our experience, a tube that is too small has the propensity to bend and kink more easily. A compromise is a 28 Fr chest tube [47, 48].

With regard to an isolated pneumothorax without any hemothorax component, the use of an even smaller pigtail catheter has been adopted by many institutions as standard therapy. These can be inserted via the Seldinger technique at either the 2nd intercostal space or the standard chest tube insertion site at the 4th intercostal space. The benefits of placing the tube in the 2nd intercostal space include the following: better evacuation (as most pneumothoraces are apical), the tube is out of the way of the patient (may be more comfortable), and in theory is safer, as one would avoid mediastinal injuries if inadvertently over-penetrating the chest wall upon placing the tube [49].

47.3.2.4 Setup of the Pleur-evac or Atrium

There are a variety of suction canister types. These originated from the 3-bottle system. It is critical to understand how the 3-bottle system works, as all modern collection chambers function similarly. In this system, one bottle functions as a collection chamber, the second functions as a water seal, and the third bottle regulates the amount of negative pressure. The authors recommend a dry-type suction (e.g., Atrium Oasis) for a couple reasons. First, the suction indicator allows care providers to easily recognize whether the chest tube is on suction. Second, there is no noise associated with the dry suction, whereas the bubbling with wet suction canisters can confuse bedside providers into thinking that the degree of bubbling is related to the amount of suction [50].

47.3.2.5 Heimlich Valves

When a patient with an isolated pneumothorax has a small but persistent air leak, resolution may be achieved by attaching a Heimlich valve to the chest tube. A Heimlich valve is a one-way valve that allows air to escape from the pleural cavity but prevents atmospheric air from leaking back in. Patients may be able to be managed at home with such an approach. The patient can later be seen in the clinic to allow more time for pulmonary healing and air leak resolution prior to remove the chest tube [51].

47.3.2.6 Thoracotomy and VATS for Hemothorax Evacuation

Less than 10% of blunt and only 15–30% of penetrating thoracic injuries will require an operation [32]. There are three operative indications for a hemothorax: hemorrhage control, retained hemothorax, and the clinical judgement of the surgeon.

The classic teaching for initial indications of operative intervention includes evacuation of over 1500 mL of blood on initial chest tube insertion or a persistent drainage of 200 mL per hour for over 4 h. Karmy-Jones et al. recommend third indication when there is over 1500 mL of blood loss in 24 h [52]. These parameters are indicative of bleeding that will not self-resolve and thus requires an exploratory operation, during which injuries to intrathoracic organs or vasculature must be addressed. The ability to measure these outputs is more difficult than described. Often, there is an immeasurable volume of blood that spills onto the patient bed upon chest tube insertion that does not get captured in the chest tube canister. In addition, if one realizes that the chest tube output is higher than usual, one does not have to wait 4 h before taking the patient to the operating room. As such, the clinical judgement of the surgeon is critical in determining whether and when operative intervention is warranted.

It is not clearly delineated who may be at higher risk for a retained hemothorax despite chest tube drainage. The rate is estimated to be roughly 29%, but risk factors may be related to initial size of hemothorax, age, and other associated injuries [53]. Instilling fibrinolytics such as tissue plasminogen activator and dornase through the chest tube was thought to be useful for breaking up and draining a retained hemothorax. However, this practice has fallen out of favor, and instead, early VATS is recommended due to its superior outcomes with regard to prevent the need for evacuation with a thoracotomy [46, 54]. Early VATS within 3–6 days of identified hemothorax has been associated with decreased incidence of complications, such as empyema, duration of ventilator days, hospital days, and need for thoracotomy [45].

47.3.2.7 VATS Pleurodesis

While the majority of pneumothoraces that an emergency surgeon addresses will relate to trauma, a subset of patients may present with a primary or spontaneous pneumothorax from ruptured subpleural blebs. Depending on the surgical capabilities of the region, it may be the responsibility of the acute care surgeon to manage and treat this pathology. For non-traumatic primary pneumothoraces, there is evidence of equivalent outcomes with needle aspiration and tube thoracostomy for the initial episode. For recurrent episodes, recommendations vary regarding surgical intervention with VATS and apical blebectomy and/or pleurodesis [55].

47.3.2.8 Post-surgical Management

Post-procedure or post-surgical chest tube management may vary by practitioner and institution. There is Level I evidence, however, by Younes and associates supporting the removal of chest tubes when the output decreases to less than 2 mL/kg/day for a hemothorax [56]. There is increasing evidence that chest tubes can be removed despite larger outputs, even up to 500 mL/day without an increase in reaccumulation or need for thoracentesis [57, 58].

For a pneumothorax, there should be no air leak detected prior to chest tube removal. Inspection for air leaks should be performed daily. To check for an air leak, the chest tube is removed from suction, the pressure in the canister equalized and the water seal chamber observed for evidence of air leakage (bubbles) with the patient's respiration. A traditional method of chest tube management is as described: with no evidence of an air leak, the chest tube may be placed off suction and on water seal for 4–6 h. A repeat CXR is then obtained to ensure a pneumothorax has not recurred prior to chest tube removal. After chest tube removal, a post-removal CXR is obtained in approximately 4–6 h to further ensure that there has not been a reaccumulation of the pneumothorax and a need for chest tube reinsertion.

Existing evidence, however, suggests that most chest tubes can be removed without a period of water seal and rates of recurrent pneumothorax are low enough (~2%) that one does not need to obtain a post-removal CXR. Avoidance of post-removal CXRs decreases hospital length of stay and the number of CXRs. It is also reasonable to forgo obtaining a CXR after transitioning from suction to water seal, as this has also been shown to be safe [59, 60]. In addition, varying textbooks will describe and emphasize removing a chest tube at either the end of inspiration or expiration, but either practice is equally safe [61].

47.3.3 Prognosis and Complications

47.3.3.1 Tube Thoracostomy Complications

The complication rate of chest tube placement is approximately 20%, with a high proportion of iatrogenesis. This is not a benign procedure and is not without risks. The chest tube can be inserted too forcefully despite its blunt tip, tearing the lung (the most common organ injured), or even worse, can enter the heart or a multitude of surrounding structures. Without tactile confirmation that the chest tube is between the ribs, it can mistakenly be placed into the subcutaneous space. Despite the blunt tip, it is easy to penetrate the lung, heart, vessels, esophagus, and even abdominal organs when placed too low. Trocar chest tubes have gone out of favor for good reason [62].

The angle of insertion is shown to have a direct correlation with the complication rate. Inexperienced proceduralists will place the chest tube perpendicular to the patient's thoracic cavity. However, the placement of a chest tube should be thought of as placing the tip of the tube in a cephalad position making the angle less than 45° between the chest tube and chest wall [63].

Complications may occur even after a successful chest tube placement. Chest tubes can become dislodged without careful monitoring or adequate dressing fixation [62]. Chest tubes can get clogged, but stripping a chest tube may not prevent this, as two-thirds of clogged chest tubes will resolve spontaneously. A major complication with a hemothorax is the inability to fully evacuate the blood. In this case, a VATS is required to prevent infection of the hemothorax and ultimately a trapped lung [45].

47.3.3.2 Persistent Air Leak

Most air leaks resolve within 5–7 days. If the air leak is small, turning the suction pressure lower or placing the chest tube to water seal (as long as the pneumothorax does not worsen) can help seal the air leak. If the leakage is persistent for over 5 days, then the general recommendation is to proceed with a bronchoscopy to evaluate the tracheobronchial tree for injury. Most air leaks from trauma are due to injuries to the lung parenchyma. Autologous blood patches, fibrin sealants, or surgical intervention with pleurodesis have been described to seal these parenchymal injuries. A more conservative approach with prolonged use of the Heimlich valve has been described for smaller leaks [64].

47.3.3.3 Tracheobronchial Injury

If there is a large air leak after tube thoracostomy and the pneumothorax is enlarged or not improved on subsequent CXRs, then a second chest tube may be required to control the air leak. A very large air leak is indicative of a tracheobronchial injury and flexible fiberoptic bronchoscopy would be the next step in diagnosis. Most injuries are found within 2 cm of the carina. A thoracotomy as well as intubation of the contralateral mainstem bronchus with single-lung ventilation may be necessary for primary surgical repair. Alternatively, commercial sealants and endobronchial one-way valves are additional treatment modalities that have been described [65].

> **Dos and Don'ts**
> - Do not wait to diagnose a tension pneumothorax radiographically.
> - Do not place a chest tube at greater than 45 degrees relative to the patient's chest wall.
> - Always ensure that chest tube connections are secure and on the desired setting.
> - Always check for air leaks when rounding on patients.
> - Always confirm chest tube placement with a CXR.

> **Take-Home Messages**
> - Use an occlusive dressing for an open chest wound.
> - A chest tube size of 28 Fr is likely adequate for drainage in the setting of trauma.
> - A dry-type chest tube canister is easier to use.
> - VATS for retained hemothorax is preferred over fibrinolytics.

Multiple Choice Questions

1. At what hemothorax depth on axial CT should you drain with tube thoracostomy?
   A. 1 cm
   B. **1.5 cm**
   C. 2 cm
   D. 3 cm

2. For a chest tube placed for a hemothorax caused by trauma, at what initial output should you take someone to the operating room for operative intervention?
   A. 500 mL
   B. 1000 mL
   C. **1500 mL**
   D. 2000 mL

3. What should the next step be if a pneumothorax is increasing in size despite tube thoracostomy already performed?
   A. Increase the negative pressure of the chest tube system
   B. **Place a second chest tube**
   C. Immediate thoracotomy
   D. Bronchoscopy

4. At what angle relative to the patient's chest wall should a chest tube be placed?
   A. Greater than 30 degrees
   B. **Less than 45 degrees**
   C. 90 degrees, perpendicular
   D. Greater than 90 degrees

5. Currently, what is thought to be the standard chest tube size required for traumatic chest injuries?
   A. 12 Fr pigtail
   B. 40 Fr chest tube
   C. 36 Fr chest tube
   D. **28 Fr chest tube**

6. Which of these is not a known potential complication of chest tube placement?
   A. Hemorrhage from intercostal vessels
   B. Chest tube placement into the liver
   C. **Development of subpleural blebs**
   D. Pneumonia

7. All the following thoracic ultrasound findings help rule out the presence of a pneumothorax except:
   A. **A pleural stripe**
   B. B-lines
   C. Lung sliding
   D. "Seashore sign"

8. A 27-year-old man is brought to the emergency department after being stabbed in the right chest. He is dyspneic and his initial vitals include a heart rate of 124, blood pressure of 88/45, respiratory rate of 30, and oxygen saturation of 82%. His GCS is 14 and breath sounds are absent in the right lung field. What is the next best step in management?
   A. Intubation
   B. **Needle decompression of the right chest**
   C. Obtain a chest X-ray
   D. Obtain an e-FAST

9. Absence of lung sliding is an ultrasound finding that can occur in all of the following except:
   A. **Pulmonary edema**
   B. Atelectasis
   C. Right mainstem intubation
   D. Pneumothorax

10. A 71-year-old woman is brought into the hospital for evaluation after a fall down four steps. She is hemodynamically normal but complains of left-sided chest pain with associated ecchymosis. An upright chest X-ray demonstrates blunting of the costophrenic angle. What is the minimum volume of fluid accumulation needed to demonstrate this finding?
    A. 50 mL
    B. 100 mL
    C. **175 mL**
    D. 400 mL

References

1. Bobbio A, Dechartres A, Bouam S, Damotte D, Rabbat A, Régnard J-F, et al. Epidemiology of spontaneous pneumothorax: gender-related differences. Thorax. 2015;70(7):653.
2. Gupta D. Epidemiology of pneumothorax in England. Thorax. 2000;55(8):666–71.
3. Shirley PJ. Trauma and critical care III: chest trauma. Trauma. 2005;7(3):133–42.
4. Liman ST, Kuzucu A, Tastepe AI, Ulasan GN, Topcu S. Chest injury due to blunt trauma. Eur J Cardio-Thorac Surg Off J Eur Assoc Cardio-Thorac Surg. 2003;23(3):374–8.
5. Sirmali M, Türüt H, Topçu S, Gülhan E, Yazici U, Kaya S, et al. A comprehensive analysis of traumatic rib fractures: morbidity, mortality and management. Eur J Cardio-Thorac Surg Off J Eur Assoc Cardio-Thorac Surg. 2003;24(1):133–8.
6. Celik B, Sahin E, Nadir A, Kaptanoglu M. Iatrogenic pneumothorax: etiology, incidence and risk factors. Thorac Cardiovasc Surg. 2009;57(5):286–90.
7. El Hammoumi MM, Drissi G, Achir A, Benchekroun A, Benosman A, Kabiri EH. Iatrogenic pneumothorax: experience of a Moroccan Emergency Center. Rev Port Pneumol. 2013;19(2):65–9.
8. Sugarbaker DJ, editor. Sugarbaker's adult chest surgery. 3rd ed. New York: McGraw Hill Education; 2020.
9. Boersma WG, Stigt JA, Smit HJM. Treatment of haemothorax. Respir Med. 2010;104(11):1583–7.
10. Richardson JD, Miller FB, Carrillo EH, Spain DA. Complex thoracic injuries. Surg Clin North Am. 1996;76(4):725–48.
11. Sassoon CS, Light RW, O'Hara VS, Moritz TE. Iatrogenic pneumothorax: etiology and morbidity. Results of a Department of Veterans Affairs Cooperative Study. Respir Int Rev Thorac Dis. 1992;59(4):215–20.
12. John J, Seifi A. Incidence of iatrogenic pneumothorax in the United States in teaching vs. non-teaching hospitals from 2000 to 2012. J Crit Care. 2016;34:66–8.
13. Azfar Ali H, Lippmann M, Mundathaje U, Khaleeq G. Spontaneous hemothorax. Chest. 2008;134(5):1056–65.
14. Light RW. Pleural diseases. Dis Mon. 1992;38(5):266–331.
15. Carr JJ, Reed JC, Choplin RH, Pope TL, Case LD. Plain and computed radiography for detecting experimentally induced pneumothorax in cadavers: implications for detection in patients. Radiology. 1992;183(1):193–9.
16. Odom SR. Chest trauma. In: Butler KL, Harisinghani M, editors. Acute care surgery: imaging essentials for rapid diagnosis [Internet]. New York, NY: McGraw-Hill Education; 2015. [cited 2021 May 3]. accesssurgery.mhmedical.com/content.aspx?aid=1108260535.
17. Blaivas M, Lyon M, Duggal S. A prospective comparison of supine chest radiography and bedside ultrasound for the diagnosis of traumatic pneumothorax. Acad Emerg Med Off J Soc Acad Emerg Med. 2005;12(9):844–9.
18. Ma OJ, Mateer JR. Trauma ultrasound examination versus chest radiography in the detection of hemothorax. Ann Emerg Med. 1997;29(3):312–5; discussion 315–316.
19. Husain LF, Hagopian L, Wayman D, Baker WE, Carmody KA. Sonographic diagnosis of pneumothorax. J Emerg Trauma Shock. 2012;5(1):76–81.
20. Kirkpatrick AW, Sirois M, Laupland KB, Liu D, Rowan K, Ball CG, et al. Hand-held thoracic sonography for detecting post-traumatic pneumothoraces: the Extended Focused Assessment with Sonography for Trauma (EFAST). J Trauma. 2004;57(2):288–95.
21. Rahimi-Movaghar V, Yousefifard M, Ghelichkhani P, Baikpour M, Tafakhori A, Asady H, et al. Application of ultrasonography and radiography in detection of hemothorax; a systematic review and meta-analysis. Emerg Tehran Iran. 2016;4(3):116–26.
22. Ball CG, Kirkpatrick AW, Laupland KB, Fox DI, Nicolaou S, Anderson IB, et al. Incidence, risk factors, and outcomes for occult pneumothoraces in victims of major trauma. J Trauma. 2005;59(4):917–24; discussion 924–925.
23. Ball CG, Ranson K, Dente CJ, Feliciano DV, Laupland KB, Dyer D, et al. Clinical predictors of occult pneumothoraces in severely injured blunt polytrauma patients: a prospective observational study. Injury. 2009;40(1):44–7.
24. Mahmood I, Younis B, Ahmed K, Mustafa F, El-Menyar A, Alabdallat M, et al. Occult pneumothorax in patients presenting with blunt chest trauma: an observational analysis. Qatar Med J. 2020;2020(1):10.
25. Ball CG, Hameed SM, Evans D, Kortbeek JB, Kirkpatrick AW, Canadian Trauma Trials Collaborative. Occult pneumothorax in the mechanically ventilated trauma patient. Can J Surg J Can Chir. 2003;46(5):373–9.
26. Kheirabadi BS, Terrazas IB, Koller A, Allen PB, Klemcke HG, Convertino VA, et al. Vented versus unvented chest seals for treatment of pneumothorax and prevention of tension pneumothorax in a swine model. J Trauma Acute Care Surg. 2013;75(1):150–6.
27. Arnaud F, Tomori T, Teranishi K, Yun J, McCarron R, Mahon R. Evaluation of chest seal performance in a swine model: comparison of Asherman vs. Bolin seal. Injury. 2008;39(9):1082–8.
28. Sharma A, Jindal P. Principles of diagnosis and management of traumatic pneumothorax. J Emerg Trauma Shock. 2008;1(1):34.
29. Shaireen H, Rabi Y, Metcalfe A, Kamaluddeen M, Amin H, Akierman A, et al. Impact of oxygen concentration on time to resolution of spontaneous pneumothorax in term infants: a population based cohort study. BMC Pediatr. 2014;14(1):208.
30. Clark SD, Saker F, Schneeberger MT, Park E, Sutton DW, Littner Y. Administration of 100% oxygen does not hasten resolution of symptomatic spon-

30. taneous pneumothorax in neonates. J Perinatol. 2014;34(7):528–31.
31. Jodie P, Kerstin H. BET 2: pre-hospital finger thoracostomy in patients with chest trauma. Emerg Med J EMJ. 2017;34(6):419.
32. Henry S. Advanced trauma life support 10th edition student course manual. 10th ed. Chicago, IL: American College of Surgeons (ACS), Committee on Trauma; 2018.
33. Clemency BM, Tanski CT, Rosenberg M, May PR, Consiglio JD, Lindstrom HA. Sufficient catheter length for pneumothorax needle decompression: a meta-analysis. Prehospital Disaster Med. 2015;30(3):249–53.
34. Chang SJ, Ross SW, Kiefer DJ, Anderson WE, Rogers AT, Sing RF, et al. Evaluation of 8.0-cm needle at the fourth anterior axillary line for needle chest decompression of tension pneumothorax. J Trauma Acute Care Surg. 2014;76(4):1029–34.
35. Zhang M, Teo LT, Goh MH, Leow J, Go KTS. Occult pneumothorax in blunt trauma: is there a need for tube thoracostomy? Eur J Trauma Emerg Surg Off Publ Eur Trauma Soc. 2016;42(6):785–90.
36. Enderson BL, Abdalla R, Frame SB, Casey MT, Gould H, Maull KI. Tube thoracostomy for occult pneumothorax: a prospective randomized study of its use. J Trauma. 1993;35(5):726–9; discussion 729–730.
37. Bou Zein Eddine S, Boyle KA, Dodgion CM, Davis CS, Webb TP, Juern JS, et al. Observing pneumothoraces: the 35-millimeter rule is safe for both blunt and penetrating chest trauma. J Trauma Acute Care Surg. 2019;86(4):557–64.
38. Brasel KJ, Stafford RE, Weigelt JA, Tenquist JE, Borgstrom DC. Treatment of occult pneumothoraces from blunt trauma. J Trauma. 1999;46(6):987–90; discussion 990-991.
39. Kirkpatrick AW, Rizoli S, Ouellet J-F, Roberts DJ, Sirois M, Ball CG, et al. Occult pneumothoraces in critical care: a prospective multicenter randomized controlled trial of pleural drainage for mechanically ventilated trauma patients with occult pneumothoraces. J Trauma Acute Care Surg. 2013;74(3):747–55.
40. Bilello JF, Davis JW, Lemaster DM. Occult traumatic hemothorax: when can sleeping dogs lie? Am J Surg. 2005;190(6):841–4.
41. Gilbert RW, Fontebasso AM, Park L, Tran A, Lampron J. The management of occult hemothorax in adults with thoracic trauma: a systematic review and meta-analysis. J Trauma Acute Care Surg. 2020;89(6):1225–32.
42. Choi J, Anand A, Sborov KD, Walton W, Chow L, Guillamondegui O, et al. Complication to consider: delayed traumatic hemothorax in older adults. Trauma Surg Amp Acute Care Open. 2021;6(1):e000626.
43. Maxwell RA, Campbell DJ, Fabian TC, Croce MA, Luchette FA, Kerwin AJ, et al. Use of presumptive antibiotics following tube thoracostomy for traumatic hemopneumothorax in the prevention of empyema and pneumonia—a multi-center trial. J Trauma 2004;57(4):742–748; discussion 748-749.
44. Bosman A, de Jong MB, Debeij J, van den Broek PJ, Schipper IB. Systematic review and meta-analysis of antibiotic prophylaxis to prevent infections from chest drains in blunt and penetrating thoracic injuries. Br J Surg. 2012;99(4):506–13.
45. Lin H-L, Huang W-Y, Yang C, Chou S-M, Chiang H-I, Kuo L-C, et al. How early should VATS be performed for retained haemothorax in blunt chest trauma? Injury. 2014;45(9):1359–64.
46. Moore HB, Moore EE, Burlew CC, Moore FA, Coimbra R, Davis JW, et al. Western Trauma Association critical decisions in trauma: management of parapneumonic effusion. J Trauma Acute Care Surg. 2012;73(6):1372–9.
47. Bauman ZM, Kulvatunyou N, Joseph B, Jain A, Friese RS, Gries L, et al. A prospective study of 7-year experience using percutaneous 14-French pigtail catheters for traumatic hemothorax/hemopneumothorax at a level-1 trauma center: size still does not matter. World J Surg. 2018;42(1):107–13.
48. Inaba K, Lustenberger T, Recinos G, Georgiou C, Velmahos GC, Brown C, et al. Does size matter? A prospective analysis of 28-32 versus 36-40 French chest tube size in trauma. J Trauma Acute Care Surg. 2012;72(2):422–7.
49. Kulvatunyou N, Vijayasekaran A, Hansen A, Wynne JL, O'Keeffe T, Friese RS, et al. Two-year experience of using pigtail catheters to treat traumatic pneumothorax: a changing trend. J Trauma Inj Infect Crit Care. 2011;71(5):1104–7.
50. Zisis C, Tsirgogianni K, Lazaridis G, Lampaki S, Baka S, Mpoukovinas I, et al. Chest drainage systems in use. Ann Transl Med. 2015;3(3):43.
51. Gogakos A, Barbetakis N, Lazaridis G, Papaiwannou A, Karavergou A, Lampaki S, et al. Heimlich valve and pneumothorax. Ann Transl Med. 2015;3(4):54.
52. Karmy-Jones R. Timing of urgent thoracotomy for hemorrhage after trauma: a multicenter study. Arch Surg. 2001;136(5):513.
53. Prakash PS, Moore SA, Rezende-Neto JB, Trpcic S, Dunn JA, Smoot B, et al. Predictors of retained hemothorax in trauma: results of an eastern association for the surgery of trauma multi-institutional trial. J Trauma Acute Care Surg. 2020;89(4):679–85.
54. Oğuzkaya F, Akçali Y, Bilgin M. Videothoracoscopy versus intrapleural streptokinase for management of post traumatic retained haemothorax: a retrospective study of 65 cases. Injury. 2005;36(4):526–9.
55. Hallifax R, Janssen JP. Pneumothorax-time for new guidelines? Semin Respir Crit Care Med. 2019;40(3):314–22.
56. Younes RN, Gross JL, Aguiar S, Haddad FJ, Deheinzelin D. When to remove a chest tube? A randomized study with subsequent prospective consecutive validation. J Am Coll Surg. 2002;195(5):658–62.
57. Paydar S, Ghahramani Z, Ghoddusi Johari H, Khezri S, Ziaeian B, Ghayyoumi MA, et al. Tube thoracostomy (chest tube) removal in traumatic patients: what do we know? What can we do? Bull Emerg Trauma. 2015;3(2):37–40.

58. Yap KH, Soon JL, Ong BH, Loh YJ. The safe volume threshold for chest drain removal following pulmonary resection. Interact Cardiovasc Thorac Surg. 2017;25(5):822–6.
59. Davis JW, Mackersie RC, Hoyt DB, Garcia J. Randomized study of algorithms for discontinuing tube thoracostomy drainage. J Am Coll Surg. 1994;179(5):553–7.
60. Pacanowski JP, Waack ML, Daley BJ, Hunter KS, Clinton R, Diamond DL, et al. Is routine roentgenography needed after closed tube thoracostomy removal? J Trauma. 2000;48(4):684–8.
61. Bell RL, Ovadia P, Abdullah F, Spector S, Rabinovici R. Chest tube removal: end-inspiration or end-expiration? J Trauma. 2001;50(4):674–7.
62. Stawicki Stanislaw PA, Kwiatt M, Tarbox A, Seamon Mark J, Swaroop M, Cipolla J, et al. Thoracostomy tubes: a comprehensive review of complications and related topics. Int J Crit Illn Inj Sci. 2014;4(2):142.
63. Hernandez MC, Laan DV, Zimmerman SL, Naik ND, Schiller HJ, Aho JM. Tube thoracostomy: increased angle of insertion is associated with complications. J Trauma Acute Care Surg. 2016;81(2):366–70.
64. Dugan KC, Laxmanan B, Murgu S, Hogarth DK. Management of persistent air leaks. Chest. 2017;152(2):417–23.
65. Mahmodlou R, Sepehrvand N. Tracheobronchial injury due to blunt chest trauma. Int J Crit Illn Inj Sci. 2015;5(2):116.

Chest Trauma

48

Joseph M. Galante and Tanya N. Rinderknecht

48.1 Introduction

> **Learning Goals (Chapter Core Messages)**
> - Chest injuries are heterogenous in pattern and severity.
> - Consideration of the traumatic mechanism and the likely associated injury patterns helps to guide timely identification and management of injuries.
> - Many chest injuries are managed non-operatively, but meticulous medical care and a clear understanding of when operative intervention is necessary are essential for optimal patient outcomes.

48.1.1 Epidemiology

Injury is a major contributor to the global burden of disease, and the leading cause of death and disability in those under age 35 [1]. Approximately one-third of patients admitted to major US trauma centers sustain serious injury to the chest, and thoracic trauma—both blunt and penetrating—has historically been a major contributing factor in approximately 75% of trauma mortality [2, 3]. Motor vehicle collisions cause the majority of major blunt thoracic trauma, with falls as the next highest contributing blunt mechanism [4]. Penetrating traumatic injuries account for a lower percentage of overall patients (approximately 20%), but have similar or higher mortality rates [5]. It is relevant to note that most studies focus on trauma patients requiring admission to the hospital, so the overall burden of thoracic trauma is likely underreported, as the literature is biased toward more extensively injured patients. Significant blunt thoracic injury is often associated with extra-thoracic injury as well, which contributes to high overall morbidity and mortality rates.

48.1.2 Etiology

Penetrating chest trauma is most commonly caused by gunshot wounds and stabbings. Blunt chest trauma is caused most commonly by motor vehicle collision (cars, motorcycles), as well as by falls, bicycle and pedestrian accidents, assaults, crush injuries, and occupational incidents, among others. Primary lung blast injury and shrapnel injury due to explosions are additional mechanisms of chest injury; although historically more common in military and conflict settings, global terrorism makes it increasingly likely that civilian physicians will encounter these entities as well.

J. M. Galante · T. N. Rinderknecht (✉)
Department of Surgery, University of California Davis Medical Center, Sacramento, CA, USA
e-mail: jmgalante@ucdavis.edu;
trinderknecht@ucdavis.edu

48.1.3 Classification

There is no single classification system for chest injury, because it can entail injury to multiple organs. The American Association for the Surgery of Trauma (AAST) does provide individual grading systems for injuries to the chest wall, lungs, heart, thoracic vasculature, and diaphragm, but these are generally used more for research communication than for clinical decision making. A separate grading system for blunt aortic injuries from the vascular literature is based on anatomic layers of the aorta; this scale is more clinically applicable and helps to guide management of these injuries [6]. Many different rib fracture scoring systems exist, but no one system is universally accepted and their clinical utility remains unclear.

48.1.4 Pathophysiology

The chest contains multiple vital organs and injuries can range from non-consequential to imminently life-threatening or life-ending. A thorough understanding of the structure and anatomy of the chest is essential to suspecting, identifying, and treating injuries in a timely fashion.

The chest wall consists of bones, muscles, and cartilage and serves both to provide the structure necessary to support respiration, and to protect the intra-thoracic contents. The lungs and the major mediastinal structures (aorta, esophagus, trachea, and heart) lie within the chest, and the diaphragm forms the inferior border of the chest, anatomically dividing it from the abdomen and functionally playing an important role in respiratory mechanics. While injury to the chest wall is common and can cause considerable morbidity, it is rarely immediately life-threatening in itself. Injury to any of the underlying intra-thoracic organs, however, can be lethal.

Traumatic mechanism dramatically affects the type and extent of the injuries in the chest. For example, a transmediastinal gunshot wound can injure multiple organs in the chest within its limited trajectory, while a high-speed MVC may spare the mediastinal structures but cause massive chest wall trauma and pulmonary contusions. In blunt trauma, consideration of both rapid deceleration mechanisms (which tend to cause tearing of organs such as the aorta and trachea at fixed points) and massive direct impact to the chest (which can change pressure differentials and lead to esophageal, tracheal, cardiac, alveolar, and diaphragmatic rupture) will help raise clinical suspicion of these serious injuries.

Regardless of mechanism, however, it is useful to consider the ultimate pathways of injury systematically. Injury to the chest can cause bleeding (massive or minor, diffuse or focal, from single or multiple organs), tamponade or tension physiology (via air or blood accumulation in the pericardial or pleural spaces), primary cardiac dysfunction (via myocardial contusion, rupture, compression, or laceration), disruption of respiratory mechanics (via diaphragmatic, chest wall, or tracheal injury), hypoxemia and/or hypercapnia (via direct pulmonary or bronchial injury), and esophageal perforation.

48.2 Diagnosis

48.2.1 Clinical Presentation (Sxs and Phys Exam)

Chest trauma and its associated injuries can present very heterogeneously, with presentations ranging from minimal symptoms to overt arrest. The Advanced Trauma Life Support (ATLS) primary and secondary surveys with adjuncts (EKG, chest X-ray, ultrasound) will identify many of these injuries, as well as external signs that should increase the clinician's suspicion for underlying injury. Patients may report pain, shortness of breath, chest tightness or pressure, among other symptoms. On exam, vital signs should be noted early and their trend followed closely; changes or significant abnormalities in heart rate, blood pressure, respiratory rate or oxygen saturation can all be indicators of life-threatening underlying injury. Physical exam findings can include wounds, abrasions, ecchymosis, tenderness, external bleeding, chest wall deformity, seat belt and steering wheel marks, distended neck veins, crepitus and subcutaneous emphysema, stridor, respiratory distress, and cyanosis, among others.

48.2.2 Tests (Labs, Imaging)

Patients should be cared for by ATLS protocol, with standard telemetry monitoring, frequent vital signs, continuous pulse oximetry, standard initial trauma labs, and arterial blood gases as needed. Chest radiograph should be done as part of the initial survey, with ultrasound as needed for additional pulmonary assessment (pneumothorax), cardiac assessment (pericardial fluid, tamponade, overall cardiac function), and concurrent abdominal hemorrhage. In the unstable patient, some interventions serve as both diagnostic and therapeutic (e.g., empiric chest tube placement after arrest, release of pericardial tamponade during emergency department thoracotomy for arrest). If the patient is stable enough, CT with intravenous contrast can be useful in delineating the extent of blunt thoracic trauma (including potential associated spine injuries), and for assessing the trajectory of penetrating injuries (particularly helpful for identifying vascular injury).

If there is suspicion for blunt cardiac injury (BCI) based on mechanism or vital signs, an EKG should be done and a troponin level sent. Echocardiography is not necessary purely as a screening tool (see below, 'Medical Management').

If there is concern for aerodigestive tract injury, the patient should undergo both endoscopic and imaging evaluation targeted at these injuries; most commonly this involves some combination of bronchoscopy, laryngoscopy, esophagoscopy, and esophagography [7].

> **Differential Diagnosis**
> Injury to all components of the chest cavity should be considered, and based on mechanism and subsequent clinical suspicion, systematically ruled out as necessary. Information about the type of weapon and some basic ballistics knowledge can help guide the penetrating trauma work up and differential diagnosis. In blunt trauma, the differential varies between high velocity (MVC) versus low velocity (fall from standing), and should also be adjusted based on the age and frailty of the patient.
> If patients present after explosions or bombings, a good history is critical to forming the appropriate differential. Physicians need to have a high index of suspicion for primary pulmonary blast injury, especially in patients who were in an enclosed space with or in close proximity to an explosion. In addition to the primary lung injury, these patients are also at risk for injuries from shrapnel, blunt trauma from structural damage, and inhalation injury or burns [8].

48.3 Treatment

48.3.1 Medical Treatment (Including IR)

48.3.1.1 Immediate Treatment

The initial treatment of all chest trauma follows ATLS guidelines. A reliable airway is confirmed (patient maintaining) or obtained (endotracheal intubation). Breath sounds are assessed bilaterally and, if absent or decreased, treated with tube thoracostomy for presumed pneumo- or hemothorax. Respiratory support is provided as needed to ensure adequate oxygenation and ventilation, with interventions ranging from simple nasal cannula to mechanical ventilation. Circulation is assessed and supported as needed, with prompt control of all identifiable bleeding as soon as possible. In addition to hemorrhage control (discussed more in the next section), the treatment of confirmed or suspected significant blood loss, especially with hypotension, includes: massive transfusion with balanced blood products, active efforts to achieve normal temperature and normal pH, targeted treatment of any underlying coagulopathy, both medication related (e.g., reversal or treatment of known anti-platelet or anti-coagulant medications) and hemorrhage related (e.g., TEG-based blood product resuscitation), and consideration of empiric tranexamic acid administration.

48.3.1.2 Ongoing Medical Treatment Considerations

Most chest trauma can be managed with supportive care and simple maneuvers, such as tube thoracostomy; historically, only about 10–15% of patients require operative intervention [3]. Meticulous medical care is essential to help patients heal from these injuries and avoid complications.

Rib fractures are the most common identifiable injury after blunt thoracic trauma, and the associated morbidity and mortality increase with a higher number of rib fractures, advanced age, and higher injury severity scores [4, 9–11]. Since the most intense pain period usually correlates with the peak inflammatory response at 24–36 h post-injury, both early and consistent attention to adequate analgesia are essential. Adequate pain control enables more active participation in respiratory therapy and pulmonary hygiene exercises, a faster normalization of respiratory mechanics, and earlier mobilization, all of which promote recovery and help prevent complications, including pneumonia. Multi-modal analgesia generally allows for the best pain control while minimizing side effects from any one class of medication, especially opioids. Early consideration of neuraxial options (epidural, continuous peripheral nerve infusion catheters, etc.) if other injuries and coagulation status allow is recommended [12].

Traumatic lung injury (blunt or penetrating) can acutely and directly affect oxygenation and ventilation. In addition, these patients are often at risk for developing acute respiratory distress syndrome (ARDS), because in addition to their lung injury, they often also require large volume resuscitation, which can lead to pulmonary edema, and they experience a massive inflammatory response to their trauma. If there is ongoing need for mechanical ventilation, lung protective ventilator management strategies are the standard of care to minimize additional barotrauma. Patients who have suffered primary lung blast injury have a high rate (about 80%) of needing mechanical ventilation, and are also at increased risk for developing pulmonary complications, including ARDS, pulmonary hemorrhage, and pneumothoraces. Care is supportive [8].

Occasionally, interventional radiology may be able to assist with control of bleeding for targets that are surgically more challenging or invasive to access (e.g., bleeding posterior intercostal artery, intra-parenchymal central pulmonary bleeding). These interventions require the patient to be stable enough to undergo cross-sectional imaging and to travel to the endovascular suite.

Blunt aortic injury occurs most commonly with deceleration injury. The injuries are most often near the takeoff of the left subclavian artery, where the isthmus creates an anatomic fixed point that is susceptible to tearing. If patients survive to the hospital, they often have a significant associated trauma burden. Initial management of these blunt aortic injuries is medical, with diligent blood pressure and heart rate control to minimize stress on the injured aortic wall. Consultation with vascular and/or cardiac surgery, depending on the location of injury, is needed to determine the patient's need for further intervention and the injury's suitability for endovascular versus open repair. Timing of the aortic repair will depend on the extent of the aortic injury and the patient's other injuries [6, 13].

BCI should be considered in any patient with significant blunt chest trauma. These injuries can range from myocardial contusion to valvular disruption and cardiac rupture; this discussion focuses on myocardial contusion. Multiple studies have attempted to determine predictive models for BCI based on other injuries, but none has shown a consistent association with any specific injury—not even with sternal fractures [14–17]. While sternal fractures—especially in isolation—do not predict BCI, high mechanism blunt trauma does place patients at risk for both sternal fractures and BCI, and they are often seen concurrently. The decision to screen is thus clinician-dependent. The Eastern Association for the Surgery of Trauma (EAST) provides useful practice guidelines for BCI: together, a normal (or unchanged from baseline) EKG and a normal troponin rule out BCI, and obviate the need for further work up or monitoring, while abnormality of either should prompt admission to the hospital with cardiac monitoring. Hemodynamic instability or persistent new arrhythmia should prompt an echocardiogram [18]. Care is generally supportive unless workup reveals anatomic trauma (e.g., valvular) or non-traumatic pathology (e.g., coronary artery disease). BCI should be approached mostly as a diagnosis of exclusion, as patients at risk for BCI often have polytrauma and have physiologic derangements from other—often treatable—causes, which should not be missed.

48.3.2 Surgical Treatment (Incl Open and MIS)

48.3.2.1 Emergency Department

Some chest injuries require urgent or emergent surgical management in the emergency department. Tube thoracostomies are placed for pneumothorax and hemothorax as necessary. Tube thoracostomy can be a life-saving maneuver in the setting of tension pneumothorax (Fig. 48.1), and can help determine the need for operative intervention in the setting of massive hemothorax. Emergency department thoracotomy can also provide access for emergent interventions in the chest, including relief of cardiac tamponade, control of cardiac, pulmonary, or chest wall hemorrhage, control of massive air leak, and limiting sub-diaphragmatic bleeding via cross-clamping of the aorta.

48.3.2.2 Operating Room

Some injuries require definitive repair in the operating room. Other chapters address cardiac, thoracic vascular, and esophageal injuries; this chapter will focus on injuries to the chest wall, lung, trachea and bronchi, and diaphragm.

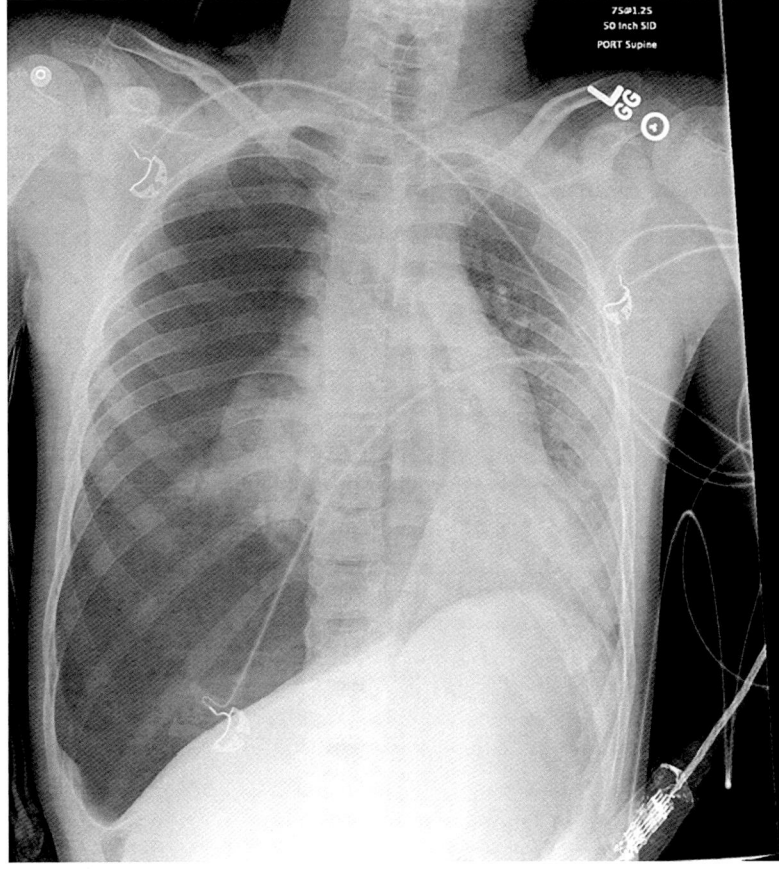

Fig. 48.1 Tension pneumothorax is an imminently life-threatening condition that can be reversed with prompt tube thoracostomy. Ideally, this diagnosis is made clinically and treated before imaging is ever completed

Chest Wall Injury

Chest wall injury includes injury to the bony and muscular structures that give the thorax its shape and structure, as well as to the intercostal blood vessels that supply these structures. Rib fractures are very common in thoracic trauma, and can have a wide spectrum of clinical presentation. They almost always cause pain, which needs to be adequately treated to avoid subsequent complications (as above), but they can also cause secondary pathology. Bony fragments from fracture sites can puncture the visceral pleura, leading to pneumothorax. Fragments or displaced segments of rib can lacerate the pulmonary parenchyma and/or intercostal blood vessels, both of which can cause bleeding. Both pneumo- and hemo-thoraces can be addressed initially with tube thoracostomy drainage, as above, and further management of lung injuries is discussed below. Rib fractures can also alter pulmonary mechanics, most commonly via pain, but occasionally due to structural compromise of the chest wall. The most serious manifestation of this is flail chest, which occurs when two or more sequential ribs are each fractured in two places, allowing for paradoxical motion of that segment of chest wall.

The indications for operative fixation of rib fractures are a topic of ongoing discussion in trauma, and wide variations in practice patterns remain. The most agreed-upon indication for surgical stabilization of rib fractures (SSRF) is flail chest. Other suggested indications, such as three or more displaced fractures, failure of non-operative management, chest wall deformities, lung herniation, a thoracic procedure for a different indication, and chronic rib non-union, all have support in various individual studies but have not been widely adopted. Benefits of SSRF range from improvement of patient-reported pain control and quality of life to decreased ventilator, ICU and hospital days, among others. These benefits have been demonstrated in both ventilated and non-ventilated patients [19–24]. Based on a 2017 review of the literature, the EAST practice guidelines conditionally recommend ORIF of the ribs in the setting of flail chest, but in non-flail rib fractures, they found no clear benefit to operative versus non-operative management (based on outcomes of decreased mortality, incidence of pneumonia, need for tracheostomy, and shorter durations of mechanical ventilation, ICU stay, and hospital stay) [25]. Relative contraindications to SSRF have traditionally included traumatic brain injury and pulmonary contusion, as both conditions often overpower the potential benefits provided by SSRF. Patient positioning for SSRF can be both limited and risky in the setting of unstable spine fractures, so these are also generally considered a contra-indication [20]. Figure 48.2 shows comminuted rib fractures pre- and post-SSRF.

Based on respiratory mechanics, ribs 3–10 are the most relevant for fixation. Fractures should be accessed through incisions that preserve blood supply and spare muscles while optimizing exposure of as many fracture sites as possible [26]. The fractures need to be a sufficient distance from costochondral and costovertebral junctions to allow for hardware placement. Technically, rib fracture fixation can be performed via both open and minimally invasive (thoracoscopic) approaches, or a combination [20, 27]. Multiple fixation methods exist, with commercial plating systems being the most commonly used. It is essential to maintain reduction of the fracture while placing the plate to optimize fracture alignment (Fig. 48.3). In general, if rib fixation is undertaken, as many fractures as are reasonably accessible should be fixed to maximize the effect of the intervention. If there is a flail segment, ideally both fractures are plated, but if only one can be accessed, chest wall stability is still improved [20].

Injury to the chest wall can also cause bleeding, both from intercostal vessels as well as from the raw, injured surfaces of bones and soft tissue. The approach to this bleeding is similar to the management of bleeding from a direct lung injury (which is discussed in the next section) and starts with a tube thoracostomy. Most chest wall bleeding will stop on its own, especially once coagulopathy is corrected and patients are warm and adequately resuscitated. Occasionally, chest wall bleeding is persistent and requires intervention. Bleeding intercostal vessels can sometimes be controlled via interventional radiology embo-

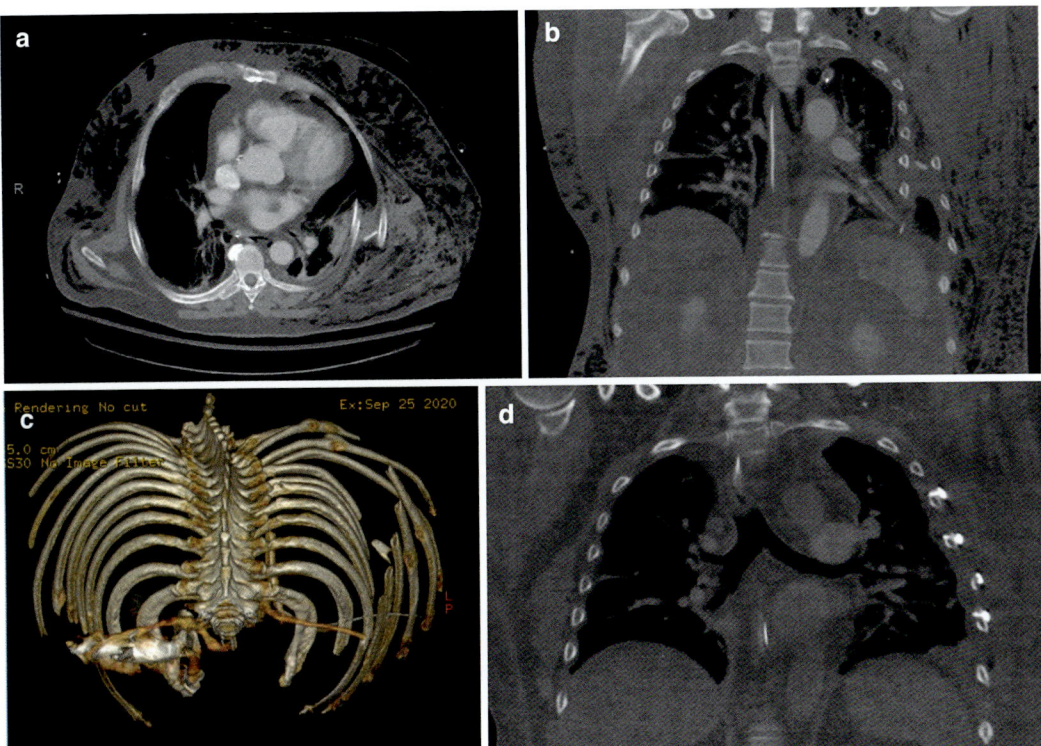

Fig. 48.2 CT scan showing markedly displaced rib fractures with associated pulmonary contusion, subcutaneous emphysema, and significant chest wall deformity (**a, b**). 3D reconstruction of the bony chest wall (shown here in cranio-caudal view—**c**) can help inform surgical planning. A post-operative CT scan (**d**) shows restored chest wall anatomy, with plates visible laterally on the ribs

lization, which is an appealing option in stable patients who do not have an additional indication for operative intervention or are at particularly high operative risk. Alternatively, intercostal vessels can be surgically ligated, with the caveat that this is often more technically challenging than anticipated based on angles of approach in the chest. Raw surface bleeding of the chest wall can be controlled with energy devices, hemostatic agents, and if necessary, packing and damage control strategies. Frequently, no active source of bleeding is identified, and patients improve with evacuation of the hemothorax and thoracostomy tube drainage.

Rarely, chest wall injury is truly destructive and includes open fractures and full thickness tissue loss of the chest wall. These injuries require operative washout and debridement, management of intra-thoracic injuries, stabilization of physiology, and then careful planning for chest wall reconstruction. Depending on the amount of tissue loss, reconstruction may require mesh and/or tissue transfer (ranging from skin grafting to flap coverage). Consultation with thoracic and/or plastic surgeons is generally recommended.

Lung Injury

Other than shock and arrest, the main indications for operative intervention in the setting of acute lung injury are ongoing hemorrhage and massive air leak.

Small injuries to the visceral pleura and the peripheral lung parenchyma can cause pneumothoraces and bleeding. Most of these injuries do not require operative intervention and will heal with tube thoracostomy drainage, aggressive pulmonary hygiene, and time [3]. More extensive injuries, and injuries to the central lung parenchyma and associated blood vessels, can cause significant bleeding. A tube thoracostomy

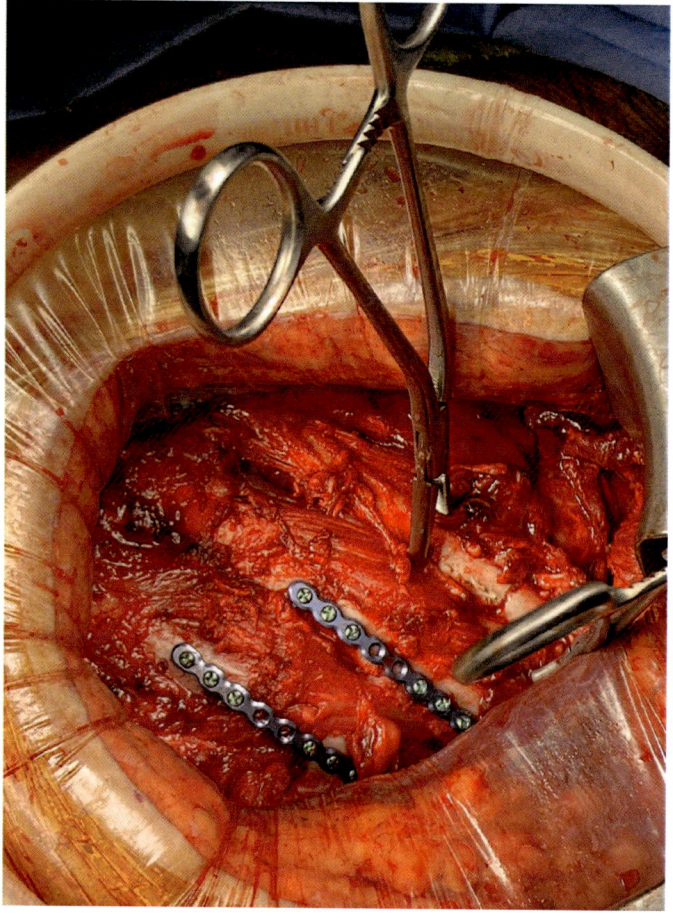

Fig. 48.3 Surgical stabilization of rib fractures. Most plating systems are designed to be used on the exterior surface of the ribs. Heavy clamps are used to manually reduce the fractures, and to hold the alignment in place while the plates are secured into the bone

should be placed, and the output from the tube can be used to help guide whether the patient requires operative intervention to control the bleeding. Classically, the amounts of 1500cc of blood output on insertion of the tube or ongoing output of 200–300cc of blood per hour for multiple hours after tube placement have been used to determine the need for thoracotomy [28, 29]. However, the decision to proceed with thoracotomy should take into account more than just chest tube output. The patient's overall injury burden and physiology, time to presentation (i.e., how much time the initial blood had to accumulate), coagulopathy, and potential for diffuse intra-parenchymal bleeding (versus a source amenable to surgical control) should all be considered. Notably, only 20–30% of patients who undergo thoracotomy for bleeding require any kind of pulmonary resection [30].

When operating for thoracic hemorrhage in the acute setting, patient positioning should be carefully considered. Supine position maintains the most options and flexibility, especially in the case of emergency or arrest, while lateral decubitus position with a posterolateral thoracotomy incision generally provides the best pulmonary and hilar exposure. Patient stability, suspected location of bleeding, anticipated need for managing the unexpected, and limitations of other injuries should all be considered. In general, unstable patients, or those with significant risk of becoming so, should be positioned supine. Location of suspected or known injuries may dramatically affect incision (and thus positioning) choice if otherwise feasible (Table 48.1) [3]. Patients whose injuries have not yet been fully defined, who likely have multiple or bilateral intra-thoracic injuries, or who will need a

Table 48.1 Surgical approaches for traumatic injuries to the lung and associated structures

Site	Sternotomy	Right thoracotomy	Left thoracotomy
Main PA	+++	0	++
Right PA	++	+++	0
Left PA	++	0	+++
Right UL	++	+++	0
Right ML	++	+++	0
Right LL	+	+++	0
Left UL	+	0	+++
Left LL	0	0	+++
Right hilum	++	+++	0
Left hilum	++	0	+++

Table modified from Meredith AV, Hoth JJ. Thoracic trauma: when and how to intervene. Surg Clin North Am. 2007; 87(1):95–118. https://doi.org/10.1016/j.suc.2006.09.014

PA Pulmonary artery, *UL* Upper lobe, *MI* Middle lobe, *LL* Lower lobe

concurrent laparotomy, pelvic intervention, or lower extremity operation, should be positioned supine. Limitations of other injuries (need for full spine precautions, or presence of external fixators, for example) need to be taken into account as well. It is worth mentioning that although video-assisted thoracoscopic surgery (VATS) has traditionally been used mostly for retained hemothorax evacuation in trauma settings, it may have a role in stable patients with thoracic trauma, as a it allows for excellent visualization of the intra-thoracic organs, facilitating diagnosis and localization of injuries, and enables possible intervention as well [31].

If physiology allows and the anesthesiologist is able, a double-lumen endotracheal tube or a single lumen tube with a bronchial blocker should be used; single lung ventilation enables better visualization of one side of the chest cavity at a time. Once in the chest, the surgeon should systematically explore all areas accessible from the chosen approach. Bleeding should be identified and temporized as able. If there is massive bleeding from the lung or hilum that cannot be controlled with compression, a hilar clamp or twist can provide temporary control, but imposes a large physiologic stress and can cause hemodynamic instability. The inferior pulmonary ligament should be released prior to hilar twist to provide mobility and avoid causing additional injury. Packing can be used as needed to help control chest wall bleeding, but requires some caution as the heart and great vessels can easily be inadvertently compressed. The internal mammary artery also deserves special attention: if it has been transected either traumatically or on surgical entry to the chest, it should be proximally and distally ligated to prevent ongoing hemorrhage. If the patient is hypotensive, the vessel may not bleed actively, but it will bleed again once the patient is resuscitated.

Upward of 80% of penetrating lung injuries can be managed with lung-sparing techniques, such as suture pneumonorrhaphy, tractotomy, and peripheral wedge resection. These techniques are simpler and generally faster than more extensive anatomic resections [31]. If the source of bleeding is accessible and can be controlled with suture ligation, the lung can be sewn closed— a suture pneumonorrhaphy. If there is bleeding from within a penetrating parenchymal wound, a stapler can be placed along the trajectory of the wound and the parenchyma stapled and divided, creating a tractotomy, which exposes the injured vessels and bronchi for subsequent suture ligation. If the tract is deep and central, the patient may require a more extensive pulmonary resection. If the injury and bleeding are relatively peripheral, a non-anatomic wedge resection can be performed with a stapler.

In blunt lung injuries that require thoracotomy, smaller areas of injury can be controlled as above, with lung-sparing techniques. Compared with penetrating injury, however, blunt injury more often requires more extensive lung resection, including lobectomy (non-anatomic or anatomic) and pneumonectomy. In a multi-center review, overall mortality rates increased with the extent of lung resection, blunt mechanism, and impaired physiology (likely representing the overall increased trauma burden) [30]. Pneumonectomy for trauma carries very high morbidity and mortality rates, and should be avoided unless all other attempts at hemorrhage control have failed [32].

If a patient is physiologically unwell and cannot tolerate a definitive procedure, damage control thoracotomy is an option. With resuscitation ongoing, the surgeon controls as much bleeding as possible with limited wedge resections, hemostatic agents and a judicious number of packed laparotomy pads. Thoracostomy tubes are placed, and the chest is closed with a temporary vacuum assisted closure device, with or without approximating the ribs with suture. The patient is transferred to an ICU for ongoing resuscitation. Definitive injury management can occur when the patient's physiology is sufficiently improved [33].

Tracheobronchial Injury
Tracheobronchial injury in the chest is not commonly identified, both because it is relatively rare and because it is often either lethal itself or associated with lethal injury patterns [34]. Injury to the thoracic trachea and proximal bronchi can occur from both penetrating and blunt insults. Both tracheal and bronchial injuries occur most commonly within 2.5 cm of the carina [35, 36]. Diagnosis is often delayed, as some injuries are clinically silent, and others have signs and symptoms that are attributed to other injures (e.g., pneumothorax) [37, 38]. While many imaging findings such as pneumomediastinum and pneumothorax are associated with but not specific for tracheobronchial injuries, modern CT technology has been shown to be very good at identifying patients with a high likelihood of tracheobronchial injury, and CT of the chest is generally considered the appropriate screening exam for airway injury [39]. If injury is suspected based on clinical or imaging findings, the airway is secured with bronchoscopic guidance (to avoid further damage to the injury), and bronchoscopy is used to confirm the diagnosis. If possible, the endotracheal tube should be placed distal to the injury to minimize air leak and, with large injuries, restore air flow to the lungs.

Tracheobronchial injuries that involve greater than 1/3 of the circumference of the trachea should generally be surgically repaired. Smaller injuries without tissue loss and with healthy, well-opposed edges can potentially be allowed to heal spontaneously. A non-operative management strategy should only be pursued if there are no signs of ongoing air leak, such as persistent pneumothorax or worsening subcutaneous emphysema. If possible, the balloon of the endotracheal tube should be positioned distal to the injury, minimizing pressurized airflow past the tracheal defect [36]. If a tracheal injury is identified intra-operatively, it should be repaired. There is also a growing interest in using endobronchial stenting as an option for some injuries, if the technology and expertise are available [40].

Operative exposure for thoracic tracheobronchial injuries is most commonly through a right posterolateral thoracotomy, which provides access to the distal trachea, right mainstem bronchus, and proximal left mainstem bronchus. If the injury is to the distal left mainstem bronchus, a left-sided thoracotomy is ideal. More proximal tracheal injuries are approached through the neck and occasionally through mini-sternotomies via splitting of the manubrium. Once exposed, simple injuries can be repaired with interrupted absorbable suture. Debridement and segmental resection are occasionally required for more destructive injuries. Avoiding tension and preserving the tracheal blood supply are essential for successful repairs. For very extensive injury, extra-corporeal membrane oxygenation may be a temporizing option to allow for repair as well [36]. If there are concurrent esophageal or vascular injuries, it is imperative to separate the tracheal repair from the other injuries with a soft-tissue buttress (most commonly pleura, pericardium, or an intercostal muscle flap) to prevent fistula formation.

Diaphragm Injury
Diaphragm injury can occur from both penetrating thoraco-abdominal trauma and blunt trauma (most commonly high speed MVC). Imaging (CXR and CT) can show diaphragm injuries very well when the defect is large and abdominal contents herniate into the chest (Fig. 48.4a, b), but smaller injuries are much harder to identify and require a high degree of clinical suspicion. With

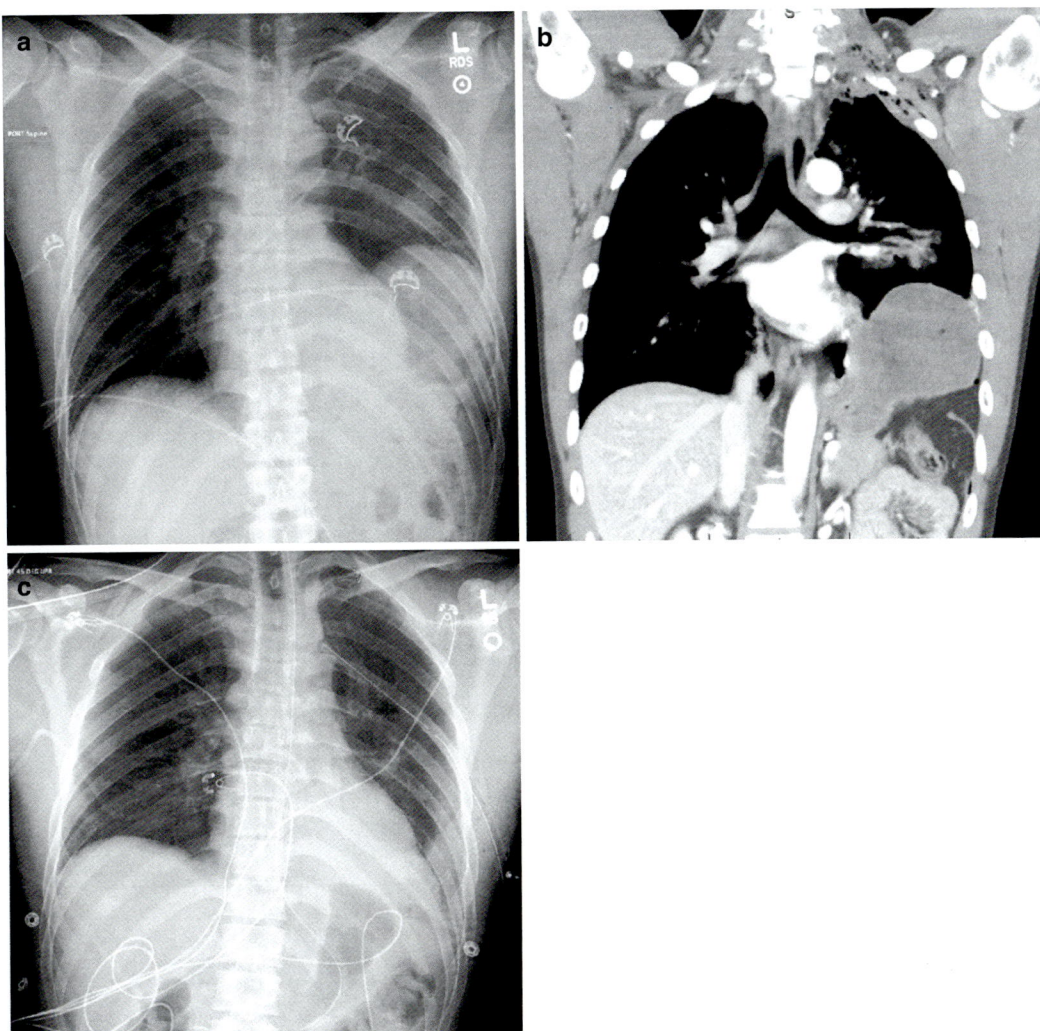

Fig. 48.4 Diaphragmatic rupture after high speed motor vehicle collision. (**a**, **b**) show the presenting chest X-ray and CT, respectively. There is a left pneumothorax, pulmonary contusion, and the stomach is seen herniated into the chest. The edge of the torn lateral diaphragm is visible on the CT scan as well. (**c**) shows the chest X-ray after repair, with abdominal contents reduced, diaphragm repaired, and chest tube in place

right-sided injuries, the liver generally prevents significant herniation of abdominal contents, making these injuries harder to diagnose on imaging. Laparoscopy can be an excellent tool for diagnosis, especially after penetrating trauma. The goals of operative intervention are to reduce any herniated contents, assess for concurrent injury to abdominal organs, and repair the traumatic diaphragmatic defect(s), thus re-establishing normal pulmonary mechanics and preventing the long-term complications of diaphragmatic hernia. Small penetrating right-sided diaphragm injuries can often be managed non-operatively, as the liver generally both prevents herniation of abdominal contents and makes access for repair more challenging. However, a bilothorax can result if there is an associated liver injury with a bile leak. In this setting, repair is generally necessary and a thoracoscopic approach is sometimes preferred [41].

Traumatic diaphragm injuries are most commonly approached via the abdomen, either via a laparoscopic or open approach, as this allows for concurrent examination of the abdominal organs for trauma. The thoracic approach is more often used for chronic hernias in the elective setting, especially for patients with prior abdominal surgery.

Once a diaphragm injury is identified, any herniated abdominal contents should be carefully reduced. Injuries to abdominal organs are managed in the standard fashion. If there is gross contamination in the abdomen, the chest should be washed out via the diaphragmatic defect to reduce the risk of post-operative empyema. A tube thoracostomy is generally placed in the ipsilateral chest cavity once the abdominal contents are reduced (Fig. 48.4c). The diaphragmatic defect can then be closed in a running or interrupted fashion. Care should be taken to avoid inadvertent injury to the heart during repair of the central tendon. The diaphragm can undergo delayed repair if damage control measures are necessary. Destructive diaphragm injuries with tissue loss may require a mesh repair.

48.3.3 Prognosis (Incl Complications and Their Management)

Prognosis after chest trauma is highly variable, based both on initial injuries in the chest as well as on overall injury burden, including extra-thoracic injuries. Patients who survive their initial injuries are at risk for a variety of complications.

48.3.3.1 Complications

Potential complications from chest wall injury include pneumonia, retained hemothorax, nonunion of rib fractures, acute and chronic pain, and potential infection of rib plating hardware. Lung injury can be complicated by prolonged air leak, recurrent pneumothorax, retained hemothorax, empyema, pneumonia and pulmonary abscess, ARDS, and ongoing bleeding related to surgical intervention (for example, from a transected internal mammary artery). Notably, retained hemothorax, prolonged air leak, and empyema may require operative intervention, because while less invasive options such as tube thora-

costomy drainage, intra-pleural therapies (lytic therapies, chemical pleurodesis), and endobronchial interventions are options, these strategies have only variable success.

Tracheobronchial injuries can result in strictures of the airway, which then predispose patients to developing pneumonia, and repairs that are not sufficiently buttressed with soft tissue can form fistulas with surrounding structures. Prolonged air leak can also occur. Diaphragm injuries can be missed early in the trauma work up, and thus allow for contamination of the chest cavity from the abdomen, leading to empyema or bilothorax, or strangulation of herniated contents. Diaphragms repairs can fail and go on to become chronic diaphragmatic hernias.

> **Dos and Don'ts**
> - DO expediently address the potentially life-threatening conditions that can be treated in the ED with tube thoracostomy
> - DONT forget to actively manage coagulopathy and temperature—not all chest bleeding has a surgical target
> - DO use mechanism of injury to help inform your suspicion for various injuries and guide your work up
> - DONT underestimate the potential morbidity over time of multiple rib fractures, especially in the elderly

> **Take-Home Messages**
> - ATLS protocol should guide the work up of all patients with potential chest trauma
> - Consideration of traumatic mechanism is essential to forming an accurate differential diagnosis
> - Many thoracic injuries can be treated with tube thoracostomy and attentive medical management
> - Injury patterns are diverse, and if operative intervention is necessary, careful

consideration of multiple variables (including organs involved, patient physiology, coagulopathy, and operative positioning, among others) is essential to optimizing outcomes
- Rib fractures are a major source of morbidity and mortality, especially in elderly or frail patients, and require proactive care to prevent associated complications

Multiple Choice Questions

1. The most common identifiable injury after blunt thoracic trauma is:
   A. Rib fracture
   B. Sternal fracture
   C. Spine fracture
   D. Pulmonary contusion
   (Answer: A)
2. Which of the following diagnostic assessments is recommended as an initial screening tool for blunt cardiac injury?
   A. Echocardiogram
   B. Electrocardiogram
   C. Cardiac catheterization
   D. Pericardial window
   (Answer: B)
3. Which of the following injuries may be associated with primary pulmonary blast injury?
   A. Shrapnel injury
   B. Inhalation injury
   C. Burns
   D. All of the above
   (Answer: D)
4. Which group is particularly at risk for increased morbidity and mortality from rib fractures?
   A. Children
   B. Male gender
   C. Athletes
   D. The elderly
   (Answer: D)
5. All of the following are essential components of the treatment of rib fractures EXCEPT:
   A. Adequate analgesia, generally multi-modal
   B. Diligent pulmonary hygiene
   C. Daily chest radiographs
   D. Early physical mobilization
   (Answer: C)
6. Despite ongoing discussion about the indications for surgical stabilization of rib fractures, most experts agree that patients will benefit from fixation in the setting of:
   A. Greater than 3 rib fractures
   B. A flail segment
   C. Pulmonary contusion
   D. Fractures of ribs 1 and 2
   (Answer: B)
7. A patient survives emergency department thoracotomy and subsequent left lower lobe wedge resection for hemorrhage control after a gunshot wound to the left chest. Prior to applying the temporary closure device to expedite transfer to the intensive care unit for ongoing resuscitation and warming, it is essential to:
   A. Ensure that the internal mammary artery has been identified and ligated both proximally and distally
   B. Confirm that laparotomy pads packed for bleeding are not compressing the great vessels or heart
   C. Place chest tubes for adequate drainage in addition to the temporary closure device
   D. All of the above
   (Answer: D)
8. Which position/incision combination allows for the best surgical access to a distal tracheal injury?
   A. Supine/Left anterolateral thoracotomy
   B. Supine/Median sternotomy

C. Right lateral decubitus/Left posterolateral thoracotomy
D. Left lateral decubitus/Right posterolateral thoracotomy
(Answer: D)

9. Which of the following is essential to the successful healing of a tracheal repair after traumatic injury?
   A. Tension-free repair
   B. Preservation of tracheal blood supply
   C. Separation from concurrent digestive tract repair with a tissue flap
   D. All of the above

(Answer: D)

10. Which of the following is not a routine part of the management of diaphragmatic injury after blunt trauma?
    A. Reduction of abdominal contents out of the chest
    B. Thoracoscopic evaluation of the lung for pulmonary contusion
    C. Assessment for concurrent abdominal organ injury
    D. Repair of diaphragmatic defect

(Answer: B)

References

1. Alberdi F, García I, Atutxa L, Zabarte M. Epidemiology of severe trauma. Med Intensiva Engl Ed. 2014;38:580–8.
2. Miller DL, Mansour KA. Blunt traumatic lung injuries. Thorac Surg Clin. 2007;17:57–61.
3. Meredith JW, Hoth JJ. Thoracic trauma: when and how to intervene. Surg Clin North Am. 2007;87:95–118.
4. Liman ST, Kuzucu A, Tastepe AI, Ulasan GN, Topcu S. Chest injury due to blunt trauma. Eur J Cardiothorac Surg. 2003;23:374–8.
5. Champion HR, Copes WS, Sacco WJ, Lawnick MM, Keast SL, Bain LW, Flanagan ME, Frey CF. The Major Trauma Outcome Study: establishing national norms for trauma care. J Trauma. 1990;30:1356–65.
6. Azizzadeh A, Keyhani K, Miller CC, Coogan SM, Safi HJ, Estrera AL. Blunt traumatic aortic injury: Initial experience with endovascular repair. J Vasc Surg. 2009;49:1403–8.
7. Penetrating neck injuries, management of—practice management guideline. https://www.east.org/education-career-development/practice-management-guidelines/details/penetrating-neck-injuries-management-of. Accessed 3 May 2021.
8. Scott TE, Kirkman E, Haque M, Gibb IE, Mahoney P, Hardman JG. Primary blast lung injury—a review. Br J Anaesth. 2017;118:311–6.
9. Shulzhenko NO, Zens TJ, Beems MV, Jung HS, O'Rourke AP, Liepert AE, Scarborough JE, Agarwal SK. Number of rib fractures thresholds independently predict worse outcomes in older patients with blunt trauma. Surgery. 2017;161:1083–9.
10. Bulger EM, Arneson MA, Mock CN, Jurkovich GJ. Rib fractures in the elderly. J Trauma Acute Care Surg. 2000;48:1040–7.
11. Ho S-W, Teng Y-H, Yang S-F, Yeh H-W, Wang Y-H, Chou M-C, Yeh C-B. Risk of pneumonia in patients with isolated minor rib fractures: a nationwide cohort study. BMJ Open. 2017;7:e013029.
12. Thoracic trauma, blunt, pain management of—practice management guideline. https://www.east.org/education-career-development/practice-management-guidelines/details/thoracic-trauma-blunt-pain-management-of. Accessed 6 Apr 2021.
13. Blunt aortic injury, evaluation and management of—practice management guideline. https://www.east.org/education-career-development/practice-management-guidelines/details/blunt-aortic-injury-evaluation-and-management-of. Accessed 27 Apr 2021.
14. Rashid MA. Cardiovascular injuries associated with sternal fractures. Eur J Surg. 2001;167:243–8.
15. Oyetunji TA, Jackson HT, Obirieze AC, Moore D, Branche MJ, Greene WR, Cornwell EE, Siram SM. Associated injuries in traumatic sternal fractures: a review of the national trauma data bank. Am Surg. 2013;79:702–5.
16. Chiu WC, D'Amelio LF, Hammond JS. Sternal fractures in blunt chest trauma: a practical algorithm for management. Am J Emerg Med. 1997;15:252–5.
17. Athanassiadi K, Gerazounis M, Moustardas M, Metaxas E. Sternal fractures: retrospective analysis of 100 cases. World J Surg. 2002;26:1243–6.
18. Blunt cardiac injury, screening for—practice management guideline. https://www.east.org/education-career-development/practice-management-guidelines/details/blunt-cardiac-injury%2c-screening-for. Accessed 12 Apr 2021.
19. Pharaon KS, Marasco S, Mayberry J. Rib fractures, flail chest, and pulmonary contusion. Curr Trauma Rep. 2015;1:237–42.
20. de Campos JRM, White TW. Chest wall stabilization in trauma patients: why, when, and how? J Thorac Dis. 2018;10:S951–62.
21. Pieracci FM, Lin Y, Rodil M, et al. A prospective, controlled clinical evaluation of surgical stabilization of severe rib fractures. J Trauma Acute Care Surg. 2016;80:187–94.
22. Pieracci FM, Leasia K, Bauman Z, et al. A multicenter, prospective, controlled clinical trial of surgical stabilization of rib fractures in patients with severe, nonflail fracture patterns (Chest Wall Injury

Society NONFLAIL). J Trauma Acute Care Surg. 2020;88:249–57.
23. Marasco SF, Davies AR, Cooper J, Varma D, Bennett V, Nevill R, Lee G, Bailey M, Fitzgerald M. Prospective randomized controlled trial of operative rib fixation in traumatic flail chest. J Am Coll Surg. 2013;216:924–32.
24. Coughlin TA, Ng JWG, Rollins KE, Forward DP, Ollivere BJ. Management of rib fractures in traumatic flail chest. Bone Jt J. 2016;98-B:1119–25.
25. Rib fractures, open reduction and internal fixation of—practice management guideline. https://www.east.org/education-career-development/practice-management-guidelines/details/rib-fractures-open-reduction-and-internal-fixation-of. Accessed 19 Apr 2021
26. Greiffenstein P, Tran MQ, Campeau L. Three common exposures of the chest wall for rib fixation: anatomical considerations. J Thorac Dis. 2019;11:S1034–43.
27. Pieracci FM. Completely thoracoscopic surgical stabilization of rib fractures: can it be done and is it worth it? J Thorac Dis. 2019; https://doi.org/10.21037/jtd.2019.01.70.
28. McNamara JJ, Messersmith JK, Dunn RA, Molot MD, Stremple JF. Thoracic injuries in combat casualties in Vietnam. Ann Thorac Surg. 1970;10:389–401.
29. Karmy-Jones R, Jurkovich GJ, Nathens AB, Shatz DV, Brundage S, Wall MJ Jr, Engelhardt S, Hoyt DB, Holcroft J, Knudson MM. Timing of urgent thoracotomy for hemorrhage after trauma: a multicenter study. Arch Surg. 2001;136:513–8.
30. Karmy-Jones R, Jurkovich GJ, Shatz DV, Brundage S, Wall MJJ, Engelhardt S, Hoyt DB, Holcroft J, Knudson MM. Management of traumatic lung injury: a western trauma association multicenter review. J Trauma Acute Care Surg. 2001;51:1049–53.
31. Petrone P, Asensio JA. Surgical management of penetrating pulmonary injuries. Scand J Trauma Resusc Emerg Med. 2009;17:8.
32. Matsushima K, Aiolfi A, Park C, Rosen D, Strumwasser A, Benjamin E, Inaba K, Demetriades D. Surgical outcomes after trauma pneumonectomy: revisited. J Trauma Acute Care Surg. 2017;82:1.
33. O'Connor JV, DuBose JJ, Scalea TM. Damage-control thoracic surgery: management and outcomes. J Trauma Acute Care Surg. 2014;77:660–5.
34. Bertelsen S, Howitz P. Injuries of the trachea and bronchi. Thorax. 1972;27:188–94.
35. Kiser AC, O'Brien SM, Detterbeck FC. Blunt tracheobronchial injuries: treatment and outcomes. Ann Thorac Surg. 2001;71:2059–65.
36. Symbas PN, Justicz AG, Ricketts RR. Rupture of the airways from blunt trauma: treatment of complex injuries. Ann Thorac Surg. 1992;54:177–83.
37. Glazer ES, Meyerson SL. Delayed presentation and treatment of tracheobronchial injuries due to blunt trauma. J Surg Educ. 2008;65:302–8.
38. Dowd NP, Clarkson K, Walsh MA, Cunningham AJ. Delayed bronchial stenosis after blunt chest trauma. Anesth Analg. 1996;82:1078–81.
39. Dissanaike S, Shalhub S, Jurkovich GJ. The evaluation of pneumomediastinum in blunt trauma patients. J Trauma Acute Care Surg. 2008;65:1340–5.
40. Grewal HS, Dangayach NS, Ahmad U, Ghosh S, Gildea T, Mehta AC. Treatment of tracheobronchial injuries: a contemporary review. Chest. 2019;155:595–604.
41. Diaphragmatic injury, evaluation and management of—practice management guideline. https://www.east.org/education-career-development/practice-management-guidelines/details/diaphragmatic-injury-evaluation-and-management-of. Accessed 3 May 2021.

Further Reading

Eastern Association for the Surgery of Trauma (EAST) Practice Management Guidelines, avaialable online at https://www.east.org/education-career-development/practice-management-guidelines.

Karmy-Jones R, Jurkovich GJ, Shatz DV, Brundage S, Wall MJJ, Engelhardt S, Hoyt DB, Holcroft J, Knudson MM. Management of traumatic lung injury: a western trauma association multicenter review. J Trauma Acute Care Surg. 2001;51:1049–53.

Meredith JW, Hoth JJ. Thoracic trauma: when and how to intervene. Surg Clin North Am. 2007;87:95–118.

Thoracic Vascular Trauma

G. Janssen, M. Khashram, S. Bhagvan, and I. Civil

49.1 Introduction

> **Learning Points**
> - Thoracic vascular trauma is uncommon but life-threatening.
> - Fluid resuscitation needs to adhere to damage control and haemostatic principles.
> - Endovascular treatment is frequently an option.

49.1.1 Epidemiology

Thoracic vascular trauma may arise from either blunt or penetrating mechanisms of injury. Depending on the nature of the society in which the injury occurs one or other mechanism may be more common. Military action leads almost exclusively to penetrating trauma, whereas societies that are highly regulated with strict gun control experience thoracic vascular injuries more commonly from blunt mechanisms, such as motor vehicle crashes and high falls. A large number of patients with thoracic vascular injury die prior to reaching the hospital or the operating room. This is usually due to exsanguination at the scene [1].

49.1.2 Etiology

49.1.2.1 Penetrating Trauma

The vast majority of thoracic vascular trauma is secondary to penetrating injury [2]. Many patients exsanguinate before they come to the hospital. Those that do arrive alive are acutely sensitive to over-resuscitation and the key to management is to obtain vascular control and some degree of haemostasis before initiating fluid resuscitation except for those in extremis [3]. Penetrating trauma involves sharp injury to structures directly in the line of the weapon and commonly involves both venous and arterial injury [4]. There is greater mortality associated with penetrating vascular injury than blunt trauma [4]. Truncal vascular injury is the most common type of penetrating vascular trauma [2].

49.1.2.2 Blunt Trauma

Blunt thoracic vascular trauma is usually a result of rapid deceleration or high energy transfer, often from a head-on collision [4]. Although vascular injury is less common with blunt trauma than penetrating, 96% of patients with blunt thoracic vascular trauma have associated chest injury

[5], and many have additional vascular or visceral injuries elsewhere. Occasionally, a blunt injury resulting in skeletal fractures can cause penetration damaging surrounding vascular structures.

Blunt thoracic trauma is a common cause of death in trauma second only to head injury. There is higher morbidity associated when vascular structures are involved [4].

49.1.3 Classification

49.1.3.1 Aorta

Penetrating

The thoracic aorta is a rare site of penetrating injury and most patients with this injury die from haemorrhage before reaching the hospital.

Blunt

Blunt aortic injury most commonly follows road traffic crashes and less commonly high falls, and requires a high level of energy transfer. Less than 10% of patients with aortic injury following motor vehicle crash survive. Even in those who reach the hospital, mortality is high, usually from associated injuries [6]. Most patients admitted with blunt aortic injury have concurrent severe intracranial or visceral injuries [7].

49.1.3.2 Arch Vessels

Penetrating

Penetrating injury to aortic arch vessels is similarly often fatal unless the injury is such that the vessel thromboses. Where this is the case, there will be evidence of end-organ ischaemia such as a cerebrovascular event or upper limb ischaemia with loss of pulses.

Blunt

Injuries to great vessels most commonly occur at the vessel origin and often involve dissection [7, 8]. Injury to the subclavian vessels is rare as they are protected by the overlying clavicle. Injuries to these vessels are more common in penetrating injuries. A road traffic crash is again implicated

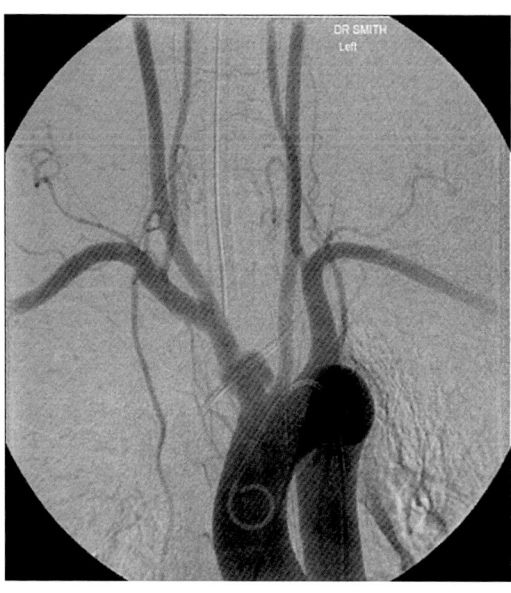

Fig. 49.1 False aneurysm of origin of the innominate artery in a patient injured in a high velocity road crash

as a prime mechanism for these injuries (Fig. 49.1).

49.1.3.3 Pulmonary Vessels

Penetrating

Injury to the pulmonary vessels is a common consequence of penetrating thoracic trauma and usually results in a haemothorax. Large vessel injury will result in a massive haemothorax requiring thoracotomy, whereas less severe injury can often be treated successfully by a thoracostomy tube.

Blunt

Pulmonary vessel injury is associated with rapid deceleration injuries and may result in either haemothorax or cardiac tamponade. It is reported that 38% of injuries to the pulmonary arteries occur from blunt trauma [9].

49.1.3.4 Vena Cava

Penetrating

Penetrating injury to the superior vena cava is associated with significant mortality and occurs more commonly than after blunt injury.

Blunt

Injury to the mediastinal venous structures is uncommon in blunt trauma and usually associated with severe concomitant injury in the chest and elsewhere.

49.1.3.5 Chest Wall Vessels

Penetrating

Damage to intercostal vessels can occur from gunshot wounds and stabbing but more commonly bleeding results from iatrogenic injury when a thoracostomy tube is inserted. The internal mammary artery may be injured with anterior chest stabbing because of its position between the ribs and when this occurs haemorrhage is usually profuse.

Blunt

Chest wall vessels (intercostals and internal mammary) are commonly injured in blunt chest trauma, but the nature of those injuries usually leads to thrombosis and haematoma rather than free haemorrhage.

49.1.4 Pathophysiology

Patients seen in the Emergency Department with thoracic vascular trauma may range in severity, from patients who are clinically stable, through to severe shock from haemorrhage [1]. As with vascular injuries in any part of the body, the consequences of the injury can be either haemorrhage or ischaemia.

49.2 Diagnosis

49.2.1 Clinical Presentation

History of the mechanism of injury may be obtained from the patient, family members, or ambulance staff. Initial assessment involves the use of the ATLS® principles. Ensuring the adequacy of the airway and adequate oxygenation are clear priorities in trauma resuscitation. Patients with thoracic vascular injuries will almost always exhibit some degree of shock and fluid resuscitation will be required [3]. An early review by a trauma or vascular surgeon is recommended [1].

49.2.1.1 Penetrating

Information regarding weapons is useful in penetrating trauma. By definition in patients with a penetrating mechanism for thoracic vascular trauma, there will be a wound. Trajectory and the type of weapon, however, may mean that the wound is not in the thoracic region. Wounds in the neck and upper part of the abdomen are not infrequently associated with thoracic injuries (Fig. 49.2).

49.2.1.2 Blunt Trauma

Speed, vehicle intrusion, seatbelt use, the height of fall, and death of others involved is useful for understanding the severity of the mechanism after blunt trauma [4].

Clinical signs raising suspicion for the presence of a blunt thoracic vascular injury include thoracic contusion, haemothorax, chest wall instability, pulse deficit between left and right upper limbs, and upper and lower limbs [1, 4].

Chest X-ray signs suggestive of a blunt thoracic vascular injury include mediastinal widening, first or second rib fractures, thoracic spinal fractures, sternal and multiple rib fractures.

49.2.2 Tests

A plain chest X-ray may demonstrate multiple signs that raise suspicion for vascular injury, including widened mediastinum, massive haemothorax, tracheal deviation, and fractures [1]. None of these signs are diagnostic, and in a stable patient, further imaging should be initiated.

CT Arteriogram is the "gold standard" for investigating thoracic vascular injury; however, this is not suitable in an unstable patient.

In an unstable patient, thoracotomy is the first line, as it is diagnostic, and has the potential for therapeutic intervention [1].

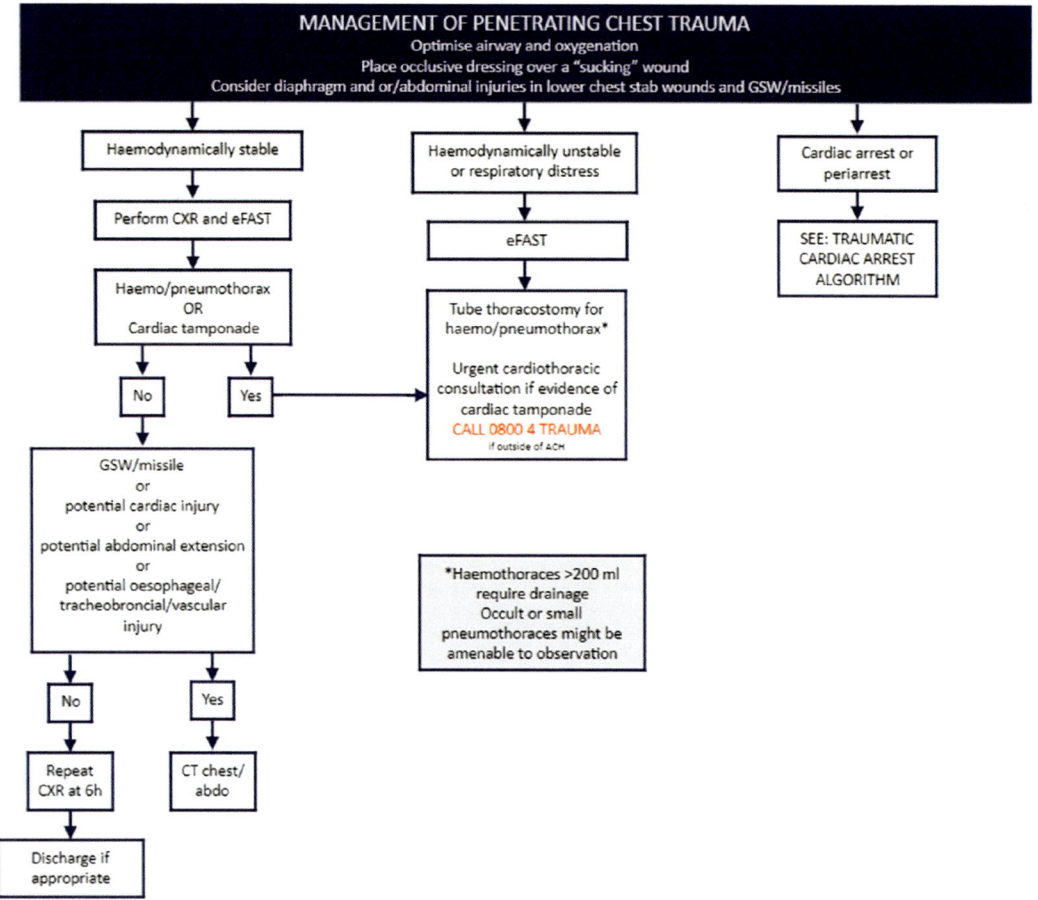

Fig. 49.2 Algorithm describing initial management of penetrating chest trauma. Penetrating thoracic trauma [Internet]. Auckland: The Northern Regional Trauma Network; [updated 2021 April; cited 2021 October] Available from: https://www.northerntrauma.co.nz/adult_trauma/penetrating-chest-trauma/

Differential Diagnosis

Thoracic vascular trauma is usually associated with a haemothorax and if associated with severe shock a thoracotomy will be required. This procedure will reveal the injury and provide an anatomic diagnosis. When it is unclear which side of the thorax contains the underlying vascular injury, a clamshell thoracotomy may be the best option. This is also the fastest way to access the thoracic cavity in a supine patient when the operator is not one who regularly operates on the chest.

If the patient has sufficient haemodynamic stability, then a CT angiogram is a useful tool to provide a diagnosis.

49.3 Treatment

49.3.1 Medical Treatment

The initial approach to a patient with a thoracic vascular injury involves haemostatic resuscitation [10]. In some cases, particularly with penetrating vascular trauma, there is the ability to arrest external blood loss. Where direct pressure is unsuccessful, the use of balloon tamponade using a Foley catheter may be helpful (Fig. 49.3)

After gaining IV access and taking blood for haematology, crossmatch and coagulation studies patients should be managed according to their physiological status. Those who are stable should receive minimal fluid resuscitation, while diagnostic imaging is undertaken [3]. The possibility

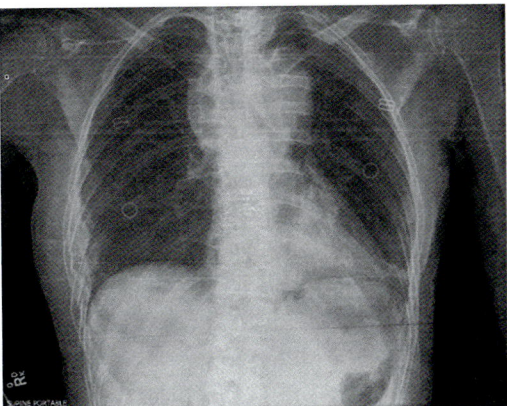

Fig. 49.3 Illustration of CXR associated with innominate artery blunt injury

of aggressive fluid resuscitation to "pop the clot" needs to be borne in mind.

49.3.2 Surgical Treatment

Some patients with thoracic trauma would require a tube thoracostomy in the Emergency Room.

Those who are unstable need to progress to the operating room while at the same time receive elements of a massive transfusion protocol consistent with their status. Viscoelastic monitoring and the use of early tranexamic acid, fibrinogen and cryoprecipitate are key elements in maintaining a haemostatic coagulation profile.

Indications for thoracotomy include penetration through the mediastinum, in-hospital cardiac arrest, cardiac tamponade, imaging confirmed vascular injury, and large volume haemothorax with persistent blood loss [1]. Thoracotomy in the Emergency department is indicated following penetrating trauma when the patient does not have a pulse, but does have other signs of life, and has received less than 5 min of CPR pre-hospital [11].

The role of endovascular therapy to treat thoracic vascular injuries surpassed open surgical repair, due to the lower morbidity and mortality [12] (Fig. 49.4).

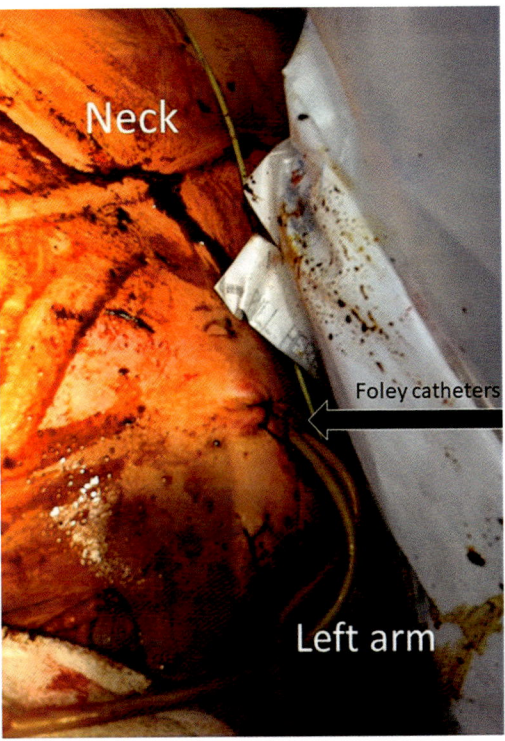

Fig. 49.4 Use of Foley catheter for direct pressure haemostasis in a subclavian artery penetrating injury

49.3.2.1 Aorta

Penetrating

Penetrating injury to the aorta is often fatal and survivors usually have a massive haemothorax and severe shock. An emergency thoracotomy and direct suture of any wound is appropriate. Occasionally, a penetrating injury to the aorta may be sufficiently proximal to cause bleeding into the pericardium and cause cardiac tamponade. In this situation, release of the tamponade will be required and direct suture should then be possible. A clamshell thoracotomy provides good access for this procedure. Depending on the segment of the aorta injured, other structures in close proximity could also be injured, such as the oesophagus, heart and thoracic duct.

Blunt

Blunt thoracic aortic injury (BTAI) can vary from intimal tears to free aortic rupture [12].

Blunt injuries are classified into four grades:

I Intimal tear
II Intramural hematoma
III Pseudoaneurysm
IV rupture (Fig. 49.5)

Depending on the location of the injury, open surgical repair is performed via a left posterolateral thoracotomy. Once the chest is opened and aorta exposed a proximal and distal clamping sites are prepared. Surgical options to maintain distal aortic perfusion to reduce the risk of spinal cord ischaemia and systemic heparinization in cases requiring full cardiopulmonary bypass should be considered.

Endovascular Repair

Due to the lower morbidity and procedural mortality with endovascular repair, TEVAR has replaced open surgery as the dominant treatment strategy [12].

Vascular access via the femoral artery and occasionally left brachial artery is attained via surgical cutdown or percutaneously. A guidewire followed by a pigtail catheter is inserted into the aorta and an angiogram is performed to locate the injury. Heparin can be given but can be avoided in some cases. A suitable sized vascular stent-graft is then deployed to cover the aortic injury with adequate proximal and distal sealing zones to exclude the injury. A completion angiogram is performed to ensure that the injury has been excluded and major aortic branches are not accidentally covered [13]. For thoracic aortic injuries around the left subclavian, coverage of the vessel origin is usually required to achieve an adequate proximal seal. In the emergency setting, coverage of the left subclavian artery, with selective revascularisation depending on the clinical condition of the patient, is recommended [14].

Indications for subclavian revascularization include an internal mammary coronary bypass graft, a dominant left vertebral artery, and a functioning left arteriovenous fistula for dialysis. In young patients, access to the femoral and iliac vessels might be challenging due to the size of the vessels, ancillary exposure of iliac vessels, and the use of a prosthetic graft as a conduit might be required.

The ideal timing for BTAI treatment should be individualized to the aortic injury grade and burden of other injuries involved. Initiation of medical therapy to optimize blood pressure and heart rate control should be the first line treatment. In cases without frank rupture (Grade 4), delaying TEVAR when possible (>24 h) has been shown to improve survival and outcomes [14, 15].

49.3.2.2 Arch Vessels

Penetrating

Penetrating injury to any of the arch vessels within the chest will result in a massive haemothorax. Stab wounds usually produce simple partial or complete lacerations, whereas gunshot wounds usually cause more extensive damage. Depending on the degree of destruction of the

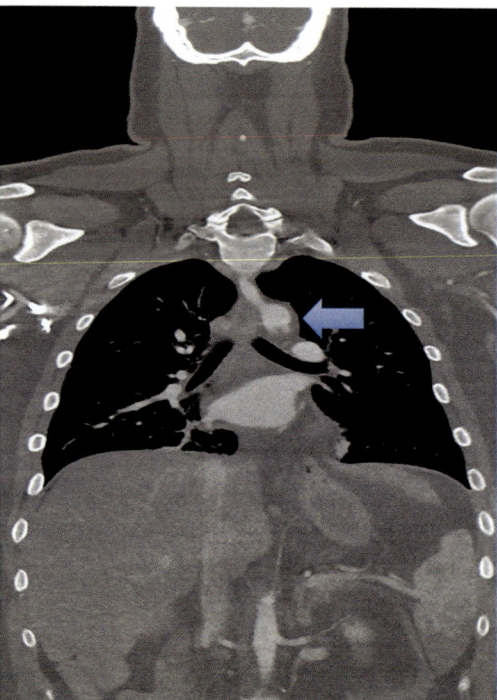

Fig. 49.5 Coronal section of a CT angiogram demonstrating a pseudoaneurysm with associated thrombus and an incidental right aberrant subclavian artery

vessel, there may be relevant vascular (pulse) or neurological deficits. In the first instance, the goal is to arrest haemorrhage and subsequently reestablishment of flow will be required. Access to the arch vessels can be problematic. The best incision is a median sternotomy, but this can be challenging to do in an emergency setting, particularly if the surgeon does not routinely undertake this procedure. A high lateral thoracotomy on the relevant side can provide access to the subclavian artery, but if the exact arch vessel injured is not known, then a central approach will be best. Extension of a median sternotomy into the neck will allow distal access to the carotid vessels if necessary.

Blunt

In blunt injury to the arch vessels (innominate, carotid, subclavian and an aberrant left vertebral artery), patients might present with mediastinal or supraclavicular haematoma, hemispheric neurologic deficit, and brachial plexus injury. Axial imaging usually directs the optimal surgical exposure to access the injured vessel(s). The left subclavian artery possesses the greatest challenge as ideal exposure depends on the location of the injured segment. The proximal part is accessed via an anterolateral thoracotomy, whereas the distal artery can be exposed via a left supraclavicular incision. Most patients tolerate subclavian artery ligation without developing upper limb ischaemia due to the rich collateral flow into the arm (Fig. 49.6).

Endovascular Repair

Endovascular treatment for arch vessel injuries has gained popularity as it avoids challenging exposures and extensive surgical dissection [12]. The treatment principles are to gain arterial access to the injury which could be approached from a transbrachial or transfemoral approach or both. The site of injury is traversed with a wire and the lesion is covered with an endovascular stent using either a self-expanding or a balloon expandable covered graft.

In situations when drainage of the hematoma is required to relieve compression symptoms, this can be performed once the bleeding has stopped.

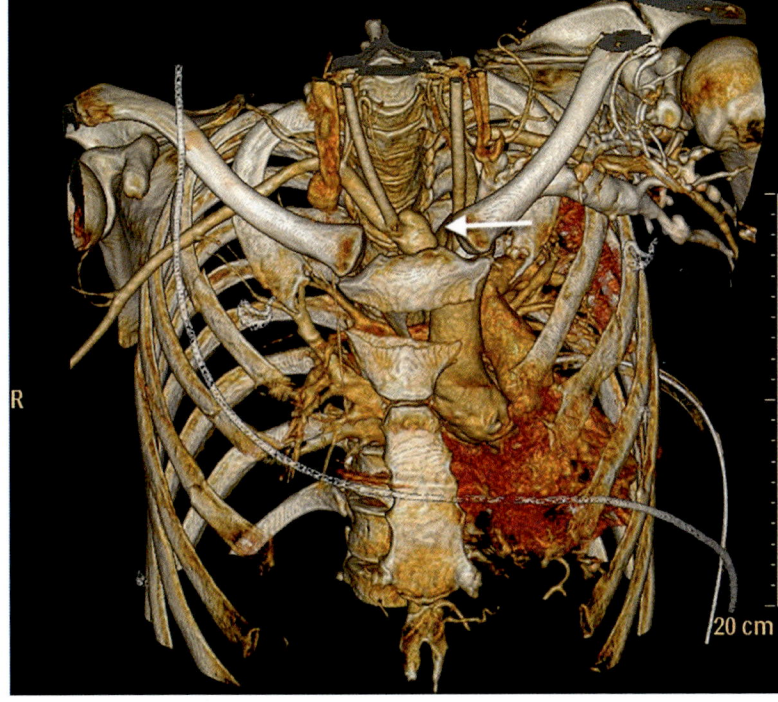

Fig. 49.6 Volume rendering CT angiogram demonstrating a bovine arch associated with a pseudoaneurysm of the inominate artery (arrowed) and manubrium fracture in a patient involved in a high-speed motor vehicle crash

For injuries around the left subclavian, coverage of the vessel origin is usually required to achieve an adequate proximal seal. In the emergency setting, societal guidelines recommend coverage of the left subclavian artery, with selective revascularisation depending on the clinical condition of the patient [13].

49.3.2.3 Pulmonary Vessels

Penetrating
Damage to the pulmonary vessels is usually associated with a missile or weapon track through lung tissue. In addition to significant bleeding, there is usually bronchial injury and an air leak. Proximal control can be obtained by hilar clamping, but direct access to the bleeding vessel can be facilitated by a tractotomy. This procedure involves dividing the lung tissue on either side of the injury with a three-row cutting stapler which creates lateral haemostasis while allowing direct access to the injury at the base of the wound. In rare situations, it may be necessary to perform a lobectomy or even a pneumonectomy in order to gain control. This should only be undertaken in extremis, as it has a high mortality.

Blunt
Blunt injury to the pulmonary vessels is associated with major intrathoracic injury, and has a high pre-hospital mortality [9]. Those who reach hospital alive, and have timely surgery without cardiac arrest have good outcomes [9]. Access to the pulmonary hilum can be obtained through a thoracotomy incision, with clamping for proximal control [9, 16]. This provides haemorrhage control, allowing time to resuscitate the patient, and performs a definitive repair of the injured vessel. If venous ligation is required, the involved lung parenchyma may need to be resected [16].

49.3.2.4 Vena Cava

Penetrating
The vena cava is infrequently injured but can also cause a massive haemothorax or cardiac tamponade if injured within the pericardium. Access can be obtained via a right thoracotomy, clamshell thoracotomy, or median sternotomy. In addition to haemorrhage control, care has to be taken to avoid air embolism. In severe shock, the vena cava will be under low pressure and air can be sucked into the vessel. Once it has been established that there is an injury, the vena cava should be kept under the surface of any bleeding until the moment repair is undertaken.

Blunt
Unlike peripheral venous injury, the intrathoracic vena cava injury is non-compressible [17]. This requires operative intervention to apply pressure for haemostasis. Access is obtained via median sternotomy [17] and the surgeon can proceed to suture, staple, or occlude the defect with a foley catheter. As with penetrating injury, care must be taken to avoid air embolism. Caval inflow occlusion can be utilized in the patient in extremis, with cardiopulmonary bypass an option when access is not possible [17].

49.3.2.5 Chest Wall Vessels

Penetrating
The location of the intercostal arteries underneath the rib is protective; however, these vessels are commonly injured in penetrating trauma. If there is arterial bleeding from this site, a deep suture under the rib is usually effective, but occasionally, where there is a posterior wound, the depth of muscle prevents a direct approach. In this situation, there is a place for selective arterial embolization.

Blunt
Blunt injury to intercostal vessels is frequently a result of laceration from rib fractures. Initial management is with placement of a thoracostomy tube. CT angiography can aid in surgical decision-making, and provide targets for interventional radiology [18]. In a stable patient, transcatheter artery embolization or video-assisted thoracoscopic surgery is viable treatment options. In the case of hemodynamic instability, thoracotomy is indicated [19].

49.3.3 Prognosis

Due to the variety of mechanisms and structures that can be injured, thoracic vascular trauma varies in its prognosis.

Patients who sustain thoracic vascular injury, and make it to hospital alive, will require ongoing treatment in an intensive care unit. Concurrent injuries need to be considered and treated with a multidisciplinary approach, guided by the trauma surgeon. Those who have early identification of injuries, and prompt management with tube thoracostomy or operative intervention in the operating room have good prognostic outcomes.

Recent evidence has shown good prognosis following endovascular intervention. The long-term re-intervention after TEVAR in trauma is relatively low, [20]; however, serious complications such as graft thrombosis, infection and migration have been reported; therefore, clinical and radiological follow-up has been recommended. The long-term impact of prosthetic stents in younger patients and the natural dilatation of the thoracic aorta in young patients remains unknown.

Patients who have injuries requiring thoracotomy in the emergency department have a high mortality rate attributable to the severity of injury, with up to 60% mortality in blunt trauma, and 40% for penetrating trauma [21].

Dos and Don'ts

Do:
- Do initiate haemostatic resuscitation measures if a patient is unstable
- Do utilise large bore tube thoracostomy in the Emergency Department
- Do consider the use of endovascular stent grafts and other percutaneous strategies
- Do CT angiography in the stable patient

Don't:
- Don't over resuscitate hemodynamically stable patients
- Don't treat grade 1 and 2 aortic injuries, interval imaging might suffice and most will heal and the aorta remodels
- Don't oversize endovascular stent grafts
- Don't forget concurrent injuries

Take-Home Messages

- CT scanning is a useful investigation in stable blunt injuries
- Grade 1 and 2 aortic injuries can be managed medically
- Beware of neck injuries that might involve thoracic vasculature
- CT angiogram that includes the brain and neck vessels can assist planning of endovascular procedures.

References

1. Mattox KL. Thoracic vascular trauma. J Vasc Surg. 1988;7:725–9.
2. Mattox KL, Feliciano DV, Burch J, Beall AC Jr, Jordan GL Jr, De Bakey ME. Five thousand seven hundred sixty cardiovascular injuries in 4459 patients. Epidemiologic evolution 1958 to 1987. Ann Surg 1989;698–705.
3. Bickell WH, Wall MJ Jr, Pepe PE, Martin RR, Ginger VF, Allen MK, et al. Immediate versus delayed fluid resuscitation for hypotensive patients with penetrating torso injuries. N Engl J Med. 1994;331(17):1105–9.
4. O'Connor JV, Byrne C, Scalea TM, Griffith BP, Neschis DG. Vascular injuries after blunt chest trauma: diagnosis and management. Scand J Trauma Resusc Emerg Med. 2009;17:42.
5. Tambyraja AL, Scollay JM, Beard D, Henry JM, Murie JA, Chalmers RTA. Aortic trauma in Scotland—a population based study. Eur J Vasc Endovasc Surg 2006;32:686–689.

6. Richens D, Kotidis K, Neale M, Oakley C, Fails A. Rupture of the aorta following road traffic accidents in the United Kingdom 1992-1999. The results of the co-operative crash injury study. Eur J Cardiothorac Surg. 2003;23:143–8.
7. Hudson HM 2nd, Woodson J, Hirsch E. The management of traumatic aortic tear in the multiply-injured patient. Ann Vasc Surg. 1991;5:445–8.
8. Wall MJ Jr, Hirshberg A, LeMaire SA, Holcomb J, Mattox K. Thoracic aortic and thoracic vascular injuries. Surg Clin North Am. 2001;81:1375–93.
9. Yanagawa Y, Ishikawa K, Nagasawa H, Takeuchi I, Jitsuiki K, Ohsaka H, et al. Traumatic pulmonary artery injury: a review of the recent literature [Internet], vol. 2. Vessel Plus; 2018. p. 1. https://doi.org/10.20517/2574-1209.2017.37.
10. Gonzalez E, Moore EE, Moore HB, Chapman MP, Chin TL, Ghasabyan A, et al. Goal-directed hemostatic resuscitation of trauma-induced coagulopathy a pragmatic randomized clinical trial comparing a viscoelastic assay to conventional coagulation assays. Ann Surg. 2016;263:1051–9.
11. Cothren CC, Moore EE. Emergency department thoracotomy for the critically injured patient: objectives, indications, and outcomes. World J Emerg Surg. 2006;24:1–4.
12. Tang GL, Tehrani HY, Usman A, Katariya K, Otero C, Perez E, et al. Reduced mortality, paraplegia, and stroke with stent graft repair of blunt aortic transections: a modern meta-analysis. J Vasc Surg. 2008;47:671–5.
13. Glaser JD, Kalapatapu VR. Endovascular therapy of vascular trauma—current options and review of the literature [Internet]. Vasc Endovasc Surg. 2019;53:477–87. Available from:. https://doi.org/10.1177/1538574419844073.
14. Lee WA, Anthony Lee W, Matsumura JS, Scott Mitchell R, Farber MA, Greenberg RK, et al. Endovascular repair of traumatic thoracic aortic injury: clinical practice guidelines of the Society for Vascular Surgery [Internet]. J Vasc Surg. 2011;53:187–92. https://doi.org/10.1016/j.jvs.2010.08.027.
15. Demetriades D, Velmahos GC, Scalea TM. Blunt traumatic thoracic aortic injuries: early or delayed repair—results of an american association for the surgery of trauma prospective study [Internet]. J Vasc Surg. 2010;52:1111–2. https://doi.org/10.1016/j.jvs.2010.08.068.
16. Alarhayem AQ, Rasmussen TE, Farivar B, Lim S, Braverman M, Hardy D, et al. Timing of repair of blunt thoracic aortic injuries in the thoracic endovascular aortic repair era. J Vasc Surg. 2021;73:896–902.
17. Miller DL, Mansour KA. Blunt traumatic lung injuries [Internet]. Thorac Surg Clin. 2007;17:57–61. https://doi.org/10.1016/j.thorsurg.2007.03.017.
18. Giannakopoulos TG, Avgerinos ED. Management of peripheral and truncal venous injuries. Front Surg. 2017;4:46.
19. Chemelli AP, Thauerer M, Wiedermann F, Strasak A, Klocker J, Chemelli-Steingruber IE. Transcatheter arterial embolization for the management of iatrogenic and blunt traumatic intercostal artery injuries. J Vasc Surg. 2009;49:1505–13.
20. Khashram M, He Q, Oh TH, Khanafer A, Wright IA, Vasudevan TM, et al. Late radiological and clinical outcomes of traumatic thoracic aortic injury managed with thoracic endovascular aortic repair. World J Surg. 2016;40:1763–70.
21. Narvestad JK, Meskinfamfrad M, Soreide K. Emergency resuscitative thoracotomy performed in European civilian trauma patients with blunt or penetrating injuries: a systematic review. Eur J Trauma Emerg Surg. 2016;42:677–85.

Further Reading

Feliciano DV, Mattox KL, Moore EE. Trauma. 9th ed. McGraw Hill; 2020.
Hirshberg A, Mattox KL. Top knife: the art & craft of trauma. TFM Publishing Ltd.; 2004.
Rasmussen TE, Tai NRM. Rich's vascular trauma. 3rd ed. Elsevier Inc; 2016. p. 73–112.

Resuscitative Thoracotomy

Ning Lu and Walter L. Biffl

50.1 Introduction

Learning Goals
- The primary objectives of RT are to release pericardial tamponade, control cardiac or intrathoracic hemorrhage, evacuate bronchovenous air embolism, perform open cardiac massage, and temporarily occlude the descending thoracic aorta.
- Survival depends on injury mechanism, anatomic location, and the patient's physiologic condition.
- RT should be performed for (1) penetrating nontorso trauma with cardiopulmonary resuscitation (CPR) of less than 5 min, (2) blunt trauma with CPR of less than 10 min, (3) penetrating torso trauma with CPR of less than 15 min, and (4) profound refractory shock (SBP <60 mmHg or CPR with signs of life).

N. Lu (✉) · W. L. Biffl
Scripps Memorial Hospital, La Jolla, CA, USA
e-mail: Lu.Ning@scrippshealth.org;
Biffl.Walter@scrippshealth.org

50.1.1 Definitions of Resuscitative Thoracotomy

The terminology used to describe resuscitative thoracotomy (RT) may be confusing due to ambiguous use of the phrase in literature. This chapter refers in general to RT performed in the Emergency Department (ED) on trauma patients in extremis. The same principles apply to that performed in the operating room (OR) or intensive care unit for acute physiologic deterioration. "No signs of life" refers to the absence of a palpable pulse, detectable blood pressure, respiratory effort, motor effort, cardiac electrical activity, or pupillary activity. "No vital signs" is defined by no palpable pulse or detectable blood pressure, but demonstrated respiratory or motor effort, pupillary reactivity, or cardiac electrical activity.

50.1.2 Historical Perspective

Emergent thoracotomy was first promoted by Schiff, in 1874, for the purpose of resuscitative open cardiac massage [1]. In 1896, Rehn performed the first successful suture cardiorrhaphy in a human [2]. Ingelsbrud then resuscitated a patient who suffered cardiac arrest during surgery [1]. After these initial successes, emergent thoracotomy was used routinely over the next 50 years for the treatment of cardiac wound and anesthesia-induced cardiac arrest.

During this period, however, resuscitative techniques improved and critical analysis of these arrests noted that most of the causes of cardiovascular collapse was from medical causes. In 1943, Blalock and Ravitch [3] promoted pericardiocentesis as the preferred treatment for post-injury cardiac tamponade. In 1956, Zoll et al. [4] introduced external defibrillation. In 1960, Kouwenhoven et al. [5] demonstrated the effectiveness of closed-chest compression. These innovations virtually eliminated the practice of open-chest resuscitation. However, beginning in the late 1960s, a role for RT was solidified in the salvage of patients with life-threatening chest wounds [6] and exsanguinating abdominal hemorrhage [7, 8].

50.1.3 Objectives of Resuscitative Thoracotomy

Then primary goals in performing RT are to do the following:

(a) Release pericardial tamponade
(b) Control intrathoracic vascular or cardiac hemorrhage
(c) Correct massive air embolism
(d) Perform open cardiac massage
(e) Temporarily occlude the descending thoracic aorta to improve perfusion to the myocardium and brain while mitigating subdiaphgragmatic hemorrhage

50.2 Diagnosis

50.2.1 Assessment of the Trauma Patient

In order to determine a patient's eligibility for RT, a rapid assessment is mandatory to determine the following:

- Mechanism of injury (blunt vs penetrating mechanism; location of penetrating injury, i.e., torso vs head/neck/extremities
- Signs of life (respiratory effort or motor activity, pupillary reactivity, cardiac electrical activity)
- Vital signs (pulse, blood pressure)
- Ultrasonographic findings (cardiac activity, pericardial fluid/tamponade)
- Evidence of a nonsurvivable injury (e.g., decapitation, massive head injury with exposed brain)

50.2.2 Indications for Resuscitative Thoracotomy

In general, the indications for RT include:

- Patients with traumatic cardiac arrest
- Patients in profound refractory shock (systolic blood pressure [SBP] <60 mmHg)

However, indications for RT have long been debated in light of poor neurologically intact survival rates among certain patient subgroups, and potential risks to trauma team members. The Western Trauma Association endorsed an algorithm [9] based on a study of survivors of RT [10], and offered the following indications:

(a) Patients without signs of life and who have undergone CPR for less than 15 min in the setting of penetrating torso trauma; 10 min in blunt trauma; or 5 min in penetrating non-torso trauma
(b) Patients without vital signs but with signs of life; those with profound refractory shock (SBP <60 mmHg)

In contrast, the 2015 Eastern Association for the Surgery of Trauma (EAST) Practice Management Guideline [11] evaluated the literature for both hospital survival and neurologically intact survival, and recommended against RT in blunt trauma patients presenting without signs of life, regardless of the duration.

50.3 Pathophysiology

50.3.1 Pericardial Tamponade

Early recognition and prompt pericardial decompression and cardiac repair are critical for survival of cardiac wounds [12]. As intrapericardial pressure rises, ventricular diastolic filling and subendocardial blood flow are restricted [13]. Compensatory tachycardia, increased systemic vascular resistance, and elevated central venous pressure allow for maintenance of cardiac output during the initial phase of hemodynamic derangement. In the intermediate phase, as increasing pericardial pressures overwhelm coronary perfusion, prevent adequate diastolic filling, and decrease stroke volume, cardiac output is finally diminished. Patients may have a normal blood pressure, but develop clinical signs of shock, including anxiety, diaphoresis, and pallor. In the final phase, as intrapericardial pressure approaches ventricular filling pressure, and coronary hypoperfusion occurs, the patient suffers profound hypotension and resultant cardiac arrest. In patients presenting in this final phase, RT is required for immediate evacuation of pericardial blood and to control cardiac bleeding [14, 15].

50.3.2 Intrathoracic Hemorrhage

Following penetrating trauma, life-threatening intrathoracic hemorrhage occurs in less than 5% of patients, even less following blunt trauma [16]. Pulmonary or great-vessel lacerations are often lethal, secondary to the significant blood flow through them, compounded by lack of containment by adjacent tissue tamponade or vessel spasm. Each hemithorax can accumulate 40–50% of the patient's total blood volume, and in a young patient, this can occur rapidly before physical signs of shock are obvious. Patients with exsanguinating thoracic wounds require RT for control of hemorrhage and survival.

50.3.3 Bronchovenous Air Embolism

Treatment of bronchovenous air embolism requires a high index of suspicion following thoracic trauma, and is likely more common that we recognize [17–19]. A classic presentation is a patient suffering penetrating chest trauma, who develops precipitous shock after endotracheal intubation and positive-pressure ventilation. This is due to traumatic alveolovenous communications causing coronary arterial air emboli, which produce global myocardial ischemia. The addition of positive pressure ventilation to intrathoracic blood loss results in increasing bronchoalveolar pressure and concomitant decreases an already low intrinsic pulmonary venous pressure. This combination of processes increases the gradient for air transfer across bronchovenous channels [20]. In blunt trauma, this can also occur in patients with pulmonary lacerations. The treatment for cardiopulmonary collapse secondary to bronchovenous air embolism requires the following maneuvers to salvage a patient in extremis: (1) immediate thoracotomy with pulmonary hilar cross-clamping to prevent further pulmonary venous air embolism; (2) Trendelenburg positioning, allowing the embolized air to accumulate in the ventricles, which can then be aspirated following thoracotomy; (3) vigorous cardiac massage, which may move air out of the coronary arteries; and (4) venting of air from the root of the aorta to prevent further flow into the coronary arteries [19].

50.3.4 Open Cardiac Massage

External chest compressions only provide 20–25% of normal cardiac output, resulting in 10–20% normal myocardial and 20–30% normal cerebral perfusion [21–23]. Normothermic patients may survive this degree of perfusion for 15 min, but rarely longer than 30 min. Trauma patients often have additional pathophysiology that decrease the effectiveness of external compressions. For those in hypovolemic (hemorrhagic) shock have inadequate intravascular volume, and those with pericardial tamponade have limited ventricular filling; and in these patients, external chest compressions are unable to augment arterial pressure or achieve adequate systemic or coronary perfusion [24]. Open cardiac massage provides better cardiac output compared to closed-chest compressions, improving cerebral and coronary perfusion [21–23, 25–28]. In normovolemic models of cardiac arrest, open cardiac massage for 30 min can achieve survival without neurologic deficits [29]. While open cardiac massage is superior to closed cardiac massage, it is not accepted as the sole indication for RT. However, expeditious thoracotomy with the adjunct of open cardiac massage is necessary for salvaging patients suffering traumatic cardiopulmonary arrest.

50.3.5 Thoracic Aortic Cross-Clamping

The objective in temporary thoracic aortic occlusion in an exsanguinating patient is redistribution of limited blood volume to increase myocardial and cerebral perfusion while limiting subdiaphragmatic hemorrhage [7, 8]. This allows for enhanced aortic diastolic and carotid systolic blood pressure, thus increasing coronary and cerebral perfusion [30, 31]. In canine studies, thoracic aortic occlusion during hypovolemic shock increases left ventricular stroke-work index and myocardial contractility [32]. Improved coronary perfusion from increased aortic diastolic pressure is presumed to account for the observed increased myocardial contractility [33]. Thus, in patients with persistent shock following cardiac repair and control of other hemorrhage, there may be some value temporary thoracic aortic occlusion. In fact, this procedure increases the return of spontaneous circulation following CPR [34, 35]. However, thoracic aortic occlusion in the normovolemic patient would be harmful due to increased myocardial oxygen demands secondary to increased systemic vascular resistance [36].

It is important to note that there are significant metabolic side-effects and a risk of paraplegia associated with thoracic aortic cross-clamping [37–39]. In hemorrhagic animal models, thoracic aortic cross-clamping reduces femoral artery systolic blood pressure by 90% [38], and abdominal visceral blood flow by 92–98% [39]. In both traumatic and elective surgical procedures, the metabolic costs of aortic cross-clamping increase dramatically when the occlusion time exceeds 30 min [40–42]. Hypoxia in distal organs induces activation of inflammatory cell adhesion molecules and mediators that have been linked to end organ dysfunction and multiple organ failure [43]. As such, the aortic clamp should be removed once sufficient cardiac function and systemic arterial pressure have been achieved. During aortic occlusion, the fullness of the heart should be observed closely as acute ventricular dilation secondary to volume overloading can precipitate cardiac failure [44]. Finally, unclamping the aorta is associated with reperfusion of the ischemic distal torso, and washout of the metabolic products can further increase inflammatory mediators in the cardiopulmonary system.

50.4 Treatment

50.4.1 Surgical Technique

50.4.1.1 Thoracic Incision
A left anterolateral thoracotomy incision is performed at the level of the fourth or fifth intercostal space (Fig. 50.1). This level of incision corresponds to the inferior border of the pectoralis major muscle; in women, the breast should be retracted superiorly. The skin, subcutaneous fat, and chest wall muscle fibers are incised with a scalpel. The length of the incision is typically described as "from the sternum to the bed," following the course of the rib as it curves upward laterally. Once the intercostal space is exposed, the intercostal muscles and parietal pleura are divided with heavy scissors, along the superior margin of the rib to avoid the neurovascular bun-

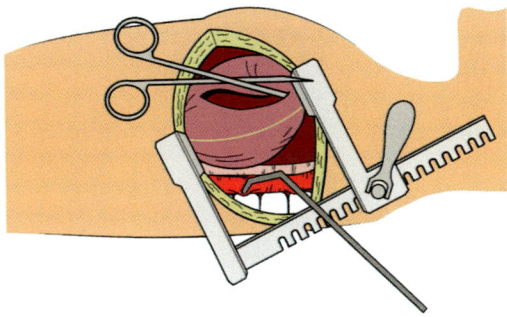

Fig. 50.1 Left anterolateral thoracotomy incision with pericardiotomy and aortic occlusion. Illustration from Eric Craig Brandt

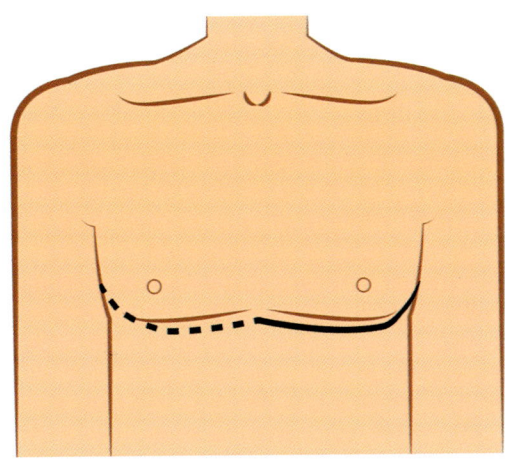

Fig. 50.2 Left anterolateral thoracotomy (solid line) with "Clamshell" extension (dotted Line). Illustration from Eric Craig Brandt

dle. In the patient in extremis, there is minimal chest wall hemorrhage until normal cardiovascular function is restored. A standard rib retractor (Finochietto) should be inserted with the handle facing posteriorly (toward the bed). As the retractor is opened, resistance can be resolved by division of any remaining intercostal muscles within the incision or transection of the costal cartilages above and below the interspace. Extension of the incision across the sternum to include a right anterolateral thoracotomy results in a "clamshell" incision, exposing both pleural cavities and the mediastinum. The sternum is transected with a Lebsche's knife and mallet. The internal mammary vessels must also be ligated when performing this "clamshell" incision. The "clamshell" and other extensions of the initial incision may be performed for improved exposure of the aortic arch or proximal subclavian/brachiocephalic vascular injuries (Fig. 50.2). In the setting of penetrating injury to the right chest, or if there is need for greater exposure of the heart or other mediastinal structures, trans-sternal extension of the incision should be performed promptly.

50.4.1.2 Pericardiotomy and Cardiac Hemorrhage Control

After the thoracotomy is performed, the next step is to release pericardial tamponade with pericardiotomy (Fig. 50.1). In the presence of tamponade, this may require a scalpel or sharp point of scissors. The pericardium should be opened widely, anterior and parallel to the phrenic nerve. Blood clots must be evacuated from the pericardium to allow for assessment of cardiac bleeding. Ventricular hemorrhage should be initially controlled with digital pressure and atrial hemorrhage may be controlled with partially occluding vascular clamps.

Cardiorrhaphy is best performed with 3-0 nonabsorbable running or horizontal mattress sutures. In the nonbeating heart, suturing should be performed prior to defibrillation and cardiac massage. Teflon pledgets are used to buttress suture repairs in the thin-walled right ventricle. Low pressure venous and atrial lacerations are repaired with simple running sutures or pursestring sutures. In the thick-walled left ventricle, a skin stapling device may be used if there is good coaptation of the edges; otherwise, a running suture is used. Wounds in proximity to coronary arteries should be repaired with a horizontal mattress suture that excludes the artery (Fig. 50.3). Posterior cardiac wounds are especially challenging, as they may require elevation of the heart for exposure in addition to optimal lighting and equipment. Massive ventricular lacerations or inaccessible posterior cardiac injuries may be better exposed with temporary inflow occlusion of the superior and inferior vena cavae. Fibrin glue may be a useful adjunct to repairs. The use of balloon catheters may inadvertently extend the injury due to traction, so their use is not recommended.

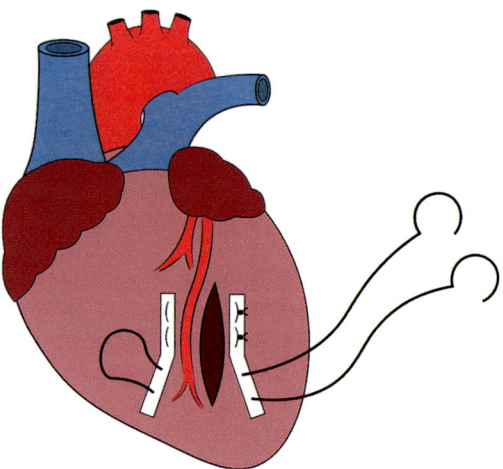

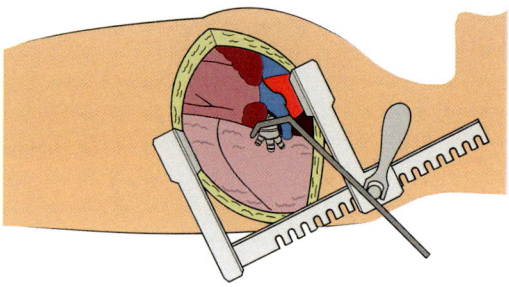

Fig. 50.4 Vascular clamp placed across the pulmonary hilum. Illustration from Eric Craig Brandt

Fig. 50.3 Cardiac laceration parallel to a coronary vessel repaired with horizontal mattress suture. Illustration from Eric Craig Brandt

50.4.1.3 Thoracic Aortic Occlusion and Pulmonary Hilar Control

Following control of cardiac hemorrhage, the descending thoracic aorta should be clamped to redistribute perfusion to the myocardium and brain. This is preferentially performed distal to the inferior pulmonary ligament. The left lung should be retracted superiorly and anteriorly. The thoracic aorta should be dissected under direct vision by incising the mediastinal pleura and bluntly separating the aorta from the esophagus anteriorly, and from the prevertebral fascia posteriorly. Placement of an orogastric tube allows for easier identification of the esophagus. It should be noted that completely encircling the aorta may avulse thoracic and other aortic branches, causing further hemorrhage. Once the aorta is properly exposed, the thoracic aorta is occluded with a large Satinsky or DeBakey vascular clamp.

The pulmonary hilum should be controlled if there is concern of bronchovenous air embolism, or if there is marked hemorrhage from the hilum or lung (Fig. 50.4). In the setting of bronchovenous air embolism, vigorous cardiac massage will also help expel air from the coronary arteries. In addition, air can be evacuated by needle aspiration of the elevated left ventricular apex and the aortic root. Definitive techniques for major pulmonary injuries are best carried out in the OR with optimal lighting and instrumentation.

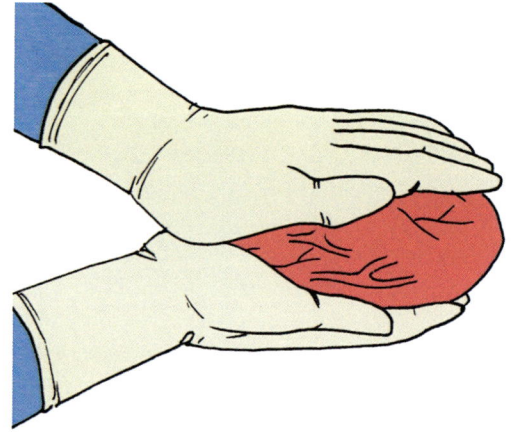

Fig. 50.5 Open cardiac massage. Illustration from Eric Craig Brandt

50.4.1.4 Cardiac Massage and Advanced Cardiac Life Support (ACLS) Interventions

If the patient remains in cardiac arrest, standard ACLS interventions including defibrillation and open cardiac massage should be performed. Open cardiac massage should be performed with wrists apposed, and ventricular compression proceeding from the apex to the base of the heart (Fig. 50.5). This method is described as a hinged, clapping motion. Given the risk of myocardial perforation by the thumb, the one-handed technique is not recommended. Intracardiac injection of epinephrine may be administered into the left ventricle with a specialized syringe. Then, after further cardiac massage to allow the vasopressors to circulate, internal defibrillation should then be performed at 30J using internal paddles.

If cardiac activity is not restored at this point, descending thoracic aortic occlusion should be performed to optimize coronary perfusion. The left lung should be retracted superiorly and anteriorly to allow for aortic cross-clamping just inferior to the pulmonary hilum. The thoracic aorta should be dissected under direct vision by incising the mediastinal pleura and bluntly separating the aorta from the esophagus anteriorly, and from the prevertebral fascia posteriorly. Placement of an orogastric tube allows for easier identification of the esophagus. It should be noted that completely encircling the aorta may avulse thoracic and other aortic branches, causing further hemorrhage. Once the aorta is properly exposed, the thoracic aorta is occluded with a large Satinsky's or DeBakey's vascular clamp.

50.4.1.5 Markers of Futility

The trauma surgeon who undertakes RT must recognize and abide by markers of futility. Failure of the patient to achieve an SBP >70 mmHg with aortic cross-clamp in place will not survive. The need for vasopressors to hold the blood pressure is a poor prognostic sign. Failure to maintain a perfusing rhythm or regain signs of life is also a sign of nonsalvageability.

50.4.1.6 Definitive Surgery

The salvageable patient should be transferred to the OR for definitive procedures.

50.4.2 Technical Complications

Technical complications of RT can involve injury of any intrathoracic structure. This includes lacerations of the heart, coronary arteries, aorta, phrenic nerves, esophagus, lungs, and avulsion of the aortic branches. Previous thoracotomy is a relative contraindication to RT, as dense pleural adhesions significantly increase the likelihood of injury to intrathoracic structures and difficulty performing all of the maneuvers described above. For survivors of RT, there are significant postoperative morbidities including recurrent chest bleeding, pericardial infection, pleural space infection, chest wall infection, and postpericardiotomy syndrome.

50.4.3 Medical Optimization Following RT

During and after RT, patient hemodynamics are in tenuous state. The combination of direct cardiac injury, ischemic myocardial insult, circulating cardiac depressants, pulmonary hypertension, and inflammatory mediators have detrimental effects on posttraumatic cardiac function. In addition, aortic occlusion produces significant lactic acidemia secondary to anaerobic metabolism. In further resuscitation, the objectives shift to cardiac function optimization and increasing tissue oxygen delivery.

The primary goal for a patient in extremis is establishing a perfusing cardiac rhythm. Asystole is not a treatable rhythm after traumatic arrest. Per the 2020 AHA guidelines, ventricular fibrillation (VF) or pulseless ventricular tachycardia (VT) requires early defibrillation, with treatment with epinephrine, followed by amiodarone (lidocaine as alternative) for refractory patients [45]. Magnesium is beneficial for torsades de pointes [45].

Throughout this resuscitative process, patients should be resuscitated with volume including no more than 1 L crystalloid, and balanced transfusion with a massive transfusion protocol (MTP), if available [46]. Resuscitation should continue until lactic acidosis has resolved and coagulopathy has been corrected. It is important to note that hypocalcemia is common in those receiving MTP secondary to citrate and serum calcium chelation [47]. For patients in hemorrhagic shock, it has also been shown that there is a decreased mortality when tranexamic acid is given within 3 h of injury, including 1 g prehospital and a repeat dose in the ED [46]. Finally, hypothermia should be avoided with trauma patients, as it is known to worsen coagulopathy [48]. Simple methods for preventing hypothermia include removal of wet clothing, warming the trauma rooms in the ED and OR, warming resuscitative fluids, and applying warming blankets. Intra-operatively, any irrigation used in the chest or abdomen should be warmed.

50.4.4 Prognosis

The overall survival rate after RT has historically been low but is dependent on numerous variables, including the mechanism of injury and physiologic condition at the time of RT. In a 25-year study reported in 2000, overall survival was 7.4% with normal neurologic outcomes in 92% of survivors [49]. More recent data suggest that overall survival may be up to 9.6% [50].

The 2015 EAST Practice Management Guideline [11] reported data on 10,238 patients in 72 studies. The overall survival was 8.5%. Of those studies reporting intact neurologic status, 86% of survivors were neurologically intact, and overall 6.1% of RT patients survived neurologically intact. Patients sustaining penetrating injuries had 10.6% overall survival, with 90% neurologically intact; in contrast, only 2.3% of blunt trauma RT patients survived, and 59% were neurologically intact (Table 50.1).

Based on the WTA study of RT survivors, the duration of prehospital CPR is a good marker of futility. Blunt trauma patients with more than 10 min of prehospital CPR and no signs of life, penetrating torso trauma patients with more than 15 min of prehospital CPR and no signs of life, and those with penetrating neck or extremity trauma and more than 5 min of prehospital CPR and no signs of life should all be pronounced dead secondary to non-existent survivorship [9, 10, 51].

50.4.5 Risks to the Trauma Team

Rapid surgical techniques, sharp instruments, and exposure to the patient's blood are involved for expeditious RT in the salvage of acutely injured patients. Even during elective OR procedures, there is up to 50% risk of contact between the patients' blood and the surgeons' skin; in fact, the rate of contact between the patients'' blood and any health care workers' blood is as high as 6% [52]. Four percent of patients admitted to the ED for trauma are HIV seropositive; however, 14% of penetrating trauma victims [53] and 30% of intravenous drug abusers [54] are HIV seropositive. Caplan et al found that 26% of acutely injured patients had exposure to HIV (4%), hepatitis B (20%), or hepatitis C (14%), with no difference comparing blunt and penetrating trauma patients [55].

While the likelihood of a healthcare worker becoming exposed to transmissible disease in the ED, in the age of post-exposure prophylaxis, the risk of contracting HIV is reduced to 1 in 1,000,000 following a percutaneous injury to the surgeon from a sharp instrument used on an HIV-positive patient [56]. In addition, there are vaccines for hepatitis B and there antiviral treatment for hepatitis C. As such, when patients have clear indications, with appropriate standard barrier precautions, RT should still be performed.

Table 50.1 Pooled outcomes following resuscitative thoracotomy among 10,238 patients in 72 studies [11]

Injury mechanism	Hospital survival	Neurologically intact hospital survival
Penetrating thoracic with SOL	21.3% (18.7–24.2)	11.7% (9.0–15.0)
Penetrating thoracic without SOL	8.3% (6.6–10.2)	3.9% (2.6–5.6)
Penetrating extra-thoracic with SOL	15.6% (10.6–21.9)	16.5% (9.7–25.5)
Penetrating extra-thoracic without SOL	2.9% (0.9–6.8)	5.0% (1.3–13.0)
Blunt with SOL	4.6% (3.0–6.9)	2.4% (1.0–4.6)
Blunt without SOL	0.7% (0.3–1.4)	0.1% (<0.1–0.6)
Overall	8.5% (8.0–9.1)	6.1% (5.5–6.6)

50 Resuscitative Thoracotomy

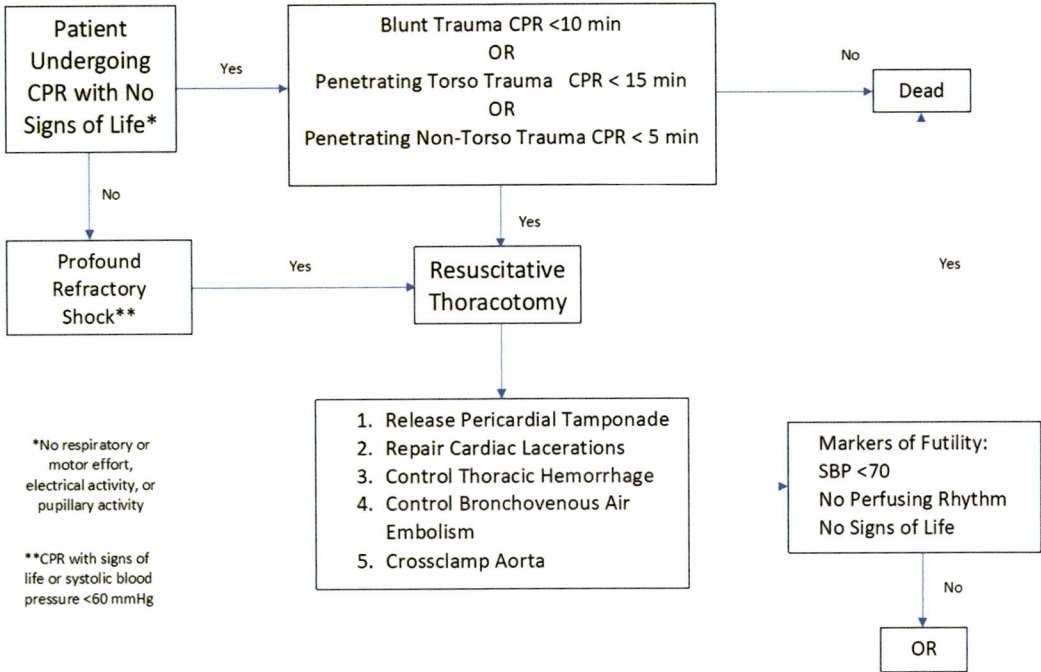

Fig. 50.6 WTA Resuscitative Thoracotomy Algorithm. Adapted from Burlew et al. [9]

50.4.6 Selective Application of Resuscitative Thoracotomy

The authors follow the WTA algorithm (Fig. 50.6).

Dos and Don'ts
- Do perform timely RT on indicated patients.
- Don't perform RT on patients who do not have clear indications, as salvabeability is near non-existent.
- Do evaluate and treat for cardiac tamponade, intrathoracic hemorrhage, air embolism, and intra-abdominal hemorrhage.
- Don't forget to assess for salvageablity prior to committing OR and other significant resources after RT.

Take-Home Messages
- The primary objectives of RT are to release pericardial tamponade, control cardiac or intrathoracic hemorrhage, evacuate bronchovenous air embolism, perform open cardiac massage, and temporarily occlude the descending thoracic aorta.
- Survival depends on injury mechanism, anatomic location, and the patient's physiologic condition.
- RT should be performed for (1) penetrating nontorso trauma with cardiopulmonary resuscitation (CPR) of less than 5 min, (2) blunt trauma with CPR of less than 10 min, (3) penetrating torso trauma with CPR of less than 15 min, and (4) profound refractory shock (SBP <60 mmHg).

Multiple Choice Questions
1. Which of the following is not an objective of RT?
   A. Release pericardial tamponade
   B. Control intrathoracic vascular or cardiac hemorrhage
   C. Stabilize fractured ribs
   D. Perform open cardiac massage
2. Which of the following is an indication for RT?
   A. SBP <60
   B. SBP = 70
   C. HR >120
   D. Agonal breathing
3. Which of the following patients has an indication for RT?
   A. Patient without signs of life and who has undergone CPR for 10 min in penetrating nontorso trauma
   B. Patient without signs of life and who has undergone CPR for less than 15 min in the setting of penetrating torso trauma;
   C. Patient without signs of life and who has undergone CPR for 20 min in penetrating nontorso trauma
   D. Patient without signs of life and who has undergone CPR for 20 min in blunt trauma
4. Pericardial tamponade can result in which of the following?
   A. Increased cardiac output
   B. Increased ventricular diastolic filling
   C. Increased intrapericardial pressure
   D. Increased subendocardial blood flow
5. Which of the following is a maneuver for treating pulmonary venous air embolism?
   A. Aortic cross-clamping
   B. Aspiration of embolized air from the atria
   C. Reverse Trendelenberg positioning of the patient
   D. Vigorous cardiac massage
6. Thoracic aortic cross-clamping
   A. Improves coronary and cerebral perfusion
   B. Decreases myocardial contractility
   C. Improves visceral blood flow
   D. Decreases circulating inflammatory mediators
7. Pericardiotomy should be performed
   A. Posterior and parallel to the phrenic nerve
   B. Anterior and parallel to the phrenic nerve
   C. Perpendicular to the phrenic nerve
   D. To achieve the smallest opening possible
8. Open cardiac massage
   A. Should be accompanied by external defibrillation
   B. Should be performed primarily with the fingertips
   C. Should be performed with the one-handed technique
   D. Should be performed with the two-handed technique
9. Which of the following is not a marker of nonsalvageability after aortic cross-clamping?
   A. SBP <70
   B. Failure to maintain a perfusing rhythm
   C. Need for vasopressors
   D. Lack of signs of life
10. Which of the following is true?
    A. Survival after RT is higher after penetrating injury compared to blunt injury
    B. Survival after RT is lower after penetrating injury compared to blunt injury
    C. Most survivors of RT are not neurological intact
    D. Duration of prehospital CPR does not correlate with futility

Answers: 1. C; 2. A; 3. B; 4. C; 5. A; 6. A; 7. B; 8. D; 9. C; 10. A

References

1. Hemreck A. The history of cardiopulmonary resuscitation. Am J Surg. 1988;156:430–6.
2. Blatchford J. Ludwig Rehn: the first successful cardiorrhaphy. Ann Thorac Surg. 1985;39:492–5.

3. Blalock A, Ravitch M. A consideration of the nonoperative treatment of cardiac tamponade resulting from wounds of the heart. Surgery. 1943;14:157–62.
4. Zoll P, Linenthal A, Norman L. Treatment of unexpected cardiac arrest by external electric stimulation of the heart. N Engl J Med. 1956;254:541–6.
5. Kouwenhoven W, Jude J, Knickerbocker G. Closed-chest cardiac massage. JAMA. 1956;173:1064–7.
6. Beall A, Dietrich E, Crawford H, Cooley D, De Bakey M. Surgical management of penetrating cardiac injuries. Am J Surg. 1966;112:686–92.
7. Ledgerwood A, Kazmers M, Lucas C. The role of thoracic aortic occlusion for massive hemoperitoneum. J Trauma. 1976;16:610–5.
8. Millikan J, Moore E. Outcome of resuscitative thoracotomy and descending aortic occlusion performed in the operating room. J Trauma. 1984;24:387–92.
9. Burlew CC, Moore EE, Moore FA, Coimbra R, McIntyre RC, Davis JW, et al. Western trauma association critical decisions in trauma: resuscitative thoracotomy. J Trauma Acute Care Surg. 2012;73(6):1359–63.
10. Moore EE, Knudson MM, Burlew CC, Inaba K, Dicker RA, Biffl WL, et al. Defining the limits of resuscitative emergency department thoracotomy: a contemporary western trauma association perspective. J Trauma. 2011;70(2):334–9.
11. Seamon MJ, Haut ER, Van Arendonk K, Barbosa RR, Chiu WC, Dente CJ, et al. An evidence-based approach to patient selection for emergency department thoracotomy: a practice management guideline from the Eastern Association for the Surgery of Trauma. J Trauma Acute Care Surg. 2015;79(1):159–73.
12. Breaux E, Dupont J, Albert H, Bryant L, Schechter F. Cardiac tamponade following penetrating mediastinal injuries: improved survival with early pericardiocentesis. J Trauma. 1979;19(6):461–6.
13. Wechsler A, Auerbach B, Graham T, Sabiston D. Distribution of intramyocardial blood flow during pericardial tamponade. Correlation with microscopic anatomy and intrinsic myocardial contractility. J Thorac Cardiovasc Surg. 1974;68(6):847–56.
14. Mattox K, Beall A, Jordan G, De Bakey M. Cardiorrhaphy in the emergency center. J Thorac Cardiovasc Surg. 1974;68(6):886–95.
15. Wall M, Mattox K, Chen C, Baldwin J. Acute management of complex cardiac injuries. J Trauma. 1997;42(5):905–12.
16. Graham J, Mattox K, Beall A. Penetrating trauma of the lung. J Trauma. 1979;19(9):665–9.
17. King M, Aitchison J, Nel J. Fatal air embolism following penetrating lung trauma: an autopsy study. J Trauma. 1984;24(8):753–5.
18. Thomas A, Stephens B. Air embolism: a cause of morbidity and death after penetrating chest trauma. J Trauma. 1974;14(8):633–8.
19. Yee E, Verrier E, Thomas A. Management of air embolism in blunt and penetrating thoracic trauma. J Thorac Cardiovasc Surg. 1983;85(5):661–8.
20. Graham J, Beall A, Mattox K, Vaughan G. Systemic air embolism following penetrating trauma to the lung. Chest. 1977;72(4):449–54.
21. Arai T, Dote K, Tsukahara I, Nitta K, Nagaro T. Cerebral blood flow during conventional, new and open-chest cardio-pulmonary resuscitation in dogs. Resuscitation. 1984;12(2):147–54.
22. Bartlett RL, Stewart NJ, Raymond J, Anstadt GL, Martin SD. Comparative study of three methods of resuscitation: closed-chest, open-chest manual, and direct mechanical ventricular assistance. Ann Emerg Med. 1984;13(9):773–7.
23. Jackson R, Freeman S. Hemodynamics of cardiac massage. Emerg Med Clin North Am. 1983;1(3):501–13.
24. Luna G, Pavlin E, Kirkman T, Copass M, Rice C. Hemodynamic effects of external cardiac massage in trauma shock. J Trauma. 1989;29(10):1430–3.
25. Bircher N, Safar P. Comparison of standard and "new" closed-chest CPR and open-chest CPR in dogs. Crit Care Med. 1981;9(5):384–5.
26. Boczar M, Howard M, Rivers E, Martin G, Horst H, Lewandowski C, et al. A technique revisited: hemodynamic comparison of closed- and open-chest cardiac massage during human cardiopulmonary resuscitation. Crit Care Med. 1995;23(3):498–503.
27. Delguercio L, Feins N, Cohn J, Coomaraswamy R, Wollman S, State D. Comparison of blood flow during external and internal cardiac massage in man. Circulation. 1965;31(suppl 1):171–80.
28. Rubertsson S, Grenvik A, Wiklund L. Blood flow and perfusion pressure during open-chest versus closed-chest cardiopulmonary resuscitation in pigs. Crit Care Med. 1995;23(4):715–25.
29. Bircher N, Safar P. Cerebral preservation during cardiopulmonary resuscitation. Crit Care Med. 1985;13(3):185–90.
30. Spence PA, Lust RM, Chitwood WR, Iida H, Sun YS, Austin EH. Transfemoral balloon aortic occlusion during open cardiopulmonary resuscitation improves myocardial and cerebral blood flow. J Surg Res. 1990;49(3):217–21.
31. Wesley R, Morgan D. Effect of continuous intra-aortic balloon inflation in canine open chest cardiopulmonary resuscitation. Crit Care Med. 1990;18(6):630–3.
32. Dunn EL, Moore EE, Moore JB. Hemodynamic effects of aortic occlusion during hemorrhagic shock. Ann Emerg Med. 1982;11(5):238–41.
33. Michel J, Bardou A, Tedgui A, Levy B. Effect of descending thoracic aorta clamping and unclamping on phasic coronary blood flow. J Surg Res. 1984;36(1):17–24.
34. Gedeborg R, Rubertsson S, Wiklund L. Improved haemodynamics and restoration of spontaneous cir-

35. Rubertsson S, Bircher NG, Alexander H. Effects of intra-aortic balloon occlusion on hemodynamics during, and survival after cardiopulmonary resuscitation in dogs. Crit Care Med. 1997;25(6):1003–9.
36. Kralovich KA, Morris DC, Dereczyk BE, Simonetti V, Williams M, Rivers EP, et al. Hemodynamic effects of aortic occlusion during hemorrhagic shock and cardiac arrest. J Trauma. 1997;42(6):1023–8.
37. Connery C, Geller E, Dulchavsky S, Kreis DJ. Paraparesis following emergency room thoracotomy: case report. J Trauma. 1990;30(3):362–3.
38. Mitteldorf C, Poggetti RS, Zanoto A, Branco PD, Birolini D, Castro de Tolosa EM, et al. Is aortic occlusion advisable in the management of massive hemorrhage? Experimental study in dogs. Shock. 1998;10(2):141–5.
39. Oyama M, McNAMARA JJ, Suehiro GT, Suehiro A, Sue-Ako K. The effects of thoracic aortic cross-clamping and declamping on visceral organ blood flow. Ann Surg. 1983;197(4):459–63.
40. Fabian TC, Richardson JD, Croce MA, Smith JS, Rodman G, Kearney PA, et al. Prospective study of blunt aortic injury: Multicenter Trial of the American Association for the Surgery of Trauma. J Trauma. 1997;42(3):374–80; discussion 380-383.
41. Gharagozloo F, Neville RF, Cox JL. Spinal cord protection during surgical procedures on the descending thoracic and thoracoabdominal aorta: a critical overview. Semin Thorac Cardiovasc Surg. 1998;10(1):73–86.
42. Katz NM, Blackstone EH, Kirklin JW, Karp RB. Incremental risk factors for spinal cord injury following operation for acute traumatic aortic transection. J Thorac Cardiovasc Surg. 1981;81(5):669–74.
43. Evans TW, Smithies M. ABC of intensive care: organ dysfunction. BMJ. 1999;318(7198):1606–9.
44. Gelman S. The pathophysiology of aortic cross-clamping and unclamping. Anesthesiology. 1995;82(4):1026–60.
45. Panchal AR, Bartos JA, Cabañas JG, Donnino MW, Drennan IR, Hirsch KG, et al. Part 3: adult basic and advanced life support: 2020 American Heart Association guidelines for cardiopulmonary resuscitation and emergency cardiovascular care. Circulation. 2020;142(16_suppl_2):S366–468.
46. Galvagno SM, Nahmias JT, Young DA. Advanced trauma life Support® update 2019. Anesthesiol Clin. 2019;37(1):13–32.
47. Giancarelli A, Birrer KL, Alban RF, Hobbs BP, Liu-DeRyke X. Hypocalcemia in trauma patients receiving massive transfusion. J Surg Res. 2016;202(1):182–7.
48. Perlman R, Callum J, Laflamme C, Tien H, Nascimento B, Beckett A, et al. A recommended early goal-directed management guideline for the prevention of hypothermia-related transfusion, morbidity, and mortality in severely injured trauma patients. Crit Care. 2016;20(1):107.
49. Rhee PM, Acosta J, Bridgeman A, Wang D, Jordan M, Rich N. Survival after emergency department thoracotomy: review of published data from the past 25 years. J Am Coll Surg. 2000;190(3):288–98.
50. Joseph B, Khan M, Jehan F, Latifi R, Rhee P. Improving survival after an emergency resuscitative thoracotomy: a 5-year review of the Trauma Quality Improvement Program. Trauma Surg Acute Care Open. 2018;3(1):e000201.
51. Powell DW, Moore EE, Cothren CC, Ciesla DJ, Burch JM, Moore JB, et al. Is emergency department resuscitative thoracotomy futile care for the critically injured patient requiring prehospital cardiopulmonary resuscitation? J Am Coll Surg. 2004;199(2):211–5.
52. Lin EY, Brunicardi FC. HIV infection and surgeons. World J Surg. 1994;18(5):753–7.
53. Kelen GD, Fritz S, Qaqish B, Brookmeyer R, Baker JL, Kline RL, et al. Unrecognized human immunodeficiency virus infection in emergency department patients. N Engl J Med. 1988;318(25):1645–50.
54. Kelen GD, DiGiovanna T, Bisson L, Kalainov D, Sivertson KT, Quinn TC. Human immunodeficiency virus infection in emergency department patients. Epidemiology, clinical presentations, and risk to health care workers: the Johns Hopkins experience. JAMA. 1989;262(4):516–22.
55. Caplan ES, Preas MA, Kerns T, Soderstrom C, Bosse M, Bansal J, et al. Seroprevalence of human immunodeficiency virus, hepatitis B virus, hepatitis C virus, and rapid plasma reagin in a trauma population. J Trauma. 1995;39(3):533–7; discussion 537-538.
56. Goldberg D, Johnston J, Cameron S, Fletcher C, Stewart M, McMenamin J, et al. Risk of HIV transmission from patients to surgeons in the era of post-exposure prophylaxis. J Hosp Infect. 2000;44(2):99–105.

Further Reading

Burlew CC, Moore EE, Moore FA, Coimbra R, McIntyre RC, Davis JW, et al. Western trauma association critical decisions in trauma: resuscitative thoracotomy. J Trauma Acute Care Surg. 2012;73(6):1359–63.

Seamon MJ, Haut ER, Van Arendonk K, Barbosa RR, Chiu WC, Dente CJ, et al. An evidence-based approach to patient selection for emergency department thoracotomy: a practice management guideline from the Eastern Association for the Surgery of Trauma. J Trauma Acute Care Surg. 2015;79(1):159–73.

Cardiac Trauma and Tamponade 51

Lena M. Napolitano

51.1 Introduction

Learning Goals
- Understand the common locations of cardiac injury and appropriate treatment based on blunt or penetrating mechanism.
- Understand that the goal of the eFAST exam in trauma is to rapidly diagnose hemopericardium in addition to hemoperitoneum.
- Understand that treatment algorithm of cardiac trauma is in part dependent on mechanism of injury (blunt vs. penetrating) and hemodynamic status (stable or unstable).

Cardiac trauma includes both blunt cardiac injury (BCI) and penetrating cardiac injury (PCI) [1–3]. It is imperative to maintain a high index of suspicion for cardiac trauma when evaluating trauma patients, as many present hemodynamically stable, and diagnostic delays may increase morbidity and mortality.

L. M. Napolitano (✉)
Department of Surgery, University of Michigan Health System, Ann Arbor, USA
e-mail: lenan@umich.edu

51.1.1 Epidemiology

51.1.1.1 Blunt Cardiac Injury
Blunt cardiac injury (BCI) refers to injury sustained due to blunt trauma to the heart, and occurs in the setting of high impact trauma [4, 5]. Mechanisms of high impact chest trauma include motor vehicle/motorcycle crashes, pedestrian struck, falls, crush injuries, assault, and sports-related injuries with direct blows to the chest. There is a wide range of BCI, from minor BCI causing transient dysrhythmias to cardiac wall aneurysm and acute cardiac wall rupture. The true incidence of BCI is unknown, but reported rates range between 8 and 71% [6]. Autopsy reports confirm BCI is present in 20% of all motor vehicle deaths. Myocardial contusion is the most common BCI, comprising greater than 60% of all BCI. Right ventricle and right atrial injury are most common. Left cardiac chamber injuries, septal, coronary artery, and valvular injuries are least common. Pericardial rupture with cardiac herniation is very rare and can be lethal [7].

51.1.1.2 Penetrating Cardiac Injury
Penetrating cardiac injury (PCI) most frequently occurs with trauma to the anterior chest. The majority of penetrating cardiac injuries are to the right ventricle. PCI can be fatal, and a majority of patients die in the prehospital setting [8–10]. Mortality is also high for those patients who

© The Author(s), under exclusive license to Springer Nature Switzerland AG 2023
F. Coccolini, F. Catena (eds.), *Textbook of Emergency General Surgery*,
https://doi.org/10.1007/978-3-031-22599-4_51

survive to trauma center evaluation [10]. A single-center review from Grady Memorial Hospital Level I Trauma Center of 271 PCI patients included 60% stab wounds, and 40% gunshot wounds, and 26% had cardiac arrest in the emergency department requiring ED thoracotomy. Cardiac tamponade was present in 52% of patients. Mortality was much higher for patients with gunshot wounds (45%) versus stab wounds (19.5%). Suture repair of cardiac injuries was most common (98%), and only 2% of patients required coronary artery repair with cardiopulmonary bypass. Risk factors for PCI mortality included ED thoracotomy, initial systolic blood pressure 90 mmHg or less, multichamber and multicavity injuries [11].

An analysis of 240 PCI cases from Bogota, Colombia [12] reported that overall mortality was 14.6%. Mortality from gunshot wounds was much higher (41.2%) than from stab wounds (11.7%). Importantly, for patients with cardiac tamponade, mortality was also significantly higher for gunshot wounds (54.5%) than for stab wounds (18%), related to challenges in surgical repair of these tissue destructive cardiac injuries.

51.1.2 Etiology

The etiology of blunt cardiac injury (BCI) is due to a direct impact to the anterior chest, high-speed sudden deceleration, compression of the chest, or a mixture of those mechanisms of injury. Motor vehicle accidents are the most common cause and can include involve many of these mechanisms of injury. Individuals struck by motor vehicles, falls, crush injuries, and seemingly innocuous trauma such as sports-related (baseball hitting a chest) or animal-related (animal kick) may also cause BCI.

Penetrating cardiac trauma (PCI) is most commonly due to stab wounds, with gunshot wounds as the second leading cause. Blast injuries (both firearm and non-firearm related) and impalements are also reported causes of PCI [13].

51.1.3 Classification

The AAST Organ Injury Scale for cardiac injuries (Table 51.1) ranges from Grade I to VI for both BCI and PCI. Grade I and II cardiac injuries are usually stable injuries; Grade III and IV injuries are unstable injuries, and Grade V cardiac injury is usually lethal.

Table 51.1 AAST Organ Injury Scale for cardiac injuries

Grade I
1. Blunt cardiac injury with minor EKG abnormality (non specific ST of T wave changes, premature atrial or ventricular contractions, or persistent sinus tachycardia
2. Blunt or penetrating pericardial wound without cardiac injury, tamponade, or cardiac herniation
Grade II
1. Blunt cardiac injury with heart block or ischemic changes without cardiac failure
2. Penetrating tangential cardiac wound, up to but not extending through endocardium, without tamponade
Grade III
1. Blunt cardiac injury with sustained or multifocal ventricular contractions
2. Blunt or penetrating cardiac injury with septal rupture, pulmonary or tricuspid incompetence, papillary muscle dysfunction, or distal coronary artery occlusion without cardiac failure
3. Blunt pericardial laceration with cardiac herniation
4. Blunt cardiac injury with cardiac failure
5. Penetrating tangential myocardial wound, up to but not through endocardium, with tamponade
Grade IV
1. Blunt or penetrating cardiac injury with septal rupture, pulmonary or tricuspid incompetence, papillary muscle dysfunction, or distal coronary artery occlusion producing cardiac failure
2. Blunt or penetrating cardiac injury with aortic or mitral incompetence
3. Blunt or penetrating cardiac injury of the right ventricle, right or left atrium
Grade V
1. Blunt or penetrating cardiac injury with proximal coronary artery occlusion
2. Blunt or penetrating left ventricular perforation
3. Stellate injuries, less that 50% tissue loss of the right ventricle, right or left atrium
Grade VI
1. Blunt avulsion of the heart
2. Penetrating wound producing more than 50% tissue loss of a chamber

51.1.4 Pathophysiology

Cardiac trauma most frequently occurs with trauma to the anterior chest.

Blunt cardiac trauma is generally caused by a direct impact to the anterior chest or direct precordial impact, high-speed sudden deceleration, compression of the chest, crush injury from compression between the sternum and the spine, hydraulic effect, blast injury or a mixture of those [14]. Motor vehicle crashes are the most common cause and can involve all three of the mechanisms above. Interestingly, sternal fractures are not associated with an increased incidence of blunt cardiac injury

Penetrating cardiac trauma is generally caused by stab or gunshot wounds to the chest.

In both BCI and PCI, the right heart, specifically the right ventricle, is the most common location of cardiac injury. The right heart is in close proximity to the anterior chest wall, given its anterior location in the thoracic cavity.

51.2 Diagnosis

51.2.1 Clinical Presentation

(symptoms + physical findings)

The clinical presentation may range from an asymptomatic patient with complete hemodynamic stability to acute cardiovascular collapse and cardiopulmonary arrest. The majority of patients are asymptomatic or complain of chest pain, which may in part be related to associated chest wall injuries. If the trauma patient presents with hypotension and shock, then cardiogenic shock related to BCI or PCI must be distinguished from other potential shock etiologies, including hemorrhagic, hypovolemic, and neurogenic shock.

The clinical presentation depends on several factors including (1) mechanism of injury, (2) time from injury to assessment, (3) extent of injury, (4) extent of associated hemorrhage and blood loss, and (5) whether hemopericardium and cardiac tamponade is present or absent. While BCI is commonly associated with thoracic trauma, it can occur in any patient with multisystem trauma.

Diagnosis requires a careful physical examination, based on the primary and secondary survey of Advanced Trauma Life Support (ATLS). After initial assessment of vital signs, airway and breathing, an evaluation of circulation and the cardiac system is required. Physical examination for anterior and lateral thoracic wounds and contusions, cardiac auscultation for muffled heart tones or dysrhythmias, and assessment for distended neck veins is required. The presence of hypotension, shock, tachycardia, dysrhythmias, and abnormal pulse examination will initiate further diagnostic evaluation for cardiac trauma.

For BCI, direct blunt trauma to the anterior thorax may be indicative of cardiac trauma. A seat-belt sign (Fig. 51.1) is a significant risk factor for BCI.

There are no clinical signs or symptoms specific to blunt pericardial or myocardial injury, but a high index of suspicion is paramount.

Some physical findings strengthen the suspicion for BCI. Clinical findings of cardiac tamponade include "Beck's triad" consisting of (1) distended neck veins, (2) muffled heart sounds,

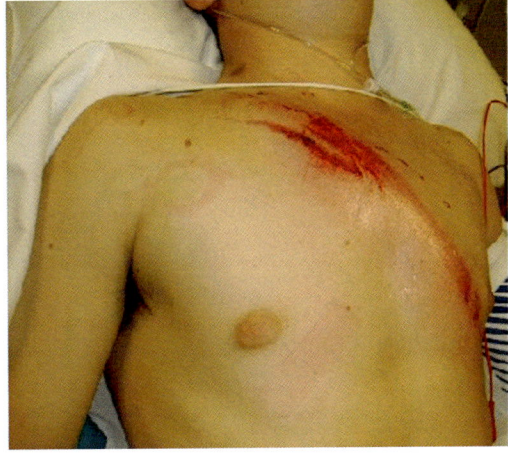

Fig. 51.1 Anterior chest "seatbelt sign", risk factor for blunt cardiac injury

and (3) hypotension. Clinical findings and classical signs of cardiac tamponade also include "Kussmaul's sign" that is paradoxical inspiratory distension of neck veins upon expiration. But these signs can be challenging to confirm in the acute trauma situation in the emergency department and sometimes are not present. The presence of decreased breath sounds on the left is associated with possible left hemothorax and is associated with possible BCI. Refractory hypotension and shock are also indicative of possible BCI.

Clinical presentation is not a sensitive tool for BCI diagnosis, and additional diagnostic testing must be pursued despite no physical findings when suspicion for BCI is high.

51.2.1.1 PCI and the "Cardiac Box"

Penetrating wounds to the precordium (the precordial area of the anterior thorax) are at risk of causing cardiac injury. Penetrating wounds in this anatomic area known as the "cardiac box" (Fig. 51.2) [15] have historically been associated with cardiac injury [16]. The "cardiac box" is an area of the anterior thorax defined as bordered superiorly by the sternal notch and the clavicles, inferiorly by the xiphoid, and the nipples laterally [17].

A recent retrospective autopsy study reported gunshot wounds not in the "cardiac box," including lateral and posterior areas of the thorax, actually had a higher likelihood of cardiac injury [18]. These data, along with the classic anatomic areas of concern, have led to the development of a more inclusive thoracic area defining possible injury. This "three-dimensional cardiac box" (Fig. 51.2) represents a modern structure for penetrating wounds that should be of highest concern for cardiac injury.

A single-center review of trauma patients with penetrating thoracic injuries ($n = 330$) confirmed that a wound location within the cardiac box was associated with a sevenfold increased risk of cardiac injury, and a threefold increased risk of requiring a thoracotomy or sternotomy. Interestingly, a subgroup analysis confirmed that stab wounds to the "cardiac box" were associated with a higher risk of cardiac injury, but this was not true for gunshot wounds [19]. Therefore, for thoracic gunshot wounds, the location of the external wound is not as important as the cardiac ultrasound findings to determine risk for PCI.

51.2.2 Tests

(lab, imaging)

Diagnosis of BCI is very challenging and controversial, as there are no definitive diagnostic criteria for BCI. There is also no accepted gold standard in the evaluation of the sensitivity and specificity of various diagnostic tests for the diagnosis of BCI [20].

Early diagnostic imaging for cardiac injury (both BCI and PCI) must include portable chest radiograph and eFAST exam with subcostal views to evaluate for hemopericardium and other significant cardiac abnormalities.

51.2.2.1 Electrocardiogram (ECG)

A normal ECG has a high negative predictive value for BCI. ECG is therefore an important screening test for hemodynamically stable trauma patients with possible BCI, and is recommended by the EAST Guidelines (Table 51.2) [21]. There is a two- to fourfold increased risk of arrhythmia (sinus tachycardia and atrial fibrillation most common) in BCI patients compared with matched controls with blunt thoracic trauma without BCI [22]. Similarly, a population-based study confirmed that BCI was associated with a threefold increased risk for cardiac conduction abnormalities during hospitalization, and both BCI and thoracic trauma had a significant association with right bundle branch block (OR 6.04 and 1.75 respectively) [23].

51.2.2.2 Laboratory Tests—Cardiac Biomarkers

Cardiac biomarkers, particularly cardiac troponin levels, may be elevated in the setting of BCI. But the utility of cardiac biomarkers in the BCI remains unclear, and they are not routinely recommended by the EAST Guidelines (Table 51.2).

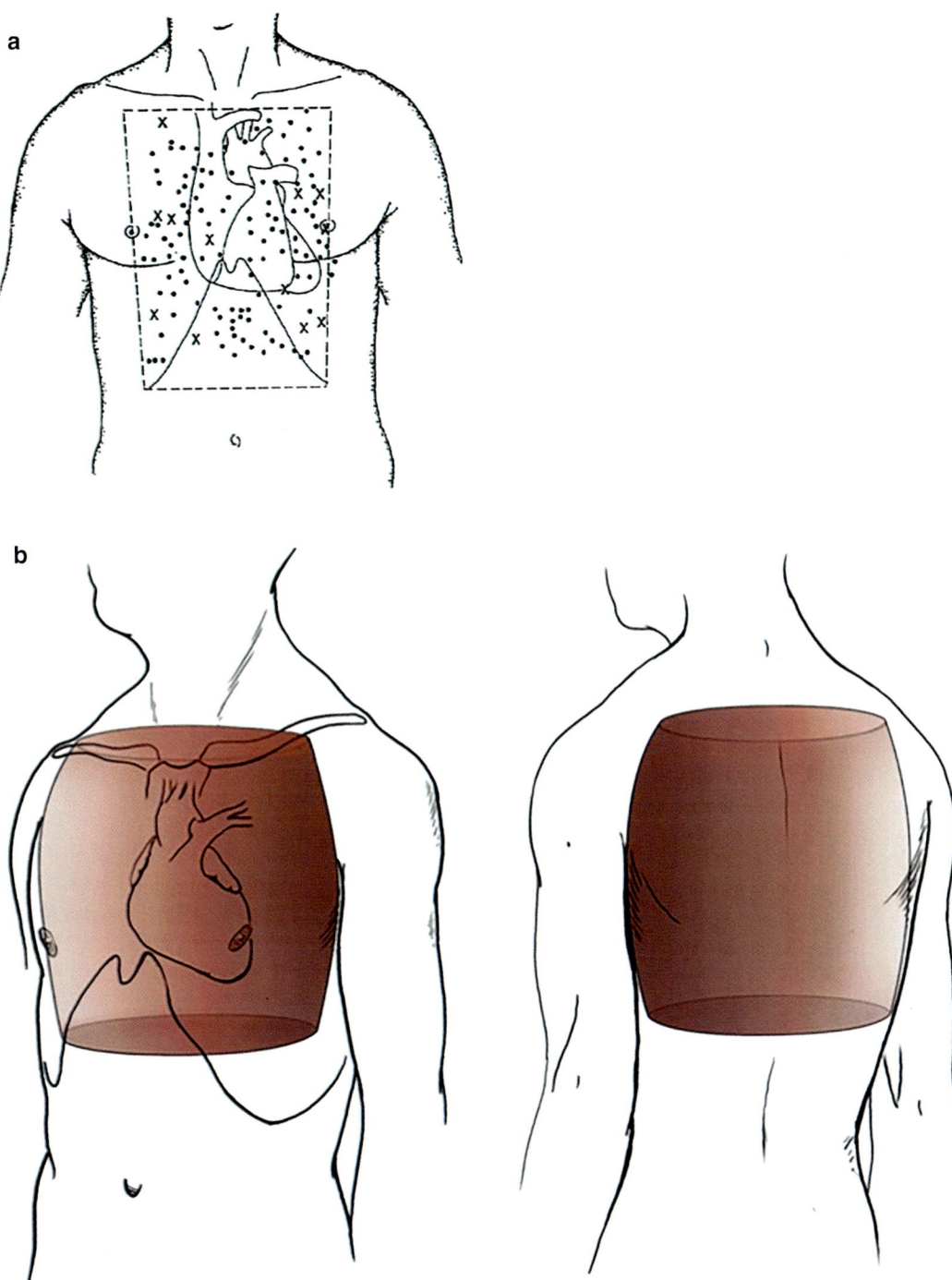

Fig. 51.2 (a) <u>**Historical "Cardiac Box"**</u> defining location of proximity wounds to the heart. X indicates wounds that produced cardiac injuries in that study. *(Reproduced with permission from Nagy K et al. J Trauma 1995;38:859).* (b) <u>**New "3-Dimensional Cardiac Box"**</u> extending laterally and posteriorly. Brighter red gradient indicates higher degree of likelihood of cardiac injury. *(Reproduced with permission from Bellister SA et al. Surg Clin N Am 2017;97:1065-1076)*

Table 51.2 EAST guideline for blunt cardiac injury (2012)

Level I	1. An admission electrocardiogram (ECG) should be performed on all patients in whom BCI is suspected (no change).
Level II	1. If the admission ECG reveals a new abnormality (arrhythmia, ST changes, ischemia, heart block, and unexplained ST changes), the patient should be admitted for continuous ECG monitoring. For patients with preexisting abnormalities, comparison should be made to a previous ECG to determine need for monitoring (updated).
	2. In patients with a normal ECG result and normal troponin I level, BCI is ruled out. The optimal timing of these measurements, however, has yet to be determined. Conversely, patients with normal ECG results but elevated troponin I level should be admitted to a monitored setting (new).
	3. For patients with hemodynamic instability or persistent new arrhythmia, an echocardiogram should be obtained. If an optimal transthoracic echocardiogram cannot be performed, the patient should have a transesophageal echocardiogram (updated).
	4. The presence of a sternal fracture alone does not predict the presence of BCI and thus should not prompt monitoring in the setting of normal ECG result and troponin I level (moved from Level 3).
	5. Creatinine phosphokinase with isoenzyme analysis should not be performed because it is not useful in predicting which patients have or will have complications related to BCI (modified and moved from Level 3).
	6. Nuclear medicine studies add little when compared with echocardiography and should not be routinely performed (no change).
Level III	1. Elderly patients with known cardiac disease, unstable patients, and those with an abnormal admission ECG result can safely undergo surgery provided that they are appropriately monitored. Consideration should be given to placement of a pulmonary artery catheter in such cases (no change).
	2. Troponin I should be measured routinely for patients with suspected BCI; if elevated, patients should be admitted to a monitored setting and troponin I should be followed up serially, although the optimal timing is unknown (new).
	3. Cardiac computed tomography (CT) or magnetic resonance imaging (MRI) can be used to help differentiate acute myocardial infarction (AMI) from BCI in trauma patients with abnormal ECG result, cardiac enzymes, and/ or abnormal echo to determine need for cardiac catheterization and/or anticoagulation (new).

https://www.east.org/Content/documents/practicemanagementguidelines/Screening_for_blunt_cardiac_injury___An_Eastern.5.pdf
Clancy K, Velopulos C, Bilaniuk JW, et al. Eastern Association for the Surgery of Trauma Screening for blunt cardiac injury: an Eastern Association for the Surgery of Trauma practice management guideline. J Trauma Acute Care Surg. 2012;73:S301–306

Measurement of their levels in conjunction with ECG evaluation may aid in BCI diagnosis, as the combination of normal ECG and normal serum troponin I ruled out the diagnosis of significant BCI [24]. Some studies have reported that elevated troponin levels have prognostic significance in BCI, with elevated troponin levels associated with higher mortality [25].

51.2.2.3 Radiologic Tests

Chest radiographs are routinely obtained and may detect chest wall injuries such as rib fractures, sternal fracture, and clavicular fracture that are commonly seen in conjunction with BCI. Chest radiographs have limited utility for the diagnosis of BCI except in confirmation of hemothorax or wide mediastinum. But chest radiographs can be very useful in PCI with confirmation of the presence and precise location of a foreign body, and associated hemothorax or pneumothorax.

51.2.2.4 Ultrasound and eFAST Exam

All trauma patients must have an eFAST exam with subcostal cardiac views (Fig. 51.3) to evaluate for hemopericardium and other cardiac abnormalities. Ultrasound imaging for detection of hemopericardium is very helpful (79% sensitive, 92% specific), except in patients with left hemothorax with a high false-negative ultrasound rate. Patients with left hemothorax require an additional diagnostic test for hemopericardium.

A single-center study ($n = 172$) reported that ultrasound had an 86.7% sensitivity for detecting

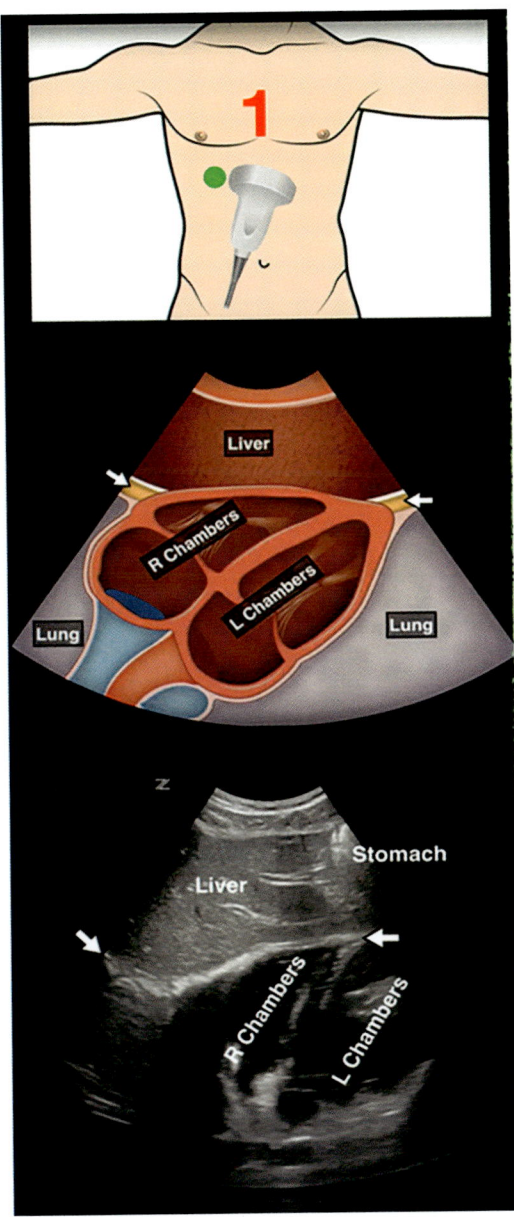

Fig. 51.3 Cardiac eFAST exam to evaluate for hemopericardium. Subcostal view of the eFAST exam. The transducer should be placed in the subxiphoid position, directed toward the patient's left shoulder. The liver is an acoustic window to image the heart

tive single-center study examined the diagnostic accuracy of chest ultrasound for the diagnosis of occult penetrating cardiac wounds in hemodynamically stable patients ($n = 141$) and reported 79% sensitivity and 93% specificity. Similarly, six false negative studies were in patients with left hemothorax [27].

A systematic review and meta-analysis of the diagnostic accuracy of ultrasound for PCI in hemodynamically stable patients (5 studies, $n = 556$) reported that, compared with pericardial window, ultrasound was 79% sensitive and 92% specific for detection of occult penetrating cardiac injuries. This meta-analysis again confirmed that the presence of a concomitant left hemothorax was common in patients with false-negative ultrasound imaging. Therefore, in PCI patients with left hemothorax, a second diagnostic test should be performed [28].

The optimal second diagnostic test for occult PCI is not studied well, but computed tomographic (CT) scan with EKG gating to reduce pulsation artifacts is currently the best standard imaging modality of cardiac injury in stable patients [29]. In the case of equivocal initial ultrasound results in patients with hemothorax, a repeat ultrasound after drainage of hemothorax can be considered, but CT imaging at present is the best adjunctive imaging test to screen for occult PCI [26]. Transesophageal echocardiography (TEE) and cardiac magnetic resonance imaging (MRI) are also possible, but TEE requires sedation and MRI may require long scanning time. In contrast, in BCI direct CT findings of myocardial contusion (myocardial hypoenhancement) are poorly sensitive, and echocardiography and cardiac MRI may also be used to evaluate for wall motion abnormalities [30].

51.2.2.5 Echocardiography

Echocardiography can be useful in the assessment of potential BCI. Transthoracic echocardiography (TTE) can be useful for the evaluation of cardiac wall motion and structural abnormalities. TTE can detect hemopericardium, pericardial, and segmental wall abnormalities or valvular dysfunction, and can be easily performed at the

hemopericardium in penetrating thoracic trauma patients who were hemodynamically stable, with a positive predictive value of 77%. Of 18 false-negatives, 11 had associated hemothorax, and 6 had pneumopericardium [26]. Another prospec-

bedside in the emergency department. But TTE can also be technically very challenging in the setting of significant chest trauma, particularly if any subcutaneous air, pneumomediastinum, or pneumopericardium are present in the trauma patient. Although transesophageal echocardiography (TEE) is more sensitive than the transthoracic route, its use is limited by its invasive nature, requirement for patient sedation or anesthesia, and its difficulty in performing acutely in the setting of severe traumatic thoracic injury.

51.2.2.6 Computed Tomography Scan

CT examinations can be very helpful in assessing potential cardiac injury in hemodynamically stable patients, particularly when performed to also assess thoracic trauma [31]. In cases of suspected cardiac trauma, ECG gating can be used to decrease both cardiac and motion artifact [32, 33]. In both BCI and PCI, CT imaging can identify hemopericardium as well as direct signs of cardiac injury including contour irregularity, focal outpouching, aneurysm and pseudoaneurysm, post-traumatic ventricular septal defect, pericardial injury, and cardiac herniation. In patients with PCI, CT imaging can greatly assist with determination of the trajectory of the stab wound or projectile, which are not apparent on physical examination. In particular, ballistic trajectories are important to assess by CT imaging, as there can be complex pathways within the thorax. Bullets can also enter cardiac chambers and can also embolize in great vessels and distally. CT imaging is a valuable tool for the evaluation of acute cardiac injury, since it is commonly performed as the initial diagnostic assessment to evaluate all other traumatic injuries in stable patients. CT findings of cardiac injury can assist in making a prompt diagnosis and providing direction for life-saving care.

51.2.2.7 Magnetic Resonance Imaging

There is a very limited role for cardiac MRI in the evaluation of acute cardiac trauma. Although the EAST guidelines recommended MRI as a potential tool to differentiate acute myocardial infarction from BCI, the recent publication of the American College of Radiology Appropriateness Criteria for Blunt Chest Trauma—Suspected Cardiac Injury Expert Panel designated MRI as "usually not appropriate" based on inadequate data and evidence [34].

Differential Diagnosis

For both BCI and PCI, the specific type of cardiac injury must be identified as early as possible, as the treatment of the cardiac injury is directly dependent on the type of injury identified. For BCI, myocardial contusion or blunt myocardial injury is the most common diagnosis, and is managed conservatively. Hemopericardium, cardiac tamponade, and cardiac rupture are rare causes of BCI, but a high index of suspicion should be maintained in blunt trauma patients who present or develop hypotension that is refractory to hemorrhagic shock management with blood product resuscitation.

Hemopericardium and cardiac tamponade are more commonly seen with PCIs. Ultrasound imaging via the eFAST approach is the ideal study for early diagnosis and confirmation of hemopericardium and possible cardiac tamponade in trauma patients (Fig. 51.4).

Cardiac tamponade is caused by pericardial fluid/blood accumulation under pressure, which results in impaired cardiac diastolic filling, reduced cardiac output and venous return, with resultant hypotension and hemodynamic instability. Additional clinical signs of cardiac tamponade include tachycardia and pulsus paradoxus, defined as an abnormal decline (>10 mmHg) in systemic arterial pressure during inspiration. Beck's triad of hypotension, jugular venous distention, and muffled heart sounds constitute the classic clinical presentation of cardiac tamponade. But the findings of Beck's triad may not be present in up to 25% of patients with cardiac injuries [35].

Other specific cardiac injuries for both BCI and PCI include atrial and ventricular lacerations and injuries, valvular injuries, coronary artery injuries, cardiac rupture, pericardial rupture with cardiac herniation, and possible traumatic ventricular-septal defect or arteriovenous fistulae.

"Commotio cordis" (Fig. 51.5) is a very rare type of BCI in which low impact trauma causes sudden cardiac arrest, and usually occurs from being struck by a projectile during sports. The pathophysiology of cardiac arrest with commotion cordis is ventricular fibrillation and cardiac arrest triggered by a blunt, nonpenetrating blow to the chest without damage to the ribs, sternum or heart, and can result in sudden death.

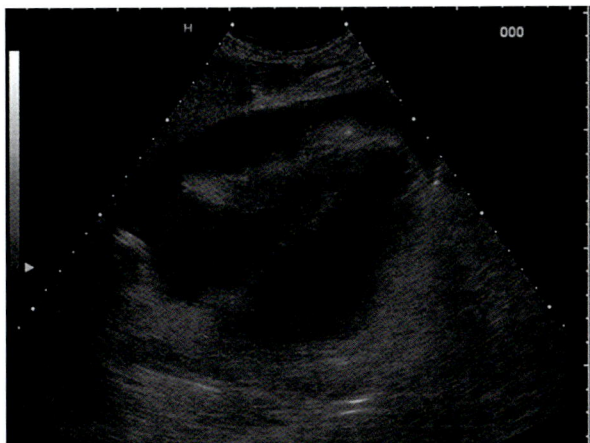

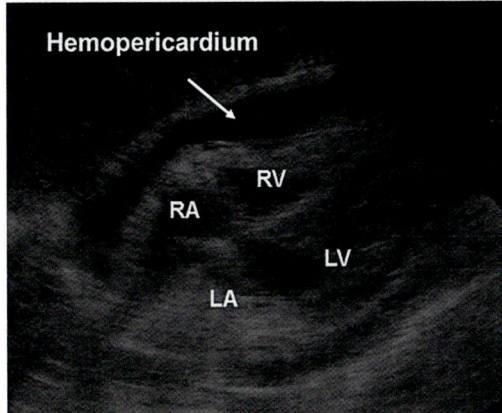

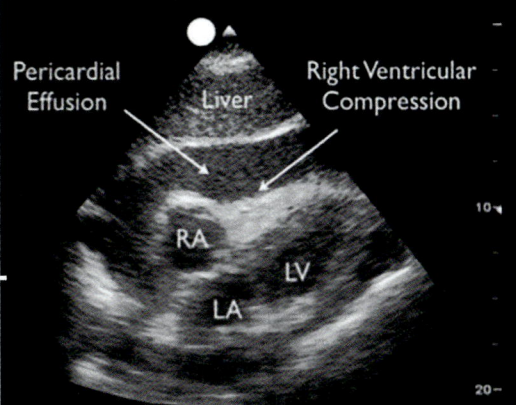

Fig. 51.4 Hemopericardium and cardiac tamponade ultrasound findings. Pericardial fluid will appear as a dark band (anechoic) that separates the bright (hyperechoic) pericardium from the heterogeneous grey myocardium. Pericardial fluid (hemopericardium if blood) is noted with compression of the right ventricle, indicative of cardiac tamponade

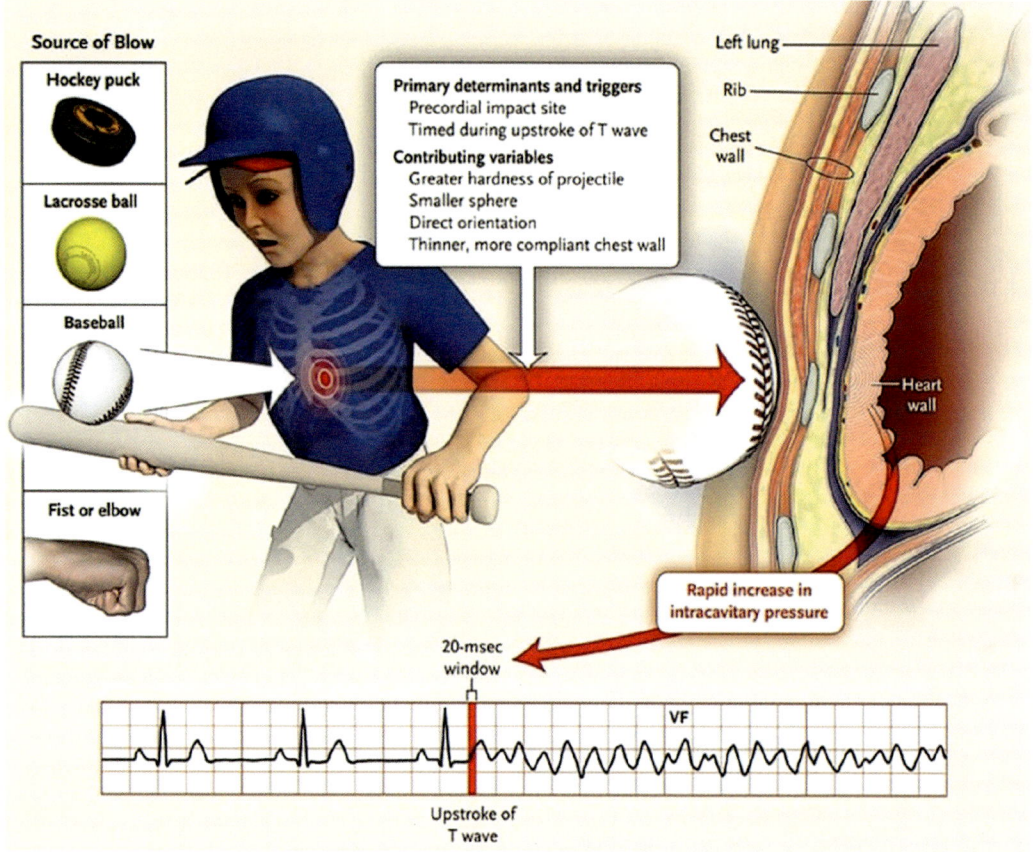

Fig. 51.5 Pathophysiology of commotio cordis. Ventricular fibrillation and cardiac arrest triggered by a blunt, nonpenetrating blow to the chest without damage to the ribs, sternum or heart. From: Maron BJ, Estes NAM. Commotio Cordis. N Engl J Med 2010; 362:917-927. DOI: 10.1056/NEJMra0910111

51.3 Treatment

The treatment algorithms for cardiac trauma depend on:

- Mechanism of injury (blunt or penetrating, BCI vs. PCI)
- Hemodynamic status (stable or unstable)

BCI Algorithm

There are a number of treatment algorithms for the evaluation and management of BCI, and a streamlined algorithm is provided for review (Algorithm 51.1) [36]. Since most BCI patients have low-risk myocardial contusion injuries, this algorithm aims to identify patients that warrant in-hospital treatment with ECG monitoring, serial transthoracic echo, or additional diagnostic studies to identify rarer blunt cardiac injuries.

One area of controversy is in BCI patients with pericardial fluid identified. There is significant variability in the treatment of these patients with pericardial fluid from blunt trauma that has been identified with ultrasound or CT imaging confirmation. Recent reports have confirmed that conservative management with observation is successful in many patients who are hemodynamically stable [37]. In contrast, those patients with hemodynamic instability must undergo operative exploration. Two suggested algorithms

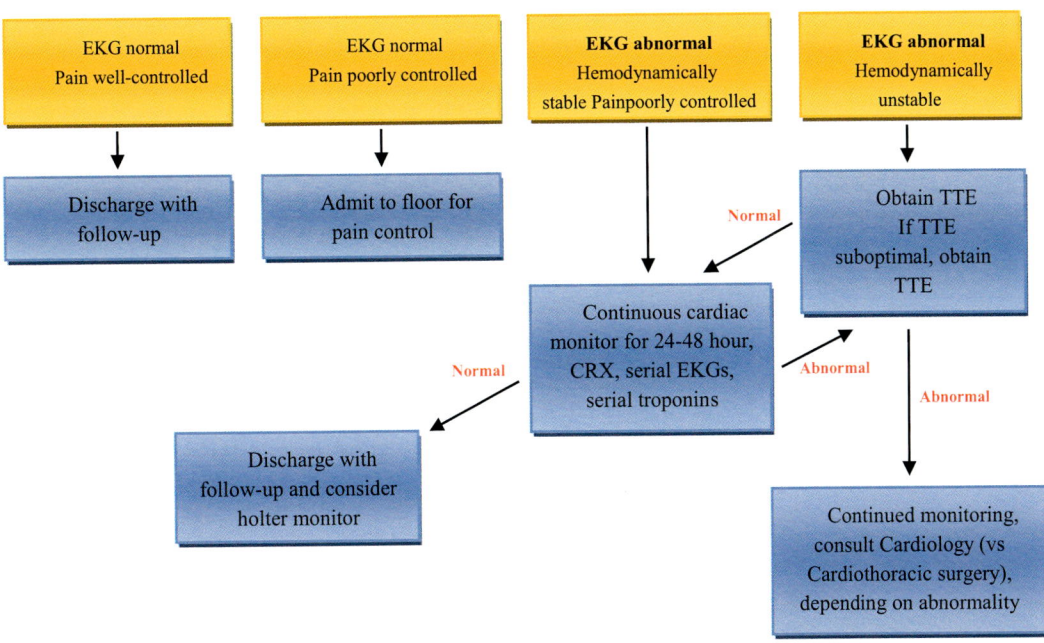

Algorithm 51.1 Treatment algorithm for blunt cardiac injury (BCI)

(Algorithm 51.2) for the management of stable patients with blunt pericardial effusion are provided for review [38].

PCI Algorithm

The treatment algorithm for patients with PCI is based upon the patient's initial vital signs (Algorithm 51.3). Management of the stable patient (SBP >90 mmHg) allows additional diagnostic evaluation with chest radiograph and echocardiography. Unstable patients (SBP <90 mmHg) require immediate surgical exploration if eFAST confirms PCI [39]. Trauma patients with loss of vital signs during initial evaluation in the emergency department are treated with resuscitative thoracotomy [40].

A controversial area of PCI management is the optimal management of PCI patients who are hemodynamically stable, with a normal physical examination, positive ultrasound confirming a small amount of pericardial blood, with no signs of cardiac tamponade or active bleeding. The current internationally accepted management algorithm has been immediate sternotomy and cardiac exploration. One study documented that 71% of such patients had a non-therapeutic sternotomy [41]. Other studies have reported similar findings [42–44]. A small randomized trial ($n = 111$) confirmed that 93% of patients randomized to sternotomy had either no cardiac injury or tangential injury. Subxiphoid pericardial window and drainage was effective

Treatment algorithms for Clinical Management of Blunt Chest Trauma Patients with Pericardial Fluid on CT Scan Imaging

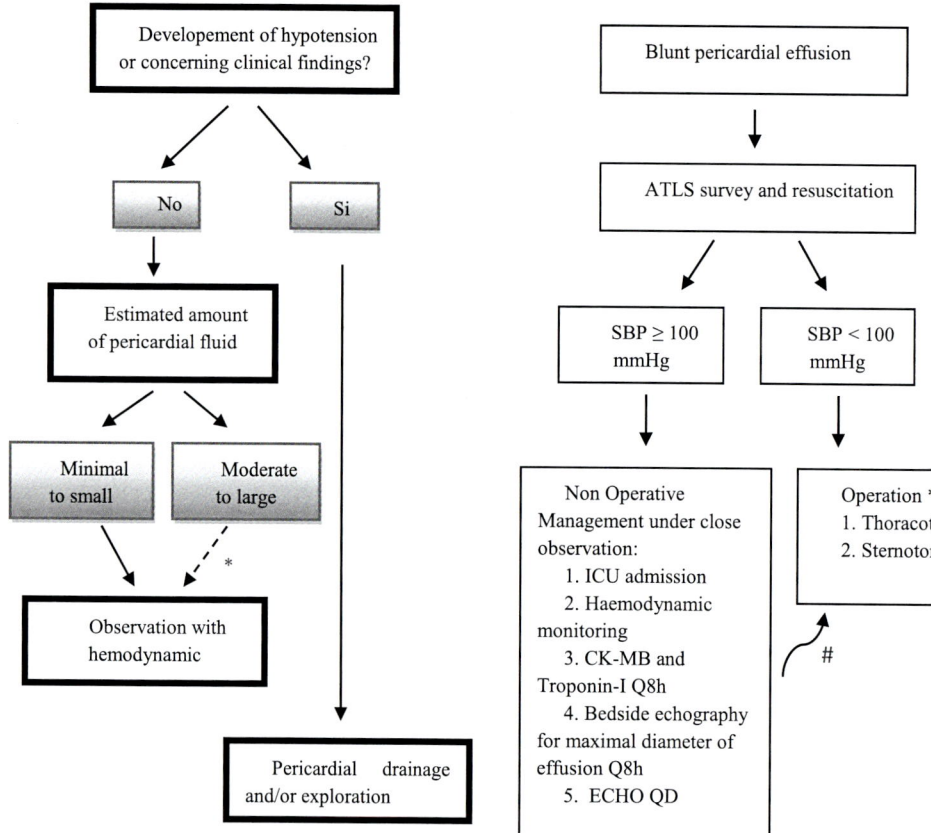

Algorithm 51.2 Treatment algorithms for clinical management of blunt chest trauma patients with pericardial fluid on CT scan imaging
*Data suggest that hemodynamically normal patients with moderate to large amounts of fluid may be observed; however, given small sample sizes, this recommendation must be confirmed in larger studies.
From: Witt CE, Linnau KF, Maier RV, Rivara FP, Vavilala MS, Bulger EM, Arbabi S. Management of pericardial fluid in blunt trauma: variability in practice and predictors of operative outcome in patients with computed tomography evidence of pericardial fluid. J Trauma Care Surg. 2017 Apr; 82(4):733. doi: 10.1097/TA.0000000000001386. PMID 28129264; PMCID: PMC5360471

**The selection of operation may depend on clinical judgment.
#Absolute indication for delayed operation: Hypotension without response to medical treatment
#Relative indications for delayed operation:
1. Increasing pericardial effusion amount
2. Presence of tamponade sign (right ventricle collapse or global hypokinesia) on follow-up ECHO
3. Increasing levels of cardiac enzymes
4. Any deterioration without other origin
From: Huang JF, Hsieh FJ, Fu CY, Liao CH. Nonoperative management is feasible for selected blunt trauma patients with pericardial effusion. Injury 2018 Jan:49(1):20–26

and safe in stable patients with hemopericardium after PCI, with no difference in mortality, and shorter ICU and hospital stay [45]. Small hemopericardium in a stable patient may not always warrant surgical treatment with a subxiphoid window or sternotomy [46, 47].

51.3.1 Medical Treatment

(interventional radiology included)

Selective nonoperative management of penetrating thoracic injury has been reported to be successful, but once PCI is identified with hemo-

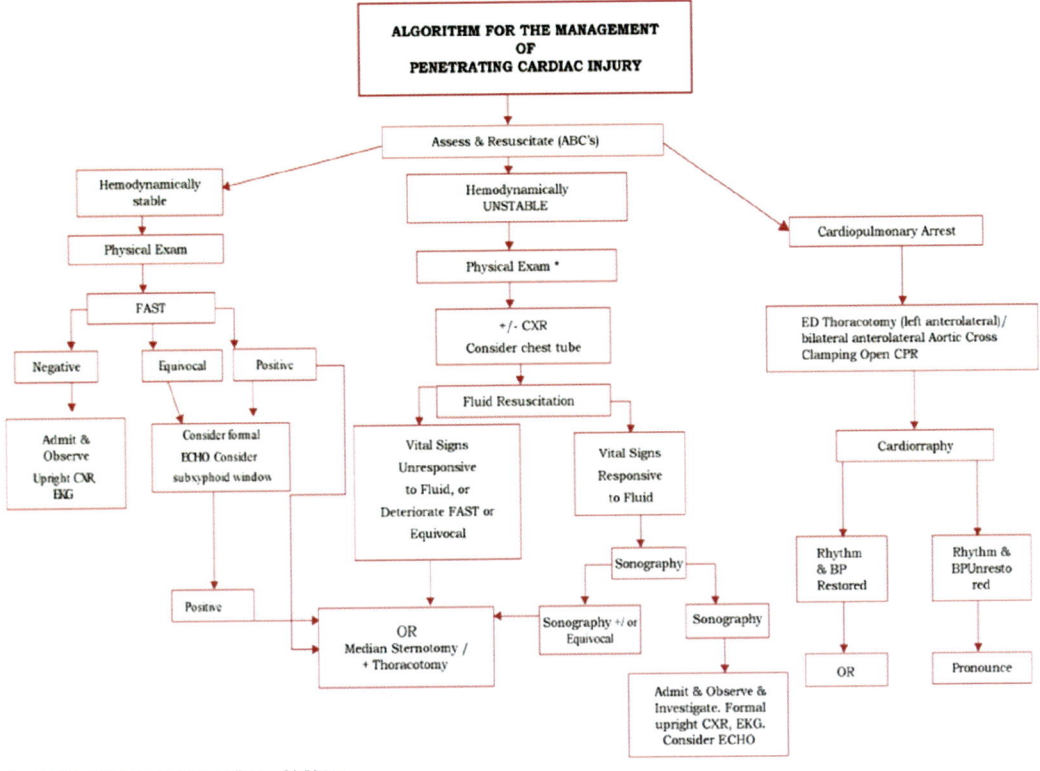

Algorithm 51.3 Treatment algorithm for penetrating cardiac injury (PCI)

pericardium, then definitive management is indicated [48]. In a single-center report of 248 patients, 14 (5.7%) required immediate emergency surgery. Nonoperative management was successful in 93.2% of patients. Mortality rate was very low at 2% [49].

Pericardiocentesis is not indicated for the treatment of hemopericardium and/or cardiac tamponade due to acute trauma. Pericardiocentesis can be considered as a treatment strategy for chronic pericardial effusions. Some patient with hemopericardium may develop pericarditis, and treatment with non-steroidal anti-inflammatory drugs (NSAIDs), colchicine and steroids can be considered.

51.3.2 Surgical Treatment

(including open and mininvasive surgical techniques)

PCI with hemodynamic instability warrants immediate surgical management. Median sternotomy is the optimal surgical access for PCI, as it provides excellent exposure of the heart and mediastinal structures. In situations where median sternotomy cannot be performed, then left anterolateral thoracotomy with clamshell extension and transverse sternotomy in the 5th intercostal space is used.

Initial management of PCIs requires prompt bleeding control which can be accomplished with direct finger pressure and occlusion of the site of injury. When digital pressure does not suffice for cardiac hemorrhage control, a Foley catheter can be placed into the cardiac site of injury with balloon inflation and tension, with subsequent suture repair around the foley catheter site. If hemorrhage control is unable to be achieved from the cardiac injury site, or cardiac arrest ensues during attempts at hemorrhage control, then initiation of cardiopulmonary bypass should be considered.

Atrial injuries can be commonly managed with application of a vascular clamp and direct suture repair using 3-0 to 5-0 polypropylene monofilament sutures dependent on the thickness of the atrial wall. For ventricular injuries, 2-0 to 3-0 interrupted polypropylene pledgeted sutures can be used in a simple or horizontal mattress manner (Fig. 51.6).

Other cardiac injuries, including intra-cardiac and valvular injuries, traumatic ventricular-septal defect, and some coronary artery injuries, will require cardiopulmonary bypass for optimal repair.

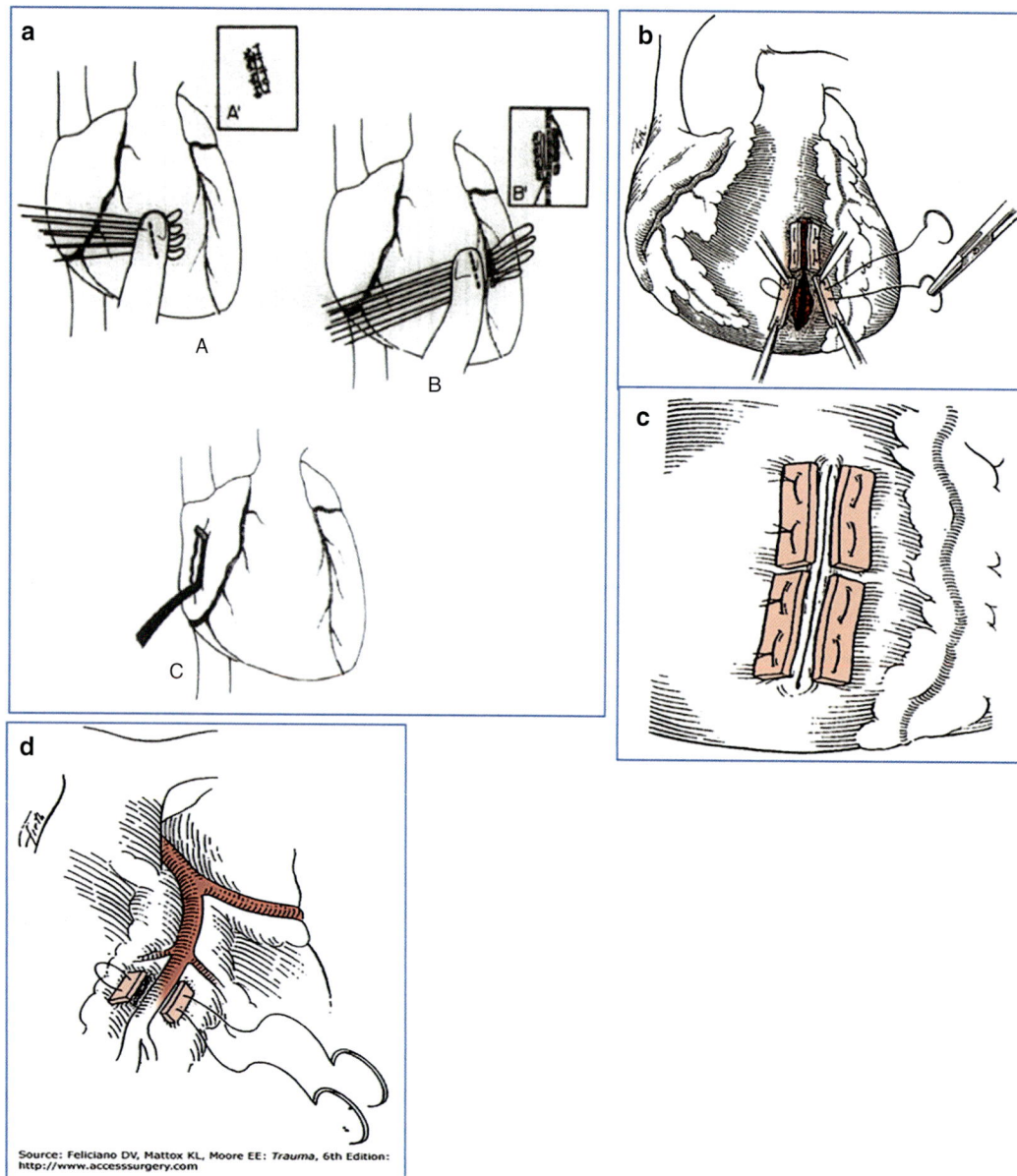

Fig. 51.6 Options for surgical management and repair of penetrating cardiac injuries (PCI):
A. Suturing of cardiac laceration underneath finger occlusion
B. Placement of horizontal mattress sutures through the myocardium
C. Control of atrial bleeding with a vascular clamp
D. Pledgeted sutures for repair of myocardial lacerations

51.3.3 Prognosis

(including complications and their management)

In general, outcomes for BCI and PCI depend on the clinical findings at presentation, particularly whether the patient is hemodynamically stable or unstable. Increased mortality is associated with higher AAST grade of cardiac injury for both BCI and PCI, with hemodynamic instability and shock, and with cardiac tamponade or cardiac rupture. A recent single-institution review of PCI outcomes reported a very high mortality rate with gunshot wounds (59%) with lower mortality for knife stab wounds (21%) [50]. For patients with "myocardial contusion" alone, based on findings of an abnormal ECG, arrhythmias or cardiac biomarkers, overall outcome is very good with no long-term sequelae [51].

> **Dos and Don'ts**
> (List what should and should not be done when treating patients)
>
> - Do—Perform eFAST to evaluate for BCI and PCI and cardiac tamponade.
> - Do—Median sternotomy is the optimal surgical access for PCI treatment.
> - Do—Use the new "3-Dimensional Cardiac Box" extending laterally and posteriorly from the original cardiac box which indicates higher degree of likelihood of cardiac injury.
> - Don't—Don't rely on Beck's triad (hypotension, jugular venous distention, and muffled heart sounds) as the classic clinical presentation of cardiac tamponade.
> - Don't—Stab wounds to the "cardiac box" are associated with a higher risk of cardiac injury, but gunshot wounds are not.
> - Don't—Don't use ultrasound alone to diagnose hemopericardium in patients with left hemothorax, as there is a high false negative rate, and these patients require additional diagnostic testing to confirm hemopericardium

> **Take-Home Messages**
> - Rapid diagnosis of cardiac injuries is imperative, with differentiation of blunt (BCI) versus penetrating (PCI) cardiac injuries
> - For BCI, there is no clear diagnostic test, but FAST exam, EKG, troponin, and transthoracic echocardiography are helpful.
> - CT scan imaging with EKG gating can identify structural injuries to the heart for both BCI and PCI.
> - The right heart, specifically the right ventricle, is the most common location of cardiac injury in both blunt and penetrating trauma.
> - For PCI, early surgical intervention can save lives, and in unstable patients with cardiac tamponade, median sternotomy is indicated as it provides optimal access to all cardiac and mediastinal structures.

> **Multiple Choice Questions**
> 1. Is it possible conservative management of heart trauma?
>   A. Yes
>   B. No
>   C. All the previous ones
>   D. **Only in selected cases**
> 2. Penetrating cardiac injuries
>   A. May be treated non operatively
>   B. Must be treated with cardiectomy
>   C. Must be managed always with ECMO
>   D. **Operative treatment is the suggested management**
> 3. Cardiac suture in penetrating trauma
>   A. **Must keep into consideration the coronary arteries damage**
>   B. Can be performed only with small stitches
>   C. Can be performed with thoracoscopy
>   D. Must be performed with glue

References

1. Bellister SA, Dennis BM, Guillamondegui OD. Blunt and penetrating cardiac trauma. Surg Clin N Am. 2017;97:1065–76. https://doi.org/10.1016/j.suc.2017.06.012.
2. Marcolini EG, Keegan J. Blunt cardiac injury. Emerg Med Clin N Am. 2015;33:519–27. https://doi.org/10.1016/j.emc.2015.04.003.
3. Warrington SJ, Mahajam K. Cardiac trauma. [Updated 2020 Jul 17]. In: StatPearls [Internet]. Treasure Island (FL): StatPearls Publishing; 2021 Jan. https://www.ncbi.nlm.nih.gov/books/NBK430725/
4. Singh S, Heard M, Pester JM, Angus LD. Blunt cardiac injury. [Updated 2021 Feb 21]. In: StatPearls [Internet]. Treasure Island (FL): StatPearls Publishing; 2021 Jan. https://www.ncbi.nlm.nih.gov/books/NBK532267/
5. Huis In't Veld MA, Craft CA, Hood RE. Blunt cardiac trauma review. Cardiol Clin. 2018;36(1):183–91. https://doi.org/10.1016/j.ccl.2017.08.010.
6. Leite L, Gonçalves L, Nuno VD. Cardiac injuries caused by trauma: Review and case reports. J Forensic Leg Med. 2017;52:30–4.
7. Chughtai T, Chiavaras MM, Sharkey P, Shulman H, Miller HA. Pericardial rupture with cardiac herniation. Can J Surg. 2008;51(5):E101–2.
8. Trinkle JK. Penetrating heart wounds: difficulty in evaluating clinical series. Ann Thorac Surg. 1984;38:181–2.
9. Sugg WL, Rea WJ, Ecker RR, Webb WR, Rose EF, Shaw RR. Penetrating wounds of the heart: an analysis of 459 cases. J Thorac Cardiovasc Surg. 1968;56:531–45.
10. Thourani VH, Feliciano DV, Cooper WA, Brady KM, Adams AB, Rozycki GS, Symbas PN. Penetrating cardiac trauma at an urban trauma center: a 22-year perspective. Am Surg. 1999;65(9):811–6; discussion 817–8.
11. Morse BC, Mina MJ, Carr JS, Jhunjhunwala R, Dente CJ, Zink JU, Nicholas JM, Wyrzykowski AD, Salomone JP, Vercruysse GA, Rozycki GS, Feliciano DV. Penetrating cardiac injuries: A 36-year perspective at an urban, Level I trauma center. J Trauma Acute Care Surg. 2016;81(4):623–31. https://doi.org/10.1097/TA.0000000000001165.
12. Isaza-Restrepo A, Bolívar-Sáenz DJ, Tarazona-Lara M, et al. Penetrating cardiac trauma: analysis of 240 cases from a hospital in Bogota, Colombia. World J Emerg Surg. 2017;12:26. https://doi.org/10.1186/s13017-017-0138-1.
13. Lateef Wani M, Ahangar AG, Wani SN, Irshad I, Ul-Hassan N. Penetrating cardiac injury: a review. Trauma Mon. 2012;17(1):230–2. https://doi.org/10.5812/traumamon.3461.
14. Schultz JM, Trunkey DD. Blunt cardiac injury. Crit Care Clin. 2004;1:57–70.
15. Nagy KK, Lohmann C, Kim DO, Barrett J. Role of echocardiography in the diagnosis of occult penetrating cardiac injury. J Trauma. 1995;38(6):859–62.
16. Evans J, Gray LA Jr, Rayner A, Fulton RL. Principles for the management of penetrating cardiac wounds. Ann Surg. 1979;189(6):777–84. https://doi.org/10.1097/00000658-197906000-00015.
17. Asensio JA, Stewart BM, Murray J, et al. Penetrating cardiac injuries. Surg Clin North Am. 1996;76(4):685–724.
18. Jhunjhunwala R, Mina MJ, Roger EI, et al. Reassessing the cardiac box: a comprehensive evaluation of the relationship between thoracic gunshot wounds and cardiac injury. J Trauma Acute Care Surg. 2017;83(3):349–55. https://doi.org/10.1097/TA.0000000000001519.
19. Kim JS, Inaba K, de Leon LA, Rais C, Holcomb JB, David JS, Starnes VA, Demetriades D. Penetrating injury to the cardiac box. J Trauma Acute Care Surg. 2020;89(3):482–7. https://doi.org/10.1097/TA.0000000000002808.
20. Shoar S, Hosseini FS, Naderan M, Khavandi S, Tabibzadeh E, Khavandi S, Shoar N. Cardiac injury following blunt chest trauma: diagnosis, management, and uncertainty. Int J Burns Trauma. 2021;11(2):80–9.
21. Clancy K, Velopulos C, Bilaniuk JW, et al. Eastern Association for the Surgery of Trauma Screening for blunt cardiac injury: an Eastern Association for the Surgery of Trauma practice management guideline. J Trauma Acute Care Surg. 2012;73:S301–6. https://www.east.org/Content/documents/practicemanagementguidelines/Screening_for_blunt_cardiac_injury___An_Eastern.5.pdf
22. Ismailov RM, Ness RB, Redmond CK, Talbott EO, Weiss HB. Trauma associated with cardiac dysrhythmias: results from a large matched case-control study. J Trauma. 2007;62(5):1186–91. https://doi.org/10.1097/01.ta.0000215414.35222.bb.
23. Ismailov RM. Trauma associated with cardiac conduction abnormalities: population-based perspective, mechanism and review of literature. Eur J Trauma Emerg Surg. 2010;36(3):227–32. https://doi.org/10.1007/s00068-009-9096-y. Epub 2010 Jan 27.
24. Velmahos GC, Karaiskakis M, Salim A, Toutouzas KG, Murray J, Asensio J, Demetriades D. Normal electrocardiography and serum troponin I levels preclude the presence of clinically significant blunt cardiac injury. J Trauma. 2003;54(1):45–50; discussion 50-1. https://doi.org/10.1097/00005373-200301000-00006.
25. Joseph B, Jokar TO, Khalil M, Haider AA, Kulvatunyou N, Zangbar B, Tang A, Zeeshan M, O'Keeffe T, Abbas D, Latifi R, Rhee P. Identifying the broken heart: predictors of mortality and morbidity in suspected blunt cardiac injury. Am J Surg. 2016;211(6):982–8. https://doi.org/10.1016/j.amjsurg.2015.10.027. Epub 2016 Jan 7.
26. Nicol AJ, Navsaria PH, Beningfield S, Hommes M, Kahn D. Screening for occult penetrating cardiac injuries. Ann Surg. 2015;261(3):573–8. https://doi.org/10.1097/SLA.0000000000000713.
27. Gonzalez-Hadad A, García AF, Serna JJ, Herrera MA, Morales M, Manzano-Nunez R. The role of ultrasound for detecting occult penetrating cardiac wounds in hemodynamically stable patients. World

28. Manzano-Nunez R, Gomez A, Espitia D, Sierra-Ruiz M, Gonzalez J, Rodriguez-Narvaez JG, Castillo AC, Gonzalez A, Orjuela J, Orozco-Martin V, Bernal F, Giron F, Rios AC, Carranza P, Gonzalez-Hadad A, García-Perdomo HA, García AF. A meta-analysis of the diagnostic accuracy of chest ultrasound for the diagnosis of occult penetrating cardiac injuries in hemodynamically stable patients with penetrating thoracic trauma. J Trauma Acute Care Surg. 2021;90(2):388–95. https://doi.org/10.1097/TA.0000000000003006.

29. Basi AJ, Restrepo C, Mumbower A, McCarthy M, Rashmi K. Cardiac injuries: a review of multidetector computed tomography findings. Trauma Mon. 2015;20(4):e19086. https://doi.org/10.5812/traumamon.19086.

30. Hammer MM, Raptis DA, Cummings KW, Mellnick VM, Bhalla S, Schuerer DJ, Raptis CA. Imaging in blunt cardiac injury: computed tomographic findings in cardiac contusion and associated injuries. Injury. 2016;47(5):1025–30. https://doi.org/10.1016/j.injury.2015.11.008. Epub 2015 Nov 19.

31. Raptis DA, Bhalla S, Raptis CA. Computed tomographic imaging of cardiac trauma. Radiol Clin North Am. 2019;57(1):201–12. https://doi.org/10.1016/j.rcl.2018.08.009. Epub 2018 Oct 31.

32. Co S, Yong-Hing C, Galea-Soler S, et. al. Role of imaging in penetrating and blunt traumatic injury to the heart. Radiographics 2011; 31:1496.

33. Restrepo C, Gutierrez F, Marmol-Velez J, et. al. Imaging patients with cardiac trauma. Radiographics 2012; 32:633-649.

34. Expert Panels on Cardiac Imaging and Thoracic Imaging, Stojanovska J, Hurwitz Koweek LM, Chung JH, Ghoshhajra BB, Walker CM, Beache GM, Berry MF, Colletti PM, Davis AM, Hsu JY, Khosa F, Kicska GA, Kligerman SJ, Litmanovich D, Maroules CD, Meyersohn N, Syed MA, Tong BC, Villines TC, Wann S, Wolf SJ, Kanne JP, Abbara S. ACR appropriateness criteria(R) blunt chest trauma-suspected cardiac injury. J Am Coll Radiol. 2020;17:S380–90. https://doi.org/10.1016/j.jacr.2020.09.012.

35. Demetriades D. Cardiac wounds. Experience with 70 patients. Ann Surg. 1986;203(3):315–7.

36. El-Menyar A, Al Thani H, Zarour A, Latifi R. Understanding traumatic blunt cardiac injury. Ann Card Anaesth. 2012;15(4):287–95. https://doi.org/10.4103/0971-9784.101875.

37. Huang JF, Hsieh FJ, Fu CY, Liao CH. Nonoperative management is feasible for selected blunt trauma patients with pericardial effusion. Injury. 2018;49(1):20–6.

38. Witt CE, Linnau KF, Maier RV, Rivara FP, Vavilala MS, Bulger EM, Arbabi S. Management of pericardial fluid in blunt trauma: Variability in practice and predictors of operative outcome in patients with computed tomography evidence of pericardial fluid. J Trauma Acute Care Surg. 2017;82(4):733–41. https://doi.org/10.1097/TA.0000000000001386.

39. https://arizonatrauma.org/penetrating-cardiac-injury/

40. Seamon MJ, Haut ER, Van Arendonk K, Barbosa RR, Chiu WC, Dente CJ, Fox N, Jawa RS, Khwaja K, Lee JK, Magnotti LJ, Mayglothling JA, McDonald AA, Rowell S, To KB, Falck-Ytter Y, Rhee P. An evidence-based approach to patient selection for emergency department thoracotomy: # practice management guideline from the Eastern Association for the Surgery of Trauma. J Trauma Acute Care Surg. 2015;79(1):159–73. https://doi.org/10.1097/TA.0000000000000648.

41. Navsaria PH, Nicol AJ. Haemopericardium in stable patients after penetrating injury: is subxiphoid pericardial window and drainage enough? A prospective study. Injury. 2005;36:745–50.

42. Thorson CM, Namias N, Van Haren RM, et al. Does hemopericardium after chest trauma mandate sternotomy? J Trauma Acute Care Surg. 2012;73(1):291; author reply 291-2. https://doi.org/10.1097/TA.0b013e3182580c28.

43. Huang YK, Lu MS, Liu KS, et al. Traumatic pericardial effusion: impact of diagnostic and surgical approaches. Resuscitation. 2010;81:1682–6.

44. Chestovich PJ, McNicoll CF, Fraser DR, Patel PP, Kuhls DA, Clark E, Fildes JJ. Selective use of pericardial window and drainage as sole treatment for hemopericardium from penetrating chest trauma. Trauma Surg Acute Care Open. 2018;3(1):e000187. https://doi.org/10.1136/tsaco-2018-000187. eCollection 2018.

45. Nicol AJ, Navsaria PH, Hommes M, Ball CG, Edu S, Kahn D. Sternotomy or drainage for a hemopericardium after penetrating trauma: a randomized controlled trial. Ann Surg. 2014 Mar;259(3):438–42. https://doi.org/10.1097/SLA.0b013e31829069a1.

46. Thorson CM, Namias N, Van Haren RM, Guarch GA, Ginzburg E, Salerno TA, Schulman CI, Livingstone AS, Proctor KG. Does hemopericardium after chest trauma mandate sternotomy? J Trauma Acute Care Surg. 2012;72(6):1518–24; discussion 1524-5. https://doi.org/10.1097/TA.0b013e318254306e.

47. https://arizonatrauma.org/category/cardiac/

48. Dayananda K, Kong VY, Bruce JL, Oosthuizen GV, Laing GL, Brysiewicz P, Clarke DL. A selective non-operative approach to thoracic stab wounds is safe and cost effective—a South African experience. Ann R Coll Surg Engl. 2018;100(8):1–9. https://doi.org/10.1308/rcsann.2018.0118. Epub ahead of print.

49. Van Waes OJF, Halm JA, Van Imhoff DI, Navsaria PH, Nicol AJ, Verhofstad MHJ, Vermeulen J. Selective nonoperative management of penetrating thoracic injury. Eur J Emerg Med. 2018;25(1):32–8. https://doi.org/10.1097/MEJ.0000000000000401.

50. Stranch EW, Zarzaur BL, Savage SA. Thinking outside the box: re-evaluating the approach to penetrating cardiac injuries. Eur J Trauma Emerg

Surg. 2017;43:617–22. https://doi.org/10.1007/s00068-016-0680-7.

51. Lindstaedt M, Germing A, Lawo T, von Dryander S, Jaeger D, Muhr G, Barmeyer J. Acute and long-term clinical significance of myocardial contusion following blunt thoracic trauma: results of a prospective study. J Trauma. 2002;52(3):479.

Further Reading

Bellister SA, Dennis BM, Guillamondegui OD. Blunt and penetrating cardiac trauma. Surg Clin N Am. 2017;97:1065–76. https://doi.org/10.1016/j.suc.2017.06.012.

Management of Cardiothoracic Surgery Complications

52

Bernd Niemann, Ursula Vigelius-Rauch, and Andreas Hecker

Learning Goals

After reading this chapter you should

- be sensitized concerning perioperative thoracic and cardiovascular complications.
- be able to indicate the right diagnostic and therapeutic measures to treat these critically-ill patients.

52.1 Perioperative Complications in Thoracic Surgery

52.1.1 Introduction

Severe perioperative complications after thoracic surgery are quite rare, but can summit in life-threatening situations with dramatically increased morbidity and mortality. Generally early complications range from dramatic bleeding to bronchopleural fistula (BPF), but more often include intrapulmonary complications like pneumonia or pulmonary edema. Late postoperative complications—in most cases—not only require a medical treatment only but can also lead to surgical revision of the situs.

52.1.2 Diagnosis and Treatment

1. Postoperative bleeding

    With 52%, postoperative bleeding is one of the most common postoperative indications for reexploration. Other reasons are bronchopleural fistula (17%) and prolonged air leak (10%). In case of a postoperative hemothorax, the drained pleural effusion diagnosed by either chest X-ray or ultrasound is characterized per definition by the hemoglobin (>5 g/dL) and the hematocrit, which should be more than half of the serum hematocrit. Independent from the cardiovas-

B. Niemann
Department of Cardiovascular Surgery, University Hospital of Giessen, Giessen, Germany
e-mail: Bernd.Niemann@chiru.med.uni-giessen.de

U. Vigelius-Rauch
Department of Anesthesiology and Surgical Intensive Care Medicine, University Hospital of Giessen, Giessen, Germany
e-mail: Ursula.Vigelius-Rauch@chiru.med.uni-giessen.de

A. Hecker (✉)
Department of General & Thoracic Surgery, University Hospital of Giessen, Giessen, Germany
e-mail: andreas.hecker@chiru.med.uni-giessen.de

© The Author(s), under exclusive license to Springer Nature Switzerland AG 2023
F. Coccolini, F. Catena (eds.), *Textbook of Emergency General Surgery*,
https://doi.org/10.1007/978-3-031-22599-4_52

cular (in-)stability any reexploration is indicated, if blood loss is >200 mL/h or 900 mL within 6 h. In most cases, bleeding sources are branches of the bronchial arteries (21%), intercostal arteries (16%), and hilar vessels (16%), while in more than one third an active bleeding cannot be detected. In cases of an initial nonoperative treatment, the hemothorax should be evacuated by video-assisted thoracoscopy surgery (VATS) in the later postoperative phase, to avoid pleural empyema.

2. Despite preoperative patient assessment improved significantly in the last decades, the incidence of myocardial infarction and/or cardiac ischemia ranges between 1 and 4% in the early postoperative phase [1]. An openable pericardial tamponade or herniation is rare, but complications possible after thoracic surgery. Arrhythmias are the most common cardiac complications. In contrast to open surgery (up to 30%), the incidence of atrial tachyarrhythmias decreased by implementation of the VATS approach (up to 12%) [1].

3. Bronchopleural fistula (BPF) is defined as a communication between the bronchial system and the pleural cavity. It is one of the most dangerous complications after anatomic lung resection and bronchoplastic reconstruction and shows highest incidence for pneumonectomy (up to 10%!) [1]. While early (<7 days) BPF in most cases is based on mechanical/technical insufficiency of stapled or hand-made sutures, the late (>30 days) BPF is caused by an impaired healing of the tissue (e.g., diabetes mellitus, and corticosteroid therapy). Table 52.1 provides the most accepted risk factors from the recent literature reviews [2].

The spectrum of BPF symptoms ranges from asymptomatic via persistent fistula via the chest tube up to pleural empyema development with fever, cough, and clinical impairment. Pleural empyema shows an air-fluid level in the conventional chest X-ray combined with chest pain. Subcutaneous emphysema and purulent sputum are alarm symptoms of patients after pneumonectomy (Fig. 52.1).

Table 52.1 Risk factors for postoperative BPF due to bronchial stump insufficiency/anastomotic leakage after bronchoplasty [2]

Risk factors of bronchopleural fistula (insufficiency of the bronchial stump or of a bronchial anastomosis)
– Chronic obstructive pulmonary disease (COPD)
– Persistent tobacco abuses
– Diabetes
– Long-term steroid application
– Preoperative radiotherapy
– Right-sided pneumonectomy
– Long bronchial stump
– Postoperative mechanical ventilation
– Postoperative chemotherapy
– R2-situation at the bronchial stump
– No plastic covering on the bronchial stump

Chest-computed tomographic (CT) is the diagnostic gold standard. Once suspected, BPF is confirmed by bronchoscopy. Therapy of small BPF can be interventional bronchoscopy, while larger fistula requires surgical reintervention (reclosure of the bronchial stump combined with coverage by an intercostal, omental or dorsal latissimus flap). Alternatively, a transmediastinal/sternal closure could be performed. The more complicated BPF after pneumonectomy could summit in an open window thoracostomy, which allows repetitive cleansing of the infected pleural cavity. After initial pleural drainage, an open (re-)thoracostomy is performed. Debridement and closure of the fistula are the initial surgical steps followed by a plastic flap construction to cover the bronchial stump. Once healed, the open window could be closed directly (after filling the pleural cavity with antimicrobial solution) or requires a plastic filling of the pleural cavity with vital tissue. In contrast to the open window thoracostomy (Clagett's procedure), modern surgical approaches include serial packing of the pleural cavity with antibiotic-soaked gauze. Vacuum-assisted closure (VAC)-techniques could also be implemented to allow both lavage, drainage, and repetitive surgical rethoracostomies [3]. In case of a massive infection of the pleural cavity, a transsternal

Clinical Signs and Symptoms of bronchial insufficiency/leakage of bronchial anastomosis

- Emphysema of the mediastinum and/or the skin
- Air leakage via chest tube
- Productive cough (pus, large amounts of fluid)
- Sudden dyspnea, chest pain
- Pneumonia of the other/non-operated side
- Collaps of the remaining lobes of the operated side
- Fever, loss of weight

Diagnostic pathway

1.) Chest x ray (Infiltration, pleural empyema, emphysema
2.) Bronchoscopy (Insufficiency of the bronchial anastomosis/the bronchial stump, aspiration of specimen for microbiological analysis)
3.) Chest CT (Localization of the empyema, pneumonia? Drainage possible?)

Therapy of an insufficiency of the bronchial stump

1.) Upper body elevation/lateral position on the affected side
2.) Drainage of pleural cavity
3.) Antimicrobial therapy, Analgesia
4.) Parenteral nutrition
5.) Discuss: Stentimplantation in cases of anastomotic leakage (after bronchoplasty) Primary/secondary closure of the bronchial stump (e.g. after lobectomy/pneumonectomy)
6.) Clagett procedure/Vacuum-assisted closure/transmediastinal resection/closure of the stump

Fig. 52.1 Algorithm for the management of bronchopleural fistula in cases of insufficiency of the bronchial stump or anastomotic leakage due to bronchoplastic suture insufficiency

mediastinal access to the central bronchi might be helpful, because this compartment should be free of infection.

If a persistent postoperative air leak (defined as a leak for more than 5 days after surgery) exists in a residual pleural cavity (typically after bilobectomy or upper lobar resection), drainage of the pleural space is indicated. Typically, a residual pleural space after resection slowly fills with the maintained lung parenchyma. In rare cases, a more complicated persistent postoperative air leak requires more invasive therapeutic approaches. Individual therapeutic options include pleurodesis and endobronchial valve implantation. A score recently implemented by the European Society of Thoracic Surgery (ESTS), which predicts the risk for air leak development after lobectomy. It includes male sex, forced expiratory volume in 1 s <80% and body mass index (BMI) <18.5 kg/m^2 as the main predictors allowing a stratification of the patients [4].

4. **Pleural empyema**

    While thoracic surgeons are confronted with parapneumonic pleural empyema in the majority of cases, pleural empyema can also occur in a preexisting postoperative cavity in up to 5% of cases. While in the exudative phase, the pleural effusion could be drained, which typically results in a re-expansion of the lung, the fibrinopurulent phase is characterized by formation of membranes and loculations, which require surgical intervention or fibrinolysis via chest tube drainage. The third phase results in an entrapped lung caused by fibrosis and scaring of the pleural space [3].

5. **Chylothorax**

    The accumulation of chylus in the pleural space caused by lymphatic leakage due to an injury of a thoracic duct occurs in 0.5 to 1% of cases. The volume drained by the chest tube can reach up to 5 L [5]. Laboratory examination of the pleural secretion reveals increased amounts of triglycerides (>110 mg/dL) and the presence of chylomicrons. First the nonoperative therapy consists of total parenteral nutrition or enteral nutrition with mid-chain triglycerides (MCT). This therapy is often combined with somatostatin application, which is recommended as an inhibitor of gastrointestinal secretions. If conservative treatment fails, surgical revision with ligation of the thoracic duct often combined with an intraoperative pleurodesis is the method of choice.

6. **Pulmonary edema and postoperative respiratory insufficiency**

    In the early postoperative phase, the patients are threatened by respiratory insufficiency often caused by changes in hemodynamic, endocrine, and immune functions due to systemic inflammatory response syndrome. Extravascular lung water (EVLW) is one maker for pulmonary edema and could be increased by alveolar capillary leakage, rapid volume resuscitation, manipulation of the lung parenchyma, and open thoracotomy. Implantation of a PiCCO (PULSION, Munich, Germany) catheter or noninvasive monitoring with ultrasound of the lungs allow monitoring of the EVLW or fluid accumulation and thus could detect success or failure of intensive care medicine in these cases [1]. Besides pulmonary edema, respiratory insufficiency could also be caused by pneumonia and atelectasis in the postoperative phase. Furthermore, failure of the patient to clear secretions form bronchi and trachea results in sputum retention, atelectasis and concomitant pneumonia. Noninvasive ventilation (NIV) has been shown to reduce respiratory failure rates in the postoperative phase after thoracic surgery significantly.

    Besides intubation the rapid detection and management of postoperative respiratory failure is life-saving. According to the revised "Berlin"-classification ARDS is classified as mild moderate and severe. Noninvasive ventilation, inhalation, bronchodilators, restrictive volume resuscitation combined with diuretics and mobilization are initial therapeutic options for these critically-ill patients. Repetitive bronchoscopies could be necessary. NIV has been proven to avoid intubations and reduce mortality after surgical intervention. If necessary mechanical ventilation should be performed according to the protective ventilation standard protocol ("lung-protective ventilation"): pressure-controlled ventilation with low tidal volume

(< 6 mL/kg/body weight), reduced peak pressure (< 30 mmHg) and elevated positive end expiratory pressure [PEEP]). While mortality could reach 100% after major thoracic surgery implantation of a veno-venous extracorporeal membrane oxygenation (VV-ECMO) system could save time and life in critical situations. Indications for urgent ECMO implantation in cases of postoperative respiratory insufficiency are hypoxemia (paO2 < 50 mm Hg, FiO2 1.0) and decompensated acidosis (pH < 7.15) [6].

7. **Lesion of the phrenic nerve**

    Both cervical or intrathoracic lesions of the phrenic nerve are possible and cause an ipsilateral elevation of the hemi-diaphragm. While a disturbance in respiratory physiology could be one further element leading to respiratory failure in the postoperative phase the reduced size of pleural cavity could result in atelectasis and pneumonia. Typical surgical interventions leading to phrenic nerve injury are thymectomy, dissection of the mediastinal lymph nodes or pneumonectomy [1].

8. **Lesion of the inferior laryngeal/recurrent nerve**

    Although every thoracic surgeon is aware of the anatomic location of the laryngeal recurrent nerves and their course around the subclavian artery (right side) or aortic arch (left side) injuries of the nerves are frequent especially in cases of expansive tumor disease and preoperative radiation or radiochemotherapy. Palsy of the recurrent laryngeal nerve occurs in 18.5 to 31% after left-sided oncologic resections, while about 50% of cases are caused by an intended resection of the nerve due to tumor infiltration, and 50% are unexpected injuries [7].

    Single-sided injury of the nerve goes in line with an increased risk for aspiration, pneumonia and vomiting (Table 52.2).

    Severe injury of both sides could require tracheostomy, laryngoplastic approaches (medialization laryngoplasty, intracorporal(?)injection, Type-I-thyroplasty with Montgomery-/Gore-Tex implantation) [2].

Table 52.2 Signs and symptoms of a palsy of the recurrent laryngeal nerve [2]

Dyspnea	98%
Shortness of breath	
Aspiration	35–63%
Hoarseness	100%
Dysphagia	6.5%
Weakness of coughing	25%

9. **Lobar torsion (with gangrene)**

    Lobar torsion is a rare, but very severe complication typically after (bi-)lobectomy. In the most common and typical scenario the middle lobe is rotated after upper lobectomy and thus bronchial and vascular connection interrupted. The infarction of the lung parenchyma can summit in septic shock with highest mortality rates. X-ray typically reveals a large opacity at the operated side of the chest. Once suspected the CT is the gold standard diagnostics to confirm the torsion of the lobe with occlusion of both bronchus and pulmonary artery. Immediate surgical reintervention with detorsion of the lobe is indicated. Depending on the macroscopic aspect of the lung parenchyma the lobectomy/pneumonectomy could be demanded.

10. **Postpneumonectomy syndrome**

    After pneumonectomy a shift of the mediastinum into the cavity, where resection was performed, typically goes in line with an obstruction of the airways. While postpneumonectomy syndrome typically occurs after right-sided resection a more dangerous shift to the right side after left-sided pneumonectomy could lead to a mediastinal rotation with compression of the right main bronchus [1]. Treatment options would be bronchial stenting or vascular reconstruction even.

52.2 Perioperative Complications in Cardiac Surgery

52.2.1 Introduction

The spectrum of postoperative adverse events can be divided into cardiovascular and noncardiovas-

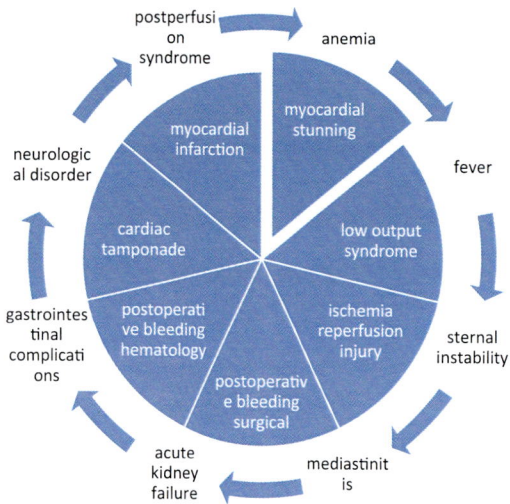

Fig. 52.2 Main postoperative complications after cardiovascular surgery (blue: cardiovascular, orange: noncardiovascular). Complications and pathophysiological alterations amplify one another

cular complications. It is important here that no sharp dividing line can be drawn, since in particular in the vulnerable direct postoperative phase, a mutual induction and perpetuation of pathophysiological factors can develop into a vicious circle that is potentially life-threatening. A close-knit therapy regimen aimed at avoiding complications is therefore preferable to complication management. However, should complications arise, immediate control is essential.

The spectrum of complications can include hemodynamic, inflammatory, metabolic and surgical causes. Figure 52.2 provides an overview of the range of complications:

52.2.2 Diagnosis and Treatment

52.2.2.1 The Main Cardiovascular Complications during the Intensive Treatment Phase

Myocardial Stunning
With prolonged extracorporeal circulation and especially prolonged myocardial ischemia/clamping time, prolonged myocardial dysfunction can occur in some patients. In addition to a reduced systolic function, there is also primarily a prolonged diastolic cardiac dysfunction. In particular, a severely hypertrophied myocardium and a reduced LVEF (<30%) are considered predisposing factors. Prolonged operative courses with long ischemia and perfusion times and myocardial protection via cardioplegia, that is difficult to establish, are intraoperative risk factors. Complete revascularization has a protective effect. Therefore, patients with poor connecting vessels or reduced coronary periphery with microangiopathy or pathologically altered coronary periphery are particularly at risk of myocardial stunning. Echocardiographic assessment of cardiac function is indicative and should be done immediately.

The therapeutic approach of positive chronotropic and inotropic therapy using β-1 receptor stimulation can be unfavorable in this case. A nonreceptor-bound increase in inotropy and a simultaneous reduction in afterload to optimize the cardiac work and load profile appear more favorable to improve diastolic and systolic function. If pulmonary hypertension is also present at the same time, the use of phosphodiesterase inhibitors or calcium sensitizers can be beneficial. Fluid and volume replacement may be necessary in this phase, but should be carried out with close monitoring of the cardiac preload and the right and left cardiac function.

Low Cardiac Output Syndrome
The low Cardiac Output Syndrome (LCOS) is a form of cardiogenic shock and as such is characterized by typical clinical signs such as a cardiac index <2L/min/m^2, a peripheral vascular resistance >1100 dyn*s*cm^{-5} and hypotension a MAP <60 mmHg, a tachycardia, a weakly palpable peripheral pulse, a pale and / or cyanotic skin, an oliguria of <0.5 mL/h lasting longer than 2 h, a metabolic acidosis, a Sc_vO_2 <60% at S_aO_2 of 98% and a lactate >2 mmol/L. The life-threatening LCOS must be recognized and treated quickly. Extended hemodynamic monitoring is expedient, if not essential, in these patients. In particular, prompt therapy should also prevent the genesis of secondary organ dam-

age. The initially symptomatic therapy must then be followed by a root cause analysis of the complex causality. Common causes are: insufficient myocardial protection during extracorporeal circulation, remaining coronary stenoses, coronary embolisms, alterations of the coronary integrity, acute myocardial infarction, incomplete revascularization, functional disorders of applied bypasses, functional disorders of heart valves, uncorrected residual valve defect, pre-existing ventricular dysfunction, pericardial tamponade, hypoxia, mechanical irritation from organs or iatrogenically introduced material. The successful therapy of LCOS is therefore directly dependent on the elimination of the underlying cause. The S3 guideline of the German Society for Thoracic, Cardiac and Vascular Surgery provides therapeutic framework conditions for this. Surgical causes of pericardial tamponade, bypass dysfunction or remaining valvular or structural vitia must be corrected surgically immediately.

In addition, the cardiac work must be made more economical through stabilization and normalization of the heart rate and/or the rhythm. The work diagram and the cardiac load parameters must be analyzed, monitored and optimized; if necessary, positive inotropic and afterload-reducing therapy may be necessary. It is important here that maximum peripheral vasoconstriction and an increase in the MAD are not expedient, but rather an optimization of the generated cardiac output. A balanced therapy with inotropes (dobutamine/PDE inhibitors/adrenaline), vasodilators (nitroprusside, nitroglycerin, alpha2 inhibitors) or vasoconstrictors (noradrenaline, vasopressin) may be necessary for this. Relative ischemia due to centralization mechanisms and excessive vasoconstriction should be avoided. In case of doubt, a balanced volume administration can lead to more favorable circulatory stabilization. If these basic measures cannot be stabilized by optimizing the cardiac afterload and distension, mechanical circulatory support systems can be used. The support of the cardiac output, the cardiac unloading and an adequate gas exchange should be ensured, which are brought about by support. Various systems are available for this, such as the IABP for increasing coronary perfusion and reducing afterload, the vv ECMO for supporting gas exchange, and the va ECMO/ECLS for supporting both—hemodynamics and pulmonary function. Newer concepts of direct ventricular unloading and hemodynamic support by microaxial pumps can be used alone or in combination with an ECMO (ECMELLA concept). However, it must be noted that mechanical circulatory support systems are not a causal therapy per se, but merely a supportive therapy as a bridge to the causal therapy or therapy decision. Figure 52.3 gives an algorithm for left heart failure.

In particular, hemodynamic conditioning of the right heart in the case of right cardiac decompensation can be challenging. Here, an optimized coronary perfusion should first be guaranteed. In addition to an increase in right ventricular inotropy, a chronotropic increase should be avoided if possible. Rather, the optimization and strict control of the right ventricular preload and the reduction of the right ventricular afterload via intravenous and inhaled vasodilators represent the basis of the demanding therapy. The exclusive assessment via the TAPSE can fail because effects on the function of the free wall and the septal retention of the right ventricle are not assessed. Extended hemodynamic monitoring with estimation of the pulmonary arterial parameters using a pulmonary artery catheter is recommended. If conservative therapy fails, supportive right ventricular microaxial pumps and right heart ECMOS can be used. Figure 52.4 gives an algorithm for right heart failure.

Postoperative Bleeding

After cardiac surgery, higher drainage quantities are possible due to the operative trauma, but also due to rheological changes due to the extracorporeal circulation, temperature fluctuations and the intensive intraoperative use of heparin and thrombocyte disorders.

Blood losses in excess of 100 mL/h require increased attention. First, physiological coagulation should be achieved; the therapeutic goal can be supported with a point-of-care diagnosis.

Frequent causes of coagulation deterioration are insufficient antagonization of heparin by

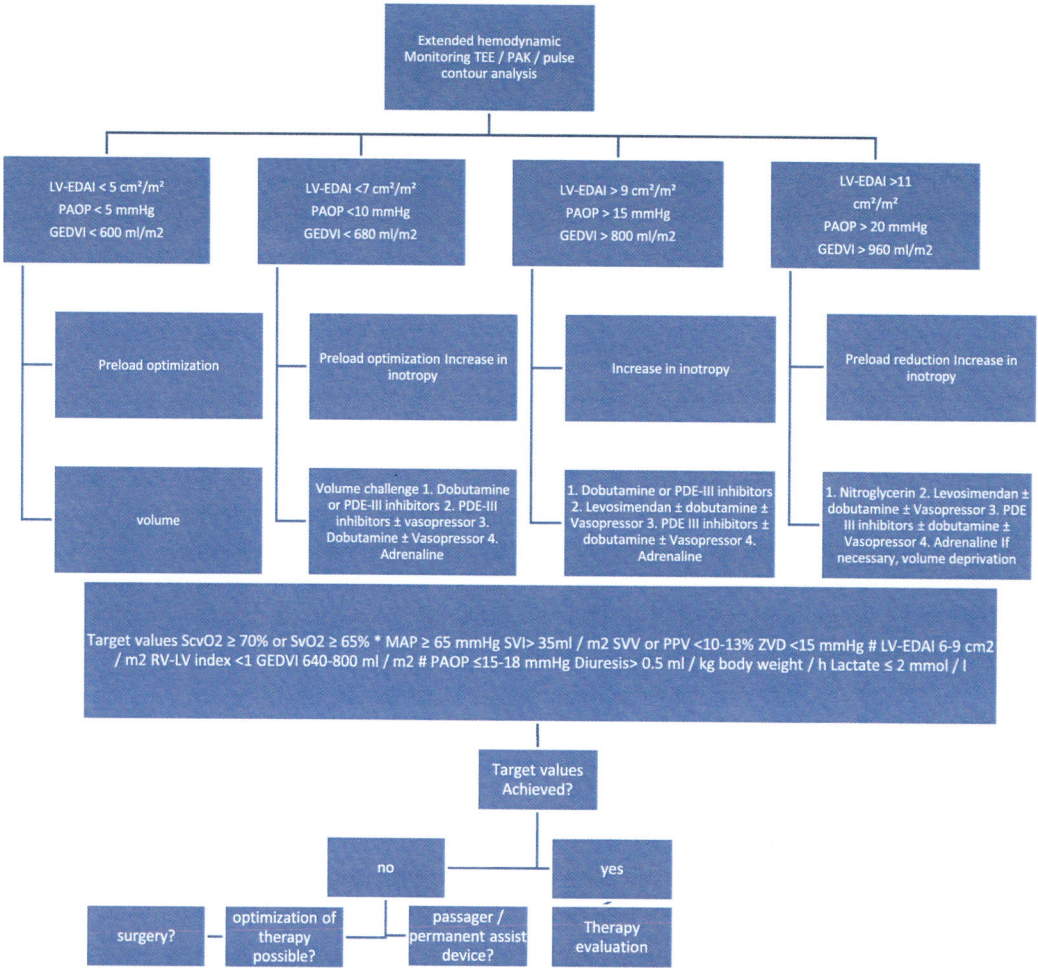

Fig. 52.3 Algorithm for the therapy of left heart failure according to Habicher, M. AWMF Register 001/016

protamine, disorders of the thrombocyte function through the extracorporeal circulation, thrombocytopenia, disseminated intravascular coagulation, increase in fibrinolysis and loss of individual coagulation factors, mostly fibrinogen. If the blood losses persist, reach a total of more than 1000 mL or exceed 3 mL/h/kg body weight, they require surgical treatment. Intramediastinal/thoracic hematomas should then be removed and surgical bleeding sources excluded or stopped. The preexisting access route should be chosen primarily, if necessary an extended access in the case of hemodynamic instability. However, while most of the bleeding is drained outward through the drainage system, some bleeding is occult if the drainage does not reach it. Regular checks of hemoglobin and hematocrit should be performed. Sudden massive blood loss, possibly accompanied by hemodynamic instability, is always an alarm sign for sudden surgical bleeding and always requires a surgical assessment and, if necessary, an immediate surgical revision. Hidden bleedings on the other hand might be difficult to recognize and might only arise attention by secondary complications such as hemothorax, cardiac tamponade or cardiac circulatory instability needing surgical revision and eventually circulatory support.

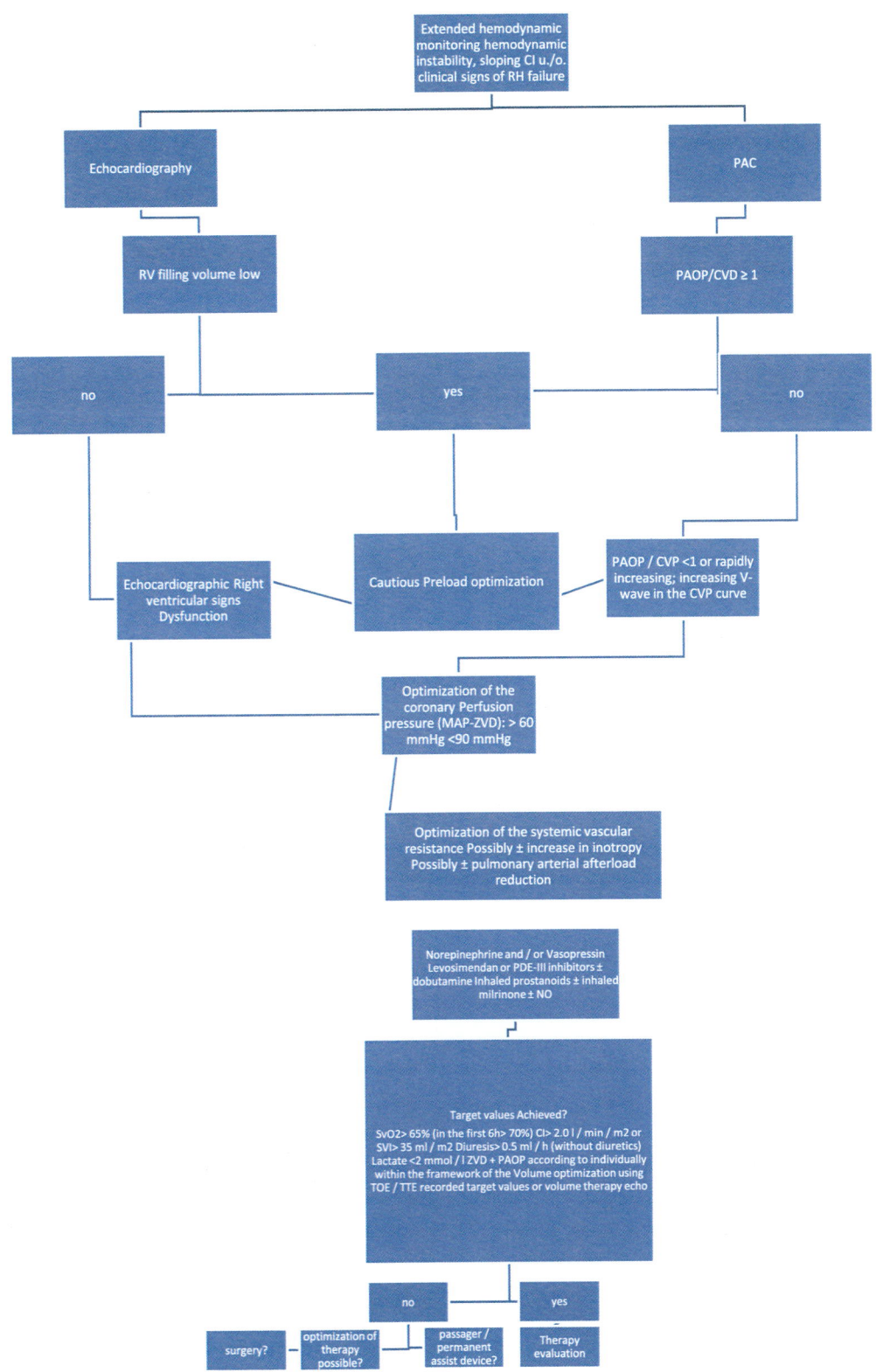

Fig. 52.4 Algorithm for the therapy of right heart failure according to Habicher, M. AWMF Register 001/016

Cardiac Tamponade

Cardiac tamponades can causally arise in the early postoperative phase from operative bleeding and diffuse bleeding in the medium-term phase from developed effusions in the sense of a postcardiotomy syndrome.

An intrapericardial effusion increased the pressure on the heart and led to a decrease in the cardiac preload, obstruction of the diastolic filling and escalation of the left ventricular end-diastolic pressure. Cardiac function is further reduced by decreasing coronary blood flow. Compensatory catecholamine release leads to heart rate increase, arterioles and veins contraction and increased peripheral vascular resistance. A central venous pressure increase is detectable. Typically, these patients do not react adequately to volume substitution and have an increased catecholamine need. The mediastinum is widened on the X-ray. Typically, there is a triad of oliguria, increase in CVP, and hemodynamic instability. TOE is indicated to find the diagnosis. The decisive factor here is first of all relieving the effusion in order to restore the hemodynamic function, but then also the causal therapy. This can be re-thoracotomy and surgical hemostasis, normalization of coagulation or, in the case of effusions that cannot be controlled otherwise, intermittent tamponade and open treatment of the thorax with secondary occlusion during the following course. In contrast, pericardial effusions due to a post cardiotomy syndrome are often slower to develop and continue to be compensated for. Nevertheless, here, too, relief may be necessary via an interventional drainage system. This should be followed by a longer anti-inflammatory therapy using nonsteroidal anti-inflammatory drugs and colchysate. Corticoids are currently only used for recurrent effusions and then over the long term.

Myocardial Infarction

Myocardial infarctions can result from embolizations, temporary occlusions from gas during open heart surgery, permanent occlusions from mechanical obstacles or dysfunctional coronary bypasses. It is not the individual measured values of myocardial necrosis parameters that are groundbreaking, but their dynamics in combination with the assessment of electrocradiographic changes, hemodynamic function, myocardial contractility and regional wall movement disorders. In addition to myocardial infarction - associated increases in necrosis parameters, these can result from cardiomyotomies, ablation therapies, myocardial sutures, and inadequate cardioplegic cardioprotection. These can be accompanied by, in some cases, deliberate increases in the necrosis parameters and make a diagnosis of a relevant myocardial infarction more difficult. Special cases are gas embolism after opening of cardiac cavities, which can lead to temporary ischemia and regress, and coronary occlusions due to sutures close to RCX in mitral valve surgery, which are then often permanent and need surgical treatment. If a relevant myocardial ischemia is suspected, a coronary angiography must provide clarity. A decision-making to be made in the cardiac team may favor surgical correction, but should also consider interventional therapy if there is a high perioperative risk for close redo surgery.

Cardiac Rhythm Disorders

Due to the spectrum of side effects of class I antiarrhythmics, therapy schemes with beta blockade, amiodarone and xylocaine are often used in cardiac surgery intensive therapy, in rare cases digitalis. A highly normal serum concentration of potassium, calcium and magnesium is often sought. Cardiac bradycardiac conduction and stimulation disorders are in many cases not perceived as problematic complications after cardiac surgery, since intraoperative epicardial pacemakers usually treat bradycardiac disorders without any problems. Severe AV blockages can occur, especially after aortic valve surgery. In the majority of cases, these regress and do not lead to permanent pacemaker implantations. After a reasonable waiting period of 5–7 days, if the symptoms persist, an implantation of a permanent pacemaker may be indicated in a maximum of 5 to 7% of patients. Malignant ventricular tachycardia arrhythmias require defibrillation therapy.

The most common postoperative irritation disorder is newly occurring postoperative atrial fibrillation in up to 40% of cases and is associated to long extracorporeal circulation, obesity, inflammation and av-valve disorders and low ejection fraction. Mostly symptoms occur during pod 2-3. Frequently, spontaneous conversions into the sinus rhythm can be seen with a balance of the electrolytes and regressive inflammatory symptoms. Drug-based rhythm-controlling therapy using amiodarone and / or beta blockade or, in the case of persistence, cardioversion is recommended, particularly if atrial fibrillation is hemodynamically relevant. With regard to further therapy, there are inconsistent schemes ranging from complete freedom from rhythmological therapy to permanent drug-based rhythm control and therapeutic anticoagulation. Ongoing studies should enable prospective data to be able to give consistent therapy recommendations.

PostPerfusion Syndrome

The postperfusion syndrome is a systemic inflammatory reaction after cardiopulmonary bypass, which is understood as SIRS (systemic inflammation reaction). It is associated with impaired kidney and lung function, hemorrhagic diathesis and increased susceptibility to infections. The patients often show edema and increased interstitial fluid as a result of capillary leakage, a partly pronounced, but initially a-bacterial leukocytosis, fever and pain symptoms. In contrast to sepsis, there is no detectable infection.

For a SIRS, the SIRS criteria should be met:

- Body temperature: <36 °C or >38 °C
- Heart rate >90/min
- Tachypnea with a respiratory rate >20/min and a $paCO_2$ ≤33 mmHg or one

Oxygenation index <200 (with mechanical ventilation)

- White blood cell counts <4000/mm^3, >12,000/mm^3 or >10% immature white blood cells

However, since the SIRS criteria have a low specificity and sensitivity, they are in many cases replaced by the SOFA Score.

In addition, some clinical parameters such as leukocytosis, leukopenia (with shift to the left), hypophosphatemia, thrombocytopenia, decrease in fibrinogen and factors II, V, X, increase in CRP and PCT, as well as an increase in interleukin-6 and -8 are groundbreaking.

The release of different cytokines and the activation of the complement system can be countered with cytokine filters within the extracorporeal circulation during the postoperative course. As a result, reductions in SIRS in the postoperative course have been described, particularly in risk collectives such as dialysis patients and endocarditis patients.

SIRS is currently understood as a multifactorial inflammatory syndrome and is therefore difficult to access by monocausal therapy. Therapy by means of radical scavengers has not shown itself to be additively profitable; anti-inflammatory therapy by means of corticoids is usually only used cautiously against the background of the side effect profile. Therapeutically, the hemodynamics, cardiac preload and central venous saturation (to 70%) should be optimized. A catecholamine-resistant vasoplegia in the context of the SIRS with a mortality of 10% in hypotension and up to 30% in vasoplegic shock is considered to be particularly relevant for prognosis. In these cases, additive vasopressors such as methylene blue and vasopressin are recommended in the literature. Ultimately, a balanced dosage must also take place here in order not to provoke reactive, drug-induced nonocclusive ischemia through vasopression within reactive vascular areas. In the case of patients who require ventilation, it is essential to ensure a lung-protective ventilation regime.

52.2.2.2 The Main Noncardiovascular Complications During the Intensive Treatment Phase

Anemia and Blood Products

Cardiac surgery operations lead to anemia due to hemodilution in the extracorporeal circulation and possibly incomplete traceability of ECC volumes, which can be exacerbated by postoperative bleeding. Diagnosis is carried out on the bedside using BGAs; centralization could simulate paleness. Clinical signs of listlessness, fatigue and dyspnea are often absent in the immediate postoperative phase due to the still existing sedation. While the therapy is a transfusion, the indication should be set very closely and follow the principles of patient blood management. Signs of underperfusion, increased volume requirements, and a persistent bleeding tendency, as well as an increased patient age can be triggers for a transfusion, but Hb limits should be set low for the indication. A preoperative treatment with erythropoietin and iron can help elective patients to reduce the perioperative transfusion requirement. Due to the difficult and urgent nature of most cardiac surgical interventions and the underlying cardiac disease itself, preoperative autologous blood donation is often not indicated.

Absolute lower Hb or Hct limit values, from which a transfusion is required, are not evident, but must individually taking the underlying disease and age into account. Hb values above 8 g/dL or Hkt values of 24 to 25% generally apply not as an indication for an erythrocyte replacement. Young patients may tolerate even lower values under certain circumstances. A substitution of platelet concentrates should only be carried out under strict indication control if clinical signs of bleeding are absent. If heparin-induced thrombocytopenia is suspected and the 4-T test is positive, an examination for antibodies should be carried out and the anticoagulant should be switched to direct thrombin inhibition. The use of plasma preparations for volume therapy is largely prohibited in the context of patient blood management and the possible complications of frequent transfusion. Optimizing coagulation therapy is also unlikely with the idea of a resulting dilutional coagulopathy in these cases.

52.2.2.3 Heparin-Induced Thrombocytopenia

Heparin-induced thrombocytopenia (HIT) is one of the most often defects of platelet function in cardiac surgery. In addition to the mechanical damage to thrombocytes by roller and centrifugal pumps and by inhibition of thrombocyte aggregation induced by ASA and other preparations, it is one of the most common complications in cardiac surgery that affect the coagulation system. Up to 10% of patients show HIT. In addition to consumption-related coagulation reduction, activation of platelet agglutination results in peripheral thrombi and vascular occlusions. It is an immunization after previous heparin therapy and the activation of the immune system when heparin is administered again. This reaction typically occurs after 5 to 14 days, but can occur immediately if the patient has been treated with heparin within the last 4 weeks. Platelet factor 4 (PF-4)—heparin complexes are recognized by antibodies. Thrombocytic activation and disseminated coagulopathy occur. The diagnosis is made after a suspicion is established by detecting the circulating antibodies. A 4-T test (Fig. 52.5) is helpful in establishing diagnoses.

If HIT II is suspected, heparin therapy must be stopped immediately. Warnings should be noted in the patient file. A therapy to inhibit coagulation by means of direct thrombin antagonization must be initiated. It should be noted that the dosage should be tailored to the patient's clinic and point-of-care diagnostics on the patient's bedside can avoid overdosing and excessive coagulation inhibition. An initial bolus administration of thrombin inhibitors has proven to be a complicating factor in many cases. If there are no bleeding symptoms, substitution of platelets should be avoided in order to avoid a further increase in thrombosis. In the case of critically low platelet concentrations, however, substitution must be considered. If a patient has HIT II before therapy with a heart-lung machine, heparinization can be carried out with thromboxane protection of the platelets, prednisolone administration, and histamine-receptor blockade. The further therapeutic course should be conducted after heparin antagonization with direct thrombin inhibition. Therapy on cardiac support systems (ECMO/ECLS/Impella) can be carried out using argatroban. Therapy can be controlled using ACT or PTT according to the usual clinic scheme.

points	2	1	0
Platelet count	> 50% drop or lowest at 20-100 / nl	30-50% drop or lowest at 10-19 / nl	<30% drop or low point <10 / nl
Platelet decline time course	Days 5-10 after administration of heparin, in case of re-exposure within 30 days <= 1 day	> 10 days, unclear course, or <1 day in the case of re-exposure after 31-100 days	<4 days without prior exposure to heparin
Manifestation of thrombosis	Proven, fresh thromboses, including skin necrosis	Suspected thrombosis, including reddening of the skin	none
Other causes of thrombocytopenia	none	possible	secure

Fig. 52.5 HIT—probability calculation via 4-T-Test. The highest possible score is 8. 8–6 points means a high probability of a HIT II, 5–4 points: medium probability, 3–0 points: low probability

Fever

On the one hand, postoperative fever can be an indication of infections and septic processes, it can be triggered by medication, it can also be a symptom of malignant hypertension, in the further course it can also be the result of strokes or be part of a B-symptomatology of previously undetected malignancies.

Any fever needs evaluation and treatment. Since infections are the most common cause, a comprehensive focus search should be carried out. This includes the clinical examination, blood cultures, exchange and microbiological examinations of all access lines, inspections and swabs of wounds, urine cultures, obtaining bronchial examination material. X-ray diagnostics and CT imaging, if necessary, and a positron emission tomography-computed tomography can support the focus search.

The most common causes include atelectasis, pneumonia, bacterial, viral and mycotic soft tissue infections, pneumonia, resorption of extensive hematoma, mediastinitis, urinary tract infection, resorption of the protein-containing coating of vascular prostheses during aortic replacement. Therapy depends on the cause. Antibiotic/antimycotic therapy, initially empirical and then specific according to the resistogram, should be carried out in the event of infections. The fever-lowering effect of steroid medication can be used, but should be weighed against the frequent cardiac risk profile. The use of hearter—cooler units might be considered.

Sternal Instability and Mediastinitis

Mediastinitis is a particularly dangerous form of deep wound infection. The incidence can be up to 5%; the mortality of up to 20% is to be assessed as critically high. Clinically, stern instability and seropurulent secretions are common. Some patients report painful cracking, and crepitation can be clinically diagnosed. It is often not possible to clearly define whether the infection is preceded by mechanical instability or, conversely, by the infection. Mechanical restlessness, possibly entertained by delirium, asymmetrical stress, COPD, poorly controlled diabetes mellitus, and diseases of the bone structure such as osteoporosis are considered to be special risk factors. The bilateral use of the mammary artery is particularly beneficial in coronary bypass surgery. Therefore, in diabetics, the skeletonized preparation of the thoracic arteriae is recommended to reduce the risk of wound healing disorders. Prophylactic measures include preoperative shaving without blades with electric razors, antiseptic washing / showering, disinfection of the skin with preoperative hair removal, chlorhexidine, alcohol-containing solutions, or iodine-containing polyvidone. The use of surgical foils can minimize contact with the skin, but an increase in the bacterial dermal exposure due to sweating should be taken into account during longer surgery. Perioperative antibiotic prophylaxis should be used. The diagnosis of mediastinitis is defined by main and secondary criteria, whereby both main and at least one secondary criterion must be met:

Main Criteria

- Infection within 30 days after surgery without an implant or within 1 year with an implant.
  - Infection of the deep tissue layers of the incision (fascia and muscles)

Secondary Criteria

- Spontaneous dehiscence (or opening of the wound by the surgeon) with at least one of the following signs: fever >38 °C, local pain or tension, abscess, or other evidence of infection found directly during surgery or by radiological examination.

The diagnosis must be treated radically. The introduced osteosynthetic material must be removed in toto. Tissue samples and smears should be taken for microbiological examination and histological assessment of possible osteomyelitis and bacterial colonization. Systemic treatment of bacterial infection should be based on a resistogram with a high tissue penetrance antibiotic. After disinfecting rinsing, the wound should be conditioned using vacuum bandage therapy. Surgical, reconstructive wound closure can be performed when the germ load is remedied and the healing tendency is optimized by granulating tissue. In the case of extensive defects, the mediastinal defect can be filled by pulling up the omentum. If wound closure is not possible as originally or if the sternum is not adapted, the defect can be covered with a muscle displacement plastic or a muscle flap plastic.

Acute Kidney Failure

After cardiac surgery, acute kidney failure often occurs as a result of previous damage, as acute to chronic kidney failure, after exposure to contrast media or as a result of cardiac dysfunction in the context of a low cardiac output syndrome. The therapeutic regimes depend on the pre-, intra-, or postrenal cause of the dysfunction. Favoring factors are the patient's high age, long extracorporeal circulation, high serum Hb concentrations, musculoskeletal necrosis, and high myoglobin concentrations (crush kidney), previous damage to the kidney, and drug therapies, for example, with aminoglycoside antibiotics. A division according to the time course differentiates early postoperative kidney failure (12–18 h postoperatively) from delayed kidney failure (72–96 h postoperatively). The early forms of kidney failure are often characterized by higher resistance to therapy, oliguria, immediate electrolyte imbalance, and uremia. Dialysis therapy is often necessary. Delayed forms, on the other hand, are characterized by a slow increase in retention parameters and are less associated with oliguria. As the prognosis is favorable, dialysis therapy is less often necessary. The basic principles of therapy are, first of all, adequate hemodynamics to increase the kidney's preload and reduce the afterload. A calculated diuretic therapy and a balanced volume supply should be carried out.

Gastrointestinal Complications

Gastrointestinal complications, which seem far removed from cardiac surgery beginners and inexperienced in particular, are in fact rare at 1 to 2% of cases, but are considered a serious and feared postoperative problem by experienced surgeons and intensive care professionals due to the high rate of complications, difficult diagnosis and high mortality in these patients. The most important complications are mesenteric ischemia, ileus, mesenteric infarction, gastrointestinal bleeding, hepatic dysfunction, ischemic cholecystitis ("intensive gallbladder"), and, less often, pancreatitis. In sedated and critically ill patients in particular, the symptoms can often be occult in the absence of pain and be overseen as they are reduced to unspecific increases in inflammation parameters, transaminases, cholestasis parameters, lipase, and amylase and lactate. The clinical examination with regard to bowel noises, gastrointestinal transport function, and peritonism is therefore particularly important. Sonographic findings can provide support, while endoscopic findings can unmask possible ischemia and sources of bleeding.

Nonocclusive Mesenteric Ischemia and Ischemic Cholecystitis (NOMI)

This organic ischemia caused by vascular spasms is observed in 1 to 2% of the cases of cardiac surgery patients. The occurrence of a NOMI is favored by the extracorporeal circulation, dialysis therapy, digitalist therapy, heart failure, and cardiac arrhythmias as well as low-cardiac output syndrome and peripheral arterial obstructive disease (PAOD). In particular, intensive, high-dose use of vasopressors appears to be pathogenetically significant. The groundbreaking diagnosis must be carried out immediately by means of CT angiography or angiography if there is any suspicion, which may be due to an otherwise inexplicable increase in lactate. Organ- and life-sustaining therapy is only possible in the early stages of the symptoms without resection of the necrotic intestine, which is usually unavoidable in the case of peritonism. Only an early diagnosis of a vascular spasm can enable organ-preserving local spasmolytic therapy using prostaglandins via a regional spasmolysis catheter inserted in the superior mesenteric artery. An adapted dosage enables regional spasmolysis and prevents a systemic effect through the hepatic first pass mechanism. Delayed diagnosis is associated with a mortality of up to 85%.

Ischemic cholecystitis is a special form of nonocclusive organic ischemia. Patients exhibit septic clinical symptoms with an otherwise not detectable infection. Due to its reduced prognosis and a possible septic shock originating from this focus, early diagnosis and therapy is live saving. The diagnosis is usually made by ultrasound. A cholecystectomy is performed therapeutically. Pre-existing cholecystolithiasis and anamnestic cholecystitis have a predisposing effect.

Abdominal Bleeding

Abdominal bleeding can be found as stress ulceration, as catheter-associated complications, as a result of vascular malformations, for example, during VAD implantation, as a result of an acquired von Willebrand syndrome or manipulation-related (transesophageal echocardiography, gastric tubes, intestinal tubes or probes). The suspicion is usually nourished by gastric efflux similar to coffee grounds—refluxes, tarry stools or blood admixture in the stool, as well as a constant drop in Hb. In addition to the administration of blood reserves adapted to the target of the transfusion, diagnostic confirmation by means of endoscopy and, if necessary, causal therapy through local hemostasis should be carried out. Surgical therapies are rather rare and are only indicated if endoscopic therapy is unsuccessful.

Hyperbilirubinemia and Hepatic Injury

In most cases, liver damage is the result of venous congestion caused by right heart failure and, with rapid hemodynamic correction, shows a prolonged course, but then also an optimistic prognosis. If the pathogenicity persists and, in addition to hepatocellular damage, there is a relevant restriction in protein synthesis, the provision of coagulation factors and a restriction in gluconeogenesis, the long-term prognosis is extremely limited. In addition to primarily hepatic damage, icterus and bilirubinemia after a transfusion must also be ruled out as a result of hemolysis and a transfusion reaction.

Neurological Disorders

Serious neurological damage caused by operations with heart-lung machines have become significantly less common. Predisposing factors are an extensive surgical procedure on the aorta, a high arteriosclerotic load and plaque formation in the aorta and the supra-aortic vessels, retrograde perfusions, watershed phenomena, pre-existing apoplexes, intraoperative cardiac arrest, endocarditis and intracardiac thrombus surgery, in particular interventional valve implantations bear a higher risk. After coronary bypass surgery, severe neurological disorders occur in about 1% of all patients. Affected patients show nonawakening after surgery, with neurological awakening failures, developing neurological failures after awakening or as severe confusion. In particular, a lack of alertness is associated with a significantly reduced prognosis, whereas focal neurological deficits and states of confusion are often only temporary phenomena with a good prognosis.

The cause can be embolisms with air, thrombi, tissue sequesters and foreign material on the one hand, but also bleeding due to pathological and/or therapeutic changes in coagulation and bleeding in pre-existing apoplexes or through rupture of aneurysms in hypertonic phases on the other. Hypotonic phases can cause temporary or manifest functional impairments in stenoses of the carotid arteries. In the case of previously known stenoses, a primary surgical correction or a concomitant correction can be carried out as a preventive measure. The diagnosis of symptoms is carried out by means of computed tomographic, contrast agent-assisted diagnosis. If the latency period is sufficiently short for diagnosis, embolectomy can have a beneficial therapeutic effect on embolectomy. In the case of bleeding with a prognostic severity, the therapeutic procedure must be coordinated with neurosurgical colleagues with regard to relieving surgical interventions to prevent entrapment or to limit therapy if the prognosis is missing. Neurorehabilitative measures can significantly alleviate symptoms and stabilize quality of life, depending on the findings.

Postoperative Delirium (POD)

A delirium is an organically caused decline from a previously attained baseline level of cognitive function. A fluctuating course, attentional deficits and generalized severe disorganization of behavior are found in different estimation among the patients. Mostly cognitive deficits, changes in arousal, perceptual deficits, altered sleep-wake cycle, psychotic features (hallucinations/delusions) are hindrances during the postoperative course and rehabilitation. Up to 80% of long-term ventilated patients and 50% of nonventilated patients show signs of delirium in varying degrees. In 20 to 30% of cases, delirium is an expression of the onset of sepsis. Delirium is by no means an unproblematic transient symptom but a dangerous diagnosis with a tripling of mortality within 6 months and a further 10% increase per day in delirium. It is problematic that identifying measuring instruments are either not used or only used inadequately or with insufficient training, so that identification of the symptoms is usually inadequate and up to 40% of cases are overlooked. A distinction is made between hypoactive (45% of cases), hyperactive delirium (5%) and the mixed forms (55%). Complicated courses are seen particularly often in hypoactive delirium. Typical rhythms of an intensive care unit with loud communications, examinations during the rest and sleep phases, alarm circuits during sleep, pain, fear, experiencing illness and a lack of day-night rhythm as well as a lack of daylight promote the initiation of delirium, so that adjustments to the treatment and Code of conduct of the staff and an equipment with natural light sources can be cheap. The day-night rhythm can be maintained using melatonin. Patients with higher age dementia, somatic comorbidity, hearing and visual disability, anemia, malnutrition, low albumin [serum], anxiety, depression, alcohol abuse, benzodiazepines, pain, mild cognitive disturbance, loneliness, minor intelligence are considered to be particularly at risk. The higher the predisposition, the lower the triggering noxa can be. It is possible to dispense with polymedication, in particular with drugs from Table 52.3. In particular, pronounced and long-lasting sedations and the use of benzodiazepines and barbiturates are obsolete these days. Adequate analgesia must be guaranteed and good preoperative and perioperative hydration and water supply seems to be the best and most potent preventive but also therapeutic.

Table 52.3 Polymedication in particular with drugs shown below promotes the development of postoperative delirium

Painbusters
- Opioids
- Nonsteroidal anti-inflammatory drugs

Sedatives/neuro-actives
- Benzodiazepines
- Anticholinergic substances: tri- and tetracyclic antidepressants, neuroleptics
- Anticonvulsives, Parkinson medication
- Antidepressants: selective serotonin-reuptake-inhibitors

Cardiacs
- Antiarrhythmics, betablocker, calcium antagonist
- Cardiac glycosides diuretics

Antibiotics
- Fluoroquinolones, macrolides, cephalosporines
- Theophylline
- Antihistamines, urological, antiemetics
- Corticosteroids

Take-Home Messages

- Both cardiac and thoracic surgical interventions bear the risk of a broad spectrum of postoperative complications.
- Cardiovascular and Thoracic surgeons are confronted with a different spectrum of disorders in the postoperative phase.
- Rapid detection of the potential complications is life-saving and essential to become an experienced surgeon.

Multiple-Choice Questions

1. Typical signs of bronchopleural fistula (BPF) are NOT
   A. Emphysema of the mediastinum and/or the skin.
   B. Productive cough
   C. Sudden dyspnea
   D. **Hematothorax.**
2. Risk factors of bronchopleural fistula are NOT
   A. COPD
   B. Diabetes
   C. Right-sided pneumonectomy
   D. **R0-situation at the bronchial stump**
3. Diagnostics of choice for bronchopleural fistula is
   A. Ventilation/perfusion scinthigraphy
   B. Chest-MRI
   C. **Chest CT**
   D. Bronchography
4. Typical complications after thoracic surgery are NOT
   A. Pleural empyema
   B. Chylothorax
   C. Lesions of the phrenic nerve
   D. **Lesion of the accsessoric nerve.**
5. Lesions of the inferior laryngeal/recurrent nerve
   A. Occur in 1% after oncologic pulmonary resections.
   B. Have dysphagia as the most common, typical symptom
   C. Are typically caused by lobar torsion
   D. **Require tracheostomy and laryngoplastic approaches in cases of injury of both sides.**
6. Myocardial stunning
   A. Is one typical complication after lobectomy
   B. **Occurs after prolonged extracorporeal circulation.**
   C. Should be treated with negative inotropic pharmaceuticals
   D. Require immediate surgical re-intervention.
7. Low cardiac Output Syndrome
   A. Is a form of septic shock.
   B. Typically goes in line with an increased cardiac index.
   C. **Has an MAP < 60 mmHg as one typical sign.**
   D. Requires immediate surgical re-interention.

8. Cardiac tymponade
   A. **Is typically caused by a postoperative bleeding in the early postoperative phase.**
   B. Requires CT-scan as the diagnostic gold standard.
   C. Should lead to immediate surgical re-opening of the chest.
   D. Leads to increased filling in the diastolic phase.
9. Nonocclusive mesenteric ischemia
   A. Has a gool prognosis
   B. Typically occurs after embolic occlusion of the superior mesenteric artery
   C. **Requires immediate surgical exploration.**
   D. Goes in line with a vasodilatation of the mesenteric vessels.
10. Main criteria for mediastinitis after cardiac surgery are
    A. Infection within 60 days after surgery
    B. Infection of the pleural cavity.
    C. **Infection of the deep tissue layers of the incision (fascia and muscles)**
    D. Superficial soft tissue infection.

References

1. Andolfi M, Potenza R, Puma FCL. Complications in thoracic surgery. In: Nistor CE, Tsui S, Kirali K, Ciuche A, Aresu GKK, editors. Thoracic surgery. Springer; 2020. p. 51–61.
2. Welter S, Cheufou D, Darwiche K, Stamatis G. Tracheal injuries, fistulae from bronchial stump and bronchial anastomoses and recurrent laryngeal nerve paralysis: Management of complications in thoracic surgery. Chirurg. 2015;86:410–8.
3. Reichert M, Hecker M, Witte B, Bodner J, Padberg W, Weigand MA, et al. Stage-directed therapy of pleural empyema. Langenbecks Arch Surg. 2017;402:15–26.
4. Pompili C, Falcoz PE, Salati M, Szanto Z, Brunelli A. A risk score to predict the incidence of prolonged air leak after video-assisted thoracoscopic lobectomy: an analysis from the European Society of Thoracic Surgeons database. J Thorac Cardiovasc Surg. 2017;153:957–65.
5. Sziklavari Z, Neu R, Hofmann HS, Ried M. Persistent pleural effusion following thoracic surgery. Chirurg. 2015;86:432–6.
6. Kösek V, Wiebe K. Postoperative respiratory insufficiency and its treatment. Chirurg. 2015;86:437–43.
7. Filaire M, Mom T, Laurent S, Harouna Y, Naamee A, Vallet L, et al. Vocal cord dysfunction after left lung resection for cancer. Eur J Cardio-thoracic Surg. 2001;20:705–11.

Acute Congenital and Acquired Heart Disease

53

Alessandro Leone, G. Murana, L. Di Marco, E. Angeli, L. Careddu, G. Gargiulo, and D. Pacini

53.1 Introduction

Cardiac surgical emergencies are broken down into two main categories: acute aortic syndromes, and surgery for acute myocardial infarctions. Emphasis is given to describe the presentation of patients with such problems, and to the salient aspects of the clinical and surgical strategies for managing each problem. An important goal of each section is focusing the critical care physician on the early recognition of cardiac surgical emergencies and providing him with some rationale for instituting an expeditious plan of therapy.

On the other hand, critical congenital heart defects are still a challenge for pediatric surgeon that requires expertise and adequate skill to manage this kind of emergencies.

53.2 Acute Aortic Syndromes

Acute aortic syndrome (AAS) is the modern term that includes aortic dissection (AD), intramural hematoma (IMH), and penetrating aortic ulcer (PAU). In the classic sense, acute aortic dissection requires a tear in the aortic intima that commonly is preceded by medial wall degeneration or cystic media necrosis [1]. Blood passes through the tear separating the intima from the media or adventitia, creating a false lumen. Propagation of the dissection can proceed in anterograde or retrograde fashion from the initial tear involving side branches and causing complications such as malperfusion syndromes, tamponade, or aortic valve insufficiency [2]; (Fig. 53.1).

IMH is a collection of blood within the tunica media of the aortic wall, without the presence of a clear intimal flap or false lumen. Many authors consider IMH as a result of the rupture of the vasa vasorum or the ischemia of the tunica media in older patients [3]. The presenting symptoms

---

A. Leone (✉)
Department of Cardio-Thoracic and Vascular Medicine, Adult Cardiac Surgery, IRCCS Azienda Ospedaliero-Universitaria di Bologna, Bologna, Italy

Cardio-Thoracic-Vascular Department, S.Orsola Hospital, University of Bologna, Bologna, Italy

G. Murana · L. Di Marco · D. Pacini
Department of Cardio-Thoracic and Vascular Medicine, Adult Cardiac Surgery, IRCCS Azienda Ospedaliero-Universitaria di Bologna, Bologna, Italy
e-mail: giacomo.murana@aosp.bo.it; davide.pacini@unibo.it

E. Angeli · L. Careddu · G. Gargiulo
Department of Cardio-Thoracic and Vascular Medicine, Pediatric Cardiac Surgery and Adult Congenital Heart Disease Program, IRCCS Azienda Ospedaliero-Universitaria di Bologna, Bologna, Italy
e-mail: emanuela.angeli@aosp.bo.it; lucio.careddu@aosp.bo.it; gaetano.gargiulo@unibo.it

© The Author(s), under exclusive license to Springer Nature Switzerland AG 2023
F. Coccolini, F. Catena (eds.), *Textbook of Emergency General Surgery*,
https://doi.org/10.1007/978-3-031-22599-4_53

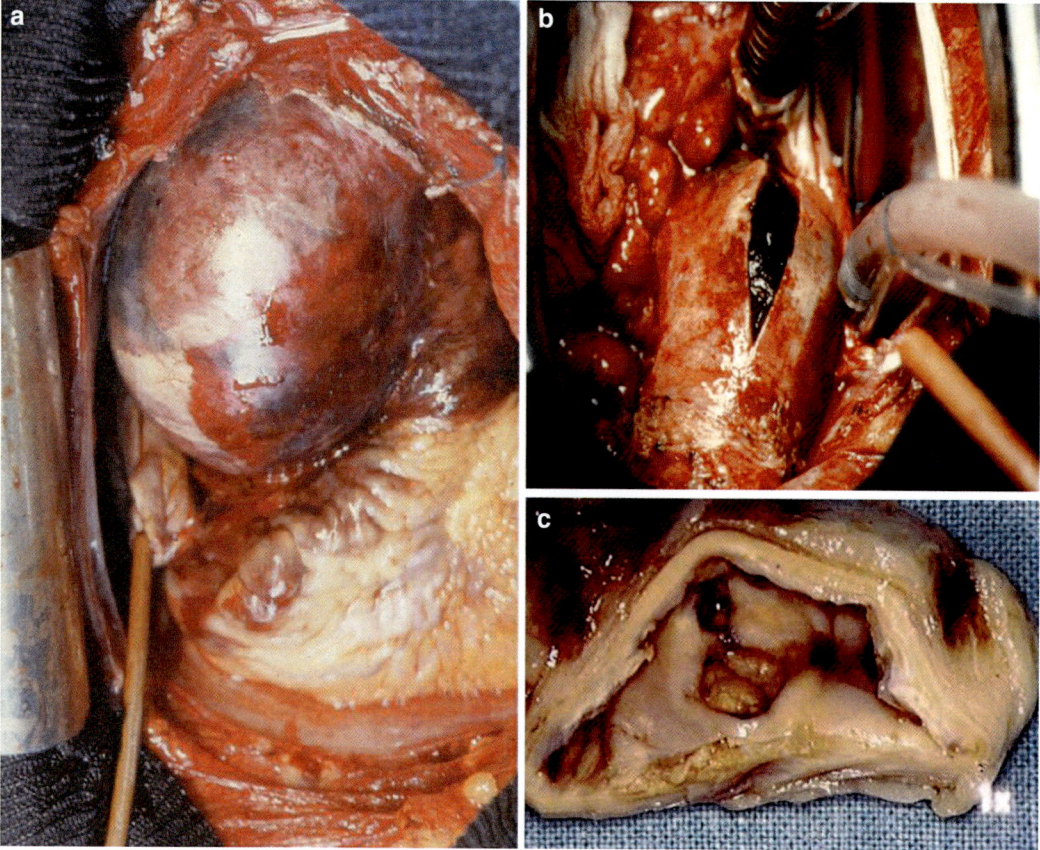

Fig. 53.1 Acute aortic syndromes: (**a**) acute aortic dissection, (**b**) intramural hematoma, and (**c**) penetrating aortic ulcer

and risk factors associated with IMH are similar to those observed in AD—chest pain and/or acute lumbar pain. In addition, an IMH that propagates in the ascending direction may lead to hemopericardium, rupture, and, in very rare cases, aortic regurgitation [4]. Whereas there is no intimal flap or false lumen associated with IMH, stroke or visceral ischemia would be uncommon accompanying complications.

PAU occurs with ulceration of an atherosclerotic plaque involving the aortic wall and blood penetrates through the internal elastic lamina to reach the tunica media. It is often associated with the formation of coexisting IMH [5].

Both acquired and genetic conditions share a common pathway leading to the breakdown in the integrity of the intima. All mechanisms that weaken the media layers of the aorta will eventually lead to higher wall stress, which can induce aortic dilatation and aneurysm formation, eventually resulting in intramural hemorrhage, aortic dissection, or rupture. The factors culminating in a clinical dissection are quite diverse. The most common risk condition for aortic dissection is hypertension, with chronic exposure of the aorta to high pressures leading to intimal thickening, fibrosis, calcification, and extracellular fatty acid deposition. Furthermore, the extracellular matrix may undergo accelerated degradation, apoptosis, and elastolysis with eventual intimal disruption, most often at the edges of plaques [1].

Marfan's syndrome, vascular Ehlers–Danlos syndrome, annuloaortic ectasia, bicuspid aortic valve, and familial aortic dissection are genetic conditions that often cause acute aortic syndromes. A common denominator to these different genetic disorders is a similar pathophysiology that includes a dedifferentiation of vascular smooth muscle cells and enhanced elastolysis of aortic wall components, leading to a compromised intima and aortic dissection [6]. Given this genetic predisposition, a detailed family history in patients diagnosed with acute aortic syndromes or sudden death is particularly important in assessing the need for family screening.

Knowledge regarding the incidence of aortic dissection in the general population is limited. Studies suggest an incidence of 2.6–3.5 cases per 100,000 person-years [2]. In a review of 464 patients from the International Registry of Acute Aortic Dissection (IRAD), two thirds were male, with a mean age for all patients of 63 years. Although less frequently affected by acute aortic dissection, women were significantly older than men, with a mean age of 67 years [6].

53.3 Clinical Symptoms and Signs

Patients with AAS often present with symptoms that cannot be associated with a specific disorder (AD, IMH or PAU), which may lead to serious outcomes [8]. Owing to low sensitivity and specificity of the clinical AAS symptoms, physicians can experience serious difficulty in making a correct differential diagnosis. Pain is the common denominator to all AAS patients; it occurs regardless of age, gender and other associated clinical conditions.

AD is one of the most frequent AAS and symptoms may be variable and can mimic those of more common conditions such as acute myocardial infarction. Therefore, it is recommended that clinicians consider this diagnosis when caring for patients with chest pain to avoid diagnostic delays that may be fatal [9]. Pain is the most frequent symptom (96% of cases) [10] and occurs abruptly, reaching maximum intensity in the early stages. Patients describe pain as lacerating, rending, and piercing. Sometimes the patient, driven by a sense of impending disaster, writhes, looking for a position that brings some relief. The pain is typically migrant and tends to follow the path of the aorta; it may radiate from the chest to the back or vice versa. Other clinical manifestations that can delay diagnosis and increase the rate of mortality [11] are acute heart failure (often caused by a severe acute AD of the ascending aorta); syncope (which is frequent during AD of the ascending aorta and generally associated with hemopericardium, rupture or stroke); and severe nausea and vomiting (which is related to the involvement of the abdominal viscera). The main objective findings of AD are hypertension (found in about 70% of patients) [10]; hypotension (in case of cardiac tamponade, aortic rupture or acute heart failure related to acute aortic insufficiency); deficit of the peripheral pulses; neurological manifestations; and physical findings of aortic valve insufficiency (in cases of dissection in the ascending direction); acute ischemia of the lower limbs or of the peripheral organs; and signs of acute myocardial infarction (if the dissection involves the ostium of one or more coronary arteries).

PAU and IMH are two AAS that may present with similar symptoms to AD, causing chest pain or intense low back pain. For this reason, diagnostic imaging is useful for clinicians, as it serves to distinguish them from AD.

PAU can be found throughout the course of the aorta, mainly at the level of the thoracic and abdominal segments. It is occasionally found incidentally during imaging; however, PAU can exhibit symptoms such as acute chest or lumbar pain, similar to AD. Physicians should be informed about the propensity to rupture of PAU, so it is important to know how to recognize it. PAU can degenerate in AD, but most patients have no associated aortic valve insufficiency, pulse deficits, or visceral ischemia.

53.4 Classification

There are several classifications with the Stanford and DeBakey anatomical classifications as the most common used. First, the Stanford classification is the most decisive for surgical treatment. It discriminates upon proximal extent between the following:

- Type A involving the ascending aorta and
- Type B affecting the descending aorta distal of the left subclavian artery, irrespective of entry site or distal extent

Second, the DeBakey classification denominates three types
- Type I starting in the ascending aorta and proceeding to the whole thoracic aorta;
- Type II with extent limited to the ascending aorta;
- Type III limited to the descending aorta equivalent to Stanford type B.

Third, AAS can be classified upon morphology and pathologic mechanism as first described by Svensson. Five entities are specified:

1. Classic aortic dissection (AD) with true and false lumen, with or without reentry;
2. Intramural hematoma (IMH);
3. Limited intimal tear with eccentric bulge;
4. Plaque rupture/penetrating aortic ulcer (PAU);
5. Iatrogenic or traumatic AD.

Fourth, orientated on the pattern of malperfusion estimating the risk of mortality, the Penn classification for type A AoD was introduced
- Penn class Aa—no ischemia (absence of ischemia);
- Penn class Ab—localized ischemia (branch vessel malperfusion producing clinical organ ischemia);
- Penn class Ac—generalized ischemia (circulatory collapse, with or without cardiac involvement);
- Penn class Ab&c—combined ischemia.

53.5 Technique of Ascending Aorta and Arch Replacement

In case of type A acute aortic syndromes, the classic aortic arch operation consists in the replacement of the ascending aorta with or without partial arch.

Effective methods of cerebral, myocardial as well visceral protection are necessary to obtain acceptable results in terms of hospital mortality and morbidity. The best method to protect the brain has demonstrated to be the bilateral antegrade selective cerebral perfusion (ASCP) with moderate hypothermia according to Kazui's technique [12]. In fact, very favorable outcomes are reported in literature indicating ASCP as the best method to protect the brain, especially when time consuming and complex arch repairs are required [13]; (Fig. 53.2).

Total arch replacement in acute type A aortic dissection (AAAD) may be an effective strategy, especially when in complex cases, the left subclavian artery re-implantation is not feasible or in case of excessive dilatation of the distal arch, in

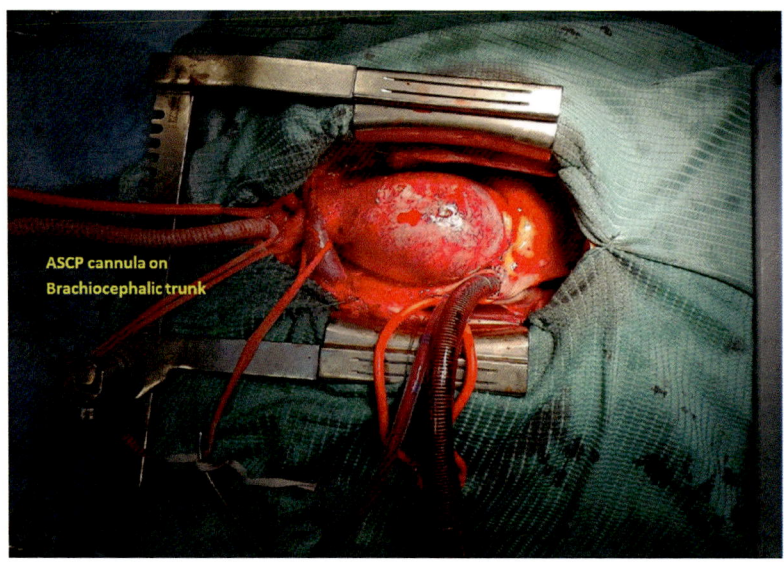

Fig. 53.2 Preparation of the extracorporeal circulation and antegrade cerebral perfusion for a total arch replacement in patient with acute type A aortic dissection: a Dacron prosthesis was used as ASCP cannulation

such cases the distal anastomosis can be performed after the left carotid artery, thus allowing a necessary landing zone for a further endovascular extension. However, the left subclavian artery must be ligated, and a carotid-subclavian bypass performed.

The elephant trunk procedure (ET) [14] can be an alternative technique for total arch replacement. This technique, in which a segment of prosthetic graft beyond the distal arch anastomosis floats freely within the descending aorta, facilitates interval repair of distal aortic aneurysms.

The ET was initially studied to facilitate the second-stage operation where the descending aorta would be replaced through left thoracotomy access, allowing an easier end-to-end anastomosis during this phase. With the increase in the experience with this technique, the indication has been progressively expanded from the arch and descending aorta aneurysm, to chronic type A, acute type B, and finally to acute type A aortic dissection.

However, in case of acute dissection, ET can present some technical difficulties due to the small dimension of the true lumen and if the false lumen is pressurized, the floating graft can result compressed. In that case, the dissected layers should be united during the anastomosis using Teflon felt strips in order to avoid tearing of the fragile tissue. Moreover, the graft should be slightly oversized so that the "ET" presses against the dissected aorta.

During years, several graft modifications occurred. Modern grafts with four side branches as well as sewing collars for the distal anastomosis simplified the ET implantation.

These modern grafts incorporate radio-opaque markers at the distal end that are helpful to identify the proximal lending zone in case of endovascular extension as second stage of the procedure.

A recent modification of the ET is the "frozen elephant trunk" (FET) technique, initially developed by some Japanese authors [15], mainly consisting in treating complex lesions of the thoracic aorta in a single-stage procedure combining endovascular treatment with conventional surgery.

The graft is composed of a proximal part consisting of vascular prosthesis and a distal part of self-expandable nitinol stent graft (Fig. 53.3).

During the early experience with this technique, the prosthesis used where basically custom made, afterward the first commercially available was the E-VITA Jotec Hybrid graft (JOTEC GmbH, Hechingen, Germany) [15], and recently the Thoraflex Hybrid multi-branched graft and distal stent (Vascutek, Renfrewshire, Scotland, UK) [16].

The technique consists in the implantation of the stented distal segment of the hybrid-prosthesis into the descending aorta through the opened aortic arch, while the proximal nonstented segment is used for conventional replacement of the upstream aorta.

Indications at the use of the FET are chronic aneurysm of the ascending arch and descending aorta, chronic dissection involving all the thoracic aorta, retrograde type A aortic dissection after TEVAR procedure, rupture of the arch, and also the chronic aneurysm involving the distal part of the aortic arch and the upper part of the descending aorta. The FET technique facilitated single-stage arch and descending aorta replacement in complex lesion, afterward the indication has been extended to selected patients with AAAD [17].

In some patients with AAAD, this technique can resolve the entire aortic pathology, especially in case of type I or retrograde dissection limited to the descending thoracic aorta. Moreover, patients with organ malperfusion and consequent visceral ischemia, such as for true lumen collapse in the thoracoabdominal aorta or for branch vessel obstruction for extending dissection into visceral arteries with narrowed true lumen compressed by false lumen, may represent another viable indication for the use of FET. In such cases, the stented part of the prosthesis can easily re-expand the compressed true lumen in the descending aorta. FET is undoubtedly a major aortic procedure and requires very accurate preoperative planning. For this reason, the assessment of the aortic anatomy is essential. In details, great care has to be taken when assessing the extent of the intimal flap, the relationship exist-

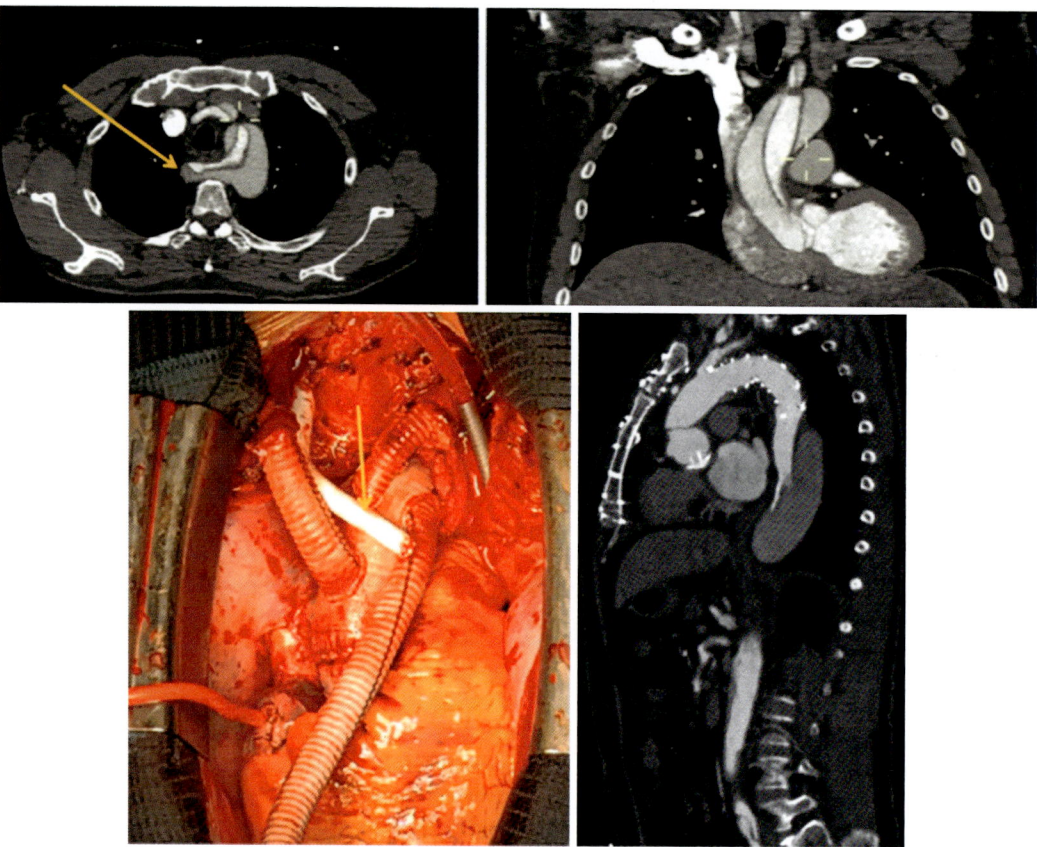

Fig. 53.3 Frozen elephant trunk technique: intraoperative and postoperative image; the arrow indicates the reimplantation of the aberrant right subclavian artery reimplantation

ing between the true and false lumen, the location of entry and re-entry tears, and the origin of visceral vessels from the false lumen. In fact, in patients with visceral arteries rising from the false lumen not communicating with the true by the presence of near re-entry tears, organ malperfusion can be a lethal complication after FET [18]. Moreover, oversizing of the stent graft is not indicated in patients with aortic dissection, whereas a 10–20% oversizing should be performed in patients with degenerative aneurysms. Furthermore, if the patients are not selected carefully, or the disease progresses into the downstream aorta, a second-stage procedure may be necessary even with FET.

Patient's conditions represent one of the most important turning point in the decision-making process, sometimes even if the anatomy of the dissection is suitable for a multi-stage or a single-stage approach, total arch replacement may be not indicated, as in patients with advanced age or in extremely poor clinical condition.

On the other hand, young patients, Marfan and patients in stable condition, can benefit more from a radical treatment of the thoracic aorta even in terms of hospital mortality and above all at long term.

53.6 Mechanical Complications of Acute Myocardial Infarction

Acute myocardial infarction (AMI) can result in ischemic, mechanical, arrhythmic, embolic, or inflammatory complications. Since the introduction of primary percutaneous coronary intervention (PCI) as the principal reperfusion strategy following acute ST-elevation myocardial infarction (STEMI), the incidence of mechanical complications has reduced significantly to less than 1%, including rupture of the left ventricular free wall (0.52%), papillary muscle (0.26%), and ventricular septum (0.17%) [19].

53.6.1 Ventricular Septal Rupture

Ventricular septal rupture (VSR) represents a defect in the interventricular septum caused by ischemic necrosis following AMI. VSR occurs following a transmural infarct, and may be subclassified into simple and complex VSR [20]. A simple VSR represents a single defect with openings in both ventricles at approximately the same level, whereas a complex VSR represents a meshwork of serpiginous channels with hemorrhage and disruption of myocardial tissue, which are more commonly found following posteroinferior AMI. AMI complicated with VSR can progress into left ventricular (LV) or right ventricular (RV) failure, cardiogenic shock, and potentially irreversible multiorgan malperfusion [21].

Echocardiography with color flow Doppler is the gold standard for diagnosis, monitoring, and planning treatment, distinguishing between papillary muscle rupture and VSR, as well as assessing LV and RV function.

Standard surgical repair of a postinfarction VSR involves using the infarct exclusion technique.

This procedure comprises a left ventriculotomy through the infarcted anterior or inferior wall, 2–3 cm parallel to the left anterior descending artery or posterior descending artery, respectively.

A bovine pericardial patch is then sutured to healthy endocardium deep in the left ventricle, to exclude the infarct and VSR from the high-pressure area of the left ventricle. This patch is then brought out through the ventriculotomy and incorporated in the closure. The ventriculotomy is closed in two layers, buttressed by Teflon strips. Using this technique, LV geometry and volume can be restored. Surgical repair of a posterior VSR is technically more difficult because of access to the inferobasal LV wall, especially involving necrotic and friable myocardium immediately after an AMI [22].

53.6.2 Rupture of Left Ventricle Free Wall

Rupture of the LV free wall occurs in 0.5% of patients following AMI and is associated with 20% mortality [19].

Approximately 50% of patients with free-wall rupture are diagnosed within 5 days of the AMI, with 90% diagnosed within 2 weeks [20].

Early free-wall rupture, seen within the first 24 h, represents a small-tear, full-thickness rupture, which is temporarily sealed by clot and fibrinous pericardial adhesions. The use of thrombolysis may result in the necrotic tissue developing into a hemorrhagic infarct, with a sudden "blow-out" rupture, which is associated with 35–60% mortality [23].

LV wall rupture requires emergent salvage surgery. The use of emergency pericardiocentesis is controversial [24]. Although emergency pericardiocentesis may provide hemodynamic short-term improvement by relieving the tamponade, it can cause a dangerous increase in blood pressure with increased tension on damaged myocardium, with the potential for extension of a small tear to a rupture.

Traditionally surgical repair is performed by direct suture of the myocardium over the infarct zone with reinforcement by Teflon felt strip, or repair using the infarct exclusion technique [22].

More recently, a bovine pericardial patch has been used over the repair, reinforced with surgical glue beneath the patch, with or without epicardial suture on the patch borders (patch and glue technique) [25].

53.6.3 Papillary Muscle Rupture and Acute Mitral Regurgitation

Acute MR is a catastrophic complication of an AMI that, if recognized, is amenable to emergent surgical intervention.

Acute MR secondary to papillary muscle rupture, however, is a life-threatening complication with a poor prognosis [26]. Papillary muscle rupture occurs in 0.25% of patients following AMI and represents up to 7% of patients in cardiogenic shock following AMI [27]. Although acute MR secondary to papillary muscle rupture is usually diagnosed between 2 and 7 days after AMI, the median time to papillary muscle rupture is approximately 13 h [28].

In the acute setting, pulmonary edema and cardiogenic shock may ensue, as there is not enough time for the left ventricle to dilate or compensate. Acute MR secondary to papillary muscle dysfunction or rupture occurs most commonly following an inferior MI, owing to the single blood supply to the posteromedial papillary muscle from the posterior descending coronary artery.

The anterolateral papillary muscle, however, has a dual blood supply (left anterior descending and circumflex coronary arteries) and, therefore, is more likely to be protected following an AMI in a single-vessel territory.

When acute MR accompanies complete papillary muscle rupture, patients may present with immediate pulmonary edema, hypotension, and, in some cases, cardiogenic shock.

Prompt diagnosis with immediate initiation of aggressive medical therapy is vital until emergent surgical intervention can be performed. Urgent cardiac catheterization needs to be performed to identify coronary anatomy, as concomitant revascularization during mitral valve surgery is associated with improved short-term and long-term outcomes.

During the operation, careful assessment of the mitral valve and the subvalvular apparatus will allow for decision making regarding repair or replacement. If there is evidence of papillary muscle necrosis or there are concerns about subtle, ongoing progression of ischemic injury, mitral valve replacement provides a definitive treatment of the failing mitral valve apparatus.

53.7 Critical Congenital Heart Disease

The prevalence of congenital heart disease is about 0.8–1% of all live births and is, therefore, one of the most common congenital malformations. Critical congenital heart defects (cCHD) are causes for acute cardiac failure in the neonate, and despite the progress in cardiothoracic surgery, they remain a principal cause of comorbidity and mortality with a mortality rate up to 25% in the first year of life. For that reason, prenatal diagnosis and initiation of adequate treatment are mandatory [29–31].

The distribution of cCHD differs from the distribution of CHDs with coarctation and aortic arch pathologies as the first risk with 30–40%, followed by transposition of the great arteries (approx. 30%). Another type of emergency is obstructed total anomalous pulmonary venous return, right ventricle stenosis, and congenital cardiomyopathy or arrhythmia [31].

Prenatal diagnostics sensitivity for critical heart defects is up to 51% but is still inadequate despite improvements in prenatal diagnostics, and postnatal clinical examinations are still a valuable diagnostic tool in neonates. However, the sensitivity of the clinical examination is less than 50% due to a possible symptom-free interval for the transition from neonatal physiology. The use of pulse oximetry screening in association with clinical examination cloud reduces this postnatal "diagnostic gap" period due to postnatal circulatory transition that is variable and influenced by several functional and anatomical aspects. Nevertheless, the transition to serial circulatory physiology might lead to a life-threatening condition in the presence of critical heart defects [31].

Basing on severe of cCHD, several classifications have been proposed; the most recent and accurate has been made by Petruz and colleagues [31]. On that base, we want to describe the major neonatal emergencies in pediatric represented by hypoplastic left heart syndrome (HLHS), transposition of great arteries (TGA), obstructed total pulmonary vein connection (oTPVC), and aortic coarctation (CoAo) without ductus arteriosus.

53.7.1 Hypoplastic Left Heart Syndrome (HLHS)

This cCHD is dependent on adequate balance in the pulmonary and systemic circulation. For that reason, the rare cases of HLHS with restrictive or closed foramen ovale (FO) at birth may not show the severe hemodynamic and rapid for [30, 31] rapid intervention in the first few hours after delivery due to rapid and progressive clinical deterioration. New strategies for improving infants' outcomes with HLHS and restrictive or closed FO are now based on delivery in operating room (OR) with neonatal ECMO implant and emergent creation of an atrial communication. Antenatal diagnosis and selection for safety delivery in such a group of fetuses are crucial to coordinate the cardiothoracic team and neonatologist for performing, in the first hours of life, all the advanced treatment the patient needs.

53.7.2 Transposition of Great Arteries (TGA)

Distinguishing between TGA with nonrestrictive atrial septal defect (ASD) from critical TGA with restrictive ASD is still challenging even in tertiary centers. Even in that case, antenatal diagnosis is crucial to perform a safe delivery and avoid significant complications. Missing a restrictive ASD/FO could become critical for the newborn that progressively decompensates before receiving the appropriate cardiac intervention.

For that reason, is nowadays a good measure to treat all babies with TGA as the FO will close at deliver, and transfer before delivery in a location where there are cardiologists available to perform the septostomy, if it is needed. This strategy has reduced the risk of newborn mortality and morbidity with TGA due to severe cyanosis at birth. Emergency treatment of TGA is percutaneous atrial septostomy (Rashkind operation). At the same time, complete correction is reserved intact septum or failure of Rashkind operation [30, 31].

53.7.3 Obstructed Total Pulmonary Vein Connection (oTPVC)

Total anomalous pulmonary venous return (TAPVR) with obstruction is the cCHD with high mortality and is still a challenging antennal diagnosis. Those neonates develop rapid respiratory distress and decompensation due to the substantial obstruction of pulmonary venous connection. Appropriate patient stabilization and early surgical treatment could result in a good prognosis. However, the high morbidity encountered when not recognized makes this condition a seriously challenging emergency for congenital heart surgeons. In fact, surgery requires reconnecting the pulmonary veins and decompressing the pulmonary circulation to allow both oxygen delivery and reduce severe pulmonary edema. Such patients could suffer from pulmonary vein stenosis during infancy or childhood, and continuous follow-up is mandatory [29].

53.7.4 Aortic Coarctation (CoAo)

Aortic coarctation (CoAo) could develop isolated or with aortic arch hypoplasia and other intracardiac defects (ex VSD). Controversies remain regarding the most appropriate timing of surgical intervention for severe coarctation. Neonates with severe CoAo could present with profound cardiogenic shock, and surgery has unique options. Moreover, patients with worse perioperative global LV function had a shorter time diagnosis to surgery than neonates with normal LV function. Most commonly, direct anastomosis with end-to-end extended is the standard strategy for the neonate with isolated CoAo. In contrast, the optimal strategy for infants with CoAo associated with other arch pathologies or intracardiac defects has yet to be generally recognized and is still based on surgeon preference. Even with surgical improvement nowadays, mortality after an emergency is still high, especially in the case of LV dysfunction [32].

Multiple Choice Questions
1. Acute aortic dissection may develop from:
   A. PAU
   B. IMH
   C. Connective tissue disorder
   D. **All of them**

2. In case of acute type A aortic dissection the most common operation performed is:
   A. Frozen elephant trunk
   B. **Hemiarch replacement**
   C. Bentall procedure
   D. Aortic valve replacement
3. Early free-wall rupture is associated with a mortality rate of:
   A. 10%
   B. 90%
   C. 20–25%
   D. **35–60%**
4. Critical congenital heart defects (cCHD) are causes for acute cardiac failure in the neonate, and they remain a principal cause of mortality with a mortality rate up to:
   A. **25%**
   B. 35%
   C. 40%
   D. 70%
5. Oversizing of the stent with the FET in acute aortic dissection:
   A. Is always indicated
   B. **Is no indicated**
   C. Only 10%
   D. Up to 20%

References

1. Larson EW, Edwards WD. Risk factors for aortic dissection: a necropsy study of 161 cases. Am J Cardiol. 1984;53:849–55.
2. Meszaros I, Morocz J, Szlavi J, Schmidt J, Tornoci L, Nagy L, Szep L. Epidemiology and clinicopathology of aortic dissection. Chest. 2000;117:1271–8.
3. Nienaber CA, Sievers HH. Intramural hematoma in acute aortic syndrome: more than one variant of dissection? Circulation. 2002;106:284–5.
4. Coady MA, Rizzo JA, Elefteriades JA. Pathologic variants of thoracic aortic dissections: penetrating atherosclerotic ulcers and intramural hematomas. Cardiol Clin. 1999;17:637–57.
5. DeSanctis RW, Doroghazi RM, Austen WG, Buckley MJ. Aortic dissection. N Engl J Med. 1987;317:1060–7.
6. Lesauskaite V, Tanganelli P, Sassi C, Neri E, Diciolla F, Ivanoviene L, Epistolato MC, Lalinga AV, Alessandrini C, Spina D. Smooth muscle cells of the media in the dilatative pathology of ascending thoracic aorta: morphology, immunoreactivity for osteopontin, matrix metalloproteinases, and their inhibitors. Hum Pathol. 2001;32:1003–11.
7. Nienaber CA, Fattori R, Mehta RH, Richartz BM, Evangelista A, Petzsch M, Cooper JV, Januzzi JL, Ince H, Sechtem U, Bossone E, Fang J, Smith DE, Isselbacher EM, Pape LA, Eagle KA. Gender-related differences in acute aortic dissection. Circulation. 2004;109:3014–21.
8. Hayter RG, Rhea JT, Small A. Suspected aortic dissection and other aortic disorders: multidetector row CT in 373 cases in the emergency setting. Radiology. 2006;238:841–52.
9. Nienaber CA, Powell JT. Management of acute aortic syndromes. Eur Heart J. 2012;33:26–35b.
10. Hagan PG, Nienaber CA, Isselbacher EM. The International Registry of Acute Aortic Dissection (IRAD): new insights into an old disease. JAMA. 2000;283:897–903.
11. Upchurch GR, Nienaber C, Fattori R, IRAD Investigators. Acute aortic dissection presenting with primarily abdominal pain: a rare manifestation of a deadly disease. Ann Vasc Surg. 2005;19:367–73.
12. Kazui T, Inoue N, Yamada O, Komatsu S. Selective cerebral perfusion during operation for aneurysms of the aortic arch: a reassessment. Ann Thorac Surg. 1992;53:109.
13. Khaladj N, Shrestha M, Meck S, Peterss S, Kamiya H, Kallenbach K, Winterhalter M, Hoy L, Haverich A, Hagl C. Hypothermic circulatory arrest with selective antegrade cerebral perfusion in ascending aortic and aortic arch surgery: a risk factor analysis for adverse outcome in 501 patients. J Thorac Cardiovasc Surg. 2008;135:908–14.
14. Borst HG, Walterbusch G, Schaps D. Extensive aortic replacement using "elephant trunk" prosthesis. Thorac Cardiovasc Surg. 1983;31(1):37–40.
15. Di Bartolomeo R, Di Marco L, Armaro A, Marsilli D, Leone A, Pilato E, Pacini D. Treatment of complex disease of the thoracic aorta: the frozen elephant trunk technique with the E-vita open prosthesis. Eur J Cardiothorac Surg. 2009;35(4):671–5.
16. Shrestha M, Pichlmaier M, Martens A, Hagl C, Khaladj N, Haverich A. Total aortic arch replacement with a novel four-branched frozen elephant trunk graft: first-in-man results. Eur J Cardiothorac Surg. 2013;43(2):406–10.
17. Di Bartolomeo R, Pantaleo A, Berretta P, Murana G, Castrovinci S, Cefarelli M, Folesani G, Di Eusanio M. Frozen elephant trunk surgery in acute aortic dissection. J Thorac Cardiovasc Surg. 2015;149(2 Suppl):S105–9.
18. Tsagakis K, Pacini D, Di Bartolomeo R, Benedik J, Cerny S, Gorlitzer M, Grabenwoger M, Mestres CA, Jakob H. Arch replacement and downstream stent grafting in complex aortic dissection: first results of an international registry. Eur J Cardiothorac Surg. 2011;39:87–93.

19. French JK, Hellkamp AS, Armstrong PW, et al. Mechanical complications after percutaneous coronary intervention in ST-elevation myocardial infarction (from APEX-AMI). Am J Cardiol. 2010;105:59–63.
20. Crenshaw BS, Granger CB, Birnbaum Y, et al. Risk factors, angiographic patterns, and outcomes inpatients with ventricular septal defect complicating acute myocardial infarction. Circulation. 2000;101: 27–32.
21. Figueras J, Cortadellas J, Soler-Soler J. Comparison of ventricular septal and left ventricular free wall rupture in acute myocardial infarction. Am J Cardiol. 1998;81:495–7.
22. David TE, Dale L, Sun Z. Postinfarction ventricular septal rupture: repair by endocardial patch with infarct exclusion. Thorac Cardiovasc Surg. 1995;110(5):1315–22.
23. Coletti G, Torracca L, Zogno M, et al. Surgical management of left ventricular free wall rupture after acute myocardial infarction. Cardiovasc Surg. 1995;3(2):181–6.
24. Fitch MT, Nicks BA, Pariyadath M, et al. Videos in clinical medicine. Emergency pericardiocentesis. N Engl J Med. 2012;366(12):e17.
25. Zoffoli G, Battaglia F, Venturini A, et al. A novel approach to ventricular rupture: clinical needs and surgical technique. Ann Thorac Surg. 2012;93(3):1002–3.
26. Kishon Y, Oh JK, Schaff HV, et al. Mitral valve operation in post infarction rupture of a papillary muscle: immediate results and long-term follow up of 22 patients. Mayo Clin Proc. 1992;67:1023–30.
27. Thompson CR, Buller CE, Sleeper LA, et al. Cardiogenic shock due to acute severe mitral regurgitation complicating acute myocardial infarction: areport from the SHOCK Trial Registry. Should we use emergently revascularize Occluded Coronaries in cardiogenic shock? J Am Coll Cardiol. 2000;36(3 Suppl A):1104–9.
28. Menon V, Webb JG, Hillis LD, et al. Outcome and profile of ventricular septal rupture with cardiogenic shock after myocardial infarction: a report from the SHOCK trial registry. J Am Coll Cardiol. 2000;36(Suppl A):1110–6.
29. Dolk H, Loane M, Garne E, European Surveillance of Congenital Anomalies Working Group. Congenital heart defects in Europe: prevalence and perinatal mortality, 2000–2005. Circulation. 2011;123(8):841–9.
30. Mitchell SC, Korones SB, Berendes HW. Congenital heart disease in 56,109 births. Incidence and natural history. Circulation. 1971;43(3):323–32.
31. Khalil M, Jux C, Rueblinger L, Behrje J, Esmaeili A, Schranz D. Acute therapy of newborns with critical congenital heart disease. Transl Pediatr. 2019;8(2):114–26.
32. Domadia S, Kumar SR, Votava-Smith JK, Pruetz JD. Neonatal outcomes in total anomalous pulmonary venous return: the role of prenatal diagnosis and pulmonary venous obstruction. Pediatr Cardiol. 2018;39(7):1346–54.

Further Reading

Di Bartolomeo R, Di Marco L, Armaro A, Marsilli D, Leone A, Pilato E, Pacini D. Treatment of complex disease of the thoracic aorta: the frozen elephant trunk technique with the E-vita open prosthesis. Eur J Cardiothorac Surg. 2009;35(4):671–5.

Erbel R, Aboyans V, Boileau C, et al. 2014 ESC Guidelines on the diagnosis and treatment of aortic diseases: document covering acute and chronic aortic diseases of the thoracic and abdominal aorta of the adult. The Task Force for the Diagnosis and Treatment of Aortic Diseases of the European Society of Cardiology (ESC). Eur Heart J. 2014;35(41):2873–926.

Slodki M, Respondek-Liberska M, Pruetz JD, Donofrio MT. Fetal cardiology: changing the definition of critical heart disease in the newborn. J Perinatol. 2016;36(8):575–80.